Watson's

Clinical Nursing and Related Sciences

Sixth Edition

Edited by

Mike Walsh

PhD BA PGCE RGN DipN

Reader in Nursing Studies,
St Martin's College,
Lancaster, UK

Baillière Tindall

Edinburgh · London · New York · Philadelphia · St Louis · Sydney · Toronto 2002

BAILLIÈRE TINDALL
An imprint of Elsevier Science Limited

First edition published 1972 by W B Saunders Company as *Medical–Surgical Nursing and Related Physiology*, by Jeanette E Watson
Second edition published 1979 by W B Saunders Company
Third edition published 1987 by Baillière Tindall as *Watson's Medical–Surgical Nursing and Related Physiology*, by Jeanette E Watson and Joan A Royle
Fourth edition published 1992 by Baillière Tindall as *Watson's Medical–Surgical Nursing and Related Physiology*, by Joan A Royle and Mike Walsh
Fifth edition published by Baillière Tindall as *Watson's Clinical Nursing and Related Sciences*, edited by Mike Walsh
Sixth edition published 2002 by Elsevier Science Limited as *Watson's Clinical Nursing and Related Sciences*, edited by Mike Walsh

ISBN 0702026077

International Student Edition 2002
Sixth Edition 2002

British Library Cataloguing in Publication Data
A catalogue record for this book is available from the British Library

Library of Congress Cataloging in Publication Data
A catalog record for this book is available from the Library of Congress

Note
Medical knowledge is constantly changing. As new information becomes available, changes in treatment, procedures, equipment and the use of drugs become necessary. The editor, contributors and the publishers have taken care to ensure that the information given in this text is accurate and up to date. However, readers are strongly advised to confirm that the information, especially with regard to drug usage, complies with the latest legislation and standards of practice.

 ELSEVIER SCIENCE your source for books, journals and multimedia in the health sciences

www.elsevierhealth.com

The publisher's policy is to use **paper manufactured from sustainable forests**

Printed in China by RDC Group Limited

Watson's **Clinical Nursing and Related Sciences**

For Baillière Tindall:

Senior Commissioning Editor: Jacqueline Curthoys
Project Development Manager: Karen Gilmour
Project Manager: Jane Dingwall
Design Direction: Judith Wright

Contents

Contributors   ix

Preface   xi

Publisher's acknowledgements   xiii

Publisher's notes   xiii

A guide to the physiology cross-referencing system   xv

Physiology for Nursing Practice (second edition) excerpt from the editors' introduction   xvii

Section one   The context of care

Chapter 1   The nature of nursing   3

Introduction; The nurse and the healthcare system; The focus of nursing; The delivery of nursing care; Documentation; Nursing ethics; The nurse as a promoter of health; Health education and health promotion: the debate; Models of health promotion; Health education and patient teaching; Summary

Chapter 2   Therapeutic communication and nursing practice   29

Introduction; The importance of communication; Barriers to effective communication; Skills for effective communication; The unpopular patient; Summary

Chapter 3   Ageing and health   41

Introduction; Demography; Contemporary policy context; Emerging trends; Normal ageing; Assessment; A profession equipped to support and work with older people; Health promotion and wellness; Summary

Chapter 4   Death, grief and loss   59

Introduction; Normal grieving; Anticipatory grieving; Sudden death; Viewing the body; Absent at the time of death; Breaking bad news; Responding to altered body image; Summary

Chapter 5   Primary health care and the management of chronic illness   75

Introduction; What is primary health care?; Primary care as an approach, activities, level of care or a philosophy; Policy and primary care; The nurse's role in primary health care;

The primary healthcare team; Chronic illness; Chronic illness management in primary care; Working with patients who live with a chronic condition; The nurse as educator; The nurse as change agent; Summary

Section two   Key clinical principles

Chapter 6   Principles of pharmacology   95

Introduction; Pharmacology and nursing practice; Classification and naming of medicines; Administration, absorption and distribution of medicines, and bioavailability; How drugs act; Inactivation, metabolism and elimination; Unwanted and adverse effects of medicines; Interactions between drugs when used together; Drug discovery, development and evaluation; Summary

Chapter 7   The management of pain   111

Introduction; Pain pathways; Psychosocial factors in the experience of pain; Assessment and evaluation of acute pain; Methods of managing pain; Summary

Chapter 8   Infection and disease   125

Introduction; Infectious agents; Interaction between host and infectious agents; The course of an infectious disease; Types of infection; Clinical characteristics of infection; Diagnostic procedures used in infection; The management of patients with an infection; Occurrence of infectious disease in populations; Infectious disease in hospital populations; Community prevention and control of infection; Human immunodeficiency virus (HIV) infection; Summary

Chapter 9   Clinical investigations   151

Introduction; Rationale for clinical investigations; Assessment and clinical investigations; Care of patients needing clinical assessment; Informed consent; Giving information; Patient anxiety and clinical investigations; Professional preparations; Essential nursing knowledge related to clinical investigations; Pre-procedure preparation; Care of specimens; Principles behind the specific types of clinical investigation; Specimens for culture and sensitivity; Investigation by means of diagnostic imaging; Health screening; Giving unwelcome news; The future; Summary

Chapter 10   The patient undergoing surgery   165

Introduction; Preparation of the patient for surgery;
Intraoperative phase; Postoperative management;
Day surgery; Summary

Section three   Caring for patients with a specific disorder

Chapter 11   Caring for the patient with cancer   195

Introduction; Prevention and early detection of cancer;
Detection and diagnosis of cancer; Treatment of cancer;
Nursing assessment and management of disease- and
treatment-related problems; Common issues in coping with
cancer; Care of the patient with advanced cancer;
Rehabilitation; Survivorship; Summary

Chapter 12   Caring for the patient with a   247
              cardiovascular disorder

Introduction; Circulation; Prevention of cardiovascular
disorders; The person with a cardiovascular disorder;
Causes and types of heart disorder; Congenital
cardiovascular defects; Disorders of cardiac muscle;
Disorders of myocardial blood supply; Disorders of
electroconduction; Heart failure; The person having
cardiac surgery; Disorders of the vascular system;
Summary

Chapter 13   Caring for the patient with a   333
              respiratory disorder

Introduction; Respiratory structures; Assessment; Specific
disorders; Patients requiring respiratory assistance; Patients
requiring mechanical ventilation; Localized airway
obstruction; Summary

Chapter 14   Caring for the patient with a   371
              haematological disorder

Introduction; Physiology; Blood disorders; Health
assessment; Erythrocyte disorders; Leucocyte disorders;
Lymphatic disorders; Haemorrhagic disorders; Transfusion
practice; Summary

Chapter 15   Caring for the patient with a disorder   435
              of the gastrointestinal system

Introduction; Overview of the structure and function of the
gastrointestinal tract; The person with a disorder of the
gastrointestinal system; Health problems in the upper portion
of the alimentary canal; Disorders of the stomach and
duodenum; Intestinal disorders; The person with faecal
diversion; Summary

Chapter 16   Caring for the patient with a liver, biliary   507
              tract or exocrine pancreas disorder

Introduction; Assessment; The person at risk of a disorder
of the liver and exocrine pancreas; Disorders of the liver;
Disorders of the gallbladder and bile duct; Disorders
of the pancreas; Summary

Chapter 17   Caring for the patient with a nutritional   537
              disorder

Introduction; Metabolism; Meeting nutritional requirements;
Recommendations for healthy eating; Factors that influence
dietary patterns; Assessment; Obesity; Undernutrition;
Undernutrition due to withholding of nutritional support;
Nutritional needs of the elderly; Cultural and religious
influence on dietary habits; Summary

Chapter 18   Caring for the patient with a disorder   561
              of the endocrine system

Introduction; Disorders of the endocrine system; The person
with diabetes; The person with a disorder of the thyroid
gland; The person with a disorder of the parathyroid glands;
The person with a disorder of the pituitary gland (hypophysis); The person with a disorder of the adrenal cortices; The
person with a disorder of the adrenal medullae; Summary

Chapter 19   Caring for the patient with a disorder   611
              of the renal system

Introduction; The renal system and urinary tract; Assessment
of renal function; Clinical characteristics of renal dysfunction;
The person with impaired renal function; The person with a disorder of the urinary system; Tumour of the bladder; Summary

Chapter 20   Caring for the patient with a disorder   665
              of the nervous system

Introduction; The nervous system; Assessment of neurological
function; The person with a neurological disorder; The
person with a cerebrovascular disorder; The person with
trauma of the nervous system; The person with a neoplasm
of the nervous system; The person with a degenerative
disorder; The person with a paroxysmal disorder; The person
with an infection of the nervous system; The person with a
peripheral nerve disorder; Summary

Chapter 21   Caring for the patient with a disorder   747
              of the senses

Introduction; Structure and functions of the ear; The person
with a disorder of the ear; Structure and functions of the
nose; The person with a disorder of the nose or nasal
sinuses; Structure and functions of the eyes; The person
with health problems related to vision; Summary

Chapter 22   Caring for the patient with a disorder   781
             of the male reproductive system

Introduction; Summary of physiology; Sexuality; Disorders of
the male reproductive system; Summary

Chapter 23   Caring for the patient with a female   797
             reproductive system disorder

Introduction; Physiology of the female reproductive tract;
Disorders of the female reproductive system; The woman
with a disorder of the breast; Summary

Chapter 24   Caring for the patient with a disorder   869
             of the musculoskeletal system

Introduction; Structure and function of bones; Structure and
function of joints; Trauma assessment; Fractures; Treatment
and nursing care required for specific injuries; Injuries to
joints; Amputation of a limb; Inflammatory joint disease;
Degenerative joint disease; Other inflammatory joint
diseases; Metabolic joint disease; Connective tissue
(collagen) disease; Infective bone disease; Osteoporosis;
Back pain; Osteomalacia; Paget's disease (osteitis deformans);
Bone neoplasms; Summary

Chapter 25   Caring for the patient with a skin or   925
             wound care need

Introduction; Pressure ulcers; Burn injuries; General skin
conditions; Summary

Chapter 26   Caring for the patient with substance   961
             misuse

Introduction; Definitions and descriptions of terminology;
Alcohol; Tobacco; Commonly abused illicit drugs;
Multidisciplinary working and service structures;
Assessment; Treatment interventions; Suicide;
Deliberate self-harm; Summary

Appendix 1   Shock, cardiac arrest and resuscitation   991
             guidelines

Appendix 2   Learning by reflection   1001

Index   1003

Contributors

Douglas Allan MN BEd RGN RMN RNT
(Chapter 20)
Programme Organiser, BSc Specialist Nursing,
Department of Nursing and Community Health,
Glasgow Calendonian University, Glasgow, UK

Dolsie Allen MSN CRNP
(Chapter 23)
Family Nurse Practitioner, Shawnee Medical Group, PC,
Family Practice Specialists, Shawnee-on-Delaware,
Pennsylvania, USA

Ann Brown RN BA MA RNT
(Chapter 10)
Principal Lecturer, Department of Nursing Studies,
St Martin's College, Bowerham Road, Lancaster, UK

Mark Collier BA(Hons) RNT RCNT ONC RN
(Chapter 25)
Nurse Consultant/Senior Lecturer – Centre for Research
and Implementation of Clinical Practice, Thames Valley
University, Ealing, London, UK

Alison Crumbie MSN BSc RGN Dip NP Dip App ScN PGCE
(Chapter 5)
Senior Lecturer/Nurse Practitioner, St Martin's College,
Bowerham Road, Lancaster, UK

Alyson Dickson RGN BSc MA
(Chapter 13)
Senior Lecturer in Nursing, St Martin's College,
Lancaster, UK

Teresa MD Finlay RN MSc CTHE
(Chapter 15)
Senior Lecturer, Autonomous Health Care Practice,
School of Healthcare, Oxford Brookes University,
Oxford, UK

Pauline Ford RGN MA(Gerontology) DHSM
(Chapter 3)
Director, RCN Gerontological Nursing Programme,
Royal College of Nursing, London, UK

Richard Hatchett RN BA(Hons) MSc CertH/Promotion
(Chapter 12)
Principal Lecturer in Cardiac Nursing, South Bank
University, London, UK

Cathryn Havard BA(Hons) DipNurs RGN CertEd(FE)
OncNursCert
(Chapter 11)
Senior Lecturer in Nursing and Programme Leader
for Cancer and Palliative Care, University of the West
of England, Glenside Campus, Blackberry Hill,
Bristol, UK

Helen L Leathard BSc PhD
(Chapter 6)
Professor of Healing Science and Pharmacology,
Department of Nursing Studies, St Martin's College,
Lancaster, UK

Sue Lee RGN BA(Hons) MSc ENB 998 & 100 FETC
(Chapters 16, 17)
Associate Head of Department Nursing Studies,
St Martin's College, Lancaster, UK

Graham Martindale RGN BSc(Hons)
(Chapter 13)
Clinical Nurse Specialist, Intensive Care Unit, Furness
General Hospital, Barrow-in-Furness, Cumbria, UK and
Associate Lecturer, St Martin's College, Lancaster, UK

Steve Morgan MA
(Chapter 26)
Practice Development Manager, Risk, Sainsbury Centre
for Mental Health, London, UK

Tara O'Neil DClinPsych Bsc(Hons)Psychol
(Chapter 26)
Dual Diagnosis Service Coordinator, Camden & Islington
NHS Mental Health Trust, Hunter Street Health Centre,
8 Hunter Street, London, UK

Lynn J Parker MSc RGN CertEd ENB 329-Infection Control
(Chapter 8)
Clinical Nurse Specialist – Infection, Sheffield Teaching
Hospital NHS Trust, Northern General Hospital,
Sheffield, UK

Miriam K Rowswell MSc BSc(Hons) RGN DipN OncCert
(Chapter 14)
Oncology Nurse Specialist – Gynaecology, Queen Mary's
Hospital, Sidcup, Kent, UK

Susan Skinner SRN ENB 904 DipNurseEd BA MAEducation
(Chapter 9)
Senior Lecturer, Neonatal Health, Anglia Polytechnic
University, Chelmsford, Essex, UK

Veronica Thomas BSc PhD DipN RGN PG DipCouns PGDip
CBT CPsychol
(Chapter 7)
Consultant Health Psychologist, Department of
Haematology, Guy's, St Thomas' NHS Trust,
Lambeth Palace Road, London, UK

Mike Walsh PhD RGN BA(Hons) DipN(London) A&ECert
(Oxford) PGCE
(Chapters 1, 2, 18, 19, 20, 21, 22, 24)
Reader in Nursing, St Martin's College, Lancaster, UK

Tina Wills RGN RMN ONC MSc Health Studies and Gerontology(Exon)
(Chapter 3)
Stroke Coordinator, East Devon Primary Care Trust, Honiton Hospital, Honiton, Devon, UK

Bob Wright Hon MSc RGN RMN Fellow of the Florence Nightingale Foundation
(Chapter 4)
Clinical Nurse Specialist – Crisis Care, Accident/Emergency Department, Leeds General Infirmary, Leeds, UK

Audrey Yandle MSc BA RGN
(Chapter 14)
Lecturer, Florence Nightingale School of Nursing and Midwifery, King's College London, London, UK

Preface

Health care in the UK today faces much the same challenges as in other advanced industrialized countries: spiralling costs, ageing populations, new and emerging health hazards such as antibiotic resistance and the spread of HIV/AIDS, and also shortages of staff, including nurses. Paradoxically, despite the shortage of nurses, we are increasingly being seen as the solution to many of the problems in healthcare delivery as new nursing roles such as the nurse practitioner and nurse-led services (e.g. NHS Direct) are being deployed across the UK. The nurse practitioner concept is over 30 years old in North America but is a recent development in the UK, whilst Australia and New Zealand are not far behind.

All these new nursing developments are underpinned by the need for high-quality education that is clinically relevant. This book is one contribution towards meeting that need. Pre-registration students – such as you the reader – need a good basic standard of education if you are to make safe and effective Registered Nurses. But that is only the beginning of your nursing journey, for you will need to combine further education with the lessons learnt from hard experience to develop your career and nursing role. It is 28 years since I sat down in my introductory class for the first time in Whitehaven, Cumbria, and I still learn something new about nursing every day. I will continue to do just that for many years. We all continue to learn 'Now and in a time yet to be', as one of my favourite poets, WB Yeats, once wrote.

This book is also intended to get you restarted on your nursing career if you have had a career break for a few years and are now returning to the profession. Health care changes at a very rapid rate and even a few years out of practice can suddenly leave you feeling both inadequate and antiquated. Fear not, as you are neither and have a wealth of experience to draw on; however, you do need to know the current thinking on a range of techniques and treatments. This book should help ease you back into clinical practice.

So, whether you are a novice or returning after a career break, I trust this book will help you on your way in the modern, complex world of health care.

Lancaster 2002   Mike Walsh

Publisher's Acknowledgements

Baillière Tindall would like to express their considerable gratitude to Dr Roger Watson, Professor of Nursing, Department of Nursing and Applied Health Studies, University of Hull, for his painstaking and invaluable work in providing the numerous physiology cross-references for this edition.

Publisher's Notes

Dosages   Every effort has been made to ensure any dosage recommendations are precise and in agreement with standards officially accepted at the time of publication. However, it is urged that you check the manufacturer's recommendations for dosage.

Case Studies   Throughout this book various Case Studies are described which aim to enhance aspects of the text by providing realistic clinical scenarios. Please note that the identity of each person described in these Case Studies is fictitious, and that any resemblance to known individuals, alive or dead, is thus entirely coincidental.

Permissions   The publishers have made every effort to clear permission to reproduce material from previously published work used in this book. However, if any material has been overlooked please bring it to our attention and we can amend at reprint.

A guide to the physiology cross-referencing system

Unlike any other clinical nursing textbook, *Watson's Clinical Nursing and Related Sciences* 6th Edition has invented a dynamic and innovative approach to directly linking key elements in clinical nursing with their corresponding, or underlying, physiological processes.

Wherever you see a word in the text written in **bold**, there will be a direct cross-reference in the margin to the relevant chapter in *Physiology for Nursing Practice* 2nd Edition, edited by Hinchliff, Montague and Watson. This cross-referencing system not only ensures that you are directed precisely and efficiently to the relevant chapter of one of the most highly respected bionursing physiology textbooks available, it also means that 'Watson's' is able to devote far more in-depth pages to clinical nursing.

EXAMPLE:

description of what the patient should know or be able to do and the factors influencing this.

Identifying educational needs and setting priorities requires assessing the patient's and family's present knowledge, how they see the patient's present level of functioning and what the desired level of competence may be. It is important to know whether they are able to look at the long-term implications or are able to focus only on what is happening today. This sort of assessment must be a continuous process, as changes occur once the patient has achieved the initial goals, coped with the impact of illness and begun to accept the changes in lifestyle.

Once learning needs have been identified, the nurse works with the patient to establish goals for learning, to determine priorities for teaching content and to select methods of teaching. Learning goals are usually divided into *short-term goals*, for immediate learning needs, and *long-term objectives*, for defining the eventual expected outcomes. The knowledge or skill to be achieved is defined, and the expected level or degree to which it will be met is stated. The final component of objective setting is defining the time in which the desired change is expected to occur. Behavioural objectives are worded in simple, basic terms that are clear to the patient and to all members of the healthcare team. They break learning tasks into small, sequential steps that can be tackled independently before the total goal is achieved.

The teaching plan must be written and placed in the patient's record. Without a written plan, other members of the healthcare team cannot actively participate in the teaching process. The plan must also be shared with the patient so that he or she can actively work towards achieving results.

Using a patient with **diabetes** as an example, behavioural objectives for the patient might be to:

- *state* the action of insulin

- *demonstrate* the technique of drawing up the prescribed amount of insulin into a syringe

- *talk about* feelings related to self-injection with insulin.

Teaching content must be accurately expressed in terms and language understandable to the patient and family, and adapted to age, cognitive ability, education and culture. The amount of time necessary and opportunities for questions, correction and repetition should be given consideration when planning teaching programmes.

Practical procedures should be broken down into a logical sequence of steps. First, the procedure should be demonstrated as a whole so that the patient is provided with an overview; then each step should be shown slowly and in detail. Time and opportunity should be allowed for practising the technique as soon as possible after the demonstration. The nurse should be aware that, in teaching any body of information, the first and last parts are recalled best; therefore, the most important points should come first and last. Repetition and receptiveness to questions reinforces learning.

Evaluation of the teaching programme and the patient's learning should be continuous. Revisions are made as indicated, and in some instances are made on the spot if the patient is not responding positively to the planned strategy. Outcomes of teaching are assessed: what effect the teaching has had, whether the objectives have been met, and whether the patient has acquired the knowledge and skills needed. Role playing or simulation may be used to assess changes in the patient's behavioural responses and in the ability to apply knowledge to real-life situations. The patient must also be an active participant in the ongoing and final evaluation of the educational plan. Observation and feedback are the primary ways in which the nurse determines whether (behavioural) change has occurred.

The process outlined above provides a framework for health education. It has not, however, referred to the many possible moral dilemmas that may be thrown up in day-to-day practice. Clarke (1993) has discussed health education with regard to the basic ethical principles of respecting the autonomy of the individual, acting to benefit the person (*beneficence*), not harming the individual (*non-maleficence*) and finally giving people what they deserve (*justice*). As she observes, health education involves choices and, if the wrong choices are made, a great deal of harm can follow; therefore the nurse must always be able to defend his or her actions ethically.

Health screening is an example chosen by Clarke, especially with regard to **cervical screening**. It is intended to be beneficial to the patient and to do no harm. But consider the stresses involved in the procedure and afterwards waiting for the results. Suppose that the woman is recalled for another smear or a mistake is made? The Health Belief Model would predict that, if the fears and anxieties generated by the procedure were too great, they might outweigh the possible advantages, leading to women failing to attend for screening at all.

It was issues such as these that led Foxwell and Alder (1993) to investigate whether a simple 10-minute nurse teaching package before screening could reduce anxiety levels. A large sample of 187 consecutive women (who were well educated and from a predominantly middle-class background) were allocated at random to either a control group that experienced the standard procedure or an experimental group that was given an additional nurse teaching presentation about the procedure. Anxiety levels after the smear were significantly reduced in the experimental group compared with the control group, suggesting that patient teaching in this case reduced anxiety. The researchers predict that this effect would be more pronounced in women who were less well educated or well informed, although this remains to be tested.

Encouraging women to attend for screening therefore generates anxiety, despite our principle of beneficence,

Diabetes:
See chapter 2.6.

Cervical cytology:
See chapter 6.3.

Physiology
for
Nursing Practice

Second Edition

SUSAN M. HINCHLIFF

SUSAN E., MONTAGUE

ROGER WATSON

 BAILLIÈRE TINDALL

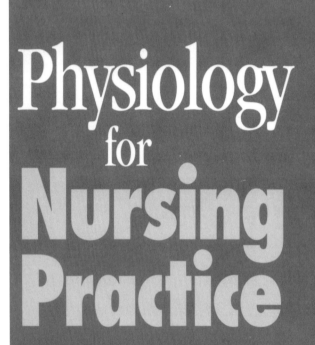

Physiology for Nursing Practice (second edition) excerpt from the editors' introduction

In the second edition of *Physiology for Nursing Practice* we have not only adapted and developed the first edition's text but also extended and reorganized the content to include important new material and to facilitate clarity and ease of use. This new content, now presented with full colour, reflects current thinking in the delivery of health care as well as the content of modern nursing and health care curricula. The content has been modified according to feedback from students who have used the first edition.

We know that pre-registration nursing students thirst for application and practice examples when learning physiology. On the other hand, registered nurses, extending their knowledge, often have rewarding experiences in class as they suddenly understand why a patient or client has a certain problem and thus the biological rationale for his or her care. This book recognizes and meets such learning needs. The second edition has been written especially for students on pre-registration diploma and degree courses in nursing and midwifery and for registered nurses and midwives following courses in specialist practice.

Although *Physiology for Nursing Practice* is written primarily for nurses, we know from experience that other health professionals will also find its content useful. It is most suitable for UK practitioners because of its terminology and focus on care practices found in the UK, and because of its use and explanation of SI units of measurement.

In preparing the text we had five main aims:

(1) to enable readers to understand the principles and mechanisms of body function, so that they can appreciate how these alter in illness;
(2) to support bioscience curricula in nursing diploma and degree level courses;
(3) to provide readers with a rational basis for assessing a patient's health problems, and for the planning, delivery and evaluation of care;
(4) to convey a sense of fascination and enthusiasm about how the body works and to motivate readers to further their studies;
(5) to express all of the above as clearly and as simply as possible but not at the expense of scientific accuracy.

We are aware that knowledge of any scientific discipline is continually being modified and extended through research. Every effort has been made to ensure that the physiology presented in this book reflects the consensus of opinion at the time of writing.

Physiology for Nursing Practice is still primarily concerned with normal, healthy body function and essentially describes how the body maintains homeostasis. Throughout the text, practice applications are highlighted to demonstrate clearly how homeostasis becomes deranged by illness and how knowledge of normal function provides a sound basis for understanding abnormality and rationale for patient/client care.

Like its predecessor the book has six major sections which, rather than following the classical systemic approach, logically illustrate the functioning of the body as a complex homeostatic system. These sections are:

1. Characteristics of Living Matter
2. Control and Co-ordination
3. Mobility and Support
4. Internal Transport
5. The Acquisition of Nutrients and Removal of Waste
6. Protection and Survival.

The introductory section, Characteristics of Living Matter, has been extended and now contains three chapters. There is a whole new chapter on the Chemistry of Life. We think the text of this chapter will, in an undaunting fashion, meet the needs of students previously unfamiliar with the subject, to equip them with crucial foundation knowledge for their applied and integrated courses. We have also incorporated new material on SI units, the organization of the body and the nature of growth, development and ageing into Section 1.

As in the first edition the remaining five sections each present a major aspect of homeostasis. As well as the new material included as a result of updating, there is an extra chapter on Stress (in Section 3) and substantial new sections on Exercise (in Section 4) and on Clinical Genetics (in Section 6). All chapters have been revised with requirements of modern nursing curricula at the forefront of each contributor's attention. All our contributors – the majority of whom are nurses – were chosen because of their knowledge of biological sciences as applied to nursing and for their reputation and experience in teaching and writing on their subject. The end result has been that their chapters all contain new content on development and ageing and focused material which supports learning in all four branches of nursing and in midwifery.

We believe that this book will be a major new resource for those involved in the care of patients. We commend it to you in the hope that through its use you will experience that same sense of fascination about how the human body works that was the inspiration for its production.

Susan M. Hinchliff
Susan E. Montague
Roger Watson
1996

Summary of key content

- Focus on the significance of homeostasis
- Increased emphasis on disturbances to equilibrium
- Entirely new chapter on the chemistry of life
- New material on developmental aspects, growth and ageing
- Extensive references to nursing literature and research

Written and edited by respected nurse educators, this edition has been fully revised and updated to reflect the changing needs of nursing students and their teachers. The text has been completely redesigned to promote understanding and critical thinking. All the illustrations appear in full colour and each chapter contains numerous opportunities for student interaction through practice examples and questions.

Text features include:

- Clear learning objectives
- Key concepts emphasized for ease of reference
- Review questions with answers
- Clinical implications and nursing care highlighted throughout
- Annotated suggestions for further reading
- For lecturers, also contains suggestions for practical activities and experiments

Susan M. Hinchliff, BA, RGN, RNT, is Vice Principal (Continuing Education), Institute of Advanced Nursing Studies, Royal College of Nursing, London, UK.
Susan E. Montague, BSc(Hons), RGN, HV Dip, RNT, is Principal Lecturer in Nursing, Division of Adult Nursing & Health Sciences, University of Hertfordshire, Hatfield, Hertfordshire, UK.
Roger Watson, BSc, PhD, RGN, CBiol, Mlbiol, is Senior Lecturer, Department of Nursing Studies, University of Edinburgh, Edinburgh, UK.

Published by Baillière Tindall ©1996

780 pages. ISBN 0-7020-1638-1

'The first edition of *Physiology for Nursing Practice* established it as a standard text. The new edition is superb.

Imaginative use of colour means that particular sections of the book can be easily found. The quality of illustrations is also very high. As an up-to-date and applied book, this would be very hard to beat.'

**** Accessibility
**** Production quality
**** User friendliness
**** Value for money

Star Guide: **** Excellent *** Good ** Fair * Poor

Nursing Standard May 8/Volume 10/Number 33/1996

The context of care

Chapter 1   The nature of nursing   *Mike Walsh*

Chapter 2   Therapeutic communication and nursing practice   *Mike Walsh*

Chapter 3   Ageing and health   *Pauline Ford and Tina Wills*

Chapter 4   Death, grief and loss   *Bob Wright*

Chapter 5   Primary health care and the management of chronic illness   *Alison Crumbie*

The context of care: Introduction

Nothing in life can ever be divorced from its context if it is to be fully understood and nursing is no exception. For a complete understanding of how to care for a patient recovering from pneumonia or a stroke, it is essential to look at the professional context within which the nurse is attempting to work, as well as at the family and wider social environment. Direct nursing care therefore depends upon a wide-ranging set of factors, which are explored in this first section of the book. It is essential that nurses know nursing and understand why nursing exists. A professional sense of self identity is crucial if nursing is to avoid merely being a collection of odd jobs that nobody else wants. At the core of that identity is the primacy of the patient.

Clinical care also depends heavily upon therapeutic communication, which is a two-way process. The word 'therapeutic' is crucial as this denotes communication as part of treatment and care. Effective communication will prevent many mishaps and improve patient outcomes. 'Effective' means not only that the patient fully understands what is being said and done but also has a part in that action and in the decision-making process. This means in turn that you as the nurse need to be a good listener. Hear what the patient is telling you and be sensitive also to the non-verbal channels of communication.

Section one of this book helps set the scene for what follows but will also allow you to make better sense of later chapters when you have read them. You are encouraged to revisit these early chapters later in your education and reflect upon their content in the light of your experience.

The nature of nursing

Mike Walsh

Introduction

The nurse and the healthcare system

The focus of nursing

The delivery of nursing care

Documentation

Nursing ethics

The nurse as a promoter of health

Health education and health promotion: the debate

Models of health promotion

Health education and patient teaching

Summary

Introduction

Large textbooks of this nature frequently start with an introductory overview of the big issues facing nursing today and a summary of the content that follows in the next thousand-odd pages. This one does not. Instead I want to start with a real person's story, a story that is not unusual for patients of her age and encapsulates many of the problems and issues that you will have to learn to deal with as a qualified nurse in the years ahead. Let me introduce you to Pat (see Case Study 1.1) and ask you to reflect upon her story as you read the rest of this introductory chapter.

Case Study 1.1   *Pat's story*

Pat was born in the 1920s at the height (or depth?) of the Great Depression. She had a brother and a sister, her father having survived the horrors of World War I as an army sergeant, wounded and invalided out of the carnage at the Battle of the Somme in 1916. She grew up in a strict authoritarian family background that was always poor, her father finding work whenever he could. She left school at 14 with no qualifications and went to work in a shop. During World War II she met her husband to be and worked in the munitions industry, suddenly finding herself employed as a draftswoman as there were insufficient skilled men to meet the demands of making Spitfire engines. She also experienced the horror of being buried alive in an air-raid shelter that took a direct hit during the blitz. Today we would understand the mental distress that followed this event and which dogged her for many years afterwards as post-traumatic stress disorder and Pat would have counselling to help her recover. In those days you were just glad to have survived and had to get on with things as best you could. After the war Pat went back to working in a soap factory as demobbed men reclaimed their old jobs. She married Bernard and had one child, working part time as a cleaner thereafter. The family was rehoused on a council estate in the 1960s.

Things began to go wrong. Both Pat's parents developed **type II diabetes**, her father had a stroke, developed gangrene in his foot, had his leg amputated and then

Type II diabetes
See chapter 2.6

developed gangrene in his other foot and died a miserable death in great pain. Her marriage fell apart when she was in her 40s, and after much argument her husband left home for another woman. Pat became depressed, began drinking heavily and took a series of overdoses, usually of the benzodiazepines that her general practitioner was supplying on an endless series of repeat prescriptions without actually seeing her. She lost the tenancy of the council house and moved to a small one-bedroomed flat. Admission to a large psychiatric hospital followed to detoxify and then to attempt to treat her anxiety and depression. Pat spent most of the next few years in one of two large psychiatric hospitals before finally being discharged to a 'half-way house', aged nearly 60. She was no longer drinking and had finally given up smoking, but had become very institutionalized. Subsequently she was discharged from care into a small council flat. Shortly afterwards, her brother died, aged 60, as a result of renal failure and multiple other complications secondary to type II diabetes, which he had also developed.

Pat now became very reclusive, refusing to leave the flat or see a doctor or any other healthcare professional. She had put on a great deal of weight during her lengthy stays in the two mental hospitals. Despite becoming increasingly disabled with osteoarthritis and having a strong family history of type II diabetes, she put on further weight after discharge. She dealt with the problems of her **obesity** and high risk for type II diabetes by denial. She had never divorced her husband (he was Catholic) and he still visited her weekly to get shopping and do odd jobs for her. Her son, who lived away from the area, also visited whenever he could and helped with shopping and odd jobs. The home help who came in twice a week was Pat's only other contact with the outside world. Her son noticed a strong odour on one visit and, despite her protestations, lifted back the bedclothes to find a gangrenous infected toe. Admission to hospital failed to save the leg and it was amputated as the diagnosis of type II diabetes was confirmed.

A short while after being discharged to a nursing home Pat was readmitted with a gangrenous ulcer on the heel of her remaining foot, caused by the foot being elevated on a footstool for long periods without any pressure relief. The other leg was amputated as, in addition, she was critically ill with septicaemia and heart failure. She was discharged to another nursing home where she was reasonably happy for a further 2 years, but then this home closed down and Pat was transferred to a third home. By now her husband had died after suffering a succession of strokes. In this final nursing home she became very disoriented and confused; she had lost her sight as a result of cataract formation and received little stimulation from the environment.

Obesity
See chapter 6.1

Finally, aged 78, Pat was admitted to hospital for the last time where she died from bronchopneumonia. Her sister survived her and she too suffers from type II diabetes.

What can we learn from Pat's story? Understanding health is clearly a great deal more than the physical process of disease. Social and psychological factors played a large part in shaping Pat's life. Her illness and care needs can be understood only in the context of the great social events that shaped the twentieth century and the lives of today's older people. How did her father's experiences in World War I and the Depression of the 1920s impact upon her upbringing? What were the long-term consequences for her mental health of her own wartime experiences? Psychological factors are also paramount in this story: witness Pat's denial of her type II diabetes and the catastrophic results that had. Yet some aspects of disease and health are beyond our control, as shown by the strong family trait of type II diabetes that dogged Pat and her family. Social isolation was a major factor in her later years whilst lack of stimulation in her last nursing home contributed to her final confusional state. Pat experienced nursing care in large psychiatric institutions, accident and emergency departments, acute hospital wards and nursing homes at various stages of her life. She was never an easy patient and presented a complex challenge whenever she came into contact with the caring system. Perhaps the nursing staff in the mental hospitals could have prevented Pat becoming so obese. Care in the community could have prevented many of her problems after discharge, but only if she had been a willing and cooperative partner in her care, which she was not. A small pressure sore, which could have been prevented, set in motion a chain of events that led to the loss of her remaining leg. These are examples of how effective nursing care improves quality of life and prevents illness.

Pat is the sort of patient you will frequently encounter: a real person with multiple interrelated problems that have physical, social and psychological origins. Nursing can make a huge difference in caring for people like Pat and that is the challenge you face in your career. This book will help you rise to that challenge and help all the Pats you will encounter in the years ahead.

The nurse and the healthcare system

There have been many changes in nursing over the past decade. Perhaps two of the most significant have been the rise of accountability and health as key concepts in nursing. Nurses have always been responsible for the care they delivered but that is not the same as being accountable. The traditional model that we largely worked with was the biomedical model with its focus on illness, not health. As Pat's story illustrates, this approach misses out a great deal that is essential to care for people who, in the majority of cases, will not be cured of their illness, only helped to live with it. This crucial shift in emphasis has led to nurses being seen as *accountable healthcare practitioners*, with a consequent growth in autonomy that is redefining our relationship with both patients and the medical profession. We need to explore how nurses fit into the healthcare system if we are to understand the implications of increased levels of autonomy and a greater focus on health.

There are various agencies that directly or indirectly control and affect your everyday nursing practice. This will become increasingly apparent to you as you progress in nursing and become more aware of the context within which you operate. The key agencies can be summarized as:

■ the higher education institution where you are educated

■ the patient and his or her family

■ the community

■ registered nurses and other healthcare professionals

■ employers and managers who run the healthcare system

■ the statutory bodies that regulate nursing.

As a student you are responsible to these agencies but when you qualify you will become fully accountable to them, except of course your university, as by then you will have qualified. Accountability means simply being able to give an account of why you did what you did, when you did it. This is very different from responsibility, which is concerned with following instructions and guidelines conscientiously, rather than acting as you see fit and then being able to justify your actions. Accountability therefore involves making decisions for yourself that you can justify. For a registered nurse to be accountable, therefore, she or he must have the necessary authority and autonomy to make decisions and act upon them, and also the necessary knowledge to make the right decisions. Full accountability comes only with registration, but even as a student you are always responsible for your actions. Initially you are likely to be most aware of your teachers and the college environment but, as you start to gain practical experience, patients, their families and staff involved in direct care will become foremost in your concerns. As your career develops, never forget that the patient is always the most important person to whom you are accountable. The patient is also a member of the wider community and increasingly becoming aware of his or her rights.

The staff involved in giving care, such as your mentor on the ward or in the health centre, are in turn accountable to those who manage the service at local, regional and national level. We are also accountable to our colleagues in other professions such as medicine. Health

service managers are in their turn accountable to the elected government of the day. But there is another major force involved in controlling practice: the United Kingdom Central Council for Nursing, Midwifery and Health Visiting, or UKCC for short. This statutory body is set to be replaced in 2002 by another body as part of a general reorganization of the bodies responsible for regulation of the health professions. However, at present, you can call yourself a nurse only if the UKCC has you on its live register.

Ultimately there are three main mechanisms for holding you accountable as a registered nurse:

1. The UKCC holds registered nurses to account via the Code of Professional Conduct.

2. The patient holds the nurse and the National Health Service to account via the civil law, which permits the patient to sue for damages should things go wrong.

3. The employer holds the nurse to account via a contract of employment, which is also enforceable by law.

In addition, no nurse or health professional is above the law, either criminal or civil, and, as we have seen in the infamous cases of nurse Beverly Allitt and Dr Harold Shipman, nurses and doctors can be convicted of murder.

Whatever country you work in, from the day you qualify, you will find yourself pulled three different ways by these competing forces of accountability: to the patient, to the national statutory body that regulates nursing and to your employer. The consequences of this tension for nursing today are explored in some depth in Walsh (2000). While it certainly presents complex problems, accountability also leads to real opportunities as increasing levels of autonomy in practice and better educational opportunities flow logically from the basic principle of accountability. This can, however, lead to potential conflict with other professional groups.

Change and the healthcare services

Changes in the delivery of healthcare services have been in response to three major social trends in the second half of the twentieth century: the explosion in scientific knowledge, the escalating costs of health services and the changing needs of the healthcare consumer population. These trends give rise to complex issues that involve economic, political, social, cultural, educational and ethical considerations.

Scientific discoveries in medicine, notably advanced medical technology, have influenced the delivery of healthcare services and nursing practice. Advances in medical technology permit intense monitoring of and interventions into human biological processes on a scale hitherto unimagined. Life and death decisions may be made on the basis of nurses' interpretations of information from high-technology equipment. These advances have led to increasing specialization within nursing, in both hospital and community settings.

Advances in computer technology, as part of the explosion in scientific knowledge, have influenced the delivery of health care. Computers have automated and consolidated information and increased the speed and efficiency of information processing. Nurses in a variety of healthcare settings are using computers to enter, store and retrieve patient information, check nursing and medical orders, and request services for their patients from other sectors of the healthcare system as diverse as pharmaceutical and social services.

Genetic engineering developments have brought in their wake very complex ethical problems and nurses have increasingly to be aware of the need to offer patients opportunities to talk through these issues in a supportive environment. Counselling skills are increasingly becoming part of the nurse's repertoire and the next chapter will explore this further.

A second trend, the rising cost of restoration to health through acute care hospitalization, in competition with other public needs and wants and in the face of finite resources, has provoked a search for alternative healthcare delivery strategies and sites. Health promotion and health maintenance through public education and community-based programmes have become widespread. Nurses have played a significant role in providing these alternatives and have been given the lead role in the NHS Direct 24-hour telephone health advice service. NHS walk-in centres are another new nurse-led innovation currently being introduced, although both these initiatives have attracted considerable criticism from organized medicine. In addition, increased attention has been given to threats to human health emanating from personal lifestyles, pollution of the environment and poor socio-economic circumstances.

The Conservative government in the UK was responsible for a marked reduction in the number of hospital beds during the 1990s and a reduction in student nurse numbers. This has belatedly been recognized as a major mistake and the Labour government that took office in 1997, after an initial period of hesitation, finally started to commit the necessary resources to reverse these trends. In the run up to the 2001 election, pre-election promises from the Conservatives signalled an intention to match Labour's expenditure on the NHS. Since the election, Labour seem to have raised the stakes and pledged even higher levels of expenditure on the NHS in a bid to bring UK health expenditure up to the EU average. However as the government are finding out to their discomfort, it takes many years to have an impact upon an organization as large as the NHS. In the short to medium term, therefore, we have to work with what we have got, which means finding smarter and more effective ways of working; this will involve challenging many traditional professional boundaries.

The care in the community policy means that elderly patients are increasingly seen as belonging in private nursing homes or being supported at home by the local social services department rather than cared for by the NHS. A major new initiative is the provision of intermediate care for older people in order to avoid acute hospital beds becoming blocked by patients whose acute medical problems have been largely resolved, but whose discharge is not possible because of predominantly social and psychological problems. Rapid response teams have also been set up in a bid to keep older people out of the hospital system. A similar community philosophy has been applied to caring for those with a learning disability or mental health problems. If such initiatives are seen purely as a cost-cutting opportunity, however, there is a danger that vulnerable groups will suffer. Community care is not necessarily cheaper and will achieve results only if the patient is a cooperative partner (reflect on Pat's story). Criticism of the care in the community policy relates to underfunding of its implementation rather than to the policy itself. It is not a means of saving money in a way that, perhaps, day-care surgery is.

A third trend, the changing needs of the healthcare consumer population, stems from changing patterns of mortality and morbidity, coupled with consumers' increased participation in their own healthcare decisions. The proportion of the population that is elderly is increasing, as is the incidence of chronic illness. The older segment of the UK population is increasingly including people from ethnic minority backgrounds born in the Indian subcontinent or the Caribbean, for whom culturally sensitive care is required. Meanwhile social disruption in other parts of the world has produced a significant number of refugees and asylum seekers who do not speak English. Their health needs must be met, despite the political rhetoric of being 'tough on bogus asylum seekers' that characterizes the main UK political parties.

Longitudinal studies show a pattern of decreasing mortality and increasing incidence of morbidity (illness) in middle-aged and older people. Previously, acute infectious diseases were the greatest threat to health; today, chronic disabling diseases, from infancy to old age, represent our major health problems. These disabling diseases are attributed to detrimental social, environmental and lifestyle factors, which are much more difficult to control than infections. Chronic illness represents a broad spectrum of diseases. Some are life-threatening, such as **heart disease**, **cancer**, **acquired immune deficiency syndrome (AIDS)** and **stroke**, while others are more physically or cognitively debilitating, such as **diabetes** (as shown by Pat's story) or **Alzheimer's disease**.

Consumers' involvement in their own health care changed considerably in the latter half of the twentieth century. In the 1970s, the women's movement and other activist groups began to assert their rights in health care. Today, consumers are much more knowledgeable about

Heart disease
See chapters 2.7 & 4.2

Cancer
See chapters 1.3 & 6.2

AIDS
See chapter 6.2

Stroke
See chapter 2.2

Diabetes
See chapter 2.6

Dementia
See chapter 2.2

health problems and interventions. More consumers want to participate actively in their health care; they seek information to make informed decisions. The formerly dependent, acquiescent patient may now prefer to be an active partner with the healthcare team members.

Nurses have responded to the changing needs of patients by focusing less on the medical emphasis of disease cure and more on the holism of patient health promotion, maintenance and restoration. Thus, the role of the nurse incorporates that of adviser, counsellor and collaborator. Nurses work in partnership with patients. Nurses increasingly provide information for patients, assisting them to examine their own values, beliefs and goals, and helping them to evaluate and choose from available courses of action.

The focus of nursing

Nursing is recognized as an emerging profession with a unique perspective on people, environment and health. It is the application of nursing knowledge to the promotion, maintenance and restoration of health for the individual and family through stressful events, which may include death and bereavement. In recent years, nursing has derived its focus not from the medical model, with its emphasis on the treatment and cure of pathological problems, but from the relationships between people, the environment and health outlined in the holistic philosophy that underpins the nursing model of care.

It is noteworthy that, from the time of Florence Nightingale, nursing has described as its focus the health of human beings. What has changed over time are the skills, scope and settings of nursing practice. Nurses maintain that care is at the core of nursing practice, but we should remember that nurses do not have a monopoly on care. Any doctor or physiotherapist would state that they care for their patients as well. The key is to understand what we mean by that little four-letter word 'care'.

This has been discussed extensively by Walsh (2000) and he concludes that, while it is axiomatic that nursing is about caring, there is uncomfortable evidence to question the commitment of some nurses to caring, especially for other nurses. The literature may be summarized by saying that caring is:

- a one-to-one interpersonal reaction. You have to recognize the person in the patient and in yourself to really care

- context dependent – the environment is crucial in the delivery of care

- about being involved and having things matter rather than performing a series of tasks in a cold, detached manner

- taking into account the person's emotional and psychological needs together with the social circumstances in which he or she lives

- about seeing things from the patient's point of view

- universal in nature: to be cared for is a fundamental human right. It is a moral imperative that the nurse discharges equally for all people.

You should reflect upon this analysis at various stages of your education. Memorable incidents occur to all nurses in their training and you will be no exception. These critical incidents can be either positive or negative but will still be valuable learning experiences if you reflect upon them critically with this view of caring in mind.

Concepts central to nursing

The patient

The patient is the recipient of nursing care and fundamentally must always be seen as a person. The patient is viewed in the context of being both a human being and being unique, with a particular make-up, experiences and responses. The person has a distinct identity, in addition to being a member of a family and community, and is in constant interaction with the environment. Interactions and responses are influenced by sociocultural background, lifestyle, values, capabilities, interests, past experiences and the patterns of behaviour laid down as a result of those experiences. These factors contribute to the uniqueness of the person, who should be regarded as having worth, dignity and the right to pursue health, happiness, love, security, purpose and freedom. The nurse considers the individual holistically by focusing the nurse–patient encounter on the total person and not merely the component parts.

The patient should always be informed about his or her health status, make informed decisions compatible with personal beliefs and values, and actively participate (as far as possible) in the care process. All people have essential basic human needs; nursing intervention may be indicated when the individual cannot independently satisfy these needs. Basic biological needs include the intake of oxygen, fluids and food, the elimination of wastes, rest, sleep, activity, and maintenance of body temperature within a definite range. Significant psychosocial needs of each person include: a sense of security, the maintenance of an identity as an individual, acceptance, a sense of being wanted and belonging, the opportunity for socializing, independence (and at times dependence and interdependence), freedom to make decisions, and opportunities to develop and use innate potential. He or she should have interests and goals and the opportunity to feel self-respect, in addition to feeling useful and having a sense of achievement.

Environment

The relationship between the individual and the environment is dynamic and influences both health and lifestyle. Within the context of nursing, the internal environment comprises everything within the skin and mucous membranes of the body. It encompasses all structural and physiological aspects of the human body and may be modified by psychological and sociocultural experiences. The external environment includes physical surroundings, patterns of relationships and interactions with family and society, outside resources, and the ways in which the individual has contact with a healthcare delivery system.

Nursing is directed towards managing the way in which the patient interacts with the environment, promoting health, preventing disease and delivering care in illness. Specific strategies and actions enabling the nurse to direct or manage the patient–environment interaction vary according to the individual, the environment and the health problem.

Health

The meaning of health is a matter of considerable controversy (see p. 14). Some nurses see health as a state, others as a process. Most recognize health as a goal to be attained and maintained. How health is perceived by the individual is influenced by cultural and educational background and by past experiences. An individual's health is measured against some yardstick or set of standards. The standard used may be absolute; for example, it may be the presence or absence of disease, or the ability or inability to function as a contributing, independent member of society. Other measurements may be relative and give greater consideration to subjective components such as the sense of well-being and quality of life but, overall, health remains an illusive concept to try to measure absolutely.

Besides the physiological and functional aspects of health, nursing is also concerned with subjective factors contributing to the quality of life and the opportunity the individual has to realize potential. Effects of the internal environment on functioning, well-being and lifestyle are readily apparent. The effects of unfavourable external environmental factors significant to health, such as polluted air, water, noise and adverse living conditions, are complex and more difficult to identify and change. Other factors related to lifestyle, such as the amount of physical exercise a person takes, dietary and smoking habits, levels of **stress** and relationships with others, can also affect health and perception of health.

Nursing

Nursing takes place within the context of the nurse–patient relationship, which is characterized as a professional or therapeutic relationship. This differs from a social relationship in that it is collaborative and is directed towards meeting the patient's goals. It may be time limited and take place within a structured and designated setting, such as a health centre or hospital. People often have preconceived ideas about the nurse as well as about how they themselves should behave as patients.

Stress
See chapter 2.7

Clarification of these perceptions may be necessary before an effective rapport can develop. The professional purpose of the relationship gives direction to the role assumed by the nurse and to the way in which the nurse applies nursing knowledge and skills. The nurse brings to the relationship respect for the person's uniqueness and integrity, and an appreciation of the patient's right to participate in or receive care. The patient, as an active participant, brings certain abilities and values, as well as a background of culture, education, experiences and needs, with the right to demonstrate and apply these in decisions and in the care process. Mutual acceptance is fundamental to the effectiveness of the nurse–patient relationship.

As the nurse develops empathy with the patient and strives to earn trust and confidence, the patient should develop trust and confidence in the nurse. With each encounter, the nurse's role is mutually agreed upon by the nurse and patient. A sincere interest and willingness to help may be demonstrated by the nurse being non-judgemental, accepting the patient, demonstrating thoughtfulness, anticipating needs, showing concern and, most importantly, by being ready to listen and answer questions. Recognition of identity by addressing the patient by name, respect for personal preferences and the demonstration of flexibility contribute to a satisfactory relationship. Appreciation of the family's concerns and each member's need for an interpretation of what is happening fosters trust and confidence. Expressing and sharing information with the family may prove therapeutic for them as well as the patient.

During the total nurse–patient relationship, the nurse's responsibilities include that of being the advocate. When acting on behalf of the patient, attempts are made to assess the situation carefully from the patient's point of view, rather than simply deciding what is 'good for' the patient on the basis of past nursing experience. As advocate, the nurse should provide information to assist the patient and/or the family to make informed decisions about the individual's health care (e.g. about a procedure, a form of therapy or a change in circumstances). Confidentiality must be respected; it is an important factor in establishing and maintaining good nurse–patient relationships. When information must be shared with other members of the healthcare team, the patient should be advised of the reasons and the advantages of communicating it to others.

The nurse–patient relationship lies at the heart of nursing and it is not surprising, therefore, to find that the UKCC, the regulatory body for nursing, makes this the cornerstone of its *Code of Professional Practice* (UKCC 1992a). This document is binding upon all nurses and sets out guiding principles for ethical and safe practice with regard to issues such as advocacy and confidentiality. You should have been issued with a copy of the code when you commenced your nurse education and are well advised to revisit the document at regular intervals. Always remember that it tells you first and foremost to safeguard the interest of individual patients and that you will always be held accountable for your actions as a registered nurse.

Rapid changes taking place in practice mean that you will find nurses in situations where in the past they did not practise. New therapeutic skills and techniques, radical changes in clinical practice (e.g. day-care surgery), shortages of junior medical staff and increasing demand for health care in the community are only some examples. The UKCC principles within the *Code of Professional Practice*, particularly concerning accountability, underpin all such new developments together with another very important UKCC document, *Scope of Professional Practice* (UKCC 1992b). This document takes the concept of accountability and uses it to show how nurses may expand and develop their roles into new areas, provided they remember that they will always be held accountable for what they do.

An exciting new development in the recent past has been the growth of the *nurse practitioner* role. This is another term bandied about loosely and which must be closely defined. The concept was developed in the USA and has several key distinguishing features. The nurse practitioner sees patients with an undifferentiated diagnosis, utilizing both nursing and medical assessment skills to arrive at a diagnosis before either initiating treatment (within protocols agreed with the relevant doctors) or referring on as appropriate. The nurse practitioner, therefore, can carry out physical examinations, take a medical history and utilize clinical decision-making skills to operate on the boundaries of nursing and medicine. She or he brings together the best of both nursing and medicine to deliver high-quality health care to the patient. There is a high degree of autonomy involved and the nurse may work in a primary care environment such as a health centre or in an acute hospital (e.g. A&E department) providing a health service that is complementary to, but different from, the conventional medical consultation. Nurse practitioners may develop clinical specialist roles in areas such as diabetes or ophthalmology. Alternatively they may work with specialist client groups such as prostitutes (such a service operates in Belfast) or farmers (see p. 17). The nurse–patient interaction, however, remains governed by the holistic philosophy outlined above; the nurse is at all times working as a nurse, remains bound by the UKCC Code of Professional Practice, and is accountable for everything that he or she does.

A very important part of the Code of Conduct reminds nurses that all patients are equal and all deserve equally high standards of care. The nurse must not be judgemental about patients and has no right to refuse to give care. As the UKCC points out, the law does not confer upon the nurse any right of conscientious objection to participation in treatment; the nurse should consider any strongly held beliefs when applying for posts in the first place. Nurses cannot refuse to care for a patient without simultaneously breaching the UKCC Code of Professional Practice and their contract of employment, whilst placing themselves at risk of a civil lawsuit for negligence.

Within different nurse–patient relationships, the nurse may find theories from other disciplines very useful in describing, explaining, making predictions about, or controlling the events that occasion the relationship. For example, the nurse may derive insights from knowledge of the psychological and physiological changes associated with ageing to assist the elderly patient; alternatively, learning theory may assist the nurse in patient teaching. Depending upon the context, theories from other disciplines have considerable relevance to nursing as descriptions, explanations and/or predictors of the relationships between patient, environment and health, and as the basis for rational nursing actions. It is, however, nursing's unique perspective that directs us to select from among the theories of other disciplines those that are useful in each nurse–patient relationship.

The growth of evidence-based practice also requires nurses to base their practice upon firm evidence. There are three sources of evidence for practice, and research is only one of them. The other two key areas are patient preferences and the practitioner's own experience of what works best. Accountable nursing practice, therefore, means that the nurse must be able to discuss the evidence base upon which practice is based. Following orders is not a valid evidence base and does not constitute accountable practice. Doing something because we have always done it or because 'Sister likes it that way' is not a sufficient foundation for professional practice and leads to ritualistic, unthinking nursing that may be positively harmful to the patient.

The delivery of nursing care

Nursing care has to be based upon the individual needs of each patient, planned with the involvement of the patient and then evaluated for its effectiveness. Consistency of care and good communication are also essential. Nursing developed the *nursing process* as a means of achieving these goals. Ford and Walsh (1994) and Walsh (1998) have, amongst others, critiqued this concept in depth. Increasingly the traditional nursing care plan derived from the nursing process is being replaced by the critical pathway, which heralds a less cumbersome, more quality-oriented approach.

The nursing process

The nursing process developed as a tool for teaching care planning and was then implemented across the whole of nursing, but unfortunately with little research to support such a major step. The result has been much criticism and a sense amongst many nurses that it is all too time consuming. It involves a series of stages that begins with assessing the patient, identifying problems, setting goals, implementing care to achieve those goals and finally evaluating the effectiveness of care given. That sounds reasonable until it is realized that this all has to be written down, in detail, for each individual patient. The writing down of copious notes, by hand, to cover each of these stages is both tedious and extremely time consuming. It leads to a great deal of documentation, which nurses feel they have not got the time for.

The critical pathway

The critical pathway is an alternative to the traditional nursing process care plan and is based upon the realization that, for most patients with the same condition, the same stages in care should be reached at the same time. Patient outcomes and the care to be delivered to achieve these goals can be pre-planned by the care team as standards whose achievement can be measured. These are then written down as a pathway the patient will follow and the patient is assigned, if suitable, to that pathway upon admission. The result is a multidisciplinary document that all the care team can use which sets out what the patient should achieve on each day. In very acute areas shorter timescales can be used, based on hours or even minutes. The pathway requires only charting by exception. In other words, the nurse (or other health professional) writes in the document only when something is different from the pre-planned care; otherwise it is merely a matter of signing to say that the care was delivered and the goal achieved as per the pathway. This document is a powerful quality assurance tool as it may be readily audited to see whether care is deviating from that which has been set as the desired standard. A more in-depth discussion of critical pathways from a nursing perspective is found in Walsh (1998).

Primary and team nursing

The nursing process and critical pathways are ways of planning and documenting care. It still remains to organize the delivery of that care. Traditionally this was done on a task basis with the nurse in charge delegating to each nurse a group of tasks to perform for all the patients. This was known as task allocation and, while it may seem an efficient way to operate, there are major problems. Patients cease to exist as whole individuals and become broken down into tasks: the holistic philosophy that distinguishes nursing from the reductionist medical scientific model is lost. Communication is very difficult and some things do not get done, whilst others may be done twice. A crucial point is the lack of accountability for any individual nurse in such a system.

Alternative methods of organizing care delivery grew out of a general dissatisfaction with this fragmented approach, and they became known as *team nursing* or *primary nursing*. In team nursing, as its name suggests, a team of nurses is responsible for care delivered to a group of patients. The team has an experienced registered nurse as its leader and patients are assigned to a team for their care. This system can work in both primary care and hospital settings. A variation on this approach, often encountered in hospitals, is patient allocation which involves patients being allocated to teams on a shift by shift basis. As the shifts change, so do the members of the teams. It is still possible for fragmented, task-centred care to occur within such a team nursing approach, but care should become more holistic as nurses and patients are able to build up more of a relationship.

The primary nursing approach is commonly understood to involve one nurse being held accountable for all care delivered to a patient 24 hours a day. She or he admits the patients, plans all care, delivers much of it while on duty, and is also responsible for discharge planning. When the primary nurse is off duty, an associate nurse carries on with care according to the primary nurse's plan. This is a simplified account but covers the main elements described by Manthey (1980), who is credited with being the first nurse fully to develop and advocate this new way of nursing. The fragmentation and task focus of traditional nursing is replaced by accountable professional care with the advantages of continuity and the opportunity to develop a good nurse–patient relationship. This is particularly important for the hospital nurse given the ever-shorter inpatient stays that characterize the rapidly changing healthcare system.

Much work has been carried out on the implementation of primary nursing and it has become clear that, as the system is implemented, a whole range of other major changes has to take place to allow the system to operate. These include increased levels of accountability for the nurse, which in turn require increased levels of both autonomy and authority. Primary nursing also requires much greater involvement of the patient and family in care. It also requires readjustments in the traditional roles of different members of the nursing team (Mead 1991). A major problem with primary nursing has been the provision of sufficient staff to make the system work and, as a result, you are far more likely to encounter team nursing when working on hospital wards.

Patient care planning

Whether a primary nursing or team nursing approach is used, patient care still has to be planned. The logical place to begin, therefore, is with patient assessment, as this always comes first.

Assessment

Assessment underpins the traditional care planning approach of the nursing process or the newer critical pathway technique. All good nursing care starts with assessment, which is a continuous process of collecting data about the patient's responses, health status, strengths and concerns. Information should be both current and historical, reflecting biological, psychological and social functioning, as well as environmental and lifestyle factors that may affect health. The patient is the primary source of data, but a variety of data sources should be used, such as the family, health records and other health professionals. A good assessment includes subjective data such as the patient's own story, their view of what is wrong and a carefully structured interview which asks questions designed to elicit information about the person's health status. Direct observation of the patient is essential, together with objective measurement of appropriate physical parameters such as vital signs, height and weight, **pulse oximetry**, **peak flows**, capillary blood glucose, urine testing, etc. Increasingly nurse practitioners are learning medical physical examination techniques such as auscultation, and combining these findings with a structured medical history to carry assessment to a new level, integrating medical and nursing skills to carry out an in-depth holistic assessment. This approach is essential if the nurse is acting as the first point of contact in seeing patients with undifferentiated diagnoses. If previous history is any guide, these skills may soon become part of normal pre-registration education rather than be the preserve of advanced post-registration courses. At the end of the assessment, it is important to confirm or validate any data and impressions with the patient. This ensures that messages conveyed by the patient are being received and interpreted accurately by the nurse.

Problem identification

Problem identification must have the patient as a focus; a correctly stated patient problem is the starting point for effective, individualized nursing care. Data obtained in the assessment need to be sorted into categories and compared with accepted norms, as defined by sciences such as anatomy, physiology or psychology, in order that actual or potential health problems may be discovered. It is also essential to seek the patient's point of view, as the patient may not agree with the nurse that a behaviour constitutes a problem; for example, the patient may see smoking as beneficial because it is perceived as reducing stress. The patient may cope with problems simply by denying they exist. Where possible, the likely cause of a problem should also be identified as this helps to focus intervention into appropriate areas.

Goal setting

Goal setting (planning) occurs when the patient and nurse identify activities to prevent, reduce or correct the patient's problems. The steps in planning are to:

- set priorities among the identified problems
- establish patient goals and outcome criteria
- identify intervention strategies
- weigh alternative actions and predict outcomes
- determine nursing interventions
- write the nursing care plan.

Once patient problems (actual and potential) have been identified, priorities are set to provide direction for nursing interventions. Knowledge, experience and, in some critical situations, intuition are applied in setting priorities. If the situation is life threatening, airway, breathing and circulation (ABC) assume priority. In many situations, priority setting involves patient and family participation to prevent conflicts arising and to enhance active cooperation in care activities.

There is no one tool or framework available that assists in making decisions on priorities of care in all situations. Emergency and life-threatening circumstances readily dictate priorities for intervention; other situations may require different considerations. Maslow's framework, which presents an ordered classification of human needs, may be used to rank patient problems (Maslow 1970). It is based on motivation theory and implies that the patient contributes to the decision. Physiological needs (for oxygen, water, food) are ranked as the most immediate priorities, followed by safety and security, love and belonging, self-esteem and self-actualization. Communicating the reasons for priorities helps in establishing mutual goals: failure to consider what is important to the patient may create conflict and delay in achieving health goals.

Goals and objectives describe the patient's expected behavioural outcomes. Each goal is derived from the identification of patient problems and the goals are directed towards the promotion, maintenance and restoration of health, the alleviation of suffering and the giving of support to the dying. Goals may be either short- or long-term statements, should be relevant to the identified problem and within the patient's capabilities and limitations. Short-term goals may be discrete steps leading to achievement of a specific long-term goal and should always reflect mutual planning with the patient. An important feature of a patient goal is that it must be measurable, otherwise how will we know whether the patient has achieved it? A 'fluid intake of 3 litres per day' represents a measurable goal which also contains a statement of the time limit (24 hours) on goal achievement, whereas a statement such as 'increase fluid intake' is too vague to be measurable as a goal and has no concept of time attached to it. Goals should therefore be stated in terms of observable behaviour and should also be realistic. Goals that are unrealistic will only discourage both patient and nurse, and are a waste of time.

Nursing intervention strategies are selected with the patient from alternatives. They are considered in the light of anticipated effectiveness in achieving outcomes, the benefits and risks involved, and the availability of resources, including people, equipment, time, finances and facilities.

Pulse oximetry
See chapter 5.3

Peak flows
See chapter 5.3

The nursing care plan should contain written statements describing the nursing interventions required to help the patient achieve the various goals outlined in the plan. They should be stated in concise, specific terms, and in the sequence in which they are to occur. They may include strategies for the promotion, maintenance or restoration of health, or for peaceful dying. The nursing interventions support the medical regimen of care and should be kept current, revised, and describe alternative plans, as necessary.

When problems are identified by the nurse that are outside the realm of nursing, a referral may be made to the appropriate member of the healthcare team. Similarly, when problems are identified that are beyond the expertise of one particular nurse, referrals may be made to other qualified nursing colleagues. These may be clinical nurse specialists, nurses practising in a special care area or specialty, or community nurses. Collaboration, cooperation and sharing of knowledge and skills provide quality and continuity of care. Medical orders and the plans developed by other healthcare workers should be integrated with the planned nursing actions to develop an overall schedule for patient care.

The critical pathway approach uses goal setting in the same way to identify desired patient outcomes. The key differences are that they are group outcomes for all patients with a common condition (e.g. myocardial infarction or undergoing breast surgery for cancer) and are placed on a timeline, giving specific deadlines by when they are normally to be achieved for all patients.

Implementation

Implementation is the performance of nursing interventions described in the nursing care plan. The scope of nursing actions include the following:

- supportive measures designed to assist with activities the patient is unable to perform and to reinforce adaptive coping mechanisms

- therapeutic measures such as breathing exercises or a dressing change

- continuous data collection and monitoring of the patient's health status

- health promotion and health maintenance activities such as teaching

- coordination of care by other members of the healthcare team

- reporting, recording and consultation.

Evaluation

Evaluation encompasses comparing the patient's health status with the goals and objectives of health care, and determining progress toward goal achievement. Evaluation is a continuous process that occurs during ongoing assessment and implementation of nursing care. When behaviour indicates that goals have been achieved, the nurse and patient either move to the next level of expectation or the relationship is terminated. If the goals are not achieved, the nurse may explore the reasons for this by questioning. For example: Were the goals realistic? Were they stated in measurable terms? Were the actions inappropriate, or did the patient's situation alter? Goals are then re-examined, modified if necessary, and priorities are re-established in relation to the patient's level of achievement and/or change in health status.

If a critical pathway is in use, the nurse or other health professional, if appropriate, will be responsible for initiating action when a goal is not achieved. Continual monitoring of outcome achievement is a powerful quality assurance tool as significant patterns may emerge showing that patients frequently fail to achieve certain goals. This, in turn, may either indicate that the goals are unrealistic or highlight a problem in the care delivery system such as inadequate preoperative respiratory assessment and preparation leading to frequent postoperative chest infections.

Documentation

The patient's health record can be used as a legal document. The nurse is accountable for ensuring that information recorded in the notes is accurate, clear, concise, factual and complete. Data collection, identification of patient problems, plan of care, interventions and results of the interventions, and evaluation of the outcome criteria are recorded. Under the UK legal system, a patient may bring a case for negligence up to 3 years after the event. The nursing staff will only have their documentation to rely on in such an instance; you are very unlikely to even remember the patient, let alone the details of their care, over 2 years later!

All members of the healthcare team should share the patient's record. Increasingly care teams are developing multidisciplinary documentation which places all the different professions' records in a single document. This greatly improves communication between different members of the care team. If the patient has a chronic condition that is managed largely in the community but still requires occasional admissions either for acute exacerbations or respite care, the patient record can be held by the patient. Some health staff find this a rather radical suggestion but it is increasingly gaining acceptance. If involving patients as partners in care is to be meaningful, why not let them look after their own notes? It means staff know exactly what community care has been given before admission, and vice versa upon discharge. It thus becomes a means of providing information about the patient's condition and the health professionals' care plans, and contributes to continuity of care. Accurate and comprehensive written documentation facilitates collaboration and cooperation among members of the various healthcare professions to ensure optimal use of resources on the patient's behalf. The record is a confidential document; it is available only to those participating in the care by permission of the patient and employer.

Nursing ethics

The moral premise of nursing practice is founded in the nurse–patient encounter, embodied in the concept of caring. Nursing practice and hence caring are underpinned by an ethical approach that in the UK is embodied in the UKCC Code of Professional Conduct (UKCC 1992a). Nurses have become increasingly aware of ethics in recent years. Hunt (1994) argues that this is a reflection of the increasing crisis of confidence amongst patients in orthodox medicine, which nevertheless still holds an excessively powerful position over patients and staff such as nurses. As nurses become more accountable and autonomous they are increasingly finding themselves caught in very uncomfortable positions, juggling a conflict of accountability between the patient on the one hand and powerful NHS managers and doctors on the other. Nurses do not make ethical decisions in a vacuum. As Holm (1997) points out, they are influenced by society at large, the environment in which they live and the healthcare system and institution within which they work. Nurses and other professionals are caught between personal, clinical and bureaucratic/legal tensions leading to many potential ethical dilemmas. However, Holm (1997) argues that these may be grouped together under broad headings such as truth telling, termination of treatment and the role of families in decision making, for which ethical guidelines and policies may be developed in advance. This should result in staff sharing their perspective and arriving at a common ethical position. This approach denies the power of medicine and preeminence of *medical* ethics in favour of a more egalitarian *healthcare* ethics. Holm is Danish and this view probably reflects the more collaborative and less hierarchical nature of Scandinavian society.

A fundamental tenet of ethical practice is truth telling. This underpins the nurse–patient relationship and empowers patients to make choices for themselves. Caring lies at the heart of nursing and nurses are clearly committed to caring. A key tenet of nursing is that of commitment which is shared by all. Tschudin (1999) describes how this demonstrates above all else that nursing therefore matters, but she also comments upon the demoralizing effect it has upon nurses when they feel their views do not matter. This erodes self-confidence, an asset often in short supply amongst nurses.

Nursing ethics rest on caring as the moral basis for both the social role of nursing as a profession, and for nursing practice. It is also underpinned by fundamental ethical principles derived from analytical philosophy (Benjamin and Curtis 1992). This ethic is governed by an appeal to principles of moral conduct. These principles of moral conduct, sometimes expressed as moral duties, include:

- *Autonomy* – the obligation to respect the personal choices another person makes
- *Beneficence* – the obligation to do good
- *Fidelity* – the obligation to keep one's word
- *Justice* – the equitable distribution of risks and benefits among people
- *Non-maleficence* – the obligation to do no harm
- *Veracity* – the obligation to tell the truth.

The principles of moral conduct have been derived from several different world views of human relationships. The world views articulate rights and obligations in human encounters through principles of moral conduct. One world view, *teleology*, argues that the goodness of an act is determined by its consequences. It further argues that the collective good takes precedence over the good of the individual: the greatest good and least harm to the greatest numbers. In contrast, a second world view, *deontology*, argues that the goodness of an act is independent of its consequences and is determined by its conformity to obligations that arise from the fact of being human. It further argues that the good of the individual takes precedence over the collective good, based on the premise that no one be treated as a means to the ends of another.

Conduct based upon any one of the principles, and not in conflict with any other principle, is morally right conduct. However, when two or more moral courses of conduct come into conflict, we have an ethical dilemma.

Nursing ethics wrestles with problems that arise when alternative courses of conduct, each moral in itself, come into conflict in a particular situation. An example in nursing practice of conflicts between alternative courses of moral conduct is the conflict between beneficence and autonomy. For example, consider the person who refuses nursing care that would greatly benefit his or her health (such as Pat). If the nurse respects the person's autonomy, the health status may be harmed. If the nurse coerces the individual into receiving nursing care, or fails to elicit consent for nursing care, the nurse violates the autonomy of the person, and possibly the law, as such an act may be construed as common assault, for which a patient may sue to obtain damages. The nurse may have to choose one over the other as a basis for the course of action.

An alternative ethical dilemma often occurs over the issue of how much information to give a patient. Nurses have traditionally identified themselves in the role of patient advocate, although authors such as Porter (1988) and Walsh (2000) have questioned the validity of this assertion. A key element of nursing involves giving information in order that a patient may make informed decisions about treatment and care. The UKCC Code of Professional Conduct requires nurses to be truthful with patients. The doctor, however, is responsible for medical decisions and may decide to withhold information about a patient's true diagnosis, typically in cases of malignant disease, or even the range of treatments that are available (e.g. in **breast cancer**). The nurse may therefore be placed in the position of having to choose between lying to the patient when asked 'What is wrong with me?' or telling the truth and contradicting the doctor in the process. There are no easy answers, except to say that nurses must be able to support their actions with sound rationales (such as the UKCC Code of Conduct), which is the essence of being an accountable practitioner. In cases of difficulty, the nurse would also derive great benefit from membership of a professional organization such as the Royal College of Nursing.

It is possible to read texts on ethics that present detailed analytical frameworks for various situations based on the principles of moral conduct outlined above. Debates in class over what to do in various situations are a good way of rehearsing the arguments and learning about the complexities of modern health care. However, when difficult ethical situations occur in practice, nurses usually have little time and are under a great deal of pressure to make a decision that they may not agree with. Under such circumstances the niceties of analytical philosophy and moral frameworks are just academic exercises. The nurse needs safe and simple solutions that will avoid harm to the patient and protect the individual nurse. Pragmatic advice is that, if in doubt, adhere to the Code of Conduct at all times with its fundamental principle that the patient's interests are paramount: tell the truth, seek an opinion from a senior colleague and do not be rushed or 'bounced' into anything. Above all, remember that *you* are accountable for *your* actions, following doctors' orders is not a defence. Document immediately what you did and why (remember that accountability is about justifying your actions). A final piece of advice is to belong to a professional organization and involve it at the earliest opportunity if you feel morally compromised.

The nurse as a promoter of health

It will be helpful to begin by defining what is meant by health and two other much-used terms: health promotion and health education. Many different definitions of each are found in the literature. It is important to realize that there is no one 'right' definition, but the definitions chosen will give you a basis for understanding the other concepts presented. Some historical perspectives will also be discussed.

Health

It is important when thinking of health not to see it just in *biological terms,* as health also has important social and psychological dimensions. Many theories of health differ

Breast cancer
See chapter 6.3

principally on how much weight they attach to these three components. A more philosophical view of health sees it as empowering people to fulfil their potential (Seedhouse 1986). This presents the nurse with a very challenging and rewarding perspective on nursing as our job is to help people achieve their maximum personal development. Health is therefore a very dynamic and positive concept that is all about the growth and development of both the individual and the society in which they live (Ewles and Simnett 1999).

The biomedical or Western scientific model of health has been summarized by Naidoo and Wills (2000) as having the following characteristics:

- *Biomedical* – it is associated with living organisms

- *Reductionist* – disease and health may be understood by breaking down the body into smaller and smaller units from systems to cells

- *Mechanistic* – the body is conceptualized as functioning like a machine

- *Allopathic* – opposing forces of health defeat the threat of disease (e.g. medication or surgery).

In reviewing this approach to health, Naidoo and Wills (2000) point out that improvements in living conditions since the mid-1800s probably had far more to do with improving health than specific biomedical interventions. These authors cite interesting statistics concerning death rates from infectious disease such as tuberculosis (TB). In 1838 the death rate from TB was approximately 4000 per million in England and Wales. By the time the causative organism had been discovered in 1882, the mortality rate from TB had already more than halved to 1750 per million. When effective chemotherapy to treat TB became available in the late 1940s the figure had dropped to 650 per million and by 1960 had fallen to 250 per million. Only a small proportion of the reduction in death rate from its 1838 levels (approximately 10%) can therefore be assigned to the introduction of effective drugs and the BCG vaccination programme. Gough et al (1994) point out that medical dominance led to the NHS becoming a disease- and hospital-focused service rather than a true health service. Despite these criticisms, the biomedical model remains the dominant approach to health care in the UK and there is a great deal of evidence to support its validity. Much of your work as a nurse will take place within the context of the biomedical model; however, we have to ask whether it is the whole story.

Aggleton (1990) offers some alternatives to the biomedical model of health. The *social–positivist* approach applies the methods of the natural sciences to social enquiry in order to identify the causes of health and illness, while *interactionist* explanations concentrate on the meanings that people give to the experiences of health and illness. Finally, there is the *structuralist* approach, which sees health in terms of how power and authority are distributed in the broader context of society; the effects of capitalism, class structure and the power of men over women are examples of how this view seeks to explain health.

We can recognize the validity of Aggleton's suggestion that there is a significant social component to health by considering the Black Report (Davidson and Townsend 1982). This was commissioned by the Labour Government in the late 1970s and was ready for publication as the new Conservative Government came to power in 1979. It found little favour with Prime Minister Thatcher but was published in paperback in 1982 and widely discussed. As a major study of the health of the UK, the Black Report proved very embarrassing for the government of the day. It pointed out that health and mortality were closely linked to social class and wealth. The investigators showed that, for a whole range of medical conditions, *mortality* (death rate) and *morbidity* (reported illness) were lowest amongst the wealthiest and highest amongst the poorest. Much research has followed in the 20 years since the Black Report, but the findings remain the same: your life expectancy and health are heavily influenced by where you are in society. Authors such as Bywaters and McLeod (1996) claim that there is substantial evidence to show that social inequalities continue to undermine health and, what is worse, during the 1990s the gap between the better off and the poorest in our society steadily widened. Research into health inequalities demonstrates that, while the biomedical model of health has much validity, it is only part of the story. Health cannot be seen in purely scientific reductionist terms, divorced from sociological and environmental factors.

Research into the interactionist approach to health described by Aggleton (1990) has also thrown up serious challenges to the conventional biomedical model. This reveals that if health is examined from the individual's perspective it may look very different from the professional's view. Helman (1994) writes of illness as something that you go to the doctor with, whereas disease is something you have when you leave the surgery. Each person is aware of their own symptoms and attaches their own meanings to these; this subjective experience is the illness. However, the medical profession has objective models of disease that when applied to the person's complaints (illness) give it a label which is the disease. There is often little relationship between the severity of a symptom as perceived by the individual when compared with the doctor's view. What may seem trivial to the person may be important to the doctor, and vice versa.

As an illustration of the many personal views of health (interactionist models) that people have, the work of Stainton-Rogers (1991) is very illuminating. Her research was carried out in the UK and her sample was biased towards professional people. She found the following personal accounts of health, some of which have already been encountered:

1. The '*body as machine*' account sees illness as natural and real, and as something that can be dealt with only by modern biomedical science.

2. The '*body under siege*' account views the body as under attack from outside forces such as stress and difficult relationships which act through the mind to affect the way the body works, in addition to biological agents such as bacteria.

3. The '*inequality of access*' account supports modern medicine but sees health as threatened by poverty and lack of access to health care.

4. A '*cultural critique*' views exploitation and oppression within modern society as determining health.

5. A '*health promotion*' account recognizes the adoption of a healthy lifestyle and the responsibility of the individual in achieving health.

6. The '*robust individualism*' account is concerned with doing whatever the person wishes and attaches little importance to health as long as freedom of choice is present.

7. The '*God's power*' account sees health as in the hands of a deity; the person therefore needs to follow religious teachings to achieve God's care.

8. The '*willpower*' account places the person in complete control of their own health and stresses the need to use 'will' to maintain health.

Setting aside criticism about the representativeness of the sample chosen by Stainton-Rogers, this work is important to you as a future registered nurse. It shows that people have a whole range of views about health and you need to explore these views with each patient before any meaningful care or health education work can take place. There are echoes of all three main approaches to health given by Aggleton (1990) in this work, but its strength is the way it shows such a wide variation in personal perspectives. A person who subscribes to the 'robust individualism' account is much less likely to pay attention to messages about health than somebody who identifies with the 'health promotion' account.

An additional factor in understanding health is the variability introduced by different cultures. The increasing globalization of the world means that any one country is likely to have significant numbers of people from other countries, cultures and religious backgrounds who will all have different perspectives on health. Research that might shed light upon this phenomenon is rather sparse in the UK. Smaje (1995) was very critical of the lack of rigorous data gathering which could provide evidence about the health of people from minority ethnic groups. What little evidence there is suggests that people in the UK who were born abroad tended to have better health than the population in their native countries but had worse mortality statistics than UK-born citizens. Of all the ethnic groups in the UK, those born in Ireland had the worst mortality statistics.

There is a complex interplay of genetic, cultural and environmental factors at work in explaining the health records of minority ethnic populations. This is illustrated by the example of diabetes, where mortality statistics for England and Wales show that the standardized mortality rate due to type II diabetes for men aged 20–69 years who were born in the Indian subcontinent or the Caribbean is three times higher than that for the general population. However, the incidence of type II diabetes is also increasing amongst the native UK population (as it is in the USA and elsewhere) because of dietary and lifestyle changes. This is what Helman (1994) describes as the 'malnutrition of the West' meaning eating larger amounts of 'junk' food of low nutritional value.

In the introduction to this section it was stated that there are many different definitions of health, and perhaps it is best to conclude with the views of the World Health Organization (WHO). In 1958, the WHO reported that 'health is a state of complete physical, mental, and social well-being, not merely the absence of disease and infirmity' (WHO 1958, p. 459). This definition was an acknowledgement that health is more than non-disease, but it has been criticized for proposing an ideal, rather than a measurable goal for which strategies for achievement can be devised. It has since been altered to present health not as a 'state' but as a 'resource':

> Health is the extent to which an individual or group is able, on the one hand, to realize aspirations and satisfy needs and on the other hand to change or cope with the environment. Health is seen as a resource for everyday life, not the objective of living, it is a positive concept emphasizing social and personal resources as well as physical capacities.
>
> (WHO 1986)

Although regarded as an improvement on the earlier definition, this has not increased its measurability and, as Gough et al (1994) point out, this is one of the main problems surrounding health debates. If it is not possible to agree what health actually is, how can we agree measures of health and therefore know when it is improving or getting worse?

This introduction to health has shown there are many definitions of health ranging from those of learned academics in medicine and the social sciences through to the everyday personal understandings that we all carry around with us. It is these latter definitions that you will have to work with as a nurse, trying to set them within the wider academic and clinical framework of health as you care for and discuss health with each patient.

Health education and health promotion: the debate

It will not surprise you that, given the difficulties surrounding the definition of health, there is little agreement about what constitutes health promotion and how this differs from health education. Naidoo and Wills (2000) give an excellent account of the debates that have taken place around this topic and you are referred to their text for a full account.

A commonsense definition of health education sees it as teaching individuals about steps they can take to enhance their health (e.g. exercise) and avoid disease (e.g. use of a condom during sex). The relationship of this activity to health promotion was described by Tones (1993) in terms of a simple formula:

Health Promotion = Health Education × Healthy Public Policy

In this view, health education is seen as empowerment which, when combined with a health-oriented public policy, leads to the promotion of health. Nurses have a key role in this process as they can make a major contribution to individual empowerment. Tones (1992) has argued that health education has three main strands:

1. Critical consciousness raising – creating an empowered population that can exert pressure on governments for change.

2. Convincing a wide range of occupational groups that they have a role in health. Examples might be teachers, local authority housing staff, the transport industry, those responsible for planning economic growth and development.

3. Direct and individual patient-focused health education such as teaching a person newly diagnosed with diabetes about managing their diet and insulin regimen.

Nurses have traditionally been involved only in the third of these options, but are beginning now to realize that they should get involved in the other areas (see Box 1.1).

Early public health strategies were related to the eradication of illness and prevention of communicable disease (see Box 1.2). Although disease prevention and health protection are still important activities, there is a danger that health promotion will remain a very limited concept if we do not look further afield than the actions outlined in Box 1.2. Naidoo and Wills (2000) observe that a disease prevention perspective does not look beyond readily identified risk factors to the real origins of ill-health such as poverty and social breakdown. This approach may define health education as merely information giving by health experts and measure success in terms of the extent to which clients follow the advice given. The 1999 Department of Health publication *Our Healthier Nation* can be criticized from this point of view. What is missing is a

Box 1.1   A nurse practitioner-led farmers' health service

Farmers are a group who face serious health problems due to the hazardous and arduous nature of their work. Their health needs have not always been met by a health service designed for a predominantly urban population. Since the mid-1990s British agriculture has been gripped by its most serious crisis for 60 years causing a dramatic increase in mental health problems and farm suicides on top of the serious physical health problems farmers and their families face. A nurse-led project in the southern part of the English Lake District and adjacent Pennines has started providing a unique health service to individual farmers by means of a mobile clinic visiting auction marts. The nurses regularly attend farming meetings to discuss issues ranging from first aid to stress management. The project has also become involved with agricultural organizations, working to raise consciousness about risks such as mental health and organophosphate poisoning. It is working with the Health and Safety Executive as well as farmers to bring about change in accident prevention work. The project is also lobbying NHS providers to make their services more appropriate for the farming community and to increase knowledge amongst health professionals about farming problems. The nurses have showed their solidarity with the farmers by joining them on protest marches. All three of Tones' modes of health education are being addressed by this project.

Box 1.2   The three levels of prevention

- *Primary* – activities to decrease the probability of illness and to protect against illness; includes both risk avoidance and risk reduction

- *Secondary* – activities for early diagnosis and early intervention to reduce the duration and severity of illness

- *Tertiary* – rehabilitation, coping with disability or chronic disease.

willingness to work with people to help them make informed choices for themselves (empowerment), as simply telling people what to do is an ineffective health education strategy. Other models for health promotion include the social model aimed at influencing key decision makers, and the community model aimed at achieving collective action in pursuit of health. The community model brings more than just health professionals into the field of health promotion as teachers, welfare workers,

workplace managers and social workers, for example, could all be involved. These models are discussed further in the next section.

Nevertheless, as Delaney (1994) observes, health education is inseparably linked to health protection and disease prevention measures. This is characterized by the WHO, which see health promotion as an umbrella concept pulling together various aspects of health and involving public policy. This clearly makes it the business of national governments. Delaney, however, discerns amongst the WHO's general statements on health promotion two specific elements: attention to *individual lifestyle* and *living conditions*.

In the UK, health promotion has been linked to health policy for some time. Various government publications since the 1970s have carried the message that many health problems are the product of lifestyles and therefore the individual is responsible for preventing much illness. That is the message from the government at policy level and the government has the power to legislate accordingly (e.g. banning smoking in public places, car seatbelt legislation).

This latter point is crucial because, as the Black Report and much subsequent work (Whitehead 1988) has shown, social constraints are very real. Advice about a healthy diet is meaningless if the person cannot afford it. The devastating psychological effects upon an individual of redundancy and unemployment may drown out completely any health education messages. The political or economic refugee with little or no English is in no position to act upon health education messages. How many healthy options (joining an exercise group or getting support from friends to stop smoking) exist for a socially disadvantaged single woman who is the head of the household with three young children to care for? Nurses need to be sensitive here to the dangers of what is known as 'victim blaming'. This occurs where society places a double burden upon the sick: it creates the conditions that lead to health problems then establishes a model of health care that makes the individual responsible for their own sickness, and even stigmatizes them for it.

Models of health promotion

There are various approaches to health promotion, and Naidoo and Wills (2000) offer an excellent discussion of these models. They summarize them as follows:

1. *The medical or preventive approach.* This method seeks to increase medical interventions that will prevent ill-health. It is medically led, makes use of epidemiological methods and screening techniques, and works on the principle that the prevention or early detection of disease is much cheaper than treating the established disease later. The success of vaccination programmes in eliminating diseases such as smallpox and polio are testimony to the power of

this approach. However, access for disadvantaged groups remains a problem.

2. *Behaviour change*. Government publicity campaigns aimed at persuading people to change their behaviour are examples of this approach. This is expert-led and targeted at the individual.

3. *The educational approach*. This method does not directly set out to persuade people to change behaviour but rather to provide knowledge and information in the hope that the person will subsequently modify their behaviour as a result of their own choice. Both the educational and behaviour change approaches suffer from disadvantages as human health behaviour is far more complex than they acknowledge and the individual may not have the resources necessary to make individual lifestyle changes, even if they wanted to.

4. *Empowerment*. This is a bottom-up approach which involves facilitating people, either as individuals or in communities, to decide for themselves what health-promoting activity they wish to participate in and to proceed to act for themselves.

5. *Social change*. This radical approach aims to change the physical, social and economic environment as a means of achieving healthier lives for people.

The nurse may be involved in any of these approaches, whether working as a practice nurse giving vaccinations, running a well woman clinic or putting up posters in the A&E waiting room. However, as Delaney (1994) has observed, nurses have tended to view health promotion as being about preventing specific diseases or promoting general good health rather than getting involved in the more contentious political and 'conditions of living' arena. Organizations such as the Royal College of Nursing do lobby government departments, often in conjunction with the medical Royal Colleges, on a range of health issues. Some nurses are also becoming involved in health promotion by empowerment when they develop new roles such as that of nurse practitioner. They are, for example, working with high levels of autonomy in community centres in certain deprived urban areas of the UK, following a precedent set by nurse practitioners in the USA 20 years ago. Delaney's observation is still valid in general terms, however, and it remains to be seen whether nurses will become more aware of the importance of political power as a key health-promoting factor. It now remains to move to the one-to-one level in which the nurse engages in health education.

Health education and patient teaching

It is axiomatic that patient education is an important function of nursing practice. As we have already seen, it can be about raising people's awareness about an issue, working on key groups of decision makers or working with the individual client. Ewles and Simnett (1999) fill in some detail by stressing that this process involves the whole person throughout their entire life, regardless of how ill or well that person may be at any one time. They see health education as helping people to help themselves, either individually, in families or in larger communities, by using a wide range of teaching techniques to achieve goals that often involve changing behaviours, attitudes and social circumstances. In the past, nurses have tended to teach patients within a disease-oriented framework rather than from a health perspective. Focusing only on the disease is a narrow and blinkered approach that ignores a wide range of social and psychological factors and is also very limited in its goals. As Seedhouse (1986) reminds us, a major theme in health education tends to be the prevention of illness rather than the creation of wellness. In his view, health is the foundation for all human achievement; this gives a much deeper significance and meaning to health education. Patient education is an interactive process whereby learning, which may subsequently be used to influence behaviour, takes place. This leads to a more humanistic view of patient education in which the nurse and patient share responsibility for learning.

Autonomy is the key to patient-centred education. In education that is medically centred, notions of compliance and a paternalistic viewpoint tend to dominate. Freire (1985) pointed out that real education must entail emancipation; that is, liberating people to make their own decisions on their own terms. Historically, however, nurses and other professionals have hesitated to allow patients the control that they need to make their own choices and decisions. At times this reluctance has stemmed from our maternalistic/paternalistic view of patients. Hospitals and other healthcare agencies have also created organizational barriers that prevent the patient from having the freedom to make decisions about health.

If we accept the validity of the patient-centred approach to health education, what are its goals? To say 'education about health' is very trite and not very helpful. Box 1.3 shows a more structured approach to individual health education and is derived from standards set by the US Joint Commissioning Authority for Health Organizations (JCAHO).

These standards emphasize the empowering nature of health education and the need to involve family members in the process, recognizing that clients do not exist in a vacuum, but have to be seen in their social context. As we have already seen, though, promoting a healthy lifestyle is possible only if the patient has access to the necessary resources.

Seedhouse (1986) commented that the meaning of health cannot be understood from a dictionary, nor is it enough to say that health is desirable and then leave the issue at that: action is needed. In his view, health

---

Box 1.3   JCAHO goals for patient education

- Facilitate the patient and family's understanding of the patient's health status, healthcare options and consequences of options selected
- Encourage patient and family participation in the decision-making process about healthcare options
- Increase the patient and family's potential to follow the therapeutic healthcare plan
- Maximize patient and family care skills
- Increase the patient and family's ability to cope with the patient's health status, prognosis and outcome
- Enhance the patient and family's role in continuing health care
- Promote a healthy lifestyle.

From Rankin and Stallings (1996).

---

education has two main, broad aims: (1) to ensure that people have a good standard of general education and (2) to develop people's powers of intellectual conception so that they can maximize the information with which they are presented. This is an enabling point of view consistent with the JCAHO standards outlined in Box 1.3. It is about giving people the tools with which to tackle their own health problems; health education is definitely not about indoctrination and propaganda.

Every patient has the right to seek information and participate in the educational plan. Simply providing information about health matters is a waste of time. The purpose of education is to encourage patients to use knowledge to modify behaviour and perform activities that will result in improved health status. The role of the nurse, therefore, is to plan learning experiences with the patient, as a component of total care, so that adults share responsibility for health. Ideally, the outcome of learning is that the patient is able to make rational decisions with respect to health, participate effectively in self-care and adjust to the realities of the lifestyle changes that are required. However, various environmental factors can seriously hinder the patient's ability to change lifestyle.

Practising health education: an example

A prime example of the importance of health education is provided by AIDS where, in the absence of any known cure or immunization programme, the main defence against the disease is education (Wellings and Field 1996). Nurses are one of the key groups that can carry out the educational function in a wide range of situations and, in view of the importance of the issue of health education and AIDS, this is worth exploring in some detail.

There are two critical goals in the global management of **HIV** infection:

- Intervention needs to be focused on the prevention of transmission of the virus into healthy individuals.
- Intervention must be focused on appropriate and humane care of individuals affected by the virus. Self-care for the person is critically important.

Despite the agreed wisdom that prevention of the spread of human immunodeficiency virus (HIV) is so important, the evidence worldwide is not encouraging as the number of new cases continues to climb remorselessly. This trend led Lifson (1994) to speculate that, with regard to preventing HIV infection, we have all lost our way and now face a growing crisis. He suggested there are five key principles involved in meeting the threat:

1. We must emphasize the viral nature of the disease and the fact that progression towards serious illness begins with infection; therefore AIDS prevention means HIV prevention.

2. The highest priority must be given to preventing the sexual transmission of HIV and other sexually transmitted diseases that facilitate its spread. This means shifting public attention away from the occasional unfortunate healthcare worker who is infected or from speculation about a protective vaccination to the reality that HIV is spread most readily by unprotected sex.

3. The problem of HIV spread amongst drug users must be tackled irrespective of political concerns or other niceties. This should include safer sex messages.

4. Prevention programmes must be planned and carried out that are sensitive to local needs, whether they be a high incidence of intravenous drug users or commercial sex workers, for example.

5. Strong leadership is needed at national and international level to ensure that HIV is tackled as the major public health threat that it is.

Health education forms the core of the first four principles, whereas the final point relates more to health promotion (see Tones' formula on p. 16). The nurse is in the front line of this campaign whether talking to a patient and family about the risks of blood transfusion before routine surgery, working as a school nurse with adolescents or in a family planning clinic.

Prevention of HIV infection is everyone's responsibility. Abstaining from or minimizing the degree of risky behaviour is an important deterrent in decreasing transmission of the virus. It is crucial that information is provided in a culturally acceptable manner and in a language that is easily understood. Previously, the weight of responsibility has fallen on individuals infected with HIV to practise safer sexual practices or to inform sexual partners of their

HIV
See chapter 6.2

HIV status. However, self-protection is equally the responsibility of a non-infected partner. Sexual relationships require individual responsibility. For individuals to be motivated to adopt a new behaviour they must perceive a certain degree of risk or vulnerability. One of the problems of preventive education is that repression and denial are often used to minimize the degree of threat to the person. Therefore, individuals do not adopt safer behaviours because they deny they are at risk.

The nurse can teach the importance of using safer sexual practices; however, it is often difficult to motivate people to change practice. It is usually more effective to focus teaching around both partners. An atmosphere that feels safe needs to be created so that individuals feel comfortable discussing intimate behaviours. Safer sexual practices need to be incorporated so that they are pleasurable and in keeping with the individual's cultural and moral values. The individual needs to understand that safer sex is used because the person wants to stay healthy, not because their partner is suspect. Attention needs to be given not only to the mechanics of sexual behaviour but also to areas of maintaining intimacy and closeness.

The key message is that unprotected sex constitutes the highest risk behaviour, in particular:

■ male to male via penetrative anal intercourse

■ male to female via penetrative anal or vaginal intercourse.

Transmission from an infected passive male to an active male or from an infected female to a male is less likely as the concentration of infectious particles is lower in vaginal or anal secretions than in semen. Intercourse during menstruation greatly increases the risk of infection. Oral sex carries less of a risk of infection, but it is still possible. The risk for a receptive male having oral sex with an infected male partner is approximately one-sixth that of having receptive anal sex, but is still very real. An infected woman can infect a man via oral sex, although there is no conclusive evidence that 'French kissing' has caused HIV transmission. Individuals are thought to be most infectious immediately after they have become infected and then subsequently at a later stage when they are showing clinical signs of AIDS (Pratt 1995). Other factors that increase the risk of infection are if the man is uncircumcized, has multiple sexual partners, there is trauma or bleeding during sexual activity, and if other sexually transmitted diseases are present.

In addition to information on safer sexual practices, the nurse also needs to provide information on the use of condoms and lubricants. Obstacles to incorporating behaviour change may include knowledge deficits, fear, lack of skill, lack of social support or inadequate resources to purchase products such as condoms. The nurse can be of vital importance in helping individuals learn how to negotiate a sexual relationship. In particular, it may be difficult to get a sexual partner to use condoms. Many people are unsure how to initiate this discussion. Among men, a variety of reasons have been cited for the underutilization of condoms, including lack of ready access, failure to plan for sexual intercourse, the use of alcohol and drugs prior to sex, beliefs that condoms impair sexual pleasure, and the belief that condoms are unnatural or immoral. These same questions have not been asked of women. It may be useful to role-play prospective situations to try to minimize these barriers (Table 1.1). When men and women are empowered with information and negotiating skill, they are less likely to place themselves in risky situations.

Table 1.1 How to talk about condoms

If your partner says	You can reply
I know I'm disease-free. I haven't had sex with anyone in months.	As far as I know I'm clean too. But either of us could have an infection and not know it.
I can't feel anything when I wear a condom. It's like shaking hands with a rubber glove.	I know there's some loss of feeling. Why don't we try putting a bit of lubricant in the tip of the condom. It'll be fun.
Condoms are messy and smell funny.	With a condom we'll be safe. Let's try some of the scented ones. This could be a whole new experience.
I think I'll lose the mood if I use a condom.	Let's try building it in as part of foreplay. We may feel a bit awkward at first but it will pass and it's fun to try new things together.
I'll lose my erection if I stop to put on a condom.	I'll help you put it on. That will help you keep it.
I love you, I wouldn't give you anything.	I love you too, and because I love you I want to protect our relationship. Many people don't know they're infected.
I just don't feel ready to use a condom.	Maybe it's better if we wait for a while until we can work this out, or maybe we can try things other than intercourse.

After Lewis and Lewis (1987).

Expectations for patient education

Patients are becoming better consumers of health care. They are better informed and they want to know more. Because of the consumer movement and greater media attention to healthcare issues, patients are aware of their rights and are more demanding about receiving information on their condition and treatment. Many want to be involved in decision making regarding their care and treatment.

Patient education is now viewed as an integral part of high-quality health care. Quality assurance is increasingly being recognized as an essential component of health care, particularly in light of the clinical governance initiative and recent high-profile failures of the NHS. The Bristol Royal Infirmary cardiac surgery scandal in 1999, the Harold Shipman murders in 2000 and the Alder Hey Hospital children's organ scandal in 2001 are just three tragic examples of what can go wrong in health care. The process of quality assurance involves setting standards for care, monitoring the achievement of those standards and taking corrective action when standards are not met. The healthcare system must have a focus on quality.

Patient education has become part of total, comprehensive patient care. To provide quality care, all of the patient's needs must be addressed, including the need to know about health education, disease prevention and health promotion. Factors such as shorter hospital stays, reduced convalescent facilities and higher incidence of chronic illness mean that more patients are being cared for at home by family carers. Family carers cannot be expected to care for ailing relatives without learning the necessary skills.

The nurse is the health professional in most contact with a patient and has a broad overview of the patient's health status; this would appear to make the nurse the ideal person to engage in health education work. While authors such as Rankin and Stallings (1996) see education as an essential part of the nurse's role, pressure of time tends to mean that patient teaching suffers as a result. Nurses have to work hard to establish the validity of patient teaching as an essential part of caring. They still have to justify longer consultation times with patients in primary care settings or setting time aside on busy wards in order to engage in patient teaching.

Giving nurses more accountability for individual patient care may also facilitate patient education, although there is a range of factors, mentioned above, that is seen as interfering with the nurse's educative role. One key factor that is missing from the discussion, however, is whether the patient is able to respond to education to make appropriate lifestyle changes. The limitations imposed upon people by poverty, culture and environmental factors have already been mentioned, while the advertizing industry spends huge sums of money persuading people to smoke, eat unhealthy food and drink more alcohol than is good for them. There is, therefore, a powerful critique of the individualist account of health that also needs to be considered. Dines (1994), in discussing the limitations imposed upon individuals, cautions against being too fatalistic. Although there are powerful forces at work in people's lives over which they have little control, individuals still retain some autonomy, and to target health education work the nurse needs to find those areas where people retain a larger degree of control. In Dines' view health education is a constrained activity as a result of such social forces, but nevertheless is worthwhile as positive results may be obtained in limited areas.

Despite such strong historical evidence that patient education can be effective, the introduction of new education programmes should be monitored for effectiveness. Health education consumes scarce resources (such as nursing time) and the evidence must be gathered to show that it is a cost-effective use of those resources.

In summary, it is clear that there are expectations placed on nurses to teach. Quality assurance standards, professional standards and a focus on risk management emphasize the nurse's role in patient education. Nurses perceive that patient education is an important component of total patient care, yet are faced with external constraints that limit their ability to teach effectively. These constraints include time restrictions, unrealistic expectations of managers, patients who are too acutely ill to learn, and workload factors. With greater expectations on the part of patients who want to learn and demand to know, the challenge is for nurses realistically to meet these expectations.

Compliance

Much time, effort and expense is devoted to patient education by health professionals. Patient education, if viewed as a total process, can be a key component in enabling patients to act on the recommendations of the health professionals. However, patients cannot carry out a treatment or recommendation that they do not understand or *do not accept*. Refer back to Pat's story, which introduced this chapter, to see the importance of this observation. The degree to which patients follow recommendations is usually called *compliance* or *patient adherence*, although *cooperation* is a better term.

Compliance should not be viewed as coercive obedience but as a negotiated agreement. In this sense, compliance is part of the helping relationship between the health professionals and patient; it is the outcome of nurse–patient communication and interaction. It may be defined as the 'Extent to which an individual chooses behaviours that coincide with a clinical prescription … achieved through negotiations between the health professional and the patient' (Dracup and Meleis 1982).

Increased attention to the area of compliance has been generated because of the impact of compliance or noncompliance on health outcomes. Rankin and Stallings

(1996) cite extensive evidence to show that a high percentage of patients do not follow the recommendations of health professionals. Non-compliance is therefore costly; it wastes medical and human resources, and may have serious consequences for the patients and their families or significant others.

Non-compliance can take many forms: failure to keep scheduled appointments, to take medications as directed, to follow recommended dietary or lifestyle change, or to follow recommended preventive health practices. Factors that may contribute to non-compliance include financial problems (inability to pay for expensive prescriptions), inconvenience (such as taking medications during working hours), religious beliefs, denial of illness, lack of family or other support, feelings of fear or shame, and feelings of helplessness or lack of control. All of these factors can impact on the patient's decision not to follow suggestions or recommendations regarding health.

The Health Belief Model is useful in determining why some patients comply and others do not (Naidoo and Wills 2000). This model theorizes that the likelihood of patient compliance varies with:

- the patient's perception of susceptibility to the disease

- the prediction of the impact of the illness on the patient's life

- the patient's perception of barriers to taking recommended action

- the patient's perception of the benefits of taking the action.

It suggests that people carry out cost–benefit analyses in which they assess the threat and cost of illness compared to the possible benefits of seeking medical help and also the costs (in the broadest sense) of obtaining that help. The fundamental question becomes 'Is it worth it?' If the answer is yes, then the person is likely to seek help and to cooperate with treatment; if the answer is no, then he or she either will not seek help or, if they do, will not follow advice and treatment requirements. Walsh (1995) has found, for example, that this model explains much patient behaviour in attending A&E departments. This should be seen as only one amongst several factors at work in determining patient behaviour. However, the model gives the nurse some important insights into health education activity as the client has first to perceive that there is a threat to themselves, and second that the potential advantages (benefits) outweigh the disadvantages (costs) in taking therapeutic action. Those who think that only gay men and drug users contract HIV will not use a condom whilst having heterosexual sex, as infection cannot happen to them. Teenage smokers cannot really imagine what it is like to be 45 years old, so they are unlikely to perceive the long-term risks of smoking as something that will affect them, however serious they may be.

It is important for nurses to understand that all individuals are influenced by their beliefs and values (attitudes) about their health or illness. Nurses are also influenced by their own beliefs and values. At times, the individual's values and the nurse's beliefs may be very different. For effective teaching to occur, the nurse has to base the educational plan on the individual's perception of what is important and achievable because beliefs are strong motivators of human behaviour.

Yet another factor influencing education is the rapport and relationship established between the nurse and patient. In the next chapter we will explore this further as we discuss the area of therapeutic communication.

Contracting

Contracting with patients has been shown to be effective in achieving cooperation. The purpose of a contract is to promote the patient's active participation in health care by assisting the patient to identify and accomplish specific goals. Contracting helps to facilitate the patient's self-esteem, as well as promoting a trusting relationship.

Contracting promotes the patient's autonomy, involvement and responsibility for health. The patient exercises the right to self-determination and ability to solve problems. Furthermore, when nurses use contracting as a strategy, they are demonstrating belief in the dignity and worth of the patient.

The steps used in developing a contract are outlined in Box 1.4.

When helping patients to adjust to major lifestyle changes, the nurse can use contracting as a method to achieve cooperation. Contracting breaks down what might be overwhelming change into small incremental steps. The patient who feels in control of what can be accomplished will be more likely to achieve the desired objective.

Influence of culture on patient education

Culture determines many of the beliefs and values held by individuals; it therefore has a strong influence on health behaviour. Conflicts can arise when the nurse and patient hold different beliefs and values about what constitutes appropriate health behaviour.

Box 1.4   Steps in developing a contract

1. Identification of the priority health concerns or needs of the patient

2. The setting of *mutual* goals

3. Writing the contract

4. Implementation of the task or activities agreed upon

5. Evaluation of the outcomes of the contract.

Assessment of the beliefs, values and practices of the patient is vital to tailoring educational interventions (Helman 1994). The patient should be assessed as an individual, so that cultural preferences come out naturally, rather than being forced into a preconceived ethnic stereotype. For example, to teach about therapeutic changes in diet, the nurse must determine the patient's preferred and current diet, and the meaning of food in the patient's life.

The nurse needs to elicit the patient's views on the illness experience. For example, in some cultures it may be undesirable for a man to be bathed by a woman, and to put the patient in this situation would jeopardize his self-esteem. Conflicts in perspectives should be acknowledged openly and clarified. The nurse cannot enforce a teaching plan that contradicts the patient's beliefs. The patient's plan may not be the nurse's first choice but it may be more acceptable than the patient rejecting all interventions.

When English is the patient's second language, it is important for the nurse to speak slowly, use simple sentence structure, avoid medical or technical jargon, provide sequential steps in teaching, and not assume that the patient understands. Even if English is the first language, jargon and abbreviations should be avoided. The nurse should also consider the educational level of the patient and, without being patronizing, speak in terms that are appropriate and readily understood by the individual.

Helping patients change

Individual health education involves the client making significant lifestyle changes. Nurses have increasingly turned to the work of Prochaska and DiClemente (1986) on change as providing useful insights into how people may be helped to change their behaviour. These authors propose that change does not happen in one 'big bang' but rather involves the person working through a series of stages in a cyclical process. The model may be summarized as described below.

Stage 1: Precontemplation

Here the person has not become aware of any health problem and is unaware of the existence of a health risk or the need for change. Consider Graham Smith, a 50-year-old bus driver who smokes 20 cigarettes a day, takes no exercise, eats a diet high in fats and processed food, weighs 12 kg more than he should for his height, and is regularly in the local pub consuming substantial quantities of beer. He sees no reason to change his lifestyle until …

Stage 2: Contemplation

Individuals are now aware of the benefits of change but have not actually decided to make any changes. They may be seeking help to make the decision to change, but so far have not decided to do anything about it. Some people never progress beyond this stage. Graham Smith has entered the contemplation stage as a result of a 'healthy heart' initiative by the bus company's occupational health nurse. She set up an exhibition in the canteen one lunch time and gave Graham a 'cardiac MOT', as she called it. It took only 10 minutes but made him aware that he really was overweight, unhealthy and had several risk factors for serious cardiac problems including raised blood pressure. He began thinking about these facts and talking to his wife. A few days later, and coincidentally, his brother was admitted to hospital, seriously ill after a heart attack. This led on to …

Stage 3: Preparing to change

At this stage the person now sees that there is a real threat and that the advantages of changing their lifestyle outweigh the costs (remember the Health Belief Model). They also perceive that change is possible and feel ready to change, although they may need support to do so. His brother's heart attack came as a great shock to Graham, especially as his brother was 2 years younger than he was. Graham realized he should be thinking in terms of another 25–30 years of active life, yet here was his closest living relation (his father died from a heart attack 12 years ago) seriously ill in hospital with something that he had been warned only that week could happen to him. As he talked with his wife she showed him some photographs from a few years ago of a much slimmer Graham turning out for the pub football team; he also considered how much money he could save by giving up smoking, just like his mate Roy had at work. 'If Roy can, I can', he concluded. It was time for action.

Stage 4: Making the change

In order to start the change process people need to make clear decisions about what they are trying to achieve and how they will do this. Key features of making a successful change are clear goals, realistic plans, support and some kind of reward for achieving those goals. Graham got his support from his wife (who did not smoke) and from the occupational health nurse who he went to see to discuss his health. He agreed with her to give up smoking completely, a realistic programme of exercise, starting with a brisk 20-minute walk three times a week, and took home a dietary advice sheet to consider with his wife. The nurse also provided him with advice about foods to avoid at the works canteen and listed the healthier options she had just succeeded in getting the company to put on the menu (an example of health education by organizational campaigning). He also made an appointment to see his GP to discuss his blood pressure problem, reassured by the occupational health nurse that the practice nurse would also be very supportive. Having made the change, Graham realized that the hardest part was sticking at it or, in other words …

Stage 5: Maintenance

Sustaining the new behaviour pattern, moving to a healthier lifestyle and staying there is the hardest part of all, as reversion or relapse may easily occur. This puts the person back to one of the earlier stages. Few people, in fact, go through all these stages in an orderly way; relapse is common, but eventually each person will have moved through each stage. So it was with Graham as he found his first attempt at giving up smoking failed after only a week. However, reassurance from the practice nurse that this does happen and does not make him a failure led to a second successful attempt. Six months later, Graham had acquired a lively Border Terrier, which needed walking three times a day, had lost 5 kg in weight, been tobacco free for 4 months, had reduced his beer intake by a third and was feeling much better with a healthier diet.

The stages of change model outlined above depends fundamentally upon client motivation for success and this must be the focus of the nurse's efforts when working with any individual. The more involved the client is in planning the changes that are to be made, the more motivated he or she will be and therefore the more likely the nurse is to be successful in promoting healthy lifestyle changes for the client. Social support networks are very important in maintaining changes once begun. The nurse must be aware of the existence of the precontemplative stage because, if the patient is in this stage, there is little chance of achieving success. Change will occur only when the client is aware of the need for change and is willing to make the effort to do so; change must therefore come from within rather than be imposed from outside by an authoritarian or paternalistic approach. Change is more likely to be maintained if it becomes part of the person's everyday routine, such as walking the dog, rather than something that involves a special effort. We also have to be realistic in understanding how much change and uncertainty a person can cope with at any one time (Naidoo and Wills 2000). If the person is going through a very turbulent period in their life such as a divorce or struggling with the effects of redundancy, or they are living in a chaotic poverty-stricken environment, it may be unrealistic to expect significant health-related changes to occur in their lifestyle.

In working through the stages of change model with a client, the nurse should pay particular attention to the following:

1. *Attitudes to health and customs.* The patient's attitudes towards health, and the degree of belief that it is possible to be in control of your own health, will influence learning. Religious and cultural beliefs influence eating habits, lifestyle and receptiveness to health care and prescribed therapy. This information is also useful to the nurse who is helping the patient to make decisions about care.

2. *Past experience of illness.* Information about past health history should be collected, including how the person coped with illness and what changes in health habits and lifestyle resulted.

3. *Physical condition.* The patient's general feeling of well-being or illness influences the capacity and readiness to learn. The ability to carry out activities of daily living and to manage tasks and procedures necessary for self-care should be assessed. **Vision, hearing, touch,** manual dexterity and mobility all need assessment because they are important to physical functioning.

4. *Emotional state.* Emotions affect an individual's readiness to learn and to respond to teaching. In illness, and when there is a permanent loss of function, patients may progress through stages of adaptation or grieving. These stages include denial, anger and resentment, recognition and acknowledgement of the problem. When recognition and acknowledgement occur the patient begins to participate in decision making.

5. *Intellectual ability.* As well as willingness and desire to learn, the patient's ability to understand the condition and solve related problems will contribute to effective learning. The length of the individual's attention span, basic knowledge and fluency in the language being used should be kept in mind when considering comprehension and learning. This is particularly important if an interpreter is being used, especially when the interpreter might be a young child acting for his or her mother.

6. *Support system.* The response of family and friends to the situation can play an important part in the patient's education. If supportive, it facilitates learning and provides reinforcement for positive changes in behaviour.

7. *Barriers to learning.* Individual deterrents to learning include sensory deficits, decreased ability to comprehend, lack of orientation to time, place and person, decreased manual dexterity and loss of physical mobility. Learning is also inhibited by lack of motivation. Severe anxiety can interfere with learning, so that worries about lack of social and financial support and resources may inhibit effective patient education. If the language or form of words used by those teaching is unfamiliar or too technical (or perhaps too patronizing), that can also act as a barrier to understanding.

It is important early in the process to establish what the learning needs of the person are. A learning need is the educational gap between the present and the desired or required level of competence. It is mutually identified by the nurse and the patient from the analyses of the data collected and the needs expressed by the patient. The identification of learning needs should include a

Senses
*See chapters
2.3 & 2.4*

description of what the patient should know or be able to do and the factors influencing this.

Identifying educational needs and setting priorities requires assessing the patient's and family's present knowledge, how they see the patient's present level of functioning and what the desired level of competence may be. It is important to know whether they are able to look at the long-term implications or are able to focus only on what is happening today. This sort of assessment must be a continuous process, as changes occur once the patient has achieved the initial goals, coped with the impact of illness and begun to accept the changes in lifestyle.

Once learning needs have been identified, the nurse works with the patient to establish goals for learning, to determine priorities for teaching content and to select methods of teaching. Learning goals are usually divided into *short-term goals*, for immediate learning needs, and *long-term objectives*, for defining the eventual expected outcomes. The knowledge or skill to be achieved is defined, and the expected level or degree to which it will be met is stated. The final component of objective setting is defining the time in which the desired change is expected to occur. Behavioural objectives are worded in simple, basic terms that are clear to the patient and to all members of the healthcare team. They break learning tasks into small, sequential steps that can be tackled independently before the total goal is achieved.

The teaching plan must be written and placed in the patient's record. Without a written plan, other members of the healthcare team cannot actively participate in the teaching process. The plan must also be shared with the patient so that he or she can actively work towards achieving results.

Using a patient with **diabetes** as an example, behavioural objectives for the patient might be to:

- *state* the action of insulin
- *demonstrate* the technique of drawing up the prescribed amount of insulin into a syringe
- *talk about* feelings related to self-injection with insulin.

Teaching content must be accurately expressed in terms and language understandable to the patient and family, and adapted to age, cognitive ability, education and culture. The amount of time necessary and opportunities for questions, correction and repetition should be given consideration when planning teaching programmes.

Practical procedures should be broken down into a logical sequence of steps. First, the procedure should be demonstrated as a whole so that the patient is provided with an overview; then each step should be shown slowly and in detail. Time and opportunity should be allowed for practising the technique as soon as possible after the demonstration. The nurse should be aware that, in teaching any body of information, the first and last parts are recalled best; therefore, the most important points should come first and last. Repetition and receptiveness to questions reinforces learning.

Evaluation of the teaching programme and the patient's learning should be continuous. Revisions are made as indicated, and in some instances are made on the spot if the patient is not responding positively to the planned strategy. Outcomes of teaching are assessed: what effect the teaching has had, whether the objectives have been met, and whether the patient has acquired the knowledge and skills needed. Role playing or simulation may be used to assess changes in the patient's behavioural responses and in the ability to apply knowledge to real-life situations. The patient must also be an active participant in the ongoing and final evaluation of the educational plan. Observation and feedback are the primary ways in which the nurse determines whether (behavioural) change has occurred.

The process outlined above provides a framework for health education. It has not, however, referred to the many possible moral dilemmas that may be thrown up in day-to-day practice. Clarke (1993) has discussed health education with regard to the basic ethical principles of respecting the autonomy of the individual, acting to benefit the person (*beneficence*), not harming the individual (*non-maleficence*) and finally giving people what they deserve (*justice*). As she observes, health education involves choices and, if the wrong choices are made, a great deal of harm can follow; therefore the nurse must always be able to defend his or her actions ethically.

Health screening is an example chosen by Clarke, especially with regard to **cervical screening**. It is intended to be beneficial to the patient and to do no harm. But consider the stresses involved in the procedure and afterwards waiting for the results. Suppose that the woman is recalled for another smear or a mistake is made? The Health Belief Model would predict that, if the fears and anxieties generated by the procedure were too great, they might outweigh the possible advantages, leading to women failing to attend for screening at all.

It was issues such as these that led Foxwell and Alder (1993) to investigate whether a simple 10-minute nurse teaching package before screening could reduce anxiety levels. A large sample of 187 consecutive women (who were well educated and from a predominantly middle-class background) were allocated at random to either a control group that experienced the standard procedure or an experimental group that was given an additional nurse teaching presentation about the procedure. Anxiety levels after the smear were significantly reduced in the experimental group compared with the control group, suggesting that patient teaching in this case reduced anxiety. The researchers predict that this effect would be more pronounced in women who were less well educated or well informed, although this remains to be tested.

Encouraging women to attend for screening therefore generates anxiety, despite our principle of beneficence,

Diabetes
See chapter 2.6

Cervical smear
See chapter 6.3

but this study suggests these adverse effects may be minimized by further health education and information giving. This is consistent with Clarke's argument that the tension between beneficence and non-maleficence shown by this example can best be resolved by the nurse engaging the patient in full and open discussion about such procedures. This is what is meant by informed consent: the patient consents but only after being given all the information. Debate still continues about how much information is required, however, for consent to be fully 'informed'. The current UK position seems to be that it is as much as the doctor thinks the patient needs to know. The furore created in 2001 by the scandal of organ removal at autopsy without parental consent, which was highlighted by the practices at Alder Hey Children's Hospital, has brought the issue of informed consent again to the fore. The medical profession's traditional view can be criticized as paternalistic and in need of a significant shift towards a more open approach.

Health education and promotion work continually throw up these dilemmas and you may find that the basic ethical principles that underpin nursing sometimes appear to contradict one another. Ultimately, the answer lies in open communication between nurse and patient, respecting the wishes of the patient at all times. Health education is set to become an increasingly important part of the nurse's role, particularly as nursing develops its community profile in response to the future shift in health care out of hospital. However, the limitations of what can be achieved, as pointed out by Dines (1994), should be borne in mind.

Summary

The practice of nursing is dynamic and evolving, shaping and being shaped by the context within which nursing practice takes place. Changes in the healthcare delivery system have influenced the scope, skills and settings for the practice of nursing. Nursing also has to be seen in the context of a movement away from the medical model and its focus on pathology and cure. Rather, the emerging focus of nursing is on people seeking health.

Nursing is growing slowly in self-confidence and developing increased levels of autonomy. Nurse theorists have provided perspectives unique to nursing that emphasize the knowledge, research, ethics and practice of the profession. These perspectives provide a framework for applying knowledge from other disciplines to the practice of nursing, delineating the nurse–patient relationship and giving individualized, planned patient care. The nursing process is one method used by nurses to provide a systematic framework for nursing care. Alternative approaches that are more flexible and make more efficient use of time are, however, now being introduced, such as critical pathways. Accountability for care is a constant theme whatever method of care planning and

documentation is used. All nursing care must rest on a sound ethical basis. Nursing ethics is premised upon principles of moral conduct, which include autonomy, beneficence, fidelity, justice, non-maleficence and veracity. The UKCC provides guidelines for the ethical practice of nursing in its code of professional conduct.

The following chapters provide the reader with the knowledge, rationale and nursing perspective for the practice of nursing. However, excellence depends upon the nurse applying the knowledge gleaned from these chapters within the fields of health promotion and nursing practice discussed in this chapter. Each nurse–patient encounter is, however, rendered unique by its context.

References

Aggleton P (1990) Health. London: Routledge.

Benjamin M, Curtis J (1992) Ethics in nursing, 3rd edn. Oxford: Oxford University Press.

Bywaters P, McLeod K (1996) Working for equality in health. London: Routledge.

Clarke J (1993) Ethical issues in health education. British Journal of Nursing 2(10): 533–538.

Davidson N, Townsend P (1982) Inequalities in health. London: Penguin.

Delaney F (1994) Nursing and health promotion; conceptual concerns. Journal of Advanced Nursing 20: 828–835.

Department of Health (1999) Saving lives: our healthier nation. London: HMSO.

Dines A (1994) What changes in health behaviour might nurses logically expect from their health education work? Journal of Advanced Nursing 20: 219–226.

Dracup K, Meleis AI (1982) Compliance: an interactionist approach. Nursing Research 31(1): 31–36.

Ewles L, Simnett I (1999) Promoting health. A practical guide. London: Baillière Tindall.

Ford P, Walsh M (1994) New rituals for old; nursing through the looking glass. Oxford: Butterworth-Heinemann.

Foxwell M, Alder E (1993) More information equates with less anxiety. Professional Nurse October: 32–36.

Freire P (1985) The politics of education, culture power and liberation. New York: Macmillan.

Gough P, Maslin-Prothero S, Masterson A (1994) Nursing and social policy. Oxford: Butterworth-Heinemann.

Helman C (1994) Culture, health and illness, 3rd edn. Oxford: Butterworth-Heinemann.

Holm S (1997) Ethical problems in clinical practice. Manchester: Manchester University Press.

Hunt G (1994) Ethical issues in nursing. London: Routledge.

Lewis HR, Lewis ME (1987) What you and your patients need to know about safer sex. RN 50(9): 53–58.

Lifson A (1994) Preventing HIV; have we lost our way? Lancet 343: 1306–1308.

Manthey M (1980) The practice of primary nursing. Oxford: Blackwell.

Maslow A (1970) Motivation and personality. New York: Harper & Row.

Mead D (1991) An evaluation tool for primary nursing. Nursing Standard 6: 37–39.

Naidoo J, Wills J (2000) Health promotion, 2nd edn. London: Baillière Tindall.

Porter S (1988) Siding with the system. Nursing Times 84(14): 30–31.

Pratt R (1995) HIV and AIDS; a strategy for nursing care, 4th edn. London: Edward Arnold.

Prochaska J, DiClemente C (1986) Towards a comprehensive model of change. In: Miller WR, Heather N, eds. Treating addictive behaviours: processes of change. New York: Plenum.

Rankin S, Stallings K (1996) Patient education; issues, principles and practices. Philadelphia: JB Lippincott.

Seedhouse D (1986) Health: the foundation for achievement. London: Wiley.

Smaje C (1995) Health: race and ethnicity. London: King's Fund.

Stainton-Rogers W (1991) Explaining health and illness. London: Harvester Wheatsheaf.

Tones K (1992) Health education; politics and practice. Geelong, Australia: Deakin University Press.

Tones K (1993) Theory of health promotion; implications for nursing. In: Wilson-Barnett J, Clark J, eds. Research in health promotion and nursing. London: Macmillan.

Tschudin V (1999) Nurses matter. London: Macmillan.

UK Central Council for Nursing, Midwifery and Health Visiting (1992a) Code of professional practice. London: UKCC.

UK Central Council for Nursing, Midwifery and Health Visiting (1992b) Scope of professional practice. London: UKCC.

Walsh M (1995) The health belief model and use of A&E services by the general public. Journal of Advanced Nursing 22: 694–699.

Walsh M (1998) Models and critical pathways in clinical nursing. London: Baillière Tindall.

Walsh M (2000) Nursing frontiers; accountability and the boundaries of care. Oxford: Butterworth-Heinemann.

Webb P (1994) Health promotion and patient education. London: Chapman & Hall.

Wellings K, Field B (1996) Stopping AIDS. Harlow: Addison Wesley Longman.

Whitehead M (1988) The health divide. London: Penguin.

World Health Organization (1958) The first 10 years of the WHO. Geneva: WHO.

World Health Organization (1986) Ottawa Charter for Health Promotion. Ottawa: WHO.

2

Therapeutic communication and nursing practice

Mike Walsh

Introduction

The importance of communication

Barriers to effective communication

Skills for effective communication

The unpopular patient

Summary

Introduction

In chapter 1 we saw that the nurse–patient relationship lay at the heart of nursing care whether the nurse was in the active role of caregiver or in a more supportive or educational role. Any relationship depends upon good communication if it is to work properly and in this chapter we will be looking at the key elements that go to make up effective communication. The chapter will seek to apply these principles in three major areas of nursing activity: assessment, patient teaching and offering psychological support. The most difficult areas of all are perhaps giving patients bad news and supporting bereaved relatives. As these are such difficult areas they have been given a chapter of their own (see Ch. 4); however, the general principles covered in this chapter are equally applicable in helping a patient and/or their family cope with bad news and bereavement.

The importance of communication

It is essential to be clear about what we mean by caring if we are to see the real importance of communication. Caring used to be seen as getting the work done, performing a series of tasks, carrying out sister's or doctor's instructions. That was largely the case when I started my nursing career back in the 1970s. If caring is defined purely in terms of physical tasks, communication with the patient becomes of less importance. This is particularly true if the patient adopts a passive attitude of 'nurse/doctor knows best' and allows staff to carry out procedures in an unquestioning way. Nurses were advised not to get involved with patients and to remain at a distance so that they could concentrate on the tasks in hand without feelings getting in the way.

We have moved on since then. The word 'care' has come to take on new meanings in the nursing literature. Care is about mutual interaction with a person (Sadler 1997) and about being connected (Wilde 1997). Care is a deliberate and intentional process that depends upon a relationship being established and maintained between nurse and patient, not a collection of jobs to be performed in a shift. Communication is therefore an essential prerequisite for connection and the building of a therapeutic relationship with the patient and their family. This relationship may last a long time for, as we shall see in Chapter 5 on chronic illness, an increasing proportion of patients receive nursing care from the same team for the same problem over periods of many years.

One particularly interesting definition of caring comes from Sadler (1997):

> Caring is an individually and socially defined creative process of using presence, described by practising nurses as multidimensional work, where a holistic connection is made with a person to meet a recognised need.

Walsh (2000) has analysed this definition and suggests the following are key components:

1. Caring means different things to different people in different situations. This is a challenge to the nursing quality of empathy as it means the nurse must ask whether she or he can *really* appreciate what it is like to be 82 years old and have suffered a fractured hip. Good communication is therefore essential to

understand the patient's individual perspective on their health status.

2. Nurses have to use their own presence in the caring situation as a therapeutic tool, and to do so creatively. By the very act of being there, you change the situation and make it different for the patient. You cannot be in the presence of the patient without communicating, even if you do not speak. Non-verbal communications such as the expression on your face or body posture will speak volumes.

3. Caring is multidimensional work: you have to draw upon the social sciences as well as the biological sciences to practise nursing care. Communication is a constant theme running through the social sciences.

4. The very phrase 'holistic connection' means that effective communication is mandatory if that goal is to be achieved. It is essential to have communication if you are to connect with the patient and begin to explore the psychological, social, ethical and spiritual dimensions of that person's needs.

5. If a need is to be recognized, it goes without saying that there has to be a two-way channel of communication that is open and working effectively.

This analysis demonstrates that communication is a fundamental theme underpinning holistic care as practised in nursing today, rather than the task-oriented approach of 20–30 years ago.

Barriers to effective communication

One of the biggest historical barriers to communication has already been referred to: the way nurses were encouraged to distance themselves from patients, as 'getting involved' was seen as detrimental to carrying out tasks. It is still possible to see nurses rapidly changing the subject if they feel uncomfortable, or resorting to bland reassurances such as 'It will be OK' or 'We do hundreds of these operations every year'. The patient's take on this might be 'How do you *know* it will be OK?' or 'You may do hundreds of operations on other people, but this is *my* operation!'. Patients who are gay or lesbian may find that sexuality is completely missing from their care as nurses avoid all mention of a partner. To care is to connect and that cannot happen across a distant void.

The problem of distancing leads into the problem of avoiding disclosure as the nurse worries that exploring an area might do more harm than good (Faulkner 1998). Medicine has been seriously criticized for this patriarchal approach of knowing what is best for the patient and telling only what the doctor thinks the patient should know. As Faulkner points out, relatives often collude in this deceit. The patient is the only person able to decide where they wish a conversation to go, and questions must be answered honestly rather than avoided and attempts made to change the topic on to safer ground. Patient care can be an emotional minefield. Feelings such as anger, fear or despair may not be far away. You need to be aware of this at all times and tread carefully – although this is no reason for not treading at all! Once expressed, a patient's feelings do need to be explored, not ignored; we will come back to dealing with such difficult emotions later in this chapter. As a student you also need to recognize when you might be getting out of your depth with a patient. It is no admission of defeat or failure to refer a patient's questions to a registered nurse because you do not know the answer. It is also essential that all the caring team should take a consistent approach to any patient to avoid confusion due to mixed messages. This requires good communication between all members of the multiprofessional team.

Dealing with a distressed patient needs even more skill than normal. However, you must recognize that communicating effectively with even the most open, stable and cooperative patient needs skill. Lack of communication skills can therefore be a major barrier. Each individual who becomes a nurse is different and so brings a unique mix of skills and life experience to nursing. Lucky is the nurse who is a born natural communicator. Most of us have to learn communication as a set of skills that we can deploy in different situations and, by reflecting on what worked and what did not as we go along, steadily improve our communication skills.

Communication is, however, a two-way process and, however good you may be, that is only half the story. Patients may not be particularly good at expressing themselves for a range of reasons, such as linguistic skills (even if English is their first language), cultural beliefs or previous life experience. A significant proportion of the population does not have English as a first language, and in some circumstances the services of a translator are required. This can be very difficult, especially if the translator is a child and the patient is the mother, as she may not wish to share intimate details with her 10-year-old son and a complete stranger.

The two-way nature of communication means that you have to be aware of the fact that the patient's perceptions may be very different from your own, especially in relation to health. Lay beliefs about health may be very different from yours. The patient may have a very different agenda for the consultation than you have. It is essential that you find out at the beginning exactly what is the patient's purpose, perceptions and levels of knowledge about their health. This can save a great deal of frustration and misunderstanding later. The patient may, for example, present at the health centre wanting a prescription or a sick note. If the practice nurse or nurse practitioner starts the consultation with a health education package in mind, the result will be a failure of communication and a waste of time. However, if the nurse establishes the reasons for the patient's presentation at the beginning of the interview, she or he can attempt to negotiate a way into health education in such a way that the patient is meaningfully engaged and a relationship established.

The old adage that 'first impressions count' has been borne out by much experimental research in the field of social psychology. Humans tend to make perceptual short-cuts and place people in stereotypical categories based upon an initial first impression. Again this works both ways. You, as a nurse, need to beware falling into that trap when you meet a patient for the first time. You must look beyond the clothes and appearance to get to know the person within the patient. By the same token, how you appear to the patient on first meeting is equally important. Uniform requirements are not as draconian as they used to be but exist for good reasons apart from your own safety and convenience. They also convey important messages to the patient and a tidy, organized appearance is more likely to generate a sense of trust in you as a competent nurse than a dishevelled uniform, straggling hair and prominent items of jewellery festooning your ears, neck and fingers.

Perceptual stereotyping is closely linked to making assumptions about people, which is another important potential communication barrier. This can work in different ways. Faulkner (1998) cautions nurses against falling into the trap of assuming that, because the last three patients with a particular problem had a similar set of concerns and anxieties, the next patient will be the same. Assumptions are also made about ethnic groups. The fact that a person belongs to a particular ethnic or religious group does not allow you to make assumptions about what they might eat, their views on privacy or who may treat them. All patients must be treated as individuals and your interaction with them will probably get off on the wrong foot if you start with a series of assumptions made based upon previous experience of patients with similar conditions or about the ethnic or religious group to which they belong.

One final point concerning barriers to communication concerns the point of communication. If the aim is to discover information (assessment), then effective communication with the patient will not have occurred if effective communication with other colleagues does not follow. Whatever you may discover about the patient is wasted if it is not passed on to other members of the care team in clear and concisely written note form as well as verbally. The reverse is also true: effective communication with the patient for teaching or support purposes can occur only if you have the correct information to pass on.

The environment in which communication occurs can have a major influence on effectiveness and therefore constitutes a major barrier. Riley (2000) expands upon this observation to point out that lack of privacy, the layout of furniture in a room, the distance between you and the patient (too far or too close), the mood or feeling in a room (stark and clinical or soft and relaxed), whether the area is quiet or noisy are all factors that can interfere with communication. There are also interpersonal factors that affect the environment and hence communication. Excessive formality on the part of the nurse together with emphasis upon status and position will inhibit communication by the patient. Sitting behind the barrier of a desk with the patient on the other side is an example of how a combination of furniture, room layout and status can interfere with communication. Brusqueness, hurrying the patient and lack of eye contact only make things worse. I once saw a midwife carry out an entire antenatal interview with her back turned to the patient, asking questions over her shoulder. The patient happened to be my wife!

In summary, therefore, the main barriers to communication are:

- distancing from the patient associated with lack of involvement
- fear of where a conversation may go and a desire to stay on safe ground
- lack of awareness of communication skills
- patient difficulties in communicating with you
- perceptions and first impressions of people
- stereotyping and making assumptions about people
- environmental factors
- interpersonal factors surrounding role and status.

Whether you are assessing the patient, engaging in teaching, or offering support and help with difficult decisions, these factors must be taken into account. Failure to do so leads to what Riley (2000) calls non-therapeutic communication. There is a range of communication techniques that, consciously or unconsciously, is used to maintain distance from a patient or to control the direction of a conversation in order that uncomfortable areas (for the nurse) are avoided. Riley (2000) has produced a comprehensive list of such techniques to avoid (Table 2.1) and we will consider some of the main ones below.

A truism in communication work is that it is not so much the message sent that counts as the message received. In other words, listening skills are crucial, particularly active listening (see p. 35). The converse of this statement is that a failure to listen properly to the patient will inhibit therapeutic communication as you will not receive the message that the patient is trying to send you. This may occur because of distractions in the immediate environment – hence the importance of environmental factors in preventing effective communication. However, there may be factors within yourself that interfere with listening. Your mind may be on something else, such as worrying about home or social matters, thinking about the next job you have to complete, concern about another patient or getting that essay completed by the deadline.

Table 2.1   Non-therapeutic communication – mistakes to avoid

Mistake	Result
Failing to listen	Do not receive message from patient
Failure to probe	Inadequate data collection
Parroting	Irritates patient who comes to doubt your competence
Being judgemental	Suggests you have a right that you do not: the right to judge the patient. Prevents establishment of good relationship with patient
Bland reassurance	Negates patient's fears, feels not taken seriously
Refusing to discuss topics	Patient feels personally rejected
Defensive attitude	Patient feels staff will stick together rather than listen to his or her complaint
Giving advice or instructions	Contradicts patient as partner in care
Stereotyping	Makes patient feel devalued as an individual
Changing topics	Tells patient that the nurse is in charge and sets the agenda rather than discuss topics the patient wants to talk about
Patronizing	Insults and devalues patient

Adapted from Riley (2000).

Whatever the distraction, if you are not giving 100% of your attention to what the patient is trying to tell you, you will not be able to obtain a good health history and carry out a full patient assessment.

To engage with a patient who is distressed and in need of psychological support, you have to focus completely on what she or he is telling you. Any apparent disinterest on your part will be quickly picked up by the patient and the therapeutic element in the dialogue will evaporate. If you are teaching a patient, it is important to check that they have learnt what you have taught them and to provide opportunities for them to question you. Another important truism is that it is not what is taught that matters, but what is learnt. You can assess what has been learnt only by listening to the patient's questions and asking questions of your own to check understanding. It all comes back to good listening.

A potential pitfall at the start of an interview is jumping to conclusions. This relates to making assumptions and stereotyping people. If you make a decision very early on about a patient's health problems or needs, you will tend to foreclose other options. Consequently you may not actually hear the messages that are being given to you as you try to interpret the patient's statements in the light of your initial judgement. You may be totally focused on what the patient is saying, but still not listening as you manipulate their words to fit your judgement or hypothesis about the problem as you see it. It is very important to maintain an open mind if you are to maintain 'open ears' and really listen to the patient's story.

A major assessment problem is failure to probe, resulting in superficial, inaccurate or confusing data. If the nurse is worried about where the interview may lead, then the result is likely to be that questions are vague, lacking in depth or even omitted altogether. There is a cultural dimension to this problem. The British are notoriously reserved, whereas other societies (e.g. North America) are much more open. A Caucasian British nurse may feel very uncomfortable trying to assess the health needs of an Asian woman and therefore conduct a very superficial interview. Areas such as feelings, emotions and sexual practices are frequently omitted from assessments even though they are directly related to the patient's health problems. Sometimes the patient gives a hint in an answer that there is a problem without initially telling the full story. The nurse who is listening carefully will detect that hint and further gentle probing can lead to the patient opening up a whole area of their life that has remained hidden until now and that can shed light on apparently unrelated health problems. Obviously the nurse needs to ask such questions gently, unhurriedly and explain the reasons for asking, giving the patient the opportunity to decline to answer. Getting the balance right between asking sensitively about difficult areas and appearing intrusive or inquisitorial comes with experience and critical reflection upon your performance.

Adherence to rigid assessment schedules will lead to inadequate assessment. A standardized interview will tend to produce standardized data, not a holistic picture of the individual patient. An assessment framework is certainly very useful to ensure all the main areas are covered for all patients. However, you must be prepared to ask questions that are not on the schedule to arrive at a full assessment of the patient's health history. Obvious physical clues that need investigating may present themselves, such as an odour or signs of bruising. The patient may reply that they do not sleep very well in response to a question about sleeping habits. You must follow that up and explore further in order to discover why they do not sleep very well. This may be a clue to severe anxiety, a depressive illness, or frequent visits to the toilet to micturate due to an enlarged prostate or difficulty breathing whilst lying flat caused by heart failure, to name but four of many possible reasons.

We have already stated that patient teaching requires the nurse to check how much the patient has learnt. This requires not only effective listening but also effective questioning to ensure there are no misunderstandings. The patient who is upset and in need of psychological support will benefit also from a gentle probing approach which invites the patient to go as far as they feel comfortable in disclosing their problems.

Allied to a failure to probe the area being assessed is a tendency to change topics if the nurse is uncomfortable with the direction the interview is taking or if she or he wishes to explore other areas that the nurse considers of more interest. This gives the message to the patient that the nurse is not interested in what the patient has to say and may lead to important information being missed. There are times, however, when time is short and there are patients who have a tendency to ramble away from the topics that you do need to assess. The skill of therapeutic communication lies in gently guiding the patient into the key areas that you want to talk about without abruptly cutting across the patient's flow of conversation. It is also helpful to promise to come back later and continue the conversation. Such promises must be kept!

A lack of awareness of communication skills can be as bad as incompetent application of such skills. A good example of this is the skill of reflecting (see p. 37); unfortunately, in unskilled hands this sometimes becomes more like parroting as the nurse continually repeats the patient's words back to them. This can be interpreted by the patient as meaning that the nurse is not really listening to what they are saying. It can also be very annoying to the patient. Either way, parroting the patient's own words back to them will interfere with effective therapeutic communication.

Jumping to conclusions has already been mentioned as a serious problem. As nurses, we have to be aware of our own human weaknesses and the tendency to be influenced by first impressions and stereotypes. Where this really becomes a problem is if it is linked to being judgemental about patients. Nurses do not have the right to sit in judgement on patients, approving or disapproving of their actions. It is very difficult to engage with a patient who you know has committed some serious crime such as rape. Your religious beliefs may make you very uncomfortable about nursing a woman having a termination of pregnancy. The patient brought to the accident and emergency department with a drug overdose may be regarded as the author of his or her own misfortunes. However, you need to remember that your UKCC Code of Professional Conduct forbids such judgemental attitudes, which will obviously interfere with your ability to communicate effectively with the patient. However difficult it may be, judgement has to be suspended and patients treated equally with unconditional regard. Negative attitudes towards the patient will adversely effect both communication and care, which – ultimately – is the purpose of nursing.

Patronizing the patient will be very harmful to any chance of achieving therapeutic communication. This clearly sends the message that the nurse is superior to the patient and may creep in unintentionally as the nurse tries to make the situation less formal. A clumsy use of humour may inadvertently have the same effect. First names should be used only when the patient has been asked for permission to do so. Terms such as 'dear', 'chuck' and 'love' should be avoided, particularly when caring for older people, as they are extremely patronizing. Patient teaching should be carried out at the correct intellectual level for the patient, which should therefore have been determined beforehand. Clearly the approach required in dealing with a retired university lecturer is different from that needed with a builder's labourer. Children will frequently be encountered in the A&E department and, once again, you should ascertain their intellectual level of functioning and developmental stage before engaging them in conversation, even if their parents are present. Children hate being patronized just as much as anybody else.

A statement commonly read in care plans and student essays is that 'The patient will be reassured'. The word reassurance is much used and abused. In many cases it is inappropriate. A moment's reflection will suggest that a few words to the effect 'It will be OK' will have little impact upon a patient facing a life-threatening illness or surgery as they have multiple complex fears and anxieties to deal with. Reassurance like this can be little more than a meaningless platitude which might insult the patient's intelligence. The patient will probably think 'How do you know?', although rarely bother to say so. Dismissing the patient's fears with such a bland reassurance negates the patient's feelings and can make them feel trivialized. Alternatively it can convey a message of not caring – almost dismissing the patient's worries as not important.

Stereotyped responses can have the same effect as bland reassurances. Stop and think of the last time a shop assistant came out with the phrase 'Have a nice day'. I suspect you were irritated by that particular American import, seeing it as a stereotyped response with no meaning behind it. The nursing equivalent might be ending a patient assessment interview with the words 'Everything will be OK and we will have you home inside 3 days'.

At best, the patient is likely to be unimpressed by this comment and it may have exactly the opposite effect from that which was intended. If something does not quite go according to plan and there are complications, your credibility will be the first casualty, closely followed by the patient's trust in anything they are told. By the same token, if a patient is anxious about their care and needs time to talk through their anxieties, they should be given that time and not quickly dismissed with bland reassurances that prevent the conversation getting into difficult areas. You have to be honest and realistic with patients when discussing progress; if you do not know the answer to a question, be honest enough to say so. Rather than hazard a guess or give vague reassurance, contact a trained member of staff or a doctor and ask them to talk to the patient.

It is only a short step from avoiding real discussion by giving bland reassurance to refusing to discuss topics with patients altogether. Such a rejection makes therapeutic communication impossible as the patient may feel that not only has their question been rejected, but so have they. When the patient asks what the chances are of something going seriously wrong with their operation, the answer should not be 'We do not discuss things like that Mr Smith', as the author once heard a nurse reply. Refusing to discuss an area of concern with a patient is as negligent and unprofessional as refusing to give a patient an injection to relieve pain. The basic principle remains that, if you do not know the answer or feel the topic lies beyond your area of expertise, you are obliged to find someone who *can* deal with the subject.

A potential problem surrounding role and status issues arises when staff become defensive in response to questions and challenges. It is possible that staff feel threatened when care is questioned and, rather than engaging in a meaningful discussion to explain what is happening and why, go on the defensive. This can lead to a rapid breakdown in communication and hostility, which can escalate into abuse and even violence from some patients or family members. Defensive responses negate the patient's right to express opinions and say what is on their mind. They can lead to suspicions of a cover-up and the opinion that the staff are withholding the truth. Differences in social status can be exaggerated by defensiveness, leading to more antagonism. I have heard several patient outbursts along the lines of 'Who do you think you are then with your white coat (or nurse's uniform)? I pay your wages through my National Insurance/tax and I want to know what is going on/why I can't have … etc'. Sometimes you can explain things repeatedly in as reasonable a way as possible and the patient just will not listen, usually indicating that a more deep-seated problem is present. However, in many cases, unnecessary friction and poor communication can be avoided if staff accept that patients are entitled to question and challenge the care they receive. This is about

putting the rhetoric of 'patients as partners in care' into practice and treating them accordingly. This means giving them equal status and not responding defensively to their questions and criticisms.

Involving patients as partners in care does not mean telling them what they should do as this negates the contribution of the patient. It is tempting to give advice and lapse into informal everyday conversation with phrases such as 'If I were you I would …' or 'What you really should do is …'. This is the common approach frequently overheard when two people are talking on the bus, in a pub or whilst having a coffee. It might be common conversation, but it is not therapeutic communication. This is being directive, not valuing the patient's contribution and always invites the rejoinder 'But you aren't me!' or 'It's OK for you to say that but …'. A therapeutic approach needs to discover the patient's view of his or her problems first and then perhaps put forward the correct health promotion message or therapeutic interventions that would be required, but in a non-directive way. This can be followed up with the simple question 'How do you feel about that?' or 'Have you considered this?' The scene is then set for a discussion and negotiation in which you are fully aware of the patient's knowledge about the topic and his or her feelings about the problem. The patient is then a fully involved, active partner rather than a passive recipient of nursing or medical advice and instruction.

This section has summarized some of the communication pitfalls and mistakes to be avoided. It now remains to move on and look at more positive aspects and the kind of skills that will facilitate therapeutic communication. These are all skills that can be learnt and must be practised if you are to achieve effective communication with patients and members of staff also.

Skills for effective communication

Starting the interaction

Every conversation has a beginning and, as first impressions are so important in human communication, you must make a good start to the interview. That means you must explain who you are and what the purpose of the interview is. It is easy for hospital patients to become confused as they see so many different people in a day. The move away from traditional nursing uniforms is to be welcomed for all manner of practical reasons, but it may leave the patient unsure who this person in a top and trousers actually is. Small print on badges is often difficult to read, so there is no substitute for a full introduction of yourself.

If you are carrying out a health assessment interview it is important to explain that you are asking questions to try to obtain a whole picture of the person's health. The patient who is coming in for surgery on their knee may be very puzzled as to why you are asking about their diet, smoking and drinking habits, sleep patterns and whether their parents are still alive. Do avoid asking unnecessary questions such as age, date of birth and address as these are available on the patient's notes or admission form. Patients find it irritating to be asked the same questions six times on the same day by six different people.

A health education session should always start with you finding out how much the patient knows already. It is necessary to explain at the beginning that you will be asking a few questions to ascertain the patient's knowledge and views about the problem. This allows the patient to understand why these questions are being asked, which in turn is more likely to result in meaningful, helpful answers.

The patient may be reluctant to begin talking and at first remain silent. This should suggest to you that the person is very anxious and unsure. Gentle prompting such as just stating their name in a questioning way (Mr Wilson … ?) and pausing may be needed to elicit an initial response, rather than repeating the initial question.

Non-verbal aspects of communication are very important at the beginning of an interview and throughout. They will be addressed below.

Asking questions

Questions are basically open or closed. An open question might be 'How can we help you today?' or 'What brings you to the surgery this afternoon?'. The response is entirely the patient's; there is no right or wrong answer nor is there a limited choice of responses. Open questions can elicit information about patient knowledge or feelings such as 'Let's recap. What can you tell me about the two different types of inhaler that you use for your asthma?' or 'How do you feel about things since getting home from hospital?'. These sorts of question allow patients to say what they want to say and are an essential characteristic of a genuine therapeutic partnership with patients.

The closed question is characterized by a limited choice of responses (frequently yes or no) or a simple factual answer (How many days is it since those stitches were put in?). They are useful for gaining factual information and when there is a sense of urgency, such as in an emergency situation (Is this patient a known diabetic?). However, they are very limiting and do not allow patients to express their feelings. Consider a patient who has just been admitted to a surgical ward. If you begin your assessment with 'Do you know why you have been admitted today?' you will discover little. However, 'Can you tell me why you think you have been admitted to hospital today?' will start to gain an understanding of the patient's perceptions and can easily be followed up with further questions.

Another example of a closed question is to ask whether the patient is in pain. All this will obtain is a yes/no response, which is of limited value. A closed question could still be used, but one that will gain far more information such as asking the patient to rate their pain on a scale of 0–5. Perhaps a better approach would be to ask how the patient is feeling as this opens up other possible responses such as anxious or worried as well as in pain. You could then focus on pain assessment with some closed questions to elicit how severe the pain is, but should use open questions to discover *where* the pain is and what the *character* of the pain is. A closed question such as 'Is the pain in your left side?' may obtain a 'yes' answer but fail to discover a highly significant finding that it is also radiating into the patient's groin, as there is no opportunity for the patient to state this. 'Tell me where the pain is … Can you show me?' is a far more useful line to follow. A trap that the unwary may fall into, in trying to avoid a closed question, is to ask 'Is the pain in your left side?'. This is a leading question as it is suggesting the answer to the patient who may agree in order not to appear difficult. Similar questions might be 'I am sure you are happy to be going home today?' or 'Is your pain a lot better since we changed your medication?'. At all times, be careful to avoid suggesting the answer when asking questions.

Active listening

This involves attending skills in which, by both verbal and non-verbal cues, you indicate to the speaker that you are receptive and paying attention to what she or he is saying. This means it is a dynamic process as you convey to the original speaker that you have heard and understood what the speaker is saying (Duxbury 1999). Active listening involves integrating non-verbal cues from the speaker and the tone of his or her voice with the actual words the person is saying. It is about listening to the person's voice and not to a stereotype that you may carry around of that *type* of person. It is possible, for example, that the tone of voice and body language do not match the content of the speech, indicating deep-seated problems that need careful exploration.

The work of Egan (1986) has been drawn upon extensively by nurses as the basis for active listening. He suggests that the following key non-verbal skills make a simple but essential framework for effectively demonstrating to the patient that you are listening to what he or she is saying:

S   *sit* squarely to your patient in order that you may engage them fully

O   adopt an *open* posture that is welcoming and receptive

L   *lean* slightly forward suggesting attention and interest

E   maintain good *eye* contact, which again shows interest

R   show a *relaxed* approach.

You do not have to sit square on to the patient, leaning forward at all times for the entire interview. This is unnatural and will probably give you backache and prove unnerving for the patient. Move around in a relaxed way but keep returning to this position for important parts of the patient's story to show maximum interest and encouragement. Sitting with your arms and legs folded gives a 'closed' message to the patient. The relaxed open posture is encouraging and facilitates patient expression.

The SOLER skills need to be practised so that they come naturally to you. If you are concentrating on getting these things right during an interview you will not be listening to the patient! They should be practised until they are second nature. Video recordings of interviews, whether real or simulated with other students, is a very effective way of learning these skills via direct feedback. A word of caution is necessary, however, as if these techniques are used incorrectly they can actually be intimidating or even provocative. You can get *too close* to the patient and inappropriate eye contact becomes *staring* at the person.

There are other important non-verbal aspects of the interview that will enhance its therapeutic value:

1. Avoid having a barrier such as a desk, bed or trolley between you and the patient.

2. Sit with your chair at an angle to the patient. This allows you to engage the patient fully by sitting square on but without being confrontational.

3. Ensure your chair is at the same level as that of the patient, emphasizing the sense of equality.

4. Do not sit with your back to the light (e.g. a window). This means the patient cannot see your facial expressions clearly and, if the light is bright, may be squinting into the light in a way that can be disconcerting.

5. Ensure privacy and quiet whilst carrying out the interview.

6. Consider carefully the delicate issue of touch. British society is not a very 'touchy feely' society, so touching the patient can be inappropriate and unwelcome. There are some circumstances when the offer of an arm to help somebody to their feet is very welcome. A hand laid gently on a patient's arm or a soft touch on the shoulder when they are struggling with painful emotions can be a very effective piece of nursing when done at the right time with the right patient. Knowing when to do this is about experience and expertise, and the expert nurse knows intuitively when to do this. As a student, watch, listen and learn.

Just as your body posture will encourage the patients to tell their story, verbal prompts and rewards will have the same effect by demonstrating your interest and appreciation of the fact that they have chosen to share what can be very painful feelings with you. Prompts include 'Go on …' or 'And then …'. Another useful technique is to turn the end of a statement into a question and put this back to the patient. For example, the patient may say 'I felt so angry at what she said', to which you reply: 'What she said …?' This demonstrates careful attention and interest on your part and encourages the patient to expand upon what could be difficult emotional experience.

One final skill is the skill of silence. Do not dominate the conversation as the interaction is for the patient's benefit. Sometimes a carefully placed silence can encourage patients to carry on with their story, especially if followed by a slight prompt such as 'Yes …' or 'And then …'. There are times when silence is all that is required. Here you are using your presence as a therapeutic tool. Being with a patient so they are not alone at a time of great distress, or even at the ultimate end of life, is an act of immense nursing care. It merely requires presence. Do not be afraid if you can think of nothing to say, just being there is enough. Such occasions arise frequently in A&E or critical care nursing, for example when a bereaved relative is alone in the relative's room, perhaps waiting for family members to arrive, numbed by the awful truth of the death of their loved one. Your presence, alone with that person, is high-quality nursing care. Words may be of little importance in such a situation.

The skills of active listening described in this section are important in assessment and teaching, but particularly so in working with a patient who is very distressed or upset and in need of psychological support.

Empathy

Empathy involves understanding the experience, behaviours and feelings of others as they experience them (Duxbury 1999) – in other words putting yourself in the other person's shoes and trying to understand how things appear to them. Empathy is both a way of being that we all possess and that grows with age and maturity, and it is a skill that can be learnt (Price and Archbold 1997). We all possess some degree of empathy and the older we are the more we are likely to possess it as a result of life experience. Student nurses may have to work on what they start out with and develop it into a valuable tool to aid communication.

Other writers are less convinced about empathy. For example, Olson (1995) observes that, while much has been written about empathy, there is little documented evidence of its efficacy in actual nursing practice. Walsh (2000) cites encouraging evidence from two small studies (Savage 1995, Olson and Hatchett 1997), which does support the view that empathy assists nursing practice. However, as Walsh observes, we really need more evidence than this to be certain that empathy is more than an espoused ideal and is actually a tool of demonstrable value.

It is essential, however, to signal to patients that you are trying to see things from their point of view to make maximum use of this technique. However, you have to be realistic. A 21-year-old student nurse cannot really empathize with a 75-year-old man who has just suffered a stroke and it would be both insulting and patronizing to the patient to suggest that she or he could. Empathy should also make you aware of the danger of ethnocentricity, which is defined by Riley (2000) as the universal tendency of people to think that their ways of thinking, acting and behaving are the only right and natural ways. How readily can you empathize with a Bangladeshi woman or a refugee from the Balkans or Kurdish Iraq? We have already stated that nurses need to beware the trap of stereotyping people according to their ethnic, cultural or religious groups. Recognition of the individual's worth is crucial but has to be seen in the context of his or her ethnic, cultural and religious background.

Empathy should also make you aware that perhaps patients are only half expressing themselves. A woman may be telling you that she is terrified of a simple operation to remove a benign lump from her breast because of her fear of needles and pain and also because her neighbour's sister actually woke up in the middle of her operation because she was not given enough anaesthetic. Pause to think and put yourself in her position: is there something else she is not telling you because it is too frightening to talk about? Empathy might suggest the woman is actually afraid she might have breast cancer, even though the lump is a benign cyst. As Duxbury (1999) explains, an empathic nurse should hear themselves thinking: 'What is this woman only half saying?'.

Empathy allows you to use two other important skills, *reflection* and *rewording*. If you are in tune with the patient you will be able to pick up on certain feelings and emotions that can be explored further. Reflecting the patient's feelings can be achieved by rewording what they are saying and putting this back to the patient in your own words. To do this you have use active listening skills to be aware of the tone of the person's voice and their nonverbal cues as well as what they are saying. The woman sitting in front of you with tears in her eyes and who is fiddling with her hands in an agitated way and yet who says 'I am OK', clearly is not OK. This distress can be gently reflected back to the patient: 'Mmmm … are you sure? How are things at home?'.

Rewording can be used on the content of speech to clarify meaning. The woman who says 'I told my husband to go to hell!' might be helped by the nurse saying 'You were really angry with him' as this allows her to clarify her feelings and signals that the nurse is on her wavelength. She may well press on to explain why she was so angry without you even having to ask why.

A useful way of reflecting feelings that involves rewording is the formula 'I think I hear what you are saying. It sounds to me like … Am I correct?'. This should be used sparingly, however, as the patient will become irritated by continual rewording and reflecting as they feel they are going round in circles and getting nowhere. It may also encourage the person to wallow in destructive or distressing emotions without moving forward to deal with those feelings constructively.

Egan (1986) offers the following useful tips in the use of empathy:

- Pause before you speak and think carefully. Do not rush into glib statements.

- Keep your responses short as it is the patient who should be doing most of the talking.

- Recognize the emotional tone of the patient through your active listening skills and pitch your responses accordingly.

Finally, it is important to not confuse empathy with sympathy. Identifying too closely with the patient may cloud your judgement. This is especially true if the patient is the same age as yourself.

Handling emotion

In the course of the interview, especially if offering support to a distressed patient, a range of emotions may be unleashed that you have to handle. These can include anger, guilt, denial and fear. This is particularly likely when talking to the relatives of a person who has just died or who is critically ill (see Ch. 4 for a discussion of bereavement and breaking bad news).

Anger may arise from several factors such as the need to blame something or somebody for a serious illness such as cancer or a stroke that has apparently come out of the blue. The patient may complain bitterly that life is not fair. The patient may be angry because of delays in treatment or cancellations, none of which are your fault but you happen to be the person on whom the patient vents their anger. If the anger is dismissed or denied and you become defensive, this is very unproductive and will probably lead to an escalation of anger that could spill over into abusive behaviour and even violence. Responding to anger with anger will only lead to an even quicker escalation and confrontation.

A more effective approach is clearly needed which has to start by acknowledging the anger expressed by patients as a real expression of their feelings. It is essential to show that you are taking their complaint seriously and then to find out exactly what the nature of the complaint is. Only by finding out what is the root cause of the anger is it possible to move forward and resolve the potential conflict. Keeping a cool head and not reacting to harsh words is not easy but it is essential if you are to defuse the situation. Patients must be allowed to have their say and ventilate their feelings as part of the defusing process. In many circumstances the anger has resulted from a lack of communication or information compounding a sense of frustration, injustice or fear. Good listening skills and defusing techniques will usually calm such situations.

However, there may sometimes be a difficult dilemma if the outburst takes place in front of very sick patients or young children in the A&E department. You need to manoeuvre the person away from such an environment, but also beware becoming isolated from the rest of the staff for your own safety. Remain visible to others and do not become penned into a corner or side room with the aggressor between you and the exit route.

When dealing with an angry person the 'SOLER' framework needs modification. You need to place distance between yourself and the person and be out of arm's reach. This is for your own safety because, if the person suddenly lashes out at you, it gives you a chance to take avoiding or blocking action. Increasing distance from the person and not leaning towards them at a time like this is also less confrontational. The best posture is with your weight slightly on your back foot and your body placed slightly oblique to the person. This gives you the best position to defend yourself if you are attacked. Eyeball to eyeball contact can be very provocative if you are handling an aggressive person: keep your gaze at about the level of the first shirt button, as this is less threatening but shows you are paying attention. If the person is under the influence of drugs or alcohol, then you are much less likely to succeed in resolving the situation; such individuals are best dealt with quickly by security and/or the police.

Guilt is not so easy to resolve as anger. It tends to be something that has accumulated over many years, sometimes quite irrationally. The best that can be done with guilt in the short term is to be aware that it may be there and could explain otherwise inexplicable behaviour. Patients can be facilitated to expand upon their feelings and talk about their guilt as part of a supportive relationship. This is particularly important in the management of long-term illness where the nurse builds up a relationship with the patient possibly over several years. Their guilt is as much a part of them as their diabetes or asthma. Guilty feelings surface particularly after bereavement and have to be worked through as part of grieving (see p. 61).

Denial is a means of coping with events by simply pretending they are not happening. I remember a woman in her sixties presenting to my A&E department protesting all the way in that she did not need to see any doctors. She had a massive fungating malignancy of the breast that was grossly contaminated and highly odorous. I can still see the look of amazement on the face of the female student who had undressed her. 'How on earth could she have pretended that there was nothing wrong?', she asked me. Denial was of course the answer.

It can be very frustrating when patients resort to such an ineffective coping mechanism. It may be the young adult who denies their **diabetes** or **epilepsy**, ignores medication

Diabetes
See chapter 2.6

Epilepsy
See chapter 2.2

Myocardial infarct
See chapter 4.2

and advice about lifestyle, and continues to present as a regular emergency admission, or the middle-aged man who denies that he has had a **myocardial infarct** and continues as before. Complete denial presents a brick wall to therapeutic intervention. However, we should not become judgemental and must treat the patient as an adult who is making his or her own decisions about their life. Maintaining communication and contact at least holds out the hope that at some stage in the future the person will come to see things differently and reach out for help as they begin to accept the truth of their situation. Therapeutic communication means that a bridge to that person can be built eventually which will do some good, even though it may be late in life and after much harm to their health. The patient who is terminally ill and yet in denial has to be handled with great sensitivity. Eventually reality will intrude and nursing must be there for that person when this occurs.

Anxiety and fear are very common human emotions. In fact they are essential for survival. However, they can become distressing and debilitating especially when bottled up inside. Cultural and social norms play a major part in the expression of such emotions, with men in northern European society often feeling unable to admit fear and anxiety. Therapeutic communication is about giving the person the room and space to admit to such feelings. It allows you to discover the focus that lies at the root of fear. Sometimes this can be dealt with directly by clearing up misunderstandings, which will alleviate fear. Sometimes the person just feels better for talking about things and realizing that they are not the only person with this problem. On other occasions patients can be encouraged and facilitated to discuss their problems with relevant family members, perhaps including referral for skilled counselling. When fear and anxiety become totally debilitating and/or irrational, specialist mental health professionals need to be involved.

The unpopular patient

Unfortunately some patients, despite all our professional ideals to the contrary, become labelled as 'difficult' or, 'manipulative'. In short they are unpopular. Significant amounts of research have been carried out on this phenomenon and Riley (2000) summarizes the following characteristics of 'the unpopular patient' by saying they are a person who:

■ argues, complains and fails to cooperate

■ states that they do not like being in hospital and want to go home

■ states that they are suffering more than nurses believe

■ suffer from conditions that should be treated elsewhere (another ward, by their GP, etc.)

- require more time and attention than the nurses believe they should have

- have complex diagnoses with difficult illness pathways involving various complications over a long time period, especially if the nurse knows little about the condition

- are considered to be of low social value and moral worth

- are stigmatized by virtue of sexual orientation, race, religion, etc.

- have an 'own fault' diagnosis such as a drug overdose or alcoholism.

You should reflect upon this list as you work your way through your education. How many patients can you identify towards whom the nursing and medical staff had a strongly negative attitude, and how many of these characteristics were present? Pause for a moment and check this list against Table 2.1 to see how many items involve the nurse using *non-therapeutic* communication techniques such as being judgemental, using stereotypes or rejecting. The problem of the unpopular patient in health care can be greatly reduced by the use of therapeutic communication, avoiding preconceptions and treating the person as a person, not as a patient with a reputation.

Summary

This chapter has been a brief introduction to key aspects of communication, which has to be effective if it is to be therapeutic. Therapeutic communication is as important as any other skill you will learn in your career – and probably more important than most. However, it needs practice and can always be improved upon. Critical reflection is one particularly effective technique that will assist you in developing this aspect of your nursing. If knowing what to do is the science of nursing and knowing how and when to do it is the art, then therapeutic communication is the essential underpinning of both the science and art of nursing.

Critical incident

Conversation overheard on a surgical ward one day involving a medical student clerking a 70-year-old man:

Student: Do you smoke?
Patient: Yes.
Student: How many?
Patient: About 20 a day.
Student: You know that is very bad for you?

Patient: Don't be daft, a fag in the morning makes me cough and clears my chest. Smoking relaxes me and makes me clear my chest with a good cough, so don't go giving me any of your medical lectures!
Student: But the cigarettes are making you cough because they are harming your chest.
Patient: But a good cough is good for me!

The medical student pursued this circular argument with the patient for a further 10 minutes, becoming increasingly frustrated and irate while the patient became increasingly annoyed. The rest of the clerking was finally concluded in a very strained atmosphere and the patient's first afternoon on the ward had got off to a bad start.

Reflection
Reflect upon the communication technique used by the medical student and how he failed to appreciate the patient's point of view. How might you have approached this patient and discussed his smoking?

See Appendix 2 for guidelines on reflection.

References

Duxbury J (1999) Therapeutic communication and the nurse practitioner. In: Walsh M, Crumbie A, Reveley S, eds. Nurse practitioners; clinical skills and professional issues. Oxford: Butterworth-Heinemann.

Egan G (1986) The skilled helper. Monterey, California: Brooks/Cole.

Faulkner A (1998) Effective interaction with patients, 2nd edn. Edinburgh: Churchill Livingstone.

Olson J (1995) Relationships between nurse expressed empathy and patient perceived empathy and patient distress. Image; Journal of Nursing Scholarship 27(4): 317–321.

Olson J, Hatchett E (1997) Nurse expressed empathy; patient outcomes and development of a middle range theory. Image; Journal of Nursing Scholarship 29(1): 71–79.

Price V, Archbold J (1997) What's it all about, empathy? Nurse Education Today 17: 106–111.

Riley J (2000) Communication in nursing, 4th edn. St Louis: CV Mosby.

Sadler J (1997) Defining professional nurse caring; a triangulation study. International Journal of Human Caring 1(3): 12–21.

Savage J (1995) Nursing intimacy. London: RCN Publications.

Walsh M (2000) Nursing frontiers; accountability and the boundaries of care. Oxford: Butterworth-Heinemann.

Wilde M (1997) The caring connection in nursing; a concept analysis. International Journal of Human Caring 1(1): 18–24.

3

Ageing and health

Pauline Ford and Tina Wills

Introduction

Demography

Contemporary policy context

Emerging trends

Normal ageing

Assessment

A profession equipped to support and work with older people

Health promotion and wellness

Summary

Introduction

This chapter explores the context of care for older people today located within and influenced by current policy. It highlights the importance of assessment as a mode of accessing nursing and provides overviews of common theoretical perspectives on ageing. Throughout, discussion is linked to a critical care pathway in which the experiences of Mr Jacob Brown are followed through a potential healthcare experience. The chapter concludes with a consideration of the context of care in relation to the ongoing development of nursing expertise in the specialty of gerontology.

Demography

There is a folk saying that 'everyone wishes to live a good long life, but no one wishes for old age'. This may relate to the fact that desire for increased longevity is usually associated with thoughts of a healthy and active old age rather than ill-health, disability, increasing vulnerability and greater dependency upon others.

Ageing takes place within a global village where the boundaries between nations and continents are blurring different lifestyles and cultures. Trends at this worldwide level reveal key challenges for the future (Kinsella 1996):

- the older population is increasing in absolute terms and as a percentage of the total population

- the fastest growing segment is the 'oldest old' – 80 years plus

- there is a declining birth rate

- people are deferring child rearing.

In 1995 the UK was one of the demographically oldest nations in Europe: 16% of its population was aged 65 years and over. In 1991 there were just under 30 people of pensionable age per 100 people aged 16–64 years. By 2011, this figure will have risen to 43 per 100, but by 2021 there will be nearly 60 people of pensionable age per 100 people of working age (Office of Population Censuses and Surveys (OPCS) 1996). This is due in part to the social phenomenon of 'baby boomers': adults approaching retirement age who are part of the postwar baby booms (Falkingham 1997). Individuals in the 1947 birth peak will be aged 60–64 in 2010, joined in retirement by people in the second birth peak of the mid-1960s in 2025, at which point there will be 1.6 million more people of retirement age than there are today.

Birth rates have always been the most important influence on the size and composition of the population. The relative size of the older age groups is due mainly to falls in the birth rate, which result in fewer children and younger people. However, in the UK, where the birth rate has been low for some time, changes in death rates at older ages are having a stronger effect on age composition. The combination of previous fertility patterns and improvements in life expectancy have resulted in increasing numbers and proportions of older people aged 85 years and over (Askham et al 1992).

Current best estimates suggest that some 60% of boys and 70% of girls born in 1981 will survive to celebrate their 75th birthday in the year 2056. If we reflect back a century, then we see that of boys born in 1881 only half reached 55 years and a mere 20% survived to 75 years. Girls fared slightly better, with 40% dying before the age of 55 years; many of these deaths occurred in infancy. Only one-third of the girls survived to 75 years (Grundy 1994). Such dramatic statistics herald a survival revolution, achieved largely through reduced infant mortality and the near eradication of infectious diseases such as tuberculosis.

Older people, in particular the very old, make up an increasingly large segment of our population. Whilst this should be a cause for celebration, it is more frequently seen as a cause for concern. Certainly it is considered to pose a major challenge to society. Most people are aware of the fears regarding the rising cost of health and social care, but there is less understanding of changing family patterns, such as the rise of divorce, the increase in the number of single parents and those living outside any form of partnership (Haskey 1995). How these factors will affect the capacity of younger generations to support the old is still not yet fully understood. Given that the most important source of practical and emotional support for older people currently is from their spouse or partner (OPCS 1996), the trend for living alone has the potential to influence future patterns of care. The world of work is also changing, with older workers becoming an increasingly significant group. Over 1 in 4 workers will be aged over 60 by the year 2020, compared with 1 in 5 in 1990. This is viewed as a positive development, with more people using a variety of skills and talents into later life (Phillipson 1997). B & Q, one of the DIY chains in the UK, has a policy of positively seeking the employment of older people, who they see as offering many skills to the consumer. This sort of initiative, along with a rise in the traditional retirement age, could encourage older people to retrain and remain in active employment for longer, if this is their choice (Moore et al 1994). This may affect the capacity for some people to take up informal caring roles, which presently support many older people. Today, it is

estimated that some six million people are involved in unpaid caring activities (Scales and Phal 1999).

In addition to family configurations and future employment trends, health will be influenced by the way in which we live. Our geographical distance from one another and the houses we occupy, in town or countryside, will affect our access to one another and to health services. The conditions of the houses people live in are important, as is the ability to get about. Living in a balanced community, where a mixture of types of people, in terms of age, class, income and household are represented, is considered to work to everyone's advantage (Russel 1999).

So, in summary, whilst there are clear reasons for celebrating our ageing society there remain some valid reasons for concern, most commonly the cost of health and welfare services for older people. People over the age of 65 years consume more than 45% of total health spending (Ranade 1993). Expenditure on such services for those aged 85 years and over is 15 times as great as expenditure on 15–64-year-olds (Grundy 1994). This raises issues for health promotion and education, which are explored later in the chapter. There are, however, less valid reasons for society's ambivalence about services for older people, as will be considered in the next section.

Contemporary policy context

Current health and social care provision

Current provision of services for older people originated in divisions of welfare that go back to the nineteenth century. They reflect the gradual extension of public sector activity and its changing historical role in relation to the individual, the workplace and the voluntary sector (Jones 1994). Healthcare policies will continue to be heavily influenced by the economic and political context in which they operate.

Community care in the UK was fully introduced in 1993 (DoH 1990), with the intention of reducing the emphasis on institutional care and promoting home-based approaches, supported by health and social services. In the vast majority of cases, older people living at home will depend largely upon their own resources, their partner, family, friends and neighbours to meet their daily living needs. Directly relevant to these needs has been the policy focus on enabling people where possible to remain in their own homes, an objective that research has shown undoubtedly matches what older people themselves prefer (Tinker 1984, Audit Commission 2000).

Practical support for carers by service providers is advocated in several policies, such as the Carers Recognition and Services Act (Department of Health/Social Services Inspectorate 1995), but concerns have been expressed that the balance of care has shifted away from state provision towards the community, resulting in stress upon the carers of some vulnerable older people (DoH 1993, Evandrou 1992).

In recent years older people's needs have been the focus of national policy, with the Royal Commission's report on long-term care (Royal Commission 1999), the establishment of national care standards (DoH 1999a), the formation of local eligibility criteria (DoH 1995), challenges to the equity of these criteria (DoH 1999b, Royal College of Nursing (RCN) 2000a), proposals for the enhancement of partnerships between health and social services (DoH 1998) and assessment (Ford and McCormack 1999, RCN 1997a,b). Currently, nursing is free at the point of delivery for all older people except those who live in nursing homes, where means testing occurs. The National Plan (DoH 2000a) proposes changes to the funding of long-term care, with entitlement to nursing care as a 'free' component. This highlights the importance of assessment and the difficulty of differentiating between nursing and personal care (Royal Commission 1999); the differentiation of nursing care and personal care could become the new 'grey' area, replacing the previous health and social care debate (Editorial 2000). The National Plan (DoH 2000a) and the Government's response to the Royal Commission's 1999 recommendations for long-term care do not define nursing care, other than to indicate that registered nurses will assess the need for nursing care. To establish a broader understanding of nursing as more than a series of tasks (RCN 1997b), nurses working with older people will need to articulate the ways in which the presence of a registered nurse provides a constant overview or supervision of the care provided. Registered nurses will also provide actual care, while they also monitor, direct, manage and supervise care (RCN 1997a).

The NHS National Plan (DoH 2000a) requires an NHS registered nurse to establish a component of the older person's care which is nursing. The hope is that these nurses will assess in a way that reflects a clear view of the complex ways in which a nurse contributes to the care and support of an older person – in essence, with a broad view of nursing that looks beyond tasks and hopefully prevents the new grey area of confusion in relation to the boundaries of nursing and personal care from developing.

In many instances older people will require input from both health and social services, which is best provided in an integrated way. The recommendations of the Royal Commission identified lack of integration as a problem and promoted good practice examples of partnership between health and social services providers. Current government policy seeks to encourage such partnerships (DoH 1998). The development of integrated services for older people has gained much support (e.g. Henwood 1999).

Primary care is currently seen as the leading partner in determining healthcare provision, which seeks to increase the decentralization of services, bringing them closer to the older person, perhaps in the form of primary care centres (Warner et al 1999). Services might be provided in more inventive ways, the National NHS Beds Inquiry (DoH 2000b) explores options which include making better use of nursing homes in the independent sector, through the provision of intermediate care facilities, for example. The National Plan aims to expand intermediate care services (DoH 2000a); this acknowledgement of the need for services for older people that afford additional time for recovery and access to appropriate expertise (Audit Commission 2000) holds promise for expansion in the primary and independent care sectors. However, all services must be mindful of the potential for ageism within the NHS (Age Concern 2000), especially if older people are seen as users of specific services, instead of accessing all services equally.

Emerging trends

Future services will be influenced both by policy and a variety of other factors. Perceptions of old age are significantly influenced by the media through exposure to images on the television, film, radio and journals, and in newspapers. Many representations of older people in the media are less than positive; they are caricatured as a cohesive whole, wrinkled and frail, or they are infantilized. Hockey and James (1993) explore a variety of media reports, which form analogies between old age and childhood, or treat the example of fit and vital old age as the remarkable exception. As older people's individuality and vitality receives a fair hearing, health professionals can draw attention to positives models of ageing.

The independence and inclusion of older people is becoming more commonplace (Help the Aged 1997). The focus for health and social care professionals is being drawn toward user consultation. Users are articulate in expressing their viewpoint and the need to listen to what older people want from services is something that should not be ignored (NHS Executive 2000) and indeed should influence policy. The ideal is not the disenfranchisement of any group, but the empowerment of all age groups within society (Warner et al 1999).

Standards of care services are becoming highly formalized, both in the independent sector, with the introduction of national required standards (DoH 1999a), and within the National Health Service, with the formation of the National Institute for Clinical Excellence (NICE). NICE was established to give new coherence and prominence to information about clinical costs and effectiveness. In addition the National Service Framework (NSF) for older people (DoH 2001) establishes standards for use within the NHS. The NSF is a complex framework with eight standards, under the four themes of:

- respecting the individual
- intermediate care

■ providing evidence-based specialist care

■ promoting an active healthy life.

The NSF seeks to guide service and practice development in the care and support of older people, these developments will be measured by the use of performance indicators and predetermined milestones for each standard. The setting of standards may in part respond to the findings of bodies such as the Health Advisory Service (2000), whose inquiry into the care of older people on acute care wards in general hospitals resulted in the following recommendations:

■ increased user consultation in relation to all aspects of their care from older people

■ the challenging of negative views about old age, from patients, their relatives and staff – particularly the belief that prospects for recovery are gloomy

■ for the poor image and profile of older people to be tackled at every level of the health and social care system

■ that the crucial role of the ward manager in creating a supportive culture of care should be developed and promoted

■ better education for staff working with older people, in all settings.

The future for older people and the nurses who work with them has the potential to be challenging and rewarding, as we all adapt to the policy changes and move into a system that could create new partnerships across organizational boundaries and, more importantly, with older people themselves.

Meeting Mr Jacob Brown

Making sense of all the issues that could relate to the health and social well-being of an older person can be challenging. As a focus for the rest of this chapter, Jacob Brown is introduced. First you meet him as ageism and the present policy context would define him. In this first scenario (Case Study 3.1) Jacob is receiving informal caring and is encouraged to stay in his home, in keeping with the community care act (DoH 1990). In the second scenario (Case Study 3.2) Jacob's situation is described as it might be with the new policy developments and in a society without ageism.

The second of Mr Brown's scenarios is tracked as he travels on a critical pathway through service provision. Later Mr Brown is met again in relation to assessment.

Case Study 3.1   *Mr Jacob Brown: scenario 1*

Mr Brown lives alone. He can't do much for himself, and his nephew, who lives in the next village, is tired of going to drop off his dinner, only to find the next day that he hasn't eaten it. Mr Brown used to be a factory storeman for a large firm, but he retired 10 years ago and does nothing now. He used to fish but has given it up, the river being a couple of miles off, and he doesn't drive now – his nephew said a man his age would be a danger behind the wheel, so the car was sold.

Jacob lost his wife many years ago from cancer and they had no children. He has lots of nieces and nephews, because he has a brother and two sisters who have been married more than once. He sees them only at Christmas because they live all over, but they telephone now and then.

He fell last year and gave himself a fright. He went to the hospital and stayed in for 2 days; since then he has lost weight and still gets giddy when he gets up sometimes. He asked the doctor about getting a bit of help but wasn't eligible to go into the nursing home, because the local criteria did not measure his needs as nursing. Jacob used to work with Bill Taylor, who lives in a residential home, but Jacob has never been there; it might be awful – you do hear things.

These days Jacob gets the paper delivered and reads that while it's light, to save on the electricity. Then he has a cup of soup and just waits for Colin, his nephew, to call. Nice lad, but he tends to be busy ferrying his two children about, so doesn't stay long. Sometimes Jacob feels miserable; the house is too big, and one day is like the next. He thinks he probably isn't good company.

In this first scenario, Jacob is seen from an ageist viewpoint:

■ His ability to work beyond traditional retirement age is not acknowledged.

■ His skills are not utilized, for the benefit of his family or local community.

■ He receives informal care from his nephew, which is not formally acknowledged.

■ He cannot maintain his lifestyle and relationships, because he is viewed as unable to drive owing to his age.

■ Screening has not been carried out to alert his general practitioner to his dizzy spells, and Jacob has not accessed expert practitioners with specialist knowledge in gerontology.

- Assessment has been carried out in light of local eligibility criteria, which does not view Jacob's needs as nursing.

- Residential care is viewed as dependent living, in an institutional setting.

Jacob has not been valued as an individual.

Case Study 3.2   *Mr Jacob Brown: scenario 2*

Mr Brown lives alone. He drives a Morris Minor, which he has had for years. On the advice of his nephew, Colin, he has a check-up from the practice nurse once a year, just to be sure he is still safe, but he's pleased to be getting around independently as he is quite a busy chap. He likes to fish at the weekend with an old work colleague, Bill Taylor. He collects Bill from the residential home where he lives and they usually go back to Bill's for a drink and a bit of a meal. If he ever needed to, Jacob thinks he would try to get a room there – you have a small bedsit and it's all self-catering, which is lovely.

Jacob decided to move last winter after he had a nasty fall; the place was too big for him and he was keeping the lights off to keep the bills down. Looking back, that fall had been a godsend in a funny way. He ended up with a black eye, but no broken bones. The hospital assessed him and a nurse came along; she explained she was part of a team, which had a doctor and social workers in it. As a result of his assessment, they found out that Jacob had high blood pressure, and he now takes something for that so doesn't get dizzy.

The assessment helped him to think about living alone in that huge house – empty since his wife's death 30 years ago – and he decided to move nearer to his nephew. He got a first floor flat near the pub, where he's a regular feature, running the pub quiz and having his tea if he's feeling lazy. Jacob also gives Colin's children lifts here and there in return for the odd Sunday lunch at their house. Jacob is pleased to have his health, because some don't.

In this second scenario, Jacob exists in a positive framework which values older people for their ability to contribute to society:

- His skills are utilized and he remains an active member of his community.

- He is able to spend time with his nephew's children, in a positive role.

- His health problems have been identified and preventive measures put in place.

- Jacob maintains his individuality and lifestyle choices.

- His future decisions will be made in collaboration with professionals.

- Residential care is viewed as communal living in a supportive environment.

Such a positive scenario demands a society in which equity and justice are central and in which individuals' ability to choose and take their own path in life is not hampered by stereotypes of old age. In the current context, however, issues of inequity for older people exist; the next section explores this in more detail.

Issues of equity

Equity is defined in *The Oxford Dictionary* as 'fairness, the application of principles of justice'. This definition suggests that everyone should have an equal voice and value in society. The question of equity for older people in health and social care has received increasing attention in recent years, largely as a result of the debate about rationing and prioritization (Grimley Evans 1997, Williams 1997). This chapter focuses on rationing as an extreme example of inequity. Rationing is defined as 'a fixed allowance, to limit or share out'.

Rationing by age polarizes perspectives. For example, Williams (1997, p. 820) cautions against the 'vain pursuit of immortality', claiming that we have reached a point at which no one must die, until everything possible has been done for them. Henwood (1999) agrees, and suggests ways in which a dignified death can be achieved; however, she also reminds us that this is a separate argument from the one that supports rationing in relation to age. For example, Grimley Evans (1997, p. 883) counters Williams' argument, stating that it is unethical to 'use age as a criterion for depriving people of health care from which they could benefit'.

There is evidence that rationing of health care does take place, for instance in end-stage renal disease (Mallick 1994) and coronary care (Dudley and Burns 1992). These findings also reflect the ageism associated with pharmaceutical and clinical research. Half of all malignancies occur in people over 70 years of age, yet people of this age are excluded from clinical trials of cancer treatment. The rationing debate is part of the wider debate about equity in health care, as the Acheson Report (1998, p. xiii) observed:

> Although average mortality has fallen over the past 50 years, unacceptable inequalities in health persist. For many measures of health inequalities have either remained the same or have widened in recent decades.

The main barriers to equity for older people are structural and attitudinal: *structural* in terms of age-segregated services and access difficulties, and *attitudinal* in terms of prejudicial ageist attitudes. Attitude refers to a person's favourable or unfavourable evaluation of an object (Yurick et al 1988).

Structural barriers to equity for older people occur as a result of the way in which services are organized within the NHS. Speed of recovery is emphasized, and older people who require time to improve and reach their maximum potential are disadvantaged. This system encourages increased dependence and loss of role and ability for older people, with a resulting resource implication (Audit Commission 2000). Structural barriers often re-enforce attitudinal barriers to equity. Older people are treated as a burden for taking up a hospital bed, labelled negatively as 'bed blockers' to be discharged quicker and sicker, making their potential for readmission more likely (Audit Commission 1997, Yates 1998).

The attitudes of some care providers towards older people have been considered by gerontologists to have a major influence on the kind of care provided and on the self-image of the older person. A recent report from Age Concern (2000) presented evidence that the NHS discriminates against older people. Many accounts from older people themselves have described the way in which they felt healthcare personnel stereotyped them; the following comment was typical of others in the report (Age Concern 2000, p. 14):

> Elderly people have the feeling that they are expendable. People are waiting for them to die. We have excellent maternity services, and services for children, psychiatry and drug abuse. Action this and action that! Action for the elderly should be equally good or better. After a long life, it is no less than we deserve. We want to feel loved and valued as we approach the end, not just fit for the scrap heap.

As can be seen, older people do not see themselves as passive recipients of care. However, the old, and particularly those aged over 75 years, are portrayed as a burden on society and a drain on our nation's resources (Birch et al 1999). This group of people is considered to be non-productive and therefore a burden to economically active younger people (Jeffreys 1989). As Stokes (1992) has identified, people are unwilling to accept the reality of ageing as it is commonly associated with physical and mental decline. Today's society is youth oriented: concepts such as energy, creativeness and beauty are valued and considered the sole prerogative of youth.

One solution could be to foster interactions between older and younger members of society, thereby developing a tolerance for the differences between generations and mutual concern. Voluntary organizations that promote foster grandparenting and schemes in schools that enable older people to assist in the classroom as teachers' aides might encourage this. Old age holds out promises as well as challenges. More contact with older

people may help younger people to look beyond the caricature of decrepitude and dependency, instead seeing lifestyles that are free from the anxieties of childcare and the pressure of full-time work.

When negative beliefs are held about older people they often result in a paternalistic welfarization of the old. This view reinforces the beliefs that older people, and particularly the very old, are dependent and require help from the state in order to function (Johnson 1997). Whilst this sort of attitude is being challenged (Birch et al 1999), there is still a belief that an increase in the numbers of older people will pose a crisis in our society. Inevitably, health and social care professionals, as members of society, are affected by such stereotypes.

As a result of these attitudes, older people are often treated as passive consumers of health and social services (Ford 1989, Heath 1993). Sometimes they are provided with disabling help. For example, most older people who sustain a **stroke** will require some form of rehabilitation to ensure that they regain maximum independence. This may take the form of being taught how to regain sitting balance, a technique that is essential in order to regain any degree of mobility. This is a skilled activity. Yet if health and social care workers have not been taught the principles of re-enablement, if older people are discharged before they have made a complete recovery, and if rehabilitation services are not available in the community, then that older person will never reach his or her potential and may even deteriorate further (RCN 1997b).

When we see people as a homogeneous group, we overlook their individual strengths and capabilities. This is as true of older people as it would be of any other group (Ford and McCormack 2000). It is worth noting that there are several generations of older people, all of whom will have had different life experiences. Within each generation there are many individuals, all different from one another. Such concepts of individuality and personal differences are not new, and if incorporated into professional practice result in rewarding practice which locates our interactions between the older person and practitioner in a person-centred way. Such person-centred approaches aim to reduce the depersonalization of older people in care settings, where images of dependency, someone to be moved and fed, abound (Ford and McCormack 2000). Person-centred assessment helps the process of really seeing the person to begin with (RCN 2000b); we will address assessment in some depth later.

Nurses working with older people aim to provide good quality care, but they also know that the reality of achieving this rarely sits comfortably alongside frameworks of patient rights which focus on the ideal – an ideal not always met within systems and buildings that do not afford the level of choices or comfort a person might experience in their own home. Barriers to equity have been discussed, which occur through structures and systems. Nurses have to operate within these structures and

Cerebrovascular accident
See chapter 2.2

may not be able to effect substantial change in them. However, by concentrating on overcoming attitudinal barriers to equity, nurses can effect a change; the concepts of respect, partnership and interdependence are often more helpful than strict adherence to principles of autonomy (British Medical Association/RCN 1995). These concepts build upon knowledge of biological and physiological perspectives of normal ageing, which are examined next.

Normal ageing

The study of **ageing** is a multidisciplinary enterprise. Each discipline and profession brings its own theoretical perspectives and methods. In this chapter it is possible only to introduce the reader to some of these theories; further reading will be recommended at the end of the chapter.

Biological, psychological and sociological theories of ageing tend to focus on different aspects of the ageing process and do not necessarily contradict one another. They make different assumptions and use concepts in different ways, posing different questions and explanations along the way. Perspectives, then, are different. This does not make them right or wrong.

Biological and physiological perspectives

While it is important to distinguish between the changes in an older adult resulting from disease or injury, exactly how we age is not yet clear. However, there are some inconclusive theories. Kyriazis (1994) claims that the theories converge into two main camps:

1. Ageing is caused by factors that damage our body, including radiation, toxic byproducts of the metabolism, random everyday damage and the genes that promote ageing.

2. The damage is not repaired properly; this may be because of a lack of metabolic energy, hormone deficiencies, lack of genetic support, failure of the immune system, and so on.

There is a lack of precise information on normal ageing processes. Much of the research has been cross-sectional (comparing average results of a group of older people with a younger group), so that the differences found in these studies between age groups may have been due, not to age, but to the effects of environment, diet or activities interacting with the groups at different points in time. In some instances it would seem that performance actually increases with age. It has been found that exercise, diet, not smoking and practising intelligence tests have produced changes in the level of fitness, heart reserve, blood pressure, memory and reaction time of some older adults (Fries 1989).

The existing knowledge related to changes with age can serve as general guidelines for care which are aimed at preserving and prolonging function. New knowledge may alter these conceptions of old age. Most older people function well at rest but their functional capacity may be altered under conditions of stress, such as illness, surgery, trauma, physical exercise and emotional stress, which may exceed the body's threshold of physiological reserves resulting in an inability to maintain homeostasis. Older people are also more likely to develop complications and to take longer to recover than younger individuals. Physiological changes may not occur until well after 70 years of age. The older person may continue to engage in all the activities of middle age with perhaps a modification of the pace of life. Table 3.1 displays physical and functional changes that occur with ageing along with key nursing implications.

Ageing **skin** is generally characterized by diminishing function and reserve capacity. Local sensation of heat, pressure and painful stimuli may be less acute. **Wound healing** is slower, and nail and hair growth declines.

Adult **bone loss** (osteoporosis) begins to take place in both sexes around the age of 40 years and is thought to be related to diet, physical activity, hormonal changes and possibly ribonucleic acid (RNA) activity.

The **neurological system** reacts more slowly with increasing age due to vision changes, decreased numbers of axons in the nerves and synapse changes resulting in slow nerve conduction. This may result in slower reflexes, decreased pain sensation and more time being required for problem solving.

There are obviously changes to the special **senses**, of which sight and hearing are the most commonly affected. Communication involves the use of symbols and motor articulation or speech. With ageing, simple reaction time is decreased and learning occurs at a less rapid rate; normal ageing, however, does not account for speech difficulties. This is more likely to be attributed to teeth alignment or breath control. Atrophy of vocal cords affecting pitch may alter speech, but generally it remains functional. There is a decreased sense of taste and smell for some individuals.

In the **cardiopulmonary system**, cardiac output drops due to fibrosis and sclerosis in the endocardium, left ventricular wall thickening and increased fat infiltration in the right atrium and ventricle. The **heart rate** slows with age and cardiovascular stress response is less efficient in the older adult. A decrease in fluids affects the removal of dust and mucus through coughing and sneezing; this predisposes the person to bronchopneumonia. Additionally there is less pulmonary elasticity and capillary action decreases, which leads to less efficiency and contributes to bacterial growth.

The **gastrointestinal system** has such a large reserve capacity that decreases in normal function can occur with little effect on physiological processes. Periodontal disease becomes the major cause of tooth loss and there is less salivary activity. The gag reflex is weaker and the cardiac

Ageing
See chapter 1.3

Skin
See chapter 6.1

Wound healing
See chapter 6.1

Bone
See chapter 3.2

Nervous system
See chapters 2.2 & 2.3

Sense organs
See chapter 2.3

Cardiovascular
See chapter 4.2

Respiratory
See chapter 5.3

Gastrointestinal
See chapter 5.1

Table 3.1   Physical and functional changes related to ageing

Changes	Nursing implications
Skin	
Decreased elasticity	Attention to skin care, nail care, position changes and hygiene
Dryness, scaling of skin	Insulatory effect of clothing
Wound healing retarded; increased vascular fragility	Avoiding exposure to sun and heat
Nails thicken, become brittle and yellow	
Thinning of hair, loss of pigmentation	
Sweat glands atrophy	
Musculoskeletal	
Decreased subcutaneous tissue, muscle mass and strength	Accident prevention and rest
Bone demineralization	Exercise programme
Joints stiffen, lose flexibility	Weight control
	Aids to movement
	Diet high in calcium, vitamin D and protein
Neurological	
Slowed reaction, especially to multiple stimuli (neurone loss)	Slower pacing of activities
Decreased temperature regulation and pain perception	Monitor trauma or illness carefully
Increased time for problem solving	Assess sudden confusional states
Decreased overall sleep time and REM sleep	5–7 hours of night sleep may be sufficient
Sense of balance declines	
Special senses	
Diminished visual activity (presbyopia); increased sensitivity to glare and difficulty adjusting to darkness	Regular vision and hearing tests
Decreased depth perception	Avoid night driving, glare
Diminished hearing activity (presbycousis)	Home safety (lighting, furniture)
Diminished colour perception (especially blue and green)	Communication techniques (auditory, visual and tactile)
Decreased sense of taste and smell	Use of yellows, oranges against contrasting backgrounds
	Use of spices/herbs and low calorie foods
	Smoke detectors
Cardiopulmonary	
Less able to increase heart rate and cardiac output with activity	Regular blood pressure readings
Blood vessels less elastic	Posture, breathing and walking exercise
Venous return less efficient	Avoid prolonged immobility; early ambulation
Peripheral oedema and pooling may occur, especially with immobility	Avoid irritants
Pulmonary elasticity and ciliary action decrease, leading to less efficient gas exchange and slowed cough reflex	Limit salt intake
	Pacing activities
	Attention to prolonged infections
	Vaccinations (pneumococcal and influenza)
Gastrointestinal (including dentition)	
Diminished saliva, digestive juices, and decreased nutrient absorption	Regular diet low in fat and calories, high in fibre and fluids
Delayed oesophageal and gastric emptying	Small, frequent servings more readily digested
Reduced muscle tone and decreased peristalsis	Discourage long-term laxative and other non-prescription drugs
Decreased blood flow to liver lessens drug detoxication	Accessible toilet facilities
Decreased taste buds	Community resources for help with meals
Teeth more brittle, some reabsorption of gum tissue	Dental and oral hygiene
	Regular dental examinations
Genitourinary (including reproductive)	
Decreased blood flow to kidneys	Encourage hydration
Bladder capacity diminishes; reduced glomerular filtration	Minimum daily 1500–2000 mL of fluid
Decrease in bladder size and sphincter control may result in incomplete emptying	Accessible toilet and hygiene facilities
Enlarged prostate, reduced testosterone, slowed erection	Avoid constipation
Atrophy and decreased lubrication of female genital tract; reduced oestrogen	Recognize drug toxicity
	Continence promotion
	Adaptation of sexual practices
Endocrine	
Decreased testosterone	Maintain normal weight
Glucose tolerance deteriorates	Limit use of fat and sugar
Temperature regulation less efficient	

Modified from Gioiella and Bevil (1985) and Taylor et al (1989).

sphincter more relaxed; this predisposes the older person to aspiration difficulties. Less gastric acid and weaker musculature leads to a need for smaller and more frequent amounts of food. Decreased intestinal peristalsis and duller nerve sensations can cause a missed signal for defaecation.

Degeneration of the **renal system** for some leads to a slowing of filtration functions. Bladder capacity decreases from about 500 to 250 mL, resulting in frequency and nocturia. For some, bladder emptying is more difficult because of a weakening of the muscles; this can lead to urine retention. Tissue changes associated with oestrogen deficiency in women result in relaxed pelvic floor muscles. In men, prostate enlargement and atrophy of periurethral structures can occur. These changes may lead to uninhibited bladder contractions (stress incontinence and dribbling).

Age-related changes to the **reproductive system** do not prevent sexual function or alter libido. Research to date has tended to concentrate on three areas: sexual performance or behaviour; changes in sexual responses with age; and sexual problems or dysfunction. It often omits consideration of older people; it is male and heterosexually oriented, and pays little attention to the experiences or feelings of older people. Older people who do not have an active sex life are likely to be lacking a partner or fear the attitudes of society, particularly if they share a sexual relationship with a partner of the same sex.

A loss of **mental function** is not a normal part of the ageing process. There is, however, less capacity for adaptation, especially in stressful or unfamiliar settings, and if the older person has impaired senses. Older people experience a decreased ability to respond to multiple or complex stimuli, so they tend to respond to the stimuli of greatest intensity. If all stimuli are of low intensity then the person may well become disinterested, which is of particular importance for those who live alone or are residing in a home or hospital.

Older people's need for personal expression and mental health support is apparent, with an estimated 650 000 plus people in the UK with some form of dementia, many of whom are older people (Audit Commission 1999), whilst 15% of older people suffer from depression (Brodarty 1993).

Older people continue to learn and problem-solve. Intellectual performance is stable but response time is slower. This results in slower absorption, processing and response to information and environmental cues. Memory is generally stable except where distractions or time pressure is present.

Psychological perspectives

Age-related psychological changes may be associated with internal stressors, such as changes in memory, sleep patterns, hearing and vision, and gastrointestinal metabolism. These and other factors may lead the older adult to feel isolated, frustrated, bored or apathetic. External stressors such as retirement, loss of a partner or friends, and diminished resources can all contribute to a loss of self-worth and independent functioning. Developmental theories seek to explain the diverse growth processes that occur with ageing.

Erikson's theory of development

Erickson's theory or 'eight stages of life' is perhaps the most well known example (Erikson 1964). Erikson is considered one of the precursors of what is known as lifespan developmental psychology (Sugarman 1986). The emphasis on integrity of the lifespan is Erikson's lasting contribution, and one that is vital to the understanding of old age (Bond and Coleman 1994). In order to understand people in late life it is necessary to see them in the context of their whole life history with the challenges of life that may or may not have been resolved at earlier stages. Clearly such an approach has several implications, namely that older people are individuals and as such will vary according to their histories. Such courses of development are likely to diverge as we age, and therefore it is likely that we become even more individual as ageing takes place.

It is likely that development occurs on a number of different fronts. Bond and Coleman (1994) point out that there is no reason to think that intellectual, physical and social development all follow the same pathway.

A third characteristic of the lifespan approach is that the reciprocal influences between the environment and the individual are recognized. This was emphasized by Erikson, who stressed the interdependence of the generations, with the old needing the young and the young needing the old. Such a model of ageing may be too idealistic: the nature of modern society makes it difficult for someone to achieve such positive qualities. Erikson does not offer a well-worked-out theory of adjustment in later life (Bond and Coleman 1994), but he points to key elements that have to be taken into account in any consideration of ageing. He raises the special issues of adjustment which older people must face.

Sociological perspectives

One starting point in analyzing the conditions of older people in society is the influence exerted by scientific theory. As the numbers of older people have increased, they have become more 'visible' and as such have become the subject of much discussion and study. From these studies various theories have emerged about ageing which frequently reflect society's perception and treatment of our older citizens.

Renal system
See chapter 5.4

Reproductive system
See chapter 6.3

Mental function
See chapter 2.2

Socially constructed life course

Concern with old age in our time has tended to focus attention on this stage of life in isolation from the entire life course. Without denying the unique rewards and challenges of this period of life, it is important to interpret it as part of the life course, and with historical context. Hockey and James (1993) contend that the recognition of old age in the twentieth century is part of a larger historical process involving the emergence of new stages of life and their societal recognition.

Disengagement theory

Disengagement theory is generally defined as a triple withdrawal: a loss of roles, a contraction of contact, and a decline in the commitment to norms and values. The theory arose from research in the USA, which was conducted on older people (Cummings and Henry 1961). The theory proposes that, independent of poor health or poverty, ageing involves a gradual decline that inevitably results in a withdrawal from interaction between individuals and society. At the same time disengagement theory suggests that society prepares older people to play fewer active roles, with the result that the ageing person slowly and inevitably withdraws, experiencing deterioration in both the quality and quantity of relationships. However, most of the evidence is ambiguous and little attention has been paid to individual variations. A further difficulty is the implicit value judgement that disengagement is a good thing for society and the individual. Blau (1973, p. 152), an American sociologist, has argued that:

> The disengagement theory deserves to be publicly attacked because it can so easily be used by the non-old, who constitute the 'normals' in society, to avoid confronting and dealing with the issue of the olds' marginality and rolelessness in American society.

Role and activity theory

Harris (1990) suggests that the major role losses associated with old age come with retirement, loss of a partner and institutionalization. Role and activity theory, developed in the 1950s and 1960s, claims that individuals play a variety of roles throughout their lives which offer them social development leading to status and identity.

This view was combined with a sense of concern about older people's abilities to use leisure, leading to the development of activity theory. This is an extension of role theory and emphasizes the importance of maintaining a range of activities. This has led to the development of pre-retirement courses and studies on the meaning of work and retirement conducted by Havighurst (1963).

Continuity theory

Developed by Atchley (1980), this theory proposes that adaptation to ageing can proceed in several directions depending on the individual's past life. Personality and adjustment to stress remain stable over the lifespan. This theory has gained support as it accounts for factors in other theories and considers individual variation.

Exchange theory

Disengagement, role and activity theories all focus on discontinuity from one phase of life to another. Exchange theory focuses on discontinuity in terms of a loss of power. Markides and Cooper (1987) argue that, implicit within this theory, is the importance of reciprocity: the ability to return favours or rewards so that the bargaining position of social relationships is maintained. The theory is based on the assumption that much social interaction may be reduced to rewards and cost. The concept of reciprocity in relationships and society in general is basic to survival, and for Ebersole and Hess (1990) the ability of older people to survive is dependent on their ability to 'barter in the market place of human relationships' in an environment of 'generational equity'. In other words, unequal patterns of exchange create dependency. Interdependence is based on concepts of time, equity, caring and sharing; in old age an increasing amount of dependency may occur. It is therefore important to maintain a strong position of reciprocity in order to avoid the erosion of self-esteem.

Essentially this is a theory about power and status, and is therefore particularly useful for nurses as it suggests that steps to correct loss of power in older people may be an important element in any therapeutic regimen. It is clearly relevant, particularly in rehabilitation and longer-term care, in which nurses are key providers. This theory relates directly to interdependence, the opportunity for giving as well as receiving.

Political economy theory

Fennell et al (1988) suggested that in the UK and the USA the process of ageing needs to be viewed in the context of advanced capitalist societies, because the way in which resources are allocated is central to the status and experience of older people. Social gerontology has become highly political, linking the political economy to a moral economy approach which questions how ideas of fairness and human values influence policy. Taking this view one can see the importance for nurses to maintain links to national policies, so that they can influence decisions that impact on older people as they are developed.

Political economy theory focuses on the structural changes and processes that affect older people. Many themes have been developed, in particular through the works of Townsend (1979, 1981), Estes (1979), and Phillipson and Walker (1986). The theory was first developed after the public spending crisis of the mid-1970s, which led to cuts in public expenditure. Much of the money had previously been targeted at older people; they subsequently were viewed as an economic burden and the subject for political attack. Political economy theory is actually a study of the interactions between government, the economy and those groups of people who may be defined socially as 'the poor' or 'the old'. Older people came to be viewed as an intolerable burden on Western economies, with demographic changes seen as causing intolerable pressure on public spending.

In this theory, it is argued that dependency in old age is not the inevitable outcome of ageing but rather the result of social structuring. The state plays a large part in this in that it determines the events of later life that create dependence, poverty or isolation (Townsend 1981). Little attention has been paid previously to the structural relationship between older people and the rest of society and the differential impact of social and economical institutions upon older people. Implicit within this theory is that ageing is a social rather than a biologically created status.

At the start of this section it was pointed out that no one theory provides all the answers, and no single theory is right or wrong. Rather they serve to guide thinking and in this way encourage nurses to explore the relationships between theory, policy and practice. A particular challenge for nurses is the development of their relationship with older people, from a basis of genuine mutual respect and valuing or reciprocity, where each gains from the other. A key factor in this relationship will be the assessment undertaken by the nurse but which, in fact, is likely to be a two-way process in which the older person will also be assessing the nurse – albeit less overtly. In this way the nurse–user relationship should seek to establish equality, with both parties bringing skills and information that are different but of equal standing.

Assessment

Assessment is a complex activity, requiring skill in its execution (Ford and McCormack 1999, Lewis et al 1999, Heath 2000). It is a multidisciplinary process which can initiate person-centred care (Kitwood 1997, Ford and McCormack 2000, RCN 2000a). The methods used to engage older people in the assessment process will call upon story telling and the use of biography (Schofield 1994, RCN 2000b). The practitioner may use a tool to guide the assessment, whilst mindful of the need always to record the individual person's needs as viewed by them. Consequently the selection of any tool intended to provide a framework for assessment should consider the following questions (Wills and Ford 2001):

- Does the tool facilitate a holistic view of the individual, which considers individual needs, wants and aspirations? Does the tool account for ethnicity and cultural context?

- Does the tool utilize biography as an essential component of assessment?

- Does the tool call for skilled application?

- Is the tool valid and reliable?

- Can the tool be completed in a reasonable time frame: does it have a practical application within the resources that exist?

- Does the tool have a common language?

- Does the tool indicate the level of input needed, i.e. personal or nursing care?

- Does the tool account for changes over time, lending itself to the fact that assessment is a continuous process?

- Does the tool maintain a focus on the individual with room for the older person's own involvement, as opposed to the professional's needs?

- Is the tool part of the multidisciplinary assessment?

Facilitation of the assessment process for older people includes the ability to respond to any sensory needs and to monitor and respond to changes as they occur (Heath 2000). Assessment provides information that is critical to the development of a plan of action that can enhance personal health status, decrease the potential for or the severity of chronic conditions, and assist the individual in gaining control over health through self-care (RCN 1997a, 2000c). In recent years the focus on assessment has intensified (Editorial 2000) as it is the gateway to continuing care and re-enablement services for many older people. The political climate, with its emphasis on eligibility criteria and the funding of nursing care, has highlighted the importance of assessment for several reasons.

The shortcomings of current approaches to assessment have been widely reported:

1. Assessment does not have an unambiguous meaning (Ford and McCormack 1999).

2. Assessment may have an underlying fiscal drive (Royal Commission 1999).

3. Assessments are disparate, with many different practitioners, organizations and health authorities using a variety of different tools, which cannot easily be compared with one another (Lewis et al 1999, Stewart et al 1999).

4. Assessments are of varying quality (Stewart et al 1999).

5. Assessments may be undertaken by practitioners without the appropriate expertise to carry them out (Ford and McCormack 1999).

6. Assessments may use formats that lose the older person's biography and individuality, thereby losing some of the richness and detail that makes the assessment a true representation of the older person (Ford and McCormack 1999, Royal Commission 1999, RCN 2000b).

There is considerable debate over which tools are best, and whether or not there should be a move towards greater standardization of assessment tools (Ford and McCormack 1999). The development of an integrated service provision, which delivers a comprehensive service to older people, is achievable through the adoption of a standardized approach to assessment. It has been advocated that there is a need to distinguish between standardized assessments and a standardized approach to assessment (RCN 2000d). The use of one standardized assessment tool and one protocol to assess all older people may overlook the individuality of the older person. However, a standardized approach to assessment adopts a common approach to assessment through specific domains that may make use of standardized tools. Such an approach should utilize assessment tools that foster a re-enablement approach. For example, the RCN assessment tool (RCN 1997a, Ford and McCormack 1999) for nursing older people has been developed by expert gerontological nurses to identify the areas where nursing is needed and provide evidence for the prescribed level of registered nurse intervention. The assessment tool aims to promote a re-enablement model of care, which maximizes the potential of the individual by building upon the abilities needed to achieve those things they consider to be important to them (RCN 1997b).

When selecting a tool to guide the assessment process the nurse needs to consider the importance of the individual's biography, with the emphasis on the older person's potential to achieve desired, realistic health choices. This maximizing of potential is one of the aims of the assessment: to determine the person's needs, wants and aspirations, and to plan healthcare interventions in accordance with these and in partnership with the older person. Assessment for older people often involves members of the multidisciplinary team, which means that all the healthcare and social services professionals should be mindful of the need to maximize the sharing of information and the avoidance of duplication.

The initiation of the nursing assessment marks the beginning of a relationship between the nurse and older person. The interview that follows requires skill in establishing trust and confidence. A considerable amount of time is required to undertake a comprehensive health assessment. It requires specific skills of the nurse such as the ability to listen patiently, to allow for pauses, to ask questions that are not often asked, to obtain information from all the available sources and to recognize normalities of late life that would be abnormal in those who are younger. The quality and speed of the assessment is an art that is born of both experience and a genuine valuing of older people in this way.

Maximizing the potential of the older person through the process of assessment, the RCN (1997b, 2000b) calls for the skilled nurse to focus on independence and ability, as opposed to dependence. The rehabilitation of older people is not a short-term intervention usually associated with acute hospitals, but a process with potential in continuing care settings (Nocon and Baldwin 1998, RCN 2000c). The RCN views this extension of the traditional view of rehabilitation (Warren 1981) as re-enablement, helping people to adapt to changes in their life circumstances. It is a shared activity between the person affected, other people close to them and multiprofessional teams. It means recognizing that older people are experts on themselves and that professionals provide expertise in their own field. Re-enablement must have a therapeutic value for the person concerned, with the ultimate aim of maximizing their social well-being. It is not time limited with set outcomes, but may cover the lifespan of the individual; its goals are person centred, selected and set in partnership with the older person (RCN 1997a,b).

Such a philosophy promotes assessment that accesses various models of care and that could take place in a variety of settings: the older person's home, the community hospital, the nursing or residential home, or acute hospital. The family and others close to the older person may naturally have key involvement, which poses a challenge in the balancing of different perspectives. Re-enablement ways of working also offer the community in which the older person lives (whether in their own home or in more formal care) the opportunity to be involved.

Assessment and Jacob Brown

Let us return to Jacob Brown, to explore how some of the principles that relate to assessment might apply to him (see Case Study 3.3).

Case Study 3.3   Assessment and Jacob Brown

Unexpectedly one night Jacob awoke, breathless and uncomfortable. When he tried to get out of bed he felt weak. He didn't want to bother the doctor, so he stayed in bed waiting for his nephew, Colin, to pop in, as he usually did. Jacob had forgotten that Colin and the family had gone away for a long weekend. By Sunday, he was very poorly, in pain, had a sore bottom and **swollen legs**, and hadn't eaten since Thursday night, although he had sipped squash. He managed to look for help and appeared, dishevelled and seemingly incontinent of urine, in the pub next door. The landlord called an ambulance, which took Jacob to casualty. Jacob wasn't making much sense at that point. He was muddling up his words and saying that he needed to get back to work and check that the building was secure.

It can be seen how Jacob's usual independent self may be lost, as his present physical condition and confusional

Oedema
See chapter 4.2

Box 3.1 Elements of Jacob's assessment and biography (adapted from Johns 1991)

- How does Jacob deal with his admission, discomfort and distress? How can his individual reaction be supported?

- What physical needs does Jacob have (breathlessness, nutrition and hydration, skin integrity)?

- What were Jacob's previous abilities and how do they match with his present abilities?

- Which people support and interact with Jacob when he is at home? How might they be a part of his recovery?

- How can Jacob be helped and supported by the nurses and the rest of the multidisciplinary team?

- How does Jacob view the future for himself and others in his life?

state take precedent in the accident and emergency department. It is important that his physical condition is treated, so that he is hydrated, and the cause of his breathlessness and discomfort discovered, but it is also important that the nurse assesses Jacob's previous lifestyle, ability and needs, so that the goals of his recovery may be matched to his desire for independence. In Box 3.1 we consider which elements of Jacob's needs might be included in an assessment, as he is admitted to hospital.

A profession equipped to support and work with older people

In the discussion about assessment it becomes apparent that the professionals working with older people need to be knowledgeable doers (Benner 1984). Reports from the UKCC (1997) on the continuing care of older people and from Age Concern (1998) regarding training and qualifications for work with older people recommend a concentrated effort to formalize and expand the qualifications of those working with this group. Heath and Ford (1999) have explored this further, describing their vision for a gerontological nurse specialist, a band of expert, skilled and knowledgeable gerontological nurses who transcend care boundaries, moving in and out of the care location anticipating and responding to need. Such nurses could be employed in any setting; what will matter is that they are able to practise at an advanced level in an autonomous way. These practitioners would continue to promote the use of evidence in the planning and implementation of practice.

Ford and McCormack (1998) do not believe that older people have more or fewer needs depending on whether they are in an acute ward, a nursing home or in their own home, and do not believe that a nurse needs more or less knowledge and skills to work in an acute ward, nursing home or the community. The establishment of gerontological nurse specialist roles, as case managers or coordinators of care services, is an achievable option for the future (RCN/BGS 2001). If a total systems approach to services for older people is to be adopted, then roles such as these, which transcend existing organizational boundaries, would appear to be essential. It seems unlikely that we will ever achieve a state where organizational boundaries do not exist; therefore, establishing roles that help older people to cross the boundaries safely and securely seems an important way forward. Some gerontological nurse specialist posts have recently been initiated in line with such a policy. How could such roles impact on the care of Jacob Brown? (See Case Study 3.4.)

Case Study 3.4　*Jacob Brown and the gerontological nurse specialist*

Whilst on the re-enablement ward for older people, Jacob met Natalie Smith, the gerontological nurse specialist, again. He knew her from the last time he had been in the hospital after his fall. She remembered him and was sorry to find him in hospital again. She knew he had moved to the flat last year, as she had visited his home. She explained to Jacob and Colin, his nephew, that Jacob had a chest infection and some heart failure. The doctor had talked to him already, so there had been time for him to think of some questions. The nurse spent lots of time talking about medication and looking after himself. She helped him plan his discharge with the nurses on the ward. Jacob had given himself and Colin a scare, so he decided to stay in the residential home until he had fully recovered, and then go home.

Natalie Smith has arranged for Bill Taylor to come in and visit him from the home today. She just popped in there to talk to the staff about Jacob's needs and sorted it out. Jacob still feels a bit washed out but he's on the road to recovery, so seeing Bill will be nice.

The post of gerontological nurse specialist, as it has been described (Ford and McCormack 1998, Heath and Ford 1999), would take a broad view of the older person's needs. This view would promote health and wellness, discussed below.

Health promotion and wellness

Kalache et al (1988) argue that the development of priorities and practices for health promotion for a nation are dependent upon the prevailing economic and cultural conditions. There are some fundamental requirements for the health of any individual, such as income, shelter and food. These need to form the basic foundation. Without them, they argue, improvement in health is merely an abstraction. Complementary requisites are: information and knowledge about health factors, skills to promote health, supportive environments that enhance health, and the opportunity for healthier choices.

It has been suggested that healthy lifestyles for older people should encompass 'self responsibility for health, nutrition, exercise, **stress** management, interpersonal relationships/support, spiritual growth and self actualization, accident and injury prevention, safe/moderate use of medications and alcohol, smoking avoidance, self care regimes for chronic illnesses and accessing preventative health services' (Burnard and Phillipson 1991, p. 320). Balanced against this view, however, is the reality of poor housing, low income and an extensive range of social difficulties that many older people face.

The importance of health promotion is reflected by the development of Health Action Zones and Health Improvement Programmes (RCN 2000e), which aim to improve the health of communities. A whole-systems approach is suggested; this has the potential to enhance the care that is already taking place, and plan future partnerships that make the most of the available skills and resources. Joint training for all disciplines, across agencies, could raise awareness for many practitioners about the potential for joint working and the sharing of case notes and information, offering opportunities to build relationships and knowledge about one another's services, with the potential benefit of more fluid referrals between agencies for older people. Working in this way could reduce the number of practitioners an older person sees, thereby avoiding duplication of effort, whilst building more meaningful relationships for the older person.

A total population approach to the organization of services for older people recognizes that those in care homes or in receipt of long-term care services are a part of the healthcare population. Currently, people in care homes do not account for a natural component of that population, other than in considerations of medical support to care homes. A total population approach would utilize Health Improvement Plans as the basis for decision making and would recognize the care needs of older people in care homes as part of that population. Resources would be allocated according to care need, rather than location of care delivery, using the total population approach. This reinforces the need for a standard approach to assessment. This changing focus on healthy communities aims to keep older people healthier for longer.

The postponement of chronic illness is something in which we all have interest. Fit and healthy older people not only enjoy a better individual quality of life, but have the resources to continue to participate in society.

Screening and health promotion for older people has been brought to the fore by recent government publications.

The White Paper on community care (DoH 1989) lists the promotion of healthy lifestyles through education and effective health surveillance and screening as its first priority for older people and for those with a disability. Screening should be based on guidelines (RCN 1990). The RCN (1990, p. 2) chose to define screening and assessment as follows:

> Screening can be defined as the process of identifying unrecognised disease or illness by application of tests, examinations and other procedures. Screening tests differentiate between apparently well people who may have a problem from those who do not. Screening is a component of the assessment process and is not in itself a means of assisting individuals to improve and maintain their health.

Health assessments give an opportunity to do more than just identify problems. Other forms of preventive activity (both medical and social) can take place. There is, for example, evidence to suggest that both breast screening and **cervical cytology** are beneficial in old age (DHSS 1986).

Health assessments provide nurses with opportunities for health promotion in general and can include subjects such as exercise, smoking, prevention of accidents, preservation of autonomy, social contact and self-care. Information can also be given regarding services and resources available in the locality.

A number of preventive practices have been found to yield important benefits for older people, and have been summarized well by Gambert and Gupta (1989). Health education programmes are shifting from a focus on disease-specific conditions and individual responsibility to developing comprehensive health promotion programmes. Such programmes are aimed at the prevention of illness and injury, and the understanding of the determinants of health, such as socioenvironmental factors. More research studies, particularly longitudinal ones that evaluate the effectiveness of various programmes, are required.

Older people who wish to manage their own health may choose to do this through the use of complementary therapies. Many of the complementary therapies involve touch, and offer the older person 30–45 minutes per session in which they can discuss their health needs as they receive treatment. This may be one of the potential advantages of these therapies, although they are not currently widely available as part of NHS provision and therefore a cost may sometimes be attached to such an option. Studies are emerging that support the use of complementary therapies, such as aromatherapy, reflexology and Reiki (a form of hands-on healing) in NHS and other care settings (Taylor 1995, Hudson 1996, Brett 1999). More research is required to see how older people might benefit from these therapies in a variety of settings and situations.

For the nurse involved in health screening programmes that include people aged over 75, certain criteria must

Stress
See chapter 2.7

Cervical cancer
See chapter 7.3

be met to ensure competence. In order to carry out such screening the nurses should therefore:

- understand the normal ageing process

- have knowledge of the social and health resources available to older people within the locality

- understand the principles of anticipatory care

- demonstrate an ability to put anticipatory care needs into practice

- recognize the need for and understand the principles of re-enablement

- undertake effective assessment procedures, particularly the assessment of ability and disability

- understand the purpose of a health check

- recognize and utilize the opportunities for health promotion

- be able to apply knowledge and expertise relating to the medical, nursing and social needs associated with old age

- have the skills pertaining to visiting older people at home, including effective communication skills

- demonstrate positive values and beliefs about older people and their needs.

The value of screening programmes for older people continues to be a subject of considerable contention (McGarry and Arthur 1999). If health checks and health promotion can help older people to achieve greater independence, then whatever the controversy regarding the 'medical' benefits of health promotion, there is likely to be a greater recognition of the rights of older people to access health screening and assessments. A case can be made for the value of paying more attention to older people's health by arguing for the broadening of the model of screening to incorporate a true health promotion approach. Nurses are in a key position to do this and as such have the potential to help older people remain active and independent for as long as possible and thereby lessen the crisis-driven, reactive, short-term approach to our ageing population.

Summary

In this chapter the demographic picture has been examined in relation to older people; this has been related to current policy with an exploration of possible future care provision. Mr Jacob Brown provided an insight into issues of equity for older people, as he travelled on a care pathway that highlighted the importance of assessment and concluded with his discharge into the care of an expert nurse. Normal ageing was reviewed from a biological, physiological, psychological and sociological perspective, and the need to maintain health promotion and wellness as perspectives in the support of older people was discussed.

Innovative new ways of working with older people were explored, and the gerontological nurse role was introduced.

As illustrated, ageing is a process of continued development and adaptation. It is now recognized that those who survive beyond 65 years are a highly diversified group, most of whom remain well and function independently until only a short time before death. Stereotypes about older people persist and frequently lead to efforts to prevent older people from reaching their full potential. Fortunately there is a growing body of knowledge about ageing, which is challenging such negative stereotypes. This increased social awareness and greater participation by older people themselves has helped to improve equity and access to services. However, for the momentum to be maintained, it is necessary for older people to use their 'vote' judiciously. Health and social care professionals should endeavour to work in partnership with older people. This will assist the process of information exchange which, in turn, should empower the older individual. There is nothing disloyal about giving older patients the facts, as with the facts they can act on their own behalf.

The future for nurses working with older people is bright, as some of the most well known innovations in nursing have been developed in services for older people (Heath and Schofield 1999). Nurses working with older people will continue to require a range of complex skills and knowledge, but these must be shared with colleagues as services for older people are increasingly provided within the community. The potential exists for the gerontological nurse specialist role to expand our knowledge about the creative ways we might develop further partnerships with older people. Policy developments look set to change the frameworks in which we support and care for older people. There is an increasing and exciting future for nurses who choose to learn the special skills and values of nurses' work with older people.

References

Acheson D (1998) Independent inquiry into inequalities in health. London: DoH.

Age Concern (1998) Training and qualifications for work with older people. London: Age Concern.

Age Concern (2000) Turning your back on us older people and the NHS. London: Age Concern.

Askham J, Barry C, Grundy E, Hancock R, Tinker A (1992) Life after 60: a profile of Britain's older population. London: Age Concern Institute of Gerontology, King's College London.

Atchley R (1980) Social forces in later life. Belmont, CA: Wadsworth.

Audit Commission (1997) The coming of age. Improving care services for older people. London: Audit Commission.

Audit Commission (1999) Forget me not: mental health services for older people. London: Audit Commission.

Audit Commission (2000) The way to go home: rehabilitation and remedial services for older people. London: Audit Commission.

Benner P (1984) From novice to expert. New York: Addison Wesley.

Birch R, Hancock R, LeGrys D, Roberts R (1999) Paying for age in the 21st century. The millennium papers. London: Age Concern.

Blau Z (1973) Old age in a changing society. New York: New Viewpoints.

Bond J, Coleman P (1994) Introduction to social gerontology, 2nd edn. London: Sage.

Brett H (1999) Aromatherapy in the care of older people. Nursing Times 95(33): 5–6.

British Medical Association/Royal College of Nursing (1995) The older person: consent to care. London: BMA/RCN.

Brodarty H (1993) Think of depression, atypical presentations in the elderly. Australian Family Physician 22(7): 1195–1203.

Burnard M, Phillipson C (1991) Self care and health in old age. In: Redfern S, ed. Nursing elderly people, pp. 316–327. Edinburgh: Churchill Livingstone.

Challis D (1999) Assessment and care management: developments since the community care. In: Royal Commission on long-term care, community care and informal care. Research volume 3. London: The Stationery Office.

Cummings E, Henry W (1961) Growing old. New York: Basic Books.

Department of Health (1989) Caring for community care in the next decade and beyond, Cmnd 849. London: HMSO.

Department of Health (1990) NHS and Community Care Act. London: HMSO.

Department of Health (1995) NHS responsibilities for meeting continuing healthcare needs. HSG(95)8. London: HMSO.

Department of Health/Social Services Inspectorate (1995) Carer's Recognition and Services Act. London: HMSO.

Department of Health (1998) Partnership in action (new opportunities in joint working between health and social services). London: HMSO.

Department of Health (1999a) Fit for the future? National required standards for residential and nursing homes for older people. Consultation document. Modernising social services. London: HMSO.

Department of Health (1999b) HSC 1999/180 EX parte Coughlan; follow up action. London: HMSO.

Department of Health (2000a) The NHS plan. A plan for investment. A plan for reform. London: The Stationery Office.

Department of Health (2000b) Shaping the future of the NHS; long term planning for hospitals and related services. Consultation document on the findings of the National Beds Inquiry. London: Department of Health.

Department of Health (2001) National service framework for older people. Modern standards and service models. London: HMSO.

Department of Health and Social Security (1986) Community care: agenda for action. London: HMSO.

Dudley N, Burns E (1992) The influence of age on policies for admission and thrombolysis in coronary care units in the UK. Age and Ageing 21: 95–98.

Ebersole P, Hess P (1990) Towards healthy ageing, 3rd edn. St Louis: CV Mosby.

Editorial (2000) Long term care; social care or health care? British Medical Journal 320: 5–6.

Erikson E (1964) Child and society. New York: Norton.

Estes C (1979) The ageing enterprise. San Francisco: Jossy Bass.

Evandrou M (1992) Changing the invisibility of carers; mapping informal care nationally. In: Laczko F, Victors C, eds. Social policy and older people, pp. 142–158. Aldershot, UK: Avebury.

Falkingham J (1997) Who are the baby boomers? A demographic profile. In: Erandou M, ed. Baby boomers ageing in the 21st century, pp. 16–22. London: Age Concern.

Ford P, McCormack B (1998) Gerontological nurses specialist conference paper. Third European Nursing Older People Conference, Harrogate, UK, 1998. Ludlow: Lang & Bussion.

Ford P, McCormack B (1999) Determining older people's need for registered nursing and continuing health care: the contribution of the Royal College of Nursing's assessment tool. Journal of Clinical Nursing 8: 731–742.

Ford P, McCormack B (2000) Keeping the person in the centre of nursing. Nursing Standard 14(46): 40–44.

Ford P (1989) Reactions to Griffiths (implications for care of the elderly). Nursing Standard 29: 19–20.

Fries J (1989) Ageing well: a guide for successful seniors. Reading: Addison Wesley.

Gambert S, Gupta K (1989) Preventive care: what it's worth in geriatrics. Geriatrics 44: 61.

Gioiella EC, Bevil CW (1985) Nursing care of the aging client: promoting healthy adaptation. Norwalk, CT: Appleton Century Crofts.

Grimley Evans J (1997) Rationing health care by age. The case against. British Medical Journal 314: 822–825.

Grundy E (1994) Live old, live well. MRC News 64: 22.

Harris D (1990) Sociology of ageing, 2nd edn. New York: Harper & Row.

Haskey J (1995) Trends in marriage and cohabitation: the decline in marriage and the changing patterns of living in partnerships. Population Trends 80: 5–15.

Havighurst F (1963) Successful ageing. In: Williams R, Tibbitts C, Donahue W, eds. Processes of ageing, pp. 88–112. New York: Atherton.

Health Advisory Service (2000) Not because they are old; an independent inquiry into the care of older people on acute wards in general hospitals. London: HAS.

Heath H (1993) Ageism: spell out the facts. Elderly Care 5(3): 34.

Heath H (2000) Assessing older people. Elderly Care 11(10): 27.

Heath H, Ford P (1999) The development of nursing with older people. In: Heath H, Schofield I, eds. Healthy ageing; nursing older people, pp. 516–517. London: Mosby.

Heath H, Schofield I, eds (1999) Healthy ageing; nursing older people. London: Mosby.

Help the Aged (1997) A life worth living. The independence and inclusion of older people. London: Help the Aged.

Henwood M (1999) The future health and care of older people: the best is yet to come. The millennium papers. Debate of the age. London: Age Concern.

Hockey J, James A (1993) Growing up and growing old. Ageing and dependency in the life course. London: Sage.

Hudson R (1996) The value of lavender for rest and activity in the elderly patient. Complementary Therapies in Medicine 4: 52–57.

Jeffreys M (1989) Growing old in the twentieth century. London: Routledge.

Johns C (1991) The Burford nursing development model of nursing practice. Journal of Advanced Nursing 16: 1090–1098.

Johnson M (1997) The meaning of older age. In: Norman I, Redfern S, eds. Mental health care for elderly people, pp. 308–314. Edinburgh: Churchill Livingstone.

Jones H (1994) Health and society in twentieth century Britain. London: Longman.

Kalache A, Warnes A, Hunter D (1988) Promoting health among elderly people: a statement from a working group. London: King Edward's Hospital Fund for London.

Kinsella K (1996) Demographic aspects. In: Ebrahim S, Kalache A, eds. Epidemiology in old age. London: British Medical Journal/World Health Organization.

Kitwood T (1997) Dementia reconsidered – the person comes first. Buckingham: Open University Press.

Kyriazis M (1994) Age and reason; theory of ageing, ageing mechanisms. Nursing Times 90(18): 60–62.

Lewis H, Wistow G, Arbott S, Cotterill L (1999) Continuing health care; the local development of policies and eligibility criteria. Health and Social Care in the Community 7(6): 455–463.

Mallick N (1994) End stage renal failure. In: Tunbridge M, ed. Rationing in health care in medicine, pp. 14–20. London: Royal College of Physicians.

Markides K, Cooper C (1987) Ageing and ethnicity. California: Sage.

McGarry J, Arthur A (1999) Can over-75 health checks identify unmet need? Nursing Standard 13(33): 37–42.

Moore J, Tilson B, Whitting G (1994) An international overview of employment policies and practices towards older workers. Research series no. 29. London: Department of Employment.

NHS Executive (2000) Advocacy: a code of practice. Mental Health Task Force User Group. London: DoH.

Nocon A, Baldwin S (1998) Trends in the rehabilitation policy. A review of the literature. London: King's Fund.

Office of Population Censuses and Surveys (1996) Living in Britain: results for the 1994 General Household Survey. London: HMSO.

Phillipson C (1997) Employment and training: planning for 2020 and beyond. In: Erandou M, ed. Baby boomers ageing in the 21st century, pp. 41–42. London: Age Concern.

Phillipson C, Walker A (1986) Ageing and social policy, a critical assessment. London: Gower.

Ranade W (1993) A future for the NHS? Care in the 1990s. London: Longman.

Royal College of Nursing (1990) Guidelines for assessment of elderly people. London: RCN.

Royal College of Nursing (1997a) Assessment tool for nursing older people. London: RCN.

Royal College of Nursing (1997b) Nursing homes, nursing values. London: RCN.

Royal College of Nursing (2000a) Rationing by stealth. A review of the legality of health authorities' continuing care policies in England and Wales. London: RCN.

Royal College of Nursing (2000b) Nursing assessment with older people: a person centred approach. Oxford: RCN Institute.

Royal College of Nursing (2000c) Rehabilitating older people. The role of the nurse. London: RCN.

Royal College of Nursing (2000d) Internal briefing paper prepared by P Ford and B McCormack. London: RCN.

Royal College of Nursing (2000e) Internal paper. Recommendations for NHS modernisation plan, with regard to the needs of older people. Gerontological nursing programme. London: RCN.

Royal College of Nursing and the British Geriatrics Society (2001) Older people's specialist nurse, a joint statement by the RCN and BGS. London: BGS/RCN.

Royal Commission on Long Term Care (1999) With respect to old age. London: HMSO.

Russel L (1999) The future of the built environment. The millennium papers. Debate of the age. London: Age Concern.

Scales J, Phal R (1999) Future work and life styles. The millennium papers. Debate of the age. London: Age Concern.

Schofield I (1994) An historical approach to care. Elderly Care 6(6): 14–15.

Stewart K, Challis D, Carpenter I, Dickinson E (1999) Assessment approaches for older people receiving social care; content and coverage. International Journal of Geriatric Psychiatry 14: 147–156.

Stokes G (1992) On being old; the psychology of later life. London: Falmer Press.

Sugarman L (1986) Life span development: concepts, theories and interventions. London: Methuen.

Taylor A (1995) Back in touch. Nursing Times 91(26): 18.

Taylor C, Lillis C, Lemone P (1989) The fundamentals of nursing: the art and science of nursing care. Philadelphia: JB Lippincott.

Tinker A (1984) The elderly in modern society. London: Longman Press.

Townsend P (1979) Poverty in the United Kingdom: a survey of household resources and standards of living. Harmondsworth, UK: Penguin.

Townsend P (1981) The structured dependency of the elderly: creation of social policy in the twentieth century. Ageing and Society 1: 5.

UKCC (1997) The continuing care of older people. UKCC Policy Paper 1. London: UKCC.

Warren MD (1981) The need for rehabilitation. In: Mattingley S, ed. Rehabilitation today in Great Britain, 2nd edn. London: Update Books.

Warner M, Longley M, Gould E, Picek A (1999) Healthcare futures 2010. Welsh Institute for Health and Social Care. London: UKCC.

Williams A (1997) Rationing health care by age, the case for it. British Medical Journal 314: 820–822.

Wills T, Ford P (2001) Assessing older people – contemporary issues for nursing. Nursing Older People 12(9): 16–20.

Yates A (1998) Social responsibility; an issue of age. In: Marr J, Kershaw B, eds. Caring for older people. Developing specialist practice, pp. 222–234. London: Arnold.

Yurick A, Spier B, Ebert N (1988) The aged person and the nursing process, 3rd edn. Norwalk, CT: Appleton & Lange.

Further Reading

For further information about the sociological changes that have occurred and have impacted on older people, including the older person's voice:

Evandrou M, ed. (1997) Baby boomers, ageing in the 21st century. London: Age Concern.

Hareven T (1995) Changing images of aging and the social construction of the life course. In: Images of ageing, pp. 119–134. London: Sage.

Johnson J, Slater R, eds (1993) Ageing and later life. London: Sage.

Phillipson C (1998) Reconstructing old age. New agendas in social theory and practice. London: Sage.

For recent policy developments for older people:

Department of Health (2001) National service framework for older people. Modern standards and service models. London: HMSO.

For an extensive background to person-centred ways of working with and assessing older people:

Heath H, Schofield I (1999) Healthy ageing, nursing older people. London: Mosby.

Royal College of Nursing (2000) Nursing assessment with older people: a person centred approach. Oxford: RCN Institute.

Wills T, Ford P (2001) Assessing older people – contemporary issues for nursing. Nursing Older People 12(9): 16–20.

For further information about normal ageing:

Audit Commission (1999) Forget me not: mental health services for older people. London: Audit Commission.

Bond J, Coleman P (1994) Introduction to social gerontology, 2nd edn. London: Sage.

Cummings E, Henry W (1961) Growing old. New York: Basic Books.

Ebersole P, Hess P (1990) Towards healthy ageing, 3rd edn. St Louis: CV Mosby.

Erikson E (1964) Child and society. New York: Norton.

Estes C (1979) The ageing enterprise. San Francisco, CA: Jossy Bass.

Fennell G, Phillipson C, Evers H (1988) The sociology of old age. Milton Keynes: Open University Press.

Gioiella EC, Bevil CW (1985) Nursing care of the aging client: promoting healthy adaptation. Norwalk, CT: Appleton Century Crofts.

Hockey J, James A (1993) Growing up and growing old. Ageing and dependency in the life course. London: Sage.

Kyriazis M (1994) Age and reason, theory of ageing, ageing mechanisms. Nursing Times 90(18): 60–62.

Markides K, Cooper C (1987) Ageing and ethnicity. Thousand Oaks, CA: Sage.

Phillipson C, Walker A (1986) Ageing and social policy, a critical assessment. London: Gower.

Sugarman L (1986) Life span development, concepts, theories and interventions. London: Methuen.

Townsend P (1979) Poverty in the United Kingdom, a survey of household resources and standards of living. Harmondsworth: Penguin.

Townsend P (1981) The structured dependency of the elderly: creation of social policy in the twentieth century. Ageing and Society 1: 5.

Williams R, Tibbitts C, Donahue W, eds (1963) Processes of ageing. New York: Atherton.

4

Death, grief and loss

Bob Wright

Introduction

Normal grieving

Anticipatory grieving

Sudden death

Viewing the body

Absent at the time of death

Breaking bad news

Responding to altered body image

Summary

Introduction

The feelings and thoughts connected with loss, grief, dying and death have always concerned people. The questions raised by life and death, and attachments and loss, have resulted in countless books, poems and songs. The expression of grief is a universal response by which people adapt to a significant loss – the loss of something that was theirs, a valued possession that had special meaning.

There are several types of loss. The most traumatic loss is that of a significant person (that is, with whom an individual had an important relationship, one that had special meaning) through death, separation, divorce or distance. Another type of loss arises from a change in a significant relationship.

Grief can also result from loss of a pet – through disappearance, separation or death – and loss of objects due to burglary or fire. Objects can be replaced but the feelings attached to them cannot. Objects have sentimental value because they are associated with a particular moment in time. People can experience loss when they move house, too – the loss of leaving a place that is familiar and the scene of special memories. People grieve if they lose part of their bodies, such as a limb, organ or their sight. The image that people have of themselves is linked with their appearance and the way the world sees them. They connect their

attractiveness with the measure of their worth and how lovable they are. Any loss of function can lead to a loss of their role as, for example, wage earner, father or mother, wife or husband.

Another kind of loss is that associated with human development and life's milestones. This can include loss of opportunity to be a mother or, in elderly people, loss of strength or physical well-being.

Previous experiences of loss may provide people with the ability to cope with a new loss. This means that what is a loss to one person may not be a loss to another. Emotional and physical well-being also give people greater resources to handle losses. Nurses meet people who have limited emotional and physical resources for handling their loss. Misuse of drugs or alcohol, and the inability to rest or sleep, all interfere with what is regarded as the 'normal' grieving process. Family attitudes to loss, and different cultural, ethnic and religious backgrounds, also influence the way people deal with loss or death.

Although most people would view loss through death as the most significant loss, this chapter looks at all areas of loss and grief. Nurses spend a lot of time helping clients come to terms with many different losses.

A person's inability to control loss causes feelings of helplessness and despair. Nurses have no control over these feelings in their clients, but they may increase their chances of encountering them if they are negligent or unable to see the warning signs.

Philosophers and scientists have attempted to understand and even control death. The fact that everyone must face their own death as well as the death of others not only creates anxiety but also gives meaning to life. A person's thoughts about death will affect the way he or she lives. These thoughts can be threatening, painful or inspirational and give deeper meaning to a relationship.

It is essential that you, as a nurse, examine your own thoughts and feelings on these difficult issues in order to help others cope with them. This chapter confronts you with some of the more painful and difficult areas of life. If you are to be an effective nurse it is important that you face up to these uncomfortable thoughts.

We can explore these life issues positively as we make use of both our personal life experiences and the example of others. This chapter also explores various theories and ideas, and looks at what has been learned over the years about the processes people go through to help them come to terms with the pain of loss.

Loss, separation and dying are very personal, individual experiences. This chapter offers some guidelines for sharing with, understanding and caring for people who are encountering these experiences. As a nurse you may feel you are intruding into someone's most private moments, but the very nature of your work means it is almost impossible to avoid such intimacy. The understanding you gain from working through the issues of loss and grief will help you to value and respect individual needs and beliefs, as well as giving you an insight into what you can actually do to help.

Working as we do in the area of health care, we are frequently in close contact with people who face or experience loss. It is not even clear towards whom we are focusing our care. It may be the patient or client, their family, significant other or friends. Occasionally we will become involved with someone who does not even know the patient but suddenly becomes involved in the patient's life; I am thinking here of the driver who fatally injures someone. A person may, just by chance in their everyday life, witness the injury or death of someone unknown to them and may then need our care. Because of the many settings in which nurses work, they may be confronted with the distress of a child who was in a patient's house, a work colleague in a factory, or friends in a hospital setting. The effect of this loss or threat of loss will differ widely in individuals and age groups, and the response will be influenced by the setting in which we are working.

As we look at death, grief and loss, and its effects upon individuals, some of the losses will be actual losses, others will involve the threat of a loss and all the ensuing fear associated with major life transitions. We will consider how the nurse responds to and supports people during this initial impact of the loss, and through that process of bereavement.

Much of our time as nurses will be spent caring for people who are physically ill. Studies have demonstrated how death, grief and loss produce many physical symptoms (Stuart and Laraia 1998) because of all the associated anxiety. Therefore, it is important, when we take a patient's history of important life events, to identify episodes of death, grief and loss which are part of any evaluation of what may be contributing factors to the illness. Dysfunctional grieving may be a major contributing factor: some studies (Parkes 1996) have identified how some bereaved groups in the population are twice as likely to become ill as the rest of the population.

Experience of loss and normal grieving are universal and are accompanied by psychological and physical reactions. Normal grieving is the process by which we adapt to loss (Worden 1993), and it is important that we help individuals to grieve as this will be the means by which the pain of the loss is healed. Loss and its significance applies to something or someone that was owned in some way, and which was valuable or meaningful. We will consider some of the theories on the process and stages of grief, how anticipatory grief may occur before the actual loss, and how dysfunctional grieving can result in serious psychological distress or illness.

Breaking bad news, and the nursing interventions and the skills to engage with the distress will be explored. Working with the distressing nature of death, grief and loss, and given our ability to identify with the client, we should also explore the support and counselling available to us locally in order to care for ourselves in this aspect of our work.

Normal grieving

An alternative term for normal grief is uncomplicated grief. It describes a range of feelings and behaviour commonly seen and experienced after a loss. A 'theorist' (Worden 1993) defines the word 'normal' in both a clinical and statistical framework; 'clinical' defines what the clinician calls normal mourning behaviour and 'statistical' refers to the frequency with which behaviour is found among a randomized bereaved population. The more a behaviour or feeling is recorded, the more it is defined as normal.

Freud (1917) described how the normal grieving process is triggered by a significant loss, and that it is a process to be expected. He went on to say that a person experiencing normal grieving loses the capacity to give attention to others, to engage in a meaningful attachment whilst the pain of the loss is consuming them. The loss takes away the ability to focus on normal everyday activities. Even as long ago as 1917, when Freud began writing about this, he indicated a period of 1–3 years before a satisfactory resolution of the difficulty would be achieved.

Another early attempt to look at normal grief reactions was the work of Eric Lindemann. He wrote his classic

Box 4.1   Lindemann's characteristics of the bereaved

■ Somatic or bodily distress

■ Preoccupation with the image of the deceased

■ Guilt relating to the deceased

■ Hostile reactions

■ Inability to function as before the loss

■ Developing traits of the deceased in their own behaviour.

Box 4.2   Bowlby's three phases of response to loss

1. Protest

2. Disorganization

3. Reorganization.

Box 4.3   Parkes' six determinants of grief

■ Mode of death

■ Nature of the attachment

■ Who was the person?

■ Historical antecedents

■ Personality variables

■ Social variables.

paper after extensive work with the relatives of victims of the Coconut Grove night club fire in which 500 people lost their lives (Lindemann 1944). From Lindemann's observations of 101 people, he described repetitive patterns in the characteristics of acute grief. These are listed in Box 4.1.

Lindemann's much-quoted study has some limitations. Parkes (1972) criticized the lack of information about how much time elapsed between the death and the interview. Despite this criticism, many of the clients I see today demonstrate much of the behaviour and describe the feelings outlined by Lindemann. As they begin to accept the loss, the grieving process begins. This was described by Worden (1993) as the grief work.

Bowlby (1980) described normal grieving as resulting from the loss of others, of part of self or of objects. Box 4.2 shows his description of the three phases of response to loss.

In the first phase, expression of anger, denial, shock and disbelief will be underlined by periods of yearning or longing for the deceased. Crying, searching to recover the loss, and appeals for help may run alongside sleep disturbances and change in appetite.

The second phase of disorganization is described as being driven by despair and depression. This will often result in social isolation because of the withdrawal and/or regression, with psychomotor retardation.

The third phase, reorganization, describes a disengagement from the attachment, a development of new interests and attachments, and a restructuring of lifestyle. This should return the individual to a level of functioning experienced before the loss, although life will be different. Parkes (1996) made a major contribution to the study of grief by identifying the determinants that influence the whole process of grief (Box 4.3).

These six determinants or predictors of grief are the circumstances surrounding a death that will influence

the outcome or resolution; they identify the difficulties that people may need to address so they can begin to process the grief.

Mode of death

If the death was from 'natural causes' such as an illness, even if it was sudden, it is likely to cause fewer problems than traumatic death. Death by injury, which damages the body, is more likely to be thought of as causing suffering and as being an injustice.

Most people will ask whether the deceased suffered or knew anything about the process or act of dying. It will be more difficult to blame others if the death was due to illness, but they may blame themselves for not having the foresight to call a doctor or ambulance sooner. The professional ability or resources in the health centre may be blamed. Much time and effort will be needed to explore the issues around this.

Death by road traffic accident, or accident at work or at home, can cause anger and a sense of injustice far greater than does natural sudden death. Things are even worse when monetary compensation is an issue: this usually falls short in that it somehow devalues the deceased. The verdict of the coroner's court or the finding of a Fatal Accident Enquiry is often discussed at length, as is the question of whether the deceased is entirely blameless in relation to his or her own death. If the deceased was not to blame, some thing or some person is usually felt to be responsible. The area of responsibility may be even wider: if a person or organization was not to blame then culture or society may be blamed. In some extremes, civilization or humankind is blamed and the bereaved person may isolate him- or herself from society, resulting in an even greater loss.

The place where the death occurred becomes an integral part of the grief. Was the deceased on home ground, or in a strange place? The pain will be greater if she or he was far away from home and alone during death. Nobody will have known the person and this underlines a recurring theme: this was someone special, a big, important part of their lives. Away, she or he was a stranger, anonymous, alone. The real identity, the person she or he was, was not apparent. The fact that many families are now scattered throughout the world presents an added dimension to grief. This is particularly difficult if friends and neighbours did not know the deceased. The nurses, friends, neighbours and family may be at a disadvantage in having no sense of who the person was. It can reduce their ability to understand and empathize.

One mode of death that produces some tremendous difficulties is suicide. The process of grieving becomes very complicated both emotionally and intellectually. The bereaved are not only sorting out their own loss but speculating about how the victim might have emerged from the difficulty had she or he remained alive. They may come up with actions that may have prevented the suicide, and this holds the potential for profound feelings of guilt.

Nature of the attachment

The strengths of the relationship, and the security or aspects of safety gained from the relationship, are useful areas to explore because they highlight vulnerability. One feeling that recurs in crisis is ambivalence, giving rise to heartache and soul searching. If there was ambivalence in the living relationship, it will certainly occur at the death in the long term. The difficulty lies in the strong sense that this feeling is inappropriate in grief: time can usefully be spent in encouraging the expression of ambivalence.

Who was the person?

Who the deceased was in relation to the client must be ascertained. The deceased's position in the hierarchy of the family is not necessarily a clue to the enormity of the loss, and we must not make assumptions. I can still remember talking to and trying to comfort the lover of a middle-aged man, whilst his wife sat in a room a few doors away saying she was now free to get on with her own life. Not only is the family relationship an issue, but how would you feel if your husband died at the home of his lover?

Historical antecedents

A previous life crisis, particularly a sudden death, will present as a major factor in coping. If I have experienced a previous life crisis with a good or reasonable outcome, then in theory this should help me. I will have programmed into my head something that identifies difficulty but removes or diminishes some fear about the outcome. This may be useful, provided I can get in touch with the previous experience. However, if the previous outcome was one of pain and suffering, the present problems are compounded. Previously unresolved loss, or failure to confront loss, may

result in its re-emergence, causing difficulty for the helper in establishing the focus of the loss.

Other recent life changes, crisis or recent depressive illness will result in more difficulty in handling the loss. Energy and resources used up in tackling these will have left the person drained or depleted of resources.

Personality variables

Positive coping with the immediate grief does not guarantee a lack of long-term problems. A personality that allows self-actualization, a feeling of some control over one's own life, and sees problems as a challenge seems to be most likely to recover.

Raphael (1984) writes that, although no specific risk factors have been demonstrated, certain personal characteristics may carry a risk of poor outcome. These include ambivalence and dependent or clinging relationships. Earlier personal experience of grief, especially childhood loss of parents, contributes to vulnerability. I have witnessed this re-emerging vulnerability in my workshops, and it would seem that this childhood loss is diminished only with difficulty. The key factors influencing outcome appear to be personality in combination with the pre-existing relationship of dependence.

Social variables

Some loss alienates and isolates, whereas other loss produces gain. The gain may be freedom to leave a group or community or restrictions, for example those of a sexist relationship. If the person left was, or felt they were, an extension of the deceased and fed from their social network, the enormity of the loss becomes apparent.

Some religions and cultures will support the bereaved, showering them with offers of help and validation of their worth. In the UK there are diverse examples of community response to death; clear confrontation of it or avoidance may be apparent. Whilst Christianity and other religions are usually assumed to be a help and support in sudden death, the bereaved may feel otherwise.

Other work (Wright 1996) highlights how the six determinants (Box 4.3) will give some indication of who is likely to need some help and support through the whole process of grief. Very early in the process, for example, major negative determinants may indicate who is at risk from dysfunctional grieving.

Kubler-Ross (1969) looks at five stages of grief in the dying patient (Box 4.4), and also suggests that this process is reflected in those close to the dying patient.

Denial is said to offer an opportunity to deal with the shock and disbelief in the short term, whilst organizing more effective defensive strategies. The use of denial has often been viewed negatively, but Davidhizar and Newman-Eiger (1998) emphasize that nurses need to appreciate the importance of denial. They indicate that it may be the only psychologically safe way of coping with the unimaginable. Some factors reduce the need for denials; for example, how much time remains to ground the eventual death in reality, and the way the information is given, will influence the extent to which individuals remain with the denial.

The anger may well be expressed in some form of protest: 'Why me?' 'Why now?'. Resentment and expressions about injustice may quickly be verbalized, and may be projected on to others – perhaps the nurses. Nurses may find this difficult to tolerate, and may take it personally.

The bargaining stage is said to be about trying to postpone the death. Some kind of agreement or deadline will be offered, to prevent or postpone the inevitable.

In the depression stage the inevitable can no longer be denied or displaced elsewhere. The reality is recognized, producing some apparent sadness and a resignation that the course of events cannot be prevented. At this time you may witness withdrawal, silence and perhaps helplessness. This is said to be part of the anticipatory grief process in the preparation for the death. Finally, in acceptance, energy to prevent the inevitable death is no longer needed. Contemplation of the death, and giving up the struggle, should indicate that the individual is more relaxed or, as often described, peaceful. This stage is thought to make the pain less acute, as emotional distress is thought to exacerbate the intensity of pain (Dossey 1994).

Anticipatory grieving

In the past, much emphasis has been placed on the importance of the opportunity to anticipate death (Kubler-Ross 1969). Parkes (1996) also highlights this in his determinants of grief. Anticipatory grieving is said to combine the beginning and the actual process of grieving, and takes place when anticipating a significant loss before the loss actually takes place. This significant loss can refer to the potential death of a significant person who is facing a terminal illness, or the potential loss of a body part where some surgery is to take place. One's own impending death, or moving away from one's permanent place, can fall into this category of grieving (Clayton et al 1973).

People experiencing anticipatory grief exhibit similar feelings and behaviour as in normal grieving. The role

of anticipatory grief has been challenged (Fulton and Gottesman 1980); it is said to have been confused conceptually with forewarning of loss and does not automatically occur after forewarning of loss. Fulton and Gottesman (1980) conclude that the usefulness of anticipatory grief is not determined by its duration or whether all the appropriate factors are present. They say it is the manner in which it is experienced and responded to by those concerned.

Some nursing research (Breu and Dracup 1978) examines the way we allow anticipatory grief to be experienced. This includes the spouse of the dying person needing to be with the patient and helpful towards them, assisting the dying person to express feelings and to be relieved of anxiety. Whilst anticipatory grieving can help a person adjust to the actual loss, Clayton et al (1973) found that post-death depression can still follow: it can be worse in the first month after the death and no better at 1 year than in those who had no opportunity to anticipate the death. This returns to the previous observation on the way it is experienced and enabled. As far as the nurse's role is concerned, being more proactive appears to be one of the ideals that can be concluded from all this research. Worden (1993) said there was little point in saying 'How can I help you?' because usually the bereaved do not know. A more assertive approach would be to say: 'I am here to talk with you and to work with you'. Offering choices or suggestions is more about enabling the process and helping them to experience the anticipatory process.

Life transitions with a capacity for grief

Other life changes or transitions can result in a loss, and may even result in a life crisis (Caplan 1964). The work of crisis intervention is underpinned by Caplan's theories and studies, which acknowledge Erikson's 1950 model of developmental (maturational) and situational (accidental) crisis (Box 4.5).

Caplan described developmental crisis as transitional periods in personality development, characterized by disturbances in affective and cognitive functioning. A sudden unexpected threat to, or loss of, basic resources or life goals

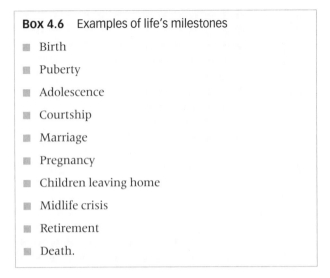

Box 4.6   Examples of life's milestones

■   Birth

■   Puberty

■   Adolescence

■   Courtship

■   Marriage

■   Pregnancy

■   Children leaving home

■   Midlife crisis

■   Retirement

■   Death.

Figure 4.1   Three routes to explore when attempting to cope with a crisis.

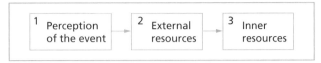

constitutes a situational crisis. Situational crises can lead to intensive periods of psychological, behavioural and physical disarray. Caplan observed that situational crises are often new to the client and that their usual coping methods do not work.

Some crises may be compounded by fitting into both categories. A 20-year-old woman, for example, may suffer the death of her husband in a road traffic accident within a month of her marriage. We cannot treat her loss, and the emotionally painful experience of the loss, without discussing the distress of this happening within a month of her marriage.

Whilst this example identifies clearly the two types of crisis, others may not be so easily identified. We need to be aware of where the client is on the developmental scale (life's milestones) in order to appreciate fully the implications of a sudden death. Placing a client's experience of loss on his life milestone graph (Box 4.6), noting the stage she or he is now at or may be heading towards or leaving, is a useful exercise. Further discussion with clients about their perception of their life situation may alter assumptions we have made about them.

Some situational crises, such as redundancy, divorce or separation, produce a loss of status and security. Again, if these are marked along the line of life's developmental crises, their overwhelming nature may be perceived. Caplan (1964) says that even individuals with relatively stable personalities can change in unexpected ways during such a crisis.

The change needed to deal with crisis may have positive aspects, highlighting the opportunities that crisis can bring. On the other hand, the crisis can result in an increased inability to cope, and lead to feelings of chaos and disorder. This leads to the view that a crisis is a transitional period offering the individual an opportunity for growth or increasing their vulnerability.

Time is another aspect to consider. A crisis cannot be tolerated for a long period because it involves intense feelings of distress and disorder which have the capacity

to damage. Nurses not only have to respond quickly but also frequent and lengthy periods of care will be necessary to prevent damage and restore equilibrium. Caplan (1964) viewed crisis intervention as a major part of preventive psychiatry. He believed that individuals could be supported and offered the right conditions to deal effectively with crisis, thereby preventing mental disorder. My aim in this chapter is to explore mechanisms for helping the patient and others use the process of grief to deal in the long term with the loss. Crisis intervention helps them to begin this process, and offers the nurse a framework to use in assisting them.

Rogers and Reich (1988) recognized the importance of reassuring and affirming a person's feelings – from the moment of impact through ongoing support – in healing the grief. The crisis model shown in Figure 4.1 provides a useful framework for intervention, identifying three routes to explore when dealing with the crisis of sudden death.

Sudden death

When a death is sudden, these three factors of crisis become even more important because the death has to be grounded in reality, and this is difficult initially.

Perception of the event

Does the client (i.e. the bereaved) understand what has happened? A realistic appraisal of the event and what led up to the death is important. Information will help this process as well as checking the client's understanding of what happened. The opportunity to see or be with the deceased will further confirm the client's perception of the reality.

External resources

The external resources available to help the client cope with this event are the second factor to work with. The disordered activity resulting from the impact of the event often makes it difficult for the client to think logically about sources of strength, comfort and support, and may actually prevent the client accessing them. The first resources to explore are usually family and friends, or other people close to or on intimate terms with the client. The person in crisis knows his or her need of them, but the disarray and distress produce fear that they will not be reached. This may be expressed clearly as: 'Please help me find my brother. He will help me, he will know what to do'. This expectation of the help to be received may

Figure 4.2   The phases of crisis.

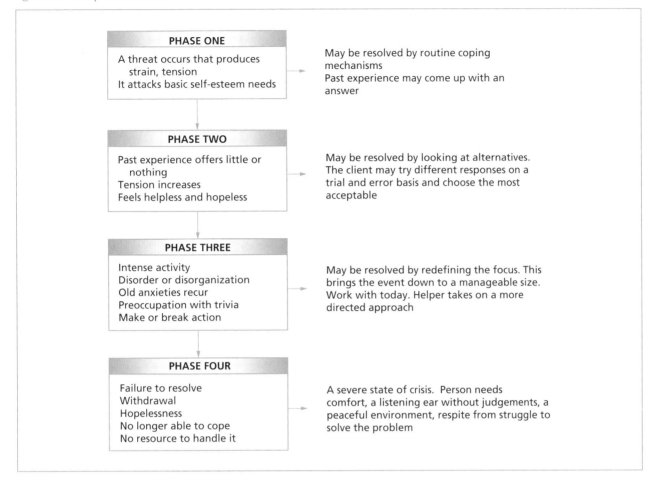

PHASE ONE

A threat occurs that produces strain, tension
It attacks basic self-esteem needs

May be resolved by routine coping mechanisms
Past experience may come up with an answer

PHASE TWO

Past experience offers little or nothing
Tension increases
Feels helpless and hopeless

May be resolved by looking at alternatives. The client may try different responses on a trial and error basis and choose the most acceptable

PHASE THREE

Intense activity
Disorder or disorganization
Old anxieties recur
Preoccupation with trivia
Make or break action

May be resolved by redefining the focus. This brings the event down to a manageable size. Work with today. Helper takes on a more directed approach

PHASE FOUR

Failure to resolve
Withdrawal
Hopelessness
No longer able to cope
No resource to handle it

A severe state of crisis. Person needs comfort, a listening ear without judgements, a peaceful environment, respite from struggle to solve the problem

well be unrealistic initially, but as time progresses – and this will help – more order will replace disorder. The external resources may also include other disciplines, caring agencies and organizations or self-help groups. It is important to be aware of local resources and the types of help available.

Inner resources

The client may be able to access inner resources in coping with the crisis, and should be helped to realize strengths and vulnerabilities. The overwhelming feeling at a time of crisis is that any forward movement is impossible; the client is rendered impotent and this increases distress. The fear produced by being immobilized is tremendously powerful; it can make one feel totally weak or lead to panic. Acknowledging inner strengths and feelings can result in activity and forward movement, enhancing potency or effectiveness. This feels positive and suggests some advance towards management of the problem. It is important for clients' self-esteem that they can ask 'What can I do about this?' and begin to look at answers and alternatives for themselves.

If we can help the client to look at and work positively with these three aspects of coping with a stressful event – perception of the event, external resources, inner resources – a crisis may be averted. Perception of the event will have strong negative content if there is denial of the meaning or the reality of the situation. Negative responses will also arise if external resources are poor or not available. The client's inability to access strengths, resources or insights within him- or herself will make exploration of the third area a non-productive exercise. One or two negative responses in these areas are likely to lead to a life crisis if the client's position remains unchanged.

The four phases of crisis

There are four recognized phases of crisis (Fig. 4.2), although individuals do not necessarily experience all phases. Using the three routes described earlier to explore ways of copying when confronted with crisis can enable the client to leave the process (i.e. begin to manage it) before reaching the final, severe stage. However, this is not a magic formula. In sudden death there is no quick answer but we can help clients to *begin* the process of managing their feelings of chaos and disorder.

Status

A sudden death can instantly or more insidiously damage a person's status. By status, I mean the position or standing in society that governs the respect or rights people receive. Their status may give them a role or place, somewhere they belong. If this is suddenly removed it leaves them vulnerable or seeking a new status:

- 'Where do I stand now?'

- 'Does this relate to what I thought I had?'

- 'This is like starting over again.'

Some people describe having to make a completely new start or an about-turn after a crisis. Image and status can be closely bound together. We have discussed how a client's place along life's milestones graph may indicate a developmental crisis; it may also highlight a threat to a client's status. For example, a shift towards retirement, or a mother's children growing up and leaving home, or the end of a woman's sexually reproductive period, indicates a new role and a change in status. If you look at a sudden death using the phases of crisis in Figure 4.2, you will see that it cannot be resolved immediately, so work needs to be done in each phase of crisis. Much of this work with a sudden death will be the concern of accident and emergency departments and critical care units, but there will be occasions when it has to be addressed on a ward, or in someone's home or other community setting.

One of the difficult elements of a sudden death is that this emergency is imposed upon clients suddenly, leading to disempowerment and loss of automony. Most therapeutic relationships result from clients asking for help for themselves: people are usually in a position to make the decision to ask for help or are referred for help with their agreement. However, in the case of sudden death the element of choice is absent and this alters the whole nature of the relationship. Family or loved ones are thrust into the position of being helpless, disempowered and needing immediate help (Wright 1999). Not only is this death difficult to grieve because of the number of negative determinants, but it can also result in post-traumatic stress disorder (Ornstein 1998).

The resulting disempowerment may mean that the nurse has to be more assertive in providing people with the conditions they need to move into the process we call grief, because many people will experience chaos and disorder in all the dimensions of their person (Box 4.7).

The theories discussed earlier suggest the need for some action on the part of the helper. They go further than this. I believe they demonstrate that the response should be clearly proactive. As we walk that line of acknowledging the unique needs of the individual, and recognizing their autonomy and choice, we may be prevented from being more proactive. If we are proactive in providing certain conditions at the time of death and

Box 4.7	The five dimensions of the person
Physical	Nausea, blurring of vision, tachycardia, weakness in legs, faint, restlessness, dry mouth and more
Emotional	A whole range of emotion can be experienced over a short timespan, for example numbness, intense sadness, helplessness, anger, frustration and occasionally rage
Cognitive	Unable to receive, retain or process information. Inability to access familiar information such as a well known telephone number
Social	May be surrounded by family and friends and feel totally alone. Unable to perceive anything as a resource
Spiritual	Loss of faith or belief. Intense distress at loss of belief in their life and in their vision for self. Too many questions and no answers. Perplexity, confusion, loss of purpose

suggesting that it would be helpful to do this or that, we could be accused of being prescriptive. An example is viewing the body.

Viewing the body

In our study on this subject (Wright 1996), relatives who were seen later spoke about the definite value of contact with the deceased. Viewing the body is especially valued by relatives not present at the point of death. The chance to say 'I am sorry I was not with you' and to affirm the death was described as providing comfort. The place where the body was viewed was also commented on.

Our study revealed that it is important to see the deceased where they died. This may be a resuscitation room or a treatment room. Some relatives viewed the body again later, in the chapel next to the hospital mortuary, but said they were most comforted by seeing the person where they had died. This seems to take the bereaved person closer to the event, which they have a strong need to feel part of. There was not one negative response to viewing the body. When my colleague, Marjorie Ashdown, and I carried out a phone-in on sudden death on local radio, most of the problems concerned the absence of a body. One woman rang to say her son was lost overboard at sea 20 years ago and she still expected him to walk through the door. Wives of pilots missing in the war talked of their difficulty at not having a body to see in order to confirm death.

The debate about bringing the bodies of the dead from the Falklands War back to Britain highlighted the focus on the deceased's body. More recently, the need to retrieve bodies after fishing boat incidents has been discussed. Raphael (1986) in her experiences with bereavement, and particularly disaster, points out that not being able to see the body contributes to later difficulties. Whilst Cathcart (1988) noted that the relatives' reluctance to see the body should be respected, she went on to say that they should be encouraged to view, and that photographs should be kept.

I am in favour of our current assertive response to viewing the body. The previous response to the question 'Should I see the body?' was often a passive one: 'If you want to' or 'It is your decision'. I have no hesitation now in saying: 'Yes, I think you should'. We can make it the most natural thing to do: 'I am sure you would want to see him, even if it's only to say goodbye'.

Occasionally I hear of someone regretting seeing the deceased, but this is unusual. More regrets and difficulties arise from not seeing the body, and later it is, of course, too late. The risk of regret seems worth taking when a beneficial outcome is most likely. A study by Jones and Buttery (1981) of relatives of sudden death victims who spent time with the body in the emergency department also concluded that the viewing process was helpful. Most people stated that the whole episode seemed like a fantasy or bad dream, and that the viewing made it a reality. Reality, whilst painful, is more manageable than fantasy. Several people in our study who did not see the deceased had difficulties with fantasies about how the body looked. Fantasies can be intrusive and are less controllable, whilst reality is preferable and frees you from bizarre and distressing images.

People in our study reported that it was helpful, if someone was blue-looking after death, for example, to have had this pointed out before viewing the body. In cases of head and facial injuries one might assume it wiser to prevent someone from seeing the body. This is not so – as long as people are told what to expect before viewing the body. If necessary, the injuries can be covered, and it need not prevent them holding the deceased's hand. Being with the deceased was certainly a major issue in our feedback from relatives. It affirmed for me that the time and effort spent with relatives and the deceased is tremendously valuable. There seems little doubt that it helps to begin the process of grief, and it is important to us as a team, in the A&E department, to have this sort of positive feedback.

In some work, advocacy (Box 4.8) is seen as an integral part of practical nursing philosophy (Seedhouse 2000). In what Seedhouse describes as a relentlessly down-to-earth guide to core central concepts in nursing, advocacy is described as a secondary purpose.

A nurse advocates for a patient if she or he is convinced that to do so is a health priority. Another interesting thought from Seedhouse (2000) is that a thorough ethical analysis is in order, to ensure that advocacy for this patient will not unreasonably compromise the health of others.

Box 4.8 Advocacy

An advocate speaks on behalf of some other person (or persons) as he or she perceives the person's interests.

There was overwhelming evidence in my study (Wright 1996) that younger women need an advocate at the time of a death. Many examples were given of male relatives and friends answering on behalf of younger bereaved women and making major decisions for them. These women later complained that we, the staff, should not have allowed this to happen. Our response is not just about choices but about more assertively facilitating an encounter with the body. This was often against overwhelming odds, with some relatives and staff being against it. For me, it was often 'putting my head on the block', inviting conflict and aggression. We know how each dimension of the person is disempowered, yet we still wait to see how things progress, perhaps waiting for them to decide what they need to do.

A death is a very personal, intimate time for individuals and families. Many nurses express the anxiety that they feel like an intruder encroaching on a private family moment. If we leave it to the families, this assumes they will know what to do and know the responses that facilitate good grief.

Absent at the time of death

Because most sudden deaths require vigorous attempts to resuscitate the patient, relatives are often not present at the time of death. Many will not be present at the hospital, and others will be kept waiting in a different room. When death is confirmed, the majority of relatives will ask whether the person suffered, whether they would have known what was happening, and whether they had said anything. Some people can place the focus more precisely on the issue most important to them and say: 'Did he ask or say anything about me?'.

Strong ambivalence is expressed at not being present at the time of death – a great need to have been there and an equally great need to run in the opposite direction. When this ambivalence has settled, many will regret or feel guilt at not having been present.

Nurses can give clear information and should not avoid answering questions. Often they will be confirming that the patient was unconscious and had no awareness of what was happening around about. At other times the nurse will be informing them that strong analgesic drugs were given to deal with the pain. Supplementary information about the nature of these drugs is helpful and can alleviate further distress. We may say, for example, 'The drug was a powerful narcotic, like morphine'. Most people have heard of morphine and understand its useful properties.

Despite all these reassurances, issues such as why they did not get to the person on time, and their helplessness in trying to facilitate this, can become prolonged difficulties for the people who are left behind. Because of the value for most people of being present at the time of death, we must not forget waiting relatives when attempts at resuscitation have failed. Some patients will continue to have a heartbeat for a short time after attempts have ceased. The relatives can be brought to the patient to spend a short time with them before they die.

The separation of family from patient has been identified as causing difficulty and often disruptive aggression in hospitals (Wright 1993). Work in a UK hospital explored whether relatives should be present while resuscitation was taking place (Doyle et al 1995). It was found that relatives may wish to be with family members who may be dying, even though resuscitation efforts are being made. Seventy people who participated in the study were taken to the resuscitation room, accompanied by a member of staff who explained what was happening. None of the participants interfered with the resuscitation efforts.

To me, this demonstrates a need for a much greater input from staff involved at the impact of a sudden death. This will result in spending much longer periods with the relatives, and in staff training and support. I have no doubt that this will enable people to re-emerge from this difficult, traumatic and distressing life crisis.

Caring for the suddenly bereaved will test all our skills of communication with people in crisis. Communication is the vehicle by which nurses establish a therapeutic relationship with clients; it involves passing on information and exchanging thoughts and feelings. This exchange influences the behaviour of others: communication is critical to the successful outcome of all nursing interventions (Stuart and Laraia 1998). Working with the immediate care of the suddenly bereaved will demand major resources of communication from the nurse, and studies highlight how the nurse can, as a result, suffer from post-traumatic stress disorder (Chandler 1993). This is particularly a problem when breaking bad news.

Breaking bad news

You may not have any control about where the bad news is given. It will certainly make a difference if you are in the patient's home as opposed to a hospital corridor, so if we can influence the conditions in which the bad news is given this will help with a difficult task. A quiet place where people are not walking through, without telephones and other disturbances, will help. Frequently the person breaking the bad news feels they have done it badly.

Communication is a dynamic, complex, continuous exchange: it is quite common to feel ineffective and at a loss as to which direction to follow (British Medical Association 1992). A study of the parents of critically ill children (Farrell and Frost 1992) found that, although the information they received was distressing and traumatic,

there was an overwhelming need to know that it was correct and honest. Euphemisms for death should be avoided: words such as 'dead' or 'died' are unequivocal. Phrases such as 'She has passed away', 'We have lost him', 'She has just gone' are open to misinterpretation.

As discussed earlier, when perception of the event is distorted or there is a possibility of denial, we must ground the event in reality. The bearer of bad news may feel they have inflicted pain on the recipient by honest, direct information. Whilst the loss is the real focus of the event, there is a need for clear, understandable information. In a situation that is outside the realms of understanding there is a need to introduce some order and remove some of the perplexity.

Honest, direct information about the death and the sequence of events, from people who do not skirt around the issues, is valued by the clients. This role involves painful confrontation and the recipient may show some cognitive disarray as a result. This leads on to the second component useful in the management of a crisis: finding some external resources.

Help to find immediate resources

Some extremely simple tasks become difficult or complicated at times of crisis. Information usually familiar to people can become difficult to locate. Family, friends or significant others, although geographically near, may seem far away. Those who are far away will cause the helplessness and frustration to intensify. For example, people familiar with telephone directories will ask you to find someone's number, because they cannot understand its sequence. It is not at all uncommon for people not be able to use the telephone or dial a number. Which persons are significant in their lives, and how you can arrange for them to join you, is an important issue. It often requires painstaking discussion to elicit where these people are.

In a large and busy hospital, it is important that relatives and friends are able to ask for a named member of staff on arrival. To arrive distressed and find that reception staff do not know who you are puts both staff and relatives in a difficult position. It also suggests that this most significant of events is not being given priority.

Prior to the arrival of others, some relatives will negotiate with the nurse as to who should give the bad news. I feel it is important that the relatives impart the information to new arrivals, and nurses must encourage this, however reluctant the relatives may be.

The arrival of other relatives and friends

The arrival of other relatives and friends will produce some intense distress and a feeling for the nurse of beginning it all again. The events leading to the death will be reviewed, perhaps more than once. The nurse may use this opportunity to evaluate how the person who was at the hospital from the start perceives and relates to the event. Allowing people to relate the events to those who join them will again confront them and allow them an opportunity to review the death.

When the story is repeated, other things may well be clarified. Other family and friends arriving may give further opportunity to spend time with the deceased. This is often a time when all the pain and anguish becomes apparent. The family may need to be alone together, but do not assume that they want to. Check first.

Loss is about more than death

Working with loss is a major part of a nurse's day, and many of the losses will have a tremendous impact on

---

Box 4.9 Some losses associated with health care

- Mastectomy
- Alzheimer's disease
- Chronic obstructive airway disease
- Prostatectomy
- Anorexia
- Stroke.

Box 4.10 Exercise 1

Many people take on traditional roles within a marriage. Copy the following lists of traditional roles on to separate sheets of paper headed 'male' and 'female'.

Male

Strong	Arranges social interaction
Wage earner	Active sexual partner
Head of the house	Decision maker
Authoritarian	

Female

Housekeeper	Manager
Loyal	Uninformed
Attractive	Submissive
Supportive	Sacrificial
Cook	Passive sexual partner

Imagine that the man loses three of his traditional male roles, for example if he is made redundant or has to stay off work for several months because of illness. How might the effect of these losses be shown in him as a person, for example in his feelings, attitudes and behaviour? Do the same for the woman losing three traditional female roles, perhaps through promotion at her work or through the demands of looking after an elderly relative.

---

people's lives. Box 4.9 lists several examples of loss associated with healthcare issues – but the list is endless.

Some losses are associated with our image, our sexuality and our status (see Exercise 1 in Box 4.10). Our image is our view of ourselves: as we grow and walk about, this image becomes well established; it becomes very important during adolescence. Young people receive messages from others and from the media about how they should look and what others will value when they see them. Many people will think that a person's body is the most important expression of who they are as an individual. At vulnerable times, like the years of growing into adulthood, we are strongly influenced by messages about our appearance from our peer group, some of whom will express values about others according to looks, body, clothes and style. These early messages are exploited by the media and advertisers, who suggest ways to achieve and maintain our attractiveness.

The ideal body image and the way you see your own body image become associated with your idea of your physical appearance. It is the body others see that demonstrates your skills and abilities; these, in turn, reveal your emotions. This means that your awareness of your own body image has important emotional consequences.

Your body image is open to change. Its shape, size, how it is structured and how it functions may alter. This can happen slowly and may not be obvious, or it may be sudden and dramatic. Your hair may gradually turn grey and lines appear on your face; you may be aware of this or choose to deny it. Some people make these changes part of their view of themselves; others deny them and then experience a sudden feeling of crisis or loss at the change. Some people undergo cosmetic surgery with high hopes that the results will change their lives. However, it is not always possible for the result of surgery to meet people's expectations, as the example about Evelyn shows (see Case Study 4.1).

Case Study 4.1

Evelyn was 50 years old and worked as a buyer of fashionable clothes for a large department store. She had to make predictions about future trends in fashion and take risks when calculating the volume of certain clothes she bought. Evelyn had always felt that her personal appearance (her body image) was very important to her overall performance and ability. She became preoccupied with the lines on her face, and when some of her fashion predictions were wrongly timed she began to worry that she was losing her ability and judgement. She told herself she was getting old and that she was no longer functioning efficiently.

Evelyn decided she needed to have cosmetic surgery to alter her image. She was sure that after surgery she would return to her former self and once again experience the energy and skill she had known when she was younger. What Evelyn failed to see was that the real problem was not her wrinkles but the fact she was out of touch with current trends. She had lost some of her former contacts, with whom she could discuss forthcoming changes in the market, and was miscalculating the moment when new styles and ideas emerged.

Because Evelyn's expectations of the outcome of the surgery were wrong, when the change in her image failed to have the expected result in her life she blamed it on poor-quality surgery. Soon she was involved in a long-standing dispute with the doctors, nurses and health authority.

How people think about the effects of an illness depends on how they cope with change. Changes in physical appearance, or in people's body image, result in changes in other areas of their lives too. Change involves leaving behind things that are familiar and accepted parts of our existence. Body image is closely associated with feelings, inner beliefs and personal goals: our own ideas of our strengths and weaknesses are the result of the way we see our image. A change in a small area of a person's body, whether internal or external, can take on great significance.

Our perception of ourselves, our body and our health is not due to media influence alone, however Watson (2000) suggests that the current medical debates about men's health are undermined and underinformed by a failure to explore men's perceptions of health and maleness.

Some work on chronic leg ulcers (Bland 1999) reveals how, along with the body breaking down, there is a breaking down of relationships with others. New, long-term relationships with healthcare professionals have to be forged, and care taken not to offend these experts. The care and management is often undertaken by district nurses and this contact may last years. This study explores the reality of living with a body that can no longer be relied upon and the enormity and significance of that loss. It is not necessarily useful that people insist the client/patient concerned is still the same and that it is all perfectly acceptable. This person is not the same: they feel different and may look different and have had to make the change between who they were and who they are now.

Responses such as 'It could be worse' are well meaning but take away from the painful consequences of the change. Clients need someone to validate their reactions and fears (Box 4.11), someone who will not try to dilute or dismiss them.

It would be easy to say that image is not important and that people value other aspects of a person much more. People say that other characteristics such as loyalty, self-determination and creativity are more important, but in practice they often place more importance on image and appearance. The advertising industry exploits this fact (see Exercise 2 in Box 4.12).

Box 4.11 Meaning of validate

To search for meaning and emotion in clients' words, and agree with them that this is how they feel.

Box 4.12 Exercise 2

Watch three advertising breaks on a commercial television channel. Describe how the product they are selling is trying to influence our perceptions of our physical image.

Altered body image may:

- threaten a person's status
- change a familiar and long-accepted part of a person
- weaken people's security by raising issues of whether they possess or have lost control of what they assumed would always be theirs
- suddenly become difficult to cope with after a long period of gradual change
- make people feel vulnerable and ill at ease with themselves, and produce grief.

Responding to altered body image

It can be useful for a client to express concern and anxiety about body image. It is a way of exploring the possible effects of the change with another person. This outward expression of inner concerns is both necessary and healthy for many clients. The nurse can use the occasion to reassure the client that she or he continues to recognize the client as a person. Certain patterns of behaviour may follow body change, including those in Box 4.13.

Passivity

If the client is passive she or he appears withdrawn and listless, simply accepting the care that is offered. Lowered morale and reduced self-esteem can lead to this sadness and withdrawal, which may result in the person not wanting to be involved in his or her own care. Demotivation and apathy will follow.

Denial

The client may show denial by refusing to touch or look at an altered part of the body, such as a colostomy, operation scar or damaged tissue. If the client has a limb amputated or a breast removed, he or she may deny its absence. For the nurse, it can be very distressing when the client resists any attempts to return attention to the loss or change. The nurse then feels that by trying to do this she or he is inflicting pain and distress on the client, and worries that this may strain their relationship.

> **Box 4.13**   Patterns of behaviour that may follow body change
>
> - Passivity
> - Denial
> - Reassurance
> - Isolation
> - Hostility.

Reassurance

The client may seek constant attention from the nurse and from his or her own family. In order to gain reassurance concerning their acceptability the client may make dismissive remarks such as 'Nobody every really fancied me anyway'. Paying the client a compliment can have a powerful effect on these occasions because it indicates that appearance or image does not take away from the attractiveness of the complete person.

Isolation

The client's isolation may be self-imposed because she or he feels unacceptable. Avoidance may be used as strategy to prevent rejection. If the client says that he or she is less acceptable to family and friends, it is easy for the nurse quickly to deny it and say it is all imagination. However, the client may have sensed the family's response correctly: it is not unusual for family members or friends to reject a client because of body changes. They make remarks like: 'He is not the person he was' or 'It has altered his personality'. This could be true, but it could be that they themselves are unable to cope with the physical changes they see in the client. Their attitude both to the physical changes and to the changes in the client's emotional state may be the reasons for their rejection.

Hostility

Feelings of hostility and anger emerge frequently when clients feel strongly about their altered or damaged body image. Their protests may be intended for someone else but may be directed at the nurse because she or he is there. If the client feels that some other person is responsible, but cannot express anger towards them, she or he may become rebellious or provocative towards the nurse.

Any of these changes in behaviour may occur after a sudden death as well as after the loss of a limb or organ or a change in appearance. The loss of some organs also results in the loss of masculinity or femininity. These losses can result in as much grief as death does.

Feelings of separation and loss associated with illness or injury remind us that we are not totally in control. We become attached to and familiar with ourselves, and feel sad if we 'lose' parts of ourselves. The bonds we develop

> **Box 4.14**   Anxiety
>
> A state or feeling of unease, uncertainty or fear resulting from an anticipated threat or danger.

> **Box 4.15**   Bowlby's three phases of loss
>
> | | |
> |---|---|
> | Protest | Characterized by the feelings of anger, disbelief, shock and yearning (great longing). The person focuses on thoughts of loss by crying, searching consciously (or unconsciously) to recover the loss and by making appeals for help. Sleep, digestion and appetite may be disturbed during this stage |
> | Disorganization | This stage is indicated by despair, depression, withdrawal, social isolation and a slowing down of physical activities. There may also be obvious signs of regression – return to an earlier, more primitive, form of behaviour |
> | Reorganization | The person breaks away from the attachment, developing new interests and attachments. Return to a level of functioning similar to that experienced before the loss |

with what is familiar, for example self and others, are threatened. If the bond is broken or continues to be threatened, we feel acute anxiety (Bowlby 1973) (see Box 4.14).

Phases of loss

John Bowlby described the loss of self (or part of self) and the loss of objects as being in three phases (Box 4.15).

Bowlby's theory is task oriented, that is, the phases he describes are demonstrated by the things people are involved in at the various stages of grief. For example, in the first phase people wander around looking for the lost one or for signs that the person may still be available; in the third phase people learn new skills. Bowlby suggests that we can recognize which phase a person is going through by looking at the purpose of the tasks they are carrying out.

Summary

Studies of social, personal and cultural responses to death highlight major changes over the centuries (Jupp and Walter 1999). Modern medicine, care and treatment has enabled many people to live at home, but most death is institutionalized.

As nurses you will become more closely involved in death, loss and dying if this trend persists. You may feel that the work discussed in this chapter involves only sadness, misery and pain, but loss and grief are part of everyday life and no one can avoid the strong feelings that surround them. You may also think you would prefer not to work with clients in such distressing situations because you find it too upsetting or difficult. Yet nurses who do tackle the issues of loss and grief find the work very rewarding. They gain great insight into the nature of relationships and the ways in which people view life and give it meaning. Many nurses find that the challenge of working with loss and grief contributes to their own personal growth. They develop a clear understanding of some of the different issues of life and gradually feel more comfortable with them. Caring for those experiencing loss, grief and separation can make an obvious difference to people's lives, be a positive experience and make a useful and meaningful contribution to care. It is a privilege to share these significant milestones of life with people, and it is not wrong to find that you actually enjoy the work. Whatever the problems, the uniqueness of each event will make it an experience to value.

Critical incident

You are accompanying a health visitor from the local health centre whilst on your community placement as a student. The health visitor is asked to visit Mary, a 70-year-old woman who is giving her GP some concern. Mary has visited the surgery regularly with numerous minor ailments over the past year. Prior to this she rarely visited her GP. The only other significant detail is that her husband died the previous year, but as it is now a year ago she is coping with that.

On entering Mary's house you introduce yourselves, and Mary appears flustered and panicky that you have arrived. She apologizes for this but says she is just preparing a meal and if you do not mind following her she will have to complete what she was doing. You all go into the kitchen and she continues chopping up carrots, puts them in a pan of water, puts the pan on the stove and turns on the gas. Mary notices you looking at a picture of an elderly man on the kitchen dresser. She walks over, picks it up and clutches it to her chest. You then have to remind her that she has not lit the gas. She is embarrassed about this and explains that she cannot concentrate very well. You notice her husband's coat hanging behind the door and two places already set at the table. The health visitor remarks how very difficult it must have been since her husband died and how the doctors were concerned about how unwell she had been recently.

Mary looks at the health visitor and at you for what seems like a long time, before saying how he just loved organizing things and that she never had to lift a finger. If they were going on holiday, every detail was decided upon by him – it was organized meticulously. She smiled and remarked how she never had to do a thing. Her friends had said they would not like that, but she said it suited her fine. She stands and ponders this.

Then, as if startled, she apologizes for not sitting you down and offering you some tea, and leads you to the sitting room. Here are more pictures of them in faraway exotic places such as India, and one of them on a kind of bobsleigh in the Canadian Rockies.

The health visitor says how she must miss him, and tears immediately well up in Mary's eyes. She apologizes and says she must not get upset, as it was now beginning to annoy people: two friends had remarked recently that she was living in the past and needed to get on with her life. She then remarks how she must be getting on people's nerves as they are visiting her less frequently, and how she is not expecting anyone to visit until the weekend (it is now Tuesday). The health visitor suggests various opportunities for Mary to socialize; she says she does not want to seem ungrateful for the suggestion but at her time of life she will not change now. She always got what she wanted from just the two of them. 'He did not like me mixing with others', she remarks, ' He says they may ask too many questions'.

You then say you are not aware of all the circumstances of his death. Mary immediately launches into all the detail. She was baking and had forgotten to get the sultanas; she apologized for this saying how it was her fault, she had not put them on his shopping list. He always did the shopping as he liked to control the money. She said she would run down to the corner shop and get some, but he was adamant that she would not. It was dusk and, as he had said to her before, 'You are too trusting, and I have told you before about talking to anyone'. He insisted he would go to the shop but then complained bitterly and became quite angry, saying how she was becoming more and more stupid and forgetful.

Mary becomes more subdued at this stage, and tearful. She says she hated it when he was angry with her and she knows it was all her fault. After half an hour she suddenly became aware that he had not returned – he should have been back after 15 minutes but she had

(Continued)

Critical incident (*Continued*)

forgotten this as she became engrossed in something on TV. She had heard the ambulance sirens but thought nothing of it. When the woman from the shop hammered on Mary's door she was frightened by the urgency of it. The woman explained that two young boys were playing football outside the shop and the ball had hit him; when they laughed he became angry and then suddenly collapsed. When Mary had arrived at the hospital she was too late.

Mary pauses then and looks away. 'He had already gone, you see, I was too late. He never got to the shop and I have not had the heart to bake since then.' When the hospital staff heard her only sister lived 200 miles away, they got her a taxi home. Eventually, the next day she thought it was, her sister arrived and took over, made all the arrangements and that was it. She agrees she is eating all right, not always sleeping very well and not very well organized. She laughs and tells you her sister said she would have to get her act together – she was her own worst enemy. Mary says she makes a point of walking down to the shops just to get out, and remarks that it is difficult to get excited about cooking for herself. She agrees the health visitor can visit her again, and if she is getting very upset or unwell she will contact her.

Reflection

From your knowledge of the grief process and negative determinants, what information did you gain that would indicate Mary is having problems with her grief process?

See Appendix 2 for guidelines on reflection.

References

Bland M (1999) Living with chronic leg ulcers. In: Madjar I, Walton JA, eds. Nursing and the experience of illness, pp. 36–57. London: Routledge.

British Medical Association (1992) A stressful shift. BMA Board of Health Science and Education teaching package. London: BMA.

Bowlby J (1973) Separation. London: Penguin.

Bowlby J (1980) Attachment and loss: loss, sadness and depression. Vol. 3. New York: Basic Books.

Breu C, Dracup K (1978) Helping the spouse of critical patients. American Journal of Nursing 78(1): 51–53.

Caplan G (1964) Principles of preventative psychiatry. New York: Basic Books.

Cathcart F (1988) Seeing the body after death. British Medical Journal 297: 997–998.

Chandler E (1993) Can post traumatic stress disorder be prevented? Journal of Accident and Emergency Nursing 1: 87–91.

Clayton PPJ, Halikas JA, Maurice WL (1973) Anticipatory grief and widowhood. British Journal of Psychiatry 122: 47–51.

Davidhizar R, Newman-Eiger J (1998) Patients' use of denial. Nursing Standard 12(43): 34–36.

Dossey L (1994) Healing words. New York: Harper Collins.

Doyle CJ, Post H, Burney RE et al (1995) Family participation during resuscitation – an option. Annals of Emergency Medicine 16(6): 673–675.

Erikson EH (1950) Childhood and society. New York: WW Norton.

Farrell MF, Frost C (1992) The most important needs of parents in critically ill children. Journal of Intensive Care and Critical Care Nursing 8(3): 104–106.

Freud S (1917) Mourning and melancholia. Cited in: Stachy J, Freud A, eds (1964) The complete works of Sigmund Freud. London: Hogarth Press.

Fulton R, Gottesman D (1980) Anticipatory grief: a psychosocial concept reconsidered. British Journal of Psychiatry 137: 45–54.

Jones WH, Buttery M (1981) Sudden death: survivors' perceptions of their emergency department experience. Journal of Emergency Nursing 7: 1.

Jupp P, Walter T (1999) The healthy society 1918–1998. In: Jupp P, Gittings J, eds. Death in England: an illustrated history, pp. 344–351. Manchester: Manchester University Press.

Kubler-Ross E (1969) On death and dying. New York: Macmillan.

Lindemann E (1944) Symptomatology and management of acute grief. American Journal of Psychiatry 101: 141–148.

Ornstein R (1998) Approach to the patient following a traumatic event. In: Stern T, Herman J, Slavin P, eds. The MGH guide to psychiatry in ordinary care, pp. 327–334. New York: McGraw-Hill.

Parkes CM (1972) Studies of grief in adult life, 1st edn. London: Tavistock.

Parkes CM (1996) Bereavement: studies of grief in adult life, 3rd edn. London: Routledge.

Raphael B (1984) The anatomy of bereavement – a handbook for caring professions. London: Hutchinson.

Raphael B (1986) When disaster strikes. London: Hutchinson.

Rogers MP, Reich P (1988) On the health consequences of bereavement. New England Journal of Medicine 319(8): 510–511.

Seedhouse D (2000) Practical nursing philosophy: the universal ethical code. Chichester, UK: John Wiley.

Stuart G, Laraia M (1998) Pocket guide to psychiatric nursing, 4th edn. St Louis: Mosby.

Watson J (2000) Male bodies – health, culture and identity. Milton Keynes: Open University Press.

Worden JW (1993) Grief counselling and grief therapy, 2nd edn. London: Routledge.

Wright B (1993) Caring in crisis, 2nd edn. Edinburgh: Churchill Livingstone.

Wright B (1996) Sudden death – a research base for practice. Edinburgh: Churchill Livingstone.

Wright B (1999) Autonomy and disempowerment at the time of a sudden death. Journal of Accident and Emergency Nursing 17(3): 154–157.

Further Reading

Aguilera DC (1997) Crisis intervention: theory and methodology. St Louis: Mosby.

Practical methods for dealing with situational and maturational crisis. Offers an explanation as to why people behave as they do around the more acute loss.

Bowlby J (1978) Separation. Harmondsworth: Penguin.

Bowlby J (1981) Attachment. Harmondsworth: Penguin.

Bowlby J (1981) Loss. Harmondsworth: Penguin.

This classic trilogy and much acclaimed work examines ways in which young children and families respond to loss. Gives a perspective on the background to the grief process.

Kubler-Ross E (1970) On death and dying. London: Tavistock.

Particularly helpful at exploring the dying process for the patient and family.

Parkes CM (1986) Bereavement: studies of grief in adult life. London: Routledge.

Long recognized as the most authoritative work of its kind.

Walker T (1999) Bereavement – the culture of grief. Milton Keynes: Open University Press.

This book looks at the social positions of the bereaved and how people find themselves caught between the living and the dead. It offers some sociological insights into this most personal of human situations.

Wright B (1996) Sudden death – a research base for practice. Edinburgh: Churchill Livingstone.

Looks at the death from the point of view of the bereaved and examines the long-term implications.

5

Primary health care and the management of chronic illness

Alison Crumbie

Introduction

What is primary health care?

Primary care as an approach, activities, level of care or a philosophy

Policy and primary care

The nurse's role in primary health care

The primary healthcare team

Chronic illness

Chronic illness management in primary care

Working with patients who live with a chronic condition

The nurse as educator

The nurse as change agent

Summary

Introduction

Over the past two decades in the UK there has been a marked shift in healthcare provision from secondary to primary care. The emphasis on primary healthcare has resulted in a vast increase in the number of nurses working in community settings and there is therefore a need for nurses to understand how health care is delivered outside the hospital. Simultaneously there continues to be a rise in the number of people with chronic health problems. The prevalence of diabetes alone looks set to rise from 1.4 million people in the UK to 3 million by 2010 (Melville et al 2000). People are living longer with chronic conditions and, because people are living longer generally, the prevalence of many of the chronic conditions is increasing.

It is in this climate that you will find yourself working as a nurse. This has relevance for all areas of nursing. Nurses working in hospital settings will be working with patients who have long-term chronic conditions, and liaison with colleagues in the community setting will be vitally important to ensure effective discharge planning. Nurses working in the community will find that they are now expected to perform aspects of care that were previously available only

in the hospital setting. The purpose of this chapter is to consider the concept of primary health care and the impact of this approach to health care on our work with people who live with chronic conditions.

What is primary health care?

In recent years we have heard a great deal of rhetoric in the media over the primary-care-led National Health Service. 'Primary-care' would appear to be a simple term and there is an assumption that we all have a shared understanding of what it means. However, there has been much debate over the definition of primary care. In 1978 the World Health Organization (WHO) stimulated an international reorientation of healthcare services towards primary health care, and at that time provided a comprehensive definition of primary care. The WHO (1978) definition of primary care is:

> … essential health care based on practical, scientifically sound and socially acceptable methods and technology, made universally available to individuals and families in the community through their full participation and at a cost that the community and country can afford to maintain at every

stage of their development in the spirit of self-reliance and self-determination.

This is a rather complex and broad definition, and further on in the document primary care is described as 'the first level of contact of individuals, the family and the community with the national health system, bringing health care as close as possible to where people live and work'. Cook (1999) suggests that this second description of primary care is more useful to nurses who work in the UK. There are, however, other perspectives that can enrich our understanding of this complex concept.

Primary care as an approach, activities, level of care or a philosophy

Primary care as an approach

Macdonald (1992) describes primary health care as an approach to the planning and delivery of health services. The primary healthcare approach encompasses comprehensive healthcare systems which include cure, prevention, health promotion and rehabilitation, with the people who receive the care as equal partners in the process (Blackie 1998). This approach also emphasizes the importance of including primary healthcare professionals in the commissioning of services. An example of this is the introduction of Primary Care Groups (PCGs) and Primary Care Trusts (PCTs) in England. The PCGs and PCTs consist of a group of healthcare professionals and lay people who make decisions about the provision of healthcare services for their population. The NHS plan (Department of Health 2000a) is a further example of the primary care approach to the delivery of health services. The plan states that patients are the most important people in the health service, and a variety of measures has been suggested to help empower and respect patients. These include the provision of more information for patients and greater patient choice. We can see the results of this approach to healthcare provision in services such as NHS Direct and walk-in centres.

Immunization
See chapter 6.2

Primary care activities

Primary care activities include, for example, community dentistry and pharmacy, community nursing, childhood immunization programmes and general practitioner (GP) services. It would not matter where these activities took place; primary care in this example would be defined by the activity rather than the approach or location. It would be possible, then, for a child to receive **immunizations** at the GP surgery or at their school. GP services can be delivered as an out-of-hours service from a base at the local hospital or by the GP travelling to a patient's home. In each

of these examples the service that is delivered to the patients is a primary care service, even though the locations may vary enormously.

Level of care

The level of care refers to the idea of the 'first contact' with health services. A patient may present to the GP surgery as a first point of contact, but they may also present to a minor injuries unit or call NHS Direct. Each of these presentations would be an example of a first point of contact, and would therefore represent primary care. This perspective demonstrates that care provided by a rapid response team in the community setting would not be primary care. The patient would first have accessed health services by contacting a healthcare professional who would then have referred the person on to the rapid response team. The team would then deliver healthcare services to the patient in his or her home, such as the administration of intravenous fluids, monitor the patient and hopefully prevent admission to hospital. In this example the nursing activity would have taken place in the community, but it does not qualify as primary care because the first point of contact was with another healthcare professional.

A philosophy of care

A fundamental feature of the philosophy of primary care is the notion that health is a basic human right. The philosophy of primary care is further defined by Vuori (1986), who states that a country can claim to practise primary care only if its entire healthcare system is characterized by an acceptance of the broad definition of health, social justice and equality, self-responsibility and international solidarity. It is clear from this definition that the active participation of people using health services is placed at the heart of the philosophy of primary care.

It is clear that there is a variety of approaches to understanding the concept of primary care. We can think of it as an approach, a group of activities, a level of care or a philosophy of care. It is evidently not defined by the place in which the activity occurs, although there is an underlying theme that primary health care involves moving service provision closer to the patient. In 1996 the Department of Health (DoH) identified the principles of good primary care in the document *Primary care: delivering the future* (DoH 1996). These are summarized in Box 5.1. It can be seen that these principles reflect the definitions of primary care discussed above, identifying the importance of focusing on the needs of the local population. There is also an emphasis on the healthcare professionals' responsibility to be knowledgeable about the patients they are working with and the conditions that present in primary care.

Quality

- Professionals should be knowledgeable about the conditions that are present in primary care and skilled in their treatment and in contributing to their prevention.

- Professionals should be knowledgeable about the people to whom they are offering services.

- Services should be coordinated with professionals aware of each other's contributions, with interprofessional working and with no service gaps.

- Premises and facilities should be of good standard and fit for their purposes, and equipment should be up to date, well maintained and safe to use.

Fairness

- Services should not vary widely in range or quality in different parts of the country.

- Primary care should receive an appropriate share of overall NHS resources.

Accessibility

- Services should be reasonably accessible when clinically needed.

- Necessary services should be accessible to people regardless of age, sex, ethnicity, disability or health status.

Responsiveness

- Services should reflect the needs and preferences of the individuals using them.

- Services should reflect the health demographic and social needs of the area they serve.

Efficiency

- Primary care services should be based on evidence of clinical effectiveness.

- Primary care resources should be used efficiently.

From Department of Health (1996), with permission.

Policy and primary care

The founding principles of the UK National Health Service have served to provide the basis for the delivery of primary care in the United Kingdom over the past 50 years. On 5 July 1948 the NHS was launched on the principles of equity and universality; the service would be comprehensive, funded by the state and managed by a consensus of professionals. In the early days there was a focus on

Figure 5.1   Organizational structure of the new National Health Service in England.

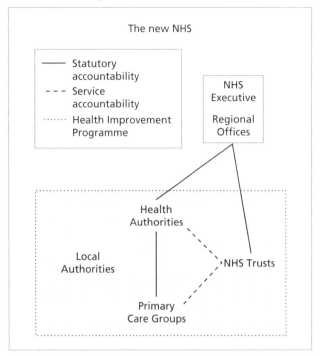

From Department of Health (1997), with permission.

hospitals as the source of administrative power. As there was concern over the use of resources, the administrative power was moved away from the hospitals to regional, area and district authorities. In the early 1980s there was an attempt to reduce bureaucracy by abolishing area health authorities; however, criticism of the inefficiency and unresponsiveness of the system continued. Towards the end of the 1980s three White Papers were released: *Promoting better health* (DoH 1987), *Caring for people* (DoH 1989a) and *Working for patients* (DoH 1989b). This provided the basis for some major reforms in the health service, with a particular shift towards primary care. The NHS and Community Care Act, 1990, provided the statutory basis for the changes outlined in the White Papers. This resulted in radical reform of the health service, with the introduction of the internal market, the development of NHS Trusts, GP fundholding and a new GP contract.

In 1997 the White Paper *The new NHS: modern, dependable* (DoH 1997) was published in England. This heralded the end of the internal market with plans to set up primary care groups (PCGs) and ultimately primary care trusts (PCTs). Typically the PCGs serve a population of 100 000 patients and one of their functions is identified as the development of primary care. They are also charged with working closely with social services and for taking responsibility for commissioning services for the local community. A diagram representing the organizational structure of the new NHS in England can be found in Figure 5.1.

As devolution had taken place during this time, Wales, Scotland and Northern Ireland put forward their own proposals for a reconfiguration of health services.

In *Northern Ireland* the document *Well into 2000: a positive agenda for health and well-being* (DHSS 1997) was published, followed by *Fit for the future* (DHSS 1999). The emphasis is on abolishing the internal market and replacing it with new primary-care-centred locality commissioning. The proposals identify Health and Social Care Partnerships, which will be made up of three to six primary care cooperatives (PCCs). The PCCs will cover communities of 50 000 to 100 000 people and their function will be to commission most health and social services for their populations, work to improve the health and well-being of their populations and improve the delivery of primary care services (DHSS 1999).

The White Paper *Designed to care* (Secretary of State for Scotland 1997) mapped out a plan for *Scotland* that had common goals with the plans for England but was based on a very different organizational structure. *Designed to care* acknowledges the NHS in Scotland as being a single organization with the emphasis on partnership and planning and the abolition of contracting and commissioning. The interface between primary and secondary care is managed through a joint investment fund and the primary care structure is made up of health boards, primary care trusts and local health cooperatives. The primary care trusts are directly accountable to the health board and they include the local health cooperatives. Participation in local health cooperatives is voluntary. *Designed to care* provided no detailed vision of the roles, structure or function of cooperatives and this has resulted in some different models developing across Scotland (Hopton and Heaney 1999). An important point to note is that the primary care trusts do not have the same commissioning power as their equivalents in England and Wales, and this has resulted in some uncertainty amongst healthcare professionals working in the primary care setting.

In *Wales* the document *Putting Patients First* (Welsh Office 1998) outlined the new roles and responsibilities of the health authorities and local health groups. In an attempt to build the NHS around the needs and wishes of the people who use it, local health groups were established to give GPs and others the opportunity to take responsibility for shaping health care to meet local needs. Local health groups have been established as subcommittees of health authorities with responsibility for commissioning local services and making decisions about resources. It is anticipated, however, that the local health groups will evolve from simply supporting the health authority to take progressively more responsibility for managing budgets, and will eventually become free-standing bodies accountable to health authorities.

Each of the organizational structures of primary care outlined above reflects a move away from centrally controlled health service provision to locally led initiatives, with power for commissioning services moving closer to the patient. In July 2000 the NHS Executive in England published the NHS plan (DoH 2000a), and this is a further example of the general shift towards a primary-care-led health service. There is evidence of the national plan operating from the perspective of a primary care approach, focusing on primary care activities, addressing the level of care and operating within a philosophy of primary care. The *primary care approach* to health services is evidenced in recommendations for improvements in curative procedures, prevention of disease, promotion of health and rehabilitation. For example, the national plan suggests that ambulance paramedics be trained to provide thrombolysis for patients who are experiencing myocardial infarction; this is estimated to save up to 3000 lives per year and should protect patients against the potential damage to their heart. There is a variety of approaches to prevention of disease, one of which is the fact that the NHS breast screening programme is being extended to include women aged 65–70 years, resulting in 400 000 more women having mammography each year. Health promotion is being implemented through a commitment to smoking cessation across the country, and rehabilitation is addressed through the promotion of independence in old age through active recovery and rehabilitation services.

There is also evidence of the plan focusing on the *activities of primary care* such as community pharmacy and GP services, and there is a pledge to increase the number of walk-in centres across the country. The *level of care* is addressed through the issue of speed of access to services. The plan guarantees that patients will have access to a primary care professional within 24 hours and to a primary care doctor within 48 hours by 2004. The plan addresses equity of access to services and closer liaison between social services and health service management. It could therefore be suggested that a *philosophy* of primary care underpins the English NHS plan, creating an exciting climate for the work of primary care nurses.

The nurse's role in primary health care

Primary care represents the context in which community nursing is delivered. The UKCC identifies eight areas of specialist practice for nurses who work in the community. There are, however, many nurses who work as generic community nurses and do not have a recordable specialist qualification; there are also others who work in roles that are not included in the eight specialty areas identified by the UKCC, and we will consider these nurses as we address the broader concept of nursing in primary care. The specialist areas of practice as defined by the UKCC are listed in Box 5.2. There is a great deal of overlap between the eight specialist areas and it is therefore difficult to identify tight definitions of each role; instead, some broad comments can be made about the type of work carried out by nurses in each of these roles.

Box 5.2   Specialist nurses in the community

- District nurses
- Practice nurses
- Community mental health nurses
- Community learning disabilities nurses
- Community children's nurses
- School nurses
- Occupational health nurses
- Public health nursing/health visiting.

District nurses tend to deliver nursing care to people in their own homes. To carry out this work, the district nurse needs to have a whole range of technical nursing skills to manage effectively patients who are increasingly being discharged early from hospital. District nurses also need to have case management skills so that they can organize the delivery of nursing care. The district nursing team needs to be able to liaise effectively with people in the hospital setting to assist with discharge planning, and with social services to help coordinate a team of people to care for people in their home setting.

Practice nurses have traditionally been employed directly by GPs to work in general practice surgeries. Practice nurses cover a whole range of healthcare activities in the surgery including travel health, cervical cytology, women's health clinics, immunizations, **diabetic** and respiratory clinics, venepuncture, coronary heart disease clinics and many more. The role of the practice nurse has developed differently in different surgeries according to the skills of the nurse and the needs of the local population. Some practice nurses have extended their work to include minor injuries clinics and telephone triage, and others visit people in their homes to deliver their specialist skills to those who could not otherwise access their services. This is an example of the way in which the role of a district nurse and a practice nurse might overlap and provides an illustration of the value of working together as a integrated team where the boundaries between roles are flexible.

Community mental health nurses are known in many parts of the UK as community psychiatric nurses. Mental health nurses may be based in a surgery or community clinic and many develop a specialty in a particular area of care, such as working with children or the elderly. Preparation for this role begins with the mental health branch following the common foundation programme of pre-registration education.

Community learning disabilities nurses work in the community setting to support people with learning disabilities in their homes. The learning disabilities nurse will have particular skills in the assessment, planning and implementation of specialist clinical nursing for individuals who have a learning disability. This may include the management of critical events such as challenging or violent behaviour. The aim of learning disabilities nurses is to maximize the clients' potential for independent living and to minimize the effects of their disability. This may involve working with families, carers and other agencies, such as social services, speech therapists and other members of the multidisciplinary team. Like community mental health nurses, community learning disabilities nurses begin their educational preparation in pre-registration courses by choosing the learning disabilities branch following the common foundation programme.

Community children's nurses assist children to stay in their own homes as long as possible, thereby avoiding admission to hospital whenever possible. Some children's nurses have become extremely specialized focusing on childhood oncology or **cystic fibrosis**, for example, and different models of practice operate in different areas of the country. In some areas community children's nurses operate an 'outreach' service where the nurses are based in the hospital and visit children at home when they are in need of their specialist skills; in other areas the nurses offer an 'in-reach' service where community-based children's nurses maintain some responsibility for children when they are in the hospital (Cook 1999). Again, nurses who wish to specialize in this area of community nursing will choose the child branch of the common foundation programme.

School nurses are responsible for the health-related needs of children at school. The school nurse is involved in health screening, health surveillance and therapeutic techniques to maintain the health of children, adolescents and the family. The nurse working in a school may act as the first point of contact for children in the school setting and will therefore need a whole range of skills associated with children's nursing, including the identification of child protection issues and methods of minimizing risk. Like all the specialist community roles, school nurses will be involved in the health education of children, and many school nurses get involved in health fayres for children and after-school activities. Some school nurses have extended their role to include the provision of clinics away from the school setting after school hours, to allow children to consult with them away from the watchful eyes of their peers. This can help to reduce embarrassment and meet the needs of children who would not have otherwise approached the healthcare system for support. This is yet another example of the fluid boundaries in the primary healthcare setting.

Occupational health nurses are specialists in the provision of services to people in their work settings. This group of nurses can be involved in a whole variety of activities including the management of clinical emergencies, the assessment of people who feel unwell at work, health promotion activities and carrying out health checks for people in the workplace. Occupational health nurses also

Diabetes
See chapter 2.6

Cystic fibrosis
See chapter 6.3

have a responsibility to interpret and apply health and safety legislation and approved codes of practice with regard for the environment, well-being and protection of those who work and the wider community.

Public health nursing/health visiting is concerned with health promotion and the prevention of ill-health (Blackie 1998). In 1977 the Council for the Education and Training of Health Visitors (CETHV) set out the principles of health visiting; these include the search for health needs, stimulation of the awareness of health needs, influence on policies affecting health, and the facilitation of health-enhancing activities. A quarter of a century later, these four principles remain important and relevant. In practice, health visitors work in a variety of settings in the community including health centres, surgeries, community halls and hostels. The health-visiting role can lead to work with travelling families and other populations that tend to have difficulty accessing mainstream healthcare services. The health visitor qualification is the only community specialist qualification that is statutory and registrable with the UKCC. A nurse cannot work as a health visitor without successfully completing a recognized course for health visiting/public health nursing.

Diabetes
See chapter 2.6

Rheumatoid disease
See chapter 3.6

There are many other nurses who work in the community and form part of the primary healthcare team; however, their roles are not captured in the eight specialist areas listed above. There are nurses who work as continence advisers, who may be based in the hospital setting but 'reach out' into the community, and others who work in the community and 'reach in' to the hospital. There are also new ways of operating in primary care such as NHS Direct, where the patient's first point of contact with the healthcare service (and often the only point of contact) is with a nurse at the end of a telephone line. The nurse on the telephone may not be one of the eight specialist community nurses, but instead will be a nurse with specialist training in telephone consultations using a computer program to guide decision making and the provision of advice. Nurse practitioners are also working in many settings where they are the first point of contact for the patient, and their role is not captured by the eight specialist areas identified by the UKCC.

In recognition of the overlap between nurses in the various specialist roles in the community setting and the need for each group to understand the role of others in the team, the educational preparation for community specialists is based on a shared core curriculum with additional specialist competencies for each of the eight areas. One of the aims of this educational approach is to enhance the possibility of nurses in the community working as an integrated team. As previously mentioned, however, there are a variety of other nurses working in primary care including nurse practitioners, continence advisers, stoma nurses and others. Healthcare professionals in primary care will also interact with nurses from specialty areas in secondary care such as respiratory health, **diabetes**, **rheumatology** and dermatology and it could be suggested that this group of practitioners should also be included in the team. The following section will focus on teamwork in primary care.

The primary healthcare team

The provision of primary health care is a complex and massive task. Recent documents from the Department of Health (DoH 1997, 2000b) have identified the need to develop the roles of healthcare professionals working in the primary care team in recognition of the fact that nurses, doctors, pharmacists and other healthcare professionals all have a great deal to offer patients, and their potential should therefore be realized. It is no longer possible for one healthcare professional to deliver all the care required by a particular population, and so it is necessary to work in teams. Working in a team can be a challenge, although it also has several potential benefits. The benefits of teamwork include the following (Pritchard and Pritchard 1994, Blackie 1998):

- Care given by a group is greater than the sum of its parts.

- Team members are better supported and have increased job satisfaction.

- Rare skills can be made more available to patients.

- Prevention and curative work can be better coordinated.

- Team members can learn from one another.

- The patient receives more efficient care when ill.

Membership of the primary healthcare team is an issue that is frequently debated. Some suggest that the team should be defined by the provision of day-to-day clinical care and therefore the team members would include the health visitor, district nurse, practice nurse and GP (Blackie 1998). Others have suggested that the team is defined by the GP and the members of staff employed by the GP, which would therefore include receptionists, practice managers, and the practice nurse, and in many cases exclude the district nurse and health visitor. Bryar and Bytheway (1996) found that there seemed to be a multiplicity of teams working together to provide primary care services. They found that the team would come together to meet the needs of different sections of the population. One team might develop around the provision of services to people with diabetes and another might emerge in relation to screening for cervical cancer. It could be suggested that a particular healthcare professional's inclusion in the primary healthcare team is determined by the needs of the patient, so you can see that the primary healthcare team is not a fixed entity: rather it is a dynamic system that has the patient at its core.

Pritchard and Pritchard (1994) state that a team can be described as intrinsic, functional or full. The intrinsic

Figure 5.2   The intrinsic team changes according to the needs of the patient.

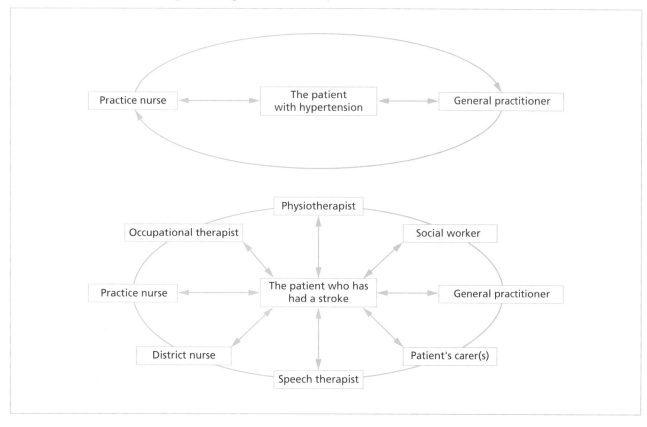

team has the patient at its core as an active participant in care. Other members of the intrinsic team will then be determined by the needs of the patient so that, in the example of a patient with **hypertension**, the team might include the patient, the practice nurse and the GP. If this particular patient had a **stroke**, membership of the intrinsic team might change to include the patient's carer, district nurse, social worker, occupational therapist and physiotherapist (see Fig. 5.2).

A functional team is defined by its purpose. An example of a functional team might be the group of people who come together to provide maternity services or healthcare services for people with diabetes. It might be suggested that the patient or the group of patients should still remain firmly at the core of the functional team as this provides the purpose for the team's existence.

Pritchard and Pritchard (1994) suggest that, on some occasions, the full team needs to gather, perhaps to make decisions related to major issues such as altering the health centre's times of opening, changing the way referrals are made between team members, or developing new protocols for the provision of health services by the team. Clearly, the full team would involve many more people than the intrinsic team; however, there are times when it is essential to include as many people as possible to make sure that the team continues to operate smoothly and that communication between team members remains effective.

Another important issue to consider here is how the team carries out its work. Teamwork can be described as multidisciplinary or interdisciplinary (integrated). The approach taken has an impact upon the healthcare professionals in the team and – more importantly – the patient's experience.

Multidisciplinary teamwork

The multidisciplinary team is the model most commonly used in primary healthcare teams. Multidisciplinary teamwork can be defined as a group of professionals providing their own expertise regardless of the techniques used by other team members. The patient in this example is perceived as a series of 'problems' to be solved. If a 75-year-old man was dying at home after surgery for gastric cancer, the district nurse might attend the patient to deal with his **wound**, the Macmillan nurse might attend to address his pain control needs and the social worker might attend to provide advice on benefits and support. An advantage of this approach is that team members tend to have a fairly clear idea of their own and others' role in the work of caring for a particular patient: roles are clearly demarcated and overlap between roles is minimized. The disadvantage is that the patient becomes split into a series of parts and some of his needs may therefore be missed. He may, for example, be experiencing depression but

Hypertension
See chapter 4.2

Stroke
See chapter 2.2

Wound healing
See chapter 6.1

because there is no mental health nurse included in the team this particular problem may be overlooked and the patient may have to struggle with his problem without assistance.

Interdisciplinary teamwork

Interdisciplinary or integrated teamwork delivers coordinated, non-hierarchical, holistic care involving the patient and family (Blackie 1998). The interdisciplinary team is focused explicitly on the patient's needs and is involved in formal, structured meetings to plan goals. If we consider the example outlined above, the team involved in the provision of care for this 75-year-old man would meet and aim to identify his needs and how best to meet them. The provision of care would then be determined by the needs of the patient, not by the make-up of the team that happened to be visiting him.

A further example might be the team's approach to the provision of care for people with **diabetes**. The team would need to meet regularly to plan a unified approach to patient education in relation to dietary advice, for example, and the ongoing monitoring of people with diabetes; some overlap of role would be expected and a unified approach would be developed. The advantage of this approach is that the patient is treated more holistically and is more likely to be able to see the value of the service provided.

A difficulty with the interdisciplinary approach is that roles between professionals can become blurred and this can cause some problems in the team as people become less clear of their own purpose within the team. A great deal of teamwork skill is required to overcome this problem. If all team members can manage to live with the lack of clear boundaries between their roles, working in a model such as this can be extremely satisfying for everyone, including the patient. All members of the primary healthcare team have an important role to play in working with people who have chronic illness, and in this area, more than most, it is vital that the team is integrated and works together effectively.

Chronic illness

As a nurse working in the primary healthcare setting you will have an important role in working with people who live with chronic conditions. The nurse working in general practice, for example, may run clinics aimed at the management and monitoring of a variety of conditions. Practice nurses run clinics for people with **asthma**, diabetes, **coronary heart disease**, **hypertension** and **epilepsy**, for instance. District nurses will frequently be working in the home with people who have any one of these conditions, and health visitors work with families with children who live with a chronic condition such as asthma, eczema or epilepsy.

Diabetes
See chapter 2.6

Asthma
See chapter 5.3

Coronary heart disease
See chapter 4.2

Hypertension
See chapter 4.2

Epilepsy
See chapter 2.2

Blood pressure
See chapter 4.2

How do we define 'chronic illness'?

Working with people who live with chronic illness is described by Funk et al (1993) as being at the heart of nursing. So, what is chronic illness and how does it differ from a condition or disease? Often these words are used interchangeably and yet there are important, although subtle, differences between the three. Illness refers to the human experience and to the perceptions of the patient and family and their responses to the symptoms and suffering caused by the disease process. Disease, on the other hand, refers to a problem that can be viewed from the medical perspective and can be defined by alterations in the structure and function of the body. A condition is a state of being and as such it describes the whole experience of a person who lives with chronic illness.

Chronic disease management, then, refers to the activities carried out in the primary care setting with patients who live with diseases such as diabetes, hypertension, epilepsy and asthma. The patient's disease is managed with the help of the healthcare professional through annual monitoring for the signs of neuropathy in the feet in diabetes, or of **blood pressure** recordings in the hypertensive patient, for example. The role of nursing, however, goes way beyond the assessment of feet and the recording of blood pressures. Because we work with people who live with these diseases, we need to consider their experience of the illness. Our nursing assessment includes a review of their understanding of the condition, how they are managing with their medications, and what involvement their family has in the process. There are many roles that a nurse can assume when working with a patient who has a chronic illness; these are explored later in this chapter.

Having considered what we mean by the terms condition, illness and disease, we now need to develop an understanding of the term 'chronicity'. Curtin and Lubkin (1998) state that it is extremely difficult to define chronicity. Many authors have attempted to capture the essence of this concept, some with simple and brief definitions and others with lengthy and complex explanations. Several of these definitions will be explored here to provide a variety of perspectives on the term 'chronic'; you may find one that you feel relates well to the people with whom you work, or two or three that capture the essence of chronic illness from your own perspective.

Kelly and Field (1996) point out that chronic illness results in the physical reality of 'bad' bodies. The body changes in chronic illness and can be seen as letting the person down. Bleeker and Mulderij (1992) speak of the body losing its silence, and Morse et al (1994) describe a body in disease. These are simple but effective comments on the experience of living with a chronic illness. The patient becomes acutely aware of his or her body. People who are without chronic illness do not experience this. The constant monitoring required in type 1 diabetes means that the patient becomes acutely aware of responses to certain foods, exercise, and simple colds and infections. People who do not have a chronic condition usually live alongside their bodies with little awareness of daily fluctuations in response to the stressors placed upon them. Clearly, chronicity involves a heightened awareness of the physical self which permeates the whole being.

Cameron and Gregor (1987) argue that chronic illness is a lived experience that involves a permanent deviation from the norm caused by unalterable pathological changes. The problem with this definition is that it labels people who have chronic illness as being abnormal. Certainly one of the important aspects of defining chronicity is the notion of permanence. Chronic conditions are not curable and this has an enormous impact upon our approach to working with people who live with chronicity. An important point to note is that most people live with rather than die from a chronic condition (Verbrugge and Jette 1994).

Several authors have offered more complex definitions of chronicity. Lyons et al (1995) state that a chronic illness is not a singular event, rather it signifies a set of complex processes that develop and endure over time. This links with the trajectory model of chronic illness outlined by Corbin and Strauss (1992), who refer to the journey of chronic illness as a trajectory, a course that varies over time and can be divided into subphases. The course of the chronic illness can be shaped and managed, and this is where we can have an impact upon the patient's experience of their disease. Funk et al (1993, p. 3) quote the 1956 definition of chronic illness by the Commission on Chronic Illness as 'being caused by pathological changes in the body that are non-reversible, permanent or leave residual disability; they may be characterised by periods of recurrence and remission and they generally require extended periods of supervision, observation, care and rehabilitation'. Curtin and Lubkin (1998, p. 6) offer a further definition of chronic illness as 'the irreversible presence, accumulation, or latency of disease states or impairments that involve the total human environment for supportive care and self-care, maintenance of function and prevention of further disability'.

It is valuable for us to develop our understanding of what it is like to live with a chronic illness because it will assist in our nursing assessment of the patient. Two important themes that seem to run through the various definitions of chronicity are the idea of the condition being permanent and that it alters the patient's awareness of his or her body. There is also a sense of *living with* the condition and being on a journey. This helps to put our interventions with patients into perspective and, as we now move on to consider the management of patients with chronic illnesses in primary care, you might want to consider how your actions could have an impact upon the patients' lived experience of their condition.

Chronic illness management in primary care

There is no doubt that a structured approach to working with people who live with a chronic condition will enhance the standard of care (DoH 2000). The structure needs to span the primary healthcare/hospital divide and should be flexible enough always to have at its centre the individual patient. The following discussion will outline the elements of a structured approach to care of the person with a chronic condition in primary health care and will go on to consider the nursing skills that you can utilize with this specific group of patients.

Setting up a register

A starting point for chronic disease management is the development of a register of patients who have the particular condition. If you work in a general practice, the patients in the practice who can be searched for are those who are identified as having the particular problem. If you are a health visitor attached to several practices, you can search your own caseload of children, for example, and identify how many of them have a particular condition. If the practice nurse finds that there are 40 patients with diabetes mellitus in her practice population when the total population is 2000, the prevalence of **diabetes** in that practice would be 2%. This is an important finding because we know that the national prevalence of diabetes mellitus is 3%; it can be as high as 10% in people over the age of 75 years and as much as 16% in the 40–65-year-old Asian population. If your practice seems to have a low prevalence of diabetes, it is worthwhile considering whether there are undiagnosed patients in the practice and therefore whether it is worth developing a screening programme to find the missing patients.

The example of a practice profile in Table 5.1 demonstrates the interesting information that can be elicited when a register is compiled. The information shown was gathered after a search for patients with **coronary heart disease** had taken place at the surgery. The healthcare team used various approaches to identify patients who had coronary heart disease. A computer search was carried out to identify all the patients who were taking nitrate medications. The nitrates are used to alleviate the occurrence of chest pain in people with ischaemic heart disease and therefore this is a good place to start. Medications used in heart failure such as digoxin were also used to identify more patients. The healthcare team also had a working knowledge of who in their care had experienced a myocardial infarction or surgery for coronary artery bypass grafting, and so this knowledge was used to identify further patients on the register. Eventually the numbers shown were presented as the practice register of people with coronary heart disease.

Diabetes
See chapter 2.6

Coronary heart disease
See chapter 4.2

Table 5.1 Ischaemic heart disease register

Age group (years)	Males	Females
0–4	0 (0)	0 (0)
5–16	0 (0)	0 (0)
17–24	0 (0)	0 (0)
25–34	0 (0)	0 (0)
35–44	0 (0)	0 (0)
45–54	3 (3)	0 (0)
55–64	5 (7)	2 (3)
65–74	10 (23)	2 (3)
75–84	8 (22)	12 (22)
85–89	3 (38)	5 (25)
⩾90	0 (0)	2 (17)
Total males	29 (5)	
Total females	23 (4)	
Total both sexes	52 (4)	

Values in parentheses are percentages of the total population in a particular age range within the practice.

Asthma
See chapter 5.3

Coronary heart
disease
See chapter 4.2

Rheumatoid
arthritis
See chapter 3.3

A list such as this, then, raises some important questions. We know that the national prevalence of coronary heart disease is 7% and yet the practice information shows a prevalence of 5%. This may be because this particular population does not have many risk factors for heart disease and therefore the prevalence is low; it may also be because the patients with heart disease have not been fully identified in the practice. It is particularly interesting to note that the prevalence in 65–74-year-old women is 3%, compared with 23% in men: the practice can now target this group for a series of health checks as there may be a number of women with undiagnosed ischaemic heart disease in this group.

The register of people with a particular condition is not only valuable for identifying undiagnosed patients who, in the case of diabetes, might benefit greatly from early diagnosis and treatment, but is also useful for structuring and evaluating a programme of care. The programme of care will depend upon the nature of the condition. For people with **asthma**, for example, the patients may be recalled for an assessment in the asthma clinic on an annual basis, or for people who suffer from psychotic illness a review of their records might take place each year to ensure that appropriate investigations have taken place for blood levels such as lithium and that a person has been identified as the main healthcare worker responsible for care.

This information has become even more important with the development of national standards such as the National Service Frameworks (NSFs) for England and Wales. The NSFs outline national standards and, once a register of people with a particular condition has been created, an assessment can be made as to the effectiveness of the care they are receiving. For example, the NSF for **coronary heart disease** states that 'general practitioners

and primary healthcare teams should identify all people with established cardiovascular disease and offer them comprehensive advice and appropriate treatment to reduce their risks' (DoH 2000b, p. 4). Clearly it is important for the primary healthcare team to identify how many people have clinical evidence of occlusive arterial disease in the practice population and then to identify who these people are so that their treatment and the advice they have received can be measured against the agreed national standards.

Call/recall systems

To manage the register of people effectively, a call/recall system should be developed. This can involve any member of the primary healthcare team; the important thing is that someone is identified as the person responsible for the system and that all members of the team involved in the care of people in a particular group feed back into the system. In the area of asthma, for example, the practice might have its own register of people who live with asthma. The health visitor might also know who in his or her caseload has been diagnosed with asthma, and the school nurse might have a similar register. The school nurse might also notice a child who seems to be short of breath in the playground and will refer potential new cases of asthma to the general practice.

The important issue is that someone in the team is reviewing the people with asthma at least annually. If the school nurse carries out the review, that information needs to be shared with the practice and the health visitor, and similarly, if the practice carries out the review the fact that a review has taken place needs to be shared with the rest of the team. In some situations patients may be reviewed in secondary care. People with **rheumatoid arthritis**, for example, are often managed by specialist nurses and/or hospital consultants, and this information needs to be fed back to the general practice. It is important that the whole healthcare team communicates, and that for each condition someone is identified as the person responsible for maintaining the call/recall system.

People with the following types of chronic condition could benefit from a register and a call/recall system:

- thyroid disorders
- diabetes mellitus
- asthma
- chronic obstructive airway disease
- epilepsy
- rheumatoid arthritis
- psychotic disorder
- coronary heart disease
- hypertension.

Figure 5.3   Audit cycle.

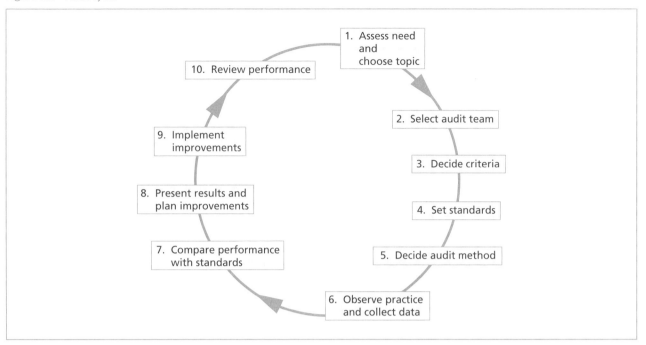

1. Assess need and choose topic
2. Select audit team
3. Decide criteria
4. Set standards
5. Decide audit method
6. Observe practice and collect data
7. Compare performance with standards
8. Present results and plan improvements
9. Implement improvements
10. Review performance

Evaluating the programme of care

Once the register and the call/recall systems have been set up, you can readily evaluate your programme of care for a particular group of people by carrying out an audit. Indeed, if you are planning to introduce a new approach to clinical practice in your area it is valuable to carry out an audit before you implement the change. In this way you can identify areas of weakness before changes are made and you will be able to use the audit to evaluate how effective your intervention has been.

The main reason for carrying out an audit is to improve patient care. The patient should always be placed at the centre of the cycle of audit so that we do not lose sight of the reasons for carrying out this activity. Carrying out an audit can also help to educate everyone involved in the process; it can enhance teamwork and help people to understand one another's roles in more depth. Audit involves several steps, which are summarized as a cycle in Figure 5.3.

Assess need and choose a topic

The first step is to identify an area of clinical practice that needs to be evaluated through audit. You can make this choice in several ways. The subject area may come to you when a patient mentions something to you in practice. For example, a patient might comment that it seems to be a long time since he had his blood pressure checked. You look back in the notes and find that it is over 18 months since the last recorded **blood pressure** reading. This patient has a history of **cardiovascular disease** and

during this consultation you find that his blood pressure is 160/95 mmHg. You are aware that the National Service Framework for **coronary heart disease** (DoH 2000b) recommends that people with established cardiovascular disease should receive advice and treatment to maintain blood pressure below 140/85 mmHg, and you therefore become concerned that your primary healthcare team might be falling short of the national standards for health care.

Alternatively, you may identify an area for evaluation by reading about standards of health care in journals or in the publications from the national organizations. You may note that Diabetes UK recommends that all people who live with diabetes in the UK should expect to have their vision checked by an appropriately qualified healthcare professional at least once a year. You may then start to ask yourself whether your practice meets this standard; you can carry out an audit to check whether you meet this standard. These are examples of the ways in which you can implement evidence-based practice in the clinical setting.

Select the audit team

There is great value in approaching an audit from a team perspective. Various members of the team will have different suggestions to offer regarding the appropriate standards to use, the methods of collecting information, and methods for improving performance once the data have been collected. Audit can be as easy as pressing a button on a computer or it may require a trawl through many sets of patients' notes. This can be very time consuming

Blood pressure
See chapter 4.2

Cardiovascular system
See chapter 4.2

Coronary heart disease
See chapter 4.2

and it may require several members of the audit team to assist with the retrieval of information. Involving the team also has the added benefit of raising the profile of whatever the subject area is and raising general awareness of the issue in the team.

Decide on criteria

A criterion is an item of care or some other aspect of clinical practice that we can use to assess quality. Each criterion should be recorded in a statement. The National Service Frameworks have helped to provide clear statements that serve as criteria for audit; for example, the coronary heart disease NSF states that all people with clinical evidence of occlusive arterial disease should have advice and treatment to maintain their **blood pressure** below 140/85 mmHg. Your primary healthcare team could identify this as the criterion and record the statement that all people with clinical evidence of occlusive arterial disease should have their most recent blood pressure recorded as 140/85 mmHg or below.

Set standards

Blood pressure
See chapter 4.2

Cardiovascular
system
See chapter 4.2

Bronchodilation
See chapter 5.3

Asthma
See chapter 5.3

Once the criteria have been identified, the standards need to be agreed by the team. A standard is a statement of the proportion of occasions or patients that must fulfil the criteria. For example, in the example of blood pressure recordings in people with coronary heart disease the team might agree that the target should be set at 80%. The National Service Framework states that the blood pressure target of 140/85 mmHg is challenging and it will not be possible to achieve this for every patient. Whilst it is acceptable, then, to set a standard that is less than 100%, practitioners should not be satisfied with any blood pressure recording over 150/90 mmHg. So the standard for the audit in this example might be recorded as '80% of the patients who are identified as having clinical evidence of occlusive arterial disease should have their most recent blood pressure recorded as 140/85 mmHg or below'.

Decide on the audit method

Clearly the method of carrying out the audit will depend upon the subject area and the criterion chosen. In the example of blood pressure recordings and the group of patients with occlusive arterial disease, a computer search could be carried out to find all the people who have blood pressure recordings that fall within the acceptable range. If the audit had been focused upon the safe transport of specimens to the laboratory, the criterion might have been that all specimens should be securely placed in a sealed bag for transport to the laboratory, the standard set might have been 100% and then the audit method might involve a review of the specimens before they are handed to the person who will transport them to the laboratory. Each specimen could be checked for the way it had been packaged for transport and whether the bag had been sealed appropriately.

Observe practice and collect data

The team needs to decide for how long they are going to collect data and/or how many data they need to acquire in order to obtain an accurate reflection of what is actually happening in practice. In computerized systems it is quite straightforward to audit all the patients on the system, and therefore our example of blood pressure recordings and **cardiovascular disease** could be carried out on the whole practice population. However, when the audit is focused on something that is not readily available on the computer, the team may need to decide to look at a sample of the overall population to gain a general impression of the standard of practice in that particular area. The question is how many instances of a particular practice does one need to observe in order to gain an accurate picture of the whole? This decision can be made by calculating the number of occurrences of the criterion, and then collecting data on the size of the sample required. In the example of the specimens for transport, the team might find that 2000 samples are sent to the laboratory annually. The team may decide to sample 10% of the specimens and would therefore need to collect data on the next 200 samples sent to the lab. It is clear that the larger the sample the more valid your results will be. You may therefore decide to sample 80% of people with diabetes when you are carrying out an audit of diabetes care, thus enhancing the validity of the results of your audit.

When you are collecting data you might also want to consider the time of year you carry out your audit. If, for example, you were looking at the use of **bronchodilators** in people with **asthma**, you might find that during the winter months there is a rise in the use of relief inhalers in this population, and again during times of high pollen counts the rate of inhaler use might increase. In a situation like this you may benefit from conducting an audit that runs over a whole year by taking the fourth week in every month to collect your data. It is important to be continually aware of threats to the accuracy of your audit. The results of your audit will inform your subsequent practice and therefore it is essential to make sure that the information you produce is accurate.

Compare performance with standards

Once the data have been collected, you are in a position to determine how close you are to the standards that you set yourself. If you find that only 50% of the people in the coronary heart disease group have a blood pressure of 140/85 mmHg or below, then you can start to search for reasons why this is so. If you find that 90% of the target group has a blood pressure in the desired range, you can be pleased that the team's performance measures up to the agreed standards; however, the cycle does not stop there.

Present results and plan improvements

An important part of the audit cycle is dissemination of your findings to other members of the team. You may choose to present the results in a report or to share your results at a meeting. Whatever the results, the team needs to be aware of them in order to analyse the findings and either seek to maintain the standard or work out a plan for improvement. If the results of your audit into blood pressure readings found that only 50% of the population had a **blood pressure** in the agreed range, the team could be invited to suggest reasons for this. It may be that people with cardiovascular disease are not systematically reviewed every 12 months, or it may be that the cardiovascular disease clinic is being held at inappropriate times for the people it is seeking to attract. It may be that not all healthcare professionals in the team were aware of the new guidelines for the management of blood pressure in this particular group and were therefore not considering this group for rigorous treatment of hypertension. Whatever the reasons identified in an area such as this, it is most likely that there will be several approaches to improving care. These need to be identified by the team, agreed upon and a plan of action should be documented.

If you found that you exceeded the standard and that 90% of the target population had a blood pressure recording in the agreed zone, you might ask yourself whether this could be improved even further and adjust the standard to 95% on the next audit occasion. You might also try to identify areas of good practice that have allowed your team to reach such a good standard. This can then be shared with other primary healthcare teams, and your findings can be disseminated with a wider group so that others may learn from your good practice.

Implement improvements

The team then needs to decide how the plans are to be implemented. You may have identified the need for more flexible surgery times or the need for different members of the team to become involved in this area of practice. For example, the primary healthcare team may have thought that the GP had sole responsibility for the maintenance of blood pressure in the group of people with cardiovascular disease, when in fact your audit identified that several housebound people had blood pressures exceeding the target and these people were being visited regularly by the district nursing team. An improvement that could be implemented might be that the district nurses assess the patients' blood pressure when they visit them at home and that they record this reading in the practice notes and speak with the rest of the primary healthcare team if the recording exceeds the acceptable limit.

Review performance

Once you have implemented the planned changes you will need to revisit the audit to see whether you have really made a difference in practice. You might carry out the same audit and compare your findings with the previous audit, or you might focus on one area of practice that was highlighted as problematic in the first audit. The cycle of audit is continuous as we strive for more effective and efficient ways of working.

Working with patients who live with a chronic condition

In addition to developing registers of people with chronic conditions, managing call/recall systems and ensuring that the existing provision meets agreed standards of care, there are many aspects of the nursing role that can have an impact upon the patients' experience of their condition. When you consider the uncertainty, stigma, grief, management of treatment regimens and alteration in family relations that are characteristic of life with a chronic illness, you can see that your role as a nurse can have an enormous impact upon the patient in a variety of ways.

It is sad to note, however, that nurses do not appear to value working with patients whose conditions are not curable (Nolan and Nolan 1995). Instead we seem to prefer to work with patients who will recover fully from their disease, and our actions with people who have a chronic condition are focused as though the patient was suffering from an acute episode of illness. Gibson and Kenrick (1998) studied a group of people who had peripheral **vascular disease** and found that the patients tended to think of the revascularization surgical approaches used as being curative and the medical team did nothing to refute this belief. In fact, the patients' vascular disease was not being cured, it was simply being managed temporarily, and therefore the patients needed to receive an approach to care that acknowledged the chronicity of their condition. Gibson and Kenrick (1998) concluded that this particular group of patients suffered from the inappropriate application of therapeutic approaches designed for use in acute episodes. It is possible that this is an example of the healthcare professionals' desire to work with people who have acute episodes of care rather than people who live with chronic conditions. As the numbers of people who live with chronic illness increase, it is possible that work in this area of practice will be recognized as a specialty in its own right. As this happens we will begin to appreciate that different approaches are required with this group of patients and nursing skills will be identified as being especially appropriate.

In your role as a nurse in primary care you have a great deal to offer a person who lives with a chronic condition. The ability to communicate effectively and to be able to listen to the patient's concerns can have a huge impact

Blood pressure:
See chapter 4.2

Vascular system:
See chapter 4.2

upon the patient and his or her family. When we make a nursing assessment of the patient with a chronic condition we need to consider the individual patient and alter our approach accordingly. It is important to remember that the patient has the most important role to play, as people who live with chronic conditions do most of the work associated with managing the illness themselves. There are, however, many roles we can take on in this situation; the exact nature of our role will be determined by the patient's individual needs at the time and the projected needs for the future. There is no doubt that we need to be clinically skilled in the area of disease management for that particular patient. When working with people who have continence problems, for example, there is no substitute for an indepth knowledge of the management of continence and the clinical application of this knowledge. In addition to the specialist knowledge required it will also be important to be able to work effectively with patients who have general needs such as the acquisition of new knowledge and skills. One of the important roles we can play in this instance is the role of educator.

The nurse as educator

Diabetes
See chapter 2.6

Blood pressure
See chapter 4.2

Cholesterol
See chapter 5.2

When a person is first diagnosed with a chronic condition they are likely to have many questions about their condition. People with diabetes might ask whether the condition is going to shorten their life, or people with asthma might want to know whether this will stop them playing sport. It is important that you discover the patient's beliefs and values, and what the most pressing questions are for him or her. If you do not address the immediate questions, the patient will not be able to internalize any of the important self-care messages you might want to pass on, and the rest of the educative role becomes meaningless. The following critical incident is based on this issue.

Critical incident

A week after I had arranged for a series of blood and urine tests, I met with Mr A to discuss the results. The blood tests had confirmed our suspicions that he had type 2 **diabetes mellitus**. I asked him whether he knew what diabetes was; he said he knew very little and did not know anyone who had the disease. I explained what was happening and began to discuss the first line of management, which is to follow the general healthy-eating guidelines. I asked him to describe his usual pattern of eating and then I began to explain in detail the approach to dietary management. I was also aware that I needed to explain to him that he should have his eyes checked, feet assessed, a follow-up for

determination of his blood sugar levels in 3 months' time, a referral to a dietician and careful monitoring of his **blood pressure** and **cholesterol** levels.

It was clear, though, that Mr A was distracted. After explaining the first step of dietary management I asked him whether there was anything that was bothering him about the diagnosis. After a short silence he asked me: 'What does this mean? Am I going to die?'. We discussed his fears and concerns, and I returned to the explanation of diabetes and the importance of monitoring and treating raised blood glucose levels and blood pressure readings. I talked about the risks of complications and emphasized all that he could do to prevent their development. The consultation ended there with a plan to meet again in 2 weeks' time to see how he was managing with his dietary changes. My plan was to review some of the areas we had discussed during this consultation and to introduce some of the topics we had not covered on this first encounter.

Reflections

I felt that this consultation was fairly straightforward. The diagnosis of diabetes was expected and I felt competent to explain this to Mr A. I was aware that it is possible to overload patients with information when they are first given the diagnosis of diabetes and I was therefore attentive to the cues Mr A was giving off. I was quite taken aback by his question 'Am I going to die?' and, knowing the statistics on the mortality rates for people with diabetes, I felt lost for an immediate answer to his question. It would have been easy to say 'Of course not!', but I did not want to reassure him falsely. I was struck by the enormity of the question and realized that there was no way he could listen to what I was saying until we had discussed his fears and concerns regarding the impact of diabetes on his life.

Questions for reflection

- How might you break the news of the diagnosis of diabetes to a patient?

- What questions could you use to learn more about the patient's concerns?

- What support mechanisms are available to Mr A?

- What would be your plan for follow-up?

- Which members of the interdisciplinary team might you include in Mr A's care?

- Identify examples of communication skills that would be helpful in addressing Mr A's needs.

See Appendix 2 for guidelines on reflection.

Figure 5.4   Teaching and learning process.

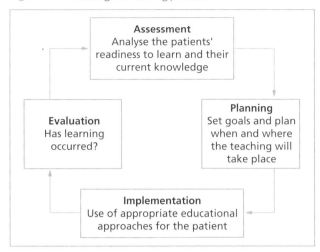

Bopp and Lubkin (1998) suggest that the teaching–learning process involves four phases: assessment, planning, implementation and evaluation (Fig. 5.4). The assessment process involves an analysis of the patient's readiness to learn. The reflection outlined in the critical incident provides an example of a patient who was not particularly ready to learn. You should also assess the patient's current knowledge about the condition, some of which might be inaccurate or based on experiences of friends or family. In working with patients who have a chronic condition it is also important to assess the family's desire to learn and the patient's willingness to include them in the process.

Planning the educational process involves deciding with the patient where and how the teaching will take place. At this point goals should be established and a period of review and evaluation can be determined.

The implementation stage of the process includes the actual act of teaching. This might take a variety of forms including one-to-one teaching in the home setting, self-directed learning through the use of the internet or other resources such as videos, leaflets, tapes or books, group sessions with local support groups, or informal learning through networks of family and friends.

After the implementation stage, evaluation of the educative process should take place. The patient and nurse can consider what the goals were at the outset and evaluate whether learning has occurred. This is part of the feedback loop and, if learning has not occurred, this information can form part of a further assessment before planning ongoing education. If learning has occurred, new goals can be set and the education can move on to different areas of interest. The learning process is summarized in Figure 5.4.

When you are working with patients to educate them about their condition and its management, it is essential to remember that you are working with an individual and not a 'diabetic', an 'asthmatic' or an 'epileptic'. No two people with diabetes will be the same and part of your assessment at the outset must include an appreciation of the individual

Box 5.3   Barriers to learning

Physical	Patient characteristics	Emotional
Pain	Age	Denial
Shortness of breath	Culture	Anger
Poor vision	Language ability	Depression
Poor mobility	Reading ability	Anxiety
Poor hearing	Motivation to learn	Withdrawal
Nausea		
Lack of energy		

characteristics of the patient. It is particularly important to take note of the patient's culture, age, readiness to learn, language ability, reading ability and motivation to learn. The patient may also be experiencing physical barriers to learning, such as pain, decreased mobility, lack of energy, breathlessness or nausea. In this state of discomfort the patient will be limited to focusing on meeting immediate basic physical needs: he or she will be less concerned about the potential long-term complications of the condition.

Bopp and Lubkin (1998) state that a patient might also experience emotional obstacles to learning. Patients may be in denial of the condition; they may be angry, depressed or withdrawn. Denial is one method of coping with a condition, particularly in the early days of diagnosis, and it is therefore important to acknowledge this and to work with the patient to accept the condition so that learning might take place at a later time. A summary of the potential barriers to learning is given in Box 5.3.

The nurse as change agent

The diagnosis of a chronic illness results in the patient and his or her family members having to prepare to make changes in their lives. Corbin and Strauss (1992) developed the trajectory model of chronic illness, which suggests that a person who has a chronic illness is on a journey that will present the patient with a variety of challenges along the way. In the same way that we identified barriers to education, Dixon (1998) points out that there may be barriers to change. Resistance to change is a most important problem that needs to be recognized in order for us to work effectively with the patient. People tend to resist change in order to maintain the status quo in their lives, and this can cause problems when change is forced upon a patient due to the nature of his or her disease. New and Couillard (1981) identified five reasons why individuals might resist change: threatened self-interest, inaccurate perceptions, objective disagreement, psychological reactance and low tolerance for change.

Threatened self-interest

If patients weigh up the cost of change and decide that it threatens their personal interests, they may become reluctant to make the change. An example of this might be when you work with a patient who has a respiratory problem, such as chronic obstructive **pulmonary disease**, and you are advising the patient to stop **smoking**. The patient considers how stopping smoking would affect his or her social life and the joy of sharing a cigarette with friends at the pub. The positive feelings associated with smoking could far outweigh the argument that shortness of breath is going to deteriorate over time if the patient does not stop smoking. In this case you would need to act in your role as change agent to point out as many benefits as possible for engaging in smoking cessation and try to eliminate the costs associated with stopping smoking, for example pointing out that the patient can still socialize with friends without using a cigarette as the focus.

Inaccurate perceptions

If a patient has an inaccurate belief about a particular change it is less likely that the change will take place. For example, if a woman who has experienced a heart attack has a perception that exercising will put a strain on her heart and therefore do it some harm, she may avoid **exercise** and remain at home in the safety of her own surroundings. In this example you would have to work with the patient to find out what her perceptions and beliefs are. Once you had determined what she understood about heart disease and the effects of exercise, you could then begin to offer her some education and support to alter her perceptions of exercise and heart disease.

Objective disagreement

In some situations a patient might have accurate information that is in disagreement with the information you have in your role as nurse. It might be that the patient has alternative information to your own and you will need to explore this to determine whether the patient's approach is not going to cause any problems. An example of this might be the breathing exercises that some patients with **asthma** use instead of salbutamol inhalers. This approach has been used in countries such as Russia and the information relating to it has been publicized in the UK. However, there is no research available in this country to date to support the use of such an approach, and you might find that you have to disagree with the patient. In a situation such as this you might need to share with the patient the best available evidence to support your approach and be prepared to support the patient if a decision to continue with the breathing exercises is made.

Psychological reactance

This describes the tendency of people to engage in behaviours that have been identified as problematic. For example, if you suggest to a young man with type 1 diabetes that drinking eight pints of beer at the weekend is going to create difficulties with **blood glucose** control,

he might begin to think of this activity as even more desirable than he had previously. You might find that he has repeated episodes of hypoglycaemia due to the alcohol consumption followed by hyperglycaemia owing to the rebound effect following a hypoglycaemic episode. Often in situations involving psychological reactance patients are unable to articulate why they are engaging in these risky behaviours, and this makes your task even more difficult because rational explanation will not help to persuade patients to alter their actions. It is important in examples such as this to continue to try to understand the patient's perspective and what his or her particular values and beliefs are concerning this behaviour. Continually encouraging the patient and reinforcing the messages you have been giving regarding the diabetes will gradually help to improve the chances of making a change in the patient's behaviour.

Low tolerance for change

Some people have more difficulty in dealing with change than others. A patient who has a low self-confidence, poor self-esteem and a poor sense of self-efficacy may feel unable to engage in the change. An example of this might be a patient who completely understands the value of exercise in reducing the risks associated with hypertension; she or he is fully able to engage in exercise but seems resistant to make the change. This might result from low self-esteem and a low tolerance for uncertainty. In this case you can encourage the patient and support them at every opportunity and, when small changes are made, praise them for what they have achieved and gradually aim to enhance their self-respect and sense of self-reliance.

In addition to the five areas listed above, Dixon (1998) points out that *alienation* is another important reason why a person might be resistant to change. This refers to the alienation between the patient and the nurse. There may be a huge gap between the client's experiential knowledge of a condition and the nurse's technical knowledge, so that the two are alienated from each other. This may result in conflict as the patient and the nurse do not understand one another. Factors that might lead to a situation of alienation include cultural, age or gender differences. You might find yourself encouraging a man to stop smoking when he has four great aunts in their nineties who have all smoked 20 cigarettes a day since they were 16. His personal experience will have provided strong messages that far outweigh the risks you might be discussing with him and therefore he will be reluctant to engage in changing his behaviour. Once again, you need to spend time understanding the patient's values and beliefs to help contextualize your messages.

Summary

A recurring theme in working with patients who have chronic illnesses is the need to understand the perspectives

Dyspnoea
See chapter 5.3

Smoking
See chapter 4.2

Effects of exercise
See chapter 4.2

Asthma
See chapter 5.3

Blood glucose
See chapter 2.6

of the patient and, on many occasions, the patient's family. Without this, our messages are meaningless and we are unlikely to be successful in helping the patient adapt to the challenges associated with their particular condition. Assess the patient thoroughly before engaging in your nursing interventions and allow the patient time to talk to express worries and concerns. Ultimately the patient has the information you need to do your job effectively; if you provide the opportunity for open communication and develop a shared understanding, your chances of success will be increased. Nurses working in the primary healthcare setting have a great deal to offer patients who live with chronic illness, both in clinical skills and approaches to managing change and providing education.

References

Blackie C (1998) Community healthcare nursing. Edinburgh: Churchill Livingstone.

Bleeker H, Mulderij K (1992) The experience of motor disability. Phenomenology and Pedagogy 10: 1–8. Cited in: Price B (1996) Illness careers: the chronic illness experience. Journal of Advanced Nursing 24: 275–279.

Bopp A, Lubkin I (1998) Teaching. In: Lubkin I, ed. Chronic illness impact and interventions, 4th edn, pp. 343–361. Sudbury, UK: Jones and Bartlett.

Bryar R, Bytheway B (1996) Changing primary health care. Oxford: Blackwell Science.

Cameron K, Gregor F (1987) Chronic illness and compliance. Journal of Advanced Nursing 12: 671–676.

Cook R (1999) A nurse's survival guide to primary care. Edinburgh: Churchill Livingstone.

Corbin JM, Strauss A (1992) A nursing model for chronic illness management based upon the trajectory framework. In: Woog P, ed. The chronic illness trajectory framework, pp. 29–38. New York: Springer.

Council for the Education and Training of Health Visitors (1977) An investigation into the principles of health visiting. London: CETHV. Cited in: Blackie C (1998) Community health care nursing. Edinburgh: Churchill Livingstone.

Curtin M, Lubkin I (1998) What is chronicity? In: Lubkin I, ed. Chronic illness impact and interventions, 4th edn, pp. 3–25. Sudbury, UK: Jones and Bartlett.

Department of Health (1987) Promoting better health. London: HMSO.

Department of Health (1989a) Caring for people. London: HMSO.

Department of Health (1989b) Working for patients. London: HMSO.

Department of Health (1990) Care in the community: making it happen. London: HMSO.

Department of Health (1996) Primary care: delivering the future. London: HMSO.

Department of Health (1997) The new NHS: modern, dependable. London: HMSO.

Department of Health (2000a) The NHS plan. A plan for investment, a plan for reform. London: HMSO. Online. Available at: http://www.nhs.uk/nhs plan

Department of Health (2000b) Coronary heart disease national service framework. London: DoH.

Department of Health and Social Services (1997) Well into 2000: a positive agenda for health and well being. Belfast: DHSS.

Department of Health and Social Services (1999) Fit for the future: a new approach. Belfast: DHSS.

Dixon E (1998) Change agent. In: Lubkin I, ed. Chronic illness: impact and interventions, 4th edn. Sudbury, UK: Jones and Bartlett.

Funk S, Tornquist M, Champagne MT, Wiese R, eds (1993) Key aspects of caring for the chronically ill. New York: Springer.

Gibson J, Kenrick M (1998) Pain and powerlessness: the experience of living with peripheral vascular disease. Journal of Advanced Nursing 27: 737–745.

Hopton J, Heaney D (1999) Towards primary care groups. The development of local healthcare cooperatives in Scotland. British Medical Journal 318: 1185–1187.

Kelly MP, Field D (1996) Medical sociology, chronic illness and the body. Sociology of Health and Illness 18: 241–257.

Lyons RF, Sullivan MJL, Ritvo PG, Coyne JC (1995) Relationships in chronic illness and disability. Thousand Oaks, CA: Sage.

Macdonald J (1992) Primary health care: medicine in its place. London: Earthscan.

Melville A, Richardson R, Lister-Sharp D (2000) Type 2 diabetes. Health Service Journal March 2000: 32–33.

Morse J, Borttorff J, Hutchinson S (1994) The phenomenology of comfort. Journal of Advanced Nursing 20: 189–195.

New JR, Couillard NA (1981) Guidelines for introducing change. In: Hein EC, Nicholson MJ, eds. Contemporary leadership behaviour: selected readings, 2nd edn. Boston: Little Brown. Cited in: Lubkin I (1998) Chronic illness impact and interventions, 4th edn. Sudbury, UK: Jones and Bartlett.

Nolan M, Nolan J (1995) Responding to the challenge of chronic illness. British Journal of Nursing 4(3): 145–147.

Pritchard P, Pritchard J (1994) Teamwork for primary and shared care, 2nd edn. Oxford: Oxford Medical Publications.

Secretary of State for Scotland (1997) Designed to care: renewing the National Health Service in Scotland. Edinburgh: Stationery Office.

Verbrugge LM, Jette AM (1994) The disablement process. Social Science and Medicine 38(1): 1–14.

Vuori H (1986) Health for all, primary health care and general practitioners (keynote address), WONCA, 1986. Cited in: Cook R (1999) A nurse's survival guide to primary care. Edinburgh: Churchill Livingstone.

Welsh Office (1998) Putting patients first. Cardiff: The Welsh Office.

World Health Organization (1978) Report of the international conference on primary health care, Alma Ata, USSR. Geneva: WHO. Cited in: Cook R (1999) A nurse's survival guide to primary care. Edinburgh: Churchill Livingstone.

Further Reading

Blackie C (1998) Community healthcare nursing. Edinburgh: Churchill Livingstone.

This book explores the meaning of primary health care, describes the NHS reforms and explains the organization of community care. It is a useful text for community nurses and student nurses as it addresses the core knowledge for nurses who work in the community setting.

Cook R (1999) A nurse's survival guide to primary care. Edinburgh: Churchill Livingstone.

This is a pocket-sized guide to primary healthcare nursing which addresses a range of issues of relevance to both student nurses and qualified staff. The book covers major policy issues, key principles of clinical care, information relating to the range of agencies operating in primary care, and valuable insights into health promotion and public health.

Crumbie A, Lawrence J (2001) Living with chronic illness. A practitioner's guide. Oxford: Butterworth Heinemann.

This book aims to equip the healthcare practitioner with the necessary knowledge and skills to manage the impact of chronicity on patients' lives. Section one is focused on developing an understanding of what it is like to live with a chronic condition and the ways in which healthcare professionals can enhance sensitivity to patients. Section two focuses on specific chronic diseases, providing an overview of the epidemiology, pathophysiology, assessment and treatment options for the patient with that particular condition.

Lubkin I (1998) Chronic illness – impact and interventions, 4th edn. Sudbury, UK: Jones and Bartlett.

This text covers a wide range of issues that influence clients and families who are living with chronic illness. Sociological, psychological, ethical, organizational and financial aspects of chronicity are dealt with in depth. A case study approach is used to add relevance to the clinical environment and to illustrate ways in which healthcare professionals can contribute to the care of people who live with chronic illness.

Lyons RF, Sullivan MJL, Ritvo PG, Coyne JC (1995) Relationships in chronic illness and disability. Thousand Oaks, CA: Sage.

This book provides a series of valuable papers focused on the dynamics of relationships of people who live with chronic illness. The impact of chronic illness on interpersonal relationships is explored and interventions such as relationship-focused coping are examined.

Key clinical principles

Chapter 6	Principles of pharmacology *Helen L. Leathard*
Chapter 7	The management of pain *Veronica Thomas*
Chapter 8	Infection and disease *Lynn J. Parker*
Chapter 9	Clinical investigations *Susan Skinner*
Chapter 10	The patient undergoing surgery *Ann Brown*

Key clinical principles: An introduction

Specific medical diagnostic labels become attached to patients as they make their way through the complex and increasingly specialised world of modern health care. However several problems are common to many patients regardless of whether they are under the care of a general practitioner, orthopedic surgeon or cardiologist. This section will address these broad themes of pain management, principles of pharmacology and infection control.

The ability to transfer and adapt skills from one clinical environment to another is an essential characteristic of high quality nursing care. The clinical themes outlined in this section will run through the rest of the book when specific conditions are discussed in a broadly systematic way. You will therefore find it useful to refer back to this section to reflect upon both your clinical experience and to expand the more detailed content of subsequent chapters. You should also remember that the principles discussed in these chapters apply with just as much validity in primary care settings as they do in the acute hospital.

Principles of pharmacology

Helen L. Leathard

Introduction

Pharmacology and nursing practice

Classification and naming of medicines

Administration, absorption and distribution of medicines, and bioavailability

How drugs act

Inactivation, metabolism and elimination

Unwanted and adverse effects of medicines

Interactions between drugs when used together

Drug discovery, development and evaluation

Summary

Introduction

Pharmacology is the study of *drugs*. A comprehensive definition of drugs is that they are chemicals that can influence the functioning of the body or its constituent tissues. In this sense hormones and neurotransmitters are included along with substances that we would normally think of as drugs, i.e. those that are foreign to the body and are produced by different organisms or by chemical synthesis. A medicine is a drug formulated for medical use, and many drugs are used in medicines. Some other substances are used recreationally or abused, some are used in the investigation of physiological processes, and others are toxins found in the environment. In this chapter, however, we will concentrate on the basic principles of those aspects of pharmacology that are relevant to nursing.

The term *pharmacotherapy* is often used to refer to the therapeutic use of medicines in the treatment of patients who are acutely ill, and the prophylactic use of drugs in chronic relapsing conditions such as asthma and inflammatory bowel disease. It can also include hormonal contraception and **menopausal** hormone therapies used by healthy people, but not recreational or abusive taking of drugs. The pharmacological principles discussed in this chapter apply equally well to all drugs, regardless of the purpose for which they are used.

The sequence in which we will cover the pharmacological content is unconventional but appropriate to the requirements for nursing practice. First, we consider how active drugs are administered and reach their intended site or sites of action. Second, we explore quite simply the various ways in which drugs can cause their actions and effects in the body and, third, we discuss ways in which the actions and effects of drugs are terminated by inactivation and elimination from the body. Specificity and selectivity of drug action are key features of the effectiveness and safety profile of any medicine. Adverse and unwanted effects of individual agents and the problem of drug interactions in people taking more than one medicine are, therefore, examined in separate sections. First of all let us look at the relationship of pharmacology to nursing practice.

Pharmacology and nursing practice

The administration of medicines has, for a long time, been an important part of registered nurses' practice that requires thought and the exercise of professional

Menopause
See chapter 6.3

Box 6.1   Group protocol

A specific written instruction for the supply or administration of named medicines in an identified clinical situation. It is drawn up locally by doctors, pharmacists and other appropriate professionals, and approved by the employer, advised by the relevant professional advisory committees. It applies to groups of patients or other service users who may not be individually identified before presentation for treatment.

(Crown 1999, p. 79)

Box 6.2   Gaining knowledge about pharmacology

Ives et al (1996) studied the actual and self-rated pharmacology knowledge of first year registered, graduate nurses in Victoria, Australia, using a postal questionnaire. The findings demonstrated that there was a very wide range of extent of knowledge of pharmacology as assessed by multiple choice questions (test scores ranged from 16% to 92%), with respondents who had participated in a graduate-year programme attaining higher test scores than those who had not. The means by which their pharmacology education had been delivered varied considerably and respondents valued their practical, clinical experience more highly than theory sessions as a means of gaining knowledge, emphasizing the importance of relating theory to practice.

Their ability to assess this is, however, questionable because self-rating of their knowledge correlated with their test scores only in relation to therapeutic effects. They overestimated their knowledge of drug administration and legal aspects by considerable margins and somewhat overestimated their knowledge of adverse effects, but underestimated their knowledge in relation to client education. These findings can, therefore, be interpreted as demonstrating that clinical experience reinforces learning of those topics that are subject to discussion and critical appraisal in the workplace. Experience has less impact, however, on topics where competence is assumed but is less subject to scrutiny by colleagues or clients.

judgement (UKCC 1992, 2000). Key roles can be grouped in three clusters:

- *Appropriate administration*: confirming the correctness of the prescription and judging the suitability of administration at the scheduled time

- *Patient support*: reinforcing positive effects of treatment and enhancing patients' and their carers' understanding of prescribed medication, so minimizing the risk of misuse of medicines

- *Evaluation of treatment*: helping assess the effectiveness of medication and recognition of adverse effects or interactions in individual patients.

More recently in the UK, *group protocols* (Box 6.1) for the supply and administration of medicines and for certain community nurses, prescribing from a nurse prescribers' formulary, have been introduced (Crown 1998, 1999). Government consultation on an Extended Nurse Prescribers' Formulary for a wider range of prescribing nurses is at an advanced stage as this book goes to press. Sound understanding of relevant pharmacology is required to underpin these aspects of professional practice. With the exception of those specifically entitled to prescribe from the Nurse Prescribers' Formularies, nurses may only supply and administer under a group protocol or administer according to a medical prescription.

Pharmacology education requirements will differ between groups of nurses, and people's requirements will depend partly upon their current employment, partly upon their career ambitions, and partly upon current and future legislation. In this short chapter I aim to provide an account of the basic principles of what I like to refer to as 'nursing pharmacology' – those aspects that are relevant to nursing practice. This is analogous to, but not identical with, clinical pharmacology – a medical specialty involving the application of pharmacology for individual patients consequent upon diagnosis, and integrated within care plans that include other therapies, or clinical investigations of new drugs as potential medicines. The application of these basic principles in nursing will be illustrated in Section 3 of this book, where particular types of medicines are included as aspects of the care provided for various groups of patients.

To provide good patient support in relation to medicines, nurses require sound and comprehensive knowledge of the actions and effects of all medicines being taken by patients in their care. They also need to know about common, clinically significant, interactions between drugs, and the reasons for which the medicines are used. Integral to this is broad familiarity with the durations of courses of treatment (for the foreseeable future, fixed-duration course or as required), dose frequency and what to do when one or more doses is or are missed. Such broad knowledge needs to be based upon secure understanding of the principles of *pharmacokinetics* (how bodies handle drugs) and *pharmacodynamics* (how drugs act upon bodies). Although retention of detailed information on a wide range of drugs is not feasible, nurses might reasonably have comprehensive understanding of medicines that are commonly encountered in their particular practice and the ability to look up appropriate information about others. Some recent, sound and relevant research demonstrates clearly that more pharmacology education correlates with better knowledge (Box 6.2) and clinical practice (Box 6.3).

The *British National Formulary* (see Further reading), or its equivalent outside the UK, is a widely available, standard source of information about currently available medicines. It is a reference book for prescribers and includes the use of many specialist terms without explaining their meaning. Medical education engenders ready familiarity with and good understanding of this clinical pharmacological language. Nurses, too, are increasingly using the *Formulary* as a reference book, so this chapter will provide clear explanations of the requisite specialist terminology.

The limited familiarity of most nurses with chemistry is a great cause of anxiety in their approach to the study of pharmacology, and yet it is unrealistic to argue the case for extensive study of this subject as a prerequisite to a career in nursing. In this chapter the principles of pharmacology will be discussed as simply as possible from the chemical point of view. The chapter on **chemistry** in Hinchliff et al (1996) provides appropriate background information.

Classification and naming of medicines

Medicines are known by a mixture of therapeutic, pharmacological and chemical classifications. None is perfect and various combinations are in common usage. The *British National Formulary* (BNF) uses primarily a therapeutic classification, but many drugs appear in multiple sections. Pharmacological classifications are really helpful because they serve as concise reminders of mechanisms of action and this can act as a key to recall of actions and effects. The chemical classifications are the most difficult for those without extensive understanding of organic chemistry, and chemical names tend to be used as labels without full understanding of their meaning. In practice, what is needed is familiarity with all the classifications in common usage, such as: opioid analgesics, non-steroidal anti-inflammatory drugs or benzodiazepine anxiolytics.

It is also important to remember the difference between *drugs* and *medicines*, as explained on p. 95. The distinction between *non-proprietary (generic or approved) names* of medicines (which specify the active ingredients, and are the names under which medicines appear in the BNF) and *proprietary (brand or trade) names* (which specify a particular pharmaceutical company's product) is also important. A useful indication of the status of a medicine's name is that non-proprietary names are treated as common nouns and have a capital initial letter only where they start a sentence. Brand names are treated as proper nouns and always have a capital initial letter and often some indication that the name is a registered trademark. For example, paracetamol is a non-proprietary (generic, British approved) name, whereas Panadol® is one particular company's brand of paracetamol. Generically named drug combinations have their name prefixed by 'co-' (combination), which draws attention to the complex nature of the medicine. Thus, co-codamol 8/500 and co-codamol 30/500 are generic names for combinations of 8 or 30 mg codeine respectively with paracetamol (500 mg). Proprietary products with the lower codeine content are available over the counter (OTC) either by the generic name, co-codamol, or as Panadeine®, Paracodol® or Parake®, whereas those with the higher codeine content are prescription-only medicines (POMs) and are marketed by different pharmaceutical companies as Kapake®, Solpadol® and Tylex®.

An individual drug may be marketed in a variety of formulations and doses under a range of brand names. Continuing the above example, paracetamol oral suspension 120 mg per 5 mL (Paediatric Mixture) is marketed by this generic name or as Cupanol® Paediatric, sugar-free; Disprol® Paediatric, sugar-free; Panadol® sugar-free; Calpol® Paediatric or Calpol® Paediatric, sugar-free. Conversely, a single brand-named medicine may contain multiple active drug ingredients, any one of which may be a source of adverse effects or interactions. Typical contents of 'cold and flu remedies' are paracetamol (antipyretic analgesic), pholcodine (antitussive, mild analgesic) and pseudoephedrine (nasal decongestant) with the addition of a sedative antihistamine for night-time use.

Administration, absorption and distribution of medicines, and bioavailability

The essentials of nursing practice in relation to the administration of medicines are summarized in Box 6.4. In the present chapter we will cover the pharmacological principles that enable understanding and make links between the practice of administration of medicines and the theory of how the active drugs reach their sites of action. Separate sections are devoted to administration

Chemistry of living matter
See chapter 1.2

> **Box 6.4** Administration of medicines
>
> The administration of a medicine involves giving:
>
> ■ the correct dose
>
> ■ to the correct patient
>
> ■ in the correct formulation
>
> ■ by the correct route
>
> ■ at appropriate time intervals.

for local action and administration for systemic action. There is an additional short section on drug access to the central nervous system because of its distinctive features and clinical significance.

Basic principles: factors influencing drug movement

Epithelial tissues
See chapter 1.1

Vascular system
See chapter 4.2

Gastrointestinal
system
See chapter 5.1

Central nervous
system
See chapter 2.2

Blood–brain barrier
See chapter 2.1

Connective tissues
See chapter 3.1

Capillaries
See chapter 4.2

Cell membrane
See chapter 1.3

Endocytosis &
Exocytosis
See chapter 1.3

The pharmacological principles are founded in physiology because, as we shall see, drug molecules enter (or are prevented from entering) the body or specific body compartments in just the same way as other molecules. A sound understanding of the properties of cell surface membranes and the functioning of various epithelia, gastrointestinal and circulatory systems, blood and the blood–brain barrier is an essential prerequisite. Relevant information can be found in textbooks such as Hinchliff et al (1996).

Types of cells and tissues through which drug molecules might need to pass include:

■ **epithelia**, such as the gastrointestinal mucosa or the skin

■ **vascular endothelium**, which is more or less permeable in different tissues, being quite readily permeable in the **gastrointestinal** mucosa and liver, but nearly impermeable in the **central nervous system** – contributing to the **blood–brain barrier**

■ **connective tissues**, especially areolar tissues and the blood.

Drug molecules move down concentration gradients from higher to lower concentrations, generally by simple diffusion. In principle they can pass through or between cells, but in practice the passage of molecules between cells (the intercellular route) is rare or constitutes only a very small proportion of drug movement. Exceptions occur in the immature gastrointestinal mucosa of infants or where **capillary permeability** is enhanced by an inflammatory reaction.

Most commonly the movement of drug molecules into and within the body depends upon their ability to cross **cell membranes**. This is determined by the phospholipid bilayer structure of the cell surface membranes and by the chemistry of the drug molecules. As noted above, we are familiar with cell membrane structure and

functioning from studying the physiology of cells, so here we need to consider the properties of drug molecules that influence their ability to cross the cell membranes. The two most important factors are *size* and *solubility*.

Size

Small molecules with suitable solubility properties can cross membranes much more readily than larger molecules of similar solubility. Molecules with very low molecular masses, such as water ($H_2O = 18$), oxygen ($O_2 = 32$) or nitric oxide, which is the active molecule released from nitrovasodilator drugs ($NO = 30$), move freely across biological membranes. In contrast, molecules with a mass of around 1000 or greater do not, regardless of their solubility properties. Specific biochemical transporters or mechanisms such as **endocytosis** and **exocytosis** are required to move these large molecules into and out of cells. Endocytosis involves the plasma membrane of the cell forming a vesicle that transports the molecule into the cell, while exocytosis involves vesicles moving molecules out of a cell by fusing with the plasma membrane and releasing the molecules on the outside of the cell.

Solubility

Between these extremes of size, it is the solubility of drug molecules in water and lipid at pHs encountered in the body that determines their ability to diffuse across cell membranes. Hydrophilic (water attracting, water soluble) molecules dissolve readily in intracellular and extracellular fluids but are unable to cross cell membranes unless they also have lipophilic (lipid attracting, lipid soluble) properties that enable them to dissolve in the lipid of the cell membranes. Equally, hydrophobic (water repelling, lipophilic) molecules dissolve readily in cell membrane lipid but are unable to dissolve in and move through the aqueous intracellular and extracellular body fluids unless they also have hydrophilic properties.

Drug molecules, like many natural hormones and neurotransmitters, combine these properties. Without going into chemical detail, this is achieved by them being relatively small molecules with a covalently bonded core consisting of atoms held together by sharing electrons. This arrangement confers lipophilic properties on the molecule. Attached to this core are various 'functional' groups that confer various degrees of water solubility. This combination of chemical properties enables most clinically used drug molecules to access the systemic circulation when administered by various routes, although the ability to cross membranes varies considerably between drug molecules, influencing their ability to penetrate into the central nervous system (CNS) and their susceptibility to metabolism and excretion. In some cases chemical 'anchors' are attached to active drug molecules to restrict their freedom of movement. For example, propionate additions help retain inhaled corticosteroids within the respiratory tract, and decanoate or enanthate additions retain antipsychotic and contraceptive agents, respectively, within oily intramuscular depots.

Blood flow

The rate of **blood flow** through various tissues, and the possible influences upon this of ageing and some diseases, can have a marked influence on drug absorption from subcutaneous and intramuscular injection sites, from applications to the skin and from the gastrointestinal tract. Vigorous exercise, for example, by increasing cutaneous blood flow, can increase the rate of absorption of insulin from subcutaneous sites, raising the blood level of the hormone and possibly leading to **hypoglycaemia**. In contrast, many elderly people who are ill and in pain have very poor cutaneous blood flow. Transdermal absorption of the analgesic fentanyl from patches can be impaired by this, leading to inadequate analgesia. Similarly, migraine is known to reduce gastrointestinal mucosal blood flow and this then impairs the absorption and, therefore, the effectiveness of migraine medication taken orally.

Administration for local action

One way of achieving selectivity in the action of drug is to administer the medicine locally to its desired site of action on or in:

- eyes
- ears
- nose
- respiratory system
- mouth and throat
- gastrointestinal system
- urinary system
- uterus or vagina
- skin and/or scalp
- cerebrospinal fluid
- other locations.

The main advantage of local application is that it is possible to achieve a pharmacologically active concentration of the drug at its intended site of action without causing unwanted or adverse effects by raising concentrations elsewhere in the body. For example, chemicals that are quite toxic can be used to kill parasites such as head lice, scabies or intestinal worms without poisoning the person needing the treatment. Similarly, corticosteroid drugs can be taken quite safely by the inhalation route for the treatment of asthma. The risk of harmful side-effects such as adrenal suppression, immunosuppression and an increased risk of osteoporosis, which could occur with systemic administration for extended time periods, can be avoided in this way.

In the sections that follow we will consider the pharmacological principles relating to local actions in the respiratory and gastrointestinal systems, and on the skin. These principles can then be applied by the reader to the localization of drug action elsewhere.

Respiratory system

There are two main aspects to achieving local action within the **respiratory system** for treatment of conditions such as **asthma** where the available drugs could produce marked or even severe unwanted effects if given systemically. One of these is to get the active agent to its site of action on the bronchial mucosa and smooth muscle, and the other is to prevent it from being removed too quickly by the pulmonary circulation. To enable the drug to reach the bronchial mucosa it needs to be inhaled as strongly as possible. *Metered dose inhalers* (MDIs) are delivery devices that help with this, but their use does need to be coordinated carefully with the timing of inhalation if an effective proportion of the active medication is to reach the bronchus rather than simply be deposited in the mouth, swallowed and inactivated. The need for skill in coordinating inhalation and MDI usage is reduced by use of *spacer devices* (used with MDIs) and *nebulizers*, but these have the disadvantage that they are cumbersome.

Diffusion of drugs from the respiratory system into the pulmonary circulation can be disadvantageous for two distinct reasons. One is loss of medication from its desired site of action resulting in reduced duration of action, which makes it necessary to give the medicine more frequently. Reduced intensity can also be compensated for by increasing the dose. The other is the risk of adverse effects on other tissues if the active agent is not sufficiently diluted in the blood to render it inactive. Acute palpitations from use of β_2-adrenoceptor stimulants (e.g. salbutamol) and long-term adverse effects of corticosteroids in asthma sufferers are problems the pharmaceutical companies have succeeded in reducing considerably. One key to success has been the use of molecules with structures that restrict their ability to diffuse across cell membranes, such as beclometasone dipropionate. Another solution has been to devise molecules, such as fluticasone propionate, that are very rapidly inactivated by the liver so that they do not persist in the general circulation. This also solves the problem of safe disposal of any fraction that is swallowed and absorbed from the gastrointestinal tract.

Gastrointestinal system

Although many medicines that are taken orally and swallowed are intended to reach the general circulation by being absorbed from the **gastrointestinal tract**, various ulcer healing agents, laxatives and anthelmintics, among

Blood flow
See chapter 4.2

Hypoglycaemia
See chapter 2.5

Respiration
See chapter 5.3

Asthma
See chapter 5.3

Gastrointestinal tract
See chapter 6.3

others, are taken orally for local action within the gut. The gut has evolved to absorb a wide range of molecular types for nutrition, so drugs that are retained within the tract or absorbed to a minimal extent are characteristically large or strongly hydrophilic (with poor lipid solubility), or both. Those taken for action in the stomach or duodenum are at risk of being flushed away very quickly by digestive secretions so they need to be administered in some way that helps them to coat and bind to the mucosal surface. Thick liquid formulations are efficacious.

With medications taken for their action within the colon there is likely to be a delay of at least 4–6 hours before they produce any effect, and this needs to be borne in mind when choosing suitable times for their administration. Lactulose and senna, for example, are relatively inert in the upper gastrointestinal tract and their effectiveness depends upon the release of active products by the action of colonic bacteria. This is why at least 6–8 hours usually elapses before the urge to defaecate is stimulated, and why these agents should be administered either at bedtime or early morning but not late afternoon or evening.

Skin and scalp

Skin
See chapter 6.1

Digestion
See chapter 5.1

The same factors that influence the passage of drugs across cell membranes also influence the rate and extent of their penetration into and through the **skin**, although the skin is thicker and a more effective waterproof barrier. Because of this, water-based treatments for skin parasites pose minimal risks of systemic toxicity, and they can be removed by washing (or bathing) after the specified treatment period. Treatments for inflammatory skin conditions such as eczema and psoriasis are generally applied as creams or oily lotions because these are partly absorbed into the epidermis and remain at their sites of action for reasonable periods without being rubbed off on to clothing. When they are removed by hand washing, they need to be reapplied. Corticosteroids and other lipid-soluble skin treatments tend to diffuse into the local blood vessels and thence into the systemic circulation. The risk of pharmacologically active concentrations being reached elsewhere in the body is minimal so long as recommended doses are adhered to.

Administration for systemic action

Systemic action is a widely used shorthand phrase to denote the potential access of drug molecules to all organs and tissues that are nourished directly from the circulatory system. It excludes the CNS, which is protected to a large extent from bloodborne chemicals by the blood–brain barrier. Routes of administration for systemic action are generally subdivided into *enteral* and *parenteral*. Other specialist routes are beyond the scope of this chapter. There are differences of opinion between various

authorities as to which group some routes belong to. The classification below is that of Laurence et al (1997). Enteral routes include:

- oral
- buccal
- sublingual
- rectal.

Parenteral (not enteral) routes include:

- intravenous
- intramuscular
- subcutaneous
- transdermal.

Oral administration

Oral administration refers to medicine being swallowed and absorbed from the gastrointestinal tract (mainly the small intestine). It is the most widely used route of administration for both prescribed and OTC medicines. Its greatest advantages lie in its familiarity, convenience and acceptability to most people and its suitability for most drugs. There is often a choice between solid (tablets, capsules, caplets) and liquid (syrup, elixir) formulations to suit people of differing ages and with differing abilities to swallow solids. *Sustained-release formulations* of some medicines are also available (Box 6.5).

The challenges to reaching effective blood concentrations by this route lie in the body's defence mechanisms against ingested foreign materials and the **digestive processes**. Nausea and vomiting are common reflex responses to the ingestion of foreign substances and serve to protect against poisoning. Because of this, the first few days of treatment with a wide range of medicines can cause nausea, with or without vomiting, in susceptible

---

Box 6.5   Sustained-release formulations

Desirable frequencies of administration for orally administered drugs are between one and three times a day, whereas many medicines, when given in safe dosages, have durations of action of only a few hours. Sustained-release formulations that retain part of a relatively large dose of a drug within the gastrointestinal tract for several hours enable twice-daily administration of medicines. These help patients who need to take one or more medicines over extended periods to accommodate these within a relatively normal lifestyle. Excessive dose frequency can impact negatively on a patient's ability to comply with their treatment even when *concordance* (agreement on treatment) has been achieved during a consultation.

individuals, but normally subsides with continued usage.

Gastric acid provides a powerful defence against ingested bacteria but inactivates some drugs, such as benzylpenicillin, which would be ineffective if administered by this route. Similarly, digestive enzymes are essential for our ability to absorb nutrients from proteins, carbohydrates and lipids, but these will also break down and inactivate protein, carbohydrate and lipid medicines, such as insulin, heparin and natural prostaglandins, which cannot, therefore, be administered orally.

Once absorbed across the intestinal mucosa into the bloodstream, the drug molecules are carried by the **portal venous system** to the **liver**, where varying proportions of the ingested dose are subject to metabolic transformations, as discussed in the section on Inactivation, metabolism and elimination (see p. 105). From an evolutionary perspective these are detoxification reactions through which the liver provides protection from foreign substances. Only after surviving into the hepatic vein do orally administered drugs become available for systemic action. The terms *first-pass metabolism* or *first-pass effect* are used to refer to the inactivation of orally administered drugs before they reach the systemic circulation.

The proportion reaching the systemic circulation is quantified as the *oral bioavailability*. It is expressed as a percentage of the dose given. For some drugs there is considerable interpatient variation in the factors that affect their oral bioavailability, either genetically determined or influenced by disease. This can necessitate careful *titration* (adjustment according to effect) of doses to achieve the best balance between beneficial and adverse effects in individual patients. Once orally administered drugs reach the systemic circulation, the rate at which they reach their sites of action will depend on the blood flow to target areas and upon their ability to cross the vascular endothelium and any other tissue barriers.

If drugs are taken orally on a fairly empty stomach their action can commence in as little as 15–20 minutes, although it will continue to increase for at least 1–2 hours. The absorption of drugs can be delayed and extended significantly if medicines are taken on a full stomach. Some medicines, such as oral flucloxacillin, need to be taken on an empty stomach to ensure full effectiveness, whereas others such as the non-steroidal anti-inflammatory drugs are best taken with food to minimize the risk of dyspepsia.

Buccal or sublingual administration

These terms refer to medications being retained in the mouth or under the tongue for local effect or to enable their rapid absorption directly into the bloodstream without being subject to first-pass metabolism. It is the second of these that concerns us here. Glyceryl trinitrate is a commonly encountered example of a drug administered in this way. It is available as tablets or aerosol spray (which can be sprayed into a patient's mouth by a carer if necessary) for rapid relief of anginal symptoms.

Rectal administration

This route of administration seems to be much less popular in the UK than in continental Europe, for socio-cultural reasons rather than pharmacological ones. It provides a non-invasive route for quite rapid absorption of drugs into the bloodstream for patients who are unable to take oral medication due to vomiting, migraine or inability to swallow. A proportion of the rectal venous drainage, which varies between individuals, is distinct from the hepatic portal system. This contributes to quite variable blood levels of drugs that are subject to substantial first-pass metabolism, with attendant risks of ineffectiveness and toxicity. A further disadvantage of this route for regular medication is the risk of causing local inflammation.

Intravenous administration

Medicines that are given intravenously reach the systemic circulation immediately and without any loss due to metabolism or barriers to diffusion. *Injection* or *continuous infusion* can be used, depending on the duration of action required. This route can be used for volumes that are too large for subcutaneous or intramuscular injection, but care needs to be taken to ensure that large doses of potentially cardiotoxic agents are given slowly enough to allow for adequate dilution in the blood before they reach the heart. Sterile precautions are required to avoid risk of infection at the site of injection.

Portal systems
See chapter 4.2

Liver
See chapter 5.2

Intramuscular administration

The intramuscular route of administration carries lower risks for cardiotoxicity and systemic infection than the intravenous route and yet can provide rapid onset of drug action because of the good blood flow through commonly used gluteal muscles or those of the upper arm. For example, it is used for opioid analgesics, antiemetics and antimicrobial drugs when rapid and reliable action is desirable. Because of the scarcity of pain-sensitive nerves in skeletal muscle, mildly irritant drugs can be given by this route. Also, volumes somewhat larger than are suitable for subcutaneous injection may be used. The intramuscular route is unsuitable for self-administration because of its inherent risks.

In addition to providing for rapid onset of action, the intramuscular route can provide for prolonged drug action through the use of depot injections. The active drug molecules or their formulations (or both) are modified to ensure very slow release of active molecules into the systemic circulation. Some antipsychotic drugs and contraceptive progestogens can be given at fortnightly or longer intervals. One disadvantage is that drugs given in this way cannot be removed if adverse reactions occur.

Subcutaneous administration

Small volumes of non-irritant formulations can be injected or infused just under the skin to achieve quite rapid systemic effects. The rate of onset of action is influenced by local blood flow, and exercise can alter the rate of absorption into the circulation. This is the least invasive route available for protein- and carbohydrate-based drugs such as insulin and heparins, and is considered suitable for self-administration by people who have received appropriate training. The duration of action, and therefore the frequency of injections, depends on the form and vehicle in which the active agent is injected. This route is commonly used for patient-controlled analgesia.

Transdermal administration

The **skin** forms a relatively impermeable barrier to many drugs, but lipophilic molecules can penetrate the skin in suitable conditions. Transdermal administration, from *patches* (adherent occlusive dressings), which release the active drug over extended time periods, is increasingly being introduced as a means of achieving relatively constant blood levels and avoiding first-pass metabolism of susceptible drugs without requiring infusions. It is used for analgesia, antiemetics or menopausal hormone therapy, and as an alternative to sublingual administration for glyceryl trinitrate.

Skin
See chapter 6.1

Central nervous
system
See chapter 2.2

Blood–brain barrier
See chapter 2.1

Bioavailability

The idea of oral bioavailability was introduced above. Bioavailability is also used to describe the proportion of drug given by any route that reaches the systemic circulation, and by this definition intravenous administration achieves 100% bioavailability. The concentration of drug at its sites of action in the tissues is, however, not necessarily the same as its plasma concentration because of *plasma protein binding*. Plasma protein binding reduces bioavailability because molecules are not free to diffuse out of the bloodstream to target tissues while they are attached to plasma proteins. Their duration of action is, however, increased by this means because the drugs are equally unavailable for hepatic metabolism or renal excretion.

Competition for plasma protein binding sites between different drugs and between drugs and natural hormones can cause adverse effects, as discussed below. In patients taking warfarin (or warfarin plus regular low-dose aspirin), intermittent use of aspirin in analgesic doses causes varying degrees of *displacement* of the anticoagulant from a large plasma protein-bound reservoir, leading to risks of bleeding episodes.

Drug access to the central nervous system

The **CNS** is quite effectively protected from blood-borne chemicals by the **blood–brain barrier**. This is formed by close apposition of vascular endothelial cells, by the high proportion of lipid (as myelin) in the brain and by selective filtration of blood solutes by the choroid plexus during the formation of cerebrospinal fluid. The ability of drugs to penetrate the blood–brain barrier and influence CNS functioning is dependent on them being strongly lipophilic. Drugs produced for actions in the CNS are either lipophilic (e.g. morphine) or they are selectively transported into the cerebrospinal fluid (e.g. levodopa).

Many drugs that are weakly or moderately lipophilic can diffuse into the bloodstream from the small intestine and reach peripheral sites of action but are relatively too hydrophilic to access the CNS in pharmacologically active concentrations. Modest differences in ability to penetrate into the CNS can have quite marked effects on the adverse effect profiles of otherwise similar drugs used for their peripheral actions. Instructive pairs to contrast in this way are propranolol with atenolol and cimetidine with ranitidine.

How drugs act

Most drugs work by activating or blocking receptors or by inhibiting enzymes that either synthesize or inactivate biological mediators. Therefore, the understanding of pharmacodynamics depends upon understanding of drug–receptor and drug–enzyme interactions, and recognition that many receptors are, or are closely linked to, enzymes. Drug–receptor and drug–enzyme interactions largely determine the quantitative relationships between concentration of drug and its pharmacological effect, and are responsible for selectivity of drug action. For the remainder of this chapter the phrase drug–receptor interaction will be used to imply drug–enzyme interaction also, because characteristics of drug interactions with both types of site are closely similar. A few drugs act independently of either of these mechanisms, and these, together with *placebo effects*, are explored in brief sections below. Some key pharmacological and related terms are defined and explained in Box 6.6.

Qualitative aspects of drug–receptor interactions

Most drugs that are used as medicines interact reversibly with receptors or enzymes, so that the degree of their action is related to the concentration of the drug in the circulation. For those drugs that have irreversible interactions with receptors or enzymes, their duration of action depends upon the rate of synthesis of new receptor or enzyme proteins, and this varies from tissue to tissue. Similarly, the effects of those drugs that act genomically (affecting genes in the cell nucleus) to stimulate the formation of new tissues or enzymes outlast the duration of the drug in the circulation.

The mechanism of action of many drugs involves interaction with receptors or active sites of enzymes, either by

---

Box 6.6   Pharmacological and related terms

Receptors are defined as those parts of a cell with which a drug or biological mediator interacts in order to produce its effect. They have evolved to mediate the actions of hormones and neurotransmitters but serve also as targets for drug action.

Enzymes, or enzyme systems, are biological catalysts that promote biochemical reactions in the body without being altered by them.

Agonist is a technical word used to describe a drug that interacts with a receptor to activate (or stimulate) it and thus produce a direct effect.

An *antagonist* is a drug that interacts with a receptor or adjacent site to interfere with the activation of the receptor by a biological mediator or other drug. It produces its effect indirectly by reducing or preventing an ongoing process as a result of *antagonizing* (inhibiting) the action of a natural hormone or neurotransmitter, or another drug.

Enzyme inhibitors also work indirectly because they increase or decrease the concentration of biological mediator available for action by inhibiting their destruction or formation respectively.

For each drug, a *therapeutic index* can be calculated from toxic and therapeutically effective doses. Where the toxic dose is only a little higher than the effective dose, the index is low. For drugs, such as digoxin, with a low therapeutic index there is limited scope for increasing the dose to obtain an increased effect without causing adverse effects.

The terms *toxicity* or *toxic dose* are not rigidly defined but tend to be used in relation to adverse effects that are serious or life threatening rather than unpleasant or inconvenient.

For some drugs (notably tricyclic antidepressants) there is a *therapeutic window* of concentrations below and above which the drug is ineffective. The reasons for this are not well established, but *receptor desensitization* (*downregulation* or *internalization*) by high drug concentrations has been postulated.

Similar mechanisms may underlie the development of *drug tolerance*, a phenomenon that occurs with opioids, benzodiazepines and glyceryl trinitrate, for example, involving progressive loss of sensitivity to the drug and requiring progressively increasing doses to maintain the desired therapeutic effect.

Box 6.7   Fundamental concept of drug–receptor interactions

Agonist + Receptor → Active drug–receptor complex
→ RESPONSE

Antagonist + Receptor → Inactive drug–receptor complex
→ NO RESPONSE

A receptor that is occupied by an antagonist cannot be activated by an agonist.

---

one will activate the mechanism (agonist), while the other (antagonist) fails to activate the mechanism and prevents access of the correct key to the activating mechanism (see Box 6.7). The selectivity or specificity of drugs for particular receptors, and whether they act as agonists or antagonists, is related to the properties of *functional groups* on covalently bonded molecular cores, and also to the molecular size.

Cell membrane receptors are complex proteins within the cell membrane. There are a number of families and superfamilies of receptor structures, such as those that regulate ion channel opening or those that are linked to intracellular G proteins and thereby regulate intracellular enzyme activities. The duration of binding of a drug to a receptor can be very short (milliseconds) when only hydrogen bonding is involved, or may be virtually permanent when covalent bonds are formed. Covalently bound drugs are rarely encountered in therapeutics because their long action tends to make dosage adjustment very difficult.

The binding sites of the receptor protein that are responsible for interactions with biological mediators or drugs have chemical properties that are specific for a single molecule or a small number of closely similar molecules. A single biological mediator or drug can have different types or subtypes of receptors in various tissues (see adrenaline-related examples in Box 6.8). As in this example, letters of the Greek alphabet are sometimes used to differentiate main receptor types, followed by subscript numbers to distinguish between subtypes. Alternatively, capital initial letters of the naturally occurring receptor activator is used (e.g. H for histamine receptors, B for bradykinin receptors, 5-HT for 5-hydroxytryptamine receptors), with subscript numbers, sometimes followed by subscript letters, indicating receptor type and subtype respectively (e.g. 5-HT_{1A}).

Quantitative aspects of drug–receptor interactions

The magnitude of response of a tissue or organ depends upon the number or proportion of receptors activated by an agonist. Receptor activation, and usually the consequent response, has been found empirically to be related

---

mimicking the action of a physiological mediator (agonist) or by blocking it (antagonist). An analogy is provided by reference to locks and keys. Two similar but not identical keys can be inserted into the same lock, but only

Box 6.8   Adrenaline-related examples of receptor subtype specificity

Adrenaline (epinephrine) acts as an agonist at α_1, α_2, β_1, β_2, β_3 receptors.

Noradrenaline (norepinephrine) acts as an agonist at α_1, α_2, β_1, β_3 receptors.

Some drug examples related to adrenaline and noradrenaline (adrenoceptor agonists and antagonists) are:

Receptor	Drug	Clinical use
α_1	Agonist: phenylephrine	Nasal decongestant[b]
	Antagonist: prazosin	Antihypertensive[b]
α_2	Agonist: clonidine	Antihypertensive[b]
	Antagonist[a]	
β_1 and β_2	Agonist: isoprenaline	Bronchodilator[b]
	Antagonist: propranolol	Antihypertensive[b]
β_1	Agonist: dobutamine	Cardiac stimulant
	Antagonist: atenolol	Antihypertensive[b]
β_2	Agonist: salbutamol	Bronchodilator[b]
	Antagonist[a]	
β_3	Agonist[a]	(lipolysis)

[a] There is currently no clinically used drug of this type; experimental tools exist.

[b] Only one important effect is listed although these substances have many actions.

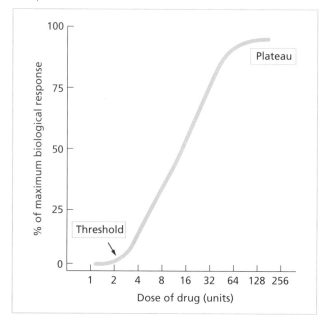

Figure 6.1   A dose–response curve. Drug dose is plotted as a logarithmic scale. The threshold is the dose of drug required to produce a measurable response. The plateau is the area of the curve where increasing the dose has no further measurable therapeutic effect.

From Clark et al (2000), with permission.

to the logarithm (base 10) of the drug concentration by a sigmoid curve (Fig. 6.1) with an approximately straight-line section between 20–25% and 75–80% of the maximum response (Neal 1997). The logarithmic relationship between concentration and response is the reason why drug doses are generally altered by doubling or halving, rather than arithmetic step increments of, say, 1 mg at a time. Ideally, therapeutic doses should give rise to free drug concentrations (in blood, interstitial fluid, cerebrospinal fluid) that are around the middle of this concentration–response curve. Owing to biological variation, low doses will be ineffective in a proportion of people and high doses may be toxic in some people. In clinical practice the range of doses recommended for adults is often quite narrow despite the wide range of variation in sizes of people, but there are different formulations and dose recommendations for infants and children aged under 12 years. For any drug with a low therapeutic index, such as cancer chemotherapeutic agents, the doses for adults can be calculated in proportion to body weight or body mass index.

Drug actions that are independent of receptor or enzyme interactions

Gastric antacids and dietary fibre are widely used examples of the few types of drug that do not interact with specific receptors.

Gastric antacids, such as sodium bicarbonate, magnesium hydroxide and calcium carbonate, neutralize gastric acid by reacting with it to produce non-irritant chloride salts (e.g. sodium chloride, magnesium chloride, calcium chloride). The quantity of acid neutralized depends upon the dose, and the action effectively ends when the drug leaves the stomach.

Dietary fibre is not absorbed from the gastrointestinal tract, and retains water with it by osmotic forces as it passes along in the lumen. Thus it increases the intraluminal bulk and stimulates increased peristalsis. Fermentation of the fibre by colonic bacteria increases the number of osmotically active particles (and carbon dioxide and water) in this organ, and thus enhances the stimulant effect here.

Placebo effects

Randomized controlled clinical trials generally show that about 30% of the population respond to inert 'treatments' (placebos) as if they had received effective medication, and also suffer side-effects. Such placebo responses are not well understood but they show us that psychological factors such as expectation of recovery, being cared for by healthcare professionals and others, or perhaps just being encouraged to rest can contribute to the diminution of symptoms. It would be unethical to treat people with placebos when effective treatments were available, but it is equally important to appreciate that placebo effects probably contribute something to the effectiveness of all pharmacological treatments. There is fuller and illuminating discussion of placebo effects in the clinical pharmacology textbooks of Grahame-Smith and Aronson (1992) and Laurence et al (1997).

Inactivation, metabolism and elimination

The rate at which a drug is inactivated (or activated) by metabolism or eliminated from the body is a major factor in determining its duration of action. This, in turn, determines the range of possible frequencies of its administration to provide a continuous therapeutic effect. Because metabolic rate in general and renal clearance and hepatic functioning in particular can be influenced by age and disease, we can understand the need for caution in particular patient groups (paediatric, elderly, those with renal or hepatic impairment). Medicines administered too frequently to people who cannot inactivate or eliminate them rapidly enough can cause adverse effects as drugs accumulate in blood and tissues.

In this section we will look first at the elimination of drugs (focusing on renal clearance, which is quantitatively the most important for the majority of systemic drugs), and then at the metabolic inactivation of drugs and their conversion into molecules suitable for excretion in urine or bile. Finally we will cover briefly some other facets of drug metabolism that are clinically important, and explain some widely used terms.

Elimination

The concentration of drug in the circulation represents not only the concentration available to act but also the concentration available for metabolism and excretion. Because of the potential impact of organ-specific disease on duration of drug action and potential toxicity, it is important to be aware of the major sites of elimination of each drug:

- the kidneys and *urinary excretion*
- excretion via the liver into *bile*, and then *faeces* or *enterohepatic circulation* (see Box 6.13, p. 106)
- *exhalation.*

There are diverse other means of eliminating locally administered medicines:

- washing the skin, or loss on to clothing
- *mucociliary clearance* from the bronchial tree
- tears from the eyes
- saliva from the mouth
- digestive and mucous secretions, and faecal elimination, clear the gastrointestinal tract
- mucous secretions and urine clear the urinary and genital tracts.

Urinary elimination of drugs or drug metabolites

The **kidneys** treat drug molecules and drug-derived molecules (metabolites) in just the same way as they handle other bloodborne solutes, being subject to:

- **glomerular filtration**
- concentration as the urine is concentrated, leading to
- various degrees of reabsorption by passive diffusion
- active **tubular secretion or absorption**.

All molecules of up to about 20 000 in molecular mass are filtered through the *fenestrated capillaries* of the glomerulus into the renal tubular fluid. Apart from large protein or glycoprotein drugs, such as insulin and heparin, and those drug molecules that are bound to plasma proteins, molecules of drugs and their metabolites are generally filtered in this way. As the tubular fluid is gradually concentrated, so too are the drug molecules, creating a concentration gradient for them between tubular fluid and the blood. Molecules that are sufficiently lipophilic to cross the membranes of the tubular epithelial cells and capillary walls will then tend to diffuse back into the blood at a rate that is proportional to the concentration gradient, and will not be excreted in the urine. More hydrophilic molecules, however, will remain in the tubular fluid and be excreted in the urine.

The rate of elimination of drugs in the urine is, therefore, determined largely by their extent of plasma protein binding and lipid solubility, with both of these factors tending to reduce the rate of excretion and prolong the duration of action. Highly lipid-soluble drugs can be eliminated in the urine only after they have been converted into more hydrophilic molecules by hepatic metabolism.

One other factor that influences the rate of urinary excretion of a few drugs is active tubular secretion. Benzylpenicillin, for example, is secreted into the urine by the epithelial cells of the renal tubules, and would have a very short duration of action unless injected in large doses, as a depot injection, or administered with probenecid, which inhibits tubular secretion.

Drug metabolism for inactivation and excretion

Drug molecules are rendered inactive and prepared for excretion in various tissues (Box 6.9). Hepatic metabolism is quantitatively the most important for the vast majority of drugs and this will be covered in more detail below.

Hepatic metabolism generally yields compounds that are less lipophilic and more hydrophilic than the parent compound. The metabolic processes detoxify ingested poisons and inactivate many medicines, although a few drugs are activated (see Boxes 6.10 & 6.11). The hydrophilic

The kidney
See chapter 5.4

Glomerular filtration
See chapter 5.4

Renal function
See chapter 5.4

Hepatic metabolism
See chapter 5.2

Box 6.9   Drug metabolism

Sites of drug metabolism:

- liver – hepatocytes
- gut – mucosal cells
- lungs – epithelial and endothelial cells
- kidney – epithelial and endothelial cells
- blood and circulation – endothelial cells, blood platelets, plasma enzymes.

Those sites in contact with the external environment are specialized to deal with foreign molecules, whereas those in contact solely with body tissues are specialized to regulate endogenous substrates, but also metabolize drugs that resemble the natural substrates.

Very few experimental studies have attempted to distinguish whether parenchymal cells or vascular endothelial cells are responsible for their metabolic capabilities in tissues, such as lungs and kidneys, with an abundance of blood capillaries.

Box 6.10   Active metabolites

Some drugs have pharmacologically active hepatic metabolites, produced by *phase 1 reactions* (see Box 6.12). The active metabolites can contribute to effect and extend the duration of action of the medicine that contains such drugs. Illustrative examples are:

Active drug	Active metabolite
amitriptyline	nortriptyline
codeine	morphine
diazepam	oxazepam

Box 6.11   Pro-drugs

Some drugs depend on metabolism to produce pharmacologically active molecules from inactive molecules at various sites following oral administration of inactive substances. Illustrative examples are:

Pro-drug	Site(s) of conversion	Active drug
cyclophos-phamide	liver	4-keto-cyclophosphamide
enalapril	liver	enalaprilat
levodopa	dopaminergic nerves[a]	dopamine
sulfasalazine	colonic bacteria	5-aminosalicylic acid

[a] Conversion of levodopa to dopamine by dopa-decarboxylase in the sympathetic nervous system is inhibited by peripheral decarboxylase inhibitors that are unable to cross the blood–brain barrier.

metabolites are more readily excreted in urine or bile than lipophilic parent compounds.

Two distinct categories of chemical reactions involved in drug metabolism are commonly referred to as *phase 1* (Box 6.12) and *phase 2* (Box 6.13) reactions. These may occur independently or sequentially, depending on the

Box 6.12   Phase 1 reactions

These reactions cause an increase in water solubility by oxidation[a], hydroxylation[a], dealkylation[a] or deamination[a] of the drug (or by various combinations of these). Many drugs, such as paracetamol, have several different metabolites.

Many phase 1 reactions are catalysed by the microsomal, *mixed-function oxidase* system, but not all oxidation reactions involve this system, for example:

- *monoamine oxidases* (in neurones and blood platelets as well as liver) inactivate many biogenic monoamines and related drugs, such as dobutamine and isoprenaline;
- ethanol is metabolized by a soluble *cytosolic enzyme*, alcohol dehydrogenase.

[a] These chemical terms refer to addition of oxygen, addition of hydroxyl groups, removal of alkyl groups and removal of amine groups respectively, all of which increase the hydrophilicity (water solubility) of the molecules. For further information about these and other chemical groups that are of biological importance, see Hinchliff et al (1996, ch. 1.2).

Box 6.13   Phase 2 reactions

These reactions involve the conjugation (joining) of drugs, or their metabolites from phase 1 reactions, to highly water-soluble entities such as sulfate, glucuronyl, acetyl groups which are available from the circulation or other hepatic metabolic processes. Morphine, for example, is converted to various conjugates.

The resulting conjugates can then be excreted in urine (which often contains a mixture of several metabolites) or bile.

Conjugates excreted in bile may undergo deconjugation by enzymes when they reach the small intestine or pass out in the faeces.

Those undergoing deconjugation may be reabsorbed into the circulation, and have their action prolonged through this process, referred to as *enterohepatic circulation*. Ethinylestradiol, the oestrogen in many oral contraceptives, has its action prolonged in this way.

available functional groups of a particular drug. The combined effect of inactivation and elimination determines the duration of action or effect of a drug in the body and this, in turn, influences the frequency of administration. The half-life of a drug (Box 6.14) is a useful indicator of the rate of its inactivation and elimination, and is used by clinical pharmacologists as a guide to frequency of administration (Fig. 6.2). The duration of therapeutic effect of a medicine can, however, also be altered by varying the dose (usually, the larger the dose, the longer its action) within limits determined by its effectiveness and safety.

Box 6.14   Half-life of drugs

The half-life ($t_{1/2}$) of a drug is the time it takes for the plasma concentration of the drug to fall by half. The concentrations of most drugs (alcohol is a notable exception) fall exponentially regardless of the size of the dose taken within the therapeutic range (see Fig. 6.2). This means that the half-life is the same irrespective of the starting concentration, and its value can be reported as a constant characteristic of that drug.

Half-life is normally measured in human volunteers at a very early stage in clinical trials, by frequent monitoring of plasma levels following a single intravenous injection.

As mentioned above, although the half-life of a drug (in minutes, hours or days) is one useful parameter of the duration of action of a drug, it is not the only factor that determines possible frequency of administration.

Figure 6.2   Drug half-life curve. In this example the drug has a half-life of 4 hours: at 4 hours the concentration has halved, and at 8 hours the concentration is half of what it was at 4 hours, etc.

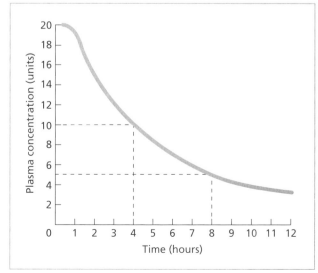

From Clark et al (2000), with permission.

Enzyme induction and enzyme inhibition

Certain drugs (including barbiturates, ethanol and phenytoin), components of foodstuffs and environmental toxins can stimulate an increase in the synthesis of mixed-function oxidase enzymes in the liver and consequently the activity of this enzyme system. The result of this *enzyme induction* is an increase in the rate of metabolism and reduction in concentration and/or duration of action of any drug or endogenous substrate. This can lead to serious drug–drug interactions (see below) and/or ineffective concentrations of drugs or hormones. For example, the effectiveness of oral contraceptives is impaired in this way by various antibacterial, antiepileptic and antifungal drugs.

For many drug groups, inhibition of specific enzymes (angiotensin-converting enzyme, cholinesterases, cyclo-oxygenases) is the mechanism of their therapeutic effect, and this has been referred to above. Some drugs, however, inhibit the hepatic mixed-function oxidase system and thus prolong and/or increase their own actions and those of other drugs or endogenous substrates. Cimetidine, for example, has been found to cause clinically significant adverse effects by enhancing the actions of various antiarrhythmic, anticoagulant and antiepileptic drugs in this way.

Unwanted and adverse effects of medicines

Nurses are well placed to help patients work out whether various signs or symptoms might be adverse effects of their medication, and whether they are mild or transient (unwanted) effects or sufficiently adverse to be a cause for concern. Anything serious or persistent, or any uncertainty, needs to be referred to the patient's doctor or other prescriber, and may merit reporting to the Medicines Control Agency and the Committee on Safety of Medicines through the yellow card system. Morrison-Griffiths et al (1998) have presented a very clear outline of this system in relation to nursing.

Unwanted and adverse effects can be part of the pharmacological activity profile of a drug, or arise from pharmacokinetic interactions with other substances being taken at the same time. The principles relating to these have been outlined above. These pharmacologically based adverse effects are generally dose related and can often be eased by reducing the dose of the medication, although some are so serious that it is essential to stop the medication immediately. Other adverse effects can be the result of immunological reactions to drugs or *haptens*. A hapten is an immunogen formed when a small molecule is attached to a larger carrier molecule. Haptens can be formed in the body from drugs or their metabolites binding covalently to tissue or plasma protein molecules. Penicillin may sometimes have this effect. Hapten formation can result in serious allergic reactions to medicines that are not dose related and are sometimes referred to as idiosyncratic.

The reader is referred to the BNF (or its equivalent) as a readily available source of detailed information on possible side-effects, cautions and contraindications for medicines.

Interactions between drugs when used together

Interactions between drugs can be pharmacodynamic or pharmacokinetic in origin. *Pharmacodynamic* interactions arise when drugs enhance or, more commonly, inhibit the actions of one another at the receptor level, and are predictable from the pharmacological profiles of the drugs. *Pharmacokinetic* interactions arise when drugs interfere with the absorption, distribution, metabolism or excretion of one another. Some examples are given above, and numerous possible drug–drug interactions are listed in an appendix to the BNF, including many that are not usually of clinical significance. Nurses will be familiar with interactions that are relatively common within their area of practice, but it is not possible to memorize all possibilities.

There is a particular risk of drug–drug interactions when patients are on multiple drug therapies. If such people develop unexpected signs or symptoms, the possibility that these might have their basis in a drug–drug interaction should always be considered, and the possible interactions of all of their treatments should be checked.

Drug discovery, development and evaluation

'They test new drugs don't they?' In a chapter under this quizzical title Freeman (1991) asserted that many people who prescribe or administer medicines have little understanding of the preclinical and clinical stages of the production of a new medicine. I am, therefore, including this section because I believe it is important that nurses should have some understanding of how medicines are discovered and tested. In fact, the introduction of a new medicine is underpinned by more rigorous regulation than is applied to any other therapy. Such rigorous appraisal is not applied to food additives, diverse complementary therapies, surgical techniques or, indeed, other orthodox therapies.

An understanding of the principles of drug discovery, development and clinical evaluation enables people to have justified confidence in the effectiveness and safety of medicines, and an appreciation of why animal studies are an essential part of this process. This contentious issue has been debated quite recently (Blake and Collins 1999). Blake, who has Friedrich's ataxia, an incurable genetic disease that affects the CNS, argued cogently for

the need for medical research that includes carefully regulated and monitored experiments on animals. Collins provided a contrasting, emotive argument that not all adverse effects of drugs are detected by animal experiments and, therefore, their use is unjustified. Such debates will undoubtedly continue.

Currently, pharmacological studies on animals almost invariably precede trials in humans. Clinical trials then proceed in four main phases:

1. *Phase 1*: safety and dose-ranging studies in healthy volunteers to establish the profile of actions and effects, half-life, and patterns of inactivation and elimination.

2. *Phase 2*: small-scale, pilot studies in patients with the disease(s) to be treated. These are 'open' trials in which both doctors and patients know the type and dose of the medication being tested. These can produce large placebo effects, at least in the short term, if the healthcare staff conducting the trials are very enthusiastic about the new treatment. Their main purpose is to discover whether or not the new treatment is effective in the illness(es) for which it was designed, and to establish what doses are effective in patients.

3. *Phase 3*: randomized controlled trials in groups of patients, in which new treatments are compared as objectively as possible with either placebo or currently available medicines, or both. Both effectiveness and safety (adverse effects) are measured and documented as accurately as possible. It is rightly regarded as unethical to use placebo controls in life-threatening or serious conditions for which there are treatments available.

4. *Phase 4*: post-marketing surveillance, in which recently licensed medicines are monitored as they are introduced to a wider population than the carefully selected groups used in phases 2 and 3. It is only at this stage that rare adverse effects are detected.

An understanding of these stages and the principles of design of clinical trials will enable nurses to evaluate claims of effectiveness and safety based on publications in journals or appearing in promotional literature. Specific information on clinical trials is provided in many textbooks of clinical pharmacology, such as that of Laurence et al (1997), and authors such as Sackett et al (1997) have produced more general guidance on interpretation of research findings to underpin evidence-based practice.

Summary

This chapter commenced with definitions of pharmacology and pharmacotherapy, followed by some consideration of the aspects of pharmacology that are particularly relevant to nursing practice. The ways in which medicines are classified on the basis of their clinical applications, pharmacological properties or chemical nature, and various combinations of these, were discussed. This led into an illustrated explanation of generic and brand naming of medicines.

The administration of medicines is an important part of nursing practice, so pharmacological principles relating to this have been covered in some detail, with a 'chemistry free' account of drug inactivation, metabolism and elimination, emphasizing how these influence the duration of drug action and therefore the necessary frequency of administration.

The topic of 'how drugs act' has been treated quite briefly, as have the subjects of drug discovery, development and evaluation, because detailed coverage of these is beyond the scope of a single chapter, although awareness of them is important. Nurses can play crucial roles in the observation and identification of adverse drug reactions and interactions, and the principal mechanisms by which these can be caused by pharmacotherapy are explained.

The chapter also includes definitions and brief explanations of many of the specialist clinical pharmacological terms used in the BNF to enable readers to use that valuable, readily available, reference book.

References

Blake A, Collins B (1999) Animal testing: for and against. Nursing Times 95(8): 32–33.

Clark J, Queener S, Burke V (2000) Pharmacologic basis of nursing practice, 6th edn. St Louis: CV Mosby.

Crown J (1998) Review of prescribing, supply and administration of medicines: a report on the supply and administration of medicines under group protocols. London: Department of Health.

Crown J (1999) Review of prescribing, supply and administration of medicines. Final Report. London: Department of Health.

Freeman J (1991) They test new drugs don't they? In: Glaxo Group Research, eds. Drug safety – a shared responsibility, pp. 13–26. Edinburgh: Churchill Livingstone.

Grahame-Smith DG, Aronson JK (1992) Oxford textbook of clinical pharmacology and drug therapy, 2nd edn. Oxford: Oxford University Press.

Hinchliff SM, Montague SE, Watson R (1996) Physiology for nursing practice, 2nd edn. London: Ballière Tindall.

Ives G, Hodge K, Bullock S, Marriott J (1996) First year RNs' actual and self-rated pharmacology knowledge. Australian Journal of Advanced Nursing 14(1): 13–18.

Jordan S, Hughes D (1998) Using bioscience knowledge in nursing actions, interactions and reactions. Journal of Advanced Nursing 27: 1060–1068.

Laurence DR, Bennett PN, Brown MJ (1997) Clinical pharmacology, 8th edn. New York: Churchill Livingstone.

Morrison-Griffiths S, Pirmohamed M, Walley T (1998) Reporting of adverse drug reactions: practice in the UK. Nursing Times 94(10): 52–54.

Neal MJ (1997) Medical pharmacology at a glance, 3rd edn. Oxford: Blackwell Science.

Sackett DL, Richardson WS, Rosenberg W, Haynes RB (1997) Evidence-based medicine. New York: Churchill Livingstone.

UKCC (1992) Standards for the administration of medicines. London: United Kingdom Central Council for Nursing, Midwifery and Health Visiting.

UKCC (2000) Guidelines for the administration of medicines. London: United Kingdom Central Council for Nursing, Midwifery and Health Visiting.

Wilson JW, Waugh A, eds (1996) Ross and Wilson: anatomy and physiology in health and illness, 8th edn. New York: Churchill Livingstone.

Further Reading

British Medical Association/Royal Pharmaceutical Society (2002) British National Formulary. London: BMA/RPS.

The BNF is published every 6 months (March and September). It contains four main sections: (1) guidance on prescribing; (2) emergency treatment of poisoning; (3) notes on drugs and preparations; and (4) appendices and indexes. The concise and current synopses of available medicines, which constitute the majority of the formulary, are written in the professional language of clinical pharmacologists. It is the hope of the author that those who have read the present chapter on Principles of Pharmacology will be able to understand this very convenient and informative reference work.

Downie G, Mackenzie J, Williams A (1999) Pharmacology and drug management for nurses, 2nd edn. Edinburgh: Churchill Livingstone.

This is a very sound basic textbook that presents quite a simple account of pharmacology and medicines management in a way that is related to nursing. Summaries of relevant physiology, immunology and pathophysiology are provided to explain how drugs work. As befits a basic textbook, there are some references to original research but no analysis of it. Useful further reading or reference lists are provided at the end of each chapter.

Hardman JE, Limbird LE, Molinoff PB, Ruddon RW, Gilman AG (1996) Goodman & Gilman's the pharmacological basis of therapeutics, 9th edn. New York: McGraw-Hill.

This substantial book contains a huge quantity of information, presented in a readable, scholarly style. The content is research based and critical/analytical where appropriate, with references to seminal, empirical research and careful selection of review articles. Although it originates in the USA, the book is intended for an international readership, and the fact that it is based on the *United States Pharmacopoeia* causes few difficulties. New editions generally appear every 5 years, so a new one is imminent.

Hinchliff SM, Montague SE, Watson R (1996) Physiology for nursing practice, 2nd edn. London: Ballière Tindall.

Of the many anatomy and physiology textbooks currently available for students of the healthcare professions, this one has the advantage of being specifically focused on nursing. Unlike the mainly functional anatomy content of 'Ross and Wilson' (Wilson and Waugh 1996), the physiology provided by Hinchliff et al contains sufficient biochemistry and chemistry to underpin 'nursing pharmacology' also.

Laurence DR, Bennett PN, Brown MJ (1997) Clinical pharmacology, 8th edn. New York: Churchill Livingstone.

This is one of many good clinical pharmacology books produced in the UK, and relating closely to the BNF. It is highly readable and, while it has much less content than 'Goodman & Gilman', it is largely evidence based, with annotated references provided as footnotes on individual pages and a fairly extensive guide to further reading at the end of each chapter.

Luker K, Wolfson D, eds (1998) Medicines management for clinical nurses. Oxford: Blackwell Scientific.

This is not a pharmacology textbook. Produced following Karen Luker's involvement in the evaluation of nurse prescribing, this book is really a manual of a wide range of related professional issues for those who are or are intending to become prescribers, and is very useful in that context. It is a multiauthor book, and the quality of evidence base, levels of referencing and extent of further reading lists varies between chapters.

Neal MJ (1997) Medical pharmacology at a glance, 3rd edn. Oxford: Blackwell Science.

This attractive, slim volume provides clear, concise summaries of all of the main aspects of basic pharmacology that are relevant to medical practice. Each topic is covered on a double-page spread, starting with a very clear diagrammatic representation of the system involved. Its disadvantage for students of nursing is that it presupposes familiarity with quite advanced chemistry (a good 'A' level grade is required for entry to medical school). Inevitably in such a condensed presentation, the style is descriptive and assertive, rather than evidence based, and the list of further reading is limited.

The management of pain

Veronica Thomas

Introduction

Pain pathways

Psychosocial factors in the experience of pain

Assessment and evaluation of acute pain

Methods of managing pain

Summary

Introduction

Before focusing on pain control it is necessary to consider the phenomenon of pain generally. If pain relief strategies are to be effective, they must integrate the knowledge of the physiological pain experience and response, opioid drug pharmacology, and the personal or psychological experience of the patient. These elements are introduced in this chapter because they are basic to the control and management of all types of pain.

Pain pathways

We now know that **pain** is mediated by free, unspecialized nerve endings. These nerve endings are present in the dermis and epidermis, and with their afferent fibres they form integral parts of single neurones, the bodies of which are situated in the posterior root ganglia associated with the spinal cord. The **receptors** are specialized for dealing with different types of noxious stimuli. The thermoreceptors respond only to heating and cooling, while some nociceptors are responsive to mechanical injury. Polymodal receptors are responsive to mechanical injury, noxious heat and chemical irritation.

It is now well established that there are two types of pathway for the conduction of pain from these nociceptors. First, there are medium-diameter nerve axons called A-delta (A-δ) fibres. These are myelinated and consequently conduct nerve impulses very quickly. Sharp, pricking pain sensations are conducted via these fibres to the brain in less than 0.1 s. The other type of fibre is known as a C fibre; this is narrower than the A-δ type and

not myelinated. As a result, conduction is much slower (1 s or more) and aching, throbbing pain sensations tend to be conducted. A painful stimulus may therefore be felt twice: an immediate sharp pain and then a duller, aching pain developing seconds later.

The afferent nerve pathways that conduct pain and other sensations away from nerve endings in the various tissues have ultimately to deliver their messages to the sensory areas of the cortex. This usually happens via a relay system involving three neurones (first, second and third order) which connect at their respective synapses. Pain impulses are conducted to the brain via the following system of neurones:

1. First-order neurone, which connects the receptor in body tissue to the spinal cord. The actual cell body of the first-order neurone is located at the posterior root ganglion and its axon synapses with the …

2. Second-order neurone, whose cell body is located in the posterior grey horn of the spinal cord. The axon of this cell crosses to the opposite side of the spinal cord and passes upwards in the spinothalamic tract. This has two components: the lateral or anterior tract. The axon terminates in the thalamus.

3. The third-order neurone, which conducts pain impulses from the thalamus to the cortex.

The information contained in the spinothalamic tract consists of rather diffuse pain and heat sensations. Associated with the spinothalamic tract is the spinoreticular tract. These ascending sensory nerve fibres are found in the anterior segment of the spinal cord and relay

Pain
See chapter 2.2

Pain receptors
See chapter 2.2

messages to the reticular formation of the brainstem. This part of the system is crucial for consciousness and awareness. Another key group of ascending nerve fibres is the dorsal column medial lemniscal pathway, which carries very precise information to the brain about touch and limb movement.

Various naturally occurring substances have been shown to play a major role in pain transmission. Substance P is a neurotransmitter found in unmyelinated fibres, and bradykinin, serotinin, histamine and prostaglandin E either excite or sensitize nociceptors.

Components of pain

Pain can be regarded as having three components: the sensory–discriminative, the motivational–affective and the cognitive–evaluative.

Sensory–discriminative

This component of pain allows the injury to be identified in time and space, and its exact extent to be determined. In addition to transmission of nociceptive stimuli, this component requires large-fibre transmission of touch and other sensory stimuli to enable the source, site and severity of the pain to be identified.

Pain transmission
See chapter 2.3

Gate control theory
See chapter 2.3

Endorphins
Enkephalins
Phantom limb pain
See chapter 2.3
(for all 3)

Referred pain
See chapter 2.3

Motivational–affective

This component produces somatic (bodily) and autonomic activity which result in various protective processes such as movement away from pain, immobilization of damaged tissue or preparation for flight. No spatial or temporal information is involved at this stage. The neural areas of the reticular formation and the limbic system are involved in the motivational–affective features of pain.

Cognitive–evaluative

This is a complex component in which response to the painful stimulus is influenced by cultural values, anxiety, attention and many other factors. These activities, which involve cortical processes, may affect the sensory–discriminative and motivational–affective dimensions. Arousal in situations of extreme danger may block the sensory–discriminative and motivational–affective components of pain. Suggestion and placebo may modulate the motivational–affective component and leave the sensory–discriminative component relatively undisturbed (Melzack and Dennis 1978).

The gate control theory of pain

Our current understanding of pain is based upon the **gate control theory** of Melzack and Wall (1965) and incorporates the three components mentioned above.

The basic idea is that within the substantia gelatinosa of the dorsal horn of the spinal cord there is a gating mechanism which controls the **transmission** of information to the brain. As a result large-diameter A-β fibres from touch and pressure receptors can inhibit the conduction of impulses through the smaller-diameter fibres that connect pain receptors with the cerebral cortex (A-δ and C fibres). Nerve impulses from the A-β fibres are preferentially conducted to the cerebral cortex, closing the gate on pain impulses in the smaller-diameter fibres. Pain impulses have to reach a certain threshold intensity to force open the gate and be conducted via the spinothalamic tract to the cerebral cortex and also to reach the reticular formation via the spinoreticular tract (Fig. 7.1).

The theory also proposes that descending fibres from the brain synapsing in the dorsal horn areas can modify the transmission of incoming pain signals. This opens up the possibility that psychological factors may play a major part in the perception of pain. Cerebral function can also be linked to physiological processes that reduce pain perception. One mechanism for doing this is secretion of chemicals that occur naturally within the body called **endorphins** and **enkephalins**, which are thought of as naturally occurring opioids. This takes place in response to stimulation from the effect of the neurotransmitter, substance P. Acupuncture is thought to stimulate the release of enkephalins, explaining its analgesic effects, whereas the placebo effect may be due to psychogenic release of endorphins. The placebo effect refers to the phenomenon whereby a patient reports a reduction in pain even though the medication that has been given has no analgesic properties.

The gate control theory also sheds light on **phantom limb pain**. Here, the patient experiences disturbingly real sensations and pain from a limb that has been amputated. This may continue for many years after amputation. Destruction of the large-diameter nerve fibres that normally input to the spinal cord from the lost limb means that their overriding effect on the surviving smaller-diameter fibres is lost, and therefore these fibres are much more sensitive than normal – hence the increased perception of pain. The brain may also interpret the input it receives from proximal, surviving sensory nerves as if the impulses were coming from the distal portion of the nerve in the limb that is no longer there. An alternative proposal is that the brain actually constructs its own virtual reality model of the body based upon neural networks within the brain. If this is true, then the loss of a real part of the body will not affect the way we perceive ourselves as this is based upon the virtual model constructed by the still intact neural networks in the brain.

A related phenomenon is that of **referred pain** in which the brain interprets pain as coming from a different part of the body to where the painful stimulus actually arises. A classic example is myocardial pain, which is often described as being in the left arm or jaw. What is

Figure 7.1 The gate control theory of pain transmission. (a) When input from the A-δ and C nerve fibres is greater than that from thick A-β fibres, the gate is open and pain is felt. (b) When input from A-δ and C nerve fibres is less than that from thick A-β fibres, the gate closes and pain is not felt. (c) The influence of the cerebral cortex via descending dorsolateral pathways closes the gate by the release of neuromodulators (e.g. endogenous opiates), neurotransmission and chemical mediators. Pain is not felt or is substantially reduced.

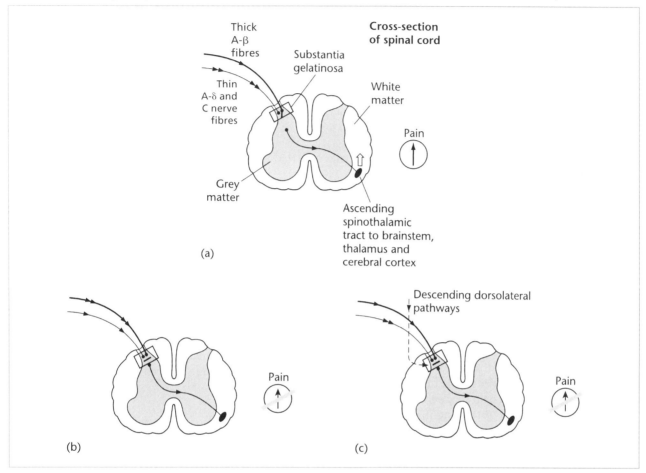

Adapted from Davis (1993).

happening here is that the damaged area and the area where the pain is perceived are both served by the same part of the spinal cord, and synapses between pain fibres from the two regions occur. The sensory nerve input from the left arm enters the spinal cord at levels T1–T5, the same levels as those from the myocardium. Synapses between the neurones that receive pain from the skin in the left arm and those neurones receiving visceral (myocardial) pain result in a shared ascending pathway to the brain. Pain impulses from the myocardium can then be perceived as coming from the left arm and the pain is said to be referred to the left arm.

Psychosocial factors in the experience of pain

Melzack and Wall (1988) argue that **pain perception** cannot be described simply in terms of stimulus intensity, and draw our attention to the complex interplay between physiological and psychological factors. In this chapter I will explore some of the psychological and social factors

that contribute to accounting for this highly individual experience. I will look at the role of sex, age, culture, personality, the meaning of the situation and needle phobia in explaining individual differences in the response to pain. An awareness of the pertinence of psychosocial factors in the experience and expression of pain is very useful to healthcare professionals because it provides them with potential insights and explanations for understanding individual reactions and behaviour to pain.

Sex differences in the experience of pain

The role of sex in an individual's response to pain has received considerable attention in the literature but the findings have not been unequivocal. In some research it seems that women report more pain or required more analgesic medication than men (Bond 1979, Taenzer et al 1986), whereas others have found the reverse pattern. Both of these findings contrast to other studies where no significant difference between males and females has been established (Streltzer and Wade 1981, Khun et al 1990).

There is therefore no research evidence to support a consistent pattern of pain appreciation related to sex.

Age differences in the experience of pain

The literature addressing the influence of age on pain experience is also not straightforward and the discussion takes account of pain experience at both ends of the developmental cycle.

Not a great deal is known about the epidemiology of pain in children (Eland 1985, Anand and Hickey 1987), and Llewellyn (1997) has argued that the reason is attributable to the fact that children's pain has little social impact. This is because the costs cannot be calculated in terms of lost work-days and benefits claimed. Consequently the incentive to investigate the extent of the problem is small (Goodman and McGrath 1991).

When considering the adult's pain experience some researchers have found that ageing is associated with enhanced analgesia, indicating that the elderly can obtain effective relief for longer periods with smaller doses of opioid analgesics than younger people (Belville et al 1971, Berkowitz et al 1975, Taenzer et al 1986, Burns et al 1989) and younger patients express greater dissatisfaction with pain relief (Donovan 1983). The picture is further complicated by the differences in the amount of pain reported by different age groups. Older people may systematically underreport the amount of pain they perceive. On the one hand, Miller and Shuter (1984) found that patients aged over 40 years reported more pain than those of a younger age group, whereas Khun et al (1990) found no relation between the amount of reported pain and age. However inconsistent these findings appear, it does seem likely that age is an important variable, which may affect the severity of pain.

Ethnic differences in the experience of pain

It is apparent from empirical studies and observations that pain experience cannot be fully explained without reference to cultural and ethnic differences. Culture seems to influence the expressiveness rather than the sensory experience itself (Melzack and Wall 1988). Cultural norms determining when and where to express pain are learnt at an early age (Peck 1986). Research on cultural differences in pain have, over the years, revealed that people from Latin origins are typically more expressive and are inclined to dramatize pain expression with excessive vocalization and posturing (Lipton and Marbach 1984). People of Scandinavian origin tend to be more stoical and are on the whole less expressive about pain (Chapman 1984). Black English people of African/Caribbean ethnicity have been found to report more pain than the white Anglo-British population (Woodrow et al 1972), but other evidence (Thomas and Rose 1991) has indicated the reverse, and that the white population is better able to tolerate pain than those born in the UK whose parents originated from the Indian subcontinent. Other studies have failed to find differences between 'Old Americans', southern US blacks, Irish, Italian and Jewish subjects in the amount of reported pain (Flannery et al 1987).

Thus it seems that the relationship between pain experience and ethnicity may be subtler than customarily thought, and that it may be possible only to describe certain responses as more or less characteristic of one group relative to another (Lipton and Marbach 1984).

Emotional states in the experience of pain

The influence of various emotional states on pain experience has been the subject of much research.

Neuroticism

Neuroticism refers to emotional stability, and studies that have used Eysenck's Personality Inventory (EPI) or Questionnaire (EPQ) to measure preoperative neuroticism have tended to find a significant positive relationship between high levels of neuroticism before surgery and pain experience after surgery in both men and women. This positive relationship between pain experience and neuroticism has been observed relatively more recently (Thomas et al 1990, 1995).

Anxiety and pain

The association between anxiety and pain is well known. Anxiety has been distinguished as:

- *state anxiety* – a transitory emotional state that varies in intensity and fluctuates over time and is associated with threatening anticipatory circumstances

- *trait anxiety* – a stable personality disposition that is said to predict state anxiety, i.e. it predisposes people to react in a highly anxious manner in stressful situations (Spielberger 1966).

It is well known that people awaiting surgery become extremely anxious and Spielberger (1973) has shown that anxiety trait remained stable in surgical patients before and after surgery, but those patients with high trait anxiety scores reacted in a highly anxious manner just before operation. In other words, patients with an anxious predisposition (trait anxiety) become acutely anxious in threatening situations.

Numerous studies have shown that both state and trait anxiety are positively correlated with the degree of pain experienced in acute and chronic pain settings (Lim et al 1983, Taenzer et al 1986, Thomas 1991, Thomas et al 1995, Seers 1997).

Overall it does appear that anxiety as an emotional state and a personality characteristic has important roles to play in the perception of pain. This consistent finding has led many researchers to attempt to reduce pain and distress by directly addressing state anxiety in the preoperative and postoperative situations.

Depression and pain

Depression, like anxiety, is also seen as a common feature of chronic pain (Romano and Turner 1985, Tyrer et al 1989, Tyrer 1992). When people experience the prolonged stress of chronic pain and feel that nothing they do helps, they may stop striving to achieve goals and come to believe that they have no control over events in their lives. In other words they learn a sense of helplessness. Depression has been found to be a common feature of chronic pain, and is characterized by withdrawal, lethargy and feelings of worthlessness.

Romano and Turner (1985) reviewed the American literature and found varying prevalence of depression in patients with pain, as well as pain in those who were clinically depressed. Similar findings were obtained by Tyrer et al (1989).

Helplessness

Learned helplessness (inability to effect change in spite of repeated efforts) is a major component of depression (Beck 1976). The psychological state of uncontrollability or helplessness is therefore a key feature of anxiety, depression and pain. There is an abundance of human and animal studies that supports the link between perceived control, anxiety, and painful or aversive events (Mandler 1972, Miller et al 1989). Psychological techniques aimed at enhancing personal control and reducing the sense of helplessness are a basic feature of an effective approach to pain control.

Needle phobia: minimizing pain because of fear

Patients may choose to minimize their pain because of needle phobia (fear of injections) or concerns about taking opioids.

Victims of needle phobia are at high risk of morbidity and death because they have a tendency to avoid health care at all costs. The use of sedatives, local anaesthetic cream such as EMLA (Frayling et al 1990) or skin coolant (Eland 1981) before injections or venepuncture is helpful in reducing pain. However, such measures are not helpful in removing the phobia because it is the sight of the needle that produces distress. Psychological interventions in the form of cognitive behaviour therapy (see p. 121) offer more effective solutions (Trijsburg et al 1992).

The role of meaning in the experience of pain

People attach meaning to their pain, and evidence suggests that such meaning may influence the ways individuals tolerate pain. The meanings associated with pain and suffering may dramatically affect the intensity and quality of the individual experience of pain. An early example of the powerful effect of meaning was described by Henry Beecher in 1956. He made comparisons between seriously wounded soldiers (during World War II) and civilians in an American hospital during peacetime and observed that, in spite their extensive wounds, the soldiers reported significantly less pain than the civilians and required less analgesic medication. Beecher suggested that the relief at finding themselves alive and removed from the line of fire was significant. For the soldiers their wounds marked release from life-threatening trauma, but for the civilians the hospitalization marked the start of personal disaster and disruption in their lives.

In a study involving 148 hospital inpatients, Copp (1974) assessed personal meanings of pain. The results showed that more than half saw pain as a challenge, something to fight and conquer, to promote self-searching and increasing understanding of others, and a quarter saw pain as weakness or punishment. These sociocultural meanings influence attitudes towards pain and resultant behaviour.

Fordham and Dunn (1994) have argued that the search for and the attribution of meaning is not only necessary for response but provides a way of coping with pain. Like pain, cancer has special meanings for people. It is commonly perceived to be uncontrollable and unpredictable, linked closely to extreme pain, suffering and death. Cassell (1982) provides an example of a patient who reported that when she believed the pain in her leg was sciatica she was able to control it with small doses of codeine. However, when she discovered that it was due to the spread of malignant disease, much greater amounts of medication were required for relief.

In another study Daut and Cleeland (1982) found that the impairment of normal activities and life enjoyment was greatest in patients who believed their pain to be caused by cancer, intermediate for those attributing pain to cancer treatment, and lowest for those who did not believe cancer was causing the pain.

Whether the pain is **acute** or **chronic**, it is closely related to the meaning the patient attaches to the pain and hence how they will cope with it. The pain of childbirth is severe and acute but the woman knows it is self-limiting. That is very different to the chronic pain of an advanced cancer, a disease that the person knows will probably lead to their death. Postoperative pain is again severe and acute, but the patient knows that eventually it should resolve and they will have a better quality of life, assuming the operation is successful. Contrast that with the chronic pain of osteoarthritis which the patient knows will not go away and is caused by disease that, while not life threatening, is progressive and disabling. Psychological factors therefore play a major

Acute and chronic pain
See chapter 2.3

role in the patient's perception of pain. Many patients adapt to chronic pain and just live with it as part of their everyday routine. They still feel the pain, but they do not show it in the same way that a person shows acute sudden pain.

Assessment and evaluation of acute pain

The efficacy of pain management strategies can be assessed and improved only if some form of measurement of the effects is made. Pain cannot be controlled properly if it is not assessed adequately. Objective **assessment** techniques have relied upon the assessment of biochemical indices such as changes in plasma concentrations of hormones, but these tend to be inaccurate, expensive and not applicable in clinical practice (Mitchell and Smith 1989). However, simple respiratory function tests may be a useful indicator of pain severity after abdominal and thoracic surgery (Chapman 1989). Posture, restlessness and facial expression can be observed and are part of the behavioural aspects of acute pain. Although an experienced observer may be able to use these indicators to make a rough assessment of the degree of pain suffered by the patient, it is widely accepted that the amount of suffering may be assessed accurately only by the patient concerned (McCaffrey and Beebe 1989, McCaffrey and Pasero 1999).

In recent years some advances have been made in the clinical measurement and evaluation of pain. A huge area of research has been devoted to the development of assessment tools, which are aimed at enhancing the person's verbal expression of their suffering so that they can convey their subjective experience. Meinhart and McCaffrey (1983) have argued that comprehensive assessment of pain should include the following information:

Assessment
See chapter 2.3

- location
- quality
- pattern
- intensity
- factors that increase the pain
- verbal statements about the pain
- non-verbal expression
- associated symptoms.

A useful tool for analysing pain as a symptom is the PQRST tool described by Walsh et al (1999). This tool can be used to analyse the nature of any symptom such as a cough or stiff knee joint and is particularly useful for analysing a patient's pain. The letters PQRST give the following framework to the assessment:

P   Provocation/Palliation – What brings on the pain? What relieves the pain?

Q   Quality – What does the pain feel like? Stabbing? Dull ache? Sharp? Throbbing?

R   Region/Radiation – Where do you feel the pain? Does it radiate anywhere?

S   Severity – See below for various pain severity rating scales. A simple approach is simply to ask the patient to rate the pain from 0 to 10, where 0 mean no pain at all and 10 the most severe pain imaginable. This should be done for the pain when at rest and when moving, if appropriate.

T   Time – How long have you had the pain? Does it vary through the day?

Pain is an intensely personal experience and no nurse can ever really know the patient's pain experience. Pain represents the limits of empathy in many cases. Unfortunately there are still many misconceptions concerning pain, and they are summarized in Box 7.1.

Unidimensional rating scales

There are a number of rating scales that are commonly used to measure pain, and these have been described as simple and reproducible. They enable the patient to express the severity of pain in a way that is quantifiable. They vary according to the nature and number of anchor points supplied, numbers, words or the presentation of visual analogue lines, and are available in a variety of languages (McCaffrey and Pasero 1999). *Visual analogue scales* (VASs) consist of a straight line with numerical, verbal or pictorial anchors and the ends representing the extreme limits of pain.

Verbal rating scales (VRSs) consist of a sequence of words corresponding to escalating pain. The more words in the scale, the more sensitive it is; however, the patient is less likely to choose the same word on different occasions even if the pain is the same.

Visual analogue scales

The VAS consists of a straight line, usually 10 cm long, with the ends representing the extreme limits of pain (Scott and Huskisson 1976). A VAS with points (either words or numbers) between the ends is known as a graphic rating scale (GRS). The patient makes a mark on the line appropriate to the level of pain she or he is experiencing.

No pain _____ Pain as bad
                                                                        as it could be

The scales may also be drawn vertically. The subject makes a mark on the line appropriate to the level of pain that is experienced. The distance from the 'no pain' end is measured, and provides the patient's intensity score. Scores obtained on the VAS and GRS show good correlation with other measurements.

Box 7.1 Misconceptions about assessment of patients who indicate they have pain

Misconception	Correction
1. The health team is the authority about the existence and nature of the patient's pain sensation	The person with pain is the only authority about the existence and nature of the pain, since the sensation of pain can be felt only by the person who has it
2. Our personal values and intuition about the trustworthiness of others is a valuable tool in identifying whether a person is lying about a pain	Personal values and intuition do not constitute a professional approach to the patient with pain. The patient's credibility is not on trial
3. Pain is largely an emotional or psychological problem, especially in the patient who is highly anxious or depressed	Having an emotional reaction to pain does not mean that pain is caused by an emotional problem. If anxiety or depression is alleviated, the intensity of pain will not necessarily be any less
4. Lying about the existence of pain, malingering, is common	Very few people who say they have pain are lying about it. Outright fabrication of pain is considered rare
5. The patient who obtains benefits or preferential treatment because of pain is receiving secondary gain and does not hurt as much as he or she says or may not hurt at all	The patient who uses pain to advantage is not the same as a malingerer and may still hurt as much as stated
6. All real pain has an identifiable physical cause	All pain is real, regardless of its cause. Almost all pain has both physical and mental components. Pure psychogenic pain is rare
7. Visible signs, either physiological or behavioural, accompany pain and can be used to verify its existence and severity	Even with severe pain, periods of physiological and behavioural adaptation occur, leading to periods of minimal or no signs of pain. Lack of pain expression does not necessarily mean lack of pain. How must the patient act for us to believe he or she has pain?
8. Comparable physical stimuli produce comparable pain in different people. The severity and duration of pain can be predicted accurately for everyone on the basis of the stimuli for pain	Comparable stimuli in different people do *not* produce the same intensities of pain. Comparable stimuli in different people will produce different intensities of pain that last different periods. There is no direct and invariant relationship between any stimulus and the perception of pain
9. People with pain should be taught to have a high tolerance for pain. The more prolonged the pain or the more experience a person has with pain, the better is the tolerance for pain	Pain tolerance is the individual's unique response, varying between patients and varying in the same patient from one situation to another. People with prolonged pain tend to have an increasingly low pain tolerance. Respect for the patient's pain tolerance is crucial for adequate pain control
10. When the patient reports pain relief following a placebo, this means that the patient is a malingerer or that the pain is psychogenic	There is not a shred of evidence anywhere in the literature to justify using a placebo to diagnose malingering or psychogenic pain

From McCaffrey and Beebe (1989), with permission.

Visual analogue pain relief scale (VAPRS)

These are comparative scales that present the extremes in amount of relief achieved. According to Skevington (1995) this approach has the advantage that all patients start from the same baseline and consequently the size of the response does not depend on the initial severity of pain. However, a big disadvantage – which outweighs its usefulness – is the absence of options to demonstrate an increase in pain. Another limitation is the fact that individual variations are masked as the scale give the impression that all patients start with the same level of pain (Skevington 1995).

No relief _____ Complete relief

Numerical rating scales

Numerical rating scales are a variation of VASs where subjects are asked to score their pain intensity from 0 to 10 or from 0 to 100. These scales are regarded as easier to score and analyse.

Picture scales

Picture scales were first developed by Frank et al (1982). The scale consists of eight line drawings of human faces experiencing different levels of pain. The drawings are presented randomly. Beyer (1994) developed *the Oucher*, a pictorial scale that makes use of happy and sad photographically represented faces for assessing pain intensity in children aged between 3 and 12 years. In addition to being ideally suited for use among children, pictorial scales are advantageous for the patient who cannot speak or understand English.

The unidimensional rating scales do not reflect the complexity of the pain experience. Reading (1984) suggests that over repeated trials patients may use single scales to reflect different components of their pain. This occurs because it is difficult for the VAS to distinguish between the intensity of sensory pain and the unpleasantness of affective pain. Attempts have been made to overcome this problem by making use of questionnaire methods in an attempt to reflect the multidimensional experience.

Pain management
See chapter 2.3

TENS
Gate control theory
See chapter 2.3

Endorphins
See chapter 2.3

Enkephalins
See chapter 2.3

Analgesic drugs
See chapter 2.3

Questionnaire methods

The McGill Pain Questionnaire (MPQ) (Melzack and Torgerson 1971) was developed from work demonstrating high agreement among patients, students and physicians on the meaning attached to pain adjectives. It consists of 78 adjectives arranged into groups. The questionnaire is intended to reflect three dimensions – sensory, affective and evaluative – with three remaining groups reflecting a sensory miscellaneous category.

The MPQ yields a number of indices: a *pain rating index* based on two types of numerical values that can be assigned to each word descriptor; the *number of words chosen*; and the *present pain intensity* based on a 1–5 intensity scale. Since its introduction the MPQ has been used extensively, and experience suggests that it provides precise information on the sensory, affective and evaluative aspects of pain experience as well as discriminating among different pain problems (Melzack 1975).

Researchers from various countries have translated the MPQ and tested its reliability and validity; it is currently available in a wide variety of languages. A shortened form of the MPQ (SF-MPQ) has been developed (Melzack 1987) for use in the clinical postoperative situation and research situations that require a more rapid acquisition of data than is possible with the standard MPQ. The data obtained with the SF-MPQ provide information on the sensory, affective and overall intensity of pain.

Methods of managing pain

Physical approaches

Transcutaneous electrical nerve stimulation

Transcutaneous electrical nerve stimulation (TENS) is a small battery-operated pack that generates impulses via electrodes that produces continuous low-intensity electrical current to the skin. One of the most obvious predictions of the **gate control theory** was that stimulation of large-diameter fibres would inhibit pain. The practical implication of this is that increasing large-diameter fibre input to the spinal cord with vibration, acupuncture and electrical stimulation can inhibit upward transmission of pain impulses. TENS controls pain by providing a continuous low-intensity electrical current that stimulates large fibres, closing the gate on the smaller-diameter pain fibres. Simultaneously, TENS is thought to stimulate the production of **endorphins**.

Acupuncture

Acupuncture is part of traditional Chinese medicine that involves the insertion of needles at specific points on the body. Acupuncture points were discovered and mapped thousands of years ago and the effects can be powerful enough to control severe pain (Schoen 1994). Acupuncture points do not necessarily have to be close to the source of the pain to be effective. The effects are produced by the release of endogenous opioids such as **enkephalins** (Heath 1997).

Pharmacological considerations in the management of pain

It is only in recent years, as we have begun to understand the physiological processes that underlie pain, that drugs have begun to be designed with predictable analgesic activity.

Analgesics can be divided broadly into two groups, anti-inflammatory and opioids, and these vary in effectiveness, site of action and incidence of side-effects.

Anti-inflammatory analgesics

Paracetamol and aspirin and are the most commonly used anti-inflammatory analgesics. They have the common property of inhibiting prostaglandin synthesis and may have a more peripheral site of action. Paracetamol is used most commonly and, although it can cause liver damage in overdose, it is safe in normal dosage. Aspirin is also an effective analgesic but has many contraindications which relate primarily to its effects on thrombotic regulation.

Non-steroidal anti-inflammatory drugs

Non-steroidal anti-inflammatory drugs (NSAIDs) are a useful group of medicines for managing pain due to inflammation such as rheumatoid arthritis and osteo-arthritis. According to Heath (1997) these drugs act per-ipherally at the site of trauma and consequently are an effective adjuvant to opioid drugs without increasing unwanted side-effects. However, they are contraindicated in patients with renal impairment and also cause gastro-intestinal bleeding and hypersensitivity reactions in situations of prolonged use. Of particular importance is the risk to asthmatic patients, who should not routinely use NSAIDs.

Opioid analgesics

Opioid analgesics are the most commonly prescribed drugs for surgical and other forms of intense acute and chronic pain. The term opioid is used to describe all drugs, natural and synthetic, which bind specifically to opioid receptors and exert an agonist action. The ability to bind to these receptors is antagonized by the opioid antagonist naloxone. It is now known that the opioid system comprises four distinct receptor subtypes: mu, kappa, delta and sigma. Mu receptors are of two kinds, m1 and m2; m1 is believed to mediate analgesia, whereas m2 receptors mediate the unwanted side-effects of respiratory depression, addiction and constipation (Melzack and Wall 1988).

Weak opioids

A number of agents related to morphine, for example codeine, dihydrocodeine and dextropropoxyphene, are used in an attempt to increase analgesia via the oral route whilst minimizing the unwanted side-effects. The main use of these drugs is for 'step up' or 'step down' treatment according to the analgesic ladder in the management of changing situations, either when simple analgesia ceases to be effective in a progressive condition or where the degree of pain no longer warrants strong opioids (Heath 1997).

Morphine

Despite the current availability of several new agonist/antagonist or partial agonist drugs, morphine – the pure agonist – remains the mainstay of the treatment of post-operative pain, sickle-cell crisis pain, cancer and other acute pain. It will be used as a practical example of the pharmacological properties of drugs of this type. Morphine is the most pharmacologically active constituent of opium; its use is dictated by intensity of pain and not brevity of prognosis (Twycross 1984). This means that morphine should be prescribed when a weaker narcotic fails to relieve pain.

Morphine and diamorphine (heroin) are agonists at mu receptors and also have some affinity for kappa receptors, although the affinity for mu receptors is nearly 100 times greater (Alexander and Hill 1988). Under some circumstances opioids may produce analgesia by a peripheral mechanism, and also act within the central nervous system.

Diamorphine is a derivative of morphine and its pharmacological properties are almost identical to those of morphine. It is readily absorbed by all routes of administration and its greater solubility allows larger doses to be administered in a single injection.

All morphine and other mu-selective opioid agonists are potent analgesics; they tend to induce euphoria and have a strong dependence liability, which makes these drugs subject to legal controls. Mu opioids are respiratory depressants and, in large doses, can cause heavy sedation. They can also produce nausea and vomiting, and cause constipation (Alexander and Hill 1988).

Morphine depresses the respiratory centre, making it less sensitive to carbon dioxide (the stimulus for normal respiration). The euphoria-inducing element of morphine is the reason for its strong addictive potential; however, there is little convincing evidence to suggest that the appropriate use of morphine to control severe pain leads to addiction. The incidence of addiction associated with therapeutic use of opiates in the adult population is generally overestimated by nursing staff (McCaffrey and Ferrell 1990).

Morphine and other mu opioids show reduced effectiveness if administered repeatedly at high doses; this is usually referred to as tolerance. When prolonged high-dose administration of mu opioids is stopped, a withdrawal syndrome develops. This can also be precipitated without stopping the opioid if a potent antagonist drug such as naloxone is given. Typically, withdrawal leads to sweating, cramps, diarrhoea, shivering and general malaise.

Alternatives to morphine

Pethidine

Pethidine is a synthetic compound that has a similar receptor-binding profile to morphine, being largely mu selective. In addition to the opioid properties shared with morphine, pethidine has atropine-like actions and is about one-eighth as potent as morphine. It has an established role in obstetrics because it is a mild stimulant of uterine contractions and appears to cause less respiratory depression in the newborn than morphine. It was also used historically to manage acute sickle-cell crisis pain but because of its short half-life and the toxic build-up of the metabolite, norpethidine, use of pethidine in this area is no longer tenable. Consequently pethidine is now contraindicated in the management of sickle-cell pain throughout the UK.

Fentanyl and alfentanil

These compounds are potent mu-selective agents and are chemically closely related to each other and to pethidine. Fentanyl is some 50–100 times more potent than morphine as an analgesic because of its lipid solubility. It has, however, a shorter duration of action, which limits

its utility. Alfentanil is similar to fentanyl but has a more rapid onset of action and an even shorter duration of action. Fentanyl has not been used generally for post-operative pain because doses that do not cause respiratory depression have a very short action. However, with the increased use of patient-controlled analgesia (PCA) fentanyl is now being used for the management of postoperative pain (Mather and Owen 1988).

Patient-controlled analgesia

From the above discussion it is clear that there is a wide range of potent medications for controlling pain, and the past three decades have seen a change in the focus of attention from seeking the perfect drug towards providing optimal drug delivery methods that integrate the personal experience of the patient. PCA offers that kind of drug delivery system, and also offers more precise control of pain.

The PCA system consists of a syringe pump and a timing device. The patient activates the system by pressing a button, causing a small dose of analgesic to be delivered into the venous system. Simultaneously a lock-out device is activated, ensuring that another dose cannot be delivered until the first dose has had time to exert its full effect. Thus, PCA is currently the ultimate patient-centred pain management technique because it allows patients to determine when and how much analgesic they receive, and secondly it allows determination of a minimum blood drug concentration associated with effective analgesic concentration and minimum side-effects, despite great interpatient variability.

Recent development of PCA technology appears to have followed two main streams. One is the development of increasingly sophisticated bedside drug delivery systems and the other is the production of smaller devices suitable for ambulatory use.

PCA as an efficient means of controlling postoperative pain

When compared to the more conventional 'PRN' (when required) method, the active involvement of the patient offered by PCA has been found to provide more effective relief (O'Connor et al 1993, Thomas et al 1995). For example, O'Connor et al (1993) found that within the first 4 hours after operation patients receiving intramuscular injections experienced 80% of the worst pain they could imagine, compared with 30% among the PCA groups.

PCA is also associated with a reduction in the length of stay in hospital (Thomas et al 1993), with findings demonstrating that patients receiving PCA are discharged on average 2 days earlier than those having intramuscular injections. This suggests that PCA promotes recovery. An explanation for this is that PCA provides an increased sense of control, which promotes a sense of well-being (Thomas and Rose 1993). The nurse should, however, ensure that the patient receives adequate antiemetic medication to prevent the continual nausea and vomiting that may be associated with PCA administration of opioids.

Psychological aspects of PCA

Although patients are generally satisfied with the effectiveness of relief obtained from PCA, effective analgesia may not necessarily be related to patient satisfaction. Some patients may prefer more nursing attention (Koh and Thomas 1994), whilst fear of overdose may result in underuse of PCA and the patient experiencing more pain than with intramuscular injections. The extent to which patients accept and use PCA is dependent on their attitudes and beliefs about pain and its relief – in other words, their psychology.

Whilst in general terms PCA does appear to be superior to intramuscular injections, this cannot be taken to mean that PCA functions optimally for all patients. For instance, Murphy et al (1993) found that a small proportion of surgical patients were unwilling to use PCA despite encouragement. Although psychological variables were not measured it is likely that this reluctance may have been influenced by psychological factors.

It is well recognized that psychological factors play a significant role in the perception and tolerance of pain as well as in the willingness to communicate the discomfort and distress caused by pain (Melzack and Wall 1988), and these factors are of utmost importance in relation to PCA (Thomas and Rose 1993). Research addressing the psychological issues concerning PCA is limited (Thomas et al 1995), but the implications from these studies suggest that, if a patient does not normally acknowledge a degree of personal control and responsibility for his or her own health, allocation to a PCA regimen may be a source of stress to the patient and prove less beneficial than more conventional methods. Further investigation is required to be able to predict patients who will benefit the most from its use.

Psychological approaches to pain management

The psychological techniques that can be used in pain management are extensive and deserve the space of a whole chapter, if not a book, and I refer the reader to Gatchel and Turk (1996). The present discussion will be confined to the role of information and cognitive behavioural therapy (CBT). As outlined in the discussion of the gate control theory, there is a close relationship between physiological and psychological factors. Thus cognitive processes (i.e. the way we think) can affect the amount and quality of pain experienced by altering the influence of the spinal gate mechanism, and directly modulate the pain experience.

Information

Eccleston (1997) suggests that pain activity in the nervous system can be interpreted as a sudden increase in information that travels quickly to the brain where it is decoded and acted upon. The decoding is known as cognition (the meaning of the pain) and the action is the resultant behaviour. Information is extremely important in helping to appraise (give meaning to sensation) and manage pain. In the acute pain situation information is used to prepare people for what to expect, whilst in the chronic pain context information is best used to counteract unhelpful and inaccurate beliefs (Williams 1997). The provision of adequate information to a person who is about to undergo surgery reduces the uncertainty and the distress and degree of pain experienced in the postoperative period.

Some typical informational control techniques have informed patients about the sensations they are likely to experience and procedures involved in the situation (Hayward 1975, Boore 1978). The extent to which information is of value depends largely on the coping styles of the patients (i.e. their normal preference for information). Thus, if a person usually copes with stress by distraction, providing detailed information about what the operation entails, what it will feel like and what the sounds represent is likely to increase anxiety and subsequent pain.

Cognitive behavioural therapy

By far the most effective psychological approach used in pain management utilizes cognitive behavioural psychology. It seeks to influence patients' perception or appraisal of events and their behaviour by addressing their concerns at cognitive and behavioural levels. The cognitive aspect recognizes the importance of the individual's personal view of the experience. The behavioural portion emphasizes active performance-based strategies to reduce pain. Behaviourally oriented training recognizes that remedial efforts towards successful coping require the practice of relevant practical skills and thinking strategies.

The central features of the CBT perspective include:

- interest in the nature and modification of patients' thoughts, feelings, beliefs and behaviours

- some commitment to behaviour therapy procedures in promoting change (e.g. graded practice, homework assignments, relaxation and relapse prevention training).

Although CBT may result in a reduction in the frequency and intensity of pain, pain relief is not the primary goal. Rather, the aim is to help patients learn to live more effective and satisfying lives despite the presence of pain (Turk and Meichenbaum 1994) (see Box 7.2).

Studies evaluating the efficacy of CBT in chronic pain have consistently revealed that it is significantly more effective in reducing pain distress and negative coping strategies, and in improving positive coping strategies, perceptions of internal control and pain self-efficacy, than an attention placebo or no-treatment control (Turner and Jensen 1993, Keefe and Caldwell 1997, Compass et al 1998, Thomas et al 1999).

The main focus of the work in CBT is to get patients to understand the relationships between their beliefs about pain, their feelings and their behaviour. The aim is to teach patients to identify unhelpful thoughts that lead to negative feelings such as anger, anxiety and depression, and to modify them. This is achieved by a technique known as cognitive restructuring, whereby patients are taught to examine objectively whether such thoughts are accurate and justified by the evidence (Turner and Keefe 1999). Another important task of the therapist is to teach patients to keep a log of their thoughts. This is achieved by providing a record sheet with four columns, for identifying a particular event that triggers such thoughts, feelings, and behavioural outcome. With respect to feelings, patients are asked to rate the intensity of accompanying emotion on a scale of 0–100%; in the example given in Box 7.3, feelings of sadness and depression are estimated to be 80%, indicating a very powerful sense of depression.

Box 7.2   Primary objectives of cognitive behavioural treatment programmes as outlined by Turk and Meichenbaum (1994)

- To combat demoralization by assisting patients to change their view of their pain and suffering from overwhelming to manageable

- To teach patients that there are coping techniques and skills that can be used to help them adapt and respond to pain and the resultant problems

- To assist patients to reconceptualize their views of themselves from being passive, reactive and helpless to being active, resourceful and competent

- To help patients learn the associations between thoughts, feelings and their behaviour, and subsequently to identify and alter automatic, maladaptive patterns

- To teach patients specific coping skills and, moreover, when and how to utilize these more adaptive responses

- To bolster self-confidence and encourage patients to attribute successful outcomes to their own efforts

- To help patients anticipate problems proactively and generate solutions, thereby facilitating maintenance and generalization.

Box 7.3   Example of thought monitoring

Event	Thought	Feeling	Behaviour outcome
Woke up with pain in right hip	There is nothing I can do to relieve the pain	Sadness, depression (80%)	Stayed in bed all day

Thought monitoring is done as homework activity, and is useful in educating patients to distinguish between thoughts and feelings. As therapy progresses, the therapist works with the patient to determine whether negative thoughts are accurate and whether alternative interpretations are possible. For example, in response to the negative thought 'There is nothing I can do to relieve the pain', the therapist helps the patient to recognize that such a thought is incorrect because relaxation is something the patient can do relieve the pain. The objective is to assist patients to recognize that negative thoughts are only one way of thinking about their situation and that with systematic examination of evidence more optimistic alternatives are possible.

Relaxation

Relaxation training appears to be an effective adjunctive treatment, used in comprehensive pain management programmes. Chief benefits include the reduction of muscle tension and pain; a decrease in the fear associated with the anticipation of pain; and an increase in confidence in coping with pain. As relaxation training emphasizes self-control, many medical centres offer this training in an attempt to reduce the need for analgesic and antianxiety medication. In evaluating the efficacy of relaxation in adults with chronic pain, McCaffrey and Beebe (1989) reported that patients rated relaxation training to be more helpful than pharmacological treatments and counselling, but less helpful than physical therapy. According to Linton (1982), relaxation is helpful because it reduces tension in patients with chronic pain. Progressive muscle relaxation is the commonest relaxation strategy used in chronic pain situations and has been found to be effective in reducing pain, anxiety and disability at 1 and 4 months' follow-up (Seers 1997).

Imagery

Focusing on a pleasant image is a useful addition to relaxation. Images can involve ourselves, the outside world and images of ourselves in the world. However, in the context of CBT strategies, images using multiple senses (seeing, hearing and touching) are likely to be most effective (Turner and Keefe 1999). For example, the patient might imagine herself lying on a Caribbean beach, and in this imagery she can imagine seeing the deep blue-green of the sea, hear children's laughter as they play in the water, feel the sun on her face, and trail her fingers in the warm sand.

As people with chronic pain frequently have imagery of the part of their body that hurts, the therapist can guide the patient (guided imagery) to soothe the pain; for example: 'Imagine that the sun is acting as a heat pad to the painful part and soothing the pain away'.

Coping self statements

Positive statements such as 'I know that can cope with this, if I remain calm and relaxed' are very helpful in countering negative thoughts such as those discussed above. As with all the strategies taught in CBT, coping self statements need to be practised over several weeks in order that they become part of a repertoire of coping skills.

Group therapy

Although CBT has been established as individual therapy, group CBT is very popular in many chronic pain management programmes. The advantages of group over individualized approaches include more efficient allocation of professional resources and the value of support from others who have similar problems (Turner and Keefe 1999). However, all group programmes take account of the individual in the group, and goals for behavioural change are developed individually with each patient.

Maintenance of gains

An important component of CBT programmes is the prevention of relapse. To maintain positive benefits, the therapist works with patients to identify early signs of obstacles or high-risk situations and develop an action plan. Through the use of role play the patient rehearses how to cope in such situations.

Summary

This chapter has considered the physiology, pharmacology and psychology of pain, which must all be taken into account when discussing pain and its control. The routine assessment of pain and its relief is an important component of any pain management strategy and, as the above discussion showed, there are many different methods of assessing pain. However, the use of a simple VAS in the absence of more comprehensive methods is recommended.

An important way of achieving effective pain control is through effective communication with the patient and the multidisciplinary team: Carr (1997) has argued that no one member of the team should assume responsibility for pain control. Therefore, the nurse needs to liaise closely with physicians, physiotherapists, psychologists and pharmacists. The development of newer methods of analgesic administration such as PCA has provided opportunities for greater relief compared with the traditional nurse-administered intramuscular injection method. Effective pain management should be seen as essential to the provision of good-quality care, but can occur only with accurate and regular assessment of the patient's pain.

References

Alexander JJ, Hill RG (1988) Postoperative pain control. Oxford: Blackwell Scientific.

Anand KJS, Hickey PR (1987) Pain and its effects in the human neonate and fetus. New England Journal of Medicine 317(21): 1321–1329.

Beck AT (1976) Cognitive therapy and the emotional disorders. New York: New American Library.

Beecher HK (1956) Relationship of significance of wound to pain experienced. Journal of American Medical Association 161: 1609–1613.

Belville JW, Forrest WH Jr, Miller E et al (1971) Influence of age on pain relief from analgesics. Journal of American Medical Association 217: 1835–1841.

Berkowitz BA, Ngai SH, Yang JC et al (1975) The disposition of morphine in surgical patients. Clinical Pharmacology and Therapeutics 17: 629–635.

Beyer J (1994) The Oucher: a pain intensity scale for children. In: Funk SG, Tornquist EM, Champagne MT, Copp LA, Weise RA, eds. Management of pain, fatigue and nausea, pp. 35–45. Basingstoke: Macmillan.

Bond MR (1979) Pain, its nature, analysis and treatment. Edinburgh: Churchill Livingstone.

Boore JRP (1978) Information a prescription for recovery. London: Royal College of Nursing.

Burns JW, Hodsman NBA, McLintock TT et al (1989) The influence of patient characteristics on the requirements for postoperative analgesia. Anaesthesia 44: 2–6.

Carr E (1997) Management of post-operative pain: problems and solutions. In: Thomas V, ed. Pain, its nature and management, pp. 156–175. London: Baillière Tindall.

Cassell EJ (1982) The nature of suffering and the goals of medicine. Oxford: Oxford University Press.

Chapman CR (1984) New directions in the understanding and management of pain. Journal of Social Science and Medicine 19(12): 1261–1277.

Chapman CR (1989) Assessment of pain. In: Nimmo WS, Smith G, eds. Anaesthesia, pp. 1149–1165. London: Blackwells.

Compass BE, Haaga DAF, Keefe FJ et al (1998) Sampling of empirically supported psychological treatments from health psychology: smoking, chronic pain, cancer and bulima nervosa. Journal of Consulting and Clinical Psychology 66: 89–112.

Copp LA (1974) The spectrum of suffering. American Journal of Nursing 74(3): 491–495.

Daut RL, Cleeland CS (1982) The prevalence and severity of pain in cancer. Cancer 50: 99–108.

Davis P (1993) Opening up the gate control theory. Nursing Standard 7(45): 25–27.

Donovan BD (1983) Patients' attitude to postoperative pain relief. Anaesthesia and Intensive Care 11(2): 125–129.

Eccleston C (1997) Pain and thinking: an introduction to cognitive psychology. In: Thomas V, ed. Pain, its nature and management, pp. 35–53. London: Baillière Tindall.

Eland JM (1981) Minimising pain associated with pre-kindegarten intramuscular injections. Issues in Comprehensive Paediatric Nursing 5: 361–372.

Eland JM (1985) The role of the nurse in children's pain. In: Copp LA, ed. Recent advances in nursing: perspectives on pain, pp. 24–45. Edinburgh: Churchill Livingstone.

Flannery RB, Sos J, McGovern P (1987) Ethnicity as a factor in the expression of pain. Psychosomatics 22: 39–50.

Fordham M, Dunn V (1994) Alongside the person in pain: holistic care and nursing practice. London: Baillière Tindall.

Frank AJM, Moll JMH, Hort JF (1982) A comparison of three ways of measuring pain. Rheumatology and Rehabilitation 21: 211–217.

Frayling IM, Addison GM, Chatergee K, Meakin G (1990) Methaemoglobinaemia in children treated with prilocaine–lignocaine cream. British Medical Journal 310: 153–154.

Gatchel RJ, Turk DC, eds (1996) Psychological approaches to pain management: a practitioners' handbook. New York: Guilford Press.

Goodman JE, McGrath PJ (1991) The epidemiology of pain in children and adolescents: a review. Pain 46: 247–264.

Hayward J (1975) Information: a prescription against pain. The Study of Nursing Care Reports, series 2, no. 5. London: Royal College of Nursing.

Heath M (1997) The use of pharmacology in pain management. In: Thomas V, ed. Pain, its nature and management, pp. 93–107. London: Baillière Tindall.

Keefe FJ, Caldwell DS (1997) Cognitive behavioural control of arthritis pain. Medical Clinics of North America Advances in Rheumatology 81: 277–290.

Khun S, Cooke K, Collins M, Jones JM, Mucklow JC (1990) Perceptions of pain relief after surgery. British Medical Journal 300: 1687–1690.

Koh P, Thomas VJ (1994) Patient controlled analgesia: does time saved by PCA improve patient satisfaction with nursing care? Journal of Advanced Nursing 20: 61–70.

Lim AT, Edis G, Kranz H et al (1983) Postoperative pain control: contribution of psychological factors and transcutaneous electrical stimulation. Pain 17: 179–188.

Linton SJ (1982) Applied relaxation as a method of coping with chronic pain: a therapist's guide. Scandinavian Journal of Behaviour Therapy 11: 161–174.

Lipton J, Marbach J (1984) Ethnicity in pain experience. Social Science and Medicine 19(12): 1279–1298.

Llewellyn N (1997) The management of children's pain. In: Thomas V, ed. Pain, its nature and management, pp. 135–155. London: Baillière Tindall.

Mandler G (1972) Helplessness: theory and research in anxiety. In: Spielberger CD, ed. Anxiety: current trends in theory and research, pp. 93–105. New York: Academic Press.

Mather LE, Owen H (1988) The scientific basis of patient controlled analgesia. Anesthesia and Intensive Care 16(4): 427–446.

McCaffrey M, Beebe A (1989) Pain: clinical manual for nursing practice. St Louis, MO: CV Mosby.

McCaffrey M, Ferrell B (1990) Do you know a narcotic when you see one? Nursing 20: 62–63.

McCaffrey M, Pasero C (1999) Pain: clinical manual, 2nd edn. St Louis, MO: Mosby.

Meinhart NT, McCaffrey M (1983) Pain: a nursing approach to assessment and analysis. New York: Appleton Century-Crofts.

Melzack R (1975) The McGill Pain Questionnaire: major properties and scoring methods. Pain 1: 275–299.

Melzack R (1987) The short form McGill Pain Questionnaire. Pain 30: 191–197.

Melzack R, Dennis SG (1978) Neurophysiological foundations of pain. In: Sternbach RA, ed. The psychology of pain, pp. 1–25. New York: Raven Press.

Melzack R, Torgerson WS (1971) On the language of pain. Anesthesiology 34: 50–59.

Melzack R, Wall P (1965) Pain mechanism: a new theory. Science 150: 971–979.

Melzack R, Wall PD (1988) The challenge of pain. Harmondsworth: Penguin Books.

Miller JF, Shuter R (1984) Age, sex and race affect pain expression. American Journal of Nursing 9: 981.

Miller SM, Coombs C, Stoddard E (1989) Information, coping and control in patients undergoing surgery and stressful procedures. In: Steptoe A, Appels A, eds. Stress, personal control and health, pp. 107–129. Chichester: Wiley.

Mitchell RWD, Smith G (1989) The control of postoperative pain. British Journal of Anaesthesia 63: 147–158.

Murphy DF, Grazioti P, Chalkiadias G et al (1993) Patient controlled analgesia for postoperative pain relief: a comparison with nurse controlled intravenous opioids. Abstracts of the Seventh World Congress on Pain, 22–27 August, p. 393. Seattle, WA: IASP Publications.

O'Connor M, Warwick P, Culpeper VE (1993) Evaluation of the effectiveness of an acute pain team. Abstracts of the Seventh World Congress on Pain, 22–27 August, p. 394. Seattle, WA: IASP Publications.

Peck CL (1986) Psychological factors in acute pain management. In: Cousins MJ, Phillips GD, eds. Acute pain management, pp. 251–274. Edinburgh: Churchill Livingstone.

Reading AE (1984) Testing pain mechanisms in persons in pain. In: Wall PD, Melzack R, eds. Textbook of Pain, pp. 195–206. Edinburgh: Churchill Livingstone.

Romano JM, Turner JA (1985) Chronic pain and depression: does the evidence support a relationship? Psychology Bulletin 97: 18–34.

Schoen AM (1994) Veterinary acupuncture, ancient art to modern medicine. Goleta, CA: American Veterinary Publications.

Scott J, Huskisson EC (1976) Graphic representation of pain. Pain 2: 175–184.

Seers K (1997) Chronic non-malignant pain: a community-based approach to management. In: Thomas V, ed. Pain, its nature and management, pp. 221–237. London: Baillière Tindall.

Skevington SM (1995) Psychology of pain. Chichester, UK: John Wiley.

Spielberger CD (1966) Theory and research on anxiety. In: Spielberger CD, ed. Anxiety and behaviour, pp. 3–21. New York: Academic Press.

Spielberger CD (1973) Emotional reactions to surgery. Journal of Consulting and Clinical Psychology 40: 33–38.

Streltzer J, Wade TC (1981) The influence of cultural group on the undertreatment of postoperative pain. Psychosomatic Medicine 43: 397.

Taenzer PA, Melzack R, Jeans ME (1986) Influence of psychological factors on postoperative pain, mood and analgesic requirements. Pain 24: 331–342.

Thomas VJ, Heath ML, Rose FD (1990) Effect of psychological variables and pain relief system on postoperative pain. British Journal of Anaesthesia 64: 388–389.

Thomas VJ (1991) Personality characteristics and the effectiveness of patient controlled analgesia. PhD thesis, Goldsmiths' College, London University.

Thomas VJ, Rose D (1991) Ethnic differences in the experience of pain. Social Science and Medicine 32: 1063–1066.

Thomas VJ, Rose D (1993) Patient controlled analgesia: a new method for old. Journal of Advanced Nursing 18: 719–726.

Thomas VJ, Rose FD, Heath ML, Flory P (1993) A multidimensional comparison of nurse and patient controlled analgesia in the management of acute post surgical pain. Medical Science Research 21: 379–381.

Thomas V, Heath M, Rose D, Flory P (1995) Psychological characteristics and the effectiveness of patient controlled analgesia. British Journal of Anaesthesia 74: 271–276.

Thomas VJ, Dixon A, Milligan P (1999) Cognitive behaviour therapy for the management of sickle cell disease pain – an evaluation of a community based intervention. British Journal of Health Psychology 4(Part 3): 209–229.

Trijsburg RW, Jelicic M, van den Broek WW, Plekker JE (1992) Behavioural treatment of needle phobia. Trijsburg voor Psychotherapie 18(6): 335–347.

Turk DC, Meichenbaum D (1994) A cognitive–behavioural approach to pain management. In: Wall PD, Melzack R, eds. Textbook of pain, 3rd edn, pp. 1337–1348. Edinburgh: Churchill Livingstone.

Turner JA, Jensen MP (1993) Efficacy of cognitive therapy for chronic low back pain. Pain 52: 169–177.

Turner J, Keefe FJ (1999) Cognitive behavioural therapy for chronic pain. In: Max M, ed. Pain: an updated review, pp. 523–535. Refresher course syllabus. Seattle, WA: IASP Press.

Twycross RG (1984) Narcotics. In: Wall PD, Melzack R, eds. Textbook of pain, pp. 515–525. Edinburgh: Churchill Livingstone.

Tyrer SP (1992) Psychiatric and psychological issues in different illnesses. In: Tyrer SP, ed. Psychology, psychiatry and chronic pain, pp. 57–69. Oxford: Butterworth Heinemann.

Tyrer SP, Capon M, Peterson DM et al (1989) The detection of psychiatric illness and psychological handicaps in a British pain clinic population. Pain 36: 63–74.

Walsh M, Crumbie A, Reveley S (1999) Nurse practitioners: clinical skills and professional issues. Oxford: Butterworth Heinemann.

Williams AC de C (1997) Psychological techniques in pain management. In: Thomas V, ed. Pain, its nature and management, pp. 108–124. London: Baillière Tindall.

Woodrow KM, Friedman CD, Siegelbaub AB, Collen MF (1972) Pain tolerance: differences according to age, sex and race. Psychosomatic Medicine 34: 548–556.

Further Reading

Thomas VJ, ed. (1997) Pain, its nature and management. London: Baillière Tindall.

This textbook provides current, scientifically based, practical information for nurses, doctors and those working in professions allied to medicine. It focuses on certain pain conditions that are known to be problematic and to represent a challenge to management approaches. The contributors to the book come from different disciplines in clinical nursing, nurse education, psychology and medicine. This variety reflects the fact that successful pain management requires the combined efforts of the multidisciplinary pain team.

McCaffrey M, Pasero C (1999) Pain: clinical manual. St Louis, MO: Mosby.

This manual also provides up-to-date, scientifically based, practical information, presented in clear manner that can be readily applied to a variety of pain populations. There are many patient examples and practical guidelines. It is written by two well known nurses who are expert pain specialists.

8 Infection and disease

Lynn J. Parker

Introduction

Infectious agents

Interaction between host and infectious agents

The course of an infectious disease

Types of infection

Clinical characteristics of infection

Diagnostic procedures used in infection

The management of patients with an infection

Occurrence of infectious disease in populations

Infectious disease in hospital populations

Community prevention and control of infection

Human immunodeficiency virus (HIV) infection

Summary

Introduction

Humans and animals are host to populations of micro-organisms that live on the skin and mucous membranes. Normally the human fetus lives in a sterile environment until birth, when the infant soon gains a complex flora of bacteria derived from maternal flora and surroundings. Certain species of bacteria regularly inhabit different parts of the body where they constitute the normal flora of the area.

Microorganisms that are capable of causing disease are termed *pathogens*. *Infection* occurs when an infectious agent multiplies within the body tissues causing adverse effects. The outcome of **infection** is determined by the ability of the microorganism to invade and overcome the host's defence mechanisms. Infection affecting specific body systems is discussed in later chapters. This chapter concerns infection in general.

Infectious agents

Microorganisms that cause infection in humans include bacteria, viruses, fungi, protozoa and parasitic worms.

Bacteria are extremely diverse single-celled microscopic organisms, usually 1–2 µm in diameter. Bacterial cells have a simple structure and are termed *prokaryotic*. They are characterized by a rigid cell wall made up of a network of carbohydrates and amino acids, called *peptidoglycan*. As it is unique to bacterial cells, peptidoglycan is a common target for antibiotics. When bacteria are viewed under a microscope they are found to occur in several distinct shapes: round (cocci), oblong (bacillus), curved rod (vibrio) or spiral (spirochaete). Staining the cells with dye distinguishes two main groups: those that stain purple are called Gram-positive and those that do not are called Gram-negative.

Some bacteria, when exposed to adverse conditions, form spores by surrounding themselves with a resistant casing. These spores are very difficult to destroy by heating or use of chemical agents. This is an important factor to consider when decontaminating used equipment.

Bacteria multiply by simply dividing into two. This process can be so rapid that, under favourable conditions, a single bacterial cell can give rise to one million cells after only 6 hours. Specimens taken for bacteriological

Infection
See chapter 6.1

analysis are usually stored in special containers and at low temperatures to prevent such rapid multiplication.

Bacteria are present in most environments. The surface of the body is populated by a wide variety of microorganisms – the **normal skin flora**. These organisms are *commensals*: they form a balance with their hosts, using them for growth and survival but not harming them. For example, the skin is a normal habitat of staphylococci, coliform bacilli are always present in the intestine, and lactobacilli inhabit the vagina. These commensal organisms may play an essential role in the body; for instance, **vitamin K**, which is necessary for **blood clotting**, is produced by the action of bacteria in the intestine. This commensal flora may cause disease if it gains access to another area of the body. For example, staphylococci may cause infection in surgical wounds and coliforms may cause urinary tract infection.

Other important organisms are rickettsiae, which are smaller than normal bacteria and are parasitic in that they can exist only within other cells. They are transmitted via tick or lice bites, producing diseases such as typhus. Chlamydia are small bacteria-like microorganisms that also only grow inside cells, and *Chlamydia trachomatis* is the major cause of non-specific urethritis in men and of cervicitis in women. Mycoplasmas are the smallest of all cells and inhabit body fluids. *Mycoplasma pneumoniae* is one cause of pneumonia.

Viruses are small infectious agents ranging in size from 0.02 to 0.3 μm. They differ from other living organisms in that they are not cells but simply a piece of either **DNA** or **RNA** surrounded by a protein coat, and sometimes a lipid envelope. They are unable to reproduce themselves but are obligate parasites of living cells in plants, animals and even bacteria. Once inside the cell, they direct the host's metabolic machinery to reproduce themselves. New viruses are released from the cell by budding out of the membrane or by causing the cell to rupture. The damage to the cells causes the symptoms of the disease in the host. Some viruses may become integrated within the host cell genome and become established indefinitely. The initial symptoms of the invasion may disappear and the virus remains dormant, only to reactivate later and produce symptoms, as in herpes simplex infection.

The many varieties or strains of virus and their intracellular location has made effective therapy more difficult. Examples of viral diseases are the common cold, influenza, measles, mumps and acquired immune deficiency syndrome (**AIDS**). There is also accumulating evidence that viruses are associated with the development of some malignant diseases.

Fungi are plants. They have complex, eukaryotic cells. Most are multicellular organisms that grow as interlacing filaments or chains. A disease caused by a fungus is called a *mycosis*, or it may be indicated by the suffix -osis, preceded by the name of the causative fungus. Thrush,

ringworm and histoplasmosis are examples of mycotic disease.

Protozoa are single-celled organisms that belong to the animal kingdom and are more complex in structure and activity than bacteria. Diseases that are caused by protozoa include malaria, giardiasis, amoebic dysentery and trichomoniasis.

Parasitic worms, or helminths, may also cause infection. The most common infections are those caused by the roundworm, pinworm and tapeworm.

Interaction between host and infectious agents

The outcome of the interaction between microorganisms and the host depends on the balance between the ability of the organism to establish infection and the host defence mechanisms. The ability of a microorganism to invade and injure host tissue is termed *virulence*.

Virulence

There are a number of ways in which microorganisms can increase their virulence. To establish infection, the organism must first be able to enter and adhere to tissue in the host. Different species are able to invade specific tissues in the host. For example, *Neisseria meningitidis* attacks the meninges of the central nervous system, while *Neisseria gonorrhoeae* and *Chlamydia trachomatis* invade epithelial cells of the cervix.

Many bacteria protect themselves against phagocytic white blood cells (see p. 376) by covering the outside of their cell with a layer of gelatinous material. This *capsule* can also help the cell to adhere to surfaces (e.g. *Streptococcus pneumoniae*). Some bacteria protect themselves from attack by the immune system by multiplying within phagocytic cells themselves (e.g. *Mycobacterium tuberculosis* multiplies within macrophages), while some viruses may lie dormant within host cells for long periods of time. Herpes simplex may persist for long periods before producing signs of infection such as cold sores and genital herpes.

Bacteria may also invade their host as a result of producing destructive substances known as *toxins* (e.g. haemolysins which destroy red blood cells). Some bacteria excrete exotoxins that give rise to serious illnesses. *Clostridium tetani*, for example, produces a toxin that, by acting on the nervous system, produces the muscular spasm associated with tetanus. Toxic shock syndrome is associated with the toxin released by *Staphylococcus aureus* when present in the vagina. Some bacteria secrete endotoxins into their cell walls. These are responsible for raised temperature and a feeling of general malaise. When bacteria are killed they may release endotoxins. These are responsible for the syndrome of septic shock characterized by high temperatures and dangerously low blood pressure (hypotension).

Skin flora
See chapter 6.1

Vitamin K
See chapter 5.1

Vitamin K and
blood clotting
See chapter 4.1

DNA and RNA
See chapter 1.2

AIDS
See chapter 6.2

Host defences

The body has several different defences to protect it from invasion by microbes or other foreign material known as *antigens*. Non-specific defences act against all types of **antigen**. The specific immune response recognizes antigens previously encountered and mounts a rapid and very specific action against them.

Non-specific defences

Barriers

The **skin** is a protective barrier against most microorganisms as long as it is intact; however, any breach such as an intravenous cannula site or a wound offers easy access for invading microbes. Mucous membranes are less resistant and may be penetrated by bacteria such as *Neisseria gonorrhoeae*, while organisms such as the influenza virus can invade mucosal cells.

Bactericidal substances in body fluids

Skin secretions contain fatty acids that inhibit the growth and survival of many pathogens. Mucous membranes secrete an external layer of mucus which traps infectious agents, preventing their adhesion to the epithelial cells. The mucus is propelled by ciliary movement (mucociliary flushing) in the respiratory tract and by coughing and sneezing.

Most body fluids have bactericidal activity. Lysozyme is present in all tissues and all body secretions except urine. It is present in high concentration in tears. It is an enzyme capable of damaging the peptidoglycan cell wall of bacteria, causing the cell to rupture and die.

Gastric juice, highly acidic at pH 2.0, is lethal for nearly all bacteria, although if large numbers of microbes are ingested they may be protected by the bulk of food eaten. Breast milk and saliva contain lactoperoxidase, which inhibits multiplication of some bacteria. It also contains an antiviral agent (distinct from antibodies) that protects the mucosa against rotavirus infections.

Normal body flora

The commensals that form the **normal body flora** help to prevent colonization and infection by pathogens. Antibiotic treatment for an infection often destroys commensals, leaving the way open for resistant strains of bacteria to flourish in their place.

Phagocytosis

Phagocytosis is the engulfment, killing and digestion of microorganisms by polymorphonuclear leucocytes, monocytes and macrophages, which originate from stem cells in the bone marrow.

Polymorphonuclear leucocytes are highly mobile amoeboid cells present in the blood. They contain granules filled with potent chemicals that enable them to kill and digest microorganisms. Every minute of the day the bone marrow produces 80 million of these cells.

Monocytes circulate in the blood and then migrate into tissues, where they develop into macrophages. They are found in connective tissues in the lungs, liver, spleen, brain and lymph nodes.

Macrophages play an important role in both the non-specific and specific defence mechanisms of the body. They rid the body of cell debris (microorganisms and worn-out cells). The vital role played by macrophages in the immune responses and the development of inflammation is discussed below.

Complement

The **complement** system is a series of about 25 proteins that work to complement the activity of antibodies in destroying bacteria, either by facilitating phagocytosis or by puncturing bacterial cell membranes. It also aids in the elimination of antigen–antibody complexes from the body.

Complement proteins circulate in the blood in an inactive form. When the first of the series is activated by encountering a microbe, it sets in motion a cascade effect. As each protein is activated, it in turn acts on the next in a precise sequence that ends in the formation of a hole in the target cell, which rapidly swells and bursts.

In addition, this cascade has other consequences: the production of vasoactive substances by degranulation of mast cells and basophils causes redness and swelling; the attraction of polymorphs to the area (chemotaxis); and the rendering of target cells attractive to phagocytes (opsonization).

Natural killer (NK) cells

These non-specific lymphocytes rid the body of what they perceive as foreign or non-self cells without having to recognize a specific antigen. They migrate from the lymphoid tissue to the site of inflammation or tumour growth where they destroy the pathogens, tumour cells or virus-infected cells.

The inflammatory response

When a microbe or other foreign material enters the body, the first line of defence is the **inflammatory response**. This is initiated by the release of histamine from mast cells in the tissues and other substances such as kinins. These cause dilatation of capillaries and an increase in vascular permeability. Polymorphonuclear leucocytes migrate to the area to phagocytose the infectious agent. In so doing, they die themselves. Macrophages appear later to mop up the debris, which consists of dead leucocytes, bacteria and necrotic tissue. If the infection is severe enough, pus may be formed. The process can be recognized by local swelling, redness, heat and pain.

Host resistance to viruses

Interferon is an important component in the defence mechanism against viruses. When certain body cells – leucocytes,

Antigens
See chapter 4.1

Skin
See chapter 6.1

Gastric juice
See chapter 6.1

Skin flora
See chapter 6.1

Phagocytosis
See chapter 4.1

Polymorphonuclear
leucocytes
See chapter 4.1

Monocytes
See chapter 4.1

Macrophages
See chapter 4.1

Complement
See chapter 6.2

NK cells
See chapter 6.2

Inflammation
See chapter 6.1

fibroblasts and T lymphocytes – are infected by some viruses, they respond by producing interferon, a group of small proteins that inhibit virus multiplication within the cells. These proteins work only in the species that produced them. Interleukins are types of interferons that aid in stimulating the antibody response (play a role in the specific immune response).

Fever

Fever is a common manifestation of the inflammatory response and often indicates that infection is present. Various products of inflammation such as the proteins and hormones released by phagocytes act upon the thermo-regulatory centre in the hypothalamus to produce an increase in body temperature.

Figure 8.1   The specific immune response. The B cells, T cells and macrophages all interact to fend off the attack from invading microorganisms.

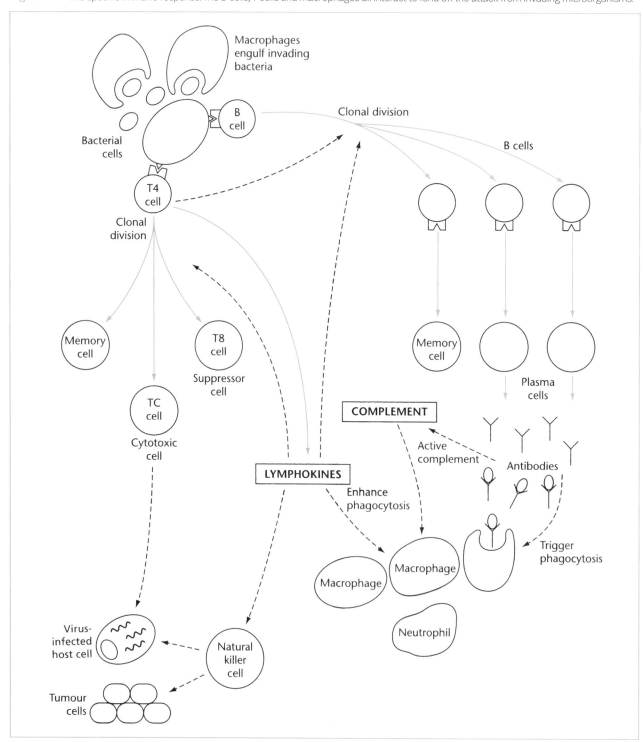

Reproduced with permission from Wilson (1995).

Specific defences

Anatomy of the immune system

The immune system consists of specialized cells and organs that are distributed throughout the body. The primary organs of the system are the bone marrow and the thymus, whereas the secondary organs include the lymph nodes, spleen and lymphatic tissue such as the tonsils.

The lymph nodes are connected by a network of small channels called **lymphatics**. Immune cells originate from the lymphoid stem cells of the bone marrow (Fig. 8.1) and differentiate into two distinct types known as T lymphocytes and B lymphocytes. The thymus gland houses the T lymphocytes which are involved in the *cell-mediated immune responses*, whilst the B lymphocytes (which originate in the red bone marrow) migrate to the lymphoid tissues where they are responsible for the production of antibodies or immunoglobulins. This is known as the *humoral response*.

The T and B lymphocytes are transported by the blood and lymph vessels. The lymph nodes filter the lymph drained from the tissues, separating out antigens and exposing them to the cells of the immune system. The spleen, like the lymph nodes, contains both T- and B-cell areas and is particularly effective in filtering out particulate antigens such as microorganisms. Removal of the spleen results in the loss of a significant part of the defences of the body.

The cells of the immune system must be able to recognize host cells to avoid attacking and destroying tissue. A marker protein on the surface of all host cells enables them to be distinguished from foreign non-self material. Autoimmune diseases are caused by the failure of the immune cells to recognize host tissue.

Cell-mediated response

When bacteria enter the body they are first ingested by macrophages. The bacterial antigen then appears on the surface of the macrophage where it is recognized by a corresponding T cell which binds with the antigen–macrophage complex. The T cell then starts to divide and produce a range of chemical mediators called *lymphokines*. The major lymphokines are interleukins and interferons, and these promote and coordinate the immune response.

Humoral response

Antibodies are secreted by the B cells, with cooperation from helper and cytotoxic killer T cells (known as T4 and T8 respectively). B cells bind with the antigen that fits their receptors. They then multiply, producing identical clone cells, which differentiate into plasma cells. The plasma cells produce large quantities of antibodies specific to the antigen for several days until they die. The antibodies are released into the circulation where they interlock with matching antigens to form antigen–antibody complexes. These complexes stimulate phagocytic activity and activate complement to destroy the bacterial cell or toxin.

The antibody production declines as the infection is overcome, plasma cells die and the cytotoxic killer T8 cells exert their control. Some activated B cells not converted to plasma cells become *memory cells*, which are stored and respond later when stimulated by exposure to the same antigen.

Antibodies are immunoglobulin molecules. They are composed of four interlinked polypeptide chains (two long or heavy chains and two shorter, light chains), shaped to form a Y (Fig. 8.2). The sections at the tips of the Y arms, called the *variable* regions, are the specific antigen-combining sites. The stem of the Y, called the *constant* region, links the antibody to complement and phagocytes. The major classes of immunoglobulins (Ig) or antibodies are labelled A, D, E, G and M, preceded by the symbol Ig (i.e. IgA, IgD, IgE, IgG and IgM) (Box 8.1).

On first exposure to an antigen there is a lag in response of a few days or weeks. IgM antibody is produced first, followed by IgG and IgA, or both. IgM levels soon decline. This is termed the *primary response*. On second exposure to the same antigen, months or even years later, antibodies are produced rapidly (the same amount of IgM but much more IgG). The prompt response is attributed to the persistence of memory cells for that specific antigen and is called the *secondary response*.

Lymphatics
See chapter 6.2

Cell-mediated immunity
See chapter 6.2

Humoral immunity
See chapter 6.2

The course of an infectious disease

The course of most infectious diseases extends over three phases: incubation, acute illness and convalescence.

The *incubation period* is the interval between the time the organism enters the body and the initial clinical

Figure 8.2   Structure of an antibody.

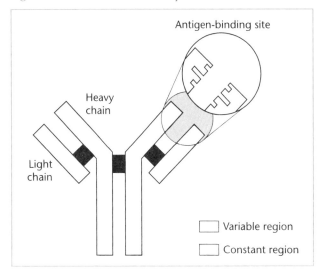

> **Box 8.1** The five major immunoglobulins
>
> ■ *Immunoglobulin G (IgG)* is the most common antibody in the blood and is able to enter the tissues. It crosses the placenta and provides protection against infection to the fetus and newborn
>
> ■ *Immunoglobulin M (IgM)* is large and tends to remain in the bloodstream where it produces an early line of attack against bacteria. It does not cross the placenta
>
> ■ *Immunoglobulin A (IgA)* is found in saliva, tears, respiratory and gastrointestinal secretions, and colostrum, as well as the bloodstream. It protects the external body openings against invasion
>
> ■ *Immunoglobulin E (IgE)* is associated with the symptoms of allergic responses
>
> ■ *Immunoglobulin D (IgD)* function is unclear but maximum levels appear in childhood.

Nausea and
vomiting
See chapter 5.1

Erythrocyte
sedimentation rate
See chapter 4.1

manifestations of an infection. During this stage the organisms multiply and host defences are mounted to counter the infection. The patient is asymptomatic but may excrete the infectious agent. If the host defences overcome the causative organisms, there may be no signs or symptoms. Sometimes a person may continue to excrete the pathogen without symptoms of the disease for a period of time. In this situation the person is said to be a *carrier*.

The *acute illness* is the stage in which the disease reaches its full intensity. The duration of acute illness varies from a few hours to weeks. It is generally predictable for the specific disease.

Convalescence is the stage during which the clinical manifestations subside. Many infectious diseases are self-limiting and recovery takes place over a short, defined period of time.

Types of infection

Certain terms may be used to describe infection. *Local* means the infection remains confined to one area. A *systemic* infection is one in which the organisms are disseminated throughout the body. If a person becomes infected by another type of organism during the course of an infection, this is termed a *secondary* infection, and the initial one is referred to as the *primary*. An infection may be *acute*, that is an intense illness of short duration, or *chronic*.

The presence of bacteria in the blood is called *bacteraemia*, but where this is accompanied by symptoms, such as fever, rigors, or chills and hypertension, this is called *septicaemia*. *Toxaemia* implies a concentration of bacterial toxins in the blood.

Clinical characteristics of infection

During the incubation period, symptoms of infection are usually general and include headache and malaise. During the acute stage the following systemic and local symptoms may occur:

■ fever, which may be preceded by chills

■ an increase in the pulse and respiratory rates

■ anorexia

■ **nausea and vomiting**

■ headache

■ apathy and fatigue

■ joint and muscle pain

■ general malaise.

The patient may appear hot and flushed, and the tongue is frequently furred and dry. There may be enlargement and tenderness of the lymph nodes closest to the site of infection.

If the infection is local, the classical symptoms are redness and heat due to vasodilatation, swelling (oedema) due to increased vascular permeability, and pain caused by the release of chemical mediators and pressure from increased tissue fluid. These symptoms are due to the inflammatory response. Inflammation is always present with infection unless the patient's immune system is severely impaired. Infection, on the other hand, is not always present with inflammation as inflammation may be caused by chemical irritants, radiation or trauma, as well as by microorganisms.

In addition to the common signs and symptoms described above, certain features characteristic of a specific infection may be present and may play an important role in the diagnosis. For example, certain infections cause a rash, while others may give rise to a marked increase in the level of a particular type of leucocyte.

Diagnostic procedures used in infection

Leucocyte count and differential

Some infections cause an increase in the number of white blood cells well above the normal, while in others there may be a decrease below the normal. An increase in a particular type of leucocyte is recognized as being characteristic of certain infections.

Erythrocyte sedimentation rate

This is a non-specific test sometimes requested as part of the diagnostic investigation. The rate at which the red blood cells settle in a specimen of blood is increased in infection and inflammation.

Identification of the causative organism

To identify the organism responsible for an infection it must be isolated from the body tissue or secretion where it is causing the infection. This is done by the following methods:

1. *Direct examination* of a specimen of sputum, blood, spinal fluid, urine, faeces, discharge or of the scrapings from a lesion. These are stained and examined under the microscope for organisms. Appearance, shape and certain staining characteristics assist in identifying different organisms.

2. *Culturing* the causative organism by inoculation of the specimen into nutrient media and allowing time for the organisms to multiply.

A pure growth of the causative organism that is isolated is tested for susceptibility to appropriate antimicrobial drugs. The results of these tests form the basis for the selection of the most appropriate, effective drug to destroy the organisms.

Antibody tests

A specimen of blood may be examined to determine the concentration of antibodies present; this is referred to as an *antibody titre*. Microorganisms act as antigens, stimulating the production of specific antibodies, and these antibody titres rise as the disease progresses (e.g. *Legionella*). Tests to detect the presence of certain antigens or antibodies may also be carried out; a known antibody is used to determine the presence of a corresponding antigen, or a known antigen is used to detect antibodies.

Skin tests

The *Mantoux tuberculin skin test* is used to determine whether an individual is immune to *Mycobacterium tuberculosis*, the cause of tuberculosis. A small amount of protein derived from mycobacterium is injected into the skin on the surface of the forearm. Swelling and redness at the site of injection within 2–3 days indicates a positive reaction. This means the individual has or has had an infection by tubercle bacilli, acquired either naturally or following bacille Calmette–Guérin (BCG) vaccination. The test is considered negative if there is no reaction. If the first test is negative, it may be repeated 6 weeks later.

An alternative skin test more commonly used in the UK is the multiple puncture test, or Heaf test. This is administered by use of a Heaf gun with a needle block of six needles that puncture the skin on firing. Puncture depth of the needles must be set to 2 mm for adults and children aged 2 years or more, and 1 mm for children under 2 years old.

The recommended site for testing is on the flexor surface of the left forearm at the junction of the upper one-third with the lower two-thirds, avoiding any eczematous areas. The skin is cleansed with an alcohol wipe only if it is visibly dirty, and is allowed to dry before undertaking the test. A small amount of tuberculin solution is dropped on to the skin at the standard test site. The Heaf gun is placed firmly on the solution and the handle is pressed until a click is heard, which indicates that the needles have been fired. Any excess fluid is wiped off the skin and the forearm checked for signs of the six puncture marks. The test is usually read at 7 days but can be read between 3 and 10 days. The heaf test is graded 0–4 and depends upon the degree of induration: 0–1 is regarded as negative; those with a grade 2 reaction are considered positive if there is no history of BCG immunization, and should be referred to the chest clinic; those with a grade 3–4 reaction should be referred directly to chest clinic (Department of Health 1996).

Collection of specimens

The examination of specimens in the laboratory plays an important part in the diagnosis and therapeutic management of an individual with infection. For accurate diagnosis it is particularly important that the sample represents the conditions that prevailed at the time of collection. The specimen must therefore not be allowed to deteriorate between collection and examination. When collecting specimens, these general procedures should be followed:

1. All specimens must be collected in a sterile, leak-proof container, which must be properly labelled with the patient's name and the source of the specimen, and submitted with a requisition form providing relevant clinical information, the date, time of collection, clinician's name and laboratory tests required. The container is usually sealed in a plastic bag to protect people handling it from contamination, should it leak.

2. The sample should be obtained from the site of infection and care must be taken to avoid contamination by normal body flora. The amount should be adequate for the number of tests required. (Check with the laboratory if unsure.)

3. Specimens should be collected before the administration of antibiotics. If this is not possible, indicate on the request form which antibiotics have been given.

4. Specimen collection should be performed with care and tact to avoid harming the patient, causing discomfort or undue embarrassment. Where patients are expected to provide a specimen themselves, they should be given clear instructions.

5. Specimens should be stored in a cool place and delivered promptly to the laboratory. If delivery is delayed, some delicate pathogens will die. Anaerobes (organisms that grow in the absence of molecular oxygen) will die when exposed to air. In addition, the normal flora of the patient may overgrow the pathogens and inhibit or kill them.

Where the suspected cause of the infection is a virus, fungus or protozoon, different techniques for specimen collection may be required and the laboratory should be contacted for advice.

The management of patients with an infection

There are two aspects to the management of a patient with infection: (1) the administration of appropriate therapy if available, and (2) supporting the patient through the illness by alleviating symptoms and monitoring for complications.

The first effective and non-toxic antimicrobial agent, penicillin, was discovered in the 1930s. Since then many other agents have been found and developed, and now a wide range of different antimicrobial drugs is available. Unfortunately many microorganisms have evolved resistance to antibiotics as a result of inappropriate use. As a consequence there is a constant race to develop new antibiotics which will replace their older and increasingly ineffective predecessors. Reacher et al (2000) have reported a 60% increase in blood isolates of microorganisms (bacteraemia) between 1990 and 1998 in England and Wales. Methicillin resistance in *Staphylococcus aureus* also rose from 1.7% in 1990 to 34% in 1998 according to these authors, indicating growth of the methicillin-resistant *S. aureus* (MRSA) problem.

The key to the management of infection is the early recognition of symptoms and identification of the causative organism. The correct drug can then be administered before the organism is able to overwhelm the host's immune defences. Viruses exist within their host cells and there are very few antimicrobial agents that are effective against them. Treatment mostly involves symptom control and supporting the patient through the acute phase of the illness, which in most cases is self-limiting.

Assessment

The clinical signs of infection may be non-specific in the early stages, and include a general malaise, headache, anorexia and arthralgia. As the infection progresses, symptoms associated with the inflammatory response may develop. The patient should be examined for these signs and for other symptoms such as purulent discharge, productive cough or abnormal respiration. Often infection will be accompanied by fever and chills. Night sweats are associated with intermittent fevers. A careful medical history can help to identify the site of the infection, and questioning about contact with an ill person, animals or travel abroad may provide vital clues regarding its cause. In the elderly the signs and symptoms of infection may be abnormal. They may not develop a fever but can often present with a history of incontinence, confusion or falling related to an underlying infection.

Once an infection has been diagnosed, there are a number of effects it may have on the body which require close monitoring.

Pyrexia. A raised body temperature is commonly associated with infection and, although it is assumed to confer an advantage to the host, the exact benefit is not clear (Mackowiak 1994). The effects of fever can be exhausting to the patient and deplete energy supplies, particularly if associated with violent shivering or rigors. The increase in metabolic rate associated with high fever may cause particular problems in the elderly.

Dehydration. High fever, sweating and diarrhoea may result in excessive fluid loss from the body. This may be exacerbated by the inability to ingest fluids or food. Severe dehydration is particularly associated with gastrointestinal infection, especially in infants and the elderly, who are vulnerable to the effects of dehydration.

Respiratory problems. Viral infections may affect the immune defences of the lungs and render them more susceptible to invasion by other microorganisms. Patients with impaired ability to clear their lungs of secretions, such as those with obstructive airway disease, are more susceptible to pulmonary infection.

Alteration in mucous membranes. The mucous membranes of the mouth are maintained by a constant flow of saliva, which removes bacteria and food debris. Saliva production is induced by chewing and is therefore reduced in the anorexic patient. The inability to ingest food and fluids, combined with fever and possibly nausea, can cause the mucous membranes to become dry and susceptible to secondary bacterial or fungal infection.

Nutritional imbalance. A severe infection may cause energy and protein depletion, particularly where a high fever increases the metabolic rate or the patient has experienced prolonged vomiting or diarrhoea.

Diarrhoea. This may be caused by the pathogen infecting the gastrointestinal tract or by an alteration in the normal flora of the bowel caused by antibiotic therapy. Children frequently manifest gastrointestinal symptoms when feverish. Severe diarrhoea may result in dehydration and cause considerable anguish and discomfort to the patient.

Nursing interventions

Planning the nursing care of a patient with infection depends on the nature of the infection. However, there are some general principles related to monitoring for complications of infection and symptom control that should be included in the plan of care.

Maintaining a normal body temperature

The **body temperature** of an infected patient requires regular assessment to monitor the progress of the infection and effect of treatment. Anti-inflammatory medication

*Temperature regulation
See Chapter 6.3*

such as aspirin may be prescribed, which will reduce body temperature. Efforts should be made to provide a cool environment by reducing the amount of bedclothes or providing a fan. Sweating may aggravate an itchy rash and this can be alleviated by bathing with warm water.

Maintaining fluid balance

The patient should be assessed for signs of dehydration. These may include dryness of the mucous membranes, concentrated urine, reduced urinary output and loss of skin turgor. Skin turgor can be evaluated by gently pinching the skin; in a dehydrated patient the skin will return only slowly to its normal position when released. Dehydration may also cause an imbalance in serum electrolytes. The patient should be encouraged to drink as much rehydration electrolyte solution as possible. Intravenous fluids may be prescribed if the patient is vomiting or the dehydration is severe.

Maintaining normal respirations

Patients at high risk of developing pulmonary complications should be carefully monitored for altered chest movements, respiratory rate, cough and shortness of breath. Regular changing of position and early mobilization help to expand and remove secretions from the lungs. Suction may be indicated if the patient is unable to remove secretions effectively. Fluid intake should be encouraged to thin the mucus and facilitate expectoration. If pulmonary function is poor, oxygenation may be indicated. The supply should be well humidified to prevent drying of secretions.

Maintaining healthy oral mucous membranes

The **mouth** should be examined regularly for signs of infection, dryness or cracking. Debris should be removed by regular cleaning using a toothbrush, toothpaste and water. Petroleum jelly can be applied to the lips to prevent cracking. The patient should be encouraged to eat, even small amounts, as soon as possible, to stimulate saliva production.

Maintaining nutrition

The nutritional status of the patient should be assessed and, where necessary, a high-protein diet provided to replace nutrients lost during the acute phase of the illness. The infection may cause loss of appetite so that meeting the preferences of the patient and providing frequent, small amounts of food may help to encourage intake. To minimize the energy demands on the body, as much rest as possible should be planned for the patient.

Maintaining bowel function

The colour, consistency and frequency of stool should be monitored. The presence of blood or mucus in the stool and history of vomiting, nausea and abdominal pain may also be of importance in the diagnosis of a gastrointestinal infection. Collection of faecal specimens for examination in the laboratory may be required.

Infection control precautions should be adhered to after contact with faeces to prevent cross-infection of other patients or staff. Gastrointestinal infection is usually self-limiting, but medication to reduce gut motility and diarrhoea may be prescribed.

Administration of antimicrobial agents

These are prescribed to destroy or control the causative organisms.

Before the administration of an antimicrobial agent, the patient should be questioned about any known allergies or drug reactions. The nurse must be familiar with the possible side-effects of the drug being used and must be alert for early signs of untoward reactions. Side-effects vary with the specific drug but generally include skin rashes, nausea, vomiting and diarrhoea.

When administering antimicrobial drugs it is important to provide adequate constant serum and tissue levels of the antimicrobial agent. To achieve this, the nurse must administer the medications at the correct time and, if given intravenously, over the prescribed time interval (e.g. 20 min). Aminoglycoside drugs (e.g. gentamicin) in particular require careful monitoring of blood levels. They can be nephrotoxic and hepatotoxic if the concentration circulating in the blood is too high. It is important to space the administration of different antimicrobial agents so that a constant serum level of the specific drug is maintained and incompatible drugs are not mixed together.

When the patient is taking antimicrobial drugs at home or is being discharged from hospital with a prescription for these agents, it is important that the patient is instructed to complete the full course of the prescribed medication and given specific instructions as to when drugs are to be taken. Times are determined by assessing the patient's daily lifestyle. The nurse should explain that antimicrobial therapy should not be stopped when the patient feels better, as this may result in relapse or enable resistant strains to develop, and that medications prescribed for a previous illness should not be substituted.

The growth of resistance is illustrated by *S. aureus*. Approximately 90% of these organisms are now resistant to penicillin in the UK and the methicillin-resistant *S. aureus* (MRSA) strain is resistant to all known antibiotics except vancomycin. Resistance is a product of evolution, as mutations that confer resistance to antibiotics are selectively bred into successive generations of bacteria. This process is aided by the incorrect prescription of antibiotics and by patients failing to complete courses that have been prescribed.

Preventing the spread of infection

Excretions and secretions may contain pathogens that are easily transmitted, especially on the hands of staff. Gloves should always be worn for handling potentially infected body fluids from a patient with infection, and

Fluid balance
See chapter 2.6

Respiration
See chapter 5.3

Mouth
See chapter 6.1

Bowel function
See chapter 6.1

hands washed before providing care to another patient. Equipment in contact with body fluids (e.g. commodes) may also transmit infection and should be carefully decontaminated before use by another patient.

Clark (2000) lists the following commonly acquired infections (hospital and community) which are resistant to antibiotics:

- wound, urine and respiratory infections due to MRSA

- septicaemia in hospital patients due to vancomycin-resistant enterococci

- respiratory infections due to penicillin-resistant *Streptococcus pneumoniae*

- food poisoning caused by multiresistant *Salmonella typhimurium* (DT 104).

Effective infection control practice can reduce the risk of a patient acquiring one of these life-threatening conditions.

Isolation precautions

Some infections spread easily from person to person. In hospital, where patients may be particularly vulnerable, isolation precautions may be necessary to prevent transmission. These precautions include the use of protective clothing for contact with infectious material and the isolation of the patient from contact with others. The precautions are intended to prevent cross-infection of other patients and to protect healthcare providers from infection. The decision to use isolation precautions depends on the infecting organism, the site and symptoms of infection, and the presence of immunocompromised patients.

Various approaches to isolation have been recommended over the years. *Standard isolation precautions* (Box 8.2) have been recommended since 1996 (Garner 1996). These are precautions to be taken with all patients regardless of their presumed infection status or diagnosis. This system combines the major features of universal precautions (transmission of bloodborne infections) and body substance isolation (transmission of infections via

---

Box 8.2   Standard precautions

These precautions apply to blood, all body secretions and excretions, areas of broken skin, and mucous membranes:

- Always wash your hands thoroughly before and after patient contact. Use plain soap

- Wear gloves if your hands will or could come in contact with any of the above substances or objects, or objects that have been contaminated with them

- Wear a gown, eye protection and a mask during procedures that may generate droplets of these substances (e.g. surgery)

- Handle with great care equipment that has come into contact with these substances and follow cleaning and disinfecting procedures closely

- Follow procedures for handling contaminated equipment such as correct labelling and packaging

- Dispose of sharps carefully and intact immediately after use into an approved disposal box

- Place potentially infective patients in a single room and notify infection control

- Mouth-to-mouth resuscitation should be used only as a last resort

- These are basic principles that need to be interpreted for individual patients.

From Springhouse Corporation (2000).

Box 8.3   Transmission-based precautions

These should be followed in addition to standard precautions when the patient is known or suspected of being infected with epidemiologically important pathogens that can be transmitted via air, droplet or contact with dry/other contaminated surfaces.

Airborne transmission-based precautions

- Nurse the patient in a single room that has monitored negative air pressure relative to surrounding area

- Limit movement in and out of the room

- Wear a face mask; this is controversial as some authors (e.g. Ward 2000) consider these to be of little value.

Droplet transmission-based precautions

- Nurse the patient in a single room (negative air pressure and ventilation precautions not necessary)

- Wear a mask when working with the patient

- Visitors to remain at least 1 metre away from the patient

- Avoid movement of the patient out of the room

- Consider extra precautions if a ventilator is needed.

Contact transmission-based precautions

- Nurse the patient in a single room

- Wear gloves and a gown whenever in the room

- Avoid movement of the patient out of the room.

From Springhouse Corporation (2000).

moist body fluids). They apply to blood, all body fluids, secretions and excretions (except sweat) whether blood can be seen or not, non-intact skin and mucous membranes. Standard precautions are used in conjunction with transmission-based precautions (Box 8.3) when patients are known or suspected to have an infection or to be colonized with pathogens that are spread by the airborne, droplet or contact route.

Isolation can affect individuals in different ways but, in general, humans, as social beings, do not like to be isolated. Isolation combined with the fear and stigma of infection can be extremely stressful. Some patients may become demanding, fussy or irritable, and the nurse must recognize these responses to isolation rather than label the patient as difficult (Knowles 1993). There can be a tendency to avoid visiting the patient because of the additional time required to put on protective clothing; this can increase the patient's fear and sense of isolation. The plan of care should, where possible, incorporate regular amounts of time spent with the isolated patient, and the precautions should be discontinued at the earliest opportunity.

Usually there is no need to limit visits by relatives, who will not have contact with infectious material and are unlikely to be as susceptible to infection as other patients.

Providing patients with information about the infection, how it is spread and how to prevent spread will help to reassure them and enable them to participate in their care (Gammon 1999).

Occurrence of infectious disease in populations

Epidemiology is the study of the occurrence and distribution of a disease within populations. An *endemic* disease is constantly present at a static level within a given population. An *epidemic* occurs when there is a definite increase in the number of cases of the disease above the normal level. A *pandemic* occurs when the epidemic extends worldwide.

The chain of infection

Microorganisms live and multiply in a *reservoir* from which they can transfer to a host. The reservoir may be in humans, animals or the environment. Viruses, in particular, are unable to replicate outside living cells and survive by passing from one human reservoir to another. Humans are a common reservoir of pathogenic microorganisms. They may be a source of infection during the incubation period, acute stage or convalescence of the disease, or may carry pathogenic microorganisms asymptomatically. Figure 8.3 illustrates stages in the transfer of pathogens between reservoir and host.

The normal flora of the body may cause disease when the host's resistance is lowered, or when the organisms are transferred to another area of the body where they are not normally found; for example, *Escherichia coli*,

Figure 8.3   The chain of infection.

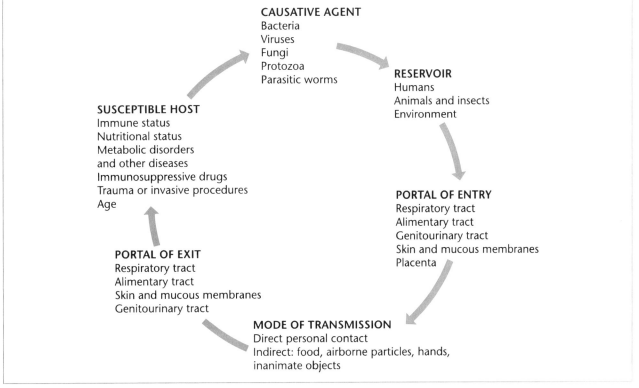

a commensal in the bowel, may cause urinary tract infection if it enters the bladder.

Organisms associated with animal reservoirs include salmonella, which commonly colonizes the intestines of poultry. A major cause of serious food poisoning are the toxins produced by *E. coli* type 0157. These lead to severe bleeding and inflammation of the intestine, and possible renal failure (Haslett et al 1999). Animals infested with parasites may be a source of disease if their flesh is eaten raw or cooked insufficiently (e.g. toxoplasmosis can be transmitted by eating cysts in undercooked meat). The most common environmental reservoirs are water, decaying organic matter and soil.

Mode of escape

The microorganism leaves the host via a portal of exit. This may be the respiratory, alimentary or genitourinary tract, or via open lesions on the skin.

Mode of transmission

Direct spread involves transmitting the microorganisms directly from the reservoir to the person (e.g. by sexual intercourse). *Indirect spread* requires an intermediary such as food, airborne particles, contaminated instruments or hands to pass the infection on.

Portal of entry to host

This may be through the respiratory, alimentary or genitourinary tracts, or via a break in the skin. In pregnancy the placenta normally acts as a barrier, preventing microorganisms from reaching the fetus. However, some organisms and viruses may cross to the placenta to cause infection in the fetus (e.g. syphilis).

Factors predisposing to infection

Factors that influence the host's resistance and susceptibility to infection include the following.

Age

Immunological maturity develops steadily during the first few years of life, and both humoral and cellular immunity are compromised in infants.

Immune changes occur in pregnancy, probably related to depression of cell-mediated immunity (Feinberg and Gonik 1991). These changes may exacerbate underlying autoimmune diseases, such as lupus erythematosus, but have little effect on the incidence of infectious disease.

The incidence of autoimmune disease and cancer increase with ageing. The elderly are more susceptible to, and have a diminished capacity to combat, infection. The thymus gland begins to atrophy at about 45 years of age, resulting in a decreased production of its hormones which play a role in the differentiation of lymphocytes. There is an increase in the number of autoantibodies in the elderly, which is believed to contribute to the pathological changes that occur with ageing. The response to

foreign antigens decreases and the elderly are not able to sustain resistance against infection.

Nutritional imbalances

Lymphoid tissue is vulnerable to excesses and deficiencies of many nutrients because of its rapid rate of proliferation. Protein and calorie deficiency can cause impaired cell-mediated immunity. Humoral immunity and phagocytosis are less affected. Inadequate dietary intake of vitamins A, B and folic acid, and of minerals such as zinc and iron, affect the components of the immune system. Without the required nutrients and energy, the production of antibodies, lymphocytes and the chemical mediators of the immune response is impaired.

Stress

Psychoneuroendocrine immunology is a developing field of study that looks at the interactions between immune function, neuroendocrine responses and life **stresses**.

Drugs

Immunosuppressive drugs are used to treat autoimmune disorders such as rheumatoid arthritis, glomerulonephritis and inflammatory bowel disease, to prevent rejection of transplanted tissue and to treat cancer. These include corticosteroids, cyclophosphamide and azathioprine. Some commonly used antibiotics may also impair immune function and increase susceptibility to infection by disrupting the normal flora. All drugs are capable of initiating a hypersensitivity reaction.

Other infections and underlying conditions

Some infections decrease the person's resistance to a secondary infection. The human immunodeficiency virus (HIV) depresses cell-mediated immunity and leaves the individual vulnerable to many opportunistic pathogens, which take advantage of the deficient immune response. Some underlying conditions affect the immune system and increase the patient's vulnerability to infection, for example carcinoma, leukaemia, liver and renal disease.

Invasive procedures and devices

These increase susceptibility to infection by bypassing defence mechanisms such as skin.

Local factors

Tissue that is poorly perfused by blood (e.g. in peripheral vascular disease) becomes anoxic and more susceptible to invasion by microorganisms. Skin lesions such as **pressure sores** and burns provide an exposed, moist area of tissue in which microbes can multiply.

Infectious disease in hospital populations

Hospital-acquired or *nosocomial* infections are infections that the patient was not suffering from, or incubating, at the time of admission to hospital. Infections may be *endogenous*, that is caused by microorganisms that colonize the body, entering another site to establish infection (e.g. Gram-negative bacilli in the intestine may cause wound infection after abdominal surgery), or *exogenous*, caused by the transmission of microorganisms from the environment or another person.

Nosocomial infections may prolong hospital stay, increasing the cost of treatment as well as causing discomfort and inconvenience to the patient. Bacteria encountered in hospital are frequently resistant to antibiotics because the widespread use of antimicrobial drugs encourages the selection and survival of more resistant microorganisms.

The principal types of infection acquired in hospital involve surgical wounds, urinary and respiratory infections. Practices to prevent the transmission of infection between patients, from patient to staff, and from staff to patient should be incorporated into routine nursing care. Healthcare workers are healthy and therefore less susceptible to infection than the patients they care for. The nurse may, however, acquire infections ranging from respiratory infections to bloodborne viruses such as hepatitis B and C, and HIV.

Control of nosocomial infections

The nurse has a responsibility to practise and promote measures that will confine microorganisms and prevent their spread to other persons.

Handwashing

The hands of staff are thought to be the most common route by which microorganisms are spread between patients. These microbes are acquired on the skin by contact with people or the environment. They do not remain on the skin for long but are readily transferred to the next person or object touched. They are also easily removed by handwashing with soap and water. Even a brief 10-second handwash is effective, but attention should be paid to exposing all parts of the skin to soap and water to ensure complete removal of transient contaminants. The actual technique of handwashing is probably of limited importance to the spread of infection. Of much greater significance is its performance on appropriate occasions (Hoffman and Wilson 1995). Unfortunately, many studies have shown that hands are frequently not washed appropriately and such omissions are commonly considered responsible for outbreaks of hospital-acquired infection (Ward 2000).

It is difficult to draw up a set of rules to cover every circumstance and it is therefore up to individual nurses to decide when they should wash their hands. The principle to be remembered is that hands should always be washed if the procedure about to be undertaken places the patient at risk of acquiring infection or if the activity just carried out could have contaminated the hands. Examples of situations where handwashing is indicated are:

- before manipulation of invasive devices (e.g. urinary catheters, intravascular devices)
- before contact with susceptible sites (e.g. wounds, pressure sores)
- before handling food
- after contact with contaminated items (e.g. soiled dressings, linen, waste)
- after using the toilet
- before leaving the ward.

A convenient alternative to washing with soap and water is alcohol handrub solutions. These can be applied quickly, without the need to walk to a handwash basin, but may not be effective if the hands are soiled, and should not be used if the hands are visibly contaminated. Alcohol handrubs are particularly useful in intensive care settings where frequent handwashing is necessary.

Surgical scrub solutions both remove transient microorganisms and reduce the resident population of microbes that normally inhabit the skin. Most of these resident microbes are not pathogenic unless they enter normally sterile tissue such as a deep wound. Surgical scrubs are useful for washing hands before performing an invasive procedure. Repeated use has been associated with skin damage (Ojäjärvi et al 1977).

Waste disposal

Waste material contaminated with body fluids could expose those who handle it to infection, and safe disposal of this clinical waste ensures that this risk is minimized. The three major groups of *clinical waste* are: contaminated materials (e.g. dressings, swabs, incontinence pads), which must be discarded into yellow plastic bags; sharps instruments, needles and scalpels, which must be discarded into puncture-resistant sharps containers; and human tissue (e.g. placenta, amputated limbs) which must be segregated from other clinical waste and collected separately. Ward (2000) cites evidence to argue, however, that contaminated waste presents no more of a biohazard than household waste, although this is a controversial point of view. Clinical waste must be disposed of by incineration. All other waste not considered contaminated or infectious is designated as household waste and can be discarded into black bags, for compaction and disposal at landfill sites (Health Services Advisory Committee 1999).

Regulations governing the safe disposal of waste are contained in the Environmental Protection Act 1990. Staff who collect waste can be put at risk by the careless actions of others, for example by the disposal of sharps into plastic bags or overfilling waste bags which subsequently spill open. Waste bags or sharps containers should be sealed securely before being taken out of the clinical area. Bags should be marked with the point of origin to help identify any breakdown in the waste disposal procedure.

Sharps: handling and disposal

Sharps include needles, scalpels, broken glass or other items that could lacerate or puncture the skin. Staff are frequently injured by sharp instruments and these injuries are a major cause of bloodborne virus transmission in healthcare settings (Heptonstall et al 1993b).

The risk of acquiring hepatitis B from a single sharps injury with a needle contaminated with infected blood is very high. As many as 1 in 4 such injuries result in the healthcare worker acquiring hepatitis B (Collins and Heptonstall 1994). Human immunodeficiency virus (HIV) is not so easily transmitted by this route, with around 0.36–2% of healthcare workers acquiring infection following an injury with contaminated blood (Royal College of Pathologists 1992, Heptonstall et al 1993a). A risk of contracting hepatitis C of between 3% and 10% is reported for healthcare workers sustaining a needlestick injury involving hepatitis C-infected blood (British Medical Association 1996). Injuries with needles often happen as they are being carried to a sharps container. Resheathing of needles is also hazardous as injury may occur if the needle misses the sheath. Carelessly discarded sharps, and overfilled or poorly assembled sharps containers that subsequently break open, are also responsible for injuries. To reduce the risk of injury from sharps they should be discarded into a designated container immediately after use, always carried in a receiver not by hand, needles should not be resheathed and syringes not disconnected. Sharps bins should be closed when three-quarters full to prevent overfilling.

During procedures where sharp instruments are passed between staff they should be placed in a receiver rather than passed directly from hand to hand.

Management of sharps injuries and other exposures to body fluid

Bloodborne viruses can be acquired through an injury with a contaminated sharp instrument or splashing of infected body fluid on to mucous membranes (eyes and mouth), or cut or broken skin. As it is difficult to identify carriers of bloodborne viruses and the source of the contaminated needle may be unknown, all such exposures must be followed up appropriately to minimize the risk of infection. This follow-up is normally carried out by the occupational health department, but by the accident and emergency department outside office hours.

Hepatitis B vaccination

There is now an effective and safe vaccine against hepatitis B. It is recommended that all healthcare workers who have direct contact with body fluids or tissues should be immunized (Department of Health 1992). Most people require a series of three injections to confer immunity and a booster dose every 3–5 years.

Linen

Microorganisms are physically removed from linen by detergent and water, and most are destroyed by the temperature of 71°C or more during the wash process. Some fabrics (e.g. patients' clothing) are damaged by high wash temperatures and are washed at a lower temperature with a chemical disinfectant added to the rinse cycle. Linen is usually sorted by laundry staff before washing. Their risk of acquiring infection can be reduced by the use of protective clothing, but guidance from the Department of Health recommends that potentially infectious linen should not be sorted before washing (NHS Executive 1995). This includes soiled linen from patients with enteric infections, bloodborne viruses and tuberculosis. Infected linen should be placed into a water-soluble plastic bag and distinguished from other linen by placing in a red outer bag. The water-soluble bag is placed directly into the washing machine, and splits open to release its contents once in contact with water.

Duvets used in clinical areas should be able to withstand a wash temperature of 71°C and should comply with Department of Health regulations on fire retardancy.

Decontamination of equipment

Equipment used between patients can present a risk of cross-infection if it is not adequately decontaminated between uses. The method of decontamination selected depends on how the equipment is used and the risk of transmission associated with it. *Sterilization* means a process that completely destroys microorganisms, including their spores. *Disinfection* is a less precise term used to describe a process that may destroy most but not all microorganisms and does not usually destroy spores. *Cleaning with detergent* removes contamination physically and along with it many microorganisms. Cleaning is an important preparation for equipment prior to sterilization or disinfection, and without it the decontamination process may be ineffective.

Selecting the level of decontamination

This depends on the intended use of the equipment. If it is used to penetrate the skin, mucous membranes or normally sterile body areas then the risk of introducing infection is high and the item must be sterile when used. Items used in contact with mucous membranes or contaminated by easily transmissible organisms can usually be disinfected, although they are more reliably decontaminated by sterilization. Equipment used on intact skin is unlikely to transmit infection and can usually be decontaminated by cleaning with detergent and water (Ayliffe et al 1993). The routine level of decontamination selected should be sufficient to destroy pathogens and a higher level of decontamination for equipment used on infected patients should not be necessary.

Methods of sterilization

The most efficient method of sterilization is *autoclaving*. If atmospheric pressure is increased, water boils at a higher temperature, sufficient to destroy even bacterial spores. In most autoclaves a pressure of 104 kPa is used to produce steam at a temperature of 121°C. This will sterilize items in 15 minutes, although the autoclave cycle includes time taken to reach temperature and cool down. In central sterile supply departments porous-load autoclaves are used to sterilize packed instruments. These create a vacuum in the chamber before the injection of steam and ensure that steam penetrates porous materials such as paper or linen wrappings. The simpler, bench-top autoclaves used in some wards, surgeries and clinics do not include a pre-vacuum stage and are therefore not suitable for the sterilization of wrapped instruments. In this type of autoclave the instruments must be separated so that steam can reach all the surfaces.

Hot-air ovens can also be used to sterilize equipment, but only those items able to withstand the high temperatures of at least 170°C for 1 hour (Department of Health 1994). Autoclave tape can be used to indicate that an item has been through an autoclave cycle, but cannot be relied upon to demonstrate sterility; the autoclave may be defective, for example.

A few *chemicals* can be used to sterilize. Ethylene oxide gas is used for heat-sensitive equipment but requires the use of specialist facilities because it is flammable, explosive and toxic. Glutaraldehyde can be used to sterilize heat-sensitive equipment (e.g. fibreoptic endoscopes) but this requires immersion for between 3 and 10 hours. Glutaraldehyde must be handled wearing heavy-duty gloves and eye protection because it is highly irritant and can cause skin reactions and respiratory symptoms in those regularly exposed.

Packed instruments will remain sterile provided the wrapping remains dry and intact. Unwrapped instruments should be stored in a sterile or clean, covered container until required, but sterility cannot be guaranteed for more than a few hours.

Methods of disinfection

As with sterilization, heat is the best method of disinfection because its effects are more predictable and more easily controlled than chemicals. Items can be *pasteurized* by heating to a temperature of between 65°C and 80°C, for between 5 and 10 minutes. This will destroy most microorganisms but not spores. In the clinical setting, pasteurization is used to disinfect bedpans, linen and crockery. *Boiling* can be used to disinfect medium-risk equipment. Items should be immersed in water at 100°C and, once the water returns to boiling, timed for 5 minutes.

Chemicals are widely used for decontamination, although to be effective they must be used appropriately. This includes ensuring the dilution is correct (if too high the chemical may be corrosive, if too low it may be ineffective);

selecting the correct chemical for the type of equipment and level of decontamination; and using freshly made solutions (diluted disinfectants are frequently unstable and cannot be stored for long periods). Most disinfectants do not penetrate organic material, and instruments must be cleaned thoroughly before immersion. The time taken to destroy microorganisms varies with different chemicals and microbes. Some (e.g. alcohol and hypochlorite) kill most microbes within a few minutes on clean surfaces. Others may take longer: immersion in glutaraldehyde for 1 hour is required to destroy some species of *Mycobacterium*.

Chemical disinfectants can be corrosive and equipment should be rinsed thoroughly after disinfection. Hypochlorites may damage some materials and should not be used to disinfect metal items or fabric. Many disinfectants are toxic and should always be handled wearing gloves and a plastic apron. Eye protection may also be necessary if there is a risk of splashing. The Control of Substances Hazardous to Health (COSHH) Regulations introduced in 1988 require an assessment to be made of every chemical used in the workplace. This should outline the hazards the chemical presents and the protection required to handle it (East 1992).

Disinfectants are frequently used unnecessarily or inappropriately. Guidance on their use should be obtained by reference to the disinfection policy or by contacting the infection control nurse.

Cleaning

A surface that is clean and dry will not easily support the growth of microorganisms, and floors, walls and furniture are not common sources of infection in hospital. Most of the microorganisms on floors can be found in dust particles that settle on horizontal surfaces. A major aim of environmental cleaning is to remove this dust, either by the use of a vacuum cleaner or dust-control mop. These devices are designed to remove the dust with the minimum of disturbance to ensure it does not become airborne. Mopping with detergent and water is of value when surfaces are soiled or exposed to spillages, for example toilets, bathrooms and kitchens. Mops need careful maintenance as they readily become heavily contaminated if allowed to stand in dirty water. They should be laundered regularly, and fresh detergent and water should be used for each cleaning task. Disinfectants will remove more bacteria from the floor than detergent but the effect is short lived and there are very few indications for their use. The frequency with which cleaning should be performed depends on the type of area and extent of use.

Nurses are commonly required to clean equipment such as washbowls, jugs and receivers. In all cleaning procedures it is advisable to wear gloves to protect the hands from contamination by microorganisms and the effects of detergent. Efficient cleaning is possible only if detergent is used to break up and remove the grease and dirt.

A clean disposable cloth and fresh water and detergent should be used for each task.

Universal blood and body fluid precautions

Concern about the risk to healthcare workers of acquiring **HIV** and the difficulties in identifying infected patients gave rise to the proposal that precautions to prevent the transmission of bloodborne viruses should be applied to all patients (Centers for Disease Control 1987, 1988). There are three routes by which healthcare workers may acquire bloodborne viruses occupationally:

- inoculation of infected blood through the skin on a contaminated needle or other sharp instrument
- contamination of mucous membranes with infected body fluid
- contamination of cut or abraded skin with infected body fluid.

Universal precautions are aimed at avoiding direct contact with body fluids from all patients at all times. They incorporate the routine infection control measures already discussed together with the use of protective clothing when direct contact with body fluid is anticipated (Box 8.4).

The selection of appropriate protective clothing depends on an assessment of the anticipated risk of exposure to body fluid during a particular procedure (Fig. 8.4). For example, assisting a patient to wash or recording their vital signs is unlikely to involve any direct contact with body fluid and therefore protective clothing is unnecessary. On the other hand, scrubbing contaminated instruments or performing a surgical procedure is likely to cause splashing of body fluid, and therefore eye protection, a mask, apron or gown and gloves need to be worn (Department of Health 1990).

The concept of universal precautions has caused some controversy. It has been suggested that where the prevalence of bloodborne viruses is low the precautions are unnecessary and should be used only with individuals known or suspected to be infected (Speller et al 1990). Others have argued that it is often difficult to identify infected individuals, and healthcare workers frequently do not detect those who practise high-risk behaviours (Centers for Disease Control 1987). Universal precautions can confer other advantages. If applied consistently they also protect the patient from other pathogens since these are most likely to be found in body fluid and transmitted between patients on the hands of staff (Wilson and Breedon 1990). The use of the same level of precaution with every patient helps to maintain patient confidentiality, which could otherwise be compromised with the use of precautions directed only at those suspected to be infected (Wilson and Breedon 1990).

Key infection control measures are listed in Box 8.5.

Figure 8.4   The selection of protective clothing: risk asessment.

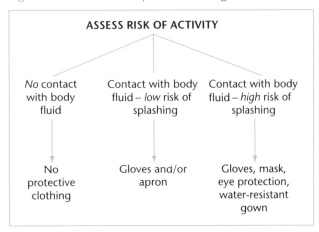

Reproduced with permission from Wilson (1995).

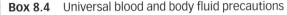

Box 8.4   Universal blood and body fluid precautions

1. Wash hands before and after patient contact and if skin is contaminated with body fluid
2. Cover cuts and abrasions with a waterproof dressing
3. Wear gloves for direct contact with body fluid and mucous membranes
4. Wear eye protection and a mask where there is a risk of body fluid splashing into the face
5. Wear a plastic apron to protect clothing from contamination with body fluid
6. Use sharps safely: place directly into sharps container, never resheathe, do not overfill container and close securely before disposal
7. Discard contaminated waste safely, either directly into the drainage system or into a clinical waste bag
8. Decontaminate equipment safely between patients
9. Disinfect spills of blood with hypochlorite and clear up using gloves and a plastic apron.

From Terence Higgins Trust (1992).

Box 8.5   Summary of key infection control measures

- Apply universal precautions
- Carry out frequent effective handwashing
- Ensure strict levels of environmental cleanliness
- Implement isolation measures as needed
- Liaise with the infection control team
- Act as a role model for patients and other staff to promote hygiene and infection control.

From Clark (2000) British Journal of Nursing with permission from Mark Allen Publishing Ltd.

Community prevention and control of infection

Community measures

In developed countries the incidence of major communicable diseases has been greatly reduced as a result of improved socioeconomic and environmental conditions, immunization programmes, and advances in epidemiology and medical treatments. In the community, measures to control infectious disease are directed at adequate sewage disposal and the provision of safe water and food supplies. Control of enteric diseases, such as typhoid fever and many other gastrointestinal infections, is largely dependent on these factors. Immunization programmes are also widely used to prevent and control the spread of many infectious diseases.

Immunization

Vaccines can be used to protect against infection by stimulating the production of antibodies. When the individual is exposed to the microorganism, the immune system can then respond quickly to prevent infection establishing.

Immunization schedules vary in different countries and in different areas depending on which diseases are more prevalent. Table 8.1 shows the recommended immunization schedule for children in the UK (Department of Health 1996). This service is provided by general practitioners and local health authorities, and is accessible to most individuals without cost.

Immunity induced artificially in this way becomes weaker over a period of months to years depending on the type of vaccine. As a result, reinforcing or booster doses of some vaccines are necessary. Records of immunization received and the date given should be kept by each individual for future reference. This is particularly important for healthcare workers, who may be exposed to a variety of infectious diseases at work and depend on vaccination for protection against infection.

Table 8.1 Schedule for routine immunizations

Vaccine	Age	
Diphtheria, tetanus, pertussis, polio, *Haemophilus influenzae* (HIB)	2 months	1st dose
	3 months	2nd dose
	4 months	3rd dose
Measles, mumps, rubella (MMR)	12–15 months	
Diphtheria, tetanus, polio, MMR	3–5 years	Booster
BCG	10–14 years	
Tetanus, diphtheria, polio	13–18 years	Booster

From Department of Health (1996), with permission.

In some instances it is possible to protect individuals who have been exposed to a pathogen by administering a booster dose of vaccine to enhance existing immunity. Rapid, short-term protection (passive immunity) can also be provided by the administration of specific antibodies (immunoglobulins). These will augment the body's immune system but will not provide lasting protection. Natural passive immunity occurs when IgG antibodies from a mother cross the placenta to the fetus and protect the newborn baby for the first few months of life.

Many measures to control infectious disease in the community are controlled by legislation and are monitored by international, European Union (EU), national and environmental health departments or local government authorities. The World Health Organization (WHO), an agency of the United Nations, monitors outbreaks of infectious disease throughout the world and institutes appropriate prevention and control measures.

Infection control in community nursing care

The principles of infection prevention previously outlined should also be applied to the nursing of patients in their own home. Their risk of infection may differ from that of hospital patients as they are less likely to acquire antibiotic-resistant organisms, less likely to have invasive devices in place, and may not be as compromised by serious illness.

Immunization
See chapter 6.2

HIV
See chapter 6.2

To minimize the risk of transmitting infection between patients, healthcare workers should:

- *wash hands before and after patient contact*

- use aseptic technique when handling or inserting invasive devices

- decontaminate equipment safely and appropriately

- discard clinical waste generated in the patient's home in the appropriate way (see p. 137).

Local authorities in the UK have a legal obligation to collect infectious waste if requested. This usually applies to waste from home dialysis patients or those known to be infected with bloodborne viruses.

It is not usually necessary to use isolation precautions with patients being nursed in their own home. Adherence to universal blood and body fluid precautions should provide sufficient protection against the transmission of infection in most instances. The family may be at risk of acquiring infection and may welcome advice on how they can reduce the risk.

Human immunodeficiency virus (HIV) infection

The **human immunodeficiency virus** (HIV) causes damage to the immune system. It is associated with a

Figure 8.5   The life cycle of a retrovirus.

spectrum of disease, ultimately presenting as acquired immune deficiency syndrome (AIDS).

A disease or illness is shaped not only by its biological qualities but also by the cultural milieu in which it exists. HIV is primarily a sexually transmitted disease and carries with it connotations of 'sin' and 'evil'. The myths and misconceptions about HIV and AIDS are widespread amongst the general public and healthcare professionals. Gallagher (1990) has shown that, even after an education programme, nurses still held irrational fears of contracting AIDS. The ramifications of AIDS are so great that Dimond (1990) has argued that there needs to be a special UK Bill of Rights for patients with AIDS to protect their position within the law.

DNA and RNA
See chapter 1.2

CD4
See chapter 6.2

Pathophysiology

The genetic information of most organisms is composed of **DNA**, and complementary molecules of **RNA** are made as templates for protein production. HIV is a retrovirus: its genetic information is RNA but it has an enzyme called reverse transcriptase, which can synthesize DNA by using RNA as the pattern (Haslett et al 1999).

The virus can infect cells that carry a protein called **CD4** on their surface. Their primary target is the T4 or T helper cells of the immune system, but it also infects macrophages, cells in the mucous membranes and the brain (Greene 1993). Once HIV has invaded a cell, the reverse transcriptase converts its RNA to DNA, which is then integrated into the DNA of the host cell (Fig. 8.5).

HIV particles are then assembled in the cytoplasm of the cell and escape by budding through the cell membrane, killing the cell in the process. As increasing numbers of T4 cells are invaded and destroyed, the body's immune system is weakened, making the individual prone to a variety of opportunistic infections, malignant diseases and neuropsychiatric complications. There is a strong association between the number of CD4+ T lymphocytes and the development of life-threatening illnesses (Table 8.2).

Transmission

HIV is transmitted by sexual intercourse, inoculation of infected body fluids through skin or on to mucous membranes, transplantation of tissues and transfusion of contaminated blood. It may also be transmitted from mother to baby, either through the placenta or during delivery. Transmission of HIV has occurred through blood, semen, vaginal fluids and occasionally breast milk.

Although HIV has been isolated in tears, urine and saliva, the concentration is extremely low and there is no documented evidence that the virus can be transmitted by these secretions (Centers for Disease Control 1987, Mok 1993).

HIV cannot be transmitted through casual contact such as hugging, holding hands, crying, shared toilet seats, etc.

Table 8.2 Centers for Disease Control classification of HIV. The system categorizes individuals using a combination of clinical conditions associated with HIV infection and CD4+ T-lymphocyte counts

Category	Examples
Clinical	
A: Asymptomatic HIV infection	
Persistent generalized lymphadenopathy (PGL)	
Acute primary HIV infection	
B: Conditions indicative of a defect in cell-mediated immunity	Candidiasis (oropharyngeal, vulvovaginal)
	Cervical dysplasia
	Constitutional symptoms (fever, prolonged diarrhoea)
	Hairy leucoplakia
	Herpes zoster
	Listeriosis
	Peripheral neuropathy
C: Conditions included in AIDS case definition	Cryptococcosis
	Cryptosporidosis
	Cytomegalovirus disease or retinitis
	Histoplasmosis
	Kaposi's sarcoma
	Lymphoma
	Mycobacterium
	Pneumocystis carinii
	Salmonella septicaemia
	Toxoplasmosis (brain)
	Wasting syndrome due to HIV
CD4+ T-lymphocyte categories	
1: $\geqslant$ 500 cells/μL	
2: 200–499 cells/μL	
3: < 200 cells/μL	

From Centers for Disease Control (1993) Morbidity and Mortality Weekly Report, with permission.

High-risk behaviours

The patterns of HIV infection and transmission vary in different parts of the world. In Africa, transmission occurs mostly through heterosexual activity, whilst in the USA and Europe infection has occurred mostly amongst homosexual and bisexual men and injecting drug users. The year 1999 saw 3300 new cases of HIV diagnosed in the UK – the highest figure on record. Even more worrying is the fact that the number of sexually transmitted diseases rose by 25% between 1998 and 1999, implying a similar increase in the rate of HIV transmission. HIV is predominantly sexually transmitted in the UK, with only 5% of cases being due to injected drug use, although the percentage in Scotland is 35% (Lipley 2000).

It is important to recognize that it is *risk behaviours* that place an individual at risk of infection rather than association with a particular group. The major route of transmission is by heterosexual and homosexual intercourse, with specific sexual practices carrying varying degrees of risk.

HIV can also be transmitted by infected blood or blood products. The use of drugs or alcohol does not specifically put a person at risk, but sharing needles to inject drugs with someone who is infected is risky because small amounts of infected blood are transmitted in the injecting equipment. Individuals who suffer from clotting disorders, who require multiple infusions of clotting factor concentrates manufactured from the pooled plasma of thousands of donors, are also at risk of HIV infection. Routine screening for HIV antibodies (available since November 1985) and heat treatment that inactivates HIV (available since 1986) have greatly reduced the risk of transmission by this route.

A small number of healthcare workers have acquired HIV following percutaneous or mucous membrane exposure to blood or body fluids. Surveillance of healthcare workers exposed to infected blood has shown that the risk of acquiring HIV is less than 1%, with the greatest risk associated with percutaneous exposure about 0.3%, or 1 case per 300 needlestick injuries (Haslett et al 1999).

An infected health worker may transmit a bloodborne virus to a patient as a result of accidental injury during a procedure such as surgery or dental practice that resulted in blood entering the patient's open tissue. Health workers who are infected with HIV may therefore be advised to avoid performing invasive procedures (Department of Health 1993).

Progression of HIV infection

The rate at which symptoms develop in people with **HIV** infection is unpredictable and varies a great deal between individuals. Some people may develop an acute illness 2–6 weeks after infection. Symptoms include fever, myalgia, arthralgia, headache, diarrhoea, sore throat, lymphadenopathy and a maculopapular rash. After about 3 months it is possible to detect antibodies to the virus in the blood; this is known as *seroconversion*.

In some cases seroconversion may take 6 months or longer. The presence of infection is detected using a test called the enzyme-linked immunosorbent assay (ELISA) and confirmed with the more specific Western blot test. Both of these tests detect antibodies to HIV in the serum.

Being tested for HIV can have far-reaching implications and place the individual under considerable stress. Issues include how the result may affect their sexual behaviour, potential problems with housing, insurance or employment, and people in whom they might confide if the test is positive. Inadequately prepared individuals may become extremely distressed, acutely anxious, severely depressed or suicidal. It is therefore crucial that the person receives professional counselling both before and after the test.

The counsellor should act as a confidential listener, questioner and source of information and support. The pre-test counselling session is an opportunity to:

- provide information about HIV infection
- explore the risks and benefits of being tested (Box 8.6)
- discuss the meanings of the test (Box 8.7)
- help the individual to develop a plan to maximize the benefits and minimize risks.

It also gives the counsellor an opportunity to assess the individual's support system and provide some preventive education related to safer sexual practices and drug use.

The counsellor can also put the individual in touch with support groups set up by people with HIV. These groups may run advice centres or alternative therapy clinics as well as providing opportunities to discuss issues with others in the same situation.

HIV disease

Current data suggest that the majority of individuals infected with **HIV** will eventually become severely immunosuppressed and develop AIDS. The main diseases associated with AIDS are unusual infections caused by microorganisms that are not pathogenic in people with a competent immune system (*opportunistic infections*) and various cancers. A case definition of AIDS has been developed by the Centers for Disease Control in the USA

HIV
See chapter 6.2

and is recognized internationally (see Table 8.2). It is estimated that 40% of HIV-infected individuals will have developed AIDS 8 years after seroconversion, 95% after 15 years. They will remain infectious throughout the course of the disease, although they are probably more infectious during the latter stages (Heptonstall et al 1993a). The progressive impairment of the immune response is caused by the gradual depletion of the CD4+ T lymphocytes, which coordinate a number of important immune functions. There is a strong association between the number of CD4+ T lymphocytes and the development of serious opportunistic illness. CD4 counts are used to monitor the progress of the disease and guide therapeutic management. In the UK, zidovudine is licensed for use in patients with a neutrophil count of less than 0.5×10^9/litre.

Usually the first clinical signs of infection are fevers, night sweats, skin rashes, diarrhoea, unexplained weight loss or respiratory symptoms (Haslett et al 1999). The type and extent of symptoms with which the individual presents will depend on the degree of immunodeficiency.

A debilitating syndrome of weight loss, diarrhoea, fever and night sweats may be caused directly by HIV or by secondary infection. The most common opportunistic infection in individuals with AIDS is *Pneumocystis carinii* pneumonia. The most common neoplasm is Kaposi's sarcoma, which is most likely to develop in homosexual

---

Box 8.6   Issues around testing for HIV

There are many things that need to be considered when planning to have an HIV test:

- It may be stressful not to know your HIV status
- Knowing whether you are HIV positive can help to make decisions about the direction of your life
- Early treatment of HIV can delay onset of AIDS
- You can protect yourself and your partner by using safer sex and/or drug use
- It may enable you to have sex with your partner without using condoms
- It may be stressful to know that you could become ill at any time
- It can be difficult to tell friends, family, partners if you are HIV positive
- You may have difficulties obtaining a mortgage or insurance
- There may be strains on your relationship with your partner if you are HIV positive
- You may need to assess the risks associated with having a baby.

From Terence Higgins Trust (1993).

Box 8.7   Facts about the HIV antibody test

The AIDS virus (usually called HIV) may cause serious disease resulting from the body's inability to fight infection. The antibody to the AIDS virus is a protein the body produces in response to an infection by the AIDS virus.

A positive test indicates that the antibody to the AIDS virus has been found in your blood. The test is not always accurate. A small percentage of persons tested may be told they have the antibody when in fact they do not. A small percentage of persons with negative test results have in fact been infected with the AIDS virus. Your blood will be tested more than once to minimize the risk of making such an error.

A positive antibody test result means that:

- your blood sample has been tested more than once and the tests indicate that antibodies to the AIDS virus are present

- you have been infected with HIV, the virus that causes AIDS, and your body has produced antibodies to it

- you should assume that you are infectious and capable of passing the virus to others.

A positive test does *not* mean that:

- you have AIDS or an AIDS-related condition

- you will get AIDS or AIDS-related complex (ARC)

- you are immune to AIDS.

A negative antibody test result means that no antibodies to the AIDS virus have been found at this time. There are three possible explanations for this:

1. You have not been in contact with the virus.

2. You have come in contact with the virus, but have not become infected. Repeated exposure to the virus through high-risk behaviour greatly increases the likelihood of your becoming infected.

3. You have been infected with the virus but have not produced antibodies yet. It may take several weeks to months to produce antibodies. A small number of persons who become infected never produce antibodies.

A negative antibody test does *not* mean that:

- you are immune to the virus

- you have not yet been infected with the virus (you may have been infected and have not yet produced antibodies)

- you should stop worrying about being infected by the AIDS virus if you participate in high-risk behaviours.

Modified from Gauthier and Turner (1989).

or bisexual men. Tables 8.3 and 8.4 outline the common opportunistic infections and neoplasms associated with AIDS.

HIV disease in women and children

HIV infection may present differently in women, with many of the symptoms being focused on gynaecological problems such as persistent and virulent yeast infections, irregular menstrual periods, pelvic inflammatory disease and cervical cancer. Women often do not have the information they require to make informed decisions about safer sex, intimacy, childcare and reproductive rights. Because women have traditionally been care providers in society, they may neglect their own health because the needs of family and significant others appear more important.

The epidemic among women follows different patterns according to the geographical area. In parts of the world where the virus was first introduced in the heterosexual population (e.g. Africa), the ratio of male to female cases is close to 1 : 1. In Europe and North America, where the epidemic began in homosexual men and intravenous drug users, the ratio of male to female cases is gradually falling from around 10 : 1 in 1987 to around 6 : 1 in 1991 (Ancelle-Park and De Vincenzi 1993).

The current evidence does not suggest that pregnancy accelerates progression of asymptomatic HIV infection to AIDS. However, it is possible that pregnancy may have adverse effects in women with advanced disease and low CD4 counts (Mandelbrot and Henrion 1993). Women who are HIV seropositive transmit the virus to their unborn child in between 13% and 35% of cases, probably *in utero* (European Collaborative Study 1991). There is no difference in rates of prematurity or low birthweight in babies born to HIV-infected women. Women who are addicted to intravenous drugs, however, commonly have premature and low birthweight babies.

Children who are born to mothers who are HIV infected are likely to carry passively acquired maternal antibodies to HIV, making an accurate diagnosis of infection difficult until the child is approximately 15 months old. Maternal antibody in the infant is usually lost at between 6 and 9 months, but may persist until 15 months. Symptoms of HIV infection usually appear when the child is between 6 months and 2 years of age (European Collaborative Study 1991).

A child with HIV infection will live approximately 2 years from the time of diagnosis. Problems associated with infection are characterized by failure to thrive and delays in development. The child is particularly prone to recurrent bacterial infections, recurrent oral thrush and chronic diarrhoea (Box 8.8). Chronic parotid swelling and pulmonary lymphoid interstitial pneumonitis, thought to be linked to the Epstein–Barr virus, are found frequently in children with AIDS. The major cause of morbidity in these children is lung disease. Children do not acquire as

Table 8.3   Common opportunistic infections in persons with AIDS

Cause	Usual site	Symptoms	Common diagnostic tests	Therapy
Protozoa				
1. *Pneumocystis carinii*	Lungs	Dry, non-productive cough, shortness of breath, fever, night sweats	Chest radiography, bronchoscopy	Trimethoprim Pentamidine Co-trimoxazole
2. *Toxoplasma gondii*	Brain	Headache, seizures, neuro-logical deficits, behaviour changes, may lead to dementia	CT scan (head) MRI scanning	Sulfadiazine Pyrimethamine
3. *Cryptosporidium*	GI tract	Profuse, watery diarrhoea, dehydration, debility	Stool cultures	Spiramycin Antidiarrhoeals Antiperistaltics
Fungi				
4. *Candida albicans*	Mouth (thrush)	Dysphagia	Visible lesions scraped and cultured	Nystatin Clotrimazole
	Oesophagus	Dysphagia (oral candida may not be present)	Endoscopy with biopsy and culture of tissue	Ketoconazole Fluconazole
5. *Cryptococcus neoformans*	Brain	Headache, fever, confusion, behaviour changes	Lumbar puncture, bone marrow aspiration	Amphotericin B
	Lungs	Non-specific cough or fever, dyspnoea	Chest radiography, sputum for culture, bronchoscopy with culture	Flucytosine
Viruses				
6. Cytomegalovirus	Eyes	Retinitis, loss of vision	Serology testing	DHPG
	Lungs	Cough, dyspnoea, fever	Bronchoscopy with biopsy and culture	Foscamet
	GI tract	Abdominal pain, ulcer, GI bleeding	Endoscopy, colonoscopy	Ganciclovir
	Spinal cord	Paraparesis, quadraparesis	Analysis of spinal fluid	
7. Herpes simplex virus	Skin	Painful cold sore clusters at mouth and perianal area	Histology and culture	Aciclovir
	Spinal cord	Paraparesis, quadraparesis	Analysis of spinal fluid	
Bacteria				
8. *Mycobacterium avium intracellulare*	Disseminated, many organs affected: liver, spleen, lungs, lymph nodes, bone marrow, GI tract	Fever, profuse sweating, productive cough, lymphadenopathy, diarrhoea, weight loss	Blood cultures, bone marrow aspiration, stool for acid-fast bacilli, endoscopy, colonoscopy with culture of biopsy tissue	Isoniazid Rifampicin Ethambutol Streptomycin Amikacin Biofazimine

Table 8.4   Secondary cancers common in patients with AIDS

Type	Site	Signs/symptoms	Diagnostic tests	Therapy
Kaposi's sarcoma	Skin	Multiple pink/purple/brown vascular lesions	Skin biopsy	Chemotherapy
	GI tract	Usually asymptomatic	Endoscopy	Radiation
	Lungs	Symptoms often same as pneumocystic pneumonia, unless pleural thickening or effusion present	Chest radiography, bronchoscopy	
Lymphomas	Brain Bone marrow GI tract	Neurological deficits according to site	CT scan Selective biopsy according to site	Radiation Chemotherapy

---

Box 8.8   Major symptoms of AIDS in children

- Failure to thrive
- Developmental delays and regressions
- Persistent or recurrent fevers, bacterial or yeast infections, diarrhoea
- Chronic lymphoid interstitial pneumonitis
- Chronic lymphadenopathy
- Hepatosplenomegaly
- Parotitis
- Chronic otitis media/sinusitis
- Opportunistic infection
- Neurological disease.

Modified from Pratt (1995).

---

many opportunistic infections as do adults, with the exception of *Pneumocystis carinii* pneumonia. Opportunistic infections presenting in the first year of life are associated with a higher mortality rate. Kaposi's sarcoma is seldom found in children. Children also present with neurological abnormalities such as acquired microcephaly, brisk tendon reflexes and abnormal electrophysiological findings. Developmental delays in motor, language and cognitive skills are also common. Some studies suggest the presence of HIV-induced embryopathy, while other studies conclude that there is not a consistently documented syndrome associated with HIV. Children with HIV infection are particularly susceptible to infectious diseases and should receive the routine immunizations outlined in Table 8.1. These vaccines are safe to give to children infected with HIV, provided the general contraindications to vaccination are not present (e.g. febrile illness, allergy to eggs (MMR), severe reaction to previous dose) (Department of Health 1996). HIV-positive individuals should not be given BCG vaccination against tuberculosis, or yellow fever vaccine.

Intravenous drug use

In developed countries, intravenous drug users are the second largest group of people infected with HIV after homosexual and bisexual men. The incidence of infection in this group has increased appreciably since the epidemic began. Infection may be complicated by poverty and social factors. Traditionally, these individuals are distrustful of medical and government establishments, making the building of a therapeutic relationship, and interventions, extremely difficult. Intravenous drug users are also not as likely to belong to formal organizations, diminishing the power of influence available through collective action. Behavioural change may be made difficult by barriers such as low educational level, alienation from sources of accurate information, and the presence of a folklore belief system that supports the activities and values of intravenous drug use.

Intervention to stop transmission of HIV through sharing of needles ideally involves reaching individuals via drug treatment centres. In reality this is often difficult to accomplish. Ideally intravenous drug users should be encouraged not to share dirty needles and syringes. In some centres this is being achieved by needle exchange programmes, where intravenous drug users are given clean needles when they return their dirty ones. If needle exchange is not possible, the risk of infection can be reduced by disinfection of the needle and syringe by boiling or flushing through with bleach solution. A suitable solution can be made by diluting household bleach 1 : 10 with water, and the needle and syringe should be flushed first in cold water until clear of blood.

Antiviral therapy

The main approach to therapy has been the use of drugs that are designed to block viral gene replication (reverse transcriptase inhibitors) or target the enzyme responsible for assembling the newly copied genetic information (protease inhibitors). Combination therapy of two or more drugs can be effective in maintaining health for long periods. Side-effects may be severe and the cost of these drugs is prohibitive for developing countries, however.

New drugs or techniques such as Compound Q or passive immunotherapy are continually being developed and tested, although access to drug trials is a controversial issue for patients.

The development of a vaccine to prevent HIV infection remains to be achieved. Retroviruses are tricky entities and difficult to understand. Clearly, the strongest weapon available against the virus is education.

Summary

This chapter discussed the main causes of infection and key preventive measures. The interaction between host and microbe determines the likely development of infection. The care of a patient with an infection centres around supporting the person through the illness, alleviating symptoms, observing for complications and administering antimicrobial therapy. Nurses must also be aware of the risks of hospital-acquired infection and take steps to protect both the patient and themselves.

In recent decades there has been a substantial reduction in many infectious diseases (e.g. measles, poliomyelitis and diphtheria). This has stemmed from increased knowledge about the interaction between host and microbial agent, and the widespread use of immunization programmes.

The decline in the many familiar infections has occurred at the same time as the growth of HIV infection. Its presentation is complicated not only by the seriousness of the illness, but also by the social and ethical challenges it provides. HIV is primarily transmitted by intimate sexual contact, exposure to contaminated blood and by a mother to her unborn infant. Care of the individual must focus not only upon the physical manifestations of the illness, but also upon the psychological and social effects. As a reliable vaccine to HIV lies a long way in the future, the only reliable mode of intervention is effective education, and hence prevention.

References

Adler MW, ed. (1991) ABC of AIDS, 2nd edn. London: British Medical Journal.

Ancelle-Park R, De Vincenzi I (1993) Epidemiology and natural history of HIV/AIDS in women. In: Johnson MA, Johnstone FD, eds. HIV infection in women. London: Churchill Livingstone.

Ayliffe GAJ, Coates D, Hoffman PN (1993) Chemical disinfection in hospital. London: Public Health Laboratory Service.

British Medical Association (1996) A guide to hepatitis C. London: BMA.

Centers for Disease Control (1987) Recommendations for prevention of HIV transmission in health-care settings. Morbidity and Mortality Weekly Report 36: 38–128.

Centers for Disease Control (1988) Update: universal precautions for prevention of transmission of human immunodeficiency virus, hepatitis B virus, and other bloodborne pathogens in health-care settings. Morbidity and Mortality Weekly Report 37: 377–388.

Centers for Disease Control (1993) Revised classifications system for HIV infection and expanded surveillance case definition for AIDS among adolescents and adults. Morbidity and Mortality Weekly Report 41: 1–19.

Clark L (2000) Antibiotic resistance: a growing and multifaceted problem. British Journal of Nursing 9(4): 225–230.

Collins M, Heptonstall J (1994) Occupational acquisition of acute hepatitis B infection by health care workers: England and Wales, 1985–93. CDR Review 4(12): R153–155.

Department of Health (1990) Guidance for clinical health care workers: protection against infection with human immunodeficiency virus and hepatitis virus. Recommendations of the Expert Advisory Group on AIDS. London: HMSO.

Department of Health (1992) Immunisation against infectious diseases. London: HMSO.

Department of Health (1993) AIDS-HIV infected health care workers: guidance on the management of infected health care workers (interim update). Expert Advisory Group on AIDS. London: HMSO.

Department of Health (1994) Dry heat sterilisers: purchase, maintenance and use. SAB(94)23. London: HMSO.

Department of Health (1996) Immunisation against infectious diseases. London: HMSO.

Dimond B (1990) AIDS and the law. Nursing Standard 4(17): 52–54.

East J (1992) Implementing the COSHH regulations. Nursing Standard 6(26): 33–35.

European Collaborative Study (1991) Children born to women with HIV infection: natural history and risk of transmission. Lancet 337: 253–260.

Feinberg BB, Gonik B (1991) General percepts of the immunology of pregnancy. Clinical Obstetrics and Gynecology 34: 3–16.

Gallagher R (1990) AIDS: the fear of contagion. Nursing Standard 4(19): 30–32.

Gammon J (1999) Isolated instance. Nursing Times 95(2): 57–60.

Garner J (1996) Guideline for isolation precautions in hospital. American Journal of Infection Control 24: 24–52.

Gauthier DK, Turner JG (1989) Anti-HIV antibody testing: procedures and precautions. American Journal of Infection Control 17: 213–225.

Greene WC (1993) AIDS and the immune system. Scientific American September, 20–110.

Haslett C, Chilvers E, Hunter J, Boon N (1999) Davidson's principles and practice of medicine, 18th edn. Edinburgh: Churchill Livingstone.

Health Services Advisory Committee (1999) Safe disposal of clinical waste. London: HMSO.

Heptonstall J, Gill OJ, Porter K et al (1993a) Health care workers and HIV: surveillance of occupationally acquired infection in the UK. CDR Review 3(11): R147–153.

Heptonstall J, Porter K, Gill N (1993b) Occupational transmission of HIV. Summary of published reports. London: PHLS AIDS Centre, CDSC.

Hoffman PN, Wilson JA (1995) Hands, hygiene and hospitals. Microbiology Digest. Public Health Laboratory Service 11(4): 211–216.

Knowles HE (1993) The experience of infectious patients in isolation. Nursing Times 89(30): 53–55.

Lipley N (2000) The forgotten epidemic. Nursing Standard 15(7): 16–18.

Mackowiak PA (1994) Fever: blessing or curse? A unifying hypothesis. Annals of Internal Medicine 120: 1037–1040.

Mandelbrot L, Henrion R (1993) Does pregnancy accelerate disease progression in HIV-infected women? In: Johnson MA, Johnstone FD, eds. HIV Infection in women. London: Churchill Livingstone.

Mok J (1993) Breast milk and HIV-1 transmission. Lancet 341: 930–931.

NHS Executive (1995) Hospital laundry arrangements for used and infected linen. HSG(95)18. London: HMSO.

Ojäjärvi J, Makelä P, Rantasol I (1977) Failure of hand disinfection with frequent handwashing: a need for prolonged field studies. Journal of Hygiene 70: 107–112.

Pratt RP (1995) AIDS: a strategy for nursing care, 4th edn. London: Edward Arnold.

Reacher M et al (2000) Bacteraemia and antibiotic resistance of its pathogens reported in England and Wales 1990–1998. British Medical Journal 320: 213–216.

Royal College of Pathologists (1992) HIV infection: hazards of transmission to patients and health care workers during invasive procedures. London: Royal College of Pathologists.

Speller DCE, Shanson DC, Aycliff GAJ, Cooke EM (1990) Acquired immune deficiency syndrome. Recommendations of a working party of the Hospital Infection Society. Journal of Hospital Infection 15: 7–34.

Springhouse Corporation (2000) Nurse practitioners clinical companion. Springhouse, PA: Springhouse Corporation.

Terence Higgins Trust (1992) How to protect yourself and others. London: Terence Higgins Trust.

Terence Higgins Trust (1993) Testing issues. London: Terence Higgins Trust.

Ward S (2000) Evidence based practice and infection control. British Journal of Nursing 9(5): 267–271.

Wilson J (1995) Infection control in clinical practice. London: Baillière Tindall.

Wilson JA, Breedon P (1990) Universal precautions. Nursing Times 86: 67–70.

Further Reading

Horton R, Parker L (1997) Informed infection control practice. London: Churchill Livingstone.

Section 2 provides practical advice for applying infection control in clinical practice. There is also a chapter on reflective practice using actual patient experience of being isolated with MRSA.

Krasner DL, Sibbold RG (1999) Nursing management of chronic wounds. Nursing Clinics of North America 34(4): 933–955.

This is an updated reference for nurses on wound management.

Wilson J (2001) Infection control in clinical practice, 2nd edn. London: Harcourt.

A comprehensive text on all aspects of infection control.

Clinical investigations

Susan Skinner

Introduction

Rationale for clinical investigations

Assessment and clinical investigations

Care of patients needing clinical assessment

Informed consent

Giving information

Patient anxiety and clinical investigations

Professional preparations

Essential nursing knowledge related to clinical investigations

Pre-procedure preparation

Care of specimens

Principles behind the specific types of clinical investigation

Specimens for culture and sensitivity

Investigation by means of diagnostic imaging

Health screening

Giving unwelcome news

The future

Summary

Introduction

The process of clinical investigation underpins every part of the health care of patients. This does not always mean that the patient is subjected to complex systems of monitoring or imaging. Clinical investigation begins when a nurse first meets the patient or client. Using clinical expertise that has come from education and experience the nurse will make a visual assessment of the patient's well-being. In addition, the nurse will listen to what the patient has to say and note the way in which the patient tells his or her story. The nurse will ultimately use all of his or her senses continuously to collect information about the patient's physical, psychological and spiritual health. This is the foundation from which further clinical assessment, using science and technology can be planned.

Technological advances in recent years have extended the precision and accuracy of clinical assessment. The complex equipment that can be utilized for diagnosis is constantly evolving to provide detailed clinical pictures, from which definitive diagnoses can be made. It must be remembered, though, that the use of this sophisticated technology follows the first examination and initial observations made by the nursing and medical staff. The equipment assists and extends the accumulation of information but it is the knowledgeable practitioner who initiates and steers the process, and ultimately interprets the results.

Rationale for clinical investigations

There should always be reasonable justification for requesting clinical investigations. When a clinical investigation is performed, there is a cost in time and money for both the patient and the health service. Anxiety is a probable additional cost to the well-being of patients while the investigation is performed and as they wait for the results.

Clinical investigations can:

- provide a snapshot with which to assess the health of a patient at a given moment in time

- be used to preclude, or confirm, a suspected diagnosis following a physical examination

- monitor the clinical status of patients as they undergo therapeutic regimens, revealing trends in health and well-being.

Assessment and clinical investigations

Few clinical investigations, used in isolation, give sufficient information on which to base clinical decisions with any certainty. The results must be evaluated using other physiological, psychological and social parameters that have an impact on the patient's health.

Lists of 'normal' reference values are commonly found in nursing textbooks and they provide useful guidelines to assess deviation from normal values and measurements. It must be remembered, however, that some values given as 'normal' may not apply to all of your patients. An example of this would be a child with congenital heart disease who has a 'normal' oxygen saturation monitor value of 92%. This compares poorly with the normal healthy oxygen saturation value, which is usually given as 99%. However, for this child a value of 92% is normal – and one the child learns to cope with.

The results of specific clinical assessments often have additional significance within a specialized hospital unit. It then becomes an essential issue of policy making to provide staff with reference list of agreed acceptable values that are applicable only for use within that hospital unit.

Whenever an abnormal value is isolated during a clinical assessment the nurse must be aware that the results may reflect factors that are associated with the patient's lifestyle rather than being a cause for concern. There are many influences acting on the body to produce deviations from expected norms. Some examples to be aware of are given below.

Food

The nutritional status of a patient has a strong influence on many tests. Dieting will produce a urine that tests positive for **ketones**, yet the presence of ketones in other circumstances (e.g. diabetes) would be a serious consideration when evaluating a patient's health. A further example is variation in **blood glucose** levels, which occur naturally in response to meal times.

Age

Ageing has a detrimental effect on all systems and tissues of the body. The person's age must always be considered when results are being interpreted (e.g. sex hormone levels).

Drugs

Drugs are designed to interfere or change physiological processes (see Ch. 6). It is therefore inevitable that they will have an impact on the results of some clinical investigations. An example of this is the decreased measured **prothrombin** time associated with oral contraceptive use.

Time of day

The importance of the biorhythms on hormone and other tissue secretions are a matter of current research. **Growth hormone** is an example of this. It is secreted in regular bursts at pre-set times throughout the day, with the largest burst of the hormone being secreted during the early part of sleep at night. As expected, the amount of growth hormone secreted and considered as a normal value will additionally be affected by the age of the patient.

Body mass

The measurement of body mass and the estimation of normal standard values will always have to be set within the considerations of age and sex. Many other additional influences will affect the measurements taken. These can include drug therapies, disturbances in metabolic rate, poor health and the appetite for food. Examples include the effects of long-term steroid therapy for a patient with inflammatory disease or young men who abuse unprescribed anabolic steroids for body building.

Geographical area

Adaptation of patients to their local environment may affect the normal values expected to be returned, when clinical investigations are carried out. For example, the lower oxygen values in air at altitude will cause the local population to have **polycythaemia** (an increased number of circulating red blood cells). This adaption makes sufficient **haemoglobin** available at the **respiratory membranes** to keep oxygen values at an adequate level.

Specimens

The conditions under which the specimen was taken, or the use of poor collection techniques, may cause the

Ketones
See chapters 1.2 & 5.2

Glucose metabolism
See chapter 2.6

Ageing
See chapter 1.3

Prothrombin
See chapter 4.1

Growth hormone
See chapter 2.6

Polycythaemia
See chapter 4.1

Haemoglobin
See chapter 4.1

Respiratory system
See chapter 5.3

results to be unreliable. For this reason results must be considered within the context of previously measured personal values or against previously measured baseline values. The nurse should use a process of individualized patient assessment and evaluation.

Care of patients needing clinical assessment

Most of us have experienced the fear and uncertainty that arises when checks are made on our own health, or on the health of our family. Some outcomes can mean a complete alteration in the opportunities that life can offer and the patterning of everyday life. Some results may cause a difficulty in the relationships with loved ones; other positive results may have financial implications that can undermine the quality of a person's life. As nurses, we must not forget that the routine blood test may take on great significance for the patient, as it may be anything but 'routine' for that person (see Case Study 9.1). Nurses must be ready to give explanations, guidance and support. They should be aware of the place that the investigation has in the planned assessment and care of the patient, and be prepared to provide a complete explanation and give some indication of the significance of the results.

Case Study 9.1 *Tom*

Tom came to the preoperative assessment unit for the necessary clinical investigations prior to a right-sided hip replacement. The operation was planned for the following week.

Tom was asked to put his arm in the correct position for blood to be taken. This was needed for grouping and cross-matching before the operation, in addition to making sure that his haemoglobin level and full blood counts were within normal limits. Tom declined to have blood taken. He said that he had had 'needle phobia' since he was a young man. He told the nurse that he declined local anaesthesia before he had dental work done and that he did not travel to any country where vaccinations were required. The nurse explained that this may mean that his operation would be postponed because the surgeon probably would not operate without knowing this vital information.

Tom remained adamant that he could not allow blood to be taken. The nurse told the medical staff, who supported her opinion that the operation would not take place. Tom visited the unit over several weeks. The nurse and Tom talked about his fear. The nurse explained about the venepuncture process and the equipment used. She asked the medical team to prescribe him some local anaesthetic cream for his arm, which he used, and became confident

that the procedure would be painless. After several visits, Tom allowed the nurse to take some blood.

It is important to give patients an explanation of the process before each investigation is carried out. The explanation must be in terms that are understandable to each patient. This clarification is important for giving patients guidance and maintaining their confidence throughout the investigative process. It is also an essential part of the process that allows patients to exercise *informed choice.* It is through the ability to understand the rationale of the clinical investigations, and the exercising of informed choice, that patients can become full partners in the planning of their care. They will be able give *consent* to the procedures needed for the clinical investigations with increased confidence. The information given must contain the reasons why the investigations are necessary and the process of the procedure. Patients must be informed of the time at which the results will be available and how they will be able to obtain them.

If you are the nurse who is to carry out the investigation, it is essential that you give yourself time to prepare before meeting the patient. The patient will appreciate a nurse who appears unhurried and is able to give appropriate support when it is needed. This initial preparation will also help should unexpected events occur while the investigation is taking place. If you are fully prepared, you can work with confidence. This helps you and the patient.

Talk to the patient throughout the procedure, reporting the progress of the techniques you are using and assuring the patient that the clinical investigation is progressing as planned. Such reassurance is especially important if the patient is experiencing discomfort and is anxious that difficulties are occurring. If it is difficult for the nurse who is carrying out the procedure to talk to the patient, a colleague must be asked to stay with the patient to give the support that is needed. The reduction of patient anxiety must be a priority for all staff.

The nurse must try to keep the patient as calm and comfortable as possible throughout the procedure, as the results of some clinical investigations may be altered by the patient feeling anxious. An environment that helps the patient to relax is also important. The procedures necessary for the test may test the tolerance of patient and it can become a difficult task for nurses to help the patient at such a personal level. The reduction of stress will improve the accuracy of many clinical investigations, especially those connected with the cardiovascular system. If the nurse observes that the patient is overly anxious, the patient should be allowed to recover his or her basal state before proceeding with the clinical assessment.

Informed consent

All clinical investigations require close interaction between the patient and the clinical practitioner. The nature of clinical investigations demands that there is a legal obligation for the patient to give consent to all investigative procedures before their instigation (McKee 1999). The United Kingdom Central Council for Nurses, Midwives and Health Visitors (UKCC 1996) states that is the patient's right to have full information about his or her own condition. As nurses work under the auspices of the UKCC, it becomes our duty to provide this information, in cooperation with the multidisciplinary team caring for this patient. This information must be truthful and unbiased, especially when the patient has to use information to make a difficult choice. The clarity and impartiality of information is especially important when a patient is giving consent to a clinical investigation that may change the course of his or her life. An example of this would be a woman who feels in good health but is advised to have screening for hepatitis C virus. A positive result from the test would confer on her a state of poor health, which will inevitably alter her perception of her own well-being. Imagine, therefore, the consequences of testing positive for human immunodeficiency virus (HIV). In the light of knowledge, the results will inevitably bring changes in her physical, psychological and spiritual life.

In all circumstances the patient must give written or verbal consent before any clinical investigation is undertaken. If the patient is unable to understand the purpose of the investigation and the process that will need to be followed for the test to be accurate, a named person, usually next of kin, will take the responsibility for giving the permission. When consenting to any investigative process the patient tacitly assumes that the person carrying out the test is competent and educated fully in the investigating procedure. This factor becomes important when the procedure is one that was originally performed by a doctor but has become part of a nurse's expanded role. Furlong and Glover (1998) argue that nurses should identify themselves as the lead practitioner in this situation as there may be legal questions to answer at a future date, if the assumption was made by the patient that a doctor was to perform the investigation and a nurse subsequently did it.

Giving information

Consent to clinical investigations can be given by the patient only if adequate information is available for him or her to make informed choices. The relevant information must be delivered in an acceptable and understandable format. It is this information that will enable the patient to cope with the process of clinical investigation and its outcome (Lowry 1995). Commonly, the patient will learn from the medical team about the clinical investigations that they are advising the patient to give consent to. The anxiety induced from such a meeting with a clinician will interfere with the amount of information the patient can recall (Lloyd et al 1999). Anxiety regarding the circumstances of the meeting, the fear of bad news and the amount of information that needs to be assimilated by the patient interferes with both the recall and comprehension of the information. It is the nurse who provides the continuing care who is in the best position to clarify the explanations for the patient. It is through the nurse providing a repetition of the facts and answering further questions that the patient is provided with a full rationale for the clinical explorations ordered.

Remembering full explanations in detail when they are given verbally is difficult for most people, and the difficulty is compounded for the patient when anxiety also becomes a barrier to listening and understanding. To help the patient with this, information leaflets to supplement the verbal explanation have become an essential tool for nurses. An information leaflet that is clearly and attractively written will provide a constant reference point and source of information for the patient. It has the additional benefit that it can be read at the patient's own speed and provide the starting point for further questions. These information leaflets should give a truthful account of the clinical investigation that they explain. A leaflet must not give a misleading account of the clinical investigation. It must be truthful when describing discomforts that are known to be expected during or after the investigation. If the information leaflet is found to be inaccurate or incomplete, the patient's confidence in other written or verbal information issued from the same source will be reduced.

Patient anxiety and clinical investigations

A 'routine' test may shatter the future hopes and ambitions of a patient. The results of the test may confirm a prognosis that is predictive of disability, sensory impairment or premature death. It may bring about changes that involve the patient adjusting his or her views on quality of life. This adaptation may become necessary in order that the patient can remain in control of events in his or her own future. The tests may cause difficulties in the relationships with those that the patient is closest to. The results of a simple, routine test performed by a nurse may lead the patient to face serious and complex difficulties. For example, a swab taken from a newborn baby with sticky eyes could produce a culture that grows the gonococcus bacterium. This is seen to have been contracted from the birth canal of the mother and can lead to a situation that is difficult to resolve at this most sensitive time. This swab result may have an impact not only on the lives of the parents but also on the early years and future life of the newborn baby.

Professional preparations

It is essential that nurses understand the principles, process and purpose of all clinical investigations that they perform, or when they give assistance during testing by another clinician. The nurse must have an understanding of the principles of the normal physiology associated with the test or have knowledge of the anatomy of the system that is being assessed. A knowledge of the normal will give the foundations on which variations found during the assessment can be identified and understood.

The accuracy of the clinical investigations will be completely dependent on the care taken by the nurse to ensure all possibilities for error are eliminated. Technology, especially when it is utilized in the clinical setting, has the potential to produce erroneous readings through the poor technique of the operator. For this reason, when the initiation of medical or nursing interventions is dependent on the information taken from the clinical investigations, it is essential that nurses are given proper clinical supervision to ensure the accuracy of testing. It is essential that the nurses have all relevant knowledge and are supervised until the technique is seen to be performed safely and competently.

Evidence that this education and supervision has taken place is especially important when professional boundaries are crossed and the nurse takes on an expanded role in order to perform a clinical investigation. A formal training period must then be instituted. Essential theoretical knowledge and practice must be tested to ensure that the nurse is performing the investigation to defined criteria. Nurses should refuse to perform a clinical investigation when they have doubts regarding their own competency or when the procedure will breach their own level of expertise. It is part of a nurse's own professional practice development to assess him- or herself, and to set his or her own standards for practice.

Learning the practical skills attached to clinical investigations may be the most straightforward part of acquiring the new skill. Competence to perform the skill will also include the interface with the patient: the ability to answer questions with assurance and empathy, and to give the patient confidence. The nurse must also be able to provide information regarding the further actions that may be necessary based on the outcome of the assessment.

To be competent to perform clinical investigations is also to be fully aware of personal safety issues when the clinical investigation is carried out. Knowledge of the risk factors for both the patient and the nurse is essential. The nurse must make provision for appropriate safety precautions for both staff and the patient.

Essential nursing knowledge related to clinical investigations

To help patients through any assessment process, nurses should ensure that they are secure in the following fundamental knowledge:

1. That they know exactly what is being measured and for what purpose; nurses must know the principles that lie behind the investigation.

2. That they have knowledge of the assessment made within the context of normal physiological function.

3. That they have given thought to how the patient can be best prepared – physically, psychologically and emotionally – to be a positive participant in the process. This point is especially pertinent when caring for children and their parents.

4. That they are aware of side-effects that can arise from the process of each clinical investigation and be prepared to prevent or counter the effect if it arises.

5. Most clinical investigation procedures have the potential to harm the assessor, or patient, through the incorrect use of equipment or procedure. The nurse must know of any specific precautionary measures that must be taken when using the equipment. Be aware of the hazards and work only within prescribed guidelines and procedures.

6. Nurses must help the patient understand that the interpretation of the results of clinical investigations is not always an easy process and that conclusions cannot be drawn from a single result. The results need to be considered using knowledge of a multiple of variables. These may include:
   a. the values being compared to the normal ranges supplied by your local policy guidelines, which may not equate to values shown in textbooks
   b. the values recorded for the patient obtained when previously investigated
   c. the values considered within the context of other clinical investigations that have an impact on the assessment taken.

7. To initiate a rapid response, nurses should ensure that a system of reporting is in place that allows the laboratory to alert staff immediately when the result obtained is life threatening for the patient.

Pre-procedure preparation

Time spent preparing for the procedure will enhance its smooth operation. Plan ahead and think through the procedure carefully. Ensure that all necessary equipment has been collected. Examine the area where the investigation is to take place and ensure that the patient, and you, will remain comfortable throughout. It is particularly important that the investigator is not placed in a position that puts any strain on the back, even for a short period of time.

There must be optimal communication with the patient throughout the procedure so, as part of the preparation, ensure that any necessary aids to understanding are available. If the patient normally need a hearing aid, make sure that they are wearing it. A translator may be necessary to allow you to communicate with the patient in a language that he or she can understand. Be additionally sensitive when the investigation requires the patient to comply with instructions that are not culturally comfortable. Be aware of the patient who has special problems associated with the investigation, for example an aversion to hypodermic needles. Alternative methods may need to be found for investigative purposes. Check that all specific preparatory test instructions have been complied with (e.g. the patient has remained nil by mouth prior to a barium meal investigation).

Instructions and assurance must be given clearly throughout the procedure, using words that the patient is clearly able to understand. Listen to what the patient says to you while the clinical investigation is proceeding. Warn of discomforts or pain, and accept the patient's word when he or she describes the pain. Patients who feel that they are experiencing an unusual degree of pain, usually suffer from increased anxiety.

Accurate records must be made once the investigation has been completed.

Care of specimens

When you are the lead nurse associated with any clinical investigation, even when it is performed by other healthcare professionals, you must ensure that:

Diabetes mellitus
See chapter 2.6

- the labels on all specimens are marked correctly and clearly

- the necessary precautions have been taken to ensure that it is a specimen that will produce valid results for the investigation

- if the specimen is to be transported, it is stored in the correct medium

- the specimen cannot be contaminated, or become a contaminant, in transit

- the forms that accompany the specimen are the correct type for the test ordered. These forms must be completed in full and contain all information requested. Omitting to complete the form may lead to a delay in the processing of the specimen. The writing must be in black ink for clear duplication of the result sheet.

Principles behind the specific types of clinical investigation

Blood tests

Specimens of blood are usually taken by venepuncture. When a small sample of blood is sufficient for testing (e.g. for capillary blood glucose measurement), a finger or heel prick will suffice.

Invasive procedures that break the integrity of blood vessels always carry risks for the patient. For this reason, the procedures must be carried out under the terms of locally agreed protocols. These policies will designate:

- the staff who are authorized to take blood from patients

- the programme of education that sets standards of practice. Staff will need to prove that they practise safely and competently when taking blood for testing

- the standards set for the procedure to ensure the safety of the client and staff.

Technique

Introducing a foreign object into a blood vessel inevitably brings a risk of infection. Aseptic technique is essential when taking all specimens of blood.

The patient's arm must be relaxed throughout the process. Some patients find venepuncture a very uncomfortable process, so supports and pillows should be used to keep the arm placed correctly. The patient's arm should also be positioned to avoid placing any strain on the nurse's back as he or she leans over to take the blood sample.

Poor technique will produce an inaccurate blood result. The most reliable blood results come from a sample of blood that has been free flowing through a wide-diameter vein.

Occlusion of the vein through prolonged use of the tourniquet or a disease process will cause stasis of the blood in the vessel. The fluid content, electrolytes and the blood gases in a blood sample taken from this vessel will not be representative of the blood that is circulating in the rest of the body.

When blood does not flow freely from a finger or heel prick, it is a temptation to squeeze the finger or heel to encourage a drop of blood to form. This not only causes intravascular fluid to move from the surrounding tissues into the blood to give inaccurate values, but is also extremely painful for the patient. Devices are now developed to reduce the pain of skin puncture when heel and finger pricks are performed. These should be available for all patients who need to have regular samples of blood taken by this method, the most obvious example being patients with **diabetes mellitus**.

Blood in specimen bottles must be *inverted* for it to mix with the container fluid, rather than shaken. Shaking the blood will damage the red blood cells and cause haemolysis. The blood will not then provide a reliable sample for testing.

Firm and prolonged pressure must be applied to the puncture site to avoid haematoma formation. This is especially relevant when the patient is having blood clotting studies carried out or is on anticoagulant therapy.

Throughout the procedure, staff must be careful to avoid coming into direct contact with the patient's blood or acquiring a needlestick injury from a contaminated needle. A health and safety policy must be in place at locations where venepuncture is carried out to allow a rapid response if an accident happens.

Other factors that affect blood values

When an intravenous infusion is in progress, blood samples should be taken from the opposite arm. The presence of the infusion fluid in the vessels may affect the measured values.

Strenuous exercise causes excessive mobilization of white blood cells from the sides of blood vessels. The picture of blood taken immediately after exercise will show an artificially raised white cell value.

When considering blood results, remember that many things besides pathology can alter them (e.g. drugs, diurnal patterns, sex and genetic make-up).

Urine testing

Reliable results from any urine test can be obtained only when the urine has been collected in a clean, dry container. The specimen must be washed, rinsed and dried to ensure that it is uncontaminated by faeces, penile or vaginal discharge, or menstrual fluid.

Technique

Urine testing requires staff to have close contact with a potentially hazardous substance: urine. For personal protection you must wear gloves when dealing with all urine specimens – at all stages of the collection and testing. Always follow local policy and procedure. Urine must be tested soon after it is voided.

For routine testing, the early morning specimen is the best specimen to collect, for the following reasons:

1. Having fasted overnight, the urine collected in the bladder will not have the recent absorption of food components to affect the overall results.

2. If the urine test is to investigate the presence of a specific substance, the quantity of that substance will accumulate in the bladder overnight.

3. The lack of fluid intake by the patient overnight will reduce the water content of the urine. This less dilute urine will hold a greater concentration of the substances investigated by testing.

The exception to the above will be the testing of the first morning urine voided by a **diabetic patient**. The early morning specimen of a diabetic patient will *not* give accurate values. This is because urine that has accumulated in the bladder overnight will not reflect the blood glucose and ketone values at the time of the urine test. The bladder will need to be emptied of the overnight urine and a specimen of fresh urine collected 1 hour later for testing.

When a nurse is collecting a specimen of urine for testing, part of the investigative procedure should include additional, pertinent, observations to give a clearer clinical picture of the patient. These observations will include:

- whether the patient reports pain or dysuria when passing urine

- whether the patient has difficulty starting the flow of urine

- how frequently the patient has to pass urine during a 24-hour period. Special note must be taken of the number of times the patient wakes during the night to use the toilet

- whether the patient has any signs of **urinary incontinence**.

The following observations should be made on the **urine** in addition to the values measured using a reagent stick:

- *The colour of the urine in the container*
  — The urine should be pale to golden yellow. A darker coloured urine may be the result of dehydration or a raised bilirubin level in the urine
  — A red-coloured urine is always alarming because of its association with blood, but a red colour may be caused by food dyes (e.g. beetroot) or harmless urates
  — Red urine may be a sign of the inherited disease porphyria
  — Injected dyes used for investigation purposes that are excreted through the kidney will also colour the urine. These dyes may be radioactive.

- *The presence of abnormal substances*
  — Urine should be clear when held up to the light
  — The nurse should look for signs of blood. It is important to observe whether the blood looks fresh, having entered the urine lower down in the **excretory system**, or is dark blood that may have been in the urine for some time. This observation will link with the reagent stick test for haemolysed or non-haemolysed blood. Fresh blood found in the urine will not contain haemolysed red blood cells in any quantity
  — Threads or casts will be visible in the urine when the urinary tract is inflamed or infected.

- *The smell of the urine*
  — The odour of the urine should not be offensive
  — **Infection** is the major cause of malodorous urine
  — Stale urine smells of ammonia.

- *Frothy urine* may indicate a high protein content.

Always label each urine specimen as the container is given to you. When more than one specimen is to be tested it is very easy to confuse the specimen and allocate the wrong results to patients.

For accurate testing, the reagent stick must be used exactly according to the instructions that are given.

Diabetes
See chapter 2.6

Urinary
incontinence
See chapter 5.4

Urine
See chapter 5.4

Lower urinary tract
See chapter 5.4

Urinary infection
See chapter 5.4

Delay in testing the urine, incorrect timing of test results or contamination of the reagent sticks will alter the results obtained.

Additional methods of obtaining a sample of urine

A specimen of urine taken from a *urinary catheter* will give fresh urine for testing almost as soon as it has left the bladder. In health, it will not contain any contaminants. A catheter specimen of urine must be drawn from the catheter tubing; a stale sample of urine drawn from the catheter bag will not provide accurate analysis or results. As the nurse will be entering a sterile area to remove the urine from the catheter tubing, it is essential to use aseptic technique for this procedure.

When an uncontaminated urine specimen is required from a patient who is not continent or is unable to comply with instructions, a *suprapubic aspiration* of urine from the bladder may be the only optional procedure. Following the palpation of a full bladder, a sterile needle is inserted into the bladder. It is inserted from a position just above the symphysis pubis and a specimen of urine is syringed back. The procedure will produce a sterile, uncontaminated specimen of urine.

A *mid-stream specimen* of urine is taken when urine is required for *culture and sensitivity* testing. The nurse and patient must work in cooperation to obtain a specimen of urine that is free from any contamination during collection. Before this urine collection, all areas of the external genitalia likely to come into contact with the urine must be washed free of contaminating organisms. The patient is instructed to produce an initial flow of urine, which is discarded. This initial urine will contain tissue debris from the **urethra** and the urinary meatus. The next, mid-part, of the urine flow is collected in a sterile container. The patient then finishes emptying the bladder and this final specimen of urine is discarded.

The collected mid-stream specimen is put into a sterile container for immediate transport to the testing laboratory. Care must be taken by the nurse, and the patient, that only the outside of any sterile container is handled during the process so contamination does not occur.

A *24-hour urine* collection may be needed. It is essential to follow local laboratory instructions when preparing for this test and while the test is underway. It is also important that, if a volume of urine is accidentally thrown away while the collection is in operation, staff admit this mistake or else the results of the test will be invalid.

Specimens for culture and sensitivity

The purpose of taking specimens for culture and sensitivity testing is to identify organisms in a specified tissue and to identify the antibiotic that will destroy the infecting bacteria.

Urethra
See chapter 5.4

When a swab or any other specimen is collected for investigation of culture and sensitivity, the sample sent for analysis must be completely uncontaminated during the collection process. Complex instructions may be required if the patient is to understand the collection protocol and to ensure that the specimen is not contaminated as it is taken or put into a container for transport. The collection protocol may be very complicated in some cases, for example a mid-stream urine specimen. Infirmity or difficulty following instructions can make adhering to the protocol very difficult for the patient to carry out alone.

An aseptic technique must be used to obtain the specimen and the nurse should wear gloves when handling the specimen container, to avoid it being accidentally contaminated with infected material. Containers and lids must be handled only using the outside surfaces.

The specimen taken should not contain any other substance that could be contaminated by bacteria, other than found in the tested tissue (i.e. food particles). Swabs are taken from tissues to collect debris and discharge directly attributed to the infecting organism. Once collected, a transport medium should be used to transport the swab to a laboratory. The laboratory slip should contain a record of recent and current antibiotic therapy.

Gram staining

Bacteria are classified into descriptive groups for identification. To identify the bacteria present on the specimen, laboratory slides are smeared with material from the collected sample. Having fixed the specimen on to the glass, colour dyes are dripped on to the slide and the bacteria that are present will take up the dye. The slides are then viewed under a microscope. Differentiation of the bacteria can then take place (Box 9.1).

Box 9.1   Microscopic differentiation of bacteria

Bacteria are typed according to the stain they have taken:

- Gram-positive organisms take the purple stain of gentian violet
- Gram-negative organisms take the red stain of eosin.

Bacteria are also typed according to their shape when seen under a microscope, for example:

- elongated-shaped bacteria are rods or bacilli
- round-shaped bacteria are cocci.

A bacterium is described as acid-fast when it stains with carbofusion after being washed with acid–alcohol solution.

Cultures

In addition to identification by microscope, a sample of the collected material is put on to a culture medium. This allows the organisms to feed and multiply under ideal conditions. From this growth, definite identification of the invasive organisms can be made.

Sensitivity

Once the identification of the infecting organism has been isolated, it is exposed to various antibiotics. From this exposure the bacteria may show:

- resistance to an antibiotic – growth is not checked

- moderate susceptibility to the antibiotic – growth is slowed

- sensitivity to the antibiotic – the bacteria are destroyed.

The most effective antibiotic against the bacterial infection can then be recommended as treatment for the patient.

Investigation by means of diagnostic imaging

With the exception of endoscopy, the following investigations are usually conducted in a radiology department. Although radiographers are responsible for the technical aspect of these clinical investigations, it is the nurse who provides the important preparatory and aftercare of patients. The patient's needs at this time are as diverse as the protocols required to be implemented by the nurse, in response to the variety of investigations. There are common factors that all patients require when they have diagnostic imaging; these are set down in the Standards of Care, Radiology Nursing, from the Royal College of Nursing (1993). This document states that patients' needs fall into the four distinct categories and it is the nurses' responsibility to respond to each:

- maintenance of physical comfort

- the need for communication and information

- the need to feel safe

- psychological support.

Ultrasonography

The patient is prepared and positioned so that the technician is able to move an electrical transducer across the skin, over the designated organ. The impulses from the transducer are changed into ultrasound waves as they travel through the internal organs. When the wave hits an internal structure, it rebounds back to the skin. The wave

Figure 9.1   Ultrasonography: echocardiogram from a normal subject in two-dimensional long-axis view. The convention that shows the position of the transducer at the top of the paper causes the heart to appear 'upside down'. Ao, aorta; IVS, interventricular spetum; LA, left atrium; LV, left ventricle; MV, mitral valve; RV, right ventricle.

From Kumar and Clark (1994), with permission.

is converted back to electrical impulses by the transducer. A computer analyses the incoming impulses and forms a visual image of the internal structures. The returned image can be processed rapidly, allowing the motion from a beating heart or from a fetus to be viewed on a monitor. Still pictures can be taken of the image as a record (see Fig. 9.1).

The clarity of the images returned will depend on the degree on pre-test preparation of the patient. Some organs require particular preparation to enhance the final pictures, and the instructions specified by the ultrasound scanning department must be followed. This preparation may give the patient some discomfort; for example, the patient may need a full bladder to give greater clarity to the image obtained. The area of skin over the site of the target organ is prepared for better penetration of the ultrasound waves. A gel is used to seal the contact between skin and the transducer to obtain a better view of the target organs.

The patient must be assured that this is not an invasive test and pre-test preparations must include a description of the test procedure.

Radiography

X-rays are used for screening and diagnostic purposes. They identify the presence of abnormal structures and lesions, and incorrect positioning of organs.

To form the required image, X-rays are aimed at the part of the body that needs investigation. As they pass through the body, the X-rays are interrupted in their track by the internal structures of the body. The X-rays that are blocked during their pathway through the body and do not reach the film make a white image on the film. X-rays that penetrate the whole width of the body form a black image. The picture that forms is a negative image of the internal tissues.

Figure 9.2   Chest radiograph.

From Kumar and Clark (1994), with permission.

The penetration of the tissues by X-rays depends on the density of the structures that are impeding their progress. A diagnostic picture of the internal organs can be built up (see Fig. 9.2), knowing that:

1. Air and spaces within the body allow the uninterrupted passage of X-rays.

2. Air-filled cavities (i.e. the lungs or flatus-filled intestines) look black on the radiograph.

3. Organs and fatty tissues become a darker grey. The shade of grey is dependent on the ability of the X-rays to penetrate the tissue mass of the organ and reach the film.

4. Water is a poor conductor of X-rays. Structures with a high water content look light on the radiograph.

5. Bones are impenetrable to X-rays. They appear white on the radiograph.

Dyes or contrast media can be used to highlight tissues and organs that would normally be poorly defined on the radiograph. Dyes are given to form an impenetrable barrier to X-rays, usually forming a thin film on the inside of the organ. The white picture that appears in contrast against the black film allows features to be seen that would not normally be visible (Fig. 9.3). Patients normally need specific instructions for preparation when dyes or contrast media are to be used. Advice regarding aftercare may also be needed until the dye has been eliminated from the body. Any instructions from the radiography department must be complied with to avoid a poor image being produced and the patient having to return for a repeated procedure and additional exposure to X-rays.

Radiological investigation is not without risk as X-rays are a form of ionizing radiation capable of damaging cellular DNA. Repeated exposure to X-rays is known to cause cell damage and disease; the procedure can therefore be hazardous for patients and staff. Protective screens and clothing must be worn by staff who need to be in close proximity to X-rays. A badge that monitors exposure to

Figure 9.3   Radiography with contrast medium: antegrade pyelography via a percutaneous catheter (small arrow) of obstructed system. A percutaneous drainage catheter (large arrow) has been inserted.

From Kumar and Clark (1994), with permission.

radiation must be worn by staff who are in frequent contact with X-rays.

The damage that X-rays can do to rapidly dividing cells explains why a pregnant woman should not be exposed to X-rays. If the slightest risk of pregnancy exists, it is essential to avoid exposure to X-rays.

If you need to accompany a patient while radiography is being performed, you need to be supportive and informative. By encouraging the patient to relax and be still, you will ease them through the procedure and ultimately obtain a good image. When mobilization or communication with the patient is difficult, the radiographer will appreciate the knowledge of the patient brought by the nurse.

Computed tomography

Computed tomography (CT) uses X-rays to make three-dimensional pictures of cross-sections of the body (Fig. 9.4). An X-ray machine revolves in an arc around the body of the patient. The pictures received reflect the varying density of the tissues met by the X-rays as they travel between the skin and the X-ray detector. A computer interprets the images received. It translates the information into pictures to show cross-sectional views of the body. From these images, tumours and other lesions, tissue damage, haemorrhage and tissue atrophy can be visualized.

Figure 9.4 Computed tomogram of the normal abdomen at the level of the liver. 1, Aorta; 2, spine; 3, top of right kidney; 4, liver; 5, gallbladder; 6, stomach; 7, pancreas; 8, spleen.

From Kumar and Clark (1994), with permission.

Contrast media can be used to improve the quality of the pictures. Contrast media may produce an allergic reaction in the patient, so the patient must be asked about any previous sensitive reactions. Full resuscitation equipment must be immediately available in case of an anaphylactic reaction. CT should not be used on a pregnant woman.

CT is a lengthy procedure and the patient is required to lie completely still while the images are produced. The patient must be safe and secure throughout, even in the midst of the technology that is surrounding them. Sedation may be needed to relax the patient and assist in keeping him or her motionless. Discussions with the patient are needed to explain the purpose of the investigation. Description of the equipment and the process may relieve some of the anxiety. All metal objects and jewellery must be removed before the procedure. Further preparation of the patient before the investigation depends on instructions from the radiography department.

Imaging with radioactive materials

These investigations are used to make an assessment of the activity of the organ under investigation.

A radionuclide or a radioisotope is given to the patient, to be absorbed by the target organ. The radioactive material has an affinity with the organ to be tested and is taken into its tissues. The radioactive substance will act as a marker as it becomes part of the activity of the target organ.

A scanner is passed across the organ and a computer analyses the amount of radioactivity emanating from the scanned tissues. When high levels of radioactivity are recorded in one area, it is described as a 'hot spot'. A low level of radioactivity is a 'cold spot'. From this analysis, the size and outline of the structure can be assessed. The position of tumours, cysts and areas of non-functioning tissue can be outlined.

Discussion with the patient needs to take place before the test is performed. The patient needs to know the length of time that the test will take to perform, the preparations that need to be made and a description of the routine that will be followed during the test. The patient's own anxieties and queries must be addressed. The patient must also be advised that the radioactive substances will be excreted in the urine. To safeguard patients and staff from this radioactive waste, local guidelines and procedures must be followed. Subsequent to investigations, precautions must be in place when the patient uses the toilet or when there is a need to dispose of a used bedpan or commode.

Endoscopy

Endoscopes have been developed to give direct access and visibility within the hollow structures of the body. Each type of endoscope is designed to enter a specified body cavity. Once in place, the operator has a direct view for examination purposes. From this biopsies can be taken via the endoscope, and cautery and other local treatments can be performed. A camera can be attached to the endoscope, and the examination findings can be recorded as photographs or on video.

Endoscopy is an uncomfortable procedure if it is performed when the patient is fully conscious. Analgesia, sedation and local anaesthetics will help the patient to cope with the procedure, but some endoscopies need to be performed under general anaesthesia (e.g. laparoscopy and arthroscopy).

The preparation of the patient will vary according to the area of body that is to be examined by endoscope. Guidelines for preparation will be set by the department that is to perform the endoscopy. The patient will need to feel supported by the nursing staff as the idea of these tests can be daunting and stressful.

After the procedure is completed the nurse must be certain that the endoscopy has not caused bleeding, either by perforating an organ or through taking biopsies. Analgesia should be given for pain or discomfort experienced as a result of the examination.

When a local anaesthetic has been given to abolish the gag reflex prior to endoscopic examination, food and fluids must be withheld until the reflex returns.

Health screening

There is a movement of national policy towards the prevention of poor health rather than its cure (Department of Health 1999). This has led to a proliferation of clinical investigations for the purpose of health screening. The motives behind health screening are impeccable, but screening does require that a 'healthy' person has to contemplate the possibility of 'ill-health' for a short time, and this brings with it uncertainty and anxiety. This may

---

Box 9.2   Screening pregnant women for HIV

The government would like all women to voluntarily be tested for HIV during the antenatal period of pregnancy. HIV testing has always been a sensitive issue because a positive result confers physiological, sociological and psychological problems on to the patient. The Department of Health (1994) produced guidelines for practice to help promote testing for HIV. The guidelines lay down standards of care that must be adhered to when HIV testing is offered.

The guidelines state that:

- the woman must give explicit consent to testing
- this consent must be obtained after appropriate pre-test discussion and information
- the woman must understand the purpose of the test, its benefits and problems for herself, partner and unborn child
- the woman must be told, at testing, when the results will be available
- the results must be confidential to the woman
- the results of the test will not affect the woman's right to determine the outcome of the pregnancy or the care of the child.

---

cause people to resist participating in health screening. It becomes important for nurses to make sure that the process of screening is easy to access, that the positive aspects of the test are made clear, and that the benefits associated with the knowledge gained from the test are emphasized to the patient. A patient who voluntarily decides to have the health assessment should be welcomed into a positive and welcoming environment. The service should also ensure that the client has to wait as short a time as possible for the test results to be returned (see Box 9.2).

Giving unwelcome news

Giving bad news to the patient, even when it follows the most minor investigation, is always difficult. The nurse who has most information and is able to answer all the patient's questions with confidence must give the results. The information will be better assimilated and accepted by the patient if the nurse knows the patient well enough to provide continuous assessment of the patient's reaction as the news is given, and is able to respond appropriately.

When the results of the clinical investigation indicate that the patient will need to be given the results in the most sensitive way possible, it is important to be fully prepared for the meeting.

The meeting must take place in a room that does not allow interruptions to conversation and where all participants can sit comfortably, with the chairs positioned to

allow good eye contact to be maintained. If possible, a close relative should also listen to what is said. The giving of information must not be hurried. Time is needed for the patient to adjust his or her self-perceptions – from a well person in command of his or her own destiny to a person who has to adjust to being 'unwell', living within the limitations that this may bring.

The professionalism and behaviour of the nurse imparting difficult news must assist the feeling of trust that the patient needs to experience in the healthcare system. The patient must leave the room feeling that he or she will receive optimal care through this most difficult time. The patient must also know the options available (informed choice) and be comfortable with the selected pathway of treatment and care (informed consent).

Nurses need support to enable patients to manage these situations effectively and with expertise. Teesdale (1995) argues that nurses require education to deal with situations that provoke patient anxiety. A nurse must be able to recognize pertinent non-verbal and verbal signs that indicate how the patient is receiving the information, and recognize the use of coping mechanisms to reduce the impact of the news.

A written record of the information given and the patient's responses must be kept to allow other staff to continue with the support of the patient. Conflicting advice or information at this time is not acceptable to the patient.

The future

Technology will continue to offer increasingly accurate measurements of biochemical values and more precise imaging of body tissues and structures. Entirely new clinical investigations that offer new dimensions in assessment will come from work developed from research into genetic and chromosome studies. These clinical investigations will carry information that has an impact not only on the patient who consents to the assessment, but on that person's family through generations to come. This brings challenges to nursing as the issues that may be raised from the tests and the questions that patients will need help to answer will be complex. The nurse is the person who is best placed to provide a continuing dialogue with the patient, who will need time to appreciate fully the results of the genetic testing and to evaluate the impact of the results on present and future family members.

Genetic assessments, especially predictive or carrier testing, will present the patient with difficult ethical problems to answer. Patients may feel a duty to comply with testing to protect the well-being of future generations of the family (Hallowell 1999). This altruistic motive for testing will not protect the patient from the psychosocial difficulties that may arise as a result of the testing. Nurses will need to be at the forefront in helping patients to find a way through the complex questions that will inevitably become part of the follow-through of the process. This opens up the question of offering counselling to patients before the test is carried out to help them come to terms with the results. Such pre-test counselling is already available for **HIV** testing.

The remarkable advances in science and technology for clinical investigation will give clinicians the highest degree of precision and accuracy of information. The questions that are associated with this type of testing are also profound. The ability to look for genetic markers that predict the onset of future disease, especially if this information is gathered from a baby or child, could have an impact on the person's total life experiences. Nurses must reflect on these issues as the technology is introduced, and they must add their voices to the debate. The nurse will be a key person who can help prepare the way for the impact of genetic testing as each new development provides a new frontier of clinical assessment. The results of each test will affect patients, their families and society. It is this holistic view of patient care that gives the nurse a powerful position in the debate.

Summary

Patients often report that it is the 'not knowing' that increases worry. Clinical investigations are part of that 'not knowing' process. The investigations are carried out to make clinical conditions known and visible. The process of investigation will exacerbate anxieties until the results confirm the fear or give joyous relief. Nurses are with patients throughout the clinical investigation process. They cannot change the outcome of the tests, but they can provide patients with information and positive support. As patients gain confidence in the care that they receive during the process of clinical investigation, they will face future treatments with more confidence, which will ultimately help them deal with their illness more positively.

Critical incident

You are caring for a woman aged 86 years. She lives on her own and, other than being a little forgetful, she copes very well. She has a hearing problem, but she is not comfortable wearing a hearing aid. She tells you that she has needed to pass urine every 2 hours for the past 4 days. You suspect that she has a urinary tract infection. A mid-stream urine test for culture and sensitivity is ordered for her. You attempt to explain to her the process of collecting the urine but she has considerable difficulty understanding the process. Using the reflective questions, consider how you might overcome this patient's (and your) difficulty.

Reflection

See Appendix 2 for guidelines on reflection.

References

Department of Health (1994) Guidelines for offering voluntary named HIV anti-body testing to women receiving antenatal care. London: DoH.

Department of Health (1999) Saving lives: our healthier nation. London: HMSO.

Fishbach F (1992) A manual of laboratory and diagnostic tests, 4th edn. Philadelphia: JB Lippincott.

Furlong S, Glover D (1998) Consent, equity and ethics in new nursing. Nursing Times 94(38): 52–53.

Hallowell N (1999) Doing the right thing: genetic risk and responsibility. Sociology of Health and Illness. A Journal of Medical Sociology 21(5): 597–621.

Hinchliff SM, Montague SE, Watson R (1996) Physiology for nursing practice, 2nd edn. London: Baillière Tindall.

Klotzko AJ (1998) The perils of knowing. Nursing Times 94(43): 32–33.

Kumar P, Clark M (1994) Clinical medicine, 3rd edn. London: Baillière Tindall.

Lloyd AJ, Hayes PD, London NJM, Bell PRF, Naylor AR (1999) Patients' ability to recall risk association with treatment options. Lancet 353: 645.

Lowry M (1995) Knowledge that reduces anxiety: creating patient information leaflets. Professional Nurse 10(5): 318–320.

McKee D (1999) The legal framework for informed consent. Professional Nurse 14(10): 688–690.

Royal College of Nursing (1993) Standards of care, radiology nursing. London: Royal College of Nursing.

Royal College of Nursing (1995) Never going to be easy: giving bad news. RCN Nursing Update. Nursing Standard 9(50).

Skirton H (1995) Psychological implications of advances in genetics – 1. Carrier testing. Professional Nurse 10(8): 496–498.

Teesdale K (1995) The nurse's role in anxiety management. Professional Nurse 10(8): 509–512.

UKCC (1996) Guidelines for professional practice. London: UKCC.

Wilson KT, Waugh, eds (1996) Ross and Wilson's anatomy and physiology in health and disease, 8th edn. Edinburgh: Churchill Livingstone.

Winchester A (1999) Sharing bad news. Nursing Standard 13(26): 48–52.

Yeo H (1998) Informed consent in the neonatal unit: the ethical and legal rights of parents. Journal of Neonatal Nursing 4(4): 17.

*HIV infection
See chapter 6.2*

Further Reading

Department of Health (1999) Saving lives: our healthier nation. London: HMSO.

An important document that provides the guidelines for the future health of the population. Within its text, the reader can interpret the need for health screening programmes and clinical testing.

Department of Health internet site. Online. Available: http://www.doh.gov.uk

This website is full of information related to patient care and health professionals.

Fuller J, Shaller-Ayres J (2000) Health assessment: a nursing approach, 3rd edn. Philadelphia, PA: Lippincott.

This book is well laid out for the reader to view and access information. The colour pictures and diagrams give additional clarity to the text. It is a detailed text but an interesting book to access.

Skinner S (1995) Understanding clinical investigations.
London: Baillière Tindall.

This book provides a clear explanation of all common clinical investigations. Using tables, flowcharts and short notes, the book clarifies the underlying principles of each investigation, shows where it links to normal physiology and indicates how disease can alter the results. It also provides links to other clinical investigations that may be useful when a particular investigation shows abnormal results.

Skinner S (1999) Understanding drug therapies. London: Baillière Tindall.

By giving a clear description of how each drug interacts with normal and abnormal physiological processes, this book explains the appropriate clinical investigations for monitoring the therapeutic value of drugs.

Wilson DD (1999) Nurse's guide to understanding laboratory and diagnostic tests. Philadelphia, PA: Lippincott.

This book contains detailed information on all the clinical investigations that a nurse is likely to meet in practice.

The patient undergoing surgery

Ann Brown

Introduction

Preparation of the patient for surgery

Intraoperative phase

Postoperative management

Day surgery

Summary

Introduction

In thinking about surgery it is tempting to focus merely on the actual surgical intervention. However, the care that contributes to the restoration and maintenance of optimal physiological and psychological status before and after the operation comprises a large portion of the total surgical treatment and is extremely important in determining the patient's progress and recovery.

Surgical operations may be classified as elective or emergency. An *elective operation* is not necessary for the patient's survival but is expected to improve the patient's comfort and health. An *emergency operation* is one that must be done with a minimum of delay in the interest of the patient's survival.

Operative procedures vary greatly. They range from one that is technically simple and uncomplicated, taking only a brief period, to a prolonged, complex, major procedure that has severe traumatic effects. Many necessary considerations and nursing measures are common to the care of all surgical patients, regardless of their particular type of surgery. The basic components of the plan of care may require modification and/or additional specific details, according to the particular operation, the individual's psychological or physiological status and the type of anaesthetic used.

Preparation of the patient for surgery

The preoperative period, which begins with the decision that an operation is to be performed, may extend over an hour to several days, weeks or months. Whenever the patient's condition permits, sufficient time should be taken for assessment and treatment so that the patient goes for surgery psychologically and physically prepared. Intelligent, conscientious, preoperative nursing contributes much to having the patient achieve an optimum condition that favours a satisfactory postoperative progress and minimizes the possibility of complications (Kanto et al 1990). When the operation is elective or essential, there is usually a period of several days or weeks during which the patient is at home awaiting admission to the hospital. A district or practice nurse may contribute to the patient's physical and psychological preparation during this time. Some of the patient's and family's questions may be answered, psychological support provided, and advice given on such matters as nutrition and rest. Possible solutions to social and economic problems that are precipitated by the impending operation may also be suggested by the district or practice nurse.

Psychological preparation

Identification of patient problems

Potential problems common to the patient before operation include: (1) anxiety and (2) lack of knowledge.

Preoperative goals are for the patient to be able to state that the level of anxiety has been reduced and to show a satisfactory level of knowledge about the operation and measures that will promote recovery. Nursing interventions are:

1. To decrease anxiety by:
   a. identifying the patient's fears and concerns
   b. assessing the effectiveness of adaptive responses

c. supporting effective adaptive responses

d. answering questions and providing information.

2. Patient teaching. The nurse should:

   a. assess the patient's understanding of the operation and events that will occur before and after operation

   b. inform the patient about the surgical procedure and the preoperative and postoperative procedures and activities

   c. teach the patient to perform deep breathing, coughing and **leg exercises**, explaining the purpose of each

   d. provide information relating to the expectations of the patient and explain the nurse's role before and after surgery.

Anxiety

Few patients face surgery without some degree of anxiety. The concerns and fears vary from one person to another: some may be anxious about the pain and discomfort, others fear possible disfigurement and incapacity, loss of control of self, or death. They may be worried because of absence from work, lack of support for dependants, lack of care for the family or disruption of plans. Many are disturbed because they simply do not know what to expect: the unknown tends to be more threatening than the known.

The patient's emotional state and physical condition should receive equal consideration. Psychological stress evokes physiological responses (release of adrenaline and noradrenaline), which may have an unfavourable effect, especially if prolonged. The emotionally disturbed patient may experience a greater problem with vomiting, urinary retention, pain and restlessness during the postoperative period (Fyfe 1999).

Assessment

The patient's concerns, perception of the surgery and usual patterns of dealing with stress should be identified. Understanding the meaning of religion to the patient may help in the selection of appropriate support for the patient and family. We live in an increasingly multiracial society, so language barriers merit consideration. Most hospitals have access to a list of available translators. It may not be necessary to involve a translator when a member of the patient's family would be more suitable, given the nature of some clinical questions and/or explanations.

Through more prolonged and intimate contact, the nurse has the opportunity to assess the patient's perception of the situation and identify attitudes and concerns. Many fears may be unrealistic, based on misinformation and misconceptions about the operation. Sexual barriers also bear recognition: it should be borne in mind, for example, that women from a Muslim background prefer, when possible, to be examined and treated by women.

Deep vein thrombosis
See chapter 4.1

The level of the patient's anxiety may be assessed by observation of behaviours such as hyperactivity, increased talking, repetition of questions, crying, physical withdrawal, decreased social interactions and insomnia. Objective signs of stress include increased heart and respiratory rates, raised blood pressure, moist palms and restless movements.

Nursing intervention

The patient is encouraged to reveal fears and concerns, which the nurse should show are accepted, reasonable and to be expected. The problems are explored and, through expressing them and receiving some explanation or available assistance, some of the apprehension may be allayed. The fact that someone expects the patient to have worries and is sufficiently interested to listen is in itself a comfort. Some patients may be reluctant to express their fears because they think of them as a personal weakness, but they may be manifesting their insecurity in other ways, such as tenseness, restlessness or withdrawal. The nurse, recognizing the problem, may initiate a discussion by saying: 'I am sure you are concerned about your operation. There may be something I could clarify for you if you would like to talk about it'. There may be the occasional patient who displays a total lack of concern; however, this person may have deep underlying concerns that are being denied as a coping mechanism. It will often be helpful to discuss strategies to help the patient to cope, and to explore family and community resources that may assist following discharge.

Unrealistic fears based on misinformation and misconceptions can be alleviated by providing factual information, both verbal and written. The patient should be kept informed as to the purpose of the operation and what is involved in the investigative and preparatory procedures. What may be expected on the day of operation and in the postoperative period is discussed. Ignorance of what is going to happen usually causes more fear and mental suffering than being advised of the facts.

Any anticipated permanent change in body function or appearance is explored, and the patient is advised as to the available assistance and how life may be managed in future; emphasis is placed on the positive aspects. For example, a patient who is being prepared for a permanent colostomy may be encouraged to see and talk with a person who has had the same operation and is living a relatively normal, active life. Patients should be referred, where possible, to nurses who have specialized in these particular problems.

It is an established practice in some institutions for an operating theatre nurse who will be involved with the patient's operation to visit the ward before the day of surgery. This has distinct advantages for the patient. It tends to lessen 'the fear of the unknown'. The visit means that when the patient is received in the operating theatre the nurses will not all be complete strangers. It also indicates an interest on the part of the staff, which is reassuring. The nurse reviews the patient's history, talks with the ward nurse, and advises the patient of the purpose of the visit. The discussion includes such matters as transport to the operating theatre, the type of room the patient will be in, any preanaesthetic checks, why staff are gowned and masked, the anaesthetic and the postoperative return to the recovery room or surgical ward. The patient is encouraged to ask questions. Even if theatre staff do not make such visits, ward staff should be exploring these areas with the patient. The visit to the ward and patient provides the theatre nurse with information about the patient that enables the theatre staff to be more fully prepared for this particular person. For example, the patient may have a disability that necessitates preparation for placement in a different position from that normally used (Matiti 1999).

Long periods in which the patient is alone should be avoided; relatives should be encouraged to visit and the nurse should 'drop in' at frequent intervals. Some form of interesting diversion may be provided. The patient may find a minister of religion a source of strength and courage. In some instances, help beyond that which the nurse can provide is needed to reduce the patient's fear. It may be necessary to consult the surgeon, anaesthetist or social worker and have one of them talk further with the patient.

Visits with other patients and socializing in the dayroom are encouraged. Most patients tend to talk readily to one another about their problems and share their preoperative fears. The fact that many of the same concerns are experienced by others seems to put them in proper perspective and make them less ominous.

Family members are kept informed, and time is taken to talk with them, answer their questions, and advise them as to how they can offer support to the patient.

Patient teaching and information giving

Assessment

The identification of learning needs includes an assessment of the patient's understanding of the surgical procedure and perceptions of the preoperative and postoperative experiences. The fact that surgery is scheduled motivates most patients to seek information, and their receptiveness to the information provided is increased. In emergency situations, life-threatening needs receive priority over detailed extensive explanations, but the patient always has the right to some information and to make *informed* decisions. A moderate degree of anxiety enhances learning, but when anxiety increases the attention span and receptiveness decrease.

Nursing intervention

The surgeon will have discussed the operation with the patient and family: why it is necessary, what it involves and the expected results. Frequently the patient and the family are so emotionally overcome at the time that they do not grasp all that has been said. Later, they want clarification of what has been said, and they usually have a number of questions. The nurse determines what information was given to them by the doctor and, in simple, understandable terms, repeats necessary information and answers their questions.

Preoperative procedures and what will be expected of the patient are discussed. Expectations for the postoperative period are outlined. The patient is advised as to where he or she will be after the operation has taken place – whether taken to a recovery room or the intensive care unit or returned to the present location.

A description of the recovery room and what occurs there is given to the patient, and the family is told that they will be permitted to visit when the patient returns to the ward. The reasons for the *frequent assessment of vital signs*, alertness and responses should also be explained.

Deep breathing is demonstrated and taught; maximal inspirations, which are held for 3–5 seconds and practised several times an hour, increase arterial oxygen saturation and prevent postoperative pulmonary complications. The technique should be demonstrated and the patient given the opportunity to practise it before operation. Use of a respirometer, to show the patient how much air is taken into and expelled from the lungs, provides incentive to practise the exercises and gives evidence of the effectiveness of the patient's efforts. The patient is taught to *cough* by supporting the area where the incision will be, taking a deep breath and expelling the air forcefully through the mouth. Coughing is encouraged after operation to facilitate the removal of bronchial secretions. Box 10.1 lists deep breathing and coughing techniques. The patient is assured that necessary assistance and support will be provided. Emphasis should be placed on *non-smoking* during the preoperative and postoperative periods; any irritation of the respiratory tract predisposes to pulmonary complications.

Postoperative *lower limb* exercises to prevent circulatory stasis and **thrombosis** are described and demonstrated. The patient is advised that he or she will be expected to get out of bed, sit in a chair and walk around the room for brief periods in the early postoperative period; early ambulation promotes normal body functioning and reduces problems such as vomiting, wind pains and urine retention. If the use of drainage tubes (e.g. chest or gastric) or special equipment such as a suction machine is anticipated, preoperative preparation includes an explanation of the purpose and procedure, and what will be expected of the patient.

Information is also given about any postoperative **pain** that may be expected, the cause of the pain and what will be done to control it. The patient is told how to participate in pain control by asking for medication before the pain becomes severe and by practising relaxation, leg exercises, ambulation and other techniques that may have worked previously in relieving pain. Relaxation techniques may

Deep vein
thrombosis
See chapter 4.1

Pain
See chapter 2.3

> **Box 10.1   Instructions given to patients about breathing and coughing exercises**
>
> *Sustained maximal inspiration*
>
> From a sitting or standing position:
>
> 1. Take a deep breath through the mouth, pushing the diaphragm down and distending the abdomen as the chest expands
>
> 2. Hold breath for 3–5 seconds
>
> 3. Breathe out slowly
>
> 4. Repeat several times each hour.
>
> *Coughing*
>
> From a sitting position:
>
> 1. Support incision with hands or pillow
>
> 2. Take a deep breath through the mouth, pushing the diaphragm down and distending the abdomen as the chest expands
>
> 3. Immediately force the air from the lungs out through the mouth
>
> 4. Expectorate secretions into a sputum pot
>
> 5. Repeat several times every 2–4 hours if secretions are present.

Urine
See chapter 5.4

Normal blood values
See chapter 4.1

Blood clotting
See chapter 4.1

Fever
See chapter 6.1

Blood pressure
See chapter 4.2

Menstruation
See chapter 6.3

Diarrhoea
See chapter 5.1

Nausea and vomiting
See chapter 5.1

Allergy
See chapter 6.2

be taught if the patient is very anxious, requests it, or if severe, prolonged pain is anticipated. Anxiety exacerbates pain, and fear of the unknown leads to anxiety. It is likely that giving information and explanations, together with answering patient questions, makes a major contribution to reducing anxiety and postoperative pain and in promoting recovery.

Group instruction in deep breathing, coughing, leg exercises and pain management can be an effective method of teaching. Group instruction saves nursing time and provides the opportunity for patients to practise techniques together and share anxieties and fears. Individual instruction is necessary to provide specific information related to the surgical experience of the individual and the family.

Physical preparation

Physical assessment

Common concerns with all surgical patients are cardiac, pulmonary and renal function; blood volume and composition; nutritional status; and fluid and electrolyte balance. Basic laboratory tests for all preoperative patients include **urinalysis**; **blood values** including haematocrit, urea and electrolytes, haemoglobin, white cell count; and bleeding or **clotting** time. An electrocardiogram is often done,

and the chest is examined by auscultation and probably radiography. Other laboratory tests, functional studies and radiographs may be done, as well as specific investigative procedures relevant to the patient's particular disorder and physiological status. These studies should be understood by the nurse so that the necessary explanation, support for the patient and appropriate adaptations to the nursing care plan can be made.

The nurse is constantly alert for signs and symptoms that might indicate a condition or change in the patient that could interfere with progress and predispose to complications. Such factors as the following are promptly reported to the doctor: a raised **temperature**; a significant change in pulse, respirations or **blood pressure**; a rash; a cough, complaint of sore throat or nasal discharge that might point to a respiratory infection; onset of **menstruation**; **diarrhoea**; **nausea and vomiting**; and a deficient food or fluid intake.

Patient history

The patient's history includes information that may be significant in responses to surgery and recovery.

Infants, young children and the elderly are less able to tolerate the stress of surgery. Obesity and nutritional deficiencies interfere with wound healing and predispose to cardiovascular and pulmonary problems. Smoking irritates the respiratory tract and increases secretions, predisposing to respiratory complications; platelet function and blood coagulation are also altered. Existing cardiovascular, renal and liver disorders and diabetes increase the potential for the development of complications after operation.

A detailed drug history related to both prescription and non-prescription medications is obtained. Acetylsalicylic acid preparations prolong bleeding. The nurse should be aware of the potential effects of previous drug therapy so that potential risks may be identified and plans made for postoperative observations and interventions for the prevention and prompt identification of problems.

History of any allergic reactions is recorded and an **allergy** alert bracelet may be placed on the patient's wrist and the chart marked appropriately to alert the surgeon, anaesthetist and nursing personnel.

Nutrition

Malnourishment may lead to many problems for the surgical patient. Protein deficiency delays healing and decreases the resistance to infection because of a slower response in antibody formation. Vitamin C also plays an important role in healing because it is necessary for the laying down of collagen fibres. It also contributes to capillary integrity. Optimal amounts of the vitamin B complex are necessary for normal glucose metabolism and for the maintenance of cellular enzymes. A deficient intake of carbohydrate depletes the liver glycogen, leaving the body without a reserve source of glucose during the period when food intake is decreased, which leads to catabolism of the body tissues.

If the patient's condition is such that ordinary solid food cannot be taken, fluids containing commercial protein concentrates and glucose may be tolerated. When oral intake is insufficient or not possible, intravenous solutions to ensure hydration and nutrition may be administered. The aim is to bring the patient to surgery with the best possible nutritional status.

There is a considerable increase in the risk of surgery in obese persons, who have a greater tendency to develop cardiovascular, pulmonary and wound complications. The excessive fat tissue frequently makes the operative procedures more difficult. The patient who is overweight is advised of the need to lose weight before operation and may be given a reducing diet assessed on an individual basis.

Fluids and electrolytes

A normal **fluid balance** is extremely important in the surgical patient: dehydration predisposes to shock, a retention of metabolic wastes and disturbances in electrolyte concentrations. The patient who has been ill for some time, particularly if the disorder is gastrointestinal, frequently has a fluid and electrolyte deficit. A record of the fluid intake and output is kept and the patient is observed for signs of dehydration. A minimum daily fluid intake of 2500–3000 mL is encouraged, unless contraindicated. Blood biochemistry studies are done to determine electrolyte concentrations, and any deficiencies are corrected by oral or parenteral preparations.

Rest and exercise

The patient awaiting an operation may find it difficult to rest and sleep because of anxiety and decreased activity. The patient's accustomed pre-sleeping habits are determined and measures that promote relaxation, such as massage, warm drinks, reading or soft music, are instituted. The doctor may be consulted regarding a prescription for a mild sedative to promote relaxation and the necessary rest.

When the patient is well enough, exercise should be encouraged. This prevents general weakness, contributes to normal fatigue and rest, and diminishes the probability of circulatory complications later.

Specific therapy

Certain treatments to correct secondary physiological disturbances or coexistent diseases may comprise a large part of the preoperative preparation. The patient who has developed anaemia because of a loss of blood or a nutritional deficiency may receive one or more blood transfusions. A course of an antimicrobial drug may be necessary to clear up some infection. A diabetic patient may require dietary and insulin therapy to bring the disease under control, lower the blood sugar, and have the urine free of sugar and ketones. The purpose of any such treatments and their significance to the operation should be explained to the patient and family.

Informed operative consent

Informed consent implies that the patient has been given information by the doctor about the nature of the operation to be done and that the patient understands that information. A *consent form* signed by the patient is also necessary for some major and invasive diagnostic procedures. It also implies that consent is given freely and that the patient has not been put under undue pressure.

In seeking consent the doctor is required to provide sufficient details and information about what is proposed to enable the patient (or parent or guardian in the case of a minor or a person with a learning disability) to form a proper decision and so give an informed consent.

The extent of the explanation given, when seeking consent, will depend on factors such as the patient's age and maturity, physical and mental state and the reason for the operation, and will also be influenced by the questions asked by the patient. Some patients request far more information than others about side-effects, complications, etc.

There is no requirement in English law that every possible complication and side-effect should be explained to the patient. The purpose of informed consent is to protect the hospital, surgeon and anaesthetist against claims of unauthorized anaesthesia and surgery, and claims related to possible adverse sequelae to the patient, and to protect the patient against unauthorized procedures (Young 1994).

When asked to sign the consent form the patient must be rational, alert and not under the influence of any drugs or alcohol that might impair comprehension and judgement.

The signing of an operative consent form must be witnessed by a medical practitioner who attests to the fact that in his or her presence the statement was read by the signatory, who stated that he or she understood and then signed the consent. If the patient is mentally competent, but unable to write, an 'X' indicating a consent is acceptable if witnessed by two signatories.

In the UK any person of sound mind who has attained the age of 16 years may give a legally valid consent to surgery. A minor's capacity to make his or her own decision depends upon the minor having sufficient understanding and intelligence to make the decision, and is not determined by any fixed age limit. Until the child achieves the capacity to consent, consent must be obtained from a parent or legal guardian (Dimond 1990).

In the case of a genuine emergency the doctor may safely proceed to do what is reasonably necessary without a formal consent, acting in good faith and in the immediate interests of the patient's health and safety. If the emergency arises in an unconscious patient, the doctor should,

Fluid balance
See chapter 2.6

if time permits, endeavour to obtain the consent of the next of kin.

When the patient is mentally ill or has a learning disability, a valid consent can be given only if the matter concerned is within his or her understanding. The relatives or responsible medical officers have no legal power to consent on the patient's behalf, although their approval should be obtained.

Immediate preoperative preparation

The following preparatory measures receive consideration the day before and on the day of operation.

Food and fluids

The patient's stomach should be empty when going to the operating theatre to prevent the possibility of aspiration of vomit. All food and fluids are withheld for at least 4–6 hours before the scheduled time for surgery, and an explanation is given to the patient. Essential oral medication (with a small amount of water) may be given during this time. If the patient's mouth becomes dry and uncomfortable, a mouthwash is given. When a patient inadvertently takes food or fluid, the anaesthetist should be promptly notified. It will probably necessitate a postponement of the operation or the passing of a gastric tube to evacuate the stomach contents (Williams 1999).

When the patient is an infant or small child, the doctor may stress the giving of clear sweetened fluids for 24 hours until 4–6 hours before operation. This is to promote an optimum glycogen reserve in the liver, as this is normally proportionately less than in the adult and will be depleted quickly.

If the patient is to receive a local anaesthetic, a light breakfast may be permitted by the doctor.

Elimination

The doctor's orders may or may not include giving the patient an evacuation enema or suppositories. If the patient has had a normal bowel movement the day before operation, this may not be considered necessary. Some surgeons prefer all patients having major surgery to have an evacuation enema or suppositories the evening before the operation to prevent constipation following surgery, when diet and activity are restricted. If the operation involves the bowel, a thorough preparation is essential in order to ensure the bowel is empty during operation. This may involve a special diet (low residue), pharmacological preparation and or bowel washouts, depending on the wishes of the surgeon.

The bladder should be empty when the patient goes to the operating theatre, especially in the case of low abdominal or pelvic surgery, as a full bladder may interfere with the surgical procedure by making the site less accessible, and may also increase the risk of accidental injury to the bladder wall. The patient is asked to void just before the preoperative medication is administered. If the patient is unable to void, the staff in the operating theatre are informed and, if necessary, catheterization is performed in the operating room before operation. If an indwelling catheter is needed, it is usually inserted in the operating room, unless otherwise ordered by the surgeon.

Local site preparation

Although the details of the preparation of the site of the operation vary according to the area and the surgeon's preference, the principles are the same. Preoperative skin care aims to have the **skin** as free as possible of dirt particles, hair, desquamated cells, secretions and organisms. Before operation the patient takes a warm bath or shower. Hair may be safely removed by depilatory cream, but abrasions and lacerations in the skin caused by a razor serve as an entry for microorganisms. If hospital policy insists that hair is shaved from the skin, it is recommended that it be done with a wet shave 1–2 hours before operation. When the skin is to be shaved, the surgeon usually specifies the extent of the area to be shaved and the time it is to be done in relation to the operation. Some research now indicates that not shaving or using a depilatory cream reduces the risk of postoperative wound infections. Walsh and Ford (1989) have discussed this research and the whole preparation for theatre, coming to the conclusion that much care is ritualistic, with little basis in sound research. Shaving skin before operation is one such ritual.

If a patient is discovered to have acne or infected lesions, the operation may be delayed until the condition has been corrected. Daily antiseptic baths or the application of an antimicrobial preparation may be prescribed.

Special preparation extending over several days may be ordered by the surgeon for some operations, such as skin grafts and orthopaedic procedures. Specific instructions for local preparation are received for any operation on the head, face and eye.

For rectal and lower bowel surgery, the patient is usually given a bowel clearance preparation such as Picolax, followed by evacuation enemas or rectal washouts until the return fluid is clear. Rectal washouts are given high and slowly, and the patient is allowed to rest after each one. Washouts should also be given early enough to make sure all fluid is expelled before the patient is taken to the operating theatre. The perineum and surrounding area are thoroughly cleansed with water and detergent after the final evacuation.

In the case of operations on the mouth or throat, unless specific preparatory instructions have been given, the teeth are cleaned and the mouth rinsed well with an antiseptic mouthwash the night before and the morning of the day of operation.

Personal care

The patient has a bath, shower or bed bath on the evening before or the morning of the operation. Prior to surgery the patient is given a clean hospital gown.

Skin flora
See chapter 6.1

The **teeth** are cleansed and an antiseptic mouthwash may be used the night before and the morning of the day of operation to make sure that all food particles have been removed. Dentures are removed because they may become displaced and interfere with respiration during induction of anaesthesia. They should be placed in an appropriate container, labelled with the patient's name, and put in the patient's locker. Any prosthesis, such as an artificial eye or limb, is removed and safely stored if it will interfere with surgical procedure. If the patient uses a hearing aid, it is usually left in place until arrival in the anaesthetic room, when it is removed and stored safely.

The hair is combed, neatly arranged back from the face, left free of hairpins, and may be secured under a cap so that it does not become soiled or interfere with the administration of anaesthetic. Coloured nail polish and make-up are removed, because checking of the colour of the lips and nail beds for cyanosis is necessary. All jewellery is removed for safekeeping. The identification wristlet should be checked to make sure it is clearly legible, secure, and the patient's name and hospital number are correct.

Medication

When the immediate preoperative orders are written, the nurse should ascertain whether there are any preceding prescriptions for medications and, if so, ask the doctor whether these preparations are to be withheld or given. The patient may have been receiving a cardiac drug, insulin or other important drugs, and the omission of such could have serious effects.

A sedative is usually given the night before operation to ensure a good night's sleep for the patient. A benzo-diazepine such as temazepam or a chloral derivative such as dichloralphenazone is commonly used. All patients receiving hypnotic preparations are instructed not to get up after taking the drug but to signal for the nurse if they want something or are unable to sleep. Frequently, simple nursing measures such as a change of position or staying with the patient briefly may reduce tension and apprehension, and promote sleep.

Approximately 45–90 minutes before operation the patient usually receives a drug to produce relaxation and allay anxiety; this is known colloquially as the 'premed' (i.e. premedication before the anaesthetic). The doctor's choice of drugs is based mainly on the patient's condition and age.

If a general anaesthetic is to be given, the patient may also receive an anticholinergic preparation such as atropine or hyoscine hydrobromide (scopolamine) to reduce salivary and respiratory secretions and to block vagal impulses that cause the bradycardia and hypotension associated with some anaesthetic agents. Scopolamine tends to make the respiratory secretions less tenacious than atropine.

All preparatory procedures should be completed before the preoperative medication is given. The patient is then left undisturbed, and quiet is maintained. A relative may remain to provide comfort and security for the patient.

A final check and recording may be made of the pulse, respirations and blood pressure about 30 minutes after the preoperative drug has been given.

Patient's notes

Treatments and any pertinent reactions of the patient are recorded, and the patient's notes, including the nurses' notes, diagnostic reports, progress notes, patient's history, relevant radiographs and/or scans and the operation consent form, are put together and taken to the operating theatre with the patient. A sheet on the front of the chart should list any factors that may be considered particularly important for the anaesthetist, surgeon and theatre staff to note. Examples are **allergies**, drug sensitivity, coexisting disease and limitation of joint movement in a limb. The latter may be significant in relation to positioning the patient on the operating room table. The patient's blood type is also noted.

Relatives are normally advised to go home while the patient is in theatre and to telephone the ward after the operation has taken place.

Emergency preoperative preparation

Preoperative preparation in emergency surgery is limited to basic essentials. When the patient is in shock or is bleeding, the haemoglobin level is checked and the blood typed immediately. An intravenous infusion is started using normal saline or a plasma expander (e.g. Haemaccel) until compatible whole blood is available.

If the patient is to have a general anaesthetic and is likely to have taken food and fluid within the last 6–8 hours, a gastric tube is passed to evacuate the stomach contents or emergency intubation is undertaken in the anaesthetic room. In the case of intestinal obstruction, a nasogastric or duodenal tube is passed and intermittent suction started in order to keep the stomach and duodenum free of fluid and gas.

As soon as possible, the patient is asked to void to obtain a specimen for urinalysis and to have the bladder empty for surgery. If the patient is unable to void, the doctor may ask for the patient to be **catheterized**, as it is important to know before operation whether the urine contains sugar or abnormal constituents that might indicate diabetes mellitus or impaired renal function.

The consent form for operation is signed, and preoperative medication is given if appropriate. Any dentures or prostheses and jewellery are removed, and the hair may be covered with a cap.

If the patient has just been admitted and is not accompanied by a relative, the nurse should be sure to obtain the name and telephone number of a family member and should notify the person as soon as possible.

Teeth
See chapter 5.1

Allergy
See chapter 6.2

Catheterization
See chapter 5.4

Evaluation of preparation for surgery

The following criteria may be used to indicate correct preparation:

1. The patient identifies concerns related to the operation.

2. The patient acknowledges feeling less anxious and shows a relaxed posture and ability to sleep the night before surgery.

3. Physical preparation of the patient is completed safely.

4. The patient expresses an understanding of the surgical procedure and the preoperative and postoperative events.

5. The patient demonstrates the ability to perform deep breathing, coughing and leg exercises, and can state their significance.

Intraoperative phase

Operating theatre procedures vary greatly from one hospital to another. The information that follows is generally applicable to most situations and may prove helpful to the nurse caring for the patient experiencing surgery. No attempt is made to present the detailed knowledge and techniques essential to nurses who are members of the operating theatre team. Anticipating surgery is a threatening and fearful experience for the patient. Some fear may be allayed if the nurse at the bedside can give the patient some information as to what will take place in the operating department. It is also important that the nurse caring for the patient in the postoperative period has some understanding of what the patient has experienced.

The operating theatre is located, constructed and equipped to promote safety and quiet, to prevent infection and to facilitate surgical procedures. It is located near the recovery room. The temperature of the room is readily controlled according to the patient's needs as well as those of the operating personnel. Windows may be absent in the operating room; air conditioning is provided by a special ventilation system which filters the air before it enters the room to remove dust and organisms and reduce the risk of infection. It also provides a higher atmospheric pressure within the operating theatre. The higher atmospheric pressure means that, when doors into the theatre are opened, air flows out of the theatre rather than in, thereby reducing the risk of airborne infection. Equipment, for example lights and tables, is designed to withstand frequent disinfection and to facilitate aseptic technique and the operation. Entry to the operating department is controlled to reduce potential transmission of organisms from the wards or outside the hospital.

All operating theatre personnel wear operating theatre gowns or suits, which are laundered by the hospital. Street clothing or ward uniforms are not permitted in the operating theatre. Personnel wear caps to cover their hair, a mask that is impervious to moisture over their nose and mouth, and antistatic footwear. A staff member with an infection (respiratory infection, local skin infection) is excluded from the operating theatre.

The incision and exposure of underlying tissues and viscera place the patient at serious risk of infection, demanding the practice of strict surgical asepsis. Everything that comes in contact with the patient's operative site must be sterile. Table covers, drapes, instruments, sutures, ligaments and swabs are sterilized and are handled only by members of the surgical team who have performed surgical scrub of their hands and arms, and are dressed in sterile gowns and gloves. Tables, lights and other equipment that do not come in contact with the wound are kept surgically clean by cleansing with a disinfectant between operations. Floors are similarly cared for.

Transfer to operating theatre

At the appropriate time, the patient is taken to the operating theatre, either in bed or on a trolley.

Before leaving the ward, the personnel responsible for transporting the patient to the operating theatre check the patient's identification bracelet with the ward staff and operating theatre list to be sure they have the right patient. The patient is lifted on to the stretcher and adequate covers are provided to keep the patient warm. Woollen blankets are not allowed within the operating theatre: wool is a potential source of static electricity. This point is particularly important as many of the gases used in anaesthesia are highly inflammable and therefore the risk of any static sparks must be avoided. Cot sides are used on the trolley. The patient is disturbed as little as possible; preoperative medication has usually been given to reduce anxiety and induce drowsiness.

Reception of the patient

The patient is taken to a waiting or holding room or area, and introduced by name to the operating theatre personnel; it is important not to leave the patient unattended. An operating theatre nurse introduces himself or herself, and proceeds to check the following data:

- The patient's response (drowsy, alert, anxious).

- Name and age. Identification is made both verbally, if the patient is responsive, and by the identification bracelet; the name is also checked with the operating theatre list.

- The operation consent form. Is it correctly signed? The type of anticipated surgery is compared with the operating theatre list and any exceptions are indicated.

- If the surgery to be performed is to be on one of paired organs (e.g. kidneys, lung) or limbs (e.g. leg, arm) or a specific unilateral area (e.g. hernia), is the correct unilateral area clearly identified?

- Special problems (e.g. allergy, rash, joint problem and limited range of motion that may interfere with positioning).

- Laboratory reports, such as urea and electrolytes, prothrombin time, **blood type**.

- Preoperative medication: what was given and the dose? Medication may be given to: allay anxiety; induce drowsiness, which lessens the amount of anaesthetic needed in the induction phase; reduce respiratory secretions; or to diminish undesirable reflex responses during induction (nausea and vomiting).

- **Vital signs**. These are entered on the operation sheet as baseline data.

Any significant observations (e.g. anxiety state; abnormal finding that is recorded, such as allergy or increased prothrombin time; or abnormal vital sign, such as tachycardia) is brought to the anaesthetist's attention before any anaesthetic is administered. A final check is made to ensure that the patient has no dentures. The hair may be covered with a cap.

If sufficiently alert, the patient is advised of the waiting period; the nurse remains close by and communicates by speaking calmly to the patient, or simply by touch if the patient is drowsy. The waiting area should be quiet: loud noises, talking and confusion arouse the patient and heighten anxiety. An overheard conversation may be misinterpreted because of drowsiness and preoperative medication.

Anaesthesia

The type of anaesthesia to be used for each patient is decided by the anaesthetist, in consultation with the patient and surgeon. The term anaesthesia implies loss of sensation which may be classified as general or regional. *General anaesthetic* agents produce reversible depression of the cerebral neurones that are responsible for awareness and responses; there is loss of sensation, consciousness, reflex responses and skeletal muscle tone. The muscle relaxation facilitates the surgery. *Regional anaesthesia* temporarily blocks the sensory receptors in the surgical area or the nerve impulses in an area of the sensory impulse conduction pathway. The patient remains conscious but may be drowsy owing to preoperative sedation.

Methods of anaesthetic administration

General anaesthesia

General anaesthesia may be produced by agents administered by inhalation or intravenous infusion. Most frequently, the current practice involves induction of anaesthesia by the intravenous injection of an anaesthetic agent such as thiopental sodium (Intraval) or propofol (Diprivan), followed by the inhalation administration of one or more anaesthetic agents.

Endotracheal intubation is almost routinely done when a general anaesthetic is to be given and the patient requires ventilating. Using a laryngoscope, a cuffed endotracheal tube or laryngeal mask is introduced into the trachea by the anaesthetist, following the intravenous induction; the chest is observed for rise and fall, and is auscultated for air entry to make sure the tube is in the respiratory tract and not in the oesophagus. When the tube is in the desired position, the cuff is inflated with air to maintain an airtight seal. Overinflation is guarded against: excessive pressure may cause necrosis of the mucosa. The tube is attached to the anaesthetic machine. This method has the advantage of the control that the anaesthetist can maintain on the amount given. Its disadvantage may be irritation of the respiratory tract and increased secretions. Suction must be readily available. Following the removal of an endotracheal tube, there may be hoarseness or loss of voice due to temporary impairment of the vocal cords, and laryngeal oedema or spasms may occur.

A laryngeal mask maintains the airway without the need to intubate. It is quick to use and avoids the need to use muscle relaxants, which can cause muscle pains after operation. This method is particularly useful for head and neck surgery and for minor procedures. It can be used for patients having laparoscopic procedures but with the proviso that it should not be used in the obese or in patients with a history of gastro-oesphageal reflux as the mask does not ensure a seal to prevent regurgitation.

Regional anaesthesia

Regional anaesthesia is produced by the following methods.

Local infiltration   This involves the injection of an anaesthetic agent into the surgical site or into the area to be manipulated. The agent makes the local receptors unresponsive to stimuli. It is used principally for minor superficial surgical procedures or pain relief.

Peripheral nerve block   This is produced by the injection of an anaesthetic agent into the area of a large nerve trunk or plexus, or into the tissues surrounding the operative site. The conduction of sensory nerve impulses is interrupted and anaesthesia is achieved. Fewer injections are required in this method, although some of the techniques are quite complex to perform.

Spinal anaesthesia   This method entails the injection of the anaesthetic agent into the subarachnoid space in the lumbar region of the spine (usually between the second and fourth lumbar vertebrae). The agent blocks impulses at the origin of peripheral nerves. The area anaesthetized is determined by the level to which the drug rises in the spinal canal as well as by the amount of the drug used. This type of anaesthesia may be used in low abdominal and lower limb surgery. Chest and high abdominal surgery would require the agent to be carried to higher levels, which would place the patient at risk of respiratory insufficiency as a result of blocking of impulses to the respiratory muscles.

Epidural or caudal anaesthesia This regional anaesthesia is induced by the injection of an agent into the extradural space of the lower part of the vertebral canal (the sacro-coccygeal region). The drug blocks impulses carried along the fibres of the cauda equina. Epidural anaesthesia may be used in rectal and perineal operative procedures and is commonly used in obstetrics during labour and delivery. Thoracic epidural anaesthesia may be appropriate for selected patients.

Topical or surface anaesthesia This is produced by the application of the agent to the skin or mucous membrane. Absorption of the agent results in a blocking of the sensory receptors. It is used principally in nose and throat procedures and comes in the form of sprays, solutions or creams. EMLA cream is particularly useful before venepuncture in children.

Anaesthetic agents

A variety of drugs are used as anaesthetic agents. Table 10.1 gives examples of anaesthetic agents used according to the method of administration. The choice depends upon the method of administration to be used, the operation to be performed, the anticipated time for the procedure, and the physiological and psychological condition of the patient.

The inhalation agents commonly used may be in the form of a gas or a rapidly evaporating (volatile) solution. They are absorbed from the lungs and reach the brain quickly via the circulation. The liquid preparations are vaporized in the anaesthetic machine, and are usually combined with oxygen for inhalation. For many years, ether and cyclopropane were popular inhalation agents but were extremely hazardous because of their inflammability and explosive potential. They have been almost entirely replaced with safer agents. Cyclopropane is still used occasionally in infants for speed of effect.

The intravenous anaesthetic agents take effect quickly and recovery is rapid. They are used for induction and for brief surgical procedures (e.g. incision for drainage of an abscess). A disadvantage of most intravenous agents is the greater difficulty in controlling the degree and depth of anaesthesia. Propofol (Diprivan) can be used as an induction agent as it provides a smooth induction, has few side-effects, and promotes a fast and immediate recovery. New infusion techniques enable propofol to be used as the agent that maintains anaesthesia, with the patient benefiting from a smooth anaesthesia and its antiemetic qualities.

Spinal anaesthetic agents depress motor and autonomic innervation as well as sensory innervation. The patient's blood pressure must be monitored at frequent intervals. A spinal anaesthetic is contraindicated for the patient whose blood pressure is labile or unstable, is in shock or likely to develop it, or has a respiratory problem. Respirations are observed closely for early recognition of the innervation block going to a level that results in impaired function of respiratory muscles. Assisted respiration may be necessary. For administration of a spinal anaesthetic, the patient is placed in a lateral position and the spine arched to increase the intervertebral spaces. The patient is then turned on to the back, and the head of the table is lowered.

The agents used in local anaesthesia are frequently combined with adrenaline (epinephrine), which constricts the blood vessels in the area. This reduces the rate at which the anaesthetic agent is absorbed into the bloodstream and the amount of bleeding in the area. The slower absorption maintains anaesthesia in the area for a longer period and prevents undesirable side-effects from rapid absorption. Local and regional anaesthesia are not

Table 10.1 Examples of commonly used anaesthetic drugs

Method of administration	Agent
General anaesthesia	
Inhalation	Volatile liquids:
	Disflurane
	Halothane (Fluothane)
	Enflurane (Ethrane)
	Isoflurane (Forane)
	Trichloroethylene (Trilene)
	Gas:
	Nitrous oxide
Intravenous	Solutions:
	Thiopental sodium (Intraval)
	Methohexitone sodium
	(Brietal sodium)
	Ketamine (Ketalar)
	Etomidate (Hyponomidate)
	Propofol (Diprivan)
Regional anaesthesia	
Local infiltration	Solutions:
	Lidocaine/lignocaine (Xylocaine)
	Prilocaine (Citanest)
Spinal	Prilocaine (Citanest)
	Cinchocaine (Nupercaine)
	Bupivacaine (Marcain)
	Lidocaine/lignocaine (Xylocaine)
Epidural	Lidocaine/lignocaine (Xylocaine)
	Bupivacaine (Marcain)
Topical or surface	Cocaine
	Lidocaine/lignocaine (Xylocaine)
	Benzocaine
	Tetracaine (amethocaine)
	(Anethaine)

usually used when there is infection in the area, because insertion of the needle tends to spread the infection.

Epidural anaesthetics may be administered over several hours. A special blunt needle is used to guard against passing through the dura mater into the subarachnoid space.

Muscle relaxants

Muscle relaxation is important in many surgical procedures. Deep anaesthesia, sufficient to produce complete muscle relaxation, may place the patient at risk of cardiac and respiratory failure. To facilitate surgery and lessen the amount of anaesthetic required, a muscle relaxant such as suxamethonium, pancuronium or tubocurarine may be given intravenously by the anaesthetist. If a muscle relaxant is given, this is brought to the attention of the nurse in the recovery room; the patient is observed closely for respiratory depression as the muscle relaxant paralyses *all* muscles, including those required for breathing.

Regional anaesthesia

Advantages

Use of regional anaesthetic techniques avoids a general anaesthetic and the associated potential complications. The patient does not lose consciousness and is able to cooperate in his or her care. There is less impact on mental abilities and cognitive functioning. The patient does not suffer from significant respiratory depression and is at less risk of developing pulmonary and embolic complications. The patient is also less likely to suffer the discomforts associated with having general anaesthesia, which can include sore throat, dizziness, and nausea and vomiting. Most patients are able to take control of their self-care soon after the operation has been completed, except in cases of spinal and epidural blocks.

Many regional anaesthetic techniques are quicker and simpler than general anaesthetics. Usually, regional anaesthesia is cheaper in terms of supplies, equipment and time compared with general anaesthesia. The analgesic effects of regional anaesthesia are also beneficial to the patient and, as the effects wear off, oral analgesics can be taken if needed.

Disadvantages

Some patients prefer not to have regional anaesthesia as they would rather not be aware of the potential frightening environment in which surgery occurs. Patients may not feel pain but will often experience other sensations such as pressure and movement. Some patients may have doubts that the regional anaesthetic will be sufficient to eliminate the pain. Many patients may not be able to cooperate with the techniques used in regional anaesthesia, especially patients who are confused, agitated or aggressive.

Regional anaesthesia is not suitable for all surgical procedures. This is usually related to the surgical site, number and volume of injections required and the timescale needed to provide a reliable nerve block. An experienced and competent practitioner is needed to use regional anaesthesia techniques correctly as there is always the possibility of a partial or failed nerve block. Some patients may find the sensations that develop following infiltration of a regional anaesthetic disturbing and disconcerting.

Other disadvantages of regional anaesthesia are related to the potential for complications relating to the actual injection technique, such as haemorrhage, nerve damage and infection (Burden 1993).

Procedure

The sequence of clinical events following injection is:

1. initial loss of autonomic function
2. loss of pain sensation
3. loss of touch and pressure sensation
4. loss of motor function.

Recovery proceeds in the reverse order. Loss of motor function may not always occur.

Duration of action is dependent on the concentration and dose of the regional anaesthetic agent and the rate of diffusion from the injection site to the nerve. This underlines the need to allow sufficient time for the anaesthetic to achieve its action before the starting procedure.

The ideal agent should be (Edwards 1994):

- non-irritant
- quick acting
- non-toxic
- have a duration of action appropriate to procedure
- leave no local after-effects.

Some common regional anaesthetic agents are listed in Table 10.2.

Nursing care

Burden (1993) lists the many considerations surrounding the nursing care of patients receiving regional anaesthesia:

- preparing the patient physically and emotionally
- organizing appropriate equipment

Muscle relaxants
See chapter 2.3

Table 10.2 Common regional anaesthetic agents

| Agent | Concentration | | Onset | Duration of action |
	Topical	Infiltration		
Cocaine	4–20%	NA	Slow	30–45 min
Lidocaine (lignocaine)	1–4%	0.5–2%	Rapid	1–2 h
Prilocaine	NA	0.5–1%	Slow	1–2 h
Bupivacaine	NA	0.25–0.75% (use in epidurals)	Slow	4–8 h

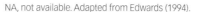

NA, not available. Adapted from Edwards (1994).

- positioning and supporting the patient during the procedure

- assisting with technical aspects of the procedure

- monitoring and evaluating the patient during the procedure

- being aware of potential side-effects of agents used.

The patient must be thoroughly prepared for the procedure, which includes giving information about the impending operation and how the procedure will be carried out and the sensations the patient will experience. The patient should be supported throughout the perioperative period by means of conversation and non-verbal communication. Any discomfort reported by the patient should be acted upon immediately. The nurse needs to be alert to signs of toxicity and allergic reactions. When the procedure is complete, the residual effects of the local anaesthetic will provide immediate analgesia, although further medication may be required in the later postoperative period.

Surgical team

The personnel required for an operation include the anaesthetist, anaesthetic nurse or operating department practitioner (ODA/P), surgical or 'scrub' practitioner(s), circulating nurse, surgeon and surgeon's assistant. The number of personnel required depends upon the surgical procedure being carried out; for example, a radiologist or pathologist may be needed.

The *anaesthetist* assesses the patient's condition and must also check all anaesthetic equipment for efficient function of all components. Having done this, anaesthesia is induced and maintained, and the patient's vital signs are monitored throughout the procedure. If special monitoring devices are to be used, the anaesthetist puts them in place before the sterile drapes are applied and prescribes necessary support during surgery, as indicated (e.g. drug to correct cardiac arrhythmia, intravenous solution).

The *scrub practitioner* performs the sterile nursing activities. These include the following:

- The setting-up and organization of the necessary tables, drapes, instruments, needles, sutures, ligatures, and special equipment appropriate to the particular surgical procedure.

- Assisting with the application of sterile drapes over the patient.

- During the operation, anticipating the necessary supplies (e.g. sutures, instruments) and having them readily available for the surgeon.

- On completion of the main operation and before wound closing, checking instruments and needles

with the circulating nurse to make sure all are accounted for.

- When the wound is closed and area is cleansed of blood, applying the sterile dressing.

- Assisting with transfer of the patient to the trolley.

The *circulating nurse* carries out non-sterile nursing activities, which include:

- Assisting with the preparation and setting-up for the operation.

- Reception of the patient and the checking of the necessary data (see Reception of the patient, p. 172).

- Providing necessary emotional support for the patient.

- Assisting with the safe transfer of the patient to the operating room table, ensuring a minimum of exposure. One arm (the one on the same side as the anaesthetic machine) is usually placed on a padded arm board and a blood pressure cuff applied so it is readily accessible to the anaesthetist.

- Being available to provide necessary equipment, drugs, etc. throughout the operation.

- Positioning of the patient for surgery and exposing the area to be prepared and draped.

- Observing for possible breaks in aseptic technique. This can occur without the personnel carrying out the sterile activities being aware of it.

- Checking needles and other instruments with the scrub nurse.

- Preparing the patient for transfer to the recovery room.

- Accompanying the patient to the recovery room.

- Giving a report of the operation and patient's condition to the recovery room nurse who takes over the care of the patient.

The *anaesthetic nurse* is available to care for the patient before induction of anaesthesia and to assist the anaesthetist as follows:

- Assisting the anaesthetist and anaesthesia induction (e.g. intravenous anaesthetic infusion) and the setting-up of monitoring devices to be used.

- Monitoring of the patient's condition throughout the operation.

- Recording medications and intravenous solutions.

Positions used in surgery

The patient is positioned to:

1. Provide the necessary accessibility and exposure for the operation.

2. Provide safety for the patient and prevent injury.

Figure 10.1 Positions used in surgery: (a) supine, (b) prone, (c) Trendelenburg, (d) reverse Trendelenburg, (e) lithotomy, (f) lateral, (g) hyperextension of the head.

3. Promote normal respiration.

4. Facilitate anaesthesia and efficient monitoring.

The position required will depend on the operation to be performed. The operating room table is designed so that sections of it may be elevated or lowered when necessary. The positions are shown in Figure 10.1 and the patient must be firmly secured for safety reasons in the chosen position. The following are the main positions:

- *Supine position* (Fig. 10.1a).

- *Prone position* (Fig. 10.1b).

- *Trendelenburg position* (Fig. 10.1c). This position is used in low abdominal and pelvic surgery; the intestines move into the upper abdomen in the head-down position, providing accessibility and greater exposure of the operative organs.

- *Reverse Trendelenburg position* (Fig. 10.1d). This position may be used in gallbladder surgery.

- *Lithotomy position* (Fig. 10.1e). This position is used for perineal, vaginal and rectal surgery. On completion of the operation, the legs are lowered slowly to prevent a rush of blood into them, which could cause a sudden fall in blood pressure.

- *Lateral position* (Fig. 10.1f). The patient is turned on to the unaffected side; sand-bags or bed-rolls are used to support the patient and maintain the position. This position may be used in chest or kidney surgery.

- *Hyperextension of the head* (Fig. 10.1g). This is used for thyroid and neck surgery, and may also be necessary for endoscopy (e.g. gastroscopy, bronchoscopy).

Potential patient problems

Table 10.3 lists the potential problems common to patients during operation.

Table 10.3   Potential problems common to the patient during surgery

Problem	Causative factors	Goals
Potential for infection	Surgical interruption of skin integrity	Infection will not occur
Potential for physical injury	Anxiety Altered level of consciousness Loss of sensation Preoperative sedation Anaesthesia Decreased mobility Altered positioning of a body part	The patient will maintain body functioning and prevent injury
Inadequate airway clearance	Endotracheal intubation General anaesthesia	
Gas exchange impaired	Altered level of consciousness Increased respiratory secretion Laryngeal oedema or spasm	The patient will maintain a clear airway and adequate respirations

Infection The patient is at risk of infection because of the surgical interruption to the integrity of the skin.

Physical injury The patient's anxiety, drowsiness from preoperative medication, and then the loss of sensation and consciousness as a result of anaesthesia produce risk of physical injury. The potential causes include:

■ No sides on the trolley.

■ Leaving the patient unattended, which may result in a fall from the trolley or operating table.

■ Malpositioning that produces nerve damage or the occlusion of a blood vessel by prolonged pressure on a part. For example, the ulnar nerve is at risk if the arm is firmly secured to an *unpadded* arm-board; the sciatic nerve may be injured if both lower limbs are not flexed together when placing the patient in the lithotomy position. Prolonged pressure on the veins of the calf of the leg may interfere with venous circulation and cause thrombus formation.

■ Hyperextension in positioning. For example, hyperextension of the arm on the arm-board may injure the shoulder, or hyperextension of the head may injure cervical nerves.

■ Insufficient people available to transfer the patient from the trolley to the table, or vice versa, or to position the patient correctly for surgery.

■ Omission of a conduction pad under the patient when electrical equipment (e.g. diathermy) is being used.

Respiratory problems Endotracheal intubation and irritating inhalation anaesthetics place the patient at risk of respiratory dysfunction. The irritation may cause excessive secretions, laryngeal oedema or spasm, or temporary impairment of the vocal cords with later hoarseness or loss of voice. Not all patients respond similarly to anaesthetic agents, and some agents may depress respirations. If the

patient has spinal anaesthesia, there is the risk of the solution going high enough in the subarachnoid space to suppress innervation of the respiratory muscles.

Nursing intervention

Risk of infection

Measures to prevent **infection** include the following considerations:

■ Knowledgeable and conscientious observance of aseptic technique should be shown by all theatre personnel.

■ Entry of personnel into the operating theatre is restricted.

■ Regulations regarding the clothing to be worn in the operating room to avoid the possible transmission of organisms by street clothes or ward uniforms should be observed.

■ Periodic throat and nose cultures are taken from operating theatre personnel, and those with positive results (especially for staphylococcus) are excluded from the operating theatre.

■ Bedding from the ward is not brought into the theatre.

■ Periodic spot-checking of sterile goods by a bacteriologist should be done to determine sterilization efficiency.

■ A large skin area (appropriate to the particular operation) is cleaned thoroughly. The procedure varies with institutions but cleansing with a surgical detergent solution followed by the application of an antiseptic agent may be the practice. In applying the antiseptic, the pooling of skin preparation solutions between two skin surfaces (e.g. the groin) is avoided because of the risk of irritation and skin damage.

Hospital-acquired infection
See chapter 6.1

- Any break in aseptic technique should be recognized and corrected promptly.

- A sterile dressing is applied securely to the wound on completion of the operation.

- In some institutions a follow-up is made of surgical patients to determine whether they remain free of infection. If infection develops, efforts are made to determine its origin. Potential sources include the operating theatre, instruments and materials used at operation, operating theatre staff and the patient's own skin flora.

Risk of physical injury

Some degree of trauma is inevitable with a surgical procedure but nursing measures should aim to minimize that trauma and prevent unnecessary injuries:

1. The patient should be lifted and positioned very gently, the limbs and head being supported adequately.

2. The covering sheet is tucked in to support the arms and the cot sides are also in place on the trolley during transfer to and from the operating theatre.

3. Similarly, when the patient is on the operating table, the appropriate restraints are necessary. A wide strap may be placed above the knees. A nurse remains with the patient during the induction and early stage of anaesthesia; extra restraint may be necessary because of restlessness. Less restlessness occurs with the rapid induction that is associated with the commonly used intravenous anaesthetic administration.

4. When positioning the patient, precautions are observed to avoid hyperextension or exposing vulnerable areas to excessive pressure and interference with blood flow. For example, having the arm-board padded, correct positioning of the arm and lower limb on the side that the patient is on when in the lateral position, and having two persons available to lift and flex the lower limbs together when placing the patient in the lithotomy position are measures that prevent injuries and complications.

5. In setting up before the operation, if the use of electrical equipment such as that for electrocautery is anticipated, the placement of a conduction pad under the patient is necessary.

Risk of inadequate respiration

The following nursing considerations contribute to the maintenance of respiratory function:

- The patient's record is checked for information that indicates the respiratory status (history, vital signs, blood gas analysis report).

- Anaesthetic equipment is kept in good condition. The anaesthetic machine is tested at frequent intervals by the engineering department; tubes, valves, pressure regulators, flow meters, chemical (soda lime) to absorb carbon dioxide, filters and tubes are checked by engineers as well as by the anaesthetist in preparation for the operation.

- Airways, suction equipment, emergency drugs and an Ambu bag are readily available.

- The patient is received with a calm, reassuring manner and the anaesthetic nurse introduces himself or herself. A quiet, confident patient has a better reaction to anaesthetic than an anxious, fearful and restless patient.

- The patient's respirations are monitored throughout the administration of the anaesthesia and operation. Equipment for taking a specimen for blood gas analysis may be required and should be at hand.

Postoperative management

All surgery has certain common effects that vary in extent and intensity with each particular individual and each specific operation. Surgery produces tissue trauma, pain, psychological reactions and loss of blood. There is an increased possibility of invasion of body tissues by pathogenic organisms through a break in the continuity of the skin or by the introduction of foreign objects into the body. In addition, there are disturbances in body functions which are due directly to the surgical procedure or indirectly to the responses of the autonomic nervous system and the adrenal glands to the associated psychological and physical stresses.

The nurse who is caring for a patient following an operation must possess knowledge and understanding of the implications of the particular operation for the patient, its possible effects on the patient's body functions, and the care and support required to assist in the return to normal with a minimum of discomfort and pain. A constant watch on the patient's clinical progress is necessary. Adverse changes and their possible significance must be recognized promptly and the surgeon alerted. If possible, the nurse who is to care for the patient in the postoperative period will have had an opportunity to become acquainted with the patient and learn something of the condition before the operation. The patient may be more confident with a nurse who is not a complete stranger, and the nurse, knowing something of the patient, is better able to evaluate the patient's reactions and condition.

Preparation to receive the patient

Most hospitals have a recovery room, either within the operating theatre department or adjacent to it, to which the patient is taken on completion of the operation. In a few instances, the patient may be returned directly to the ward unit. The recovery room has several distinct advantages: constant surveillance is provided by a staff experienced in immediate postoperative care and whose attention is undivided; proximity to the operating theatre reduces the distance the patient is transported in this critical period; equipment necessary for emergencies is concentrated in the area and is in immediate readiness; and one nurse may care for two or three patients, a situation that would not be possible on the ward where each patient is in a different location. The patient remains in the recovery room until consciousness is fully regained and vital signs are stabilized.

The patient who has had major surgery or who has developed serious complications may be transferred directly from the operating theatre to an intensive care unit, where the intensive type of care given in the recovery room may be extended for several days. The advantages of such a unit are similar to those of the recovery room, but the latter provides a briefer period of care.

In the surgical unit to which the postoperative patient is to go, certain basic preparations are made to receive the patient. The bed is made up and the top bedding folded to one side to facilitate the transfer of the patient; a draw sheet or transfer sheet may be placed on the bed to facilitate moving and turning of the patient. The bed may have cot sides in place, ready for use in the event that the patient becomes restless and confused during recovery from the anaesthesia.

Basic equipment to be assembled at the bedside includes a sphygmomanometer, stethoscope, thermometer, vomit bowl, tissues, face flannel, recording charts and drip stand. Suction apparatus, a portable emergency respirator (Ambu bag with oxygen) and an emergency tray with cardiac and respiratory drugs, sterile syringes and needles, tourniquet, alcohol swabs, oropharyngeal airway (e.g. a Guedel airway) and endotracheal tubes should be readily available.

Equipment most likely to be needed because of the nature of the operation should also be assembled in readiness for prompt use. For instance, if the patient is having gastric surgery, equipment for gastric suction or aspiration will be necessary.

The bed area is tidied; unnecessary equipment and objects are removed, and the call button is tested to make sure it is in order should assistance be required.

Transfer of the patient from the operating theatre

On completion of the operation, the patient is dried if the skin is moist with perspiration, and a clean gown and sheet are applied. The patient is then lifted, gently and without unnecessary exposure, by a sufficient number of persons to provide adequate support and prevent strain on any part of the body, particularly the operation site. When the bed is used, the patient is placed in the lateral or semiprone position, and the cot sides are raised. If the transfer is to a trolley, the dorsal recumbent position is more likely to be used and cot sides must be raised for safety. Sufficient covers are used to ensure warmth and protection from draughts. The head is extended and an oropharyngeal airway is probably in place to facilitate breathing. If the patient is on his or her back, the lower jaw must be held up and forward to prevent the tongue from obstructing breathing. The anaesthetist and a nurse accompany the patient to the recovery room. Along with immediate treatment orders, the nurse taking over receives a report on what was done, the patient's condition and anything special for which to be alert.

Immediate postoperative care

The discussion presented here deals with general postoperative considerations applicable to most surgical patients. Modifications and additional care related to specific surgery are included in later sections.

The purpose of *nursing intervention* in the immediate postoperative period is to:

1. Assess cardiovascular and respiratory functions, level of consciousness, physical activity, emotional responses, level of pain, if any, and level of comfort.

2. Maintain adequate ventilation.

3. Maintain adequate circulation.

4. Identify and evaluate potential or actual complications and initiate emergency treatment promptly if indicated.

5. Protect the patient from injury.

Assessment

When the patient is received in the recovery room, an immediate check is made of the respirations, pulse, blood pressure, colour of the skin and mucous membranes, condition of the skin (warm or cold, dry or moist) and the level of consciousness. The wound area is examined for bleeding and drainage. If there is a catheter or other type of drainage tube, it is checked for patency. These initial observations and the patient's preoperative vital signs serve as a comparative baseline which assists the nurse later in recognizing favourable and unfavourable changes and in making decisions as to actions. Cardiac arrhythmia, weak pulse, a decrease or fluctuations in the systolic blood pressure, abnormal respiratory rate and volume, and bleeding in the wound area should be reported promptly to the doctor.

The vital signs are recorded every 15 minutes for a minimum of three recordings and observation is made of the patient's colour, skin condition and operative site for any untoward signs; the patient's responses are noted at frequent intervals (Kean 2000).

The fluid intake and output are recorded accurately until normal fluid and food intake and normal urinary elimination have been resumed (Starritt 1999).

Glasgow coma scale
See chapter 22

Blood pressure measurement
See chapter 4.2

Maintenance of adequate ventilation

Inadequate ventilation (*hypoventilation*) is a common problem in the immediate postoperative period for the patient who has had a general anaesthetic, and it may lead to serious respiratory complications. Hypoventilation implies that the volume of air being moved in and out of the **alveoli** (air sacs of the lungs) with each respiration is below normal. It leads to a decrease in the vital capacity and surfactant activity, resulting in a decrease in blood oxygen concentration. Pulmonary secretions increase and, if retained, may obstruct a bronchial tube, resulting in the collapse of a segment of the lung (**atelectasis**). Bronchitis or **pneumonia** may develop, because retained secretions provide an excellent medium for the growth of pathogenic organisms. Postoperative hypoventilation and airway obstruction may result from: (1) central nervous system depression by the anaesthetic agent(s); (2) the depression of respiratory muscle activity by a muscle relaxant; or (3) partial airway obstruction caused by the tongue or lower jaw blocking the pharyngeal area, excessive mucus secretion or laryngeal oedema. Laryngeal oedema may develop if endotracheal intubation was used by the anaesthetist.

Hypoventilation may be recognized by: (1) abnormally slow or shallow respirations; (2) audible moist, gurgling respirations, indicating excessive secretions; (3) wheezing, or 'crowing' respirations (stridor); (4) râles or non-entry of air into an area detected by auscultation; or (5) restlessness, **cyanosis** and rapid pulse rate that are characteristic of hypoxaemia.

Measures to promote adequate ventilation include the following:

1. During unconsciousness, unless contraindicated by the nature of the operation, the patient is placed in a lateral or semiprone position without a pillow under the head. This position lessens the danger of aspiration of mucus and vomit, and of the relaxed tongue and lower jaw 'falling back' to block the pharynx. The head is hyperextended to facilitate free entry of air and expiration. A firm pillow may be placed at the patient's front and back, if necessary, to maintain the desired position. The knees are flexed to reduce strain, and the uppermost limb is flexed to a greater degree than the lower one. The arm that is uppermost is supported on a pillow so that chest expansion is not restricted. If the patient must be kept on the back, an oropharyngeal airway may be necessary during the unconscious period to prevent occlusion of the airway.

2. Excessive secretions may be removed by pharyngeal suction. The suction catheter is in place, the hole is occluded by the thumb, and suction established. The catheter is rotated and withdrawn slowly. If the secretions are beyond pharyngeal suction, tracheal suction may have to be undertaken.

3. Oxygen may be administered as a supportive measure and to prevent hypoxaemia. It may be given by nasal cannulae, nasal catheter or mask (see p. 361). **Oxygen therapy** is usually continued until the patient is conscious and able to take deep breaths on command.

4. If hypoventilation persists, the concentration of blood gases is determined. Mechanical ventilatory assistance may be necessary.

Aspiration of vomit may occur in the unconscious patient. If vomiting occurs, the head should be kept low, turned to the side, and the mouth and pharynx cleared of secretions by suctioning. If aspiration occurs, tracheal suctioning is done to remove the secretions.

Maintenance of adequate circulation

The patient's pulse, **blood pressure** and skin colour are assessed every 5–15 minutes and the surgical area is checked for signs of bleeding. Hypotension, shock, cardiac arrhythmias and haemorrhage are complications that may occur in the immediate postoperative period and during the next few days.

Hypotension results from the anaesthetic agents, reactions to drugs, cardiac arrhythmias, inadequate ventilation, and also from moving the patient. After an operation it is common for the patient's blood pressure to be slightly lower than usual. Systolic pressures below 90 mmHg and pulse rates below 60 or above 110 per minute require prompt intervention.

Shock is a circulatory failure that results in an inadequate perfusion of tissues and organs. This failure at the microcirculatory level reduces the delivery of oxygen and other essentials to a level below that required for normal cellular activities. It may develop during or immediately after operation, or it may develop more slowly and become evident several hours afterwards.

Early manifestations of shock are a decrease in blood pressure, restlessness, inappropriate anxiety, ashen pallor, cold moist skin, rapid weak pulse and decreased pulse pressure. Air hunger becomes apparent as the patient takes rapid, deep respirations. Shock is serious and immediately life threatening; prompt recognition and action are necessary to prevent the condition from becoming irreversible.

Haemorrhage may occur as a result of a slipped ligature, an increase in blood pressure opening up previously collapsed vessels, or the dislodgement of a clot that plugged a severed vessel.

The haemorrhage may become evident externally at the site of operation, or it may be concealed internally and manifested and recognized only by changes in the vital signs and the patient's general appearance and complaints of weakness. Loss of blood causes a fall in blood pressure and hence shock.

The dressing should be checked frequently for signs of bleeding and the body area checked for swelling or

Bronchial tree
See chapter 5.3

Atelectasis
See chapter 5.3

Pneumonia
See chapter 5.3

Cyanosis
See chapter 5.3

Oxygen therapy
See chapter 5.2

Blood pressure measurement
See chapter 4.2

Hypotension
See chapter 4.2

Shock
See chapter 4.2

Haemorrhage
See chapter 4.2

distension. Blood from the incision may run down under the patient and not be apparent on the dressing; it is discovered only by sliding a hand under the patient in the area of the surgery. Any suspicion of haemorrhage must be reported immediately. The dressing should be reinforced and the patient returned to the operating theatre for ligation of the blood vessel(s).

A **cardiac arrhythmia** may develop and is usually caused by the anaesthetic agent or is secondary to cardiac surgery. If the arrhythmia was present before operation, usually no intervention is necessary. However, ventricular arrhythmias may lead to cardiac arrest and require continuous monitoring and immediate intervention. Cardiac arrest, although rare, requires rapid, emergency treatment. A cardiac arrest trolley and emergency drugs are always kept available in the recovery room area. External cardiac massage and artificial respirations with a bag mask device must be initiated immediately. The cardiac arrest is due to failure of the heart muscle to contract, or to ventricular fibrillation. For details of cardiopulmonary resuscitation see Appendix 1.

Protection of the patient from injury

While emerging from anaesthesia, the patient may be restless. Cot sides are used on the bed or trolley to protect the patient. The nurse remains until the patient is conscious and ensures that tubes and essential equipment are not dislodged. The patient is addressed by name and given a simple, direct explanation of where he or she is and what is happening in order to help orientation to the situation as well as reducing fear.

Cardiac arrhythmias
See chapter 4.2

Return of the patient to the surgical unit

When the patient returns to the surgical unit, the nurse from the recovery room provides an assessment of the patient's condition and information about the surgical procedure and postanaesthetic events.

Assessment

The patient is immediately assessed for level of consciousness, pain and discomfort, and vital signs. The dressing is checked for signs of bleeding, and drainage and tubes are observed for patency. Equipment is connected, the cot sides raised and the call button placed within reach of the patient. If the patient is alert and the vital signs are stable, an assessment is made half hourly and then at hourly intervals, and then extended to 2–4-hour intervals over the next 12–14 hours.

Fluid intake and output should be recorded until normal fluid and food intake and normal urinary elimination have been resumed.

The patient is positioned comfortably, maintaining normal body alignment. When a spinal anaesthetic has been given, the bed is kept flat and no pillow is used. This position should be maintained until sensation and motor ability have returned to the lower limbs and the systolic

pressure is over 90 mmHg. The family may visit briefly if they wish.

Treatment

The surgeon's orders for specific treatment are noted immediately. For instance, oxygen, intravenous infusion, appropriate drainage system, special positioning and observations, and drug therapy may be ordered by the surgeon.

Any drainage tubes that are to be connected to an appropriate bottle or a suction system must receive prompt attention as they are usually clamped during transit from the operating theatre. If drainage is not quickly established, the tube may become blocked, or sufficient pressure may be built up within the body cavity to cause serious effects. For example, if a gastrointestinal tube remains clamped following gastric or duodenal surgery, distension may cause a leakage of secretions into the peritoneal cavity and may result in peritonitis.

Evaluation

Criteria for successful care in the immediate postoperative period include the following:

1. The patient is conscious, opens the eyes spontaneously and, in response to speech, makes verbal responses that indicate orientation to time, place and person, and responds appropriately to commands.

2. Blood pressure, pulse, temperature and respirations are stable and within the normal range for the patient.

3. There are no complications or, if there were any, they have abated or are controlled.

Continuing postoperative care

Table 10.4 lists patient problems that might occur after operation.

Nursing interventions during the ensuing postoperative period may be summarized as follows:

1. Promote comfort and control pain.

2. Maintain fluid and electrolyte balance and adequate nutrition.

3. Assist a return to normal patterns of elimination.

4. Encourage increasing levels of activity.

5. Promote wound healing.

6. Maintain ventilation.

7. Maintain circulation.

8. Decrease patient anxiety.

9. Prepare patient for discharge and self-management.

Table 10.4   Potential problems common to the patient after operation

Problem	Causative factors	Goals
Pain	Surgical intervention Nausea and vomiting Abdominal distension Anxiety	The patient will state he or she is free of pain
Dehydration and electrolyte imbalance	Decreased oral intake Fluid loss during surgery via drainage tubes Altered gastrointestinal activity	Minimum fluid intake of 2.4 litres per day Electrolytes within normal limits
Alteration in patterns of elimination	Decreased fluid volume Immobility Pain Surgical intervention Altered sensation	Patient will return to normal pattern of elimination once bowel function returns
Reduced mobility	Pain and discomfort Weakness Immobility	Short term. Patient will sit out of bed within 4–12 h; will not develop complications of immobility (deep vein thrombosis, pressure sores, chest infection); will walk to bathroom within 4–12 h (with assistance)
Potential for infection	Decreased level of consciousness Inadequate airway clearance Decreased sensation Impaired skin integrity Decreased mobility	No infection will occur and wound will heal without complications
Inadequate respiration	Respiratory irritation from anaesthesia Pain and discomfort Decreased mobility	Respiratory rate 12–20 per minute; breathing to be of normal depth and pattern
Inadequate circulation	Effects of anaesthetic Surgical intervention Increased fluid loss Decreased mobility	BP systolic > 90 mmHg; pulse regular, within range 60–90 b.p.m.
Anxiety	Fear of unknown Lack of knowledge Pain and discomfort Diagnosis	The patient is able to talk about concerns and fears
Insufficient knowledge about health care	Lack of knowledge and skill	The patient will verbalize an understanding of the factors involved in improving health after discharge

Promotion of comfort and control of pain

Problems common to many postoperative patients include pain, nausea and vomiting, indigestion pains and apprehension.

Pain

Pain at the operation site is to be expected because of the unavoidable tissue trauma in surgery. Inadequate control of postoperative pain may cause restlessness and contribute to shock and injury to the operation site (Haynes 1999).

Assessment of postoperative **pain** includes data on the nature, duration and location of the pain and the patient's perception of the cause (Sjostrom 1999). Pain is not always incisional in origin; it may result from abdominal distension, a full bladder, decreased circulation due to immobility, pressure or muscle spasms. The most reliable guide to the severity of pain being experienced by the patient is what the patient says. The use of a simple scale from 0 to 5, where the patient rates the pain from 0 (no pain) to 5 (the most severe imaginable) is therefore recommended in assessing pain (see Ch. 7 and Fig. 11.3). The surgeon usually orders an analgesic such as papaveretum, pethidine or buprenorphine to be given every 4 hours if required (p.r.n.) for the first 24–48 hours, or analgesics may be given by continuous infusion, using a pump that allows accurate control of the rate of infusion. The patient should be kept free of pain by the administration of analgesia before the pain becomes severe. The use of patient-controlled analgesia (PCA) delivered by such pumps

Pain
See chapter 2.3

can greatly improve pain control (see Ch. 7). The nurse needs to use judgement, however, in the administration of analgesics, because narcotics tend to depress respiration (Sjostrom 2000). When the pain is adequately controlled the patient tends to relax muscles and participate more effectively in deep breathing and coughing exercises. The use of analgesics is more hazardous in older persons, in patients with some respiratory insufficiency (e.g. chronic bronchitis or emphysema) and in young children.

The patient's position is changed and deep breathing, coughing and necessary treatments are carried out following the drug administration so that the patient may derive maximum benefit. After the first day or two, the dose of the analgesic is usually reduced or a milder drug is substituted.

Prevention of strain on the operation site by good positioning and support with a pillow contributes to the prevention and relief of pain. For instance, a patient with a pendulous abdomen who has had abdominal surgery may suffer less discomfort if the strain on the wound is relieved.

Occasionally a patient may complain of a backache or pain in a shoulder which may have been caused by prolonged immobilization during surgery. Gentle massage may provide relaxation and relief. If the lower limbs are causing discomfort, the patient is encouraged to do a few simple movements such as flexing the toes, feet and legs. Massage is never used, but a change of position and support under the full length of the limbs may be helpful. Massage of the lower limbs is discouraged because of the danger of dislodging a thrombus that may have formed as a result of venous stasis. Relaxation techniques, music, sensory stimulation by massage and guided imagery may also be used to lessen the discomfort (Nendick 2000).

The patient should be encouraged to practise techniques that were taught before operation and to inform the nurse about the type and severity of pain and the effectiveness of interventions. The patient who understands the course of the pain and participates in planning and carrying out pain control measures is usually less apprehensive and more tolerant of the discomfort.

Nausea and vomiting

Surgical patients may experience some **nausea and vomiting** immediately after the operation as a result of the toxic effects of the anaesthetic, pain, anxiety and the handling of viscera in abdominal surgery (Jolley 2000). Assistance is provided by having a kidney dish available, holding the patient's head, providing a mouthwash and wiping the patient's mouth. If the patient is still under the influence of the anaesthetic or drugs, precautions are taken to prevent aspiration by turning the patient's head to the side and if necessary using suction to make sure the vomit is removed from the mouth and pharynx. Oral fluids are usually withheld, and the patient is kept quiet and disturbed as little as possible. An antiemetic drug such as metoclopramide may be administered. Vomit bowls should be emptied promptly and soiled linen changed.

Vomiting that persists beyond 24 hours after the operation should be reported as it may indicate a complication or intolerance to the analgesic being used.

Flatulence and abdominal distension

Patients who have had abdominal surgery may experience some pain and distension which are caused by an accumulation of gas in the gastrointestinal tract. Most of the gas is air that is swallowed during nausea or when the patient is tense and fearful. The depressing effects of anaesthetics and drugs, handling of the intestine during surgery and the lack of food intake in the tract may contribute to a reduction in peristalsis. Distension persists until bowel tone returns and peristalsis resumes. The discomfort may be relieved by the insertion of a rectal tube for a brief period or by an enema. When the distension is high, a nasogastric tube may be passed and suction decompression used (see Ch. 15). If the distension persists, it may indicate a serious complication such as paralytic ileus, bowel obstruction or peritonitis (see Ch. 15). Frequent turning, early ambulation, and normal fluid and food intake are helpful in re-establishing normal peristalsis and preventing distension and gas pains. The patient is usually kept nil by mouth (NBM) until bowel sounds are audible on auscultation, indicating the return of peristalsis.

Mechanical intestinal obstruction, paralytic ileus and peritonitis are serious complications that may develop after abdominal surgery. Nursing care of patients with gastrointestinal complications is discussed in Chapter 15.

Apprehension

The postoperative patient may be apprehensive and concerned about his or her condition; this anxiety is likely to cause restlessness and aggravate discomfort and pain. An explanation of what has taken place and what may be expected may relieve some concern. The patient is also told that the nurse is close by and will be able to help. Having a family member visit or remain quietly by the bedside may be helpful. It may be necessary for the nurse to spend as much time as possible with the patient and to provide repeated explanations and reassurance until the patient regains sufficient confidence and control. If the patient is worried about the findings at operation, it may be helpful to have the surgeon advise as to the condition and the prognosis.

Maintenance of fluid and electrolyte balance and nutrition

A blood transfusion will probably be given during a major operation or immediately afterwards to replace the blood loss or to combat shock if the blood pressure falls below 90 mmHg. Before the transfusion is started, the blood is checked by two persons to be certain that the label bears the patient's name, is the correct blood type and is within the expiry date. The blood bank labels the blood with the

Nausea and vomiting
See chapter 5.1

patient's name and identification number after making sure it is the right type and is compatible. The blood should be used within 30 minutes of being taken from the fridge, and blood warming apparatus should therefore be used if the patient is to have a rapid transfusion of more than 1 unit of blood. The patient is observed for signs or symptoms of untoward reactions such as a chill, fever, dyspnoea, pain in the lumbar region or chest, or a fall in blood pressure.

Symptoms of a reaction are usually manifested during the infusion of the first 50–100 mL of each unit of blood. The rate of flow will depend on the reduction in the patient's vascular volume, blood pressure and cardiac function. It is usually considerably slower in an elderly person.

If a reaction is manifested, the transfusion is stopped and the doctor is notified immediately. In some situations, the blood and equipment are then returned to the blood bank for examination to determine the cause of the reaction.

Oral fluid and food are restricted during the period of nausea and vomiting, and after abdominal operations. Intravenous infusions of electrolyte and glucose and/or saline solutions are given to meet the patient's daily requirements, and to maintain normal **fluid** and electrolyte balance. Frequent rinsing of the mouth and cool, moist compresses laid over the lips will help with the patient's discomfort of thirst.

As soon as fluids are permitted, sips of water are given and gradually increased in amount. The intake is then progressively increased, as can be tolerated, through fluids and soft diet to general diet. The resumption of a normal diet as soon as possible promotes normal gastrointestinal functioning, and the patient is less likely to experience abdominal distension, gas pains and constipation. Normal nutrition also favours wound healing, maintenance of strength and a sense of well-being.

In the case of a patient who has had surgery on the alimentary tract (gastric or intestinal), all oral intake is withheld until peristaltic activity is established. Palpation and auscultation of the abdomen will reveal the return of peristaltic movement, as will passage of flatus and bowel sounds, usually about the second or third day after gastrointestinal surgery.

Electrolyte balance may be assessed by monitoring serum levels and determining the extent and type of fluid loss. Sodium and potassium depletion occurs with blood loss during surgery and through loss of gastrointestinal secretions in vomiting or nasogastric suctioning. Chloride is also depleted with a loss of gastric secretions. Potassium chloride is often added to intravenous solutions administered to the patient after operation.

The postoperative patient may be rather indifferent to food, but can be encouraged to take more by the offering of small amounts of foods for which the patient has indicated a preference. Foods and fluids are often not taken simply because the patient is weak and finds the effort expended in reaching and feeding too exhausting. The necessary assistance should be provided until the patient regains sufficient strength. The amounts of food and fluid taken are recorded until a normal diet is resumed.

Promotion of normal elimination

The patient who is adequately hydrated will usually void within 6–8 hours of operation. The total **urinary output** on the operative day will be less than the fluid intake because of fluid loss during operation and vomiting and fluid retention; fluid retention is due to the increased secretion of antidiuretic hormone that occurs with major surgical trauma and stress. The fluid and electrolyte balance usually returns to normal by 48 hours after operation.

The postoperative patient may have a temporary inability to void because of a depression of the bladder sensitivity to distension; the impulses that produce the desire to void and the reflex emptying are not initiated. The inhibition may be due to the anaesthetic, drugs or trauma in the region of the bladder. The recumbent position, nervous tension and fear of pain may also contribute to urinary retention. The patient may have the desire to void but is unable to do so because of spasm of the external sphincter. When the bladder becomes distended, a small amount may be voided frequently, but the bladder is not emptied; this is referred to as retention with overflow. Restlessness, complaints of pain or a feeling of pressure in the pelvic area, and a palpable fullness above the symphysis pubis are associated with retention.

Distension and stagnation of urine predispose to inflammation and infection of the bladder. If the patient has not voided for 12 hours, close monitoring is instituted and efforts are made to induce voiding. If possible, the patient is assisted out of bed to assume the normal, accustomed position. If the patient is not well enough to be out of bed, a bedpan or a commode by the edge of the bed may be used unless contraindicated. Opening taps to produce the sound of running water or pouring warm water over the vulva of the female patient may be helpful. The male patient may be permitted to stand at the side of the bed to use a urinal. The amount of fluid the patient has had since last voiding should be noted. Catheterization may be ordered if the patient's bladder is distended and retention is prolonged. Strict asepsis and gentleness are necessary in the passing of a catheter to avoid trauma of the mucous membrane and the introduction of infection.

In major abdominal and pelvic surgery, an indwelling catheter may have been passed in theatre and left in place for 2 or 3 days to avoid pressure from a full bladder on the internal operation site. An indwelling catheter may also be used to determine hourly secretion of urine if the patient is in shock or has some renal insufficiency due to disease.

As the bowel is usually empty at the time of operation and food intake is restricted for 2–3 days, bowel elimination is not an immediate postoperative concern. The patient, probably accustomed to a daily bowel movement,

Fluid balance
See chapter 2.6

Micturition
See chapter 5.4

may be worried unless advised that the delay is to be expected and will not be harmful.

If a normal diet is quickly re-established, a laxative or enema may not be necessary. Some doctors order a mild laxative, glycerine suppository or a small enema 2 days after operation. Early ambulation and being allowed to go to the toilet or use a commode help in re-establishing normal **bowel elimination**.

Increase the level of activity

Bed rest and inactivity predispose to problems of flatulence and abdominal distension, retention of urine, loss of strength, joint stiffness, and respiratory and vascular complications. Gastrointestinal peristalsis is sluggish, venous stasis occurs and respirations are shallow.

To minimize these potential difficulties, some activity and frequent change of position are promoted. Venous stasis and the resultant danger of thrombus formation, particularly in the lower limbs, may be prevented by stimulating the circulation with foot and leg exercises. These are usually commenced 8–10 hours after the operation

and done every 2–3 hours until the patient is up and walking. Alternating active flexion and extension of the toes, dorsal and plantar flexion of the feet, and flexion and extension of the legs and thighs are carried out under the direction of the nurse.

If early ambulation is not possible and the surgeon approves, self-care and the following exercises are included as soon as the patient's condition permits:

1. Flexion and extension of the head.

2. Flexion and extension of the fingers, hands, forearms and arms.

3. Abduction, adduction and external rotation of the arms at the shoulders.

4. Contraction of the abdominal muscles.

The purpose of self-care and the exercises are explained to the patient, who may otherwise feel resentful and consider due care is not being offered. The proposed activities stimulate circulation and respiration, and prevent contractures and loss of strength (Fig. 10.2).

Constipation
See chapter 5.1

Figure 10.2   Bed exercises for postoperative patients.

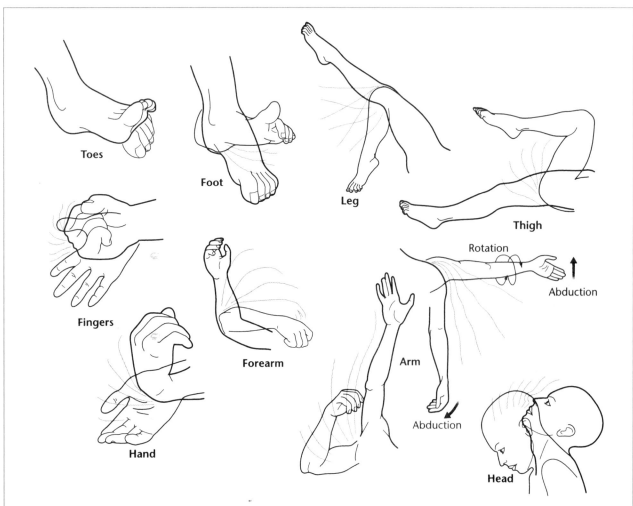

Early ambulation

Within 6–12 hours after major surgery, if the vital signs are stable and the general condition satisfactory, the patient is assisted out of bed and encouraged to walk about. At first the patient may take only a few steps, but movement can be increased progressively as the patient feels stronger and more secure. This early ambulation promotes the return of normal physiological activities such as gastro-intestinal peristalsis, reduces the incidence of respiratory and circulatory complications, prevents the loss of muscle tone and may improve the patient's morale.

The patient is likely to be cautious and weakened the first time out of bed and will need assistance and support. The height of the bed is lowered, and the patient is turned to a lateral position near the edge of the bed with the legs and thighs flexed. The patient is then slowly assisted to the sitting position and the legs are put over the side of the bed. A change in position from supine to sitting or standing may produce postural hypotension. The patient's pulse rate and rhythm and respirations are determined at this point and a check is made for pallor, feelings of dizzi-ness or light-headedness. The patient remains in the sit-ting position until the pulse and respirations stabilize. The erect position may then be assumed, with the nurse available for support if needed.

Equipment such as an intravenous drip stand should not interfere with ambulation. Intravenous bags can be placed on movable stands and pushed by the nurse or patient. When equipment cannot be disconnected, the patient is assisted to walk within the confines of the bed area.

Sitting in a chair may be relaxing and more comfort-able for the patient than lying in bed, but does not replace ambulation and should not be prolonged. When sitting, patients are encouraged to elevate their legs to prevent venous stasis in the lower limbs and lower abdomen.

The patient is encouraged to use a commode or go to the toilet while up, to promote normal bladder and bowel elimination. Precautions against overactivity are neces-sary when the patient is up more frequently for longer periods because the reparative processes are still going on within the body.

Early ambulation is contraindicated or delayed when there is shock, haemorrhage or cardiac insufficiency.

Wound care

The objectives in wound care are for the wound to remain uninfected and heal firmly with a minimum of scar tis-sue. When the edges of a wound are in close apposition, **healing** usually takes place by primary intention. A mild inflammatory reaction with fluid and cellular exudate occurs during the first 24 hours. The patient's temperature is usually slightly raised and the wound edges will be swollen, red and warm. The gap between the incised edges is bridged within 2–3 days as epithelial cells migrate across the wound and help to seal it. During the next 10 days, a collagen network forms and regeneration begins.

The area will be highly vascular and red in appearance and the edges slightly elevated. The supportive network is usu-ally adequate for the sutures to be removed in 5–10 days, unless absorbable sutures have been used for wound clos-ure. The strength of the wound increases over the next few months and the tissue shrinks and becomes pale. With no complications, the scar will have the appearance of a thin white line in about 6 months.

On completion of the operation, the incision is covered with a sterile dressing, which is usually transparent, and the area is inspected frequently during the immediate postoperative period for signs of drainage or bleeding. If the dressing becomes moist with serous drainage, it is reinforced by the application of sterile pads without disturbing the initial dressing. Should bright blood be evident, the doctor is notified promptly. The sutures are removed in 5–10 days, depending on the type of suture, rate of healing, etc. If clips or staples have been used to close the wound, these may be removed slightly earlier.

A drain may have been inserted at the time of surgery to allow the escape of serum or a body fluid such as bile. An accumulation of fluid within the tissues increases pain, delays healing and increases the risk of infection. The tube may pass through the incision or a separate small stab wound. Precautions are necessary when mov-ing or bathing the patient in order to prevent dislodge-ment of the tube and closed drainage system. The drain is usually removed when the surgeon is satisfied that drainage has ceased; this is commonly about 24–48 hours after operation.

Physiology for Nursing Practice Second edition

Wound healing see chapter 6.1

Infection see chapter 6.1

Infection

Infection is manifested by fever, increased pulse rate, general malaise and redness, swelling and tenderness of the wound area. Spontaneous purulent drainage occurs unless the infection is deep, in which case the surgeon may remove a suture and probe the area to facilitate drainage. A swab of the first discharge is taken for culture to determine the causative organism. An antimicrobial drug is administered. Even though the wound is infected, strict aseptic dressing technique is used to prevent the introduction of a secondary infection. When the soiled dressings are removed they are immediately placed in a bag for disposal, and precautions are taken to avoid con-tamination of the bedding and other objects in the envir-onment so that the transmission of infection to others is prevented.

Haematoma

A small amount of bleeding around the wound site will be drained off if a wound drain has been left *in situ*. A collection of blood in the surgical wound may occur, however, and is usually due to impaired blood clotting. Patients receiving anticoagulant therapy or aspirin for a period of time before operation are more at risk of develop-ing a haematoma. The wound edges are elevated and dis-coloured. If the haematoma is small and causing minimal discomfort, it may be left to be absorbed. If the swelling interferes with vital functions, causes discomfort and/or impairs healing, the surgeon evacuates the clot by needle aspiration or reopening the wound.

Dehiscence

Excessive strain on a wound, such as occurs in prolonged abdominal distension or severe coughing, wound infection, malnutrition and general debilitation, may cause separation of the edges of the incision; this separation is called *dehiscence*. Resuturing or the application of adhesive strips (Steri-strips) may be used to pull the edges together.

Evisceration

If there is some separation of all the tissue layers (skin, fascia and peritoneum) in an abdominal wound, protrusion of a loop of intestine on to the surface of the abdomen may occur. This is referred to as *evisceration*. It is usually sudden, and the patient experiences 'something giving way' and a warm sensation on the skin surface due to the escape of peritoneal fluid and viscera. The surgeon should be notified and sterile dressings, moistened with sterile normal saline, are applied to the exposed intestine. If a large portion of the bowel is eviscerated, a sterile towel moistened with the saline will provide better protection. The patient is requested to lie very still, and the head and shoulders and the lower limbs are slightly elevated to reduce the strain on the abdominal wall. Someone remains with the patient to provide reassurance. As the patient will probably be returned to the operating theatre, an anaesthetic and operation consent form is signed after the surgeon has explained what is necessary, and the family is notified. The anaesthetist or surgeon is advised as to when the patient last took food and fluid so that necessary precautions are taken to prevent aspiration.

Maintenance of ventilation

As soon as consciousness is regained, the patient is encouraged to do the deep breathing and coughing exercises that are taught before operation. Sustained, maximal inspirations are carried out several times each hour. The patient is positioned to allow for maximum chest expansion and is coached by the nurse to take a deep breath, hold it for 3–5 seconds and then breathe out slowly. Coughing exercises are carried out with the incision supported by the patient or nurse. A sitting position is best for both activities. The patient's level of pain is assessed before beginning coughing activities, and medication is given to alleviate the pain if indicated. Pain, fear and lack of understanding of the importance of deep breathing and coughing activities interfere with patient compliance. Alleviation of pain, provision of support and coaching of the patient in carrying out the exercises are necessary for effectiveness.

The patient is turned from side to side frequently to allow full expansion of both lungs and the drainage of secretions. Early ambulation is essential to promote respiratory functioning and prevent complications caused by hypoventilation and the retention of secretions.

Respiratory complications

The respiratory complications seen most often after operation are hypoventilation, atelectasis, pneumonia and pulmonary embolism. Whatever the disorder that develops, the common denominator is hypoxia and hypercapnia. An oxygen deficiency affects the entire body. Hypoxia may be manifested by headache, restlessness and irritability, and then apathy, dullness and clouded consciousness. The pulse rate increases and arrhythmias may develop. The respiratory rate increases as the carbon dioxide level rises.

As noted earlier in this chapter, *hypoventilation* occurs frequently in the immediate postoperative period as a result of respiratory centre depression by drugs or the anaesthetic agent. If the patient does not hyperventilate periodically, atelectasis may develop due to decreased vital capacity and surfactant activity.

Obstruction of a bronchial tube by aspirated material or a plug of mucus results in **atelectasis**, the collapse of the portion of the lung distal to the obstruction. If the collapsed area is large, the patient becomes dyspnoeic and cyanosed, the respirations are rapid and shallow, chest expansion is decreased on the affected side and intercostal retraction may be evident. The pulse rate and temperature are raised. On examination there is percussion dullness and an absence of breath sounds in the area. Trapped secretions tend to harbour organisms, leading to infection (pneumonia) in the collapsed area.

A chest radiograph may be ordered to determine the extent of the area involved. Frequent deep breathing, coughing and turning are required. Percussion of the chest by a physiotherapist to dislodge the mucus is done several times daily. Increased fluid intake and humidification of the inspired air are used to promote liquefaction of the secretions so they can be raised more easily. Endotracheal (deep) suction may be used, depending upon the location of the collapsed area and the amount of secretions in the tracheobronchial tree. If the mucous plug cannot be dislodged, bronchoscopic aspiration may be necessary. An antimicrobial preparation is prescribed to combat infection.

Pneumonia may develop independently of atelectasis. Any secretions retained in the alveoli and bronchial tubes readily become infected. The patient usually develops a cough and may complain of chest pain. The temperature, pulse and respirations are increased, and the sputum becomes purulent and streaked with blood.

Prevention of postoperative respiratory complications begins with the preoperative preparation. Recognition of even a very mild respiratory infection is important and should be reported. Unless the operation is an emergency, it is deferred until the infection has cleared up. A good nutritional status contributes to the patient's resistance

Ventilation
See chapter 5.3

Atelectasis
See chapter 5.3

Pneumonia
See chapter 5.3

to infection, and smoking should be discouraged. It is extremely important that the patient's stomach be empty when receiving an anaesthetic, to decrease the danger of aspiration of vomit.

Postoperative nursing measures that contribute to the prevention of respiratory complications include the following:

- Lateral or semiprone positioning of the patient during recovery from general anaesthesia to prevent obstruction of the airway and promote drainage of secretions and vomit.

- Use of suction when necessary to remove secretions from the pharynx and mouth.

- Frequent deep breathing, coughing and change of position.

- Avoiding exposure to persons with a respiratory infection.

- Early ambulation.

- Prompt recognition and reporting of adverse signs and symptoms.

Maintenance of circulation

As soon as consciousness is regained and the vital signs are stable, the patient is encouraged to move about in bed, do limb exercises and begin ambulation. Hypotension may result from sudden changes in position during the immediate postoperative period; a change in position should be made slowly and the patient's responses monitored closely. Physical and emotional support are necessary.

Vascular complications that may develop during the postoperative phase include deep vein thrombosis, thrombophlebitis and embolism.

Deep vein thrombosis and thrombophlebitis

Deep vein thrombosis (DVT) is the formation of a clot in the veins due to a stasis of the blood (see Ch. 14). It develops most often in the lower limbs – hence the importance of early mobilization. Frequent foot and leg exercises play an important role in the prevention of DVT in the bed patient.

The thrombus formation is a 'silent' process; there may be some tenderness in the calf of the leg which is accidentally discovered on pressure, or a positive Homan's sign (pain on stretching of the calf muscle), but there are no evident signs or symptoms. If DVT is suspected or recognized, the patient is placed at rest with the foot of the bed elevated. An anticoagulant (e.g. heparin) is usually prescribed to prevent enlargement of the thrombus. The condition is very dangerous because the clot may be carried along in the bloodstream and eventually may block an artery in the lungs, causing a pulmonary embolism (see below). As a precautionary measure the surgeon may order an elastic compression stocking (such as thrombo-embolic deterrent stockings), which usually remain in place until just before the patient is discharged or resumes a normal level of activity. The nurse removes and reapplies them twice daily to give the necessary skin care.

Thrombophlebitis is due to trauma, infection or chemical irritation of the wall of a vein, initiating a local inflammatory reaction and clot formation. In this instance the clot is fairly firmly attached to the wall of the vein. The condition is quickly recognized because the surrounding tissue becomes oedematous, reddened and painful, and there is an increase in temperature and pulse.

The patient may be kept on bed rest with the affected limb elevated. External heat may help to relieve the pain caused by vasospasm, and an anticoagulant may be ordered to prevent enlargement of the thrombus. The affected limb is handled very gently and is never massaged, in order to avoid dislodging the clot and the possibility of an embolism.

Pulmonary embolism

This is a serious vascular postoperative complication that compromises the individual's gas exchange and the volume of blood returned to the left side of the heart. Embolism involves the transport by the bloodstream of a detached blood clot (thrombus) or mass of 'foreign' material (tissue, fat globules, air) to a site remote from its origin or point of entry into the vascular system. It is most often a thrombus, which eventually lodges in a vessel, obstructing the flow of blood and causing an infarction in the area.

Deep vein thrombosis.
See chapter 4.1

A frequent site of embolism is a pulmonary artery, and the size of the artery occluded determines what happens to the patient. If it is a large pulmonary artery, the patient may experience sudden severe chest pain and respiratory distress and collapse, and die immediately. If a smaller pulmonary artery is blocked, the patient experiences chest pain, dyspnoea, coughing and an increase in temperature, pulse rate and respirations. Blood-streaked mucus may be expectorated. If it is a relatively large infarction, shock develops rapidly. In a few hours an area of dullness may be detected by percussion, and auscultation may reveal an area in which there are no breath sounds, as the alveoli in the infarct gradually collapse. Chest radiography is carried out and the blood pH and gas (oxygen and carbon dioxide) concentrations are determined frequently.

Oxygen is administered and an analgesic such as morphine sulfate may be ordered to relieve the patient's pain and anxiety. An anticoagulant (heparin) is given by intravenous infusion.

Postoperative embolism occurs more often following pelvic surgery, prolonged bed rest, fractures and orthopaedic surgery. It develops more readily in elderly persons and in those with varicosities or a history of a recent leg injury. It is also suggested that women who have been using an oral contraceptive are predisposed to embolism.

Frequent foot and leg exercises and early mobilization are important measures in the prevention of embolism.

Decreasing patient anxiety

Nursing measures to decrease the patient's anxiety should be specific to the individual patient. What does the surgery mean to the patient? How does the patient perceive the postoperative events and activities? What are the implications for the individual in terms of body image, future lifestyle changes, and social and family functioning?

An opportunity should be provided to discuss the patient's concerns and perception of the surgical experience. Immediate and long-term problems are identified and assistance planned. An explanation of what to expect and what is happening at the present time and correction of misconceptions decrease the patient's anxiety and help the development of realistic plans for the future.

When the patient is faced with new and unfamiliar activities, including getting out of bed for the first time or walking with complex equipment attached to the body, the nurse should stay with the patient and provide both physical and emotional support.

Preparation for discharge from hospital

Surgical patients remain in the hospital for a much shorter period now than they did a few years ago. Early ambulation, self-care and early resumption of a normal diet hasten recovery and help to maintain the patient's strength, making a shorter period of hospitalization possible.

As the reparative processes continue, the patient and family receive instructions as to the amount of activity permitted and the necessary rest required. Instructions given will depend on the type of operation but in general patients should be encouraged to take some exercise (e.g. walking) daily and need more rest than usual. The nurse should give explicit advice to each patient, in terms the patient will understand, which should be specific for each patient's needs. 'Activity' and 'rest' mean different things to different people. If dressings or treatments are required, the patient and a family member are taught how these are carried out, or a referral may be made for a district nurse to visit. The doctor may give the patient some idea of when work may be resumed before discharge from hospital, or it may not be decided until the initial follow-up examination.

Evaluation

Criteria for successful postoperative care include the following:

1. The patient is free from pain and discomfort, as shown by verbal expression and participation in physical activities and ability to rest and sleep.
2. The fluid intake and electrolyte concentrations are normal for the patient.
3. The patient is taking a nutritionally balanced diet.
4. Urinary and bowel elimination are re-established and normal for the patient.
5. The patient is ambulatory, active and participating in care.
6. The incision is clean, dry and intact.
7. Vital signs are normal for the patient.
8. No manifestations of complications are present.
9. The patient and family demonstrate an understanding of the required care during convalescence and the resources available.

Day surgery

Day surgery involves admission, surgery and discharge all on the same day and continues to grow in popularity both in the UK and USA. As day surgery increases, attention will have to be given to its impact on community services and the workload of general practitioners and community nurses. Patient satisfaction with day surgery is generally high, but there are concerns about the lack of information and poor postoperative pain relief. Ghosh and Sallam (1994) reported that 73% of day-case patients rated their experience as first class. Some negative comments were reported: these included 10% worried about postoperative pain relief and 8% had concerns about the information given before operation. This study also showed that, while patient contact with the community services and the day surgery unit was minimal in the immediate postoperative period, the most frequent reason for contact was pain control.

Accurate patient information in day surgery is vital if patients are going to go home feeling well and confident. Common concerns amongst day surgery patients focus on how to prevent wound infections, how long to stay off work and how their sex life will be affected and for how long. Written preoperative information to be given to patients should first be tested on a sample group to check it is readily understood.

Day surgery requires different arrangements to conventional surgery, particularly in relation to the use of theatre time, ward occupancy and staffing. Ideally a waiting area close to the theatre should be available so that patients who do not need premedication can walk to the operating room. The postoperative phase requires initial intensive nursing to ensure optimal symptom and pain control. Some hospitals have developed dedicated day surgery units that are self-contained, with their own operating theatre, ward, staff and clinical director. These dedicated units may be purpose built or may be converted from existing ward areas. Stand-alone units are a further alternative to be considered when planning a day surgery service. These units are separate from hospitals and provide all the services for the day surgery patient under one roof.

> **Box 10.2** Patient selection for day surgery
>
> - Patients requiring general anaesthetic should be generally healthy
>
> - Upper age limit is usually 65–70 years
>
> - All patients must be accompanied home and must not drive for 48 hours after general anaesthesia
>
> - Patients should not go home on public transport
>
> - Housing must be adequate for a comfortable recovery
>
> - Patients must have access to an inside toilet
>
> - An adult must be available to provide care overnight and during the day
>
> - Patients should live within a 1-hour car drive from the unit
>
> - Patients should not operate machinery, cook, sign documents or make important decisions for 24 hours after operation.
>
> Adapted from 'Report of the working party on guidelines for day case surgery' revised edition March 1992. Copyright The Royal College of Surgeons of England 1992. Reproduced with permission. A copy of the full guidelines can be obtained by calling +44 (0)20 7405 3473 or sending an email to library@rcseng.ac.uk.

Patient selection is a vital element in ensuring the patient is well enough to go home on the same day. Clinical criteria must be developed to avoid cancellations and overnight stays. The nurse has an important role to play in the assessment of the potential day-case patient (Coll 1999). Day surgery units now use a variety of methods to assess patients, from an assessment by the community nurse to a visit to an assessment clinic in outpatients or the day-case ward. Guidelines for assessment, produced by the Royal College of Surgeons (1992), are given in Box 10.2.

The introduction of the short-acting anaesthetic propofol (Deprivan) is making patients with chronic illnesses eligible for day surgery where in the past they would have been discounted. Propofol allows long procedures to be undertaken on a day-case basis; patients wake up quickly with few hangover effects.

Discharge

Day-case units have developed criteria for discharge and many units have determined that, once these criteria have been met, the nurse can release the patient. Discharge criteria focus on a number of elements that must be fulfilled, or an overnight stay has to be considered:

- Patient must be fully oriented and aware.

- Patient must be mobile and able to ambulate as well as the preoperative level.

- Patient should be able to eat and drink with little nausea and vomiting.

- Patient should be relatively pain-free and have sufficient analgesics for home use.

- Patient must be accompanied by an adult.

- Patient should feel ready to go home.

If patients fail to attain these criteria, an overnight stay is usually required. This can cause a problem in a hospital that has reduced its inpatient capacity and has few empty beds. Common reasons for admissions can usually be defined as either anaesthetic or surgically related. Those that are related to anaesthesia include nausea and vomiting, dizziness and pain. Surgical reasons are usually bleeding or a surgical problem encountered at operation. Community services such as the patient's GP and practice nurse must be notified of the events affecting their patients. If the surgery and recovery from anaesthesia has gone as planned, the GP must be informed as soon as possible, usually by fax or a letter given to the patient, to enable the patient's care in the community to continue smoothly and problem free. If the patient has been admitted for overnight stay or longer, the relatives and GP should be contacted at the earliest opportunity and a full explanation given.

Given the effective working of the multidisciplinary team in the community and the day-case unit, using the new advances in anaesthetics and surgery, day-case provision seems rapidly to be becoming the acceptable method of delivering elective surgery across a wide variety of specialties. Nursing care has to be flexible, safe and consistent. Nurses working in day surgery need to develop excellent communication skills and be able to function in a multidisciplinary team. The nursing profession as a whole has to recognize that day surgery is no longer the backwater it once was and that nursing excellence is developing in the day surgery units of a large number of hospitals.

Summary

Surgery and the effects of anaesthesia constitute major stressors to the person that affect not only physiological, but also psychological and social, functioning. The nurse has a major role in preparing the patient for operation and in ensuring that the recovery from anaesthesia is safe and free from complications. Good preoperative care can greatly reduce potential postoperative problems, and the role of the nurse in ensuring a pain-free recovery is crucial.

References

Burden N (1993) Ambulatory surgical nursing. Philadelphia: WB Saunders.

Dimond B (1990) Legal aspects of nursing. London: Prentice Hall.

Edwards B (1994) Local and regional anaesthesia. Emergency Nurse 2(2): 10–14.

Fyfe ADS (1999) Anxiety and the preoperative patient. British Journal of Theatre Nursing 9(10): 452–454.

Ghosh S, Sallam S (1994) Patient satisfaction and postoperative demands on hospital and community day services after day surgery. British Journal of Surgery 81: 1635–1638.

Haynes C (1999) Emergence delirium: a literature review. British Journal of Theatre Nursing 9(11): 502–510.

Jolley BA (2000) Postoperative nausea and vomiting: a survey of nurses' knowledge. Nursing Standard 14(23): 32–34.

Kanto et al (1990) Preoperative preparation. Nursing Times 86(20): 39–41.

Kean M (2000) A patient temperature audi within a theatre recovery unit. British Journal of Nursing 9(3): 150–156.

Matiti M (1999) Dignity: a study of preoperative patients. Nursing Standard 14(13–15): 32–35.

Royal College of Surgeons (1992) Guidelines for day case surgery. London: Royal College of Surgeons.

Sjostrom B (1999) Strategies in postoperative pain assessment: validation study. Intensive Critical Care Nursing 15(5): 247–258.

Sjostrom B (2000) Strategies used in postoperative pain assessment and their clinical accuracy. Journal of Clinical Nursing 9(1): 111–118.

Starritt T (1999) Patient assessment in recovery. British Journal of Theatre Nursing 9(12): 593–595.

Walsh M, Ford P (1989) Nursing research, rituals and rational action. Oxford: Heinemann.

Williams JR (1999) Preoperative fasting: putting research into practice. Nursing Standard 13(39): 33–35.

Young A (1994) Law and professional conduct in nursing. London: Scutari.

Caring for patients with a specific disorder

Chapter 11   Caring for the patient with cancer   *Cathryn Havard*

Chapter 12   Caring for the patient with a cardiovascular disorder   *Richard Hatchett*

Chapter 13   Caring for the patient with a respiratory disorder   *Alyson Dickson and Graham Martindale*

Chapter 14   Caring for the patient with a haematological disorder   *Miriam Rowswell and Audrey Yandle*

Chapter 15   Caring for the patient with a disorder of the gastrointestinal system   *Teresa Finlay*

Chapter 16   Caring for the patient with a liver, biliary tract or exocrine pancreas disorder   *Sue Lee*

Chapter 17   Caring for the patient with a nutritional disorder   *Sue Lee*

Chapter 18   Caring for the patient with a disorder of the endocrine system   *Mike Walsh*

Chapter 19   Caring for the patient with a disorder of the renal system   *Mike Walsh*

Chapter 20   Caring for the patient with a disorder of the nervous system   *Douglas Allan*

Chapter 21   Caring for the patient with a disorder of the senses   *Mike Walsh*

Chapter 22   Caring for the patient with a disorder of the male reproductive system   *Mike Walsh*

Chapter 23   Caring for the patient with a female reproductive system disorder   *Dolsie Allen*

Chapter 24   Caring for the patient with a disorder of the musculoskeletal system   *Mike Walsh*

Chapter 25   Caring for the patient with a skin or wound care need   *Mark Collier*

Chapter 26   Caring for the patient with substance misuse   *Steve Morgan and Tara O'Neill*

Caring for patients with specific disorders: An introduction

This is the final and largest section of the book and involves a systematic review of the human body and the various problems that can turn a person into a patient. In reading these chapters remember that most of the person's career as a patient takes place outside the hospital, at home with friends and family supported by the primary healthcare team. You should also remember that it is not uncommon for patients to have more than one problem at once, a tendency that increases with age. In using the book, therefore, you will find it helpful to think of patients that you have cared for at any given time. You will also find that you may well have to refer to more than one chapter in this section, and of course refer back to the previous section on clinical principles. Complicated? Yes it is, but that reflects the complexity of clinical practice and a very important skill you will develop in your education is the ability to think of the whole rather than just the component parts. Being able to see the big picture is the hallmark of quality nursing care and is the key skill that helps mark out the unique contribution of the registered nurse to patient care.

Caring for the patient with cancer

Cathryn Havard

Introduction

Prevention and early detection of cancer

Detection and diagnosis of cancer

Treatment of cancer

Nursing assessment and management of disease- and treatment-related problems

Common issues in coping with cancer

Care of the patient with advanced cancer

Rehabilitation

Survivorship

Summary

Introduction

The nature of cancer

Cancer is not only a disease but also a series of experiences that profoundly affect the daily living of both the person who has the cancer and those who share the experience. Cancer is a collective term for many different diseases, each carrying a different prognosis and with a variety of consequences for the individuals concerned. While many are very serious and potentially life threatening, advances in the main treatment modalities of surgery, radiotherapy, chemotherapy and increasingly bone marrow transplantation have resulted in the effective management of clinical manifestations, over variable periods of time. In other cases, the initial treatment effects a permanent cure with no recurrence of the primary disease within an individual lifespan. Increasingly, cancer is understood as a journey (National Cancer Alliance 1996) that people undertake from diagnosis, through varying amounts of treatment aimed to eradicate disease or to provide effective control and symptom management in advanced disease. At all stages of the journey, people need support and care from nurses who are knowledgeable about the causation and prevention of cancer,

therapeutic regimens and supportive care, and the physiological and psychological impact of cancer.

Carcinogenesis

In order to begin to understand cancer, it is necessary to have a thorough knowledge of the normal functioning of the cell and **cell division**. Although there has been an increase in knowledge and understanding of cancer based on recent advances in molecular biology and genetics, the exact cause of many human cancers remains unknown. A number of mechanisms that occur either alone or in combination cause abnormalities in cell growth and multiplication of cells and lead to the development of a cancer. This malignant transformation, or *carcinogenesis*, results broadly from a two-stage process.

The first stage is known as *initiation* or genetic alteration of the cell. This occurs through errors in the replication of **DNA**, leading to errors of various types:

- point mutations involve the deletion, substitution or addition of one or a few bases of DNA (e.g. a codon)

- genomic mutations involve the deletion, substitution or addition of a larger strand of DNA

■ chromosomal mutations involve the same disorders of long segments of DNA.

The majority of cancers arise as a result of these *somatic* disorders but approximately 5–10% are as a result of an inherited predisposition (McKusick 1998).

The second stage of the process, or *progression*, occurs as a result of deregulation of the normal functions of the cell. This is caused by *oncogenes*, mutated forms of protooncogenes which commonly have an important cell regulatory function. Mutated oncogenes can cause excessive cell mutiplication by 'switching on' the cell's own growth cycle. This is often combined with a loss of *tumour suppressor gene* activity, the normal function of which is to inhibit cell proliferation and growth.

Another mechanism that exists to prevent uncontrolled cell division is the process of *apoptosis* or cell death via the protein p53. Disruptions in the gene involved in the p53 may mean that abnormal cells can avoid cell death, and continue to divide and replicate. When the various control mechanisms either alter or fail, abnormal tissue growth occurs.

Controversy has centred around the question of what stimuli induce the transformation in the DNA of a cell necessary to cause cancer. Genetic, environmental, lifestyle and viral factors have all been implicated as components of carcinogenesis (Varmus and Weinberg 1993).

Single gene disorders are known to predispose to cancers of the haematopoietic and lymphoreticular system. Risks among relatives of patients with certain cancers have been shown to be statistically higher than in comparable control families or in the general population (Eeles 1995). The influences of environmental factors have been difficult to separate from a possible genetic aetiological component but, in general, these familial patterns appear to reflect the genetically transmitted susceptibility to neoplasia. For example, a female carrier of the *BRCA1* or the *BRCA2* gene has a 40–85% lifetime expectancy of the development of breast cancer, depending on ethnicity (Ford et al 1998). It is hoped that further research on oncogenes, which have the potential to cause cancer when activated, will provide answers to the aetiology of cancer and lead to more effective preventive, diagnostic and treatment techniques.

An excessive concentration of certain hormones appears to influence the change of some normal cells to malignant ones. Such cancers are said to be *hormone dependent* and manifest changes in growth activity when the concentration of particular hormones is altered. For instance, the ovarian oestrogenic hormones favour the growth of some breast cancers, while androgens (male hormones) tend to suppress their progress. Whether the hormone is the primary incitant in hormone-supported cancer in humans or whether it simply produces a tissue susceptibility to viral, chemical or physical carcinogens is not known.

Causative factors

The development of most cancer diseases is due to or enhanced by some factors in the environment. Certain chemical and physical agents and some viruses are recognized to have a causative or contributory role. Carcinogenic chemical agents include asbestos, vinyl chlorides, aniline dyes and benzene. Many of these have been recognized as a result of the high incidence of cancer associated with occupational exposure to the specific chemical. For example, persons working with an aniline dye, which may be absorbed through the skin and excreted in the urine, show a high incidence of urinary bladder cancer. A causative relationship has also been established between asbestos and lung cancer. Insecticides and herbicides are highly suspect, and animal growth-stimulating hormones and some food additives are being investigated as potential carcinogens.

Cigarette smoking as a cause of cancer of the respiratory tract, and a contributor to cancer of the bladder, has also been well documented. Air pollutants and involuntary or passive smoking are also suspect, especially in relation to lung cancer. Research has indicated that there is usually a relatively long latent period between exposure to chemical carcinogens and the development of cancer.

Diet has also been implicated as a possible factor in tumour induction. To date, epidemiological and animal studies have provided the bulk of available information. High levels of dietary fat, nitrosamines and coffee, and deficiencies of fibre and certain micronutrients (e.g. vitamins A and C, riboflavin and selenium) in the diet, have been associated with the development of cancers in humans (World Cancer Research Fund 1997).

Significant physical carcinogens include excessive exposure to the sun's rays, radiation and chronic irritation. A large proportion of skin cancers are attributed to excessive exposure to the sun's rays. Fair-skinned individuals with less natural pigmentation of the skin, and those whose occupation keeps them outdoors (e.g. farmers), appear to be more susceptible to neoplastic changes in the dermal cells as a result of excessive sun exposure. X-rays and radioactive substances have proved beneficial in the diagnosis and treatment of some diseases, but repeated radiation exposure may lead to malignant neoplasia. The adverse effects may not be seen for a long period after irradiation, as the effects can be cumulative. Repeated exposures to even very low doses may eventually be of pathological significance, hence the importance of radiological protection measures for all staff working in diagnostic radiography departments.

Chronic irritation of an area and repeated tissue destruction and repair are also thought to be contributory factors in the development of cancer.

Scientists have established that various types of RNA and DNA tumour viruses produce some forms of malignant neoplasia in experimental animals. The successful isolation of human viruses in some patients with leukaemia strongly supports the aetiological role of viruses in malignant disease, but the exact viral action in producing cancer is not known. Viruses are suspected in the development of some forms of leukaemia, lymphoma and nasopharyngeal cancer, as well as Hodgkin's lymphoma. Viruses are known to cause warts and mucosal papillomas in humans, and the human papilloma virus has been associated with cancer of the cervix.

Knowledge surrounding the complexity of the immune system and the immune response is of increasing importance in understanding the development and spread of cancer. Considerable attention and support is being given to the concept that the abnormal cells contain substances that are foreign to the host's normal body cells and are therefore antigenic. These antigens prompt an immune response in the host that controls the development, growth and spread of the disease. There is evidence that spontaneous regression and disappearance of cancers have occurred when the host's immune mechanisms have destroyed the cancer cells. If the host's immune response is deficient, the abnormal cells multiply rapidly, invade surrounding tissues and spread to distant areas. It has been observed that there is a higher incidence of cancer in persons with an inadequate immune response, which may be due partly to primary immunodeficiency disease, immunosuppressive drugs, radiation exposure or the ageing process.

The role of the immune system in the development of cancer is not fully understood, yet it is known that cancer 'runs in families' and that some people appear to have a greater prevalence and therefore risk of contracting cancer. Tumour immunity is mediated by a variety of immune mechanisms, including humoral antibodies, T and B lymphocytes, killer (K) lymphoid cells, natural killer (NK) cells (which can act on tumour cells without specific immunization) and macrophages.

Stress and cancer

Prolonged high levels of glucocorticoid secretion reduce the immune and inflammatory responses of the body. Depressed cellular immunity appears to result in impaired surveillance for abnormal cells and thus malignant cells are able to multiply and spread. **Stress** also affects the body's ability to combat infection and affects protein breakdown and synthesis mechanisms.

Investigation of immune factors in cancer continues, with the hope of determining why the patient's defence mechanisms fail and of providing information that aids in cancer prevention, detection and treatment (Gore and Riches 1995).

Differences between benign and malignant growths

Cancer often presents as a lump or *tumour*, which may be palpable or detectable only via a radiograph or scan.

In the vast majority of cases, the lump will be *benign*; new growths (neoplasms) or tumours that are benign are a frequent occurrence. They do not generally pose a threat to life unless in an anatomically difficult position, in which case there may be serious effects on neighbouring structures through obstruction of blood vessels and pressure. The growth of a benign neoplasm is slow and tends to be expansive rather than invasive; the mass remains localized and is frequently encapsulated, and the cells may show little abnormality compared with those of the normal tissue from which they originated. Some benign lesions tend to become malignant if left untreated; examples are polyps in the intestine, papillomas of the bladder and larynx, and pigmented moles. Furthermore, some tissues may display cytological changes of malignancy but without any invasion of other structures (e.g. carcinoma *in situ* of the cervix).

Benign tumours do not spread to other sites and it is usually possible to eradicate all disease by surgical removal of the mass. In contrast, *malignant* tumours or cancers are a distinct threat to life because of their ability to proliferate destructively into surrounding tissue and to other parts of the body.

Table 11.1 summarizes some of the differences between benign and malignant tumours.

Cancer may develop from any type of cell and in any body part or organ. Cancer begins as a *localized* disease, but over a period of time will spread and *invade* surrounding tissues. In the more advanced stages of the disease, cells become detached from the neoplasm and are carried by lymph or blood vessels to other parts of the body, where more cancer develops. Malignant cells may also spread by *implantation* or seeding within a body cavity. The serous fluid in the pleural or peritoneal cavities carries the tumour cells through the cavity. Cells carried in the lymph may be trapped in lymph nodes near the original site, producing disease in the nodes and causing what is known as *regional involvement*. Eventually these areas of disease disseminate cancer cells to other parts; this process is described as *metastasis*. Some tumours, such as basal cell carcinomas and gliomas, rarely metastasize, whereas others, such as melanomas and lung carcinomas, metastasize widely and are less invasive. Specific and predictable patterns of lymphatic and/or haematogenous spread have been identified clinically for many tumours. For example, testicular tumours generally favour the **lymphatics** as an initial route of spread. Once entry into the lymphatic channels has occurred, vascular spread follows: the lungs are the most common distant target organ for this particular tumour.

Many tumours have been observed to have unique patterns of metastasis that may include not only those common target organs but some more unusual sites as well. It was once thought that metatasis was a chaotic random event (Dudjak 1992, Vile 1995). However, it appears that the preferential distribution of metastasis

Stress
See chapter 2.7

Lymphatic system
See chapter 6.2

Table 11.1   Differences between benign and malignant tumours

	Benign	Malignant
Cells	Relatively normal and mature	Little resemblance to normal; poorly differentiated, atypical in size and shape, non-uniform and immature
Growth	Slow and restricted. Non-invasive of surrounding tissue; expansive, pushing aside normal tissue	Usually rapid and unrestricted. Invasive of surrounding tissue
Spread	Remains localized. Usually encapsulated	Metastasizes via blood and lymph streams
Recurrence	Rarely recurs	Frequently recurs
Threat to host	Prognosis favourable. The effect depends on the size and location. May cause pressure on vital organs or obstruct a passageway, which is usually corrected by surgical excision of neoplasm	Threatens life by reason of its local destructive proliferation and formation of secondary neoplasms in other structures. Prognosis more favourable with early diagnosis and treatment, when cells show less departure from the normal and there is no metastasis

Figure 11.1   Incidence of the ten commonest cancers for men in the UK, 1997.

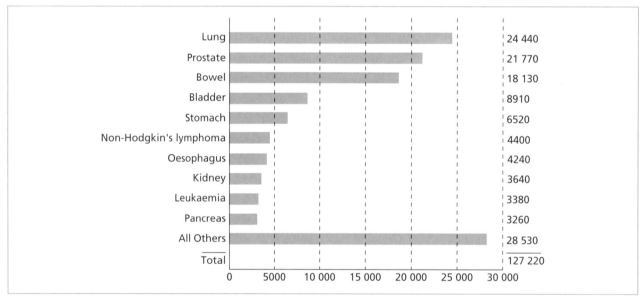

Data from Cancer Research Campaign (2001) with permission from Cancer Research UK.

is not random and is probably related to tumour cell characteristics that promote growth in some organs and not in others. Certain properties on the surfaces of tumour cells are probably responsible for the organ specificity of metastatic cells. In addition, it is thought that, although tumour cells may lodge in the capillary beds of multiple organs, certain microenvironmental characteristics determine whether tumour growth will be supported. Furthermore, as many as 70% of individuals will have *micrometastases* (disease that is not yet detectable at diagnosis) and this has major implications when planning treatment (Davidson and Sacks 1995).

Incidence and trends

It is estimated that 1 in 3 people in the UK will develop cancer during their lifetime. However, it is likely to be later in life as 70% of all new cancers are diagnosed in people aged 60 years or more (Cancer Research Campaign 2001). Cancer accounts for an increasing number of deaths – second only to heart disease in the UK. The factors that contribute to this include:

- a greater number of people living to an older age

- the increased risk of developing certain cancers due to exposure to specific carcinogens (e.g. cigarette smoke, environmental pollutants)

- increased identification through new and improved diagnostic procedures

- a decrease in deaths from acute infectious diseases.

Only a few types of cancer predominate, and details of the ten commonest cancers for men are shown in Figure 11.1 and those for women in Figure 11.2. Cancer *incidence* refers to the number of new cancer cases arising in a

Figure 11.2   Incidence of the ten commonest cancers for women in the UK, 1997.

Cancer	Incidence
Breast	38 000
Bowel	16 180
Lung	14 430
Ovary	6820
Uterus	4850
Stomach	3960
Non-Hodgkin's lymphoma	3910
Bladder	3810
Pancreas	3450
Melanoma	3270
All others	32 720
Total	131 400

Data from Cancer Research Campaign (2001) with permission from Cancer Research UK.

specified period of time. An individual's risk of developing cancer depends on many factors such as smoking, behaviour, diet, occupation and genetic inheritance, and it may be also correlated with the implementation of prevention and early detection programmes.

Cancer *prevalence* refers to the number of people with a history of cancer who are alive at any given time. It is estimated that approximately 1% of the population are alive with a history of cancer, many of whom will be elderly and thus requiring care and support in both hospital and community.

Prevention and early detection of cancer

Some cancers can be prevented by the avoidance of recognized carcinogens and by altering health behaviours. *Primary prevention* of cancer is activity taken to prevent the occurrence or reduce the risk of cancer in healthy persons. Activities in this area of health promotion include identifying risk factors for individuals and groups; counselling regarding risk factor reduction and cancer prevention activities; and implementing cancer prevention programmes (Glasel 1985).

In occupations where carcinogenic substances, such as asbestos, chromium, ether, vinyl chloride and benzene, are used, regulations are necessary to protect employees and communities from carcinogenic hazards. In addition to protective measures for those in a high-risk situation, workers need to develop an understanding of the risks and the precautions that should be observed. They should be aware of early symptoms that must be reported promptly, and receive regular examinations. Some industries may produce and release hazardous substances that could affect many citizens in the community. Governments are becoming more aware of such hazards and are requiring protective measures. Individuals who develop cancer as a result of industrial exposure may be eligible to receive compensation via government compensation schemes.

In recent years, government bodies and cancer societies have instituted intensive campaigns to alert the public to high-risk factors and to behaviour changes that may modify their risk of developing cancer. The European Commission has developed a European Code Against Cancer (Heller et al 1989), and this summarizes ten ways in which to reduce personal risk factors (Box 11.1). In the UK, the National Cancer Plan (Department of Health 2000) identifies both strategies and resources for increasing the rate of prevention and early detection.

Secondary cancer prevention is focused on early diagnosis, of which early detection and screening are the major components. Screening and detection programmes are concentrated on some of the most common cancers, including cancers of the breast, cervix, colon and rectum, prostate, skin and oropharynx. Cancers that are detected early and remain localized are more likely to be treated successfully. Delay in detection and treatment diminishes the chance of cure and survival, because it permits the growing tumour to invade surrounding tissues and metastasize to other areas of the body.

Seven important early symptoms that are stressed in public education are:

1. Unusual bleeding or discharge from any body orifice
2. A lump or thickening in the breast or elsewhere
3. A sore that does not heal
4. A persistent change in bowel or bladder habits
5. A persistent cough or hoarseness

6. Indigestion or difficulty in swallowing

7. An obvious change in a wart or mole.

Awareness of these seven signs, knowledge of the environmental and lifestyle factors that predispose to cancer, and access to community resources for information about cancer prevention and early detection provide opportunities for individuals to utilize screening and other services aimed at early detection. However, the provision of appropriate services and information is not the only factor in ensuring uptake of screening services. McKie (1993a,b) concludes that the beliefs and attitudes of target groups have a significant effect on uptake and that all health promotion strategies should take this into account.

Box 11.1   European Code Against Cancer

Certain cancers may be avoided

1. **Do not smoke**
   Smokers, stop as quickly as possible and do not smoke in the presence of others

2. **Moderate your consumption of alcoholic drinks,**
   i.e. beers, wines or spirits

3. **Avoid excessive exposure to the sun**

4. **Follow health and safety instructions,**
   especially in the working environment concerning production, handling, or use of any substance which may cause cancer

Your general health will benefit from the following two commandments which may also reduce the risks of some cancers:

5. **Frequently eat fresh fruits and vegetables and cereals with a high fibre content**

6. **Avoid becoming overweight**
   and limit your intake of fatty foods

More cancers will be cured if detected early

7. **See a doctor if you notice a lump or observe a change in a mole or abnormal bleeding**

8. **See a doctor if you have persistent problems,**
   such as a persistent cough, a persistent hoarseness, a change in bowel habits or an unexplained weight loss

For women:

9. **Have a cervical smear regularly**

10. **Check your breasts regularly**
    and, if possible, undergo mammography at regular intervals above the age of 50

From Heller et al (1989).

Angiography
See chapter 4.2

CT scan
See chapter 2.2

Detection and diagnosis of cancer

Unless discovered through routine screening procedures, most cancers remain undetected until the patient begins to experience signs and symptoms secondary to the cancer, such as weight loss, bleeding, an unexplained lump, a sore that does not heal, pain or fatigue. A wide variety of diagnostic procedures may be used in determining the presence, type and extent of a cancer. Accurate and speedy diagnosis is essential to ensure an appropriate and effective treatment approach. The impact of a diagnosis of cancer is profound, and reactions to the initial shock may include disbelief, acute distress or downright denial. Northouse (1984a), in a study of patients with breast cancer, discovered that many viewed the period between investigations and starting treatment as being more stressful than actually being on treatment.

The detection and staging of cancers through various imaging techniques has become progressively more refined and of greater diagnostic value with the introduction of new techniques. Common tumour imaging techniques are listed below and are described more fully in Chapter 9:

- plain radiography
- **angiography**
- mammography
- barium studies
- **computed tomography** (CT)
- ultrasonography
- nuclear medicine imaging
- magnetic resonance imaging (MRI).

Biopsy and histological examinations

Progressive refinement of equipment and techniques enables a great deal of information to be gained with minimal invasion, but eventually a sample of tissue is required. A biopsy obtains tissue for histological examination and thereby allows a pathological diagnosis. The confirmation or exclusion of malignancy is the most common indication for biopsy; however, inflammatory and infective tissue may also have characteristic microscopic appearances. When malignant tissue is found, the type of cancer and the degree of differentiation of the cells can be determined. Samples of tissue may be obtained by aspiration (a technique that involves removing a small plug of tissue using a needle and syringe) or by open excision of a section of tissue under local or general anaesthesia. For lesions that are impalpable, biopsies are easily performed under CT or ultrasonographic guidance.

Clonogenic assay involves the growth of human tumour cells on a special culture medium to predict specific chemotherapy for the individual patient. Culture and sensitivity assays of human tumour cell responsiveness to chemotherapeutic agents provides for more effective drug treatment of cancer.

Exfoliative cytological tests involve the microscopic examination of smears of secretion or fluid taken from a body cavity. Cells are shed continuously from the epithelial surface tissue of the body cavities; this process is referred to as exfoliation or desquamation. Neoplastic cells may be detected before there are any other recognizable signs or symptoms, resulting in successful early treatment. Specimens may be taken from the cervix, vagina, respiratory tract, mouth, oesophagus, stomach, urinary tract, prostate, and the pleural and peritoneal cavities.

Endoscopy

By inserting an endoscope into a body passage, the area can be inspected directly and a biopsy obtained. This method of examination may be used in the larynx, bronchus, oesophagus, stomach, colon, sigmoid, rectum and bladder.

Laboratory studies

Some haematological and serological tests are used to refine the diagnosis or to follow the progress of the malignancy. For example, the serum acid phosphatase level is used in investigation for carcinoma of the prostate; it is raised when the disease is present. Blood and plasma cell evaluations are important in diagnosis and assessment of malignant disease of the bone marrow and reticuloendothelial system.

Tumour markers

Tumour markers are substances produced by tumours or by the host in response to the presence of tumour. Tumour markers are useful in staging disease, following response to treatment and predicting recurrent disease. A broad range of tumour markers exists, including antigens, antibodies, genes, enzymes and hormones. Limitations in the clinical usefulness of most tumour markers are the lack of sensitivity and lack of proportionality, i.e. presentations of the marker are irregular or fail to reflect the true tumour burden.

Some of the more useful markers used today are β human chorionic gonadotrophin (β-hCG), the level of which is raised in women with choriocarcinoma and in men with testicular carcinoma. β-hCG is useful in following tumour size and in detecting recurrent disease. Cancer antigen 125 (CA-125) is present in women with ovarian cancer; it is proportional to tumour burden and is used to follow patients with disease and in detecting recurrence.

Once all available information has been obtained, it is possible to classify the cancer and confirm its grade and stage.

Cancer classification: grading and staging

All cancers have certain common characteristics, but there are also marked differences from one type to another because of the type of tissue involved, the location, and the degree to which the cancer cells depart from normal. They also differ as to signs and symptoms, effects on the host, rate of growth and patterns of metastasis, form of treatment used, and the response to treatment.

Cancers are classified according to the type of **tissue** or cells from which they arise. There are four main tissue types; these, and some examples of tumours arising from them, are outlined in Table 11.2. In addition, there are some cancers whose origin is uncertain, and some whose cells bear no resemblance to any normal tissue. These are called anaplastic tumours.

Cancers are *graded*, using a numerical system of three or four grades, with the higher numbers indicating a greater degree of undifferentiation and a more aggressive type of tumour. Internationally recognized classification systems are used to facilitate commonality of approach in diagnosis and treatment. An example of this is the *TNM system* (Hermanek et al 1997) which has been developed

Physiology for Nursing Practice

tissue
see chapter 1.1

Table 11.2 Tumours arising from the four main tissue types

Tissue type	Examples of tumour descriptions
Epithelial	Benign tumours arising from epithelial tissue are known as papillomas. Malignant tumours are named according to the cells of origin, e.g. basal cell carcinomas, cell squamous carcinomas, transitional cell carcinomas, adenocarcinomas
Connective tissue Muscle	All malignant tumours of connective tissue and muscle are called *sarcomas* and then subdivided according to tissue of origin, e.g. rhabdomyosarcoma (striated muscle), leiomyosarcoma (smooth muscle), osteosarcoma (bone)
Lymphoid and haemopoietic tissues	Classification of tumours of the haemopoietic and lymphoid systems is quite complex but includes *leukaemias*, which arise from granular leucocytes or monocytes, and *lymphomas (Hodgkin's or non-Hodgkin's)*, which arise from lymphocytes
Neural tissue	There are two main cell types: nerve cells (neurocytes) and the various supporting cells (neuroglia) Tumours are named according to their tissue of origin, e.g. gliomas, astrocytomas

cooperatively by the International Union Against Cancer (UICC) and the American Joint Committee for Cancer Staging (AJCCS).

Staging refers to the clinical evaluation of the extent of the cancer. The staging system takes account of primary tumour size, local and regional lymph node involvement, and evidence and extent of metastatic deposits. Roman numerals I–IV are used to indicate the stage, with the highest numerals indicating most extensive disease.

Despite an increasingly sophisticated range of techniques to assist the process of diagnosis, there are occasions when it is impossible to detect the primary site or differentiate between a primary or secondary deposit. This period of diagnosis can be extremely stressful and is the beginning of the journey through treatment and, hopefully, to recovery. There is increasing evidence to suggest that people newly diagnosed with cancer have a strong need for information and to be involved in the decision-making process. In a study by Beaver et al (1996), it was identified that the extent of desire for active participation varied considerably, although there was a uniform desire for information. The role of nursing is central at all stages of the journey and involves participation in the delivery of care and monitoring individual responses to treatment.

Treatment of cancer

Once a diagnosis has been made, a combination of treatment approaches is used to maximize the likelihood of cure. The concept of cure in cancer is expressed in terms of 5-year survival from initial diagnosis and treatment. Surgery has been the mainstay of treatment for solid tumours, but increasingly surgery is used in combination with chemotherapy and radiotherapy. It is now known that some tumours are far more sensitive to particular therapies. The developing knowledge around chemotherapy and radiotherapy sensitivities enables the development of treatment protocols that are designed for specific tumours and disease stage in order to achieve maximum effect. All treatments need to balance the likelihood of survival against attendant levels of toxicity, and patients need to be fully informed about treatment choices and likely outcomes. Treatment decisions in physiological terms are made on the basis of:

- tumour location
- growth rate
- metastatic potential
- general physical status.

Increasingly, quality-of-life issues and personal preference form part of the dialogue between the individual and the cancer team (Degner et al 1997, Langenhoff et al 2001). However, there is evidence to suggest that individuals may be strongly in favour of undergoing radical treatment, regardless of side-effects, despite the reservations of healthcare professionals (Slevin et al 1990).

Surgery

The role of surgery in the treatment of cancer includes tissue diagnosis through biopsy; staging of disease; curative treatment through excision, amputation or surgical diversion; palliation; and reconstruction.

Diagnostic procedures

Establishing a tissue diagnosis through biopsy can be done by *incisional* biopsy, where a small portion of tissue is removed and examined, or by *excisional* biopsy, whereby the whole tumour is removed (e.g. full or partial removal of a breast lump, usually under local anaesthesia). *Needle* biopsies use a needle to aspirate fluid or tissue and are easily done under local anaesthesia.

Although advances in imaging and endoscopic procedures have largely precluded the need for it, surgery can be utilized to determine the stage of disease where other diagnostic methods are not satisfactory. A diagnostic laparotomy is the most common example. Surgery may also be used to excise 'bulky' disease, for example residual lymphatic tissues that have been treated by chemotherapy or radiotherapy, to establish that there is no focus of active disease left.

Curative surgery

Surgery is still a definitive treatment for many cancers, particularly solid tumours, and definitive surgery needs to encompass both removal of the tumour mass and a safe margin of tissue around it. Many cancers can be removed and cured by local excision (e.g. skin cancers). Others require more radical block dissections involving not just removal of tumour, but also regional lymph nodes and any other involved contiguous structures. Examples are radical neck dissection, radical mastectomy and radical nephrectomy. Within the abdomen and pelvis, radical excisions may involve diversions of bladder or bowel and creation of stomas. Cancer *in situ* can be treated with cryosurgery, endoscopy or carbon dioxide laser. Increasingly, surgery is used in combination with other treatment modalities, and this may affect the timing and extent of the operation (Davidson and Sacks 1995). For example, wound healing may be a problem if there has been previous radiotherapy, and respiratory function may be affected by certain chemotherapy drugs (e.g. bleomycin), which may effect an individual's suitability for operation.

Prophylactic surgery

Surgery has a limited but important role in preventing the development of cancer, for example removal of the colon and rectum in the case of familial polyposis coli and hereditary non-polyposis colorectal cancer (Church 1996). Rather more controversial is the issue of prophylactic mastectomy for women with a high risk of developing breast cancer due to the inherited *BRCA1* or

BRCA2 gene. Here, the potential efficacy of the operation needs to be balanced against the impact on self-image, sexuality and a variety of psychosocial factors (Hartmann et al 1999).

Ablative surgery may be undertaken to remove hormonal influences on tumour growth through procedures such as oophorectomy, adrenalectomy and orchidectomy.

Palliative surgery is performed to improve the quality of life for the patient, rather than as a curative procedure. Examples of palliative surgery include neurosurgical management of pain (e.g. cordotomy, nerve blocks) (Brant 1995) and pinning of pathological fractures. It may also be used to bypass an obstruction in the bowel, which is a common complication of advanced ovarian cancer, or in the drainage of abscesses and control of local disease (e.g. fungating wounds). Surgery often plays a role in the management of oncological emergencies such as haemorrhage and spinal cord compression.

Reconstructive surgery

In recent years, major advances and improvements have been made in reconstructive surgery. Reconstruction utilizing skin, tissue and bone grafting is now often done simultaneously with the excisional procedure. These advances have dramatically improved the appearance and functioning of patients undergoing head and neck, orthopaedic, and radical abdominal and pelvic operations. Reconstructive breast surgery is an option for women who have had a mastectomy (Neill et al 1998).

Caring for people undergoing surgery

Caring for people undergoing surgical treatment for cancer offers unique challenges and requires understanding of the emotional and psychsocial impact of a cancer diagnosis and the ability to provide high-quality technical supportive care. In the diagnostic phase, people are frequently and understandably anxious, and need opportunities to express their fears. They also require information regarding diagnostic procedures and the possible treatment options should a diagnosis of cancer be confirmed (Degner and Russell 1988).

The person who is receiving definitive treatment may experience radical changes in functioning and/or appearance as a result of surgery. Such treatment may occur very close to the time of diagnosis, when patients are only just beginning to cope with the impact of diagnosis on physical and emotional health. Nursing involvement needs to take account of this and include exploration of reactions and concerns, the provision of information on disease and treatment, and teaching for self-care in relation to postoperative recovery and alterations in functioning. The timing and manner of information given are important factors in developing a therapeutic relationship between nurse and patient. Equally important is comprehensive discharge planning and referral to appropriate resources. Increasingly, people with cancer have access to

a range of clinical nurse specialists with specific expertise, such as breast care nurses, colorectal nurses, and head and neck specialist nurses. Community support groups and voluntary organizations may be helpful in enabling individuals to cope with cancer and lifestyle adaptation. Some people may have specific and ongoing needs for specialist equipment and rehabilitation, for example those who have undergone amputation or stoma formation. With progressively shorter stays in hospital, nursing is playing an increasingly important role in planning and coordinating continuing care in the community, as many cancer treatments move from an inpatient to an outpatient basis. While this may be valued by many people, Fallowfield (1998) notes that, for some women with breast cancer, early discharge may not be so helpful because the woman has to make many physiological and psychological adaptations in relative isolation.

Chemotherapy

Chemotherapy is the use of chemicals (cytoxic agents) in the treatment of cancer. Essentially, these are drugs that work by disrupting cellular replication, either by inhibiting the synthesis of DNA or by otherwise damaging the DNA. Although a more recent development in cancer care, this modality is now well established and is becoming an increasingly prominent treatment.

History and development

During World War II exposure of soldiers to nitrogen mustard gas produced bone marrow hyperplasia and atrophy of the lymph glands. In the next few years nitrogen mustard was developed as a chemical and, when given to patients with lymphoma, resulted in short-term therapeutic responses. These results stimulated further development and testing of chemicals in the treatment of cancer. In the late 1940s nitrogen mustard and methotrexate were the first two drugs recognized as chemotherapeutic agents. Since then, many thousands of chemicals have been tested for antitumour effects; currently there are a few dozen chemotherapeutic agents commonly used in the treatment of cancer.

Role of chemotherapy in the treatment of cancer

Chemotherapy is increasingly being used in combination with other modalities in the treatments of all forms of cancer. As a systemic therapy, it is used primarily for primary or secondary disease that is disseminated throughout the body. However, it may also be used locally, for example the instillation of cytotoxic agents directly into the bladder for the treatment of superficial tumours. For chemosensitive cancers such as Hodgkin's lymphoma, testicular cancer, acute lymphocytic leukaemia in children, Ewing's sarcoma and choriocarcinoma, chemotherapy is a primary and potentially curative mode of treatment and is the *definitive* treatment. When patients have relapsed after being treated with another modality, the term *salvage* chemotherapy is sometimes used to describe the subsequent treatment that will hopefully result in regaining control of disease. *Adjuvant* chemotherapy is the term used when cytoxic drugs are used after removal of the primary tumour to remove any micrometastatic disease, and this is an approach commonly used in the management of breast cancer. *Neoadjuvant* chemotherapy refers to the use of cytotoxic therapy to reduce or 'debulk' the size of a primary tumour to make it more easily resectable.

Patients whose cancers cannot be controlled or cured may benefit from *palliative* chemotherapy, which may be effective in shrinking the tumour mass, thus relieving obstruction or pressure on nerves or the lymphatic system. In this way, pain or other distressing symptoms may be managed and controlled more effectively.

Principles of action and treatment regimens

An understanding of the sequence of phases through which cells must pass as they replicate is fundamental to an understanding of how cytotoxic drugs act and the principles of treatment regimens.

Some drugs are *cell cycle specific*, i.e. they work at specific phases of the **cell cycle**, whereas others work throughout the cell cycle and are therefore *cell cycle non-specific*. Cell cycle-specific agents sustain their major cytotoxic effect during a particular phase of the cell cycle, such as mitosis. Cell cycle-non-specific agents act on resting and dividing cells, making the cells unable to divide or repair damage. Cancer cells that are in the process of reproducing are most likely to be affected, but normal cells are affected too. The effects are most obvious on rapidly dividing cells such as those of hair, mucous membranes and the haemopoietic system. However, normal cells are much more able to recover.

The method and time of action of individual agents has important implications for the combination of drugs used in chemotherapeutic treatment regimens. Drugs may be given as single agents, but they are most often given in combination to maximize the effect on malignant cells. However, the value of any cytotoxic agent may be limited by *tumour resistance*, when there is little or no response to drug therapy.

Classification of chemotherapeutic agents

Cytotoxic drugs may be classified as alkylating agents, antimetabolites, plant alkaloids, antibiotics, hormones, steroids, immune agents or miscellaneous.

The *alkylating agents*, also known as anitmitotic drugs, act within the nucleus of the cell and alter the DNA molecules, resulting in inhibition of cell growth and reproduction. Their activity is not specific to any one stage of the cell cycle, although reproducing cells are more vulnerable.

The *antimetabolites* resemble substances that are essential to cellular activities, and which are therefore taken up by cells. These preparations are sufficiently different from normal metabolites to alter metabolism and inhibit growth and reproduction. They function at a specific phase of the life cycle of the cell.

The *plant alkaloids* currently in use are derived from periwinkle plants. They block cell reproduction during metaphase.

Certain *antibiotics* have been found to be of value in inhibiting some types of neoplastic cells. They act by interfering with DNA and/or RNA synthesis of the cells.

The *hormones* used in the treatment of cancer alter the synthesis of RNA and protein in the tissues that contain steroid-binding receptors. Adrenal corticosteroids are commonly used because they suppress cell reproduction through inhibition of cellular protein synthesis.

Clinical trials

New drugs are introduced frequently, and the search continues for a drug that will be selective and prove toxic to malignant cells without damaging normal tissues. The clinical evaluation of drugs has three clearly defined phases:

- *Phase I*: assessment of maximum tolerated dose, best route of administration and side-effects
- *Phase II*: assessment of the efficacy of treatment in a group of patients with a single tumour type
- *Phase III*: the drug is tested in clinical trials against existing drugs or other forms of treatment.

In all forms of chemotherapy treatment, and especially when drugs are being administered within a clinical trial, informed consent is essential. Patients require sufficient information to make an informed choice and nurses have an obligation to ensure that this is available in a form that is accessible to patients with different information needs.

Administration of chemotherapy

Chemotherapeutic agents may be administered by several routes: oral, topical, intravenous, intramuscular, subcutaneous, intra-arterial, intrathecal and intracavitary.

Preparation, handling and disposal

Rigorous preparation, handling and disposal of chemotherapeutic agents is necessary because of the biohazardous nature of these chemicals. Drugs used in the treatment of cancer are very toxic. The Health and Safety at Work Act 1974 and the Control of Substances Hazardous to Health (COSHH) Guidelines 1988 offer a good general framework for the management and containment of risk. The RCN guidelines (1998) give specific guidance for nurses involved in administration. Specific instructions as to the preparation, handling and disposal of agents should be identified by the nursing and pharmacy departments, and guidelines are prepared by the

Cell cycle
See chapter 1.3

health authority. Current safety guidelines for the preparation of chemotherapeutic agents recommend the use of a laminar airflow hood and protective clothing in order to prevent exposure to the agents of the person preparing the drugs.

Personnel who are administering chemotherapy must also take precautions to prevent self-exposure or environmental contamination. As a minimum, personnel administering chemotherapy wear surgical latex or polyvinyl chloride gloves. All materials used in the preparation and administration of chemotherapeutic agents must be disposed of as biohazardous waste. Following the administration of the prescribed agents, a patient's body fluids will contain metabolic waste products. These should be regarded as potentially hazardous and nurses should employ safe handling techniques when involved in direct patient care.

Intravenous administration of chemotherapeutic agents requires careful selection of the vein because of the need for repeated administration. Many chemotherapeutic agents are extremely irritating to tissue and may cause thrombosis of the vein. Some agents (vesicants) may cause necrosis of tissue if infiltration occurs. Agents classified as irritants will cause irritation in the vein and pain if not diluted sufficiently before adminstration, and if infiltrated into the tissue will cause pain without necrosis (see Table 11.3). The injection site should be observed frequently for signs of redness or swelling and the patient questioned as to pain, tenderness or burning. Prompt identification and management of site infiltration or *extravasation* is important to prevent excessive and unnecessary tissue damage. Extravasation of a vesicant drug is an acute emergency, and treatment includes the administration of specific antidotes for the drug and the application of ice packs to the site to decrease the spread of the drug. Nursing actions taken need to be fully documented and the incident fully recorded and reported (How and Brown 1998).

Intra-arterial administration of chemotherapy is used to deliver chemotherapy directly into an artery that supplies the malignant area. The drug circulates through the affected part in high concentration before it becomes diluted in the general circulation. An arterial catheter is introduced under fluoroscopy. For example, in liver cancer, the organ may be infused with the drug of choice via a small catheter introduced into the hepatic artery. As it is intra-arterial, pressure is required to overcome the arterial blood pressure. Normally, a pump is used to deliver the drug at a prescribed rate. For patients receiving a series of intra-arterial treatments, an arterial port may be surgically implanted rather than introducing a temporary catheter for each treatment.

Intrathecal administration may be given where there are tumour cells in the central nervous system (CNS). Chemotherapy given by other routes is not usually able to cross the blood–brain barrier, and therefore tumour cells present in the CNS are unaffected by the drug. Presence of tumour cells in the CNS is documented by examination of spinal fluid. Intrathecal therapy may also be given prophylactically to patients with leukaemia who are at high risk for development of CNS disease. This type of therapy may be given either by lumbar puncture or through a ventricular reservoir called an Ommaya reservoir, which is surgically implanted in the right frontal region of the skull.

Intracavitary administration of chemotherapeutic agents is usually done following aspiration of fluid from a body compartment such as the intrapleural space or the peritoneal cavity. Patients who develop malignant pleural effusions may have chemotherapy instilled in the pleural cavity through a thoracotomy tube. The resulting sclerotic changes in the lining of the pleural cavity may prevent the reaccumulation of fluid in the pleural space. Intraperitoneal chemotherapy allows direct contact of the drugs with the tumour in the peritoneal cavity. Direct delivery of the chemotherapy to tumour cells maximizes the effect of the chemotherapy while minimizing the systemic side-effects of the drugs. Intraperitoneal chemotherapy is most commonly used in the treatment of ovarian cancer.

Devices for the administration of chemotherapy

For patients receiving long-term or repeated courses of chemotherapy, a right arterial catheter may be inserted through the chest wall and into a large vein. A portion of the catheter remains outside the body and the exit site is covered with an occlusive dressing. The greater blood volume in the large vein and the right atrium dilutes the medication, and thus decreases irritation to the vessel walls. The risk of extravasation into tissue is decreased and the peripheral veins are preserved. A right atrial catheter such as a Hickman catheter allows for greater patient mobility as it can be left in indefinitely and sealed with a cap between treatments. These may be single, double or triple lumen, and are either open or closed (e.g. Groshong type with a slit valve), and thus venous access is assured for both chemotherapy, intravenous fluids and medications, as well as blood products. Patency of the line is maintained by flushing with a dilute solution of heparin on a daily basis when the catheter is capped off.

Peripherally inserted central catheters (PICCs) are inserted via the antecubital fossa and threaded through the veins of the upper arm until the tip rests in the superior vena cava. PICCs do not require a surgical procedure for insertion, and increasingly this procedure is carried out by experienced nurses (Gabriel 1996). PICCs are ideal for short-term venous access but, as with other central venous devices, they do require the patient and/or carers to take on much of the maintenance of the device themselves. Richardson (1992) noted that patients valued being able to care for themselves whilst undergoing

Table 11.3 Chemotherapeutic agents: side-effects and toxicities

Chemotherapeutic agent	Side-effects					Toxicities											
	Bone marrow depression	Nausea and vomiting	Mucositis	Diarrhoea	Alopecia	Dermatological	Hepatic	Cardiac	Pulmonary	Renal	Haemorrhagic cystitis	Neurotoxic	Ototoxic	Reproductive	Irritant	Vesicant	
Alkylating agents																	
Cyclophosphamide	+++	++	+		++	+			+		+			+			IADH
Busulfan	+++	++	+		+				+					+			Addisonian-like syndrome
Melphalan	+++	++	+		++				+					+			
Chlorambucil	+++	++			+				+					+			
Cisplatin	+	+++			+					+		+	+	+			Anaphylaxis-like reaction
Dacarbazine	+++	+++	++	+	+		+							+	+		Flu-like syndrome starting 7 days after treatment
Mechlorethamine	+++	+++	+	++			+							+		+	Tinnitus, thrombophlebitis
Thiotepa	++	++			++	+								+	+		
Ifosfamide	+++	+++			++					+	+	+		+			
Antimetabolites																	
Cytosine arabinoside	+++	++	++	+	++	+						+		+			Conjunctivitis
5-Fluorouracil	+++	+++	+++	+++	++	+		+				+		+			Fever
6-Mercaptopurine	++	++	+	+	+	+	+							+			
Methotrexate	+++	++	+++	+++	+	+	+		+	+		+		+			Photosensitivity
6-Tioguanine	+++	+	+++	+++	+	+	+					+		+			

						Other
Nitrosureas						
BCNU	+++	+++	+	+++	+	Facial flushing
CCNU	+++	+++	++	+++	+	
Streptozocin	++	+++	+	++	+	Glucose intolerance
Antibiotics						
Actinomycin D	+++	+++	+++	+++	++	Fever, anaphylaxis
Bleomycin	+	++	+	++	+++	Red urine
Daunorubicin	+++	++	++	+++	++	Red urine; flare reaction at site of injection
Doxorubicin	+++	+++	+++	+++	+++	Red urine; flare reaction at site of injection
Epirubicin	+++	++	+	+++	++	Red urine; flare reaction at site of injection
Mithramycin	+++	+++	++	++	++	
Mitomycin C	++	++	+	++		
Plant alkaloids						
Vinblastine	+++	+	+	++	+	
Vincristine	+	+	+	++	+	IADH
Vindesine	+++	++	++	+++	++	Fever, malaise
VP-16	++	++	+	++	+	Hypotension, allergic reactions
Miscellaneous						
L-Asparaginase	+	+	+	+	+	Pancreatitis, anaphylaxis
Hydroxyurea	+++	++	+	++	++	
Procarbazine	+++	+++	++	+	+	
Mitozantrone	+++	++	+	++	+	

+ + +, Major toxicity, dose limiting; + +, less frequent or less severe; +, rarely causes or mild. IADH, increased secretion of antidiuretic hormone.

treatment, and clearly this would need to be with appropriate guidance and support.

An alternative to central venous catheters is the more recent introduction of totally implanted central venous ports. These ports are implanted under the subcutaneous tissue and the catheter attached to the port is inserted into a central vien. Access to the port is established by inserting a needle through the skin down into the port. As with the external catheters, patency is maintained by flushing with heparin before the needle is removed from the port. Ports require flushing only once a month. Implanted ports are advantageous to patients as much less self-care is required. There is no need for a dressing and there is no interference in activities of daily living as a result of having a port. Although not widely used, implanted ports are also available for implantation in the small veins of the forearm.

Ambulatory chemotherapy

The development of a range of venous access devices and more effective agents and regimens for managing side-effects has enabled many more people to receive chemotherapy at home (Dougherty et al 1998). For many patients, this may foster independence and a greater sense of control, but for others the absence of immediate access to clinical staff may be anxiety provoking. Careful consideration needs to be given to the patient's individual circumstances and needs, and a good learning programme established. Caring for people who are receiving chemotherapy, regardless of the setting, requires a high level of technical skill and knowledge, and understanding of psychosocial and pysiological responses to disease and treatments.

Side-effects and toxicities

Because chemotherapy has a systemic action, it affects the growth and division of both cancer cells and normal cells. Consequently, a wide variety of generalized side-effects and toxicities is associated with chemotherapeutic agents. As the side-effects vary with different drugs, it is essential that the nurse knows the chemotherapeutic agent given, the possible side-effects of that particular drug, their significance, how they are manifested (see Table 11.3). Treatment regimens and dosages are carefully calculated based on the nature, size and extent of the tumour and the age, general health and height : weight ratio of the individual.

The side-effects that are most commonly experienced by patients receiving chemotherapy include:

- bone marrow depression, leading to leucopenia, thrombocytopenia and **anaemia**

- mucositis

- **nausea and vomiting**

- **diarrhoea and constipation**

Anaemia
See chapter 4.1

Nausea and vomiting
See chapter 5.1

Diarrhoea and constipation
See chapter 5.1

- hair loss (alopecia)

- fatigue.

A more detailed discussion of these, along with appropriate nursing interventions, can be found on pages 221–227.

Second primary malignancy

A rare long-term complication of cancer chemotherapy is the development of a second primary malignancy, most commonly acute non-lymphocytic leukaemia (Fraser and Tucker 1988). This has been documented in relation to patients treated with chemotherapy for multiple myeloma, ovarian cancer and Hodgkin's disease. Combination treatment with chemotherapy and radiotherapy may also influence this process, although the exact mechanism is not fully understood. Treatment regimens are under continuous review to maximize the antitumour effect and minimize exposure to treatments that may induce a second cancer.

Radiotherapy

Radiotherapy is the controlled use of ionizing radiation, which damages cellular DNA and thus causes cell death. Radiotherapy for cancer began shortly after the discovery of X-rays at the turn of the century. Unfortunately, in the early era of radiotherapy, it was a rather crude treatment as little was known or understood about the effects of radiation on tissues or therapeutic doses. As a result, the outcome was often fatal due to over-radiation, with recurrence from under-radiation occurring at the other extreme.

Since that time, research has greatly expanded the knowledge and development of radiation as an effective treatment modality for cancer. Today, radiotherapy is precisely calculated to deliver the correct dose to the area treated, while sparing the surrounding normal tissues. However, as Eardley (1986) stated, fears and misunderstandings are known to be common and therefore an important aspect of care is to provide accurate information about treatment while encouraging the expression of any anxieties or concerns.

Radiotherapy is one of the three most commonly used cancer treatment modalities, with over 50% of people having radiotherapy as some part of their treatment.

The aim of radiotherapy may be *curative*, as in treatments for skin cancer, carcinoma of the cervix or Hodgkin's disease. For other lesions, cure or eradication is not possible, and *control* of the cancer for periods ranging from months to years may be the aim. Recurrent breast cancer, some soft tissue sarcomas and lung cancer are examples of cancer controlled by radiotherapy in combination with surgery or chemotherapy. *Palliation* may be another goal of radiotherapy. Relief of pain, ulceration or bleeding, prevention of pathological fractures, and return of mobility can be achieved with radiation to metastatic lesions from a variety of tumours including breast, lung and prostate tumours. Palliative radiotherapy is also given for the relief of CNS symptoms caused by brain metastasis or spinal cord compression. Haemorrhage, ulceration and fungating lesions can be reduced effectively, and in some cases eliminated, by palliative radiotherapy. It may also be used to prevent the emergence of potentially symptomatic lesions before they become a problem. Examples include the treatment of a mediastinal mass that threatens to produce superior vena cava obstruction, and treatment of a vertebral lesion when spinal cord compression is impending.

The type, duration and method of delivery of radiotherapy depends upon many factors and is tailored to individual requirements. Curative regimens may continue over many weeks and be very exhausting for the patient, whereas doses given for palliation may be very low and are sometimes delivered in a single treatment.

Principles of action

Radiation is given in the form of X-rays, gamma rays or electrons. When a radiation beam strikes an atom, it frees electrons from that atom – a process known as *ionization*. This process requires energy, and this comes from the radiation beam or *source*. Energy is thus transferred to the newly released electrons which then interact with neighbouring atoms and cause further ionizations, until all energy is dissipated. It is this ionization that accounts for the biological and chemical changes resulting from radiotherapy treatments.

Cellular function is disrupted first by damage to the DNA so that the cell is unable to repair itself, and secondly through the formation of free radicals which disrupt the chromosome structure. The radiation affects both cancer and normal cells, but the normal cells are more able to recover. Withers (1992) describes the cellular response to radiation, which may be summarized as the four Rs:

- *Repair* – some cells are able to repair themselves, but not all

- *Redistribution* – resting cells re-enter the cell cycle

- *Repopulation* – cells move into spaces and become less hypoxic

- *Reoxygenation* – as the total cell population becomes depleted, those that are left have more space, become better oxygenated and are therefore more susceptible to radiation.

This response forms the basis of radiotherapy treatments that are planned to give the maximum dose to the tumour with minimal effects on normal tissues. The radiation dose is defined as the amount of energy absorbed per unit mass of tissue and is measured in Gray (Gy). The total treatment dose is delivered in *fractions*: the small,

sublethal damage that occurs after each fraction allows normal cells to be repaired before the next fraction of treatment.

There is considerable variablity in the degree of radiosensitivity of different tissues, with eyes, lungs, ovaries and testes being very sensitive and others, such as bone, connective tissue, liver, thyroid and thyroid, less so. The least radiosensitive tissues are those that are composed of cells that do not reproduce, such as brain, spinal cord and muscle.

A number of chemical and thermal modifiers of radiation are currently being studied in clinical trials. Developments in such approaches could make many tumours that are now considered radioresistant amenable to control with radiotherapy (Noll 1990, Wotjas 1990). Similarly, a great deal of activity is being directed towards devising effective protocols that combine radiotherapy and chemotherapy followed by surgery, which then may be more conservative, for example in patients with advanced head and neck cancer (Urba et al 1994).

Methods of administration

The ionizing beams used in radiotherapy are either electrically produced or come from naturally occurring or manufactured radioisotopes. The use of external-beam irradiation is often referred to as *teletherapy*, and the accuracy of tumour dose is achieved by the use of two or more radiation fields.

Treatment planning is a meticulous and often lengthy affair, using a *simulator* machine and frequently CT or MRI to enhance the accuracy of planned tumour dose. When the final plans have been made, it is important that the same dose is delivered at each treatment. This is achieved by the positioning of the treatment source with reference to body contours and ensuring that this is consistent at each treatment. The treatment area is usually marked on the skin and the person needs to remain completely still during the actual treatment. When sensitive structures are adjacent to the treatment area, it may be necessary to immobilize the individual and thus the treatment area further by use of moulds, plaster casts, etc. This may be a particularly traumatic aspect of the planning and subsequent treatment period, and probably beyond most people's previous knowledge and experience. Careful preparation and exploration of individual fears or concerns is vital at all stages, with continual review and reassessment once treatment has started.

External-beam radiotherapy is delivered via a series of fractionated doses and the conventional fractionation is in 2-Gy treatment doses. This is usually delivered 5 days per week over a 4–6-week period, depending on the total dose required. However, there is some research evidence to suggest that some tumours have the opportunity to grow whilst treatment is being delivered. For this reason there is increasing interest in *continuous hyperfractionated accelerated radiotherapy* (CHART), which uses two or three treatment fractions in a day over a shorter period of time overall (e.g. 2–3 weeks). Clinical effectiveness has yet to be fully demonstrated in prospective randomized trials, but early results appear promising (Souhami and Tobias 1995). Hall (1995) emphasizes the importance of patient education and understanding of potential side-effects in enabling patients to tolerate such treatment regimens.

Another form of treatment involves the use of *sealed* radioactive sources which are placed close to a tumour; this is called *brachytherapy*. In this case, a high dose is received by the tumour and less by the surrounding tissues. Sources can be implanted directly into small tumours, such as those in the tongue, lip or breast, or placed in body cavities via the use of applicators as in treatments for cervical and uterine cancers. Some radioisotopes or *unsealed* sources may be administered orally or parenterally, for example iodine-131 for the treatment of thyroid tumours and strontium-89 for multiple bony metastases.

Radiation safety principles

All hospitals and other institutions that use X-ray equipment and other radioactive sources operate within national guidelines and local policies for radiation protection. Hospitals that have extensive equipment and facilities for radiotherapy treatment will have a medical physics department and radiation protection team who are responsible for the maintenance and storage of equipment and radioactive sources. There will also be a radiation protection service which, amongst other activities, monitors the amount of radiation to which nurses and other workers are exposed. Personnel are provided with monitoring badges which measure the amount of radiation exposure. The dose received is calculated at regular intervals, with records kept of the cumulative dose. The badge itself provides no protection at all; it simply measures exposure. In order to ensure accurate reading, the badge should be worn only by the designated individual, kept within the working environment and changed at the designated time.

When caring for people using an internal source of radiation, all precautions need to be taken to reduce exposure to radiation. Three principles are important in taking adequate radiation precautions:

■ *Time* – spend as little time as possible near the source

■ *Distance* – keep as far away as possible from the source

■ *Shielding* – protect self and the environment.

The principle of *shielding* is more readily employed in the handling of displaced radioactive sources, excreta collection and disposal, and disposal of linen, dressings and equipment contaminated with radioactive solutions. Because shielding from gamma radiation requires 6-mm thick lead or 10-cm thick concrete, it is usually impractical to expect that much physical care can be given from behind such a shield. The lead aprons used in diagnostic radiology are not of sufficient thickness to stop gamma

rays and cannot protect the caregiver from exposure when caring for individuals with radium or caesium sources. For example, in the rooms of patients with encapsulated sources there should be a special container into which the sources can be placed if they become dislodged. If a source does dislodge, nurses must use 12-inch forceps and not the hands to place it in the container provided. Contaminated linen, equipment, dressings and excreta are usually a safety hazard only when metabolized radiation therapy is employed (e.g. iodine-131). The decontamination of these items is necessary before disposal or reuse.

Hospitals that offer brachytherapy treatments should have specially designed facilities that offer a high degree of protection to staff and where patients can stay for the duration of treatment. The extent of safety precautions that are necessary during use of internal sources is dictated by the energy of the isotope. The medical physics team will calculate the maximum amount of time that individual nurses can safely spend in contact with the patient. This needs to be clearly documented and displayed via appropriate notices and signs. Necessary treatments and care should be well planned and expedited to minimize the time spent at the bedside, while still providing for the person's needs.

Effects of radiation on body tissues and organ systems

Several specific components determine the effect of radiation on tissues: the *dose*, the fractionation, time and volume, and the area treated. Dose–time–volume interrelationships are as follows: (1) the greater the dose, the shorter the time of onset of any reaction; and (2) the larger the treatment area, the more potentially severe the reaction.

Except for those systemic effects that are described on pages 211–212, radiation side-effects are seen only in the tissues and organ systems that are within or immediately adjacent to the treatment field. Thus, an individual receiving treatment to the mediastinum will not develop radiation-induced diarrhoea, nor will an individual receiving treatment to an abdominal field lose scalp hair. Similarly, individuals undergoing brachytherapy will develop reactions to treatment that vary with the site, dose, volume and energy of the source. Side-effects from radiation will vary from individual to individual and therefore careful monitoring and an individualized plan of care needs to be developed and implemented.

Both the immediate, or *acute*, effects of treatment and the *late* effects must be considered in any discussion of the effect of radiation on tissues. In general, acute effects are seen within the first 6 months after treatment and are due to cell damage in which mitotic activity is altered in some way. If acute effects are not reversible, late or permanent tissue changes occur. These late effects can be attributed to the organism's attempt to heal or repair the damage caused by the radiation. These may be quite debilitating and cause a great deal of distress, such as brachial plexus damage following treatment for breast cancer (Ash 1999).

General side-effects of radiotherapy

The skin

The outer layer of **skin** (epidermis) is composed of several layers of cells, with mature non-dividing cells at the surface and immature dividing cells at the base. Normal mature cells are constantly being shed from the skin surface and replaced by new cells from the basal layer. This continuous state of reproductive activity accounts for the high radiosensitivity of skin. Although the skin may be the primary site of radiation (as in skin cancer), it is also irradiated when any other site within the body is treated because radiation must pass through whatever tissues it encounters before reaching the target site. To assess pathophysiological changes and plan care accordingly, it is helpful to think in terms of cross-sectional anatomy. The entry point for external radiation is known as the *portal*. The radiation then passes through all tissues and organs encompassed in the treatment volume, and *exits* on the opposite side of the body.

Acute radiation reactions begin after a dose of 4–5 Gy. Erythema, which acts and feels like sunburn, can occur within hours or up to 1 week after the first treatment, depending on the daily dose and type of machine used. Depending on the equipment used, skin at the exit portal may also be affected. Erythema usually reaches its peak of severity near the completion of treatment.

Radiation skin reactions are caused by the inflammatory response that results from the breakdown of basal cells in the epidermis. *Erythema* may be the only manifestation, or the skin reaction may progress to dry and then moist desquamation. A *dry desquamation* is characterized by drying and scaling of the skin, whereas *wet desquamation* is characterized by a weeping of the skin. This reaction is due to the upper layers of the skin having been shed, leaving the derma exposed. Healing may be slow, but is usually complete and leaves minimal evidence of the acute damage except for the changes in pigmentation. Fibrosis and atrophy may occur after high doses, as may ulceration and necrosis, although such changes are uncommon with modern equipment and techniques.

It is important to note that skin in certain areas, such as the groin, gluteal fold, axilla and under the breasts, usually exhibits a greater and often earlier reaction to radiation owing to the natural warmth, moistness and friction in these areas. An inappropriate term for this type of reaction is a radiation 'burn', as this term implies accidental or unexpected damage, neither of which should take place in a controlled therapeutic setting.

Hair

Radiation affects all rapidly growing cells; the hair roots are no exception. **Hair**, after receiving threshold doses, becomes loose and may be pulled out painlessly or fall out spontaneously. Generally this occurs during treatment or shortly thereafter; regrowth generally occurs in 2–3 months. Hair loss may be permanent if high doses of radiation are given to the area. The loss of hair is traumatic to most people regardless of whether they are prepared for this change in body image. The needless fear of this loss is equally traumatic, and if patients are receiving treatments to areas that do not include the scalp they should be reassured that hair loss will not occur as a result of treatment.

Haematopoietic system

Bone marrow and lymphoid tissues are highly radiosensitive. The greatest effect is on the stem cells, while mature non-dividing blood cells in the circulating bloodstream are relatively insensitive to radiation. When large areas of bone marrow in the adult are irradiated, including the ilia, vertebrae, ribs, skull, long bones and sternum, the number of circulating mature red blood cells, white blood cells and platelets decreases because production is suppressed. This reaction is more severe if previous or concomitant chemotherapy has been given. It is sometimes necessary to interrupt treatment for a few days to allow the bone marrow to recover.

Gastrointestinal system

The gastrointestinal tract, from mouth to rectum, is lined with mucous membrane that contains layers of cells. A large proportion of these cells are undifferentiated and mitotic, and are thus extremely sensitive to radiation. Oral mucous membrane may develop mucositis, usually after 2–3 weeks of fractionated radiation therapy. The mucous membrane will initially have increased redness, which will progress to yellowish-white patches. These patches will eventually become a pseudomembrane covering large areas of the **mucosa**. Salivary function is altered, and the patient may experience soreness, pain on swallowing, hoarseness, dryness, or changes in the sense of taste. If the oesophagus, stomach or bowel are within the irradiated field, the patient may experience **nausea**, **vomiting** or **diarrhoea**. When the oesophagus is within the field, painful swallowing, dryness and spasms may occur. Abdominal irradiation is frequently associated with nausea, with greater exposures causing vomiting, abdominal cramping and diarrhoea. These can lead to electrolyte imbalances, dehydration and weight loss. If the anal sphincter is in the field of radiation, the distressing symptom of *tenesmus* (painful ineffectual straining) also sometimes occurs.

Respiratory system

Acute radiation pneumonitis may be asymptomatic or cause a hacking cough or mild chest discomfort. With moderate levels of radiation, acute changes such as shortness of breath may subside after 3–4 weeks. Large doses (75% of lung tissue exposed to 20 Gy or more) will often

Skin
See chapter 6.1

Hair
See chapter 6.1

Haematopoietic
system
See chapter 4.1

Mucosa
See chapter 5.1

Nausea and vomiting
See chapter 5.1

Diarrhoea
See chapter 5.1

cause permanent damage, with the degree of disability related to the amount and condition of remaining untreated lung tissue.

Reproductive system

The germinal cells of the **testes** are very sensitive to even small doses of radiation. Small doses will cause temporary halting of sperm production; 5–10 Gy will probably cause permanent sterility. The secretion of testosterone is not affected, thus sexual characteristics are unchanged.

Radiation to the **ovaries** produces either temporary or permanent sterility, depending on the age of the person being treated and the dose of radiation. Permanent sterilization will occur at doses of 6–12 Gy, and older women are sterilized at lower doses than younger women. In addition to sterility, hormonal changes (especially loss of oestrogen production) and early menopause may occur.

Systemic effects

Generalized symptoms that commonly appear during radiation treatment are fatigue, weakness, headache, nausea and anorexia. These symptoms are more frequently discussed in the nursing literature than the medical literature, and their aetiology is not well understood. One suggested cause of generalized symptoms is the rapid breakdown of cells destroyed by radiation. Cell breakdown would release toxic metabolites and endproducts, which accumulate faster than they can be excreted. These chemicals may act as toxic foreign proteins, causing some degree of shock. Others suggest that these symptoms result from an increased metabolic rate, from the body's attempt to restore homeostasis, or from the emotional stresses of daily treatment for a life-threatening illness.

Late effects

These complications may appear several months to a few years after the completion of treatment. Most late complications reflect diminished vascular supply and increased fibrosis in heavily irradiated areas. Unlike acute reactions, these complications are often chronic, and nursing management is symptomatic and based on the degree of functional impairment. The late complications of radiation therapy are summarized in Box 11.2.

Caring for people receiving external radiation therapy

During a course of radiation therapy, certain treatment-related side-effects can be expected to develop, most of which are site specific as well as dependent on volume, dose fractionation, total dose and individual differences. Many symptoms do not develop until approximately 10–14 days after the start of treatment, and some do not subside until 2 weeks or more after treatment has ended. Patients need to be assessed regularly while on treatment. In particular, the skin over the area receiving radiation as well as the exit portal needs to be examined

Testes
See chapter 6.3

Ovaries
See chapter 6.3

Box 11.2   Late effects of radiation therapy

Skin

- Fibrosis, atrophy and pigmentation changes over irradiated areas; telangiectasia
- Acute recall reaction may occur after the administration of certain antineoplastic drugs such as dactinomycin

Gastrointestinal system

- Oral fibrosis, decreased taste acuity or the loss of taste sensation, xerostomia, dental caries, chronic enteritis, intestinal fistula formation

Lung

- Radiation pneumonitis (acute or chronic)

Blood and bone marrow

- Anaemia
- Leukaemia

Eyes

- Cataracts

Thyroid

- Hypothyroidism
- Thyroid cancer

Reproductive system

- Temporary or permanent sterility
- Premature menopause in women
- Fertility may return to normal depending on the dose of irradiation administered to the gametes and age

Urinary system (bladder)

- Reduced capacity
- Chronic bleeding

Central nervous system

- Transient or widespread demyelination

---

regularly, and discussions held about fatigue, weakness and nutritional problems.

The care management described in the following sections reflects the general consensus from the literature and the current evidence base for practice. A particularly useful text for further reading is the *The Royal Marsden Manual of Clinical Nursing Procedures* (Mallet and Dougherty 2000). Specific approaches and treatments may vary from institution to institution, and between different medical practitioners.

Skin reactions

Because moisture may enhance skin reactions, the person being treated should be advised to keep the skin in the treated areas as dry as possible. Bathing or showering is permissible, but long periods of soaking are inadvisable. Treated skin should be bathed gently with tepid water and gently patted (not rubbed) dry. Lines or markings placed on the skin to guide treatment should not be removed until the radiographer advises the patient to do so. It may therefore be necessary to wash carefully rather than have a bath or shower, to avoid washing off the markings. Although protocols vary (Campbell and Lane 1996) general guidelines to follow for care of the skin within the treatment site include:

1. Keep the skin dry.

2. Avoid using soaps, powders, lotions, creams, alcohol and deodorants on skin over the treatment area. (As well as being an irritant, many such preparations contain metallic elements that may cause scattering of radiation beams.)

3. Wear loose-fitting cotton clothing next to the treatment area.

4. Do not apply tape to the treatment site if dressings are applied.

5. Shave with an electric razor only. Do not use preshaves or aftershaves.

6. Protect the skin from exposure to direct sunlight, chlorinated pools and temperature extremes (avoid cold packs, hot-water bottles or heating pads).

Such precautions are necessary throughout the course of treatment and until any skin reaction has disappeared afterwards.

Specific measures that are useful in treating skin reactions include the use of a light dusting of cornflour for pruritus from erythema and dry desquamation. If moist desquamation and denuded areas appear, a thin layer of an appropriate topical agent (e.g. hydrocortisone cream) may be applied, followed by a non-stick dressing to protect the clothing and skin. The radiation oncologist or oncology clinical nurse specialist should always be consulted regarding general skin care measures or those appropriate to the individual experiencing a skin reaction. Outpatients should be given explicit directions for managing at home; written directions are very helpful in addition to the verbal instructions.

It should also be remembered that individuals are often treated by parallel opposing portals and that only one of these portals may be marked to indicate the field. This means that, in addition to the clearly marked portal on the person's abdomen or chest (for example), there may be a corresponding field on the posterior that needs the same careful attention.

Care of the hair and scalp while receiving radiation to the scalp includes very gentle brushing and combing and infrequent shampooing. Some centres request that patients do not shampoo at all, whereas others suggest a once a week cleaning. Permanent waves or hair colouring are contraindicated because of the potential harm to the irradiated skin of the scalp. Individuals being treated in the neck and facial areas should also avoid any procedures on the hair that involve the use of harsh chemicals because such substances may run down on to treated skin. As with irradiated skin in general, the scalp should be treated with care and caution for several months to a year or more after all healing has taken place. The top of the head, forehead, ears and neck may exhibit sensitivity to the sun and need to be protected from sunburn with a cap or wide-brimmed hat.

Bone marrow depression

When large volumes of active bone marrow are irradiated (especially the pelvis or spine in the adult), the effect on the marrow can be quite significant. Other areas of concern when large fields are treated include the sternum, ribs, long bones and skull. During simulation and treatment planning, provision is made for shielding as much of this active marrow as possible without compromising the treatment; thus the majority of people receiving therapy are able to tolerate a course of treatment without experiencing bone marrow depression. None the less, complete blood cell counts need to be done at regular intervals for all individuals receiving radiation therapy. Particular attention should be paid to this when individuals are receiving concomitant chemotherapy or have had extensive chemotherapy before irradiation. The nursing management of bone marrow depression is outlined in Box 11.6 (p. 222).

Mucositis and xerostomia

Mucositis is an alteration in the mucous membranes of the oral cavity that manifests as inflammation, desquamation and overt ulceration. The mucous membranes of the oral cavity sustain a great degree of trauma on a daily basis. The cells of these tissues must be highly proliferative to replace those that are continually damaged by thermal, mechanical, chemical and microbiological stressors. Radiation has the greatest effect on cells that have a rapid rate of cell division. Because cells are damaged and cell replication is disrupted due to the effect of radiation, there is an inadequate supply of new cells to maintain the integrity of the oral mucosa, and signs and symptoms of mucositis appear. Factors such as poor nutritional status, poor oral hygiene, or any other factor that causes dryness and/or trauma of the mucous membranes, increase the severity and the duration of mucositis.

Xerostomia (dry mouth) may result from radiation to the salivary glands or portions of them. Xerostomia results in difficulty talking, eating and swallowing, and can be very distressing (Feber 1995).

Radiation caries

Although it is a potential late effect of irradiation to the mouth and oropharynx, radiation caries can be greatly reduced or avoided by proper care before, during and after a course of treatment. Absence of or a decrease in saliva and the altered pH produced by treatment promote tooth decay. Before the start of therapy, a thorough dental examination and prophylaxis should be carried out. If extensive decay and general poor dentition exist, full mouth extraction is usually the treatment of choice. However, if teeth are in good repair, a vigorous preventive programme should be initiated to protect them from the late effects of radiation. This would include brushing the teeth with a soft-bristled brush several times a day, and a daily application of fluoride gel.

Oesophagitis and dysphagia

When the oesophagus is located in the treatment field, inflammation and ulceration of the mucous membranes may occur. This condition produces difficulty in swallowing as well as a great deal of discomfort, which patients experience as a severe and constant pain located in the substernal area.

Nausea and vomiting

Nausea and
vomiting
See chapter 5.1

Diarrhoea
See chapter 5.1

Of the potential side-effects from radiation therapy, nausea and vomiting are probably the most distressing to the person being treated. Although **nausea and vomiting** are not common, the fear that they will occur causes great stress in many individuals. As with other side-effects, treatment site and dose are the variables to be considered, along with pre-existing conditions related to chemotherapy and sites of disease. The patient's emotional state and apprehension about the disease and treatment are sometimes responsible for nausea when treatment is unlikely to be the cause. Generally, the person receiving radiation therapy can be expected to experience some degree of nausea when treatment is directed to any of the following: abdomen, large pelvic fields, whole brain irradiation. However, the majority of patients experience little or no difficulty with this side-effect. When nausea does occur, it can usually be controlled by antiemetics administered on a regular schedule and by adjusting the eating pattern so that treatment is given when the stomach is relatively empty. Delaying intake of a full meal until 3–4 hours after treatment is also helpful because nausea, if it occurs, will usually appear 1–3 hours after treatment.

Diarrhoea

Diarrhoea, like nausea and vomiting, is not an expected side-effect in most individuals receiving radiation therapy. However, it does occur if areas of the abdomen and pelvis are treated after about 20 Gy have been given. Some individuals experience only an increase in their usual number of bowel movements, whereas others develop loose, watery stools and intestinal cramping. For most individuals with radiation-induced diarrhoea, a low-residue diet (e.g. starchy foods, white bread, bananas or apples, and avoiding caffeine, whole grains, high fibre, most fruits and juices, and fried, spicy or pickled meats) and perhaps a prescription of loperamide hydrochloride are usually sufficient.

Anorexia

Anorexia occurs frequently among individuals receiving radiation therapy, regardless of the treatment site. Like fatigue, anorexia is probably related to the presence in the person's system of the waste products of tissue destruction. Other possible causes for anorexia include anaemia, inactivity, medications, alterations in the person's ability to ingest and digest foods, and psychological factors. The cause often cannot be identified clearly, and therefore the symptom must be treated by utilizing all the techniques known to encourage adequate intake. A self-perpetuating cycle of anorexia, weight loss, weakness, inactivity and more anorexia may develop if the symptom is untreated. Fluid intake should be encouraged to promote elimination of the products of tissue breakdown.

Fatigue

Fatigue or malaise is common among most individuals during the course of radiotherapy and for varying periods after treatment is completed. More detailed information on the nursing assessment and management of fatigue in the individual with cancer is outlined in Box 11.11 (p. 227).

Tenesmus, cystitis, urethritis

Although infrequent, tenesmus, cystitis and urethritis do occur in some individuals receiving pelvic irradiation. Tenesmus of the anal or urinary sphincter produces a persistent sensation of the need to evacuate the bowel or bladder. Relief can sometimes be obtained from gastrointestinal and urinary antispasmodic and anticholinergic agents. The problem may persist, however, until after the course of treatment has ended. Cystitis and urethritis resulting from radiation to the bladder areas are distressing to the person being treated. A clean voided urine specimen for culture and sensitivity should be obtained and appropriate antibiotic therapy instituted if indicated. Usually, infection is not found and treatment consists of urinary antispasmodics for symptomatic relief. A high fluid intake is encouraged.

Caring for people receiving internal radiation

As patients who are receiving internal radiation therapy need to maintain a high level of self-care and sustain isolation for a period of time, a careful and detailed explanation of the treatment and subsequent care is required. They need to know what they will experience when the radiation source is applied or administered, and any restrictions on physical activities need to be explained and planned for. Box 11.3 outlines the points to be considered

Box 11.3 Preparation and information for patients receiving internal radiation

Preparation for internal radiation needs to include the following elements.

General

- Ensure that patient demonstrates knowledge and understanding before treatment
- Explain why nurse can spend only limited time with patient
- Use booklets, audiovisuals, demonstrations with instruments and models if appropriate
- Reassure concerning fears of radiation
- Stress importance of adhering to safety regulations and regulations governing visiting time and proximity to patient
- Explain guidelines for visitors to patient and family (local policies will dictate arrangements for specific treatments)
- Visitors should check at nursing station before entering the room
- No visitors under 12 years of age
- No pregnant visitors
- Visitors are restricted to a 30-minute period each day
- Visitors should sit at the end of the bed to decrease their exposure to the radiation.

Removal of the applicator or source

- Explain to patient that there is usually little or no discomfort associated with removal
- Radioactive material is removed first and placed in a portable lead safe
- There may be a noticeable odour from gynaecological packing when it is removed. Explain that this is always expected but will not persist
- Inform patient that they may feel weak or dizzy if they have been required to lie flat for several days, as is the case with some gynaecological treatments, and may require assistance with mobilization.

Other points

- Description of the procedure for inserting applicators and sources
- Possible change in appearance
- Anticipated pain or discomfort and measures available for relief

- Potential short-term and long-term side-effects and complications specifically related to the procedure
- Strategies for coping with the possible isolation and boredom that are sometimes the most difficult part of treatment with radioactive source by planning for suitable activities such as reading, listening to music, handicrafts, television, video, etc.
- Radiation precautions observed by hospital personnel:
  — reassure patient that personal care needs will be met but that the nurses' time at the bedside and in the room will be restricted because of the presence of the radioactive sources
  — discuss strategies for self-care and provide appropriate resources.

in preparing and informing individuals who are to receive internal radiation.

Patients who have internal sources of radiation are usually very sensitive to the fact that they can cause harm to others. This causes an increase in anxiety, especially as they have no way of detecting that this harm is occurring. They are also anxious about the harm the radiation is doing to their own normal tissues. This anxiety may be allayed by explaining the controls designed to protect others and also clarifying and reinforcing information about treatments and side-effects. It is also important for patients to know that they are no longer radioactive when the source has been removed.

Family members also often have a difficult time during internal radiation because of the enforced separation. Again, increased information and support may be helpful in allaying concerns and fears. Some family members may find it difficult to contemplate exposure to radiation despite explanations of radiation protection measures, in which case telephone communication can be encouraged. Box 11.4 outlines the general nursing measures for the care of patients receiving brachytherapy.

Bone marrow transplantation

Conventional treatment of cancer consists of the use of surgery, chemotherapy and/or radiation therapy to eradicate all tumour cells. Doses of chemotherapy and/or radiation therapy are often limited because of toxicity to the patient's bone marrow. Many believe that, if bone marrow toxicity could somehow be minimized, chemotherapeutic doses could be increased to levels that would cure the patient of the malignancy. If the patient's own marrow or that of a compatible donor could be

Box 11.4 General nursing care measures for the patient receiving internal radiation

Pain

- Assess for type of pain, intensity and location

- Use special mattresses to promote comfort and minimize skin lesions

- Administer analgesics as required and monitor effectiveness

- Plan pain management strategies incorporating psychological, cultural and spiritual factors that may influence pain

- Ensure that patients who have difficulty sleeping because of pain or position required by implants obtain sleep medications

- Minimize dysphagia and mucositis through the use of soft or liquid diet, pain medications or topical anaesthetic as ordered, and careful oral hygiene after removal of head and neck implant

- Explore non-pharmaceutical approaches to pain management and isolation (e.g. relaxation and guided imagery).

Nausea and vomiting

- Prevent nausea and vomiting wherever possible by use of antiemetics, administered regularly if required, and appropriate diet

- If vomiting occurs, monitor head and neck patients for dislodgement of radiation sources or aspiration of vomit; monitor patients with cervical or uterine implants for dislodgement.

Psychological issues

- Provide support and comfort as much as possible within restrictions of radiation safety precautions

- Avoid showing fear of radiation; avoid making patient feel 'untouchable'

- Make time spent with patient quality time and focus complete attention on patient in this period

- Encourage open communication and exploration of fears of altered body image, loss of sexual function, and provide specific information about actual and potential sexual problems

- Explore any specific anxieties and concerns related to current treatment and fears for the future, fear of death, etc

- Consider referral to clinical nurse specialist, social worker, psychologist or minister of religion, as indicated.

Dislodgement

- Patients with gynaecological implants need to remain in bed for the duration of the treatment

- Prevent bowel movements during implant (gynaecological only) by ensuring clean bowel before procedure and providing a low-residue diet and antidiarrhoeal agents. Ensure patient is not constipated prior to return home (laxative may be needed)

- Implement care measures and treatment to avoid vomiting, constipation or diarrhoea

- If dislodgement occurs, notify radiation safety officer immediately; follow radiation safety procedures.

Long-term complications (fibrosis, stricture, adhesions, dyspareunia, etc.)

- Head and neck implant: provide saliva substitute and encourage consumption of fluids before eating. Gradually advance diet from liquid to soft to solid foods. Explore issues related to body image and personal and social roles

- Gynaecological implant: explore issues of sexuality and provide information about resuming sexual activities, and practical advice regarding use of a vaginal dilator, creams and lubricants.

Bone marrow transplantation
See chapter 4.1

introduced into the body and successfully engrafted, then doses far higher than those used conventionally might become possible. This is the rationale for **bone marrow transplantation** (BMT), which has evolved over the past 30 years from an experimental procedure to an established and effective treatment for selected patients. These would usually be people with acute lymphoblastic leukaemia and acute and chronic myeloid leukaemias. However, in the past decade the number of recipients of marrow transplantation has increased and BMT is now being used as a treatment for an expanding list of malignant and non-malignant haematological diseases. It is also used in the treatment of metabolic disorders such as Batten's disease.

There are three sources of donor bone marrow:

1. *Autologous* – patient's own

2. *Syngeneic* – from an identical twin

3. *Allogeneic* – usually from a sibling but occasionally from an unrelated, but tissue-type-identical, donor.

In the latter case and, as with any other organ transplant, histocompatibility testing must be carried out using human leucocyte antigen (HLA) typing and the mixed lymphocyte culture (MLC).

Once a source of marrow has been identified, the recipient is prepared for the transplant which involves:

- a thorough physiological and psychosocial assessment

- insertion of a central venous catheter to maintain venous access

- a conditioning regimen to achieve total immunosuppression using high-dose chemotherapy and total body irradiation

- bone marrow harvest.

The actual infusion of the marrow itself is similar to a blood transfusion and takes place over 2–3 hours. To the patient, this may seem like quite an anticlimactic event compared with the intense pretransplant procedures.

After infusion of the marrow, there follows the period of *engraftment* when the patient's bone marrow is recolonized by the new, healthy, stem cells. Until this occurs, the patient has no marrow function and is therefore at great risk from infection in general and a whole range of side-effects, including stomatitis, bleeding, and hepatic, cardiac, renal, neurological and psychological complications. A particularly dangerous complication is graft-versus-host disease (GVHD), which occurs when immunologically competent T lymphocytes are introduced into a host who is immunologically incompetent and therefore incapable of rejecting this foreign invasion. The donor T lymphocytes mount an attack against various host cells causing various degrees of damage, especially to epithelial tissues (Caudell 1991).

A more recent development is the use of peripheral blood stem cell transplants (PBSCTs). This type of transplant involves stimulating an individual's circulating peripheral stem cells in one of several ways, such as the administration of a chemotherapeutic agent or cytokines. The collection of the stem cells is then managed through apheresis. The advantages of this method of transplant include more rapid haematological recovery from treatment, reduced cost due to being able to achieve collection and harvest on an outpatient basis, as well as less support needed for the patient in terms of antibiotics, platelets and blood transfusions following treatment (Crouch and Ross 1994).

For these reasons, higher-dose chemotherapy or accelerated radiotherapy over a shorter timescale, with their concomitant bone marrow suppression, can now be offered to a wider range of people, particularly those with solid tumours, because of the availability of stem cell rescue.

For a fuller discussion of BMT and the care of patients with haematological disorders, see Chapter 14.

Biological response modifier therapy

Bone marrow transplant is an attempt to manipulate the immune system to enable support or cure for cancer. Biological response modifiers (BRMs) are a group of agents whose primary site of action is also the immune system. These are naturally occurring molecules, often cytokines (e.g. interferon), that are capable of enhancing the immune response and therefore of being incorporated into cancer treatment. Depending on the BRM, this may occur by:

- regulation and/or augmentation of the immune response

- cytotoxic or cytostatic activity directed toward cancer cells

- inhibition of metastasis, differentiation or maturation.

As a result of advances in recombinant DNA technology, highly purified BRMs are now produced in large quantities and are available for use in cancer therapy. BRMs are unique in their ability to regulate or enhance the immune response. In contrast to chemotherapeutic agents and radiation therapy, which exert a direct effect on cancer cells, BRMs activate the body's natural defences with a potentially greater antineoplastic activity and reduced toxicity. However, despite a great deal of initial interest and much experimental evidence, there are few clear indications for use. Similarly, tumour vaccines using irradiated autologous and allogeneic tumour combined with various biological stimulants (e.g. bacille Calmette–Guérin (BCG)) have been tried but with little success. Melanoma is one form of cancer that is potentially amenable to treatment with vaccines because it has an intrinsic immunogenicity (i.e. an ability to generate an immune response in the individual). The full potential of these agents is yet to be realized, but with increasing knowledge and understanding of molecular and vaccine biology, future developments are anticipated (Gore and Riches 1995).

A complete account of the immune system and how it relates to BRM therapy is beyond the scope of this chapter, but Table 11.4 summarizes the principal actions, potential indications, and commonly reported toxicities and side-effects for several of the BRMs. Because the majority of BRMs are still under investigation, this information continues to evolve. In addition, optimal dosages have not yet been determined, so recommended dose ranges are not included.

The side-effects associated with BRMs are variable in their onset and intensity. Side-effects and toxicities vary with the agent, the dosage schedule, the dose and the patient. It is important to note that not all BRMs, or even the same BRM at the same dose, produce the same side-effects. The side-effect most unique to BRM therapy is a set of symptoms collectively known as *flu-like syndrome*. These symptoms include fever, chills and rigors, fatigue, anorexia, hypotension, myalgia, arthralgia and headache, and managing these side-effects represents a major challenge for both nurses and patients (Rieger 1995).

Table 11.4 Biological response modifier therapy: actions, potential indications and side-effects

Postulated mechanism of action	Potential indications	Toxicity and side-effects
Colony stimulating factors (CSFs) GM-CSF: stimulates production of neutrophils, macrophages, eosinophils and, in the presence of erythropoietin, red blood cells G-CSF: stimulates neutrophil production M-CSF: stimulates macrophage production EPO (erythropoietin): stimulates maturation of erythrocytes	Not directly tumoricidal. Research indicates they may be useful for cancer treatment because they: ■ decrease duration of neutropenia that often results from chemotherapy ■ enable higher doses of chemotherapy to be given since CSFs can alter the dose-related toxicity of myelosuppression ■ decrease bone marrow recovery time following bone marrow transplants or radiation therapy-related suppression of marrow. In clinical studies, CSFs have shown activity in the treatment of leukaemias, including chronic lymphocytic leukaemia, hairy cell leukaemia, myelodysplastic syndrome, and neutropenia secondary to chemotherapy	Flu-like syndrome: fever, chills, fatigue/weakness, myalgia/arthralgia, headache Gastrointestinal: nausea, diarrhoea, vomiting, anorexia Other: facial flushing
Tumour necrosis factor (TNF) *In vitro*: binds to receptors on tumour cells and is directly tumoricidal or tumoristatic *In vivo*: precise mechanism of action is unclear. TNF may be directly cytotoxic or it may cause vascular endothelial damage in tumour capillaries resulting in haemorrhage and necrosis of tumour cells. TNF may also work through immune cell activation as it has been found to augment natural killer T-cell activity and to enhance B-cell proliferation	Many clinical trials are underway to determine the efficacy of TNF. TNF may be helpful in treating metastatic adenocarcinomas including colorectal, hepatic and bladder carcinomas	Flu-like syndrome: fever, chills, fatigue/weakness, myalgia/arthralgia, back pain Gastrointestinal: nausea, vomiting, diarrhoea, anorexia Non-specific: severe pain at tumour site
Monoclonal antibodies (MAbs) Application of MAbs is based on the knowledge that all cells (including tumour cells) have antigens present on their surface that are specific to that cell type MAbs may be used alone or bound to radioisotopes, toxins or chemotherapeutic drugs to stain, destroy or identity cells with specific antigens on their cell surface	May be used in the treatment of cancer as well as for diagnostic purposes. In clinical trials MAbs have shown activity in the treatment of leukaemia, lymphoma, metastatic breast and colorectal cancer, ovarian, renal, bladder and prostate cancer	Flu-like syndrome: fever, chills, headache, fatigue, malaise, myalgia Gastrointestinal: nausea, diarrhoea, vomiting Skin: generalized erythema, urticaria, pruritus Anaphylaxis (rare, but severe and life threatening)
Interferons (IFNs) *Antiviral*: IFNs stimulate cells infected with viruses to produce proteins that interfere with viral replication *Antiproliferative*: IFNs slow the reproduction of cells. Although the mechanisms are not well understood, possible contributing factors include inhibition of DNA and protein synthesis of cancer cells and prolongation of the cell cycle	Have shown some activity in the treatment of hairy cell leukaemia, AIDS-related Kaposi's sarcoma, multiple myeloma, nodular cutaneous T-cell lymphoma and chronic granulocytic leukaemia	Flu-like syndrome: fever, chills, headache, fatigue, malaise, myalgia Gastrointestinal: nausea, diarrhoea, vomiting, anorexia, taste alterations, xerostomia Neurological/psychological: mild confusion, somnolence, irritability, poor concentration Haematological: neutropenia and thrombocytopenia

(Continued)

Table 11.4 *(Continued)*

Postulated mechanism of action	Potential indications	Toxicity and side-effects
Immunomodulatory: depending on the type of IFN, different aspects of the immune system are stimulated or augmented. Examples include: T-cell activation, increased phagocytic and cytotoxic activity of macrophages and mature natural killer cells		

Interleukins (ILs)

Interleukins are among the most important regulatory substances produced by lymphocytes and monocytes. Seven types of IL have been isolated and identified; however, other than IL-1, IL-2, IL-3 and more recently IL-4, little is known about their biological effects. Much work is still taking place in clinical trials The ILs appear to act by causing proliferation and stimulation of T and B lymphocytes, assisting in the synthesis and secretion of lymphokines (e.g. interferon, CSFs) and/or enhancing natural killer T-cell activity	Have shown some activity in the treatment of metastatic renal cell carcinoma, malignant melanoma, and non-Hodgkin lymphomas	Administration of interleukin results in multisystem toxicities that may be life threatening. Toxicities are related to dose and schedule Flu-like syndrome: fever, chills, headache, fatigue, malaise, myalgia Gastrointestinal: nausea, diarrhoea, vomiting, anorexia, taste alterations, xerostomia Skin: dryness, erythematous rash, pruritus, desquamation Neurological/psychological: confusion, irritability, impaired memory, sleep disturbances, depression Cardiovascular: capillary leak syndrome, peripheral oedema, ascites, arrhythmias, hypotension Pulmonary: dyspnoea, pulmonary oedema, ascites, arrhythmias, hypotension Renal: oliguria, anuria, azotaemia, increased serum creatinine and blood urea nitrogen levels

GM-CSF, granulocyte–macrophage colony stimulating factor.

Collectively, BRMs have the potential to manifest toxicities in virtually every body system. Box 11.5 lists some suggested nursing measures for patients receiving BRMs.

Complementary therapies

The term 'complementary' has been used widely in recent years to encompass any and all therapies that may be described as being outside orthodox or conventional medical practice. Other words used include alternative, traditional, natural, fringe and unorthodox, and even in some instances quack. The term 'unproven methods' is used in many medical papers, reflecting the concern of many orthodox medical practitioners that most of the therapies are 'unproven' by scientific research methods. A report by the British Medical Association (BMA) in 1993 opted for the term 'non-conventional' and distinguished between non-invasive, essentially self-help therapies

(e.g. yoga and massage) and those involving direct intervention (e.g. acupuncture). Generally, 'complementary therapies' may be viewed as those that are used *alongside* orthodox medical treatments and 'alternative therapies' as those that are used *instead* of conventional treatment approaches.

Whatever terminology is used, it is clear that there is an increasing interest in the use of the wide range of alternative and complementary therapies that is available. Some may be formulated specifically for the person with cancer, whereas others have wide application in both health and illness. To differing degrees, all therapies aim to enhance health and well-being by stimulating the self-healing capacities of the body. Such therapies include dietary manipulation, herbal medicines, immunizations, vitamin therapies and psychological techniques. People who seek these treatments are often terminally ill and may be particularly attracted to therapies that appear to offer the possibility of respite, or even cure. Often the

---

Box 11.5   Suggested nursing measures for patients receiving BRMs

Observe for presence and severity of symptoms. Provide information and reassurance:

- Encourage and answer questions

- Provide support and clarification of information to assist in decision-making process

- Reinforce explanation of specific agent, including mode of action, method of administration, side-effects and self-care strategies

- Provide written materials

- Include family or significant others in teaching session

- Help patient to anticipate and deal with flu-like symptoms

- Educate patient and family to report subtle symptom changes

- Participate with other team members in evaluating patient's understanding of and ability to participate in a clinical trial.

Minimize discomfort and maintain optimal mobility level and nutritional status:

- Administer narcotics, antihistamines and prostaglandin inhibitors as ordered, to manage flu-like symptoms

- Suggest strategies for developing effective coping skills such as relaxation and imagery

- Explore and implement measures to maintain level of mobility, pattern of daily activities, appropriate use of medications, application of heat

- Provide warmth during chills

- Allow for rest periods throughout the day

- Assess nutritional status and evaluate dietary intake regularly

- Provide specific suggestions for managing anorexia, nausea and vomiting, and taste changes.

---

drive to try alternative treatment regimens, which may be quite rigorous and demanding, comes from the family or significant others. While a patient may not experience any physical harm from this type of therapy, they may be at risk of being given unrealistic hope, leading to emotional distress, and of being financially burdened by the high cost of some therapies.

Some people may turn to unproven methods because of dissatisfaction with conventional medical treatment. There is often a degree of tension between conventional and unconventional practitioners, with the former believing that the latter are of no proven value and that they may lead patients to abandon potentially effective treatment regimens (Souhami and Tobias 1995).

Conversely, promoters of unproven methods may attack the medical and scientific community and be reluctant to share information about the methods employed. In either case, practitioners may be equally dogmatic, and perhaps a more constructive approach is to seek to combine elements from both. The Foundation for Integrated Medicine (1997) outlines a strategy for taking forward the integration of complementary and alternative therapies into mainstream health care. At one centre in the UK, a variety of complementary therapies and self-help techniques is offered alongside conventional treatments (Burke and Sikora 1993), and the effectiveness of this supportive care programme is under continuous evaluation.

There are many problems inherent in research into the effectiveness of complementary therapies. Conventional medicine tends to utilize the experimental design approach and incorporates such techniques as randomized controlled trials. However, as Ersser (1995) notes, this approach is not always helpful or possible in assessing the varied and individual response to therapies. Research methods that utilize or incorporate a qualitative approach may be more useful here. The difficulty of uncontrolled variables is a major challenge to researchers in this area and there has been limited rigorous evaluation of complementary therapies for people with cancer. Cawley (1997a) reviewed 14 studies that aimed to evaluate the effectiveness of massage and found that comparisons were problematic because of the differences in study designs and parameters.

To become a competent practitioner in most of these therapies, several years of training and practice is required. However, some essential elements of certain of these practices may be successfully incorporated into nursing practice and there is growing enthusiasm for this among many nurses (Trevelyan and Booth 1994). Some health authorities have developed operational policies to clarify roles and responsibilities, and to ensure good standards of practice.

It is understandable that, when faced with a potentially life-threatening disease, a person may seek out any avenues that appear to offer hope, comfort and even survival. For many individuals, complementary therapies and alternative treatments offer an opportunity to regain some choice and control over a life disrupted by disease and the unpleasant side-effects of conventional treatment. The issue of personal control in health is a recurring theme in many studies, such as that undertaken by Montbriand (1993), which explored the use of alternative therapies by 400 people with cancer.

Through knowledge and understanding about alternative and complementary therapies, and empathic discussion, nurses may play a key role in guiding the patient away from desperate measures and towards helpful coping strategies and supportive therapies.

Nursing assessment and management of disease- and treatment-related problems

There is a wide range treatment and disease-related problems of cancer, and these are discussed in this section along with suggestions for appropriate nursing management strategies. Although some needs and problems appear to be primarily physical, all aspects of cancer care and treatment also have psychosocial and emotional implications. Through an understanding of the meaning and significance of cancer-related problems, nurses can work in partnership with individuals to explore and identify effective coping strategies.

Bone marrow depression

Leucopenia is the depletion of white blood cells that often develops as a result of chemotherapy and sometimes radiotherapy, and that makes the patient very susceptible to infection. If a marked decrease in white blood cells below a normal range is identified, nursing measures need to be instituted to minimize the risk of infection. These include the implementation of protective isolation systems and processes to protect the patient from sources of infection. Regimens vary from centre to centre, but broadly include dietary restrictions, effective personal and oral hygiene, and the administration of various prophylactic pharmaceutical agents. The use of invasive procedures, and breaks in the normal protective mechanism such as the skin and mucous membranes, may potentiate the risk of infection. Patients with severe leucopenia are in a potentially life-threatening situation through the development of septicaemia and possibly septic shock. The most common sites of infection are the blood, respiratory tract, alimentary tract, skin and genito-urinary tract. An increase in temperature above 38°C is the most common sign of infection in a neutropenic patient. In most situations antimicrobial treatment is initiated immediately and continued until the patient has recovery of the bone marrow and is apyrexial.

Anaemia may be manifested by weakness, tiredness, pallor and shortness of breath. Chemotherapy-induced anaemia is usually a gradual process and may not be evident for several weeks after initiating chemotherapy. If patients are symptomatic due to anaemia, transfusion of packed red cells will be given until marrow recovery.

Thrombocytopenia increases the risk of the patient bleeding because of the impairment of the blood clotting process. Signs of thrombocytopenia include ecchymoses, petechiae, blood in the urine or stool, vaginal bleeding or evidence of bleeding in other organs or systems. The sclera is a common site of haemorrhage. When the platelet count drops below 50×10^9/L spontaneous haemorrhage may occur, and this risk increases when the counts drop below 20×10^9/L. Platelet transfusions are given to support the patient until his or her own bone marrow starts to produce adequate numbers of platelets.

Nursing management of patients with bone marrow depression includes prevention and management of infection and bleeding, patient education, close monitoring, and implementation of preventive nursing care measures. These are outlined in Box 11.6.

Gastrointestinal problems

Nausea and vomiting

Nausea and vomiting are two of the most common and distressing sequelae of cancer and cancer therapy. Inadequate control of nausea and vomiting results in complications such as dehydration, anorexia, malnutrition and metabolic disturbances. The distress associated with nausea and vomiting is one of the most feared and disruptive side-effects of chemotherapy, to the extent that it may cause patients to be unable or unwilling to continue treatment (Richardson 1991, Rhodes et al 1995). Different cytotoxic agents have different emetogenic potential, so knowledge of these and details of patients' specific chemotherapy regimens are an essential part of the assessment process. However, in recent years there has been increased effort to develop pharmacological and non-pharmacological methods to prevent and control nausea and vomiting. In particular, the serotonin antagonists, (e.g. ondansetron and granisetron) have had a significant effect in minimizing acute chemotherapy-induced nausea and vomiting.

The symptoms of nausea and vomiting may result from a wide variety of physiological causes other than cancer chemotherapy. Causes include mechanical obstruction of the gastrointestinal tract, increased intracerebral pressure as a result of the tumour, fluid and electrolyte imbalances (hypercalcaemia, hyponatraemia, hypokalaemia, volume depletion), radiation therapy (particularly to the abdomen, pelvis, back and brain) and pharmacological agents (antibiotics, narcotics).

Nursing care is directed at the prevention and active management of nausea and vomiting, and Richardson (1991) advocates the value of encouraging individuals to develop effective self-care strategies. Other interventions centre around the management of nutrition, hydration and comfort while the patient experiences nausea or vomiting; these are summarized in Box 11.7.

Mucositis (stomatitis)

The terms *mucosititis* and *stomatitis* are often used interchangeably to describe the inflammation, desquamation and ulceration of the oral mucous membrane that occurs as a result of either systemic chemotherapy or localized radiotherapy. The fast-growing epithelial cells of the mouth

Leucopenia
See chapter 4.1

Anaemia
See chapter 4.1

Thrombocytopenia
See chapter 4.1

Nausea and vomiting
See chapter 5.1

Box 11.6   Nursing care of the person with bone marrow depression

Leucopenia and infection

Assessment

Assess the patient for signs and symptoms of infection:

1. Fever > 38°C, hypotension, chills

2. Monitor the respiratory and genitourinary systems, skin and mucous membranes, and sites of peripheral and central venous catheters for infection

3. Monitor white blood cell counts and the differential daily. A neutrophil count of less than $1 \times 10^9/$L substantially increases the risk of infection

4. Monitor for signs and symptoms of sepsis.

Patient problems and goals

- The major problem is the potential for infection and consequently the goal is that the person will not develop infection

- The onset of infection will be identified as soon as defining signs and symptoms appear

- Patient/significant other will notify appropriate member of the health team when symptoms occur

- Patient/significant other knows the signs and symptoms of infection and is able to monitor and report on them

- Patient will be protected from nosocomial infection during the period of hospitalization.

Nursing intervention

1. Monitor temperature 4-hourly or more frequently

2. Minimize exposure to potential sources of infection:
   a. persons with transmissible diseases
   b. stagnant water (flower vases, respiratory equipment, humidifiers)
   c. faeces of animals

3. Instruct the patient in maintaining good hygiene:
   a. handwashing after toileting and before meals
   b. daily shower or bath

4. Maintain integrity of skin and mucous membranes:
   a. prevent injury of rectal mucosa by avoiding enemas, suppositories and rectal thermometers
   b. promote oral hygiene and prevent injury to oral mucosa by avoiding heavy brushing
   c. use an electric razor
   d. avoid injections if at all possible

5. Avoid use of invasive equipment such as indwelling urinary catheters

6. Practise protective measures:
   a. wash hands before and after caring for neutropenic patients
   b. keep equipment in contact with the patient clean
   c. institute protective isolation (single room, strict handwashing, exclude fresh fruits and vegetables from diet, no potted plants) when the neutrophil count is $<1 \times 10^9/$L

7. Administer antibiotics, antifungal and antiviral agents on time

8. Devise effective patient education and information on signs and symptoms of infection, self-care measures, how to take an oral temperature, and to notify healthcare providers if infection is suspected.

Thrombocytopenia and bleeding

Assessment

1. Monitor the platelet count daily

2. Monitor for signs and symptoms of bleeding, especially petechiae, bleeding gums, bruising, epistaxis, blood in urine, stool, emesis, heavy menstruation, intracranial bleeding, oozing from i.v. sites or other wounds.

Patient problems and goals

- The principal potential problem is that of bleeding and the patient goal is therefore that bleeding will not occur

- Signs and symptoms of minor and serious bleeding will be detected and reported

- Patient/significant other can list measures to prevent bleeding.

Nursing intervention

1. Avoid use of medications that alter platelet production and function, i.e. aspirin and aspirin-containing products, anticoagulants, non-steroidal anti-inflammatory agents

2. When the platelet count is $<50\,000/$mm³ institute measures to prevent trauma and possible bleeding:
   a. avoid activities that could cause physical injury
   b. use electric razors to shave
   c. avoid rectal manipulation including enemas, suppositories, rectal temperature
   d. blowing of the nose should be gentle to avoid epistaxis

(Continued)

Box 11.6   *(Continued)*

3. Avoid injections. If necessary, use a small needle and apply pressure after the injection for 3–5 minutes or until bleeding stops

4. Minimize venepunctures as much as possible

5. Administer platelet transfusions as prescribed.

Box 11.7   Nursing care of the person with nausea and vomiting

Assessment

1. Assess factors that may be causing or contributing to nausea and vomiting

2. Assess the onset, duration, frequency and intensity of nausea and vomiting:
   a. amount and character of emesis
   b. impact of nausea and vomiting on nutrition and fluid and electrolyte balance

3. Assess previous response to emetic therapies

4. Monitor intake, output and fluid balance

5. Monitor effectiveness of antiemetic therapy.

Patient problems and goals

■ The potential problem of nausea and vomiting indicates a goal that nausea and vomiting will not occur

■ Patient will be able to maintain adequate hydration and nutrition.

Nursing intervention

1. Administer antiemetic drug therapy at least 1 hour before emetic treatments and at regular intervals around the clock as long as the nausea persists in order to prevent or minimize nausea and vomiting. If the patient is unable to tolerate oral antiemetics, administer antiemetics by rectal suppository, intravenously or sublingually. Commonly used antiemetics include phenothiazines, butyrophenones, steroids, metoclopramide, benzodiazepines and serotonin antagonists

2. Use combinations of antiemetics with different mechanisms of action when one agent is not effective

3. Maintain adequate hydration either orally or intravenously

4. Encourage a bland, cold diet or a clear liquid diet

5. Counsel the patient to avoid eating 1–2 hours before and after chemotherapy or other treatments that cause nausea and vomiting

6. Eliminate noxious sights, smells or other stimuli that may exacerbate nausea

7. Provide frequent oral hygiene using water or normal saline

8. Utilize techniques such as visual imagery, relaxation and hypnosis to prevent and control nausea and vomiting

9. Educate the patient and family regarding self-care measures to relieve nausea and vomiting.

---

and gastrointestinal tract are particularly susceptible to damage, either by direct action on cell metabolism and replication or indirectly as a result of generalized bone marrow suppression and increased susceptibility to infection and bleeding. Loss of **saliva**, or *xerostomia*, exacerbates other problems and is a key problem, particularly for patients undergoing radiotherapy to the head and neck. *Oesophagitis* may also develop if the effects of treatment result in damaging or destroying epithelial cells in the oesophagus. As Gamble (1998) noted, the distress of mucostis is often underestimated and patients require considerable support to cope with symptoms. Nursing care is directed at managing comfort, nutrition and hydration, preventing infection and promoting oral hygiene.

Careful assessment of the oral cavity is essential when mucositis is an expected side-effect of treatment. Eilers et al (1988) developed an oral assessment guide and this has formed the basis of many subsequent assessment tools, all of which include inspection of the lips, mucous membranes, gingiva and tongue for evidence of inflammation, desquamation, ulcers and infection, as well as moistness and evidence of debris. The amount and viscosity of the saliva needs to be noted as it becomes thick, ropy and viscous with severe mucositis, contributing to the dryness of the oral cavity and difficulty in eating. The patient's ability to eat, speak, swallow or wear dentures may be severely impaired. While the patient may experience mild burning at the onset of stomatitis, a severe case is extremely painful and may require systemic narcotic analgesic management – usually a continuous morphine infusion.

Infection is a potentially serious problem when mouth ulcerations exist. The fungus *Candida albicans* is frequently the cause of lesions and inflammation, or may be a secondary infection when the oral mucosa is damaged by chemotherapy or radiation. Candidiasis presents as white patches on the tongue and buccal mucosa. When the patches are scraped off, a reddened ulcerated surface is apparent. Herpes simplex infection on the lips develops into painful vesicles that rupture and become encrusted. Gram-negative infections may occur in the mouth, as can

Saliva
See chapter 5.1

Box 11.8   Nursing care of the person with mucositis

Assessment

Assess the lips and oral cavity daily using a light source:

1. Inspect for red inflamed areas, ulcerations, bleeding and oedema

2. Note degree of moistness of tissues; amount and viscosity of saliva

3. Note presence of pain, difficulty eating or swallowing, difficulty talking

4. Assess for evidence of infection (fungal, viral, bacterial), particularly in areas of ulceration, and on the tongue and palate.

Patient problems and goals

■ When the problem of mucositis occurs the goal should be that the patient will have a normal oral mucosa and experience no discomfort

■ Patient will be able to express understanding of oral hygiene measures and perform them after meals and at bedtime.

Nursing intervention

1. Teach the patient an oral hygiene regimen or assist if the patient is dependent:
   a. self-inspection of the mouth and oral cavity
   b. follow regimen a minimum of four times a day or every 4 hours while awake
   c. brush teeth with a soft toothbrush and floss once daily
   d. if platelets $< 50 \times 10^9$/L, or gums are bleeding or painful, utilize a foam-tipped applicator or gauze to clean and discontinue flossing
   e. use a non-irritating toothpaste or baking soda to brush
   f. avoid commercial mouthwashes as they contain alcohol and are drying and irritating to oral mucosa. Do not use lemon and glycerin as this combination is drying and irritating
   g. use normal saline or diluted baking soda (5 mL in 500 mL water) as a mouthwash; increase frequency of rinsing if oral tissues are dry or saliva production is decreased
   h. a solution of 1 : 4 hydrogen peroxide and normal saline or water may be used as a mouthwash to help clean debris from the mouth
   i. lubricate the lips using a water-soluble lubricant or lanolin

2. Control pain:
   a. use a topical analgesic such as Xylocaine. Use as a mouthwash or apply to painful areas with a swab. Numbness lasts approximately 20 min, which may aid the patient with eating and drinking. Ensure foods and drinks are not hot as sensation is impaired with topical analgesics
   b. utilize systemic analgesic therapy when the patient experiences continuous severe pain. A continuous intravenous infusion of morphine will ease pain until healing begins

3. Promote adequate hydration and nutrition

4. Counsel the patient to:
   a. alter diet to soft or liquid to reduce mechanical irritation
   b. avoid salty, spicy, acidic or hot foods as they are chemically irritating
   c. try high-protein nutritional supplements
   d. maintain hydration of 3000 mL per day. If the patient is unable to swallow, intravenous hydration may be necessary

5. Manage infection:
   a. monitor temperature 4-hourly if the patient has ulcerations or signs of infection
   b. increase frequency of oral hygiene to at least every 4 hours
   c. administer topical and systemic antibiotics and antifungal agents as prescribed.

Taste
See chapter 24

Pseudomonas infections. The risk of systemic infection is of great concern. Ulcerated areas act as a port of entry for pathological organisms into the body, which may cause sepsis. Therefore, maintenance of good oral hygiene during periods of mucositis is essential in order to minimize the risk of infection. Specific nursing measures in the care of the patient with mucositis are outlined in Box 11.8.

Taste alterations

Alterations in **taste** can occur as a result of cancer treatment. The types of taste alterations include *dysgeusia*, which is an unpleasant taste perception; *ageusia*, an absence of taste; and *hypogeusia*, a decrease in the acuity of taste sensation.

Surgical treatment for cancer in the oral cavity, particularly the tongue, salivary glands, nasal area and trachea, may cause hypogeusia and ageusia. Mucositis and infections in the oral cavity may also contribute to alterations in taste. Taste alterations caused by chemotherapy include metallic and bitter taste sensations, and an increased

Box 11.9 Nursing care of the person with taste alterations

Assessment

1. Assess for the presence, type, onset, degree and duration of taste alterations

2. Assess for contributing factors (poor oral hygiene, oral infection)

3. Assess for any change in nutritional status and, in particular, which foods cause dysgeusia.

Patient problems and goals

■ The problem of taste alterations leads to the goal that the patient will report normal taste sensations or an absence of unpleasant tastes.

Nursing intervention

1. Eliminate foods that cause the patient unpleasant taste sensations. High-protein foods such as meat commonly cause dysgeusia. Use other sources of protein such as eggs, cheese, fish, nuts, legumes and milk products

2. Experiment with seasonings and flavourings to enhance taste

3. Experiment with foods that mask bitter or metallic tastes (mint, lemon)

4. Promote adequate oral hygiene; keep the oral mucosa moist.

threshold for the sweet sensation. The chemotherapeutic agents most commonly associated with taste alterations include cyclophosphamide, nitrogen mustard, 5-fluorouracil, vincristine, methotrexate and dacarbazine. Taste alterations vary widely amongst patients in terms of severity and duration. Changes due to chemotherapy and radiation usually return to normal within weeks to months.

Nursing care is directed towards maintaining nutrition and hydration, and assisting patients to adapt their diet during periods of taste alteration. Assessing the presence of taste changes and informing patients of this possibility are important nursing actions in order to assist with coping with taste alterations. Detailed nursing care of the patient with taste alterations is outlined in Box 11.9.

Anorexia, weight loss and cachexia

Anorexia and *weight loss* are common problems for many patients with cancer. Many factors may contribute to anorexia, including side-effects of therapy, nausea, taste changes, pain, fatigue and stomatitis. Weight loss is also related to an increased demand of the tumour on host tissue, resulting in loss largely from muscle rather than

fatty tissue. The combination of changes in metabolism and inadequate intake results in nutritional deficiencies that impair the body's ability to repair and heal, as well as affecting the patient's quality of life.

Cachexia involves both weight loss and anorexia, and is the wasting syndrome that is often associated with advanced cancer. Although not inevitable, many people with cancer are affected by it, particularly those with advanced disease (De Wys 1985).

Comprehensive assessment as to the nature, cause and consequences of nutritional deficiences is essential, and will enable realistic goals of care to be determined. If patients are able to eat, food intake and nutrition status may be enhanced by:

■ providing information about nutrition and calorific values

■ encouraging choice of favourite foods, particularly those that have a high protein content

■ eating small meals often

■ using antiemetics and analgesics effectively

■ maintaining good oral hygiene.

Oral food supplements are frequently employed and, where this is not possible, enteral feeding via a nasogastric or percutaneous route may be used. Parenteral (intravenous) feeding may also be an option, particularly as an adjunct to major surgery, although its general use in cancer care is controversial.

As well as being a physiological necessity, eating and drinking have a wider social significance, and the inability to engage in these activities represents a significant loss for both the individual and their carers. Jones et al (1993) interviewed 207 bereaved carers and identified that there were 144 instances where concerns about anorexia or weight loss were voiced. Any interventions that enhance comfort and enjoyment may result in a significant enhancement of quality of life.

Constipation.
See chapter 5.1

Constipation

Constipation may be induced by a variety of causes, including nutritional deficits, particularly a lack of fibre, immobility, or administration of the chemotherapeutic agents vincristine and vinblastine (Cimprich 1985). The vinca alkaloids cause smooth muscle neurotoxicity, and consequences in the bowel range from mild constipation to paralytic ileus. Chemotherapy is usually interrupted during periods of ileus. Opioid analgesics frequently cause constipation due to decreased peristalsis in the bowel. Regular administration of stool softeners and bulk laxatives will help to prevent constipation, as will an increase in fluid and fibre intake. This, of course, may be difficult if the patient is also experiencing mucositis and other gastrointestinal symptoms, and thorough assessment and planning of appropriate interventions will be required.

Diarrhoea

Diarrhoea may cause fluid and electrolyte imbalances and contribute to the weakness and fatigue that patients experience. Nutrition may be severely hampered. Diarrhoea is also irritating to the perianal skin surfaces and may cause skin breakdown. Nursing actions are focused on maintaining adequate hydration and nutrition, promoting comfort and hygiene, and returning bowel function to normal. Specific nursing care measures for the patient with diarrhoea include maintaining fluid intake at a minimum of 3000 mL per day, a low-residue diet, care of the perianal region and use of antidiarrhoeal medication.

Alopecia

Alopecia, or hair loss, is a side-effect of radiotherapy to the head, when some of the loss may be permanent, and of cytotoxic chemotherapy, when the loss may be total but is temporary. The degree of toxicity of different drugs in this regard varies (see Table 11.3) but, as many are used in combination, hair loss is an inevitable consequence of many regimens. The emotional impact of this may vary between individuals but is frequently considerable because of the visibility of the change. As Freedman (1994) noted, hair is associated with a person's identity and thus loss of hair is also linked with the loss of self. It is also a visible and long-lasting sign of treatment for a disease that individuals might otherwise wish to keep private, or share only with a chosen few. On a practical level, the protective functions of hair are also lost (i.e. conservation of heat, protection from the sun, and the filtering out of airborne particles from the eyes and nose). Scalp cooling may be offered in some centres, although this is not effective in all cases and can be quite a lengthy and uncomfortable process, so careful assessment and evaluation is required (Dougherty 1995).

Nurses are well placed to help patients prepare for hair loss and to develop effective coping and self-care strategies to manage the changes in body image and self-concept. Specific nursing care interventions for patients experiencing hair loss are outlined in Box 11.10.

Diarrhoea
See chapter 5.1

Fatigue

Fatigue or lack of energy are symptoms that occur frequently and are experienced by virtually every person with cancer (Richardson 1995). Fatigue is well known to individuals with cancer and may precede or accompany the illness; it may serve as a marker of disease progression and recurrence. A multitude of factors may contribute to fatigue, including surgery, chemotherapy, radiotherapy, disturbances in sleep and rest patterns, inadequate nutrition, mood disturbances (Wickham et al 1990) and symptom distress.

Box 11.10   Nursing care of the person with alopecia

Assessment

1. Assess the patient's understanding of the potential for hair loss and expected timeframe for regrowth

2. While the patient has hair loss, inspect the scalp for dryness, and the eyes and nasal area for irritation.

Patient problems and goals

■ Patient/significant other expresses an understanding of hair loss and its temporary nature

■ Patient/significant other is able to express feelings regarding hair loss and demonstrate continued interest in self-care and grooming.

Nursing intervention

1. Information about the potential hair loss including the expected onset, duration and severity

2. Advice about and monitoring of self-care measures:
   a. regular cleansing of the scalp with a mild shampoo (unless contraindicated by radiotherapy treatment)
   b. restriction of the use of harsh chemicals on the hair and avoidance of extreme heat or brushing

3. Discussion of possibilities for coping with hair loss: wigs, turbans, scarves and hats. A net or turban may be helpful during periods of heavy hair shedding. A photograph taken before hair loss may assist the patient in selecting a wig most suited to them

4. Suggestions about the application of make-up help to create eyebrows and improve appearance when eyebrows and eyelashes are lost

5. Provide opportunities to discuss feelings and reactions to hair loss and its effects on body image and self-concept.

Fatigue in patients with cancer is a complex phenomenon and clearly involves physical, psychological and emotional elements. Nursing interventions focus on exploring individual experiences and on ameliorating and devising strategies to adapt lifestyle, conserve energy, maintain optimum activity, and promote adequate nutrition and rest. Specific nursing care measures for patients experiencing fatigue are outlined in Box 11.11.

Box 11.11 Nursing care of the person with fatigue

Assessment

1. Assess factors that may be contributing to fatigue: nutrition, sleep/rest patterns, treatment, symptom distress

2. Assess pattern of fatigue: onset, duration, severity, ameliorating and exacerbating factors, and impact on lifestyle.

Patient problems and goals

■ The problem of fatigue leads to the setting of a goal, in conjunction with the patient, that the patient will achieve adequate periods of rest in order to pursue key interests and activities.

Nursing intervention

1. Assist patient to pace activities according to energy level. Include periods of mild activity in daily routine. Obtain assistance for activities that are fatiguing (e.g. housework, childcare)

2. Promote adequate rest and sleep pattern

3. Control symptom distress, particularly pain, nausea and vomiting, fever, diarrhoea

4. Meditation, progressive muscle relaxation and guided imaging may promote relaxation and increase energy.

Box 11.12 Suggested nursing interventions for patients experiencing breathlessness

■ Detailed assessment and identification of factors that ameliorate or exacerbate breathlessness

■ Encourage the prioritization of activities, and plan activities in advance to minimize expenditure of effort

■ Include planned rest periods, particularly with more demanding activities, which should be scheduled at hours of the day when breathing is the easiest

■ Review exertion caused by eating and suggest smaller, more frequent, meals of soft, easy-to-chew foods

■ Position patient for maximal respiratory excursion using pillows (i.e. sitting upright)

■ Improve air circulation with fans; open windows

■ Maintain adequate humidity to decrease dry airway and thick secretions

■ Liaise with physiotherapist regarding chest physiotherapy and breathing retraining techniques to encourage diaphragmatic breathing

■ Spend time with patient to understand the impact and meaning of breathlessness for them and their carers

■ Provide information on causation and significance of symptoms

■ Administer low doses of narcotics, sedatives, bronchodilators and oxygen therapy, as ordered. Steroids or antimuscarinic agents (such as atropine) may be helpful in some situations.

Dyspnoea
See chapter 5.3

Breathlessness

Breathlessness (**dyspnoea**) is an uncomfortable awareness of breathing and serves as a stimulus for actions that may relieve respiratory insufficiency, such as clearing the airway, removing constrictive clothing, or breathing rapidly and deeply. Whilst the symptom should be viewed first as a warning of disease and a signal to investigate and treat the underlying medical condition, breathlessness is a discomfort that can be relieved regardless of its pathophysiological basis.

Breathlessness is experienced as a result of many underlying conditions that may coexist in people with cancer. Respiratory failure, particularly pneumonia, is a frequent cause of death among patients with cancer, and breathlessness may also occur in a variety of other terminal conditions (e.g. sepsis, cardiac failure or severe anaemia). Specific causes of breathlessness for people with cancer are largely related to primary or secondary tumours that result in obstruction to the upper airways; pleural effusion (fluid in the pleural cavity) or a generalized lymphangitis within the lungs.

Whenever possible, the root cause should be investigated and may be treated by surgery, radiotherapy or chemotherapy. Otherwise, drug treatment with bronchodilators and/or respiratory depressants may help to prevent and alleviate acute episodes. Physiotherapy, which assists with the removal of secretions, and techniques for breathing 're-training' to encourage diaphragmatic breathing are helpful. Corner et al (1995a) proposed a model for the management of breathlessness which views the functional, emotional and sensory elements as inseparable and which employs a variety of non-pharmacological measures to enhance coping skills.

Breathlessness is a frightening experience and patients may fear they will choke or will just stop breathing and die. Patients may experience panic attacks and extreme anxiety, which exacerbate the physiological impairment and lead to even more dysfunctional breathing patterns.

The experience of being with someone who is acutely breathless is also extremely frightening, particularly in the home or other areas without immediate access to medical or nursing services. Suggested nursing measures for the patient experiencing breathlessness are listed in Box 11.12.

Pain

Pain is the symptom most frequently associated with cancer and is one of the most feared consequences of the disease and treatment. The assessment and management of pain and other symptoms in patients with cancer is one of the major activities in cancer care, although Hanks (1995) suggests that only 10–15% of pain is managed adequately. Effective pain management involves sound knowledge of the pathophysiology of cancer pain, pain assessment strategies and pain management principles, including the use of pharmaceutical and non-pharmaceutical measures.

Definition and description

Even though a person may experience pain and knows how it feels to hurt, it is difficult for both the observer and the sufferer to define and describe pain adequately. Pain is commonly divided into two subtypes: acute and chronic. Acute pain is characterized by a well defined time of onset and is associated with subjective and objective signs indicating activation of the sympathetic nervous system (e.g. sweating, paleness, tachycardia, hypertension, grimacing, crying and anxiety). Chronic pain, on the other hand, is defined as the persistence of pain for longer than 6 months. In general, the onset of chronic pain is less well defined. In addition, patients with chronic pain no longer exhibit the signs and symptoms usually associated with pain. In fact, the patient with chronic pain often shows very few signs of distress; often the suffering is hidden beneath a brave, stoical face. After long periods of unrelieved pain, the face no longer reveals anxiety – but exhaustion and depression. The lack of outwardly obvious signs and the depressed, sleepy face is often misinterpreted and the patient's complaints of severe pain discounted.

Patients with cancer may experience either acute pain, chronic pain, or acute pain superimposed on chronic pain. The type of pain experienced is determined by the stage of the disease, the type of treatment the patient is receiving, and any other predisposing medical or surgical conditions.

Nature of cancer pain and pain pathways

In order to focus attention on the complexity of pain as a somatic and psychological experience, Saunders and Baines (1983) introduced the notion of 'total pain'. The suffering experienced by the patient with cancer pain is derived from a variety of sources. Anger, anxiety, depression, isolation, fearful memories, boredom and other psychosocial factors can lower a patient's pain threshold. On the other hand, a positive outlook, a supportive family, empathy from nurses and doctor, forgiveness, diversion and sleep may raise the pain threshold and decrease the pain experience.

Pain
See chapter 2.3

Pain assessment
See chapter 2.3

> **Box 11.13**   Pain syndromes in patients with cancer
>
> *Pain caused by cancer*
>
> - Metastatic bone disease
> - Compression or infiltration of nervous structures
> - Compression or infiltration of veins, arteries, lymphatics
> - Rapid tumour growth causing stretching of pain-sensitive structures
> - Obstruction of a hollow viscus, such as bowel
> - Ulceration of pain-sensitive mucosal surfaces.
>
> *Pain caused by anticancer therapy*
>
> - Surgery
> - Chemotherapy
> - Radiation therapy.
>
> *Coincidental pain*
>
> - General debility
> - Joint stiffness
> - Pressure sores
> - Constipation.

An understanding of pain pathways and pain control mechanisms is essential to the understanding of cancer pain management, and these are outlined in Chapter 7.

Aetiology of cancer pain

As shown in Box 11.13, the pain of cancer can have multiple causes, including the cancer itself, the treatment, and concomitant non-malignant disease or factors unrelated to cancer or therapy.

Assessment

The phase of **assessment** is possibly one of the most important steps in good pain management, and accurate assessment is based on trust; McCaffrey (1979) stresses the importance of trust and belief in the patient's report of the severity and nature of the pain. As Lanceley (1995) noted, pain is deeply personal and the extent of the disease shown on examination of radiograph or scan does not necessarily reveal the extent of the pain. Lack of belief can accentuate the patient's feelings of helplessness and hopelessness, and may also lead to stoical under-reporting or anxious over-reporting of the experience. Either reaction aggravates the spiral of mistrust, anxiety and pain.

At the initial pain interview and as part of an ongoing nursing assessment, it is important to explore the key elements of a pain history, as outlined in Box 11.14 utilizing the PQRST symptom analysis tool.

Box 11.14   Components of the pain history

Provocation/Palliation

- What brings on the pain? What relieves the pain?

Quality

- Describe the pain in your own words (e.g. dull, sharp, aching, throbbing, burning).

Region/Radiation

- Location of pain. Does it spread anywhere?

Severity

- How severe is the pain? (Consider using an instrument such as a vertical or linear visual analogue rating scale to assist the patient in describing the intensity of pain and to track response to pain management strategies over time. See Fig. 11.3 and Ch. 7.)

Timing

- How long have you had it? Does it come and go, or is it always there? How long does each spasm last?

In addition to the PQRST analysis, the following should also be ascertained.

Impact of pain on daily life

- On sleep – Does pain disturb your sleep? (N.B. Patients with pain may adapt to it so they sleep)

- On mood – Does the pain cause you to be depressed or discouraged?

- On activity – How has pain affected your activities: ambulation, self-care, job, social life, etc.?

Knowledge and/or fears about use of analgesics to treat chronic pain

Meaning of pain

- What does patient think is causing the pain? What does patient think should be done about it?

Previous therapies

- Which drugs (or other therapies) have helped and which have failed to relieve the pain? Analgesic history should include: dose, frequency, regular or p.r.n., patient's view of drug efficacy, duration of use, side-effects, reason for discontinuation.

Measurement of pain

Although the experience of pain is not open to direct external measurement, several instruments have been developed to assist the patient in describing the intensity of pain. Measurement tools are advantageous because they facilitate:

- clarity and consistency in interpretation and communication of the pain. Verbal or written statements of a patient's exact numerical pain ratings are likely to be more consistently reported among health team members than a word description, such as 'a lot of pain'

- quantification of the effectiveness of an intervention. For example, if a patient's pain is the most severe at a rating of 9 and 2 hours after analgesia it is still at 7, it is evident that more effective interventions are needed.

Examples of some instruments are given in Chapter 7. However, the type of scale used is less important than:

- the consistency with which it is used

- the patient's understanding of the scale

- the clarity with which the scale assigns a score to the pain experience.

For example, a rating of 5 is meaningless unless it is followed by a statement of the scale used, for example: 5 on a scale of 0–10 (0 = no pain, 10 = worst pain), or 5 on a scale of 0–5 (0 = no pain, 5 = worst pain).

Some patients are unable to use a numerical scale to rate their pain; the numbers do not make sense to them or it is too hard for them to apply numbers to their experience. In this case, the following choice of descriptive words may be helpful for the patient to use:

- no pain

- a little pain

- a lot of pain

- too much pain.

These four phrases may then be converted to a 0–3 scale for documentation and communication among health team members: 0 = no pain, 1 = a little pain, 2 = a lot of pain, 3 = too much pain.

Some form of recording or tracking of the characteristics of the patient's pain and the response to therapy is essential for adequate management of the problem. Not keeping pain records when dealing with a patient in pain is like trying to treat hypertension without recording blood pressure.

The flow sheet allows ongoing evaluation of pain. The only safe and effective way to administer an analgesic is to monitor the patient's response to the medication and make changes based on these responses. The flow sheet is a tool that allows quick documentation of such responses along with easy retrieval of information for continuous evaluation. An example of a flow sheet that may be used by the patient or by the nurse is given in Figure 11.3.

Figure 11.3   Pain flow sheet.

Date/time	Pain rating on a scale of _ _ _ _ _ _	Respiratory rate	Accompanying symptoms/ level of consciousness/ other observations	Analgesic
NAME: _____				

Code key for accompanying symptoms:

1 Nausea	**3** Vomiting	**5** Constipation	**7** Drowsiness
2 Confusion	**4** Hallucinations	**6** Fatigue/weakness	

Pharmacotherapeutics

Administration of systemic analgesics, psychotropic **drugs** and anti-inflammatory agents is probably the most practical and widely used method for relieving cancer pain. Twycross and Lack (1990) have suggested a realistic clinical plan for 'graded pain relief': initially, a pain-free, sleepful night; next, comfort at rest in bed or a chair during the day; and finally, freedom from pain on movement.

The choice of analgesic will depend partly on whether the individual is suffering chronic or acute pain, or a combination of both. Acute pain in a person with cancer (e.g. postoperative, recent fracture, painful diagnostic procedure) might call for an intramuscular injection of a standard dose of a relatively short-acting opioid. Further analgesia would be on a p.r.n. basis because pain intensity is likely to change rapidly. However, if the individual is already taking large amounts of opioid analgesia for chronic pain, this would need to be taken into account in an acute situation.

Chronic cancer pain, on the other hand, demands a different approach. Analgesics should be given regularly (around the clock) with the dose and choice of medication matched to pain intensity. Pain severity is determined by listening to the patient's report of pain and observing the

degree of relief obtained from previously administered drugs.

As part of the Worldwide Cancer Pain Relief Programme, the World Health Organization (WHO 1986) has advocated a three-step analgesic ladder. This concept is illustrated in Figure 11.4. However, in patients with very severe pain, it may be necessary to administer high doses of strong opioids initially, with or without other adjuvant drugs. The European Association for Palliative Care Expert Working Group (1996) has produced some useful guidelines for the use of morphine in cancer pain. Once control has been established, it is possible to maintain effective pain relief but with lower doses or different combinations of drugs.

Principles of therapy

1. *Use the oral route whenever possible*. The oral administration of opioids gives more consistent and prolonged analgesia, and avoids the toxicity that may occur with parenteral administration. The oral route eliminates parenteral injections, enables the patient to maintain control of the drugs and allows mobility for home care and travel. However, when injections are required, subcutaneous administration of morphine, either continuously via a syringe driver or

Drugs
See chapter 2.3

Figure 11.4 Analgesic ladder. NSAIDs, non-steroidal anti-inflammatory drugs.

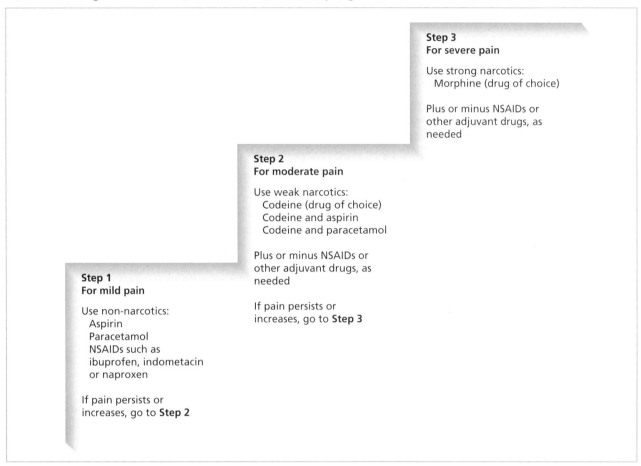

Step 3
For severe pain

Use strong narcotics:
  Morphine (drug of choice)

Plus or minus NSAIDs or
other adjuvant drugs, as
needed

Step 2
For moderate pain

Use weak narcotics:
  Codeine (drug of choice)
  Codeine and aspirin
  Codeine and paracetamol

Plus or minus NSAIDs or
other adjuvant drugs, as
needed

If pain persists or
increases, go to **Step 3**

Step 1
For mild pain

Use non-narcotics:
  Aspirin
  Paracetamol
  NSAIDs such as
  ibuprofen, indometacin
  or naproxen

If pain persists or
increases, go to **Step 2**

by regular intermittent injection, should be used in preference to the intramuscular route as it is much less painful for the patient.

2. *'Round the clock' dosing.* Most narcotics have a duration of analgesic action of 4–6 hours; therefore, control of chronic pain requires 4–6 doses spaced equally throughout the 24-hour period.

3. *Never p.r.n.* Continuous pain requires continuous analgesia and the aim of therapy is to prevent the resurgence of pain rather than repeatedly to treat it. This anticipation breaks the vicious cycle of pain–despair–more pain which causes dose escalation. While p.r.n. orders may be needed for 'breakthrough' pain, the basis of control must be regular scheduling. The individual and family members will need advice and information about the rationale for using a preventive approach.

4. *Wake the patient.* A patient with chronic pain often sleeps despite severe pain. Sleep does not indicate pain control. On initiating therapy, the patient should be woken until pain has been consistently controlled for 2–3 days and their confidence has been restored. Once pain is well controlled, some centres give a larger dose at bedtime (e.g. one and a half times or

twice the daytime dose), often allowing the patient to sleep throughout the night free of pain.

5. *Titrate the dose individually.* There is no standard or set dose of opioids in cancer pain, and there is great variation between individuals in analgesic efficacy. The correct dose is that which gives pain relief for at least 3 hours, or preferably 4 hours or more. As pain changes through various stages of disease and treatment, the dosage must be adjusted to match pain intensity.

6. *Consult.* Consult with nursing and medical experts in pain management when usual interventions are unsatisfactory and before pain becomes intractable.

Co-analgesics

Several drugs, while not true analgesics in the pharmacological sense, act to relieve pain, either alone or in combination with analgesics. These co-analgesics may be used in the treatment of all types of cancer pain but are particularly important for pain that is relatively unresponsive to morphine. Even when a narcotic is being used, the addition of a co-analgesic may often result in better pain control with fewer side-effects. Examples of co-analgesics include the steroids (e.g. prednisolone, dexamethasone), major tranquillizers (e.g. haloperidol) and tricyclic antidepressants (e.g. amitriptyline).

It should be noted that, to gain effective relief, the required dosage for all drugs may be much higher than that which doctors and nurses are accustomed to prescribing and administering in other areas of clinical practice.

Non-pharmacological measures

Cancer pain usually requires systemic analgesic therapy. However, in many situations non-drug measures may be extremely important adjuncts. Box 11.15 lists some of the

---

Box 11.15 Co-analgesics and non-pharmacological measures in cancer pain

For bone pain

- Full doses of non-steroidal anti-inflammatory drugs (e.g. indometacin, diclofenac, naproxen, aspirin), if tolerated

- Radiotherapy – usually to specific sites of localized metastasis, but in widespread disease upper or lower hemi-body irradiation may be given

- Bisphosphonates (e.g. pamidronate, clodronate).

For nerve compression

- Corticosteroids

- Anaesthetic nerve blocks

- Transcutaneous electrical nerve stimulation (TENS).

For nerve destruction

- Anticonvulsants

- Tricyclic antidepressants (e.g. amitriptyline)

- Corticosteroids

- Nerve blocks/epidural blocks

- TENS.

Other modalities

- Positioning

- Massage, warm or cold compresses

- Air fluidized therapy (e.g. Clinitron bed)

- Physiotherapy and occupational therapy; collars, corsets, splints, slings (for extra support), elastic stockings, compression cuffs transfer aids, walking aids, hydrotherapy, etc.)

- Distraction, relaxation, imagery.

(Note: The response to these modalities may be limited when used alone, but they can be useful when most pain has been controlled by other means, as above.)

---

co-analgesic and non-pharmacological measures that may be helpful in relieving cancer pain.

It is very important periodically to reassess the adequacy of pain control and to consider reasons for loss of previously adequate pain control. Cancer pain is seldom static: new pains develop and old pains re-emerge. Changes in the site or intensity of pain require thorough reassessment and review, not just an increase in the dose of the current analgesia.

Control of opioid side-effects

Constipation

If not carefully monitored and prevented, **constipation** may be just as difficult to control as the pain itself. The constipation associated with opioids occurs because the morphine binds to receptors in the gastrointestinal tract, causing decreased peristalsis and diminished secretions (Cimprich 1985, Campbell et al 2001). In patients with

---

Box 11.16 Management of common side-effects associated with narcotic analgesics

Constipation

- Record bowel movements daily

- Rectal examination to rule out impaction (in presence of diarrhoea or faecal incontinence, this also rules out overflow impaction)

- Start patients on a bowel regimen containing appropriate doses of bowel stimulants and faecal softeners but avoid bulk laxatives

- Maintain adequate fluid intake; encourage prune and other fruit juices if liked

- Provide increased fibre in patient's diet as tolerated.

Nausea and vomiting

- Pre-empt nausea. Use an appropriate antiemetic with every dose, or every other dose, of narcotic

- Nausea is worst when beginning narcotics and as the dose is increased. Once a stable dose has been reached, antiemetic medication may be decreased.

Sedation

- Sometimes this is a difficult side-effect to avoid

- The patient/family should be taught that transient sedation frequently occurs when opioids are commenced

- Continuing drowsiness may indicate a need to decrease narcotic dose or change to less sedating co-analgesics (e.g. anti-inflammatory agent).

Constipation
See chapter 5.1

cancer, decreased liquid intake, less exercise and a low-fibre diet all aggravate the problem. As in pain control, the aim of bowel care should be to prevent rather than treat the problem. Some suggestions for preventing and managing this problem are given in Box 11.16.

Nausea and vomiting

When opioids are initiated, **nausea and vomiting** may occur as a side-effect. When a person is first started on oral morphine, a prescription for an antiemetic should be obtained in case nausea or vomiting should develop. The risk of nausea and vomiting often decreases a week or two after morphine is started, so that for some people the antiemetic may be phased out.

Drowsiness and sedation

When morphine is initiated, transient sedation frequently occurs. This is partly a direct drug effect on the CNS, but the exhaustion and sleep deprivation as a result of chronic pain are other major factors. When pain is finally relieved, the patient may sleep for long periods, but general drowsiness usually clears 2–5 days after a steady dose is achieved. Continuing drowsiness may indicate a need to decrease the dose and/or add less sedating co-analgesics. Sedation may also be a sign of disease progression and not always a side-effect of therapy.

Management of oncological emergencies

Patients with cancer of all types may present with emergency conditions related to their disease or treatment. The appropriate management will depend upon the nature of the underlying disease, previous therapy and likely long-term prognosis (Falk and Fallon 1997).

Tumour lysis syndrome

Tumour lysis syndrome can occur in the treatment of tumours that have a large number of tumour cells, such as acute leukaemia or lymphoma, which are very sensitive to chemotherapy. As large numbers of malignant cells are killed by the chemotherapy, cell lysis releases large amounts of nucleic acids and intracellular ions into the bloodstream. This can cause *hyperuricaemia* (raised levels of uric acid in the blood) which, when excessive, leads to *hyperuricaemic nephropathy* and severely affects renal function. Other metabolic imbalances such as hyperkalaemia, hyperphosphataemia and hypocalcaemia may also occur as a result of massive cell lysis. Additional risk factors exist for those who are over the age of 65 years, those who have pre-existing renal disease, and those who are being treated with nephrotoxic drugs.

Prophylactic treatment includes careful monitoring of renal function and biochemical parameters in conjunction with increased fluid administration, diuresis, alkalinization of the urine and administration of the drug allopurinol.

Hypersensitivity reactions

Hypersensitivity reactions may occur in response to some chemotherapeutic agents. The agents that most commonly produce hypersensitivity reactions are bleomycin and L-asparaginase. Patients with lymphoma who are receiving bleomycin are more likely to have hypersensitivity reactions than non-lymphoma patients, and in about 6% of cases these may be as severe as an *anaphylactic reaction*. L-Asparaginase produces mild reactions in about 25% of patients, but about one-third of patients will have more severe reactions after they have had five doses or more. Intramuscular administration of L-asparaginase has been shown to decrease the incidence of hypersensitivity reactions. The administration of test doses for bleomycin and L-asparaginase to assess patient sensitivity is recommended.

Hypercalcaemia

Hypercalcaemia is a potentially fatal metabolic condition that occurs in approximately 8–20% of patients with cancer (Dietz and Flaherty 1990). Hypercalcaemia is caused by increased bone resorption, which results from tumour invasion of bone, increased levels of parathyroid hormone, prostaglandin or osteoclast-activating factor. Patients at greatest risk are those with bone metastases (commonly from breast, prostate, lung or renal tumours) which cause extensive bone destruction and release of calcium into the extracellular fluid.

The effects of hypercalcaemia in the body are seen in the gastrointestinal, neuromuscular, cardiac and renal systems. Gastrointestinal changes include anorexia, nausea, vomiting, constipation, abdominal pain and dehydration. Neuromuscular changes are confusion, lethargy, convulsion and hyporeflexia. The heart may be affected, leading to rhythm disturbances such as bradycardia and tachycardia. Polyuria, polydipsia and renal failure are signs of renal dysfunction (Heys et al 1998). Diagnostic studies will show a raised serum calcium level (normal values 2.13–2.63 mmol/L). A calcium level of 3.25 mmol/L requires emergency interventions, which include:

- rapid hydration, in order to promote renal excretion of calcium, and diuretic therapy

- intravenous mithramycin, which inhibits osteoclast activity

- calcitonin, which inhibits bone resorption and promotes urinary excretion

- bisphosphonates (e.g. pamidronate, clodronate, etidronate), which inhibit the release of bone calcium

- steroids, which decrease the release of cytokines that can stimulate osteoclastic activity

Oral phosphate may be used to control chronic or mild hypercalcaemia.

Nausea and vomiting
See chapter 5.1

Hypercalcaemia
See chapter 2.6

Specific nursing care measures are related to prescribed treatment regimens and include close monitoring of intake and output, weight, oedema, respiratory distress, confusion and disorientation, maintenance of personal hygiene and elimination, and the overall enhancement of comfort.

The urgency of the treatment depends not only on the serum calcium level but also on an assessment of the individual's general health, symptoms and overall prognosis. In some circumstances, acute treatment may not be appropriate, and treatment and care will be related to effective symptom control and helping the patient and family to cope with issues related to death and dying. As current rehydration regimens are shorter than previously, patients will spend less time in an acute setting. This may be an advantage for many patients, particularly those with a poor prognosis, but it also makes significant care demands on family and community-based services. Monitoring of early signs and symptoms of recurrence of hypercalcaemia is an important aspect of care, and patients, families and carers will need advice and information regarding significant signs and symptoms. An oral fluid intake of 3 litres per day is required to maintain hydration and promote the excretion of calcium. Assessment of practical and social support requirements, and liaison with other care agencies, is necessary to ensure that patients and family feel secure and supported.

Spinal cord compression

Spinal cord compression is caused by either primary or, more frequently, secondary tumours which lead to vertebral destruction and compression of the spinal cord or cauda equina. The resultant impairment of venous return and arterial flow leads to ischaemia and subsequent destruction of neurological tissue.

Metastatic spinal tumours of the breast, lung and prostate are the most common cancers causing cord compression, accounting for over 50% of instances (Heys et al 1997). Signs and symptoms include central back pain close to the site of compression which is not relieved by lying down, motor weakness (weakness, foot drop, ataxia), sensory loss (paraesthesia, numbness, tingling), and abnormal bladder and bowel sphincter control. The degree of sensory and motor loss is dependent on the level of the cord compression. Diagnosis is made through both clinical signs and radiological investigation.

Early detection is important, and treatment must be instituted rapidly to preserve as much neurological function as possible. Radiation therapy, surgical decompression or a combination of both may be recommended. Steroids are used immediately after diagnosis to decrease inflammation, relieve pain and increase neurological function. Chemotherapy may be used for extremely chemosensitive tumours (e.g. lymphomas), where a rapid effect may be seen.

Nursing care includes monitoring and evaluation of neurological status (sensory and motor function), vital signs and degree of pain. Assistance with self-care may be necessary if the patient is experiencing motor and sensory deficits. Assessment of skin integrity and the institution of measures to prevent skin breakdown are essential in patients experiencing sensory and motor deficits. Maintenance of regular bowel habits may require starting a bowel maintenance regimen (laxatives, suppositories). Loss of voluntary micturition control may result in distension, retention, urinary overflow and urinary tract infections. Patients may require intermittent catheterization if unable to void. Checking of residual urine after voiding is necessary. Rehabilitation following the acute phase may be indicated if the patient suffers permanent deficits.

Superior vena cava obstruction

Superior vena cava obstruction is a rare but distressing complication of primary or secondary disease in the thoracic cavity. Pressure from tumours or enlarged lymph nodes causes partial or complete obstruction of the vena cava, resulting in venous congestion in the head, arms and upper chest. The onset is usually insidious with increasing breathlessness, feelings of fullness in the head and neck, and upper body swelling. As the symptoms become more acute there may be stridor, cough, hoarseness, facial swelling and progressive cyanosis, a situation that is distressing and frightening for patient, family and carers. Radiotherapy is often the treatment of choice, and usually starts with one or more high doses followed by a course of lower doses, depending on tumour histology and clinical signs. Chemotherapy may be useful for chemosensitive tumours and is often used in combination with radiotherapy (Stewart 1996).

Nursing care is related to assistance with medical interventions, the alleviation of symptoms, and the provision of information and psychological support.

Other emergencies

Other emergencies may occur related to the cardiovascular system (e.g. cardiac tamponade, pericarditis). Erosion of major arteries may result in sudden catastrophic haemorrhage unless vascular surgery can be undertaken very swiftly.

A rare but life-threatening and distressing emergency is that of upper airway obstruction. Gradual onset may be followed by symptoms of acute breathlessness and stridor. A combination of radiotherapy and steroids is usually the most effective form of treatment, or possibly laser therapy to an obstructing lesion in the trachea.

In any such emergency, a combination of efficient clinical skills and a calm, empathic approach is required to help alleviate the distress and anxiety of the patient and the concerns of family and friends.

Spinal cord
See chapter 2.2

Superior vena cava
See chapter 4.2

Common issues in coping with cancer

Coping with cancer is a complex, multidimensional and ongoing process for the person with cancer and their family. From discovery of disease, through complex treatment regimens, rehabilitation and dying, many challenges are faced by individuals and their caregivers. There is an increasing awareness that, in addition to quality medical care, patients need emotional care and support and an opportunity to express feelings and responses to the experience of cancer (Barraclough 1994). An individual's perception of the threat posed by their disease is an important factor in determining their adjustment to it. It is possible that a positive mental attitude may have a significant effect on disease outcome, particularly in patients with early non-metastatic cancers (Greer et al 1990). Overall, there is an increasing recognition of and interest in the interaction of mind and body and the related responses of the immune system. This has given rise to the evolving study of *psychoneuroimmunology* (PNI).

Grief and loss

Grieving by the person with cancer may be due to the loss of a body part or body function, loss of independence, loss of role in the family and/or society, and the threat to life. The loss may be partial or complete, temporary or permanent, but the meaning to the individual will to a large extent depend on personal beliefs, characteristics and circumstances. There is a great need to make sense of things and to find ways to adapt to the change and disruption to life, however devastating and fundamentally unacceptable. In advanced cancer, adjustment to imminent death is clearly a major focus of the grief, but other issues that cause distress may be related to the loss of independence or the effect that illness and death will have on the family. The work of Kubler-Ross (1973) has had a major influence on shaping thinking and understanding about grieving; five stages grieving are described:

1. denial
2. anger
3. bargaining
4. depression
5. acceptance.

It is recognized that these categories are neither mutually exclusive nor sequential, but rather that the individual may move between the stages identified. Behaviours characteristic of the various stages include: shock, disbelief, denial, crying, rage, frustration, anger, sorrow, detachment, acceptance, calmness, and return to realistic functioning and reattachment. Similarly, individuals do not necessarily move through these phases progressively or within a given period of time but fluctuate in their reactions, varying in the time spent in any given phase.

This model has been criticized as being oversimplistic and too focused on the ultimate goal of 'acceptance' – the implication being that if this is not achieved, the person has somehow failed. In later writings, the model has been refined into three stages – initial, chronic and acceptance – and the acceptance is now viewed as desirable, not essential. The danger of labelling of behaviours in this way is that it may lead to stereotyping of patient responses and superficial understanding of complex phenomena. However, it does provide a framework for guiding understanding of what is happening to the individual and their significant others.

The extent to which there is *openness* about progress and care management issues at all stages of the cancer journey may vary considerably depending on the individual practitioners involved and the practice and culture of the care environment. In particular, the transition from active and palliative care and communication about death and dying still appear to be very challenging for many nurses and doctors. In their early and significant work, Glaser and Strauss (1968) proposed the concept of the 'dying trajectory' and the notions of certain and uncertain death at known or unknown times. The extent to which imminent death was acknowledged or discussed, they described as 'open' or 'closed' awareness and this was perceived to be orchestrated and maintained by staff. As a result, the support required by individual patients to develop effective coping styles was often not forthcoming. Although there has been a move towards a much greater climate of openness since this time, it is still an area of complexity and difficulty, and it is therefore not surprising that nurses may find such communication problematic (Wilkinson 1991). However, providing opportunities for listening, quiet discussion and the use of touch may help the individual to express feelings of grief, sorrow, anger or frustration.

Grieving is a normal process that requires understanding and support, but rarely direct intervention. Counselling and help from skilled, experienced workers may be necessary when grieving is delayed or one stage is prolonged, or the patient is not able to resolve grief. Problems may also arise when the patient and family members are at different stages of the grieving process at a given time. They may require help to understand the responses and feelings of one another and why conflicting emotions are occurring.

Need for information and knowledge

Advances in cancer treatment are encouraging: patients are living longer and the occurrence and duration of remissions of the disease are increasing. The period of hospitalization for most people with cancer is relatively short in relation to the overall illness experience. Responsibility for day-to-day care then rests to a large extent with the individual and the family, who require knowledge, skills and resources to manage the person's home care successfully. Understanding of the care plan and reasons for it also facilitates patient and family participation in decision making regarding treatment and care, and provides them with a sense of control and involvement in what is happening to them.

A teaching plan for health management needs to take into account the patient's and family's perspectives. What are their major concerns about hospital and home-care management? What knowledge and skills do they possess? What resources exist within the family and neighbourhood? What healthcare and social services are available in the community? How does the patient learn best? What barriers exist to learning?

Teaching sessions need to include supervised practice of care as well as information giving, so that the appropriate knowledge and skills are developed to enable procedures to be carried out safely and effectively.

Written information given to the patient and family enhances learning and facilitates recall. The use of videos, slides and pictures helps the patient and family to envisage a technique or problem being discussed. Group sessions may be useful to provide basic information and to promote sharing and discussion of experiences, but all patients and families require some individualized sessions to explore issues that are unique to their particular situation.

An assessment and evaluation of home circumstances needs to be undertaken and referral to the primary care team other agencies where appropriate. In most areas, specialist nursing services and hospital or community-based symptom control teams are available to advise and support patients and the staff involved in home care. Volunteers may be able to assist with transport, social visits and day-to-day activities.

Sexual and reproductive changes

The experience of cancer and its subsequent treatment inevitably affects an individual's sexuality to a greater or lesser extent. This may be as a result of altered body structure and function resulting from the disease process and/or therapy; change in self-concept, body image or sense of attractiveness; lack of knowledge or understanding of the effects of treatment/disease; and prolonged hospitalization and its associated lack of privacy.

Reproductive capabilities will be directly affected if there is surgical removal of the uterus, ovaries or testes, but surgery that involves the colon, rectum and genito-urinary structures may also cause physiological changes such as impotence, retrograde or lack of ejaculation, dyspareunia, sterility and decreased libido. Chemotherapy and radiotherapy can cause changes in function in relation to sexual response, fertility and fetal development. Sperm banking can be offered to men whose treatment plan may result in sterility. Effective birth control should be used during treatment and for 2 years after treatment to avoid teratogenic effects of treatment.

Fatigue, pain, decreased physical mobility, sterility, impotence and alterations in body structures resulting from the cancer or therapy may be barriers to sexual expression. Confrontation with a potentially fatal disease may expose previous sexual and relationship difficulties, but it can also provide an opportunity for couples and individuals to reassess their values and relationship (McElveen-Hoehn and McCorkle 1985). They may find that sexual expression enhances the feelings of being alive and human, and that it may serve to allay fears and provide comfort to both partners.

Open communication regarding sexuality is enhanced when trust and respect are part of the nurse–patient relationship. Unfortunately there is evidence to suggest that, whilst ideally placed, many nurses are often embarrassed or uncomfortable in discussing aspects of sexuality (Wilson and Williams 1988). Continuing professional development could provide opportunities for nurses to explore personal feelings and constraints, and develop effective approaches in this sensitive area.

General approaches that are helpful are:

- conveying a willingness to discuss the topic and providing privacy

- exploring physical and psychological issues related to disease and treatment

- providing accurate and manageable information and correcting any misinformation

- using open questions to explore and elicit fears and concerns.

Some patients and their partners may require specific information on measures available to compensate for the changes resulting from the disease or treatment (e.g. use of a lubricating gel when vaginal secretions are decreased; alternative positions and ways of expressing physical love). Complex problems may be referred to an appropriate specialist who can provide counselling and support for the patient and partner.

Altered body image and self-concept

Physical changes may result from the cancer itself, surgical removal of a body part, or the effects of chemotherapy or radiation treatment. The loss of a limb, a mastectomy, mandibular resection, loss of hair, changes in skin pigmentation, skin rashes and weight loss are examples of visible changes in the body with which many cancer patients are faced. Body image is concerned with both body perception and body attitudes (Cronan 1993, Rafferty 1995).

Actual changes in body structure and function can be assessed objectively, but how the individual perceives these changes and how they influence his or her responses is entirely subjective and thus difficult to measure. The patient with a disturbance in body image may exhibit:

- decreased socialization

- denial of the changes and avoidance of looking at the affected body part or of looking into a mirror

- refusal to touch the affected part
- avoidance of physical contact with close family members or friends
- expression of fears of rejection
- expression of feelings of hopelessness and helplessness
- preoccupation with the change.

Grieving for the lost part or previous physical appearance occurs before the patient can adjust to the changes, whether they are temporary, permanent, actual or perceived. Acceptance and understanding of this and exploration of the meaning of the loss to the individual concerned will be helpful in establishing rapport and empathy.

The cause of the physical changes and what may be expected should be explained and personal fears and concerns explored. Practical suggestions as to how physical changes and appearance may be managed are useful and these may involve the use of make-up, wearing a wig, or clothing cover defects or scars, so long as this is acceptable to them. However, over-concentration on practicalities may conceal the need to explore and develop more cognitive strategies to deal with the loss and facilitate adjustment. Moorey and Greer (1989) advocate the notion of 'adjuvant' psychological therapy to provide individuals with a different range of skills and support in order to sustain the impact of disease and treatment.

Other practitioners advocate the value of therapeutic touch and in particular massage therapy in helping individuals to experience their body in a more positive way, particularly those who have undergone mutilating surgery (Corner et al 1995b).

Psychosocial and emotional responses to cancer

The experience of cancer may evoke a range of complex emotional and behavioural responses, and some common experiences and suggestions for interventions are outlined in this section. Good communication and interpersonal skills will always be effective in developing empathy and enhancing patient care. However, some patient needs may be beyond the experience of the general nurse and the need for specialist help should be recognized and facilitated.

Anger and hostility

Anger is a common and appropriate response to the insults imposed by cancer and its treatment on bodily and personal integrity. Anger can have enormous adaptive value, allowing patients to mobilize inner resources of strength, determination and hope. Adaptive anger is generally not directed at anyone in particular. Dysfunctional anger, on the other hand, is more diffuse and intense, and may feel out of control to the patient. Dysfunctional expressions of anger may include self-destructive behaviour, refusal of treatment, and displacement on to family members, healthcare providers and others. Such exaggerated anger can isolate the patient from important sources of personal support. Providing quality nursing care to an angry patient is not easy and nurses may become afraid and defensive, and withdraw. This increases the patient's anger and a vicious circle begins. The patient manifesting anger is not likely to feel grateful or express gratitude for the care given and it can be difficult to accept and tolerate the anger and work with the patient to clarify and validate its sources. However, because anger is usually a defence against deeper feelings of hurt and fear, an understanding of this will enable nurses to work gently and compassionately towards strategies for resolution.

The patient needs to be encouraged to move beyond the anger to problem-solving strategies in order to cope with the situation that caused the feelings; however, these actions will not magically eliminate the patient's feelings of anger. The patient will continue to need to express anger as it is experienced.

Some patients are so angry that trust is not possible. This usually occurs when the anger is not dealt with and a very unhealthy system of interaction develops. Some patients have had such negative experiences in other institutions or situations that trust develops very slowly, if at all. Giving as much choice and control as possible, rather than setting strict limits, and providing continuity of care via a named nurse or key worker may be helpful.

Anxiety and fear

Anxiety has been described, with depression, as the most common psychosocial reaction experienced by persons with cancer (Lynch 1995). Anxiety is an unpleasant feeling of dread, and may be caused by an unconscious conflict between an underlying drive and the reality of the environment. The anxious person is unaware of the specific cause of his or her feelings. Anxiety is a different emotion from fear. Fear is an unpleasant feeling caused by a threat in the environment that is specific and can be identified.

Patients with cancer are justifiably fearful and anxious about many things: pain, death, abandonment, dependency, recurrence. Some fears are based on inaccurate information and can be relieved by providing that information. Other fears, such as the anticipation of unrelieved pain, require exploration and reassurance where possible, along with a description of measures that will be taken to provide for the relief of pain.

Death is a real possibility for many patients and, as identified above, both staff and patients may find it difficult to discuss death openly. Anxieties about the actuality of death are hard to allay, but the anxiety may be related more to the process of dying than to death itself. Patients may fear that they will be abandoned, and exploration of particular fears and concerns, along with information about services and facilities available, may be helpful.

Depression

Depression, sadness, despair and hopelessness in response to losses can be thought of as natural consequences of the actual or potential disruption of a close attachment or important goals. As cancer represents the potential loss of not only life, but also of body parts and functions, roles and relationships, depression has been identified as one of the most common responses to cancer.

The depressed patient often moves, thinks and speaks slowly; motivation and energy are often very low. Patients who are extremely depressed have little desire or energy to express feelings or make decisions.

People tend to either avoid the depressed person or attempt to 'cheer them up' with happy, bubbly, enthusiastic talk: both actions may drive patients further within themselves. A better strategy is to try to encourage patients to talk about their thoughts and feelings. If very withdrawn, remaining silently with the patient for periods interspersed throughout the day can sometimes be helpful.

Sometimes patients can feel very depressed and conceal the feeling behind a facade of 'normal' happy behaviour. This type of depression is a serious drain on the patient's available energy. Signs of this depression will be much more subtle but many of these patients admit to feeling depressed if asked. One of the difficulties in detecting depression in people with cancer is disentangling the symptoms of depression from those of the disease or its treatment.

Various forms of psychological therapy, with or without antidepressant medication, may be used to manage depression. For some individuals, a sense of greater well-being may be induced through use of complementary therapies such as massage, art therapy, reflexology or relaxation.

Uncertainty and loss of control

The uncertainty and predictability of the course of terminal illness can create enormous stresses. Most people are accustomed to a certain amount of predictability in their daily lives and in the way their bodies function. Cancer creates havoc. How will treatment turn out? When will new symptoms develop? How and when will death come? Uncertainty places enormous constraints and demands on the patient.

The feeling that one's internal environment is out of control often generates a frightening sensation of helplessness and vulnerability. Deep shame may arise from concerns about loss of physiological control. Some patients fear that they will not be able to control their emotions under the stress of cancer.

Serious illness such as cancer often serves to diminish, at least temporarily, a patient's sphere of control. In addition, the patient is often required to give up certain usual roles and responsibilities and to accept the care of others. For patients whose self-esteem and sense of personal worth derives from attending to others, the need to be taken care of may cause great conflict. In addition, work, finances and family issues may be negotiated without the patient's involvement. It is hard for individuals to maintain any sense of 'health' when being treated for cancer, even when the treatment is aimed at cure. McWilliam et al (1996) explored the effectiveness of a health promotion intervention for people with chronic illnesses, including cancer, and found that individuals employed a number of strategies to promote a sense of health. These included drawing on friends and family, maintaining a sense of control, and reframing expectations of life and self.

Family issues

The patient's family suffers as a result of temporary or permanent changes in the patient's capacity to fulfil family and career roles, the increased stress on family members, role transitions, and changes in responsibilities.

Northouse's review (1984b) of the impact of cancer on the family provides a framework for understanding family responses and problems in coping with cancer. In the *initial phase* the three major potential problems for family members are: (1) feeling excluded from the receiving of care and participation in care; (2) communication with hospital staff and others; and (3) managing emotional distress. Family members may feel despair, isolation, vulnerability and helplessness, uncertainty, confusion and shock (Hilton 1993, Northouse and Peters-Golden 1993). Feeling excluded from care may occur as professional caregivers focus on the care of the patient. Families may encounter difficulty in obtaining information from professionals and are frequently in the position of having to initiate contact and requests for information. Communication within the family may be affected as it is common that family members are unsure how to discuss a diagnosis of cancer and their concerns. Emotional tension in the family may be exhibited by anxiety, agitation or guilt. A sense of helplessness and loss of control is common at this time.

During the *adaptation phase* the family deals with adjusting to changes in roles and lifestyles, meeting the needs of well family members, and living with uncertainty. Changing role responsibilities in the family may cause the patient to feel dependent on others and to worry about being a burden, while other family members may have had little preparation to assume homemaking or extended parenting roles. Financial resources may be affected by the loss of ability to work. The needs of well family members may be neglected because of the focus on the ill member. Coping with uncertainty about the future is a challenge for all family members. Some families may have open communication about fears and uncertainties, whereas others may be closed in order to try to prevent worry.

During the *terminal phase* the family deals with communicating about death among family members, providing care and support to the dying person, and dealing with feelings of loss and separation. Very little discussion about death may occur among family members, which may be an effective coping mechanism for some people.

Caring for the dying family member may cause considerable strain on the family in terms of physical care and emotional support. Families have learning needs in terms of physical aspects of care, pain control and increased dependency. Feelings of grief and loss are paramount in this phase. Family members may feel helpless, abandoned and anxious.

Intervention strategies for families fall into three categories (Northouse 1984b):

1. assessing the needs of the family members

2. providing support to families

3. providing families with information and assistance.

The family can be informed of available community resources for patient care and social services. Referral for counselling may be appropriate when the family is facing long-term disruption and when the ability of the family to cope is actually or potentially inadequate. Family members are encouraged to seek help from those they consider to be helpful and appropriate for them. Continuing help and support should be readily available from the nurse, doctor, social worker, pastoral counsellor, hospital chaplain, friends and relatives. Continuity in those giving care does much to facilitate communication and long-term planning.

It is important that family members spend time together as well as resuming socialization outside the home. In the hospital setting, measures are taken to provide privacy and opportunity for the family to be together as a unit.

Care of the patient with advanced cancer

The care of the patient with advanced cancer in the terminal phase of their disease is directed towards the relief of symptoms and improving the quality of life, as opposed to quantity of life. Palliative care seeks to provide a holistic approach, focusing not only on the physical symptoms of disease but the psychosocial and spiritual needs of the patient as well, and extending this care to the family and significant others. Care may be provided within an institution (i.e. hospital, nursing home, or hospice) or within the home. Increasingly, patients may experience care in all these settings at various times, depending on symptoms and therapy needs, and the availability of support systems and carers.

There are a number of symptoms that are common to patients with advanced disease, related largely to alterations in comfort and physical or psychosocial distress. *Pain* is a factor for many people with advanced cancer, but Twycross (1997) identified that, although 75% of people admitted to a hospice reported pain, 25% did not. However, pain is feature of terminal phase of illness for many people to a greater or lesser extent, and increasing severity of pain may be perceived as signifying advance of the cancer. The pain contributes to the physiological and psychological factors that, in turn, enhance its severity. Loss of sleep and rest due to pain increases the patient's fatigue. Anorexia, nausea and vomiting associated with the pain contribute to nutritional deficiencies and weight loss. Mobility is restricted by the pain, increasing the potential for skin breakdown, constipation, muscle weakness and chest complications. The patient may exhibit anxiety, irritability, anger and withdrawal. Adequate pain control requires the cooperative efforts of the patient and the care team, and is a central goal of palliative care.

Opioid drugs are usually the first choice for most forms of severe cancer pain, with or without other adjuvant drugs. Concurrent administration of oral laxatives and careful monitoring of bowel movements is necessary to avoid opioid-induced constipation. This largely avoidable condition is a cause of great distress to patients and is a common cause of admission to hospice or hospital.

Even in the terminal phase of disease, many pathological processes can be modified through the selective use of mainstream cancer therapies. Radiotherapy is particularly helpful for the treatment of bone pain and for reducing a tumour mass that is causing pain and pressure symptoms. Occasionally chemotherapy may be useful in reducing tumour bulk and associated pain, but the value of this would need to be weighed against side-effects such as hair loss, weakness and the general malaise associated with most forms of chemotherapy. Surgical interventions such as wound debridement, bypassing of abdominal obstruction, and the fixation of fractures are all commonly undertaken for patients with advanced disease. Again, careful consideration needs to be given to the possible consequences of such interventions, for instance anaesthetic risks, impaired healing due to malignancy and malnutrition, and full informed consent obtained.

People who are terminally ill respond and cope in a variety of ways. They are grieving for a range of actual and potential losses, while still trying to maintain hope. While the hope is not likely to be for a cure, hope remains to achieve short-term goals, to have a painless death, or to participate in a particular event or family occasion (Herth 1990, Fleming 1997).

Frequent *emotional responses* are denial, anxiety, fear, depression, withdrawal, acceptance, resignation and anger. Denial may assist the individual to protect himself or herself from the painful reality of dying and to preserve hope. There are certainly degrees of denial and, while it is a useful protective response, it may also interfere with problem solving and communication between patient and family or patient and caregivers. Fear is a response to perceived danger, whereas anxiety is a feeling of distress and discomfort. Sources of anxiety for the patient may be spiritual in nature, fear of death, or fear of the dying process and what may be ahead. The person may respond to a terminal illness by withdrawal and depression as he or she disengages from relationships and surroundings. Acceptance and resignation to disease may fluctuate over time. They are dynamic in nature and may be observed in concert with other responses. Sadness and a sense of aloneness may be apparent at this time. Anger may be felt in response to actual and expected losses, and sometimes to the helplessness that patients experience.

The experience of families caring for individuals in the terminal phase of illness were explored in a study by Addington-Hall and McArthur (1995). Families described a number of symptoms that caused distress to a greater or lesser extent, and pain was reported as being 'very distressing' for over 60%. Other items that caused distress were breathlessness, dry mouth or thirst, nausea and vomiting, loss of appetite, and constipation. Over half reported that they were unable to get all the information about their dying relative that they needed. Wright and Dyck (1984) identified that families want to be assured of patient comfort and may wish to be physically close to the dying person and to spend as much time as possible with them.

Davis and Oberle (1990) identified six dimensions of the role of the nurse in palliative care and described them as follows:

■ preserving integrity

■ valuing

■ connecting

■ finding meaning

■ doing for

■ empowering.

This study was based on the experience of a community-based palliative care nurse and as such represents the perception of the professional practitioner. Clearly the quality of the caring relationship is a key factor in facilitating effective palliative care, but family units will have their own coping styles and perception of needs and required services. For example, popularly held beliefs that nurses can assist patients by encouraging the sharing and ventilation of feelings, encouraging crying and talking about negative feelings may not be perceived as supportive behaviours by those they are supposed to help. This is not to say that the opportunity to express such feelings may not be of great value to certain individuals at certain times, but respect for privacy is equally important (Pedder 1995).

Following the death of a person at home, the withdrawal of previously frequent community nursing services may be an additional loss for those who are left to sustain. Continued visits by the community nurse may be helpful in re-establishing daily life and expressing grief. Referral to specialist bereavement counselling services may be appropriate for some individuals to provide support and guidance during the period of mourning and reorganization.

However, caring for people who are dying is extremely demanding and nurses need to be realistic about how far they can actually help and support family caregivers in their grief and loss. Strategies to prevent care fatigue and to foster positive personal coping behaviours need to be addressed at an individual and an organizational level (Mathers 1995).

Spiritual issues

Cawley (1997b), in a review of the concept of spirituality, suggests that it may be beyond standard definition or expression in words but involves the individual's attempt to find meaning and purpose in life and encompasses the concepts of faith, hope and love.

Kim et al (1984) view distress of the human spirit as a disruption in the life principle that pervades a person's entire being and that integrates and transcends their biological and psychological nature. Factors related to the spiritual distress of the patient with cancer may include: challenged belief and value system, loss of sense of purpose, a feeling of remoteness from God, loss of faith, questioning of moral–ethical nature of therapy, a sense of guilt or shame, intense mental suffering, unresolved feelings about death, and anger toward God (Kim and Moritz 1982).

Expression of distress of the human spirit is very individualized. Behaviours that may indicate spiritual distress include: struggles with the meaning of life and death, seeking of spiritual assistance, expressions of anger and/or guilt, crying, withdrawal, sleep disturbances, questioning the meaning of suffering, fear of ability to endure suffering, views of illness as a punishment from God, questioning or refusing therapy, and seeking unorthodox therapy (Kim and Moritz 1982).

Some patients may find the confrontation with their values and religious beliefs to be a rewarding and reassuring experience, but for others it may be a source of considerable distress. Helping a person to address the spiritual aspects of their life offers a unique but, for many, a very challenging opportunity. Burnard (1993) emphasizes the need for nurses to explore their own beliefs and understanding about spirituality before seeking to embark on this with others. The assessment of spiritual care needs is an important area of care, but Ross (1997) suggests that this is often neglected by nurses, possibly as a result of varying degrees of spiritual distress on their own account.

Recognizing spiritual distress in others should be within the scope of all nurses' professional practice, but realistically there may be different levels of comfort and expertise in encouraging the patient to express feelings of support or conflict related to spiritual needs. If the person has a particular religious observance, a religious adviser known and respected by the patient may be a more appropriate person to explore these issues. In general terms, the practice of religious observances can be facilitated by providing privacy for prayers or personal discussions, encouraging attendance at a place of worship, or arranging for visits and observances at the bedside.

Rehabilitation

Until recently, the term 'cancer rehabilitation' was seldom found in cancer nursing literature. Perhaps the view of cancer as a terminal disease has conflicted with the concept of rehabilitation. Often, little thought is given to rehabilitation of the patient with cancer compared with those with other conditions such as cardiac disease or stroke, with needs not therefore identified or resources allocated. However, improvements in early detection, treatment and supportive care have led to an increased number of people surviving and living with cancer.

Rehabilitation is a process that maintains or restores a person to an optimal level of functioning and effectiveness within the limitations of their disease or disability in terms of their physical, mental, emotional, social and economic potential. It affords an opportunity to redefine what is a meaningful life, and Dietz (1981) has identified four different phases of rehabilitation in cancer care.

The *preventive phase* may include such things as aggressive pulmonary hygiene to prevent pneumonia in a patient undergoing chemotherapy, or thorough, systematic oral care to decrease discomfort and the chance of infection with stomatitis. For a patient receiving radiotherapy, for example, preventive rehabilitation may also include teaching realistic expectations for daily energy expenditure so that unnecessary fatigue is avoided and the daily plan can meet the individual's priorities. In cases of bereavement, support can assist family members in integrating the loss within the larger context and re-establishing meaning in their lives.

The *restorative phase* of the rehabilitation process may include mobilization and prosthesis fitting after an amputation of a leg because of an osteosarcoma, or bowel and bladder management after a cord compression from spinal metastases. Bowel and bladder management after a colostomy or urostomy would also be restorative care as the individual learns to manage a new way of meeting elimination needs. Counselling can assist with adjustment to the changes imposed by illness, and family adjustment, and can restore a sense of self-esteem, coherence and emotional balance.

The *supportive phase* is characterized by persistence of the disease and the continuing need for treatment and supportive therapies. The goal of rehabilitation is to limit functional changes where possible and enable the individual to adapt to long-term symptoms such as breathlessness.

The *palliative phase* of the rehabilitation process includes those measures used to provide comfort, symptom control, emotional support and family support during the terminal phase of the illness.

A variety of disease and cancer treatment-related problems amenable to rehabilitation approaches have been identified, including decreased mobility, problems with activities of daily living (including weakness), pain, nutritional problems, financial and vocational problems, appearance, lymphoedema, respiratory difficulties, swallowing disorders, communication, transportation, and difficulties in individual and family psychological adjustment.

The rehabilitation team may include a doctor, rehabilitation nurse, specialist nurses (e.g. breast or stoma care nurse), physiotherapist, occupational therapist, speech therapist, orthotist, prosthetist, vocational counsellor, nutritionist, psychologist, social worker and minister of religion. Not every, or even most, patients will need all the resources available. However, it would seem likely that almost all people with cancer will need the services of at least one of the team members at some stage during the cancer experience.

Assessment of needs and goal setting are key aspects of rehabilitation, centred around an individual's functional ability. The aim is to foster independence through positive adaptation to the changing circumstances imposed by the disease or treatment.

The assessment and interventions relative to many of the rehabilitation needs of people with cancer have been addressed in other sections of this chapter. The principles and philosophy of rehabilitation should be an integral part of cancer care practice.

Survivorship

Early detection and effective multimodal therapies have increased significantly the numbers of cancer survivors. Historically, cancer survivors have been defined as individuals 'cured' of their disease, with the 'cured' state commencing 5 years after diagnosis. The burgeoning population of survivors has given emphasis to the need to address quality of survival and the psychosocial consequences of cancer and its treatment. Long-term survivors may experience problems ranging from minor short-term difficulties to major psychosocial crises.

Fear of recurrence is probably the most common concern for all cancer survivors. Fear of relapse may present in a variety of forms, ranging from general uneasiness about the aetiology of mild to moderate or intermittent symptoms, to pronounced anxiety that interferes with daily life. As time passes, anxiety concerning recurrence may decrease, although a heightened sense of vulnerability to illness is often a feature of the survivor's experience. Not knowing when and whether cancer will reappear often negatively affects the survivor's sense of control over his or her life (Burnet and Robinson 2000).

The need for close, ongoing evaluation after the cessation of therapy mandates an ongoing relationship between the patient and the healthcare team. These relationships may engender both ambivalence and anxiety. As patients are nearing the end of treatment, they may feel elated over the prospect of discontinuing therapy, while at the same time being fearful of distancing themselves from the team that has helped them to get to this extended survival stage. Fear of detecting recurrence or other problems can lead to hypochondriasis, avoidance of doctors and pronounced anxiety about attending follow-up examinations.

Attempts to minimize memories of the treatment experience and to return to usual life tasks may not be easy. The transition from a sick role to a healthy role may be challenged by physical symptoms, negative expectations from those within the patient's work and social circle, and social stigma. The survivor's family may also worry about the possibility of relapse and the difficulties of social reintegration, and may respond with over-protectiveness and pervasive anxiety. On the other hand, family members may be hesitant to discuss mutual concerns about the recurrence of cancer because these concerns can trigger their own sense of insecurity about the future. Many survivors encounter ongoing socio-economic impediments to full recovery, including difficulties regaining financial and work-related stability.

Because of the prevailing perception that cancer results in a painful, lingering death, most patients' immediate reaction to the diagnosis is the expectation of a shortened lifespan. Once successful completion of therapy is achieved, hope for continued survival often supersedes thoughts of death. Many survivors experience a greater appreciation of life, value reprioritization and a greater sense of generalized well-being as a reaction to the possibility of dying younger than expected.

The availability of wellness-oriented follow-up clinics, education, counselling and supportive services, as well as advocacy, community action and policy development, are crucial to the achievement of quality survival. Further research is required to identify needs, and to develop and evaluate model programmes encompassing both professional and peer support.

Summary

Although cancer remains a major healthcare problem and a very fearsome, isolating illness for the patient and family to confront individually, significant progress continues to be made in the diagnosis, treatment and control of the numerous forms of cancer. New approaches to early diagnosis of cancer, new techniques to treat cancer, new measures to ameliorate distressing manifestations of cancer and its treatment, and new approaches to improve the quality of life for cancer survivors will continue to emerge.

Cancer nursing is integral to all these developments (Krishnasamy 1996) and, as such, will continue to be one of the most challenging fields in health care. This chapter has sought to provide an overview of the nature, treatment and experience of cancer, and of the many ways in which nurses may be involved in providing care and supporting individuals at all stages of the cancer journey. As the body of scientific knowledge and nursing knowledge continues to expand, there are opportunities and requirements for nurses to maintain and develop their professional education and knowledge base. The Calman Hine Report (Department of Health 1995) identified the need for nurses involved in caring for people with cancer to be appropriately qualified, and subsequent directives regarding the standard for the accreditation of cancer services have specified the required qualifications and level of service provision.

Peer review and clinical audit provides an opportunity for nurses and other staff to evaluate and monitor service provision. Reflection on practice is an increasing feature of professional nursing, and Johns (1996) believes that reflection offers nurses an opportunity explore and develop greater understanding about the experience of practice and reaffirm caring values. As this could be a difficult or painful process at times, an effective system of clinical supervision needs to be available and accessible.

Recent policy initiatives have also led to the more widespread development of specialist nursing roles in various aspects of cancer care. In line with policy directives, these tend to be related to site-specific diseases (e.g. breast, lung, colorectal; gynaecology; head and neck), and the requirements of the roles may vary considerably depending on location and individual perceptions. However, a common feature of all is the increased level of support offered to people with cancer and the opportunity for nurses to pursue research and provide an evidence base for practice.

There is increasing interest in all aspects of practice development in cancer care, particularly that which actively involves the perceptions and experiences of healthcare users and specialist nurses in the research process (Krishnasamy and Plant 1998). Caring for people with cancer is complex and challenging but also extremely rewarding, as it offers so many opportunities to enhance the experience of patients undergoing treatment and also for personal and professional growth and development.

References

Addington-Hall J, McArthur M (1995) Dying from cancer – results of a national population-based investigation. Palliative Medicine 9: 295–305.

Ash DV (1999) Breast irradiation injury litigation and RAGE. Clinical Oncology 11: 138–139.

Barraclough J (1994) Cancer and emotion: a practical guide to psycho-oncology, 2nd edn. Chichester: Wiley.

Beaver K, Luker K, Glynn Owens R, Leinster SJ, Degner L (1996) Treatment decision making in women newly diagnosed with breast cancer. Cancer Nursing 19: 8–19.

Brant JM (1995) The use of access devices in cancer pain control. Seminars in Oncology Nursing 11: 203–212.

British Medical Association (1993) Complementary medicine: new approaches to good practice. London: BMA.

Burke C, Sikora K (1993) Complementary and conventional cancer care? The integration of two cultures. Clinical Oncology 5: 220–797.

Burnard P (1993) Giving spiritual care. Journal of Community Nursing 1: 16–18.

Burnet NG, Robinson L (2000) Psychosocial impact of recurrent cancer. European Journal of Oncology Nursing 4(1): 29–38.

Campbell J, Lane C (1996) Developing a skin-care protocol in radiotherapy. Professional Nurse 12(2): 105–108.

Campbell T, Draper S, Reid J, Robinson L (2001) The management of constipation in people with advanced cancer. International Journal of Palliative Nursing 7(3): 100–119.

Cancer Research Campaign (2001) Facts on cancer. London: CRC.

Cassileth BR, Lusk EJ, Guerry P et al (1991) Survival and quality of life among patients receiving unproven as compared with conventional cancer therapy. New England Journal of Medicine 324: 1180–1185.

Caudell K (1991) Graft-versus-host-disease. In: Whedon MB (ed.) Bone marrow transplantation: principles, practice and nursing insights, pp. 160–182. Boston: Jones and Barrett.

Cawley N (1997a) A critique of the methodology of research studies evaluating massage. European Journal of Cancer Care 6: 23–31.

Cawley N (1997b) An exploration of the concept of spirituality. International Journal of Palliative Care 3: 31–36.

Church JM (1996) Prophylactic colectomy in patients with hereditary nonpolyposis colectal cancer. Annals of Medicine 28: 479–482.

Cimprich B (1985) Symptom management: constipation. Cancer Nursing 8(1 Suppl): 39–43.

Corner J, Plant H, Warner L (1995a) Developing a nursing approach to managing dyspnoea in lung cancer. International Journal of Palliative Care Nursing 1: 5–11.

Corner J, Cawley N, Hildebrand S (1995b) An evaluation of the use of massage and massage with essential oils on the well-being of cancer patients. International Journal of Palliative Care Nursing 1: 67–73.

Cronan L (1993) Management of the patient with altered body image. British Journal of Nursing 2(5): 257–261.

Crouch MA, Ross JA (1994) Current concepts in autologous bone marrow transplantation. Seminars in Oncology Nursing 10(1): 12–19.

Davidson T, Sacks NPM (1995) Principles of surgical oncology. In: Horwich A (ed.) Oncology: a multidisciplinary textbook, pp. 101–115. London: Chapman & Hall.

Davis B, Oberle K (1990) The dimensions of the supportive role of the nurse in palliative care. Oncology Nursing Forum 17: 87–95.

Degner L, Russell A (1988) Preferences for treatment and control among adults with cancer. Research in Nursing and Health 11: 367–374.

Degner L, Khristjanson L, Bowman D et al (1997) Information needs and decisional preferences in women with breast cancer. Journal of the American Medical Association 112(18): 1485–1497.

De Wys WD (1985) Management of cancer cachexia. Seminars in Oncology 12: 452–460.

Dietz J (1981) Rehabilitation Oncology. New York: Wiley.

Dietz KA, Flaherty AM (1990) Oncologic emergencies. In: Groenwald SL, Frogge MH, Yarbro CH (eds). Cancer nursing: principles and practice, 2nd edn. Boston: Jones & Bartlett.

Department of Health (1995) A policy framework for commissioning cancer services. London: The Stationery Office.

Department of Health (2000) National cancer plan. London: The Stationery Office.

Dougherty L (1995) Scalp cooling to prevent hair loss in chemotherapy. Professional Nurse 11: 507–509.

Dougherty L, Viner C, Young J (1998) Establishing ambulatory chemotherapy at home. Professional Nurse 13: 356–358.

Dudjak L (1992) Cancer metastasis. Seminars in Oncology Nursing 8(1): 40–50.

Eardley A (1986) Expectations of recovery. Nursing Times 23 April: 53–54.

Eeles R (1995) Developments in the study of familial breast cancer. Nursing Times 91(5): 29–33.

Eilers J, Berger A, Petersen M (1988) Development, testing and application of the oral assessment guide. Oncology Nursing Forum 15(3): 325–330.

Ersser SJ (1995) Complementary therapies and nursing research: issues and practicalities. Complementary Therapies in Nursing and Midwifery 1: 144–150.

European Association of Palliative Care Expert Working Group (1996) Morphine in cancer pain: modes of administration. British Medical Journal 312: 823–826.

Falk S, Fallon M (1997) ABC of palliative care: emergencies. British Medical Journal 315: 1525–1528.

Fallowfield L (1998) Early discharge after surgery for breast cancer: might not be applicable to most patients. British Medical Journal 317: 1264–1265 (editorial).

Feber T (1995) Mouth care for patients receiving oral irradiation. Professional Nurse 10(10): 666–669.

Fleming K (1997) The meaning of hope in palliative care patients. International Journal of Palliative Care 3: 14–18.

Freedman TG (1994) Social and cultural dimensions of hair loss in women treated for breast cancer. Cancer Nursing 17: 334–341.

Ford D, Easton DF, Stratton MR et al (1998) Genetic heterogeneity and penetrance analysis of the *BRCA1* and *BRCA2* genes in breast cancer families. American Journal of Human Genetics 62: 676–689.

Foundation for Integrated Medicine (1997) Integrated healthcare: a way forward for the next five years? London: FIM.

Fraser MC, Tucker MA (1988) Late effects of cancer therapy: chemotherapy related malignancies. Oncology Nursing Forum 15(1): 67–77.

Gabriel J (1996) Peripherally inserted central catheters: expanding UK nurses' practice. British Journal of Nursing 5: 71–74.

Gamble K (1998) Communication and information: the experience of radiotherapy patients. European Journal of Cancer Care 5: 153–158.

Glasel M (1985) Cancer prevention: the role of the nurse in primary and secondary cancer prevention. Cancer Nursing 8(1 Suppl): 5–12.

Glaser B, Strauss AL (1968) Time for dying. Chicago: Aldine.

Gore M, Riches PM (eds) (1995) Immunotherapy of cancer. Oxford: Churchill Livingstone.

Greer S, Morris T, Pettingale KW, Haybrittle JL (1990) Psychological response to breast cancer and 15 year outcome. Lancet 335: 49–50.

Hall D (1995) New ideas on fractionation and accelerated radiotherapy. Nursing Times 91(12): 42–43.

Hanks GW (1995) Problem areas in pain and symptom management in advanced cancer patients. European Journal of Cancer Care 31a: 869–870.

Hartman LC, Shaid DJ, Woods JE et al (1999) Efficacy of bilateral prophylactic mastectomy in women with a family history of breast cancer. New England Journal of Medicine 340: 77–84.

Heller T, Davey B, Bailey L (1989) Reducing the risks of cancers. London: Hodder and Stoughton.

Hermanek O, Hutter RUP, Sobin LH, Wagner G, Wittlekind C (eds) (1997) UICC TMN atlas, 4th edn. Berlin: Springer.

Herth K (1990) Fostering hope in terminally ill people. Journal of Advanced Nursing 18: 538–548.

Heys SP, Currie D, Eremin O (1997) The management of patients with advanced cancer III. European Journal of Surgical Oncology 23: 361–365.

Heys SP, Smith IC, Eremin O (1998) Hyperkalcaemia in patients with cancer: aetiology and treatment. European Journal of Surgical Oncology 24: 139–142.

Hilton BA (1993) Issues, problems and challenges for families coping with breast cancer. Seminars in Oncology Nursing 9(2): 88–100.

How C, Brown J (1998) Extravasation of cytotoxic chemotherapy from peripheral veins. European Journal of Oncology Nursing 2: 51–58.

Johns C (1996) Visualising and realising caring in practice through guided reflection. Journal of Advanced Nursing 24: 1135–1143.

Jones R, Hansford J, Fiske J (1993) Death from cancer at home: the carer's perspective. British Medical Journal 306: 249–251.

Kim MJ, Moritz DA (eds) (1982) Classification of nursing diagnosis. New York: McGraw-Hill.

Kim MJ, McFarland GK, McLaine AM (1984) Pocket guide to nursing diagnosis. St Louis, MO: Mosby.

Krishnasamy M (1996) What do patients identify as supportive and unsupportive behaviours of nurses – a pilot study. European Journal of Cancer Care 5: 103–110.

Krishnasamy M, Plant H (1998) Developing nursing research with people. International Journal of Nursing Studies 35: 79–84.

Kubler-Ross E (1973) On death and dying. New York: Macmillan.

Lanceley A (1995) Wider issues in pain management. European Journal of Cancer Care 4: 153–157.

Langenhoff BS, Krabbe PFM, Wobbes T, Ruers TJM (2001) Quality of life as an outcome measure in surgical oncology. British Journal of Surgery 88(5): 643–652.

Lynch M (1995) The assessment and prevalence of affective disorders in advanced cancer. Journal of Palliative Care 11: 10–18.

Mallet J, Dougherty L (2000) The Royal Marsden manual of clinical nursing procedures, 5th edn. London: Blackwell Scientific.

Mathers P (1995) Learning to cope with the stress of palliative care. In: Penson J, Fisher R (eds) Palliative care for people with cancer, 2nd edn, pp. 296–308. London: Arnold.

McCaffrey M (1979) Nursing management of the patient with pain. Philadelphia: Lippincott.

McElveen-Hoehn P, McCorkle R (1985) Understanding sexuality in progressive cancer. Seminars in Oncology Nursing 1: 56–62.

McKie L (1993a) Women's views of the cervical smear test. Implications for nursing practice – women who have not had a smear. Journal of Advanced Nursing 18: 972–979.

McKie L (1993b) Women's views of the cervical smear test: implications for nursing practice – women who have had a smear. Journal of Advanced Nursing 18: 1228–1234.

McKusick V (1998) Mendelian inheritance in man. Baltimore, MD: Johns Hopkins University Press.

McWilliam CL, Stewart M, Brown JB, Desai K, Coderre P (1996) Creating health with chronic illness. Advances in Nursing Science 18: 1–15.

Montbriand MJ (1993) Freedom of choice: an issue concerning alternate therapies chosen by patients with cancer. Oncology Nursing Forum 20: 1195–1201.

Moorey S, Greer S (1989) Psychological therapy for patients with cancer: a new approach. Oxford: Heinemann Medical Books.

National Cancer Alliance (1996) 'Patient-centred services?' What patients say. Oxford: NCA.

Neill KM, Armstrong N, Burnet CB (1998) Choosing reconstruction after mastectomy – a qualitative analysis. Oncology Nursing Forum 25: 743–750.

Northouse L (1984a) Mastectomy patients and the fear of cancer recurrence. Cancer Nursing 4: 213–220.

Northouse L (1984b) The impact of cancer on the family: an overview. International Journal of Psychiatry in Medicine 14(3): 215–242.

Northouse LL, Peters-Golden H (1993) Cancer and the family: strategies to assist spouses. Seminars in Oncology Nursing 9(2): 74–82.

Pedder M (1995) The role of the nurse in bereavement care. Progress in Palliative Care 3: 219–223.

Rafferty D (1995) Body image: using women who have had breast surgery as a case study. International Journal of Palliative Nursing 1: 195–199.

Rhodes V, Johnson M, McDaniel R (1995) Nausea, vomiting and retching: the management of the symptom experience. Seminars in Oncology Nursing 11: 256–265.

Richardson A (1991) Theories of self-care; their relevance to chemotherapy-induced nausea and vomiting. Journal of Advanced Nursing 16: 671–676.

Richardson A (1992) Studies exploring self-care for the patient coping with cancer treatment: an overview. International Journal of Nursing Studies 29: 191–204.

Richardson A (1995) Fatigue in cancer patients: a review of the literature. European Journal of Cancer Care 4: 20–32.

Rieger PT (1995) Patient management. In: Rieger PT (ed.) Biotherapy. A comprehensive overview, pp. 195–220. Boston, MA: Jones and Bartlett.

Ross L (1997) The nurse's role in assessing and responding to patients' spiritual needs. International Journal of Palliative Care 3: 37–41.

Royal College of Nursing (1998) The administration of chemotherapy. Clinical practice guidelines. Oxford: RCN.

Saunders C, Baines M (1983) Living with dying. Oxford: Oxford University Press.

Slevin ML, Strubbs L, Plant HJ et al (1990) Attitudes to chemotherapy: comparing views of patients with cancer to those of doctors, nurses and the general public. British Medical Journal 300: 1458–1460.

Souhami R, Tobias J (1995) Cancer and its management, 2nd edn. Oxford: Blackwell Science.

Stewart IE (1996) Superior vena cava syndrome: an oncologic complication. Seminars in Oncology Nursing 12: 312–317.

Trevelyan J, Booth B (1994) Complementary medicine: for nurses, midwives and health visitors. London: Macmillan.

Twycross RG (1997) Introducing palliative care, 2nd edn. Oxford: Radcliffe.

Twycross RG, Lack S (1990) Therapeutics in terminal care. Edinburgh: Churchill Livingstone.

Urba SG, Forastiere AA, Wolf GT et al (1994) Intensive induction chemotherapy and radiation for organ preservation in patients with advanced resectable head and neck carcinoma. Journal of Clinical Oncology 12: 946–953.

Varmus H, Weinberg RA (1993) Clues to the origin of cancer. In: Varmus H, Weinberg RA. Genes and the biology of cancer, pp. 45–66.

Vile R (1995) The metastatic cascade. In: Vile R. Cancer metastasis: from mechanisms to therapy, pp. 1–20. Chichester: John Wiley.

Wickham R, Blesch KS, Paice J et al (1990) Fatigue and its correlates in breast and lung cancer patients. Oncology Nursing Forum 17(2 Suppl): 146.

Wilkinson S (1991) Factors which influence how nurses communicate with cancer patients. Journal of Advanced Nursing 16: 677–688.

Wilson ME, Williams HA (1988) Oncology nurses' attitudes and behaviours related to sexuality of patients with cancer. Oncology Nursing Forum 15: 49–53.

Withers RH (1992) Biological basis for radiation therapy for cancer. Lancet 339: 156–159.

World Cancer Research Fund (1997) Food, nutrition and the prevention of cancer: a global perspective. Washington: American Institute for Cancer Research.

World Health Organization (1986) Cancer pain relief. Geneva: WHO.

Wright K, Dyck S (1984) Expressed concerns of adult cancer patients' family members. Cancer Nursing 7(5): 371–374.

12 Caring for the patient with a cardiovascular disorder

Richard Hatchett

Introduction

Circulation

Prevention of cardiovascular disorders

The person with a cardiovascular disorder

Causes and types of heart disorder

Congenital cardiovascular defects

Disorders of cardiac muscle

Disorders of myocardial blood supply

Disorders of electroconduction

Heart failure

The person having cardiac surgery

Disorders of the vascular system

Summary

Introduction

The care of people with a cardiovascular disorder utilizes a significant amount of nursing skill and resources. This is because cardiovascular disease remains one of the highest causes of morbidity and mortality in the Western world. Many conditions are chronic rather than curable, and in recent years nursing has adapted to more closely monitor and augment the health status of those with a cardiovascular condition. This has included the emergence of nurse-led clinics in the community and hospital settings, chest pain clinics and nurse-led thrombolysis. The latter allows specially trained nursing staff to administer thrombolytic (clot-busting) drugs to a set protocol, when a patient is suffering a myocardial infarction (MI) due to a blocked coronary artery. Such innovative approaches to traditional practice illustrate how nursing is developing and adapting to meet the needs of patients more fully. The government-initiated National Service Framework for Coronary Heart Disease, released in 2000, endorsed such practice, providing set standards to encourage the implementation of evidence-based practice and more equitable access to definitive treatments and care.

Circulation

Normal cellular activity is dependent upon a constant supply of oxygen, nutrients and certain chemicals, as well as the removal of metabolic waste products. Specialized organs are necessary for the processes of oxygenation, nutrition and excretion, as well as a transportation system between these organs and cells throughout the body. This transportation of materials to and from tissue cells by the propulsion of blood through a closed system of tubes is the process referred to as circulation.

Circulatory structures

The circulatory system consists of the heart and the vascular system.

Heart

The **heart** is a hollow, cone-shaped, muscular organ lying obliquely in the thoracic cavity. Approximately two-thirds of it is situated to the left of the midline. The upper border (or base) lies just below the second rib. The lower border (or apex) is directed downward, forward and to the left, and lies on the diaphragm at the level of the fifth intercostal space in the left midclavicular line.

Pericardium

The **pericardium** is a strong, non-distensible sac which loosely encloses the heart and attaches to the large blood vessels at the base of the heart and to the diaphragm at the apex. Although the pericardial sac is firm and considered non-extensible, it does extend in response to the gradual, sustained stretching imposed by enlargement of the heart (*hypertrophy*).

Heart walls

The **walls of the heart** are composed of three layers of tissue:

1. The *epicardium* forms the outer layer of the heart and is the visceral layer of the pericardium.

2. The *myocardium* is the middle layer of tissue. This is composed of involuntary striated muscle fibres which interlace, branch and anastomose. This layer of muscle is responsible for the heart's contractile force.

3. The *endocardium* is a thin layer of endothelial cells lining the interior surface of the heart's chambers which covers the heart's valves. This layer creates

a smooth surface, reducing friction between moving blood and the walls of the heart.

Heart chambers

The right and left sides of the heart each consist of two **chambers**, an *atrium*, which receives incoming blood, and a *ventricle*, which ejects blood into the arteries.

The atrial myocardium is much thinner than that of the ventricles, and the left ventricular wall is thicker than that of the right. This difference is related to the fact that the atria are required to deliver the blood only to the ventricles. The right ventricle pumps blood through the lungs to the left atrium, forming the circuit referred to as the *pulmonary circulatory system*. The left ventricle must provide sufficient force to carry blood through all parts of the body and return it to the right atrium. This latter circuit is referred to as the *systemic circulatory system*.

Cardiac valves

Normal circulation requires the flow of the blood in one direction only. This is maintained in the heart by a set of four **valves**: two atrioventicular and two semilunar.

The right atrioventricular (AV) valve is located between the right atrium and ventricle. It has three cusps and is called the *tricuspid valve* (Fig. 12.1). The left AV valve, situated between the left atrium and ventricle, has two cusps and is called the *mitral valve*. These valves open into the ventricles but are prevented from opening into the atria by fine tendinous cords (*chordae tendineae*).

The *semilunar valves* guard the openings from the ventricles into the pulmonary artery and aorta, and are called

Heart:
See chapter 4.2

Pericardium
See chapter 4.2

Heart walls
See chapter 4.2

Heart chambers
See chapter 4.2

Heart valves
See chapter 4.2

Figure 12.1 The valves of the heart.

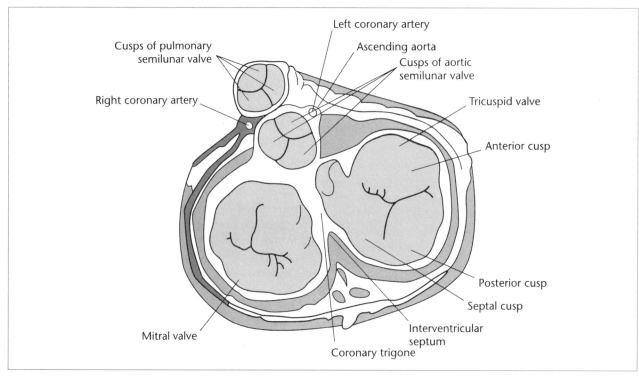

the pulmonary and aortic valves, respectively. Each consists of three pocket-like pouches arranged around the origin of the artery, with the free borders being distal to the ventricle.

Electrical conduction system

The heart is a unique organ because it has an electrical **conduction** system to maintain its rate and rhythm of activity.

The *sinoatrial (SA) node* is a small mass of specialized tissue located in the upper portion of the right atrium near the superior vena cava inlet (Fig. 12.2). It is responsible for initiating impulses for a rhythmic heartbeat.

The *atrioventricular (AV) node* lies in the lower part of the right atrium in the interatrial septum. It conducts electrical impulses from the atria to the ventricles. A bundle of fibres called the *bundle of His* proceeds from junctional tissue at the AV node into the ventricular septum, where it divides into two, forming the left and right bundle branches. The left bundle branch further divides into the anterior (superior) and posterior (inferior) divisions (Fig. 12.2). As it descends, each bundle branch gives rise to a network of fine fibres which are known as the *Purkinje fibres*. They are distributed to the ventricular myocardial cells.

Coronary artery system

The **coronary artery system** (Fig. 12.3) provides the myocardium with its blood supply. There are two main coronary arteries, the left and right. The left main coronary

Conduction
See chapter 4.2

Coronary circulation
See chapter 4.2

Figure 12.2   The electrical conduction system.

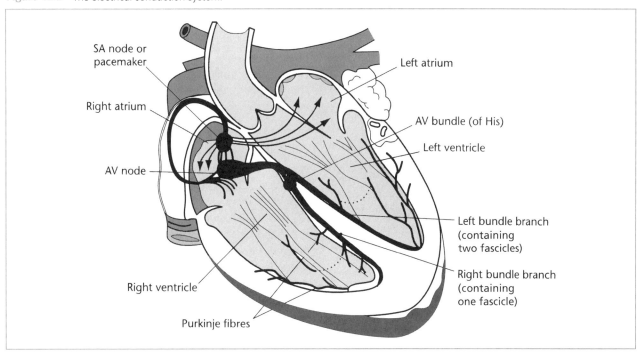

Figure 12.3   The coronary artery system.

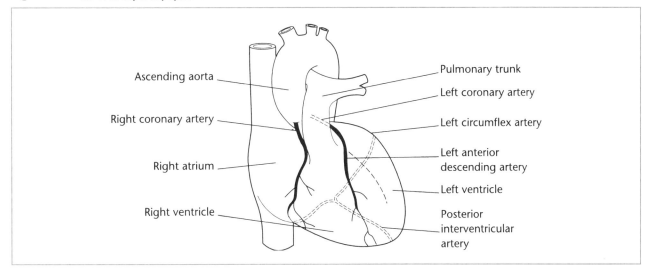

Figure 12.4   Artery–arteriole–capillary–venule–vein sequence in the circulation.

Cardiac muscle
See chapter 4.2

Vascular system
See chapter 4.2

Arteries
See chapter 4.2

Capillaries
See chapter 4.2

Veins
See chapter 4.2

artery divides into the anterior descending artery (LAD) and the circumflex artery. The large arteries divide and subdivide to form a network of smaller arteries and capillaries throughout the heart muscle. The blood is returned to the right atrium through a system of progressively enlarging veins which terminate in the coronary sinus.

The **myocardium** requires a large blood supply because it must work continuously and adapt its activity to the varying needs of tissues throughout the body. The coronary vessels dilate to increase the supply when demands are increased. They also dilate when there is an increase in the carbon dioxide concentration of the blood and a decrease in the pH.

Vascular system

The blood travels from the heart through arteries, arterioles, capillaries and veins back to the heart (Fig. 12.4). The structure of each type of vessel is modified according to its function and location.

Arteries and arterioles

The large **arteries** carry blood away from the heart, and branch and subdivide many times. Their structure varies with their size, the larger ones being more elastic and less muscular. Elasticity is an important property of these vessels; with the ejection of blood from the heart, the vessel distends and on recoil exerts a slight pressure on the contained fluid, helping to force it forward. If resistance is offered to the flow of the blood, normally the arteries can stretch to accommodate the increased volume of blood, and the pressure of the blood remains within the normal range.

The smallest arteries emerge as arterioles, which have walls composed mainly of a well developed muscular coat over the endothelium. The muscle tissue may contract or relax to decrease or increase the amount of blood passing through the arterioles (vasoconstriction or vasodilatation). This feature of the arterioles gives them an important role in determining arterial blood pressure and in controlling the blood flow into the capillaries.

Capillaries

Each arteriole channels its content into microscopic endothelial tubes, the **capillaries**, which anastomose with one another to form a capillary bed. The exchange of fluids, gases and nutrients to maintain and regulate cell activity takes place as the blood passes through the thin capillary walls, usually by diffusion.

The number of capillaries through which blood is passing at any given time is adjusted locally to meet the needs of the tissues in the area. A small proportion of the blood is located in the capillaries in resting states; the volume increases as tissue activity increases. This adjustment is possible because some capillaries have at their origin a ring of plain muscular tissue which forms a precapillary sphincter allowing for closure of its capillaries when they are not needed.

Venules and veins

The collecting part of the vascular system originates in venules which drain the capillaries and progressively unite and enlarge to form **veins**. They differ from arteries in several ways: (1) they carry blood toward the heart; (2) their walls are much thinner and less elastic with the result that they collapse when empty; (3) the contained blood is under a much lower pressure; and (4) many of the veins have valves.

The structure of veins changes as they increase in size; more muscle and fibrous tissue appear in the walls but, in comparison with arteries, the muscle fibres are sparse. The thinner walls of the veins are readily compressed by skeletal muscle contraction; this assists the blood along its course toward the heart. Backflow toward the capillaries is prevented by one-way valves.

Physiology of circulation

Normal circulation through the cardiovascular system is dependent upon an appropriate pressure gradient throughout the system, an adequate volume of blood, a closed system of unobstructed tubes and a set of valves to ensure flow in one direction only.

Role of the heart in circulation

The pressure that drives the blood through the circulatory system originates in the heart and is augmented slightly by the elastic recoil of the large arteries. A continuous succession of alternate myocardial contractions and relaxations, occurring rhythmically on an average of 60–70 times per minute, pumps the blood through the body.

Impulse origin and conduction in heart contraction

The cells of the myocardium are of two types: those that contract when stimulated and those that originate and **conduct** impulses. The ability to originate and conduct impulses is referred to as the *electrical activity* of the heart. The heart has three electrical properties:

1. *automaticity*, or the ability to initiate an electrical impulse
2. *excitability*, or the ability to respond to an electrical impulse
3. *conductivity*, or the ability to transmit an impulse from one cell to another.

Contraction of the myocardium is dependent upon impulses that arise within the myocardium itself. The structures capable of generating and conducting impulses within the myocardium form the *conduction system*. They are the SA node, tracts of conducting fibres originating with the SA node, the AV node, the bundle of His, bundle branches and the Purkinje fibres.

The rate at which impulses are normally fired varies in the different areas: the SA node originates approximately 60–80 impulses per minute and is referred to as the dominant pacemaker. Impulses arising in the SA node are quickly conducted through the atria, initiating their contraction. At the same time, impulses are transmitted to the AV node where they are delayed; this delay allows for completion of atrial emptying and ventricular filling. From the AV node and junctional tissue they travel through the bundle of His and along the right and left bundle branches and the widely distributed Purkinje fibres to the ventricular contractile fibres, initiating their contraction.

Electrophysiology

Electrical currents in cardiac cells are produced by ion movement across the cell membrane. There is a marked difference in the intracellular and extracellular concentrations of ions, the most important of which are sodium and potassium. During the resting state the inside of the cardiac cell is negatively charged while the outside is positively charged, and the membrane is referred to as *polarized*.

During *depolarization*, the cell membrane becomes permeable to sodium ions, which rapidly shift inside the cell. This sudden influx of sodium reverses the transmembrane potential and potassium ions move out of the cell.

Repolarization, or return to the normal resting potential, occurs as the inside of the cell gradually resumes its negative electrical charge. During this time a stimulus of greater than normal intensity could reactivate the cell.

There is then a period of stable resting potential which remains until the next wave of excitation.

During **depolarization**, ions move into and out of the cell because of differences in concentration gradients on either side of the cell membrane. During repolarization, however, an active transport system is required to pump out the sodium ions that have entered the cell and to pump in an equivalent amount of potassium ions. This mechanism is known as the 'sodium pump' and requires energy.

The cardiac cycle

The succession of events that occurs with each heart beat is called the **cardiac cycle**. This consists of the relaxation and contraction of the atria and ventricles, and the opening and closing of the cardiac valves, in a sequence that permits the filling and emptying of the heart chambers. Contraction of the atria or ventricles is called *systole*; their relaxation is known as *diastole*.

At the start of the cardiac cycle, the atria in diastole fill with blood received from their inlet vessels. In the early part of the relaxation period, the AV valves are closed, but as pressure builds up in the atria it becomes greater than that in the ventricles, forcing the AV valves open, and the blood starts to flow through into the ventricles. Atrial diastole is followed in a fraction of a second by contraction (atrial systole), to complete the emptying of the two upper chambers, and the atria again enter their diastole.

During the filling and contraction of the ventricles the blood floats the AV valve cusps up, closing off the AV openings and preventing a regurgitation of blood into the atria. In order to receive the blood from the atria, the ventricles must be in diastole and, at this time, the semilunar valves are closed. With ventricular filling, the intraventricular pressure builds up until it exceeds that in the aorta and pulmonary artery, with the result that the semilunar valves open, allowing blood to flow into the arteries. The ventricular muscle contracts, and the ventricles are emptied.

During ventricular systole, the papillary muscles also contract, exerting tension on the fine tendons (chordae tendineae) inserted on the AV valve cusps. This prevents the cusps from opening into the atria. If this control were not placed on the AV valves, there would be a backflow into the atria, especially with the ventricular contraction. The ventricles relax following their systole and emptying. This results in the pressure being greater in the arteries than in the ventricles, thus potentially allowing the backflow of blood into the ventricles. Closure of the semilunar valves prevents blood from re-entering the ventricles, however. The cardiac cycle is now completed.

The cycle in a heart beating approximately 70 times per minute is completed in 0.7–0.8 s. The length of each phase of the cycle varies: atrial diastole lasts approximately 0.7 s, whereas its systole is approximately 0.1 s. Ventricular diastole is about 0.4–0.5 s, and its systole takes about 0.3 s. Following the ventricular contraction

Conduction
See chapter 4.2

Depolarization
See chapter 4.2

Cardiac cycle
See chapter 4.2

there is a brief period, approximately 0.4 s, in which the entire myocardium is relaxed. The ventricular diastole overlaps the atrial diastole.

Cardiac output

The performance of the heart as a pump can be described in terms of **cardiac output** (CO). This is the volume of blood pumped by each ventricle in 1 minute. It is equal to the stroke volume (SV) or the volume of blood pumped by a ventricle in one beat, multiplied by the number of heart beats in a minute (the heart rate; HR). In an adult, the CO varies from 4 to 8 litres per minute, and the SV averages 60–80 mL. Thus, *cardiac output* is dependent on *heart rate* and *stroke volume* (CO = SV × HR).

Heart rate

The number of heart beats per minute varies in different people and under different conditions. The average normal rate for an adult is 70 beats per minute, but it may range from 60 to 90. Several factors influence the **heart rate**. In the infant a rate of 110–130 is normal. It becomes progressively slower as the child grows older; by the early teens it is usually about 80. Muscular exertion produces a marked increase, especially in an individual unaccustomed to physical exercise. The rate usually increases during emotional reactions, with fever, and in the lower atmospheric pressures found at high altitudes.

Stroke volume

Stroke volume is influenced by preload, contractility and afterload.

Preload

This is the pressure of blood contained in the ventricle at the end of diastole. Another term to describe this pressure is *left ventricular end-diastolic pressure*, which is related to the volume of blood in the ventricle at the end of diastole.

Contractility

The **contractile** or inotropic state of the myocardium is the ability of the heart to contract. If the heart is undamaged and is in a condition to respond, the strength of the heart beat is determined mainly by the length of the muscle fibres when contraction begins. Stretching of muscle fibres, within limits, increases the strength of their contraction. The length or stretching of the myocardial fibres is dependent upon the volume of blood entering the heart. This principle is known as *Starling's law of the heart*.

The inotropic state of the heart is also affected by local and circulating catecholamines, the rate and rhythm of ventricular contractions, physiological depressants such as acidosis or myocardial hypoxia, the amount of ventricular substance and certain drugs such as digoxin and/or caffeine.

Afterload

Afterload describes the force against which the ventricle is working, or the resistance to the ejection of blood. This resistance is also called *impedance* and is reflected in the tension that ventricular muscle develops during systole.

Cardiac reserve

The ability of the heart to increase its output commensurate with increased tissue activity and needs is called **cardiac reserve**. The normal heart is capable of forwarding the volume of blood delivered to it and of responding to an increased demand without difficulty. It does this without causing prolonged breathlessness, tachycardia or palpitations.

For example, in strenuous exertion, the cardiac output may increase to a volume 13 times greater than the output during rest. This is achieved by an increase in the heart rate and stroke volume. An increase in the cardiac output also occurs in high environmental temperature, emotional responses such as fear, anger or other excitement, after a heavy meal and in the later months of pregnancy.

Regulation of cardiac activity

Certain **nervous**, chemical and mechanical factors play an important role in the action of the heart.

Nervous influence

The heart muscle is capable of generating its own impulses for contraction, but nerve impulses from the parasympathetic and sympathetic divisions of the autonomic nervous system may modify the rate and strength of the contractions. Vagal or parasympathetic innervation has an inhibitory effect on cardiac activity; it slows the heart rate and decreases the force of the atrial contraction by reducing the excitability of the pacemaker (SA node) and the conductivity of the AV node and conducting system. Sympathetic stimulation increases the heart rate and the strength of heart contractions.

Chemical influence

Normal, rhythmic heart contractions are greatly dependent upon an optimal concentration of potassium, sodium and calcium in the extracellular fluid. These minerals play an important role in the excitability of the cardiac muscle cells and their contraction.

Other chemicals of significance in heart action are oxygen and carbon dioxide. Any deficiency of oxygen is quickly reflected in a deterioration of heart action. The myocardium is much more sensitive to oxygen lack than skeletal muscle. The pulse becomes rapid, weak and irregular. With an excess of carbon dioxide in the blood, as may occur in respiratory insufficiency, heart action is impaired. Conduction is slowed, the relaxation period is prolonged and the contraction is briefer than normal.

Cardiac output
See chapter 4.2

Heart rate
See chapter 4.2

Stroke volume
See chapter 4.2

Contractility
See chapter 4.2

Cardiac reserve
See chapter 4.2

Nervous control
See chapter 4.2

Mechanical influence

The principal mechanical influence on cardiac activity is the stretching of the myocardial fibres by the volume of blood entering the chambers. Stretching of muscle fibres increases the strength of their contraction. An increase in arterial blood pressure also demands a greater force of contraction: the heart muscle must release a greater amount of energy to perform its function because of meeting greater resistance (afterload).

Blood pressure and pulse

Blood pressure

Blood pressure may be defined as the pressure exerted laterally on the walls of the blood vessels. It varies in different parts of the circulatory system, being greatest in the large arteries, with a progressive decrease as the blood continues on through the smaller arteries, arterioles, capillaries and veins. The pressure is highest in the aorta and lowest in the large caval veins that enter the heart. Blood pressure at any point in the vascular system is dependent upon the force with which the heart pumps the blood out of the ventricles, the volume of blood in the system, the elasticity of the arteries, and the amount of resistance to the flow of the blood from one portion of the circulatory system to the next.

Arterial blood pressure

The blood pressure of greatest clinical interest is that in the arteries. The pulsatile nature of heart activity causes fluctuations in the pressure. With each contraction of the left ventricle a volume of blood is pumped into the aorta, which is already filled with blood. This causes an appreciable increase in the pressure of the blood and stretches the aortic walls. The higher pressure produced by the ventricular systole is referred to as the *systolic blood pressure*. The lower pressure that occurs during the ventricular diastole is dependent upon the recoil of the large arteries and is known as the *diastolic blood pressure*. The difference between these two pressures is called the *pulse pressure*. Pulse pressure varies inversely with the elasticity of the arteries. Rigid vessels with a loss of ability to distend and recoil produce a higher systolic pressure and a lower diastolic pressure, resulting in an increased pulse pressure.

Factors that determine arterial blood pressure

Arterial blood pressure is influenced by the strength of the heart beat, volume of blood, elasticity of the vessels and the resistance offered to the flow of blood. Resistance offered to the flow of blood is dependent mainly on the calibre of the arteries and the viscosity of the blood.

Normal variations in arterial blood pressure occur under the influence of factors such as age, exercise, emotion and weight.

During infancy and childhood, blood pressure is lower than later in life. In the newborn infant systolic pressure is approximately 55–90 mmHg; the diastolic is approximately 40–55 mmHg. This gradually increases throughout childhood, reaching adult level about puberty. Usually in the fifties, the systolic pressure begins to show a slight increase, which progresses with age – corresponding to the loss of elasticity and thickening of the walls of the arteries characteristic of the ageing process.

Physical exertion is accompanied by a rise in the arterial blood pressure due to the increased venous return and the increased production of metabolites such as carbon dioxide and lactic acid. The systolic pressure may increase by as much as 60–70 mmHg in strenuous exercise.

Emotions may also cause an increase in blood pressure: the more excited, anxious, angry or fearful a person becomes, the higher the blood pressure goes. Vasoconstriction is increased due to sympathetic innervation and the release of adrenaline into the bloodstream.

Blood pressure increases with increased bodyweight, especially after middle age. This is of significance in our present-day society in which obesity and hypertension have a high incidence.

Venous blood pressure

The pressure of the blood is reduced slowly but progressively from the time it leaves the capillaries until it reaches the right atrium.

Venous blood pressure is influenced by cardiac strength, blood volume, respirations and posture. The blood enters the venous system under a pressure of approximately 10 mmHg. The walls of the veins continue to offer some resistance and the blood, particularly in the lower parts of the body, must travel a considerable distance before reaching the heart. The laws of physics tell us that pressure is inversely proportional to frictional resistance and the length of the tube. As a result, venous blood pressure is dissipated progressively, and by the time it reaches the right atrium is very low: 0–10 cmH$_2$O (0–1 mmHg). Obviously, if the left ventricular systole is weak and the blood starts out at a lower than normal arterial pressure, it will tend to move more slowly in the veins towards the heart.

Pulse

Each ventricular contraction ejects a volume of blood into the aorta, producing an increase in the blood pressure which causes an expansion of the artery. During ventricular diastole, the elastic recoil of the aorta moves the blood into the next portion of the artery, which stretches and then recoils. This alternating expansion and recoil spreads along the whole arterial system, producing a pulse wave. Each pulsation corresponds to a heart beat and is the result of the impact of the ejected volume of blood on the arterial wall. The pulsations occur in the

Blood pressure
See chapter 4.2

Arterial blood
pressure
See chapter 4.2

Venous blood
pressure
See chapter 4.2

arteries of the pulmonary circulatory system as well as in the systemic circulation.

Prevention of cardiovascular disorders

In the UK, cardiovascular disease is a national health problem of considerable proportions. This is particularly true now that an increasing proportion of the population is over the age of 60 years, an age group with a high prevalence of cardiovascular disease in which the incidence amongst women approaches that in men. Cardiovascular disease is also the main cause of premature death and handicap in the UK. Approximately half of the deaths from cardiovascular disease in the UK each year are from coronary heart disease. The term **coronary heart disease** (CHD) encompasses a group of clinical conditions ranging from asymptomatic disease to angina, acute myocardial infarction (MI) and sudden death. *Ischaemic heart disease* (IHD) is the official term used in the International Classification of Diseases; it is virtually synonymous with coronary heart disease.

Coronary heart disease
See chapter 4.2

One in four men and one in five women die from CHD, with CHD causing more than 135 000 deaths in the UK a year (British Heart Foundation Statistics Database 2000). CHD is also the underlying cause of a substantial number of hospital admissions. Myocardial infarction (heart attack) and sudden death are the most conspicuous manifestations of the problem, but far more people suffer less dramatic but still significant consequences including chest pain (angina), syncope, decreased exercise tolerance, anxiety and other psychological complications. Side-effects and the consequences of treatment can also cause problems for some. Reduced mobility, for example, may result in a loss of previous lifestyle affecting all aspects of daily life including work, social activities, roles within the family and financial security. The social and economic consequences of the disorder are thus far reaching and extend beyond the personal effects on those who suffer and their families. It has been estimated that the total economic burden of CHD is now £10 000 million each year. This is more than double that for any other disease where a comparable analysis has been carried out (British Heart Foundation Statistics Database 2000). Virtually every man, woman and child in the UK will be affected in some way by heart disease as a consequence of knowing or being related to a sufferer or being a sufferer themselves.

Not surprisingly, CHD is a significant feature in government health policy. The White Paper *Saving lives: our healthier nation* has set targets for a 40% reduction in deaths from CHD and cerebrovascular accident (CVA) in those under 75 years of age by the year 2010 (Department of Health 2000). In addition the National Service Framework for Coronary Heart Disease (Department of Health 2000b) has created a 10-year programme for improving services for CHD. Standards have been set for the whole of CHD-related care, from cardiac health promotion, emergency care, specialist cardiology services and surgery through to rehabilitation.

The nurse's role in prevention of cardiovascular disorders

The nurse has many opportunities to contribute to the prevention of cardiovascular disorders. Whether the work is in the hospital, clinic, home, industry or school, the role may be participation in health screening, education or provision of care. In addition, the emerging roles of nurse consultant and nurse-led clinics offer greater autonomy in the practice area of cardiovascular nursing. In order to recognize and fulfil the responsibilities in the preventive programme, the nurse must be informed and must make a personal effort to keep abreast of new knowledge. In addition to an understanding of the role of the heart in supplying all the cells throughout the body with materials essential to their survival and activities, a knowledge of how this function may be impaired by various pathological processes is necessary. This information serves as the basis for the recognition of excessive demands on the heart and circulation, significant signs and symptoms, and the need for medical attention. It also provides the basis for explanations and appropriate health education as well as for the planning and provision of safe and effective care.

Risk factors have been identified in large-scale epidemiological studies as clinical variables that are statistically associated with the manifestation of heart disease, particularly ischaemic heart disease (IHD). These factors are presumably involved in the pathogenesis of atherosclerosis of the coronary arteries. The presence of multiple risk factors increases exponentially the likelihood of developing IHD, although individuals may live for many years with multiple risk factors and no manifestations of heart disease.

The nurse can play a very important role in facilitating health promotion, assessing potentially detrimental health patterns, and identifying and undertaking strategies to prevent or correct these behaviours.

Risk factors for ischaemic heart disease

Risk factors can be classified as either *non-modifiable*, such as age, sex, family history and culture, or *modifiable*, such as hypertension, hyperlipidaemia, cigarette smoking, diabetes mellitus, obesity, lack of physical activity and personality characteristics.

Nurses need to be aware of the far-reaching psychological and social consequences of cardiovascular disease, both for the individual and for their partners and families. Individuals may be aware that they are at risk, but having the ability to change their lifestyle is dependent on a variety of factors, including: their perception of the significance of the problem; their belief that action they take will reduce the risk; self-esteem; role within the family and society; time and financial constraints and support from others. Nurses need to consider their role in health education. Providing the patient with all the facts is not in itself a guarantee of them changing to and maintaining a healthy lifestyle. The individual needs to be able to make an informed choice about his or her own behaviour with the support of the healthcare team. The attitude of the nurse is likely to be important here. It may be necessary to prioritize risk factors in order to make compliance more likely. Someone who is overweight and smokes may be more likely to succeed in making appropriate changes if they are advised to concentrate on stopping smoking initially, even though this may lead to an initial weight gain.

Non-modifiable risk factors

Age Ischaemic heart disease is more prevalent in **older** people. Thus, the older the individual, the greater the likelihood of developing cardiovascular disease.

Sex Men have a higher incidence of IHD than women, although this difference diminishes as age increases. Women have a dramatically increased incidence of IHD after the menopause.

Family history A history of IHD among blood relatives is associated with an increased risk of cardiovascular disease and a poorer prognosis when it develops.

Culture In the 1980s, it became clear that mortality from CHD differed significantly between ethnic groups in England and Wales. More recent figures still illustrate that southern Asians (people from India, Bangladesh, Pakistan and Sri Lanka) demonstrate a much higher premature death rate from CHD than average. The rate is 46% higher in men and 51% higher in women (British Heart Foundation Statistics Database 2000). Interestingly, in the African–Caribbean population the incidence of CHD is lower than average, although the presence of cerebrovascular accident (CVA), hypertension and diabetes is high (British Heart Foundation Statistics Database 2000). Other groups with an increased mortality rate include Irish, Scottish and Polish-born immigrants (Balarajan 1991).

Modifiable risk factors

The modifiable risk factors known to play a part in ischaemic heart disease include:

- cigarette smoking
- hyperlipidaemia
- hypertension
- diabetes mellitus
- obesity
- lack of physical activity
- high alcohol intake
- personality characteristics.

Hypertension

Raised systolic and diastolic blood pressure is a significant risk factor for cardiovascular disease including IHD, CVA and heart failure. It is estimated that 14% of deaths from CHD in men and 12% in women are due to high blood pressure (this is defined as a systolic pressure of 140 mmHg and over, or a diastolic pressure of 90 mmHg and over) (British Heart Foundation Statistics Database 2000). Discussion of the nurse's role in the management of **hypertension** can be found later in this chapter.

Hyperlipidaemia

Blood lipids include cholesterol, triglycerides, phospholipids and free fatty acids. Cholesterol and triglycerides are of clinical significance and are transported in plasma as lipoproteins. There are four major classes of lipoproteins, containing varying proportions of protein and the three blood lipids:

1. *Chylomicrons* are mainly of dietary origin and are 85% triglycerides.

2. Very low-density lipoproteins (VLDLs) contain 50% triglycerides.

3. Low-density lipoproteins (LDLs) carry 75% of the total plasma cholesterol.

4. High-density lipoproteins (HDLs) remove excess cholesterol from body cells and transport it to the liver for elimination.

Age
See chapter 4.2

Hypertension
See chapter 4.2

High levels of HDLs protect against the development of coronary atherosclerosis, although it is uncertain how this occurs (Tortora and Grabowski 2000).

Hyperlipoproteinaemia may be secondary to another disease such as obstructive liver disease, due to an excessive intake of saturated fats and cholesterol in the diet, or may result from a primary or familial disorder. Determination of serum cholesterol and triglyceride levels will detect hyperlipoproteinaemia in most cases and is less costly than other laboratory procedures. However, in some instances, further studies may be warranted. Control of hypercholesterolaemia is directed toward lowering the serum cholesterol levels by diet, and in some instances by medications.

By modifying the dietary intake of fats, carbohydrate and calories, the blood lipid levels of most patients with primary hyperlipidaemia can be lowered. The contribution of diet to the prevention of coronary atherosclerosis is controversial but evidence suggests that this approach might be worthwhile. Lowering blood cholesterol levels by 1% reduces the risk of IHD by about 2–3% (Law et al 1994).

The results from clinical trials are remarkably consistent. It is estimated that a long-term reduction in serum cholesterol concentration of 0.6 mmol/L (10%), which can be achieved by moderate dietary change, lowers the risk of IHD by 50% at age 40 years, falling to 20% at age 70, the full effect of reduction being achieved after 5 years (Law et al 1994). Long-term treatment with lipid-lowering drugs has also been shown to be safe and improves the survival rate of patients with IHD (Scandinavian Simvastatin Survival Study Group 1994). Lipid-lowering therapy with a drug called a statin, to lower the cholesterol concentration to less than 5 mmol/L (low-density cholesterol to below 3 mmol/L) or by 30%, whichever is the greater, is now recommended in the National Service Framework for Coronary Heart Disease (DoH 2000b).

Current guidelines on an appropriate diet to maintain a healthy heart include the following (British Heart Foundation 1999):

■ Reducing the level of fat eaten and replacing some saturated fats with polyunsaturated and monounsaturated fats. This can be achieved by eating more starchy foods such as pasta, bread, rice, cereals and potatoes. A high-fibre diet will also reduce the amount of cholesterol absorbed from the intestine into the blood.

■ Eating at least five portions of fruit and vegetables a day. These should be of different types.

■ Eating oily fish two or three times a week. This may help to reduce the level of triglycerides, which are linked to fatty deposits in the lining of vessel walls (atheroma).

■ Reducing the amount of salt consumed. There is a clear link between a high salt intake and high blood pressure. As a nation we eat about 10 g of salt per day; this should be at least halved. Salt is found in many foods, but notably processed foods, ready-made meals, and snacks such as crisps and peanuts. Food labelling for salt is complex because it may appear as 'sodium' and contain other chemicals such as sodium bicarbonate. A sodium content of less than 0.2 g per 100 g on the label is generally recommended (Hatchett 2001).

■ Keeping a healthy weight. This will reduce the workload on the heart and help to reduce any hypertension.

Dietary education is a combined function of the doctor, nurse and dietician. The dietician is the primary person involved if the diet is complex, but the nurse also needs to be informed so that teaching can be reinforced. Some patients may require much support and understanding to continue on their diets, especially if drastic changes in eating habits are needed. Adherence will probably be greater if the diet is adjusted as much as possible to individual tastes.

Involving the spouse or the person who buys and cooks the food may make dietary change more likely. The diet needs to be perceived as lifelong rather than a short-term response to an acute event. The social significance of food should not be ignored – the individual does not want to perceive themselves as a social outcast at the meal table.

Lipid-lowering drugs that may be prescribed include atorvastatin, pravastatin and simvastatin.

Cigarette smoking

Approximately 28% of men and 27% of women in the UK smoke cigarettes (DoH 1999). The proportion is highest in the 16–24 age group and declines with age (DOH 1999). Within the various ethnic groups, males from the Bangladeshi and Caribbean communities show particularly high smoking rates: 49% and 42% respectively (British Heart Foundation Statistics Database 2000).

For both men and women, cigarette smoking is one of the major risk factors for cardiovascular disease. The risk of morbidity and mortality is dramatically greater for smokers than for non-smokers, particularly in people under the age of 50 years and those who have other risk factors.

Research has indicated that there are a number of compounds in cigarette smoke that are harmful (Khosla et al 1994). Nicotine stimulates catecholamine secretion which, in turn, promotes platelet aggregation, increased heart rate, blood pressure and oxygen consumption. Carbon monoxide also appears to increase platelet adhesiveness and reduce oxygen supply which, in the presence of coronary lesions, may increase the incidence of angina pectoris.

Macleod Clark et al (1990) have shown that there is a best time to intervene to maximize the chance of successfully stopping patients smoking – ideally after the first coronary event.

There are a number of strategies to facilitate smoking cessation:

■ Providing information that is tailored to the individual's needs (Box 12.1). A patient who has already experienced a recent cardiac condition may be more receptive to messages on the impact of smoking on the heart and health. Nurse–client interaction has been shown to be more effective than written self-help materials (Rice et al 1994).

■ Eliciting social support can be beneficial. Family members and friends can discuss their roles in helping the person to stop smoking.

■ Self-help efforts may be beneficial. Discussing with the individual behaviours that are associated with the activity and how to avoid these situations, at least initially when attempting to stop, can be helpful. Social and psychological reinforcers that contribute to smoking behaviours can be very powerful in preventing successful cessation.

■ A gradual reduction of the number of cigarettes smoked can be a successful strategy, but current

Box 12.1 Advice for smokers

1. It is best to choose a day or a date to stop smoking. Most people are more successful with this method, rather than cutting down slowly.

2. Tell patients that they are making a major decision: i.e. a 65-year-old who smokes two packets of cigarettes a day may forfeit 6 years of life but can regain 4 of those years by stopping smoking.

3. If a patient resumes smoking, provide reassurance that stopping smoking is like any other new skill: several tries may be necessary.

4. If the patient has one cigarette, inform the patient that this does not mean immediate dependence; however, emphasize that it should not become habitual.

5. Inform patients that withdrawal symptoms are generally most severe 2–4 days after stopping and symptoms slowly subside during the following week, but reach a second peak about 10 days after stopping, before slowly tapering off permanently. Emphasize that symptoms will be short lived and can often be countered by planning for them.

6. Advise patients that any weight gain almost never exceeds 2.5–3 kg (5–10 lbs), and that very few ex-smokers maintain the added weight for more than 1 year. Suggest an exercise programme.

advice focuses upon choosing a particular day or date to stop as the most successful approach. The person is then advised to keep busy, to alter usual routines that may be linked to smoking, to drink plenty of fluids, to become more active and to treat themselves with the money saved.

- Pharmacological strategies, including the use of nicotine chewing gum, may be useful when a strong addiction is present. When chewed, this gum replaces the nicotine provided by cigarettes to a certain extent.

- Cessation programmes are often available in the individual's community. The nurse should be aware of these programmes and facilitate the patient's referral as appropriate.

Diabetes mellitus

Cardiac disease is prevalent in individuals with glucose intolerance, particularly women. In post-mortem studies, people with type II **diabetes** have been found to have more extensive coronary artery lesions, which are more diffuse and involve a greater number of vessels than those found in sex-matched controls. Previously undetected diabetes is found in about 5% of coronary patients admitted to hospital (Oswald et al 1984).

Obesity

Being overweight is a weak independent risk factor for IHD. However, obesity is a major indicator for increased risk of cardiovascular disease as it is associated with many other risk factors. Surveys demonstrate that obesity is increasing in the UK (DoH 1999, British Heart Foundation Statistics Database 2000). Overweight men also have an increased likelihood of hypertension, hyperlipidaemia and diabetes mellitus (Shaper 1987). These risks can be reduced by weight loss.

Physical activity

There is now strong evidence that physical activity is important in the prevention of obesity and high blood pressure. Those with heart failure are now being encouraged to participate in supervised exercise programmes to improve functional status. Levels of physical activity are low in the UK, with only 37% of men and 25% of women meeting the activity guidelines suggested by government. This is 30 minutes of moderate intensity exercise on five or more days of the week, such as brisk walking, cycling or climbing stairs (British Heart Foundation Statistics Database 2000). Exercise should be enough to produce breathlessness, but should be enjoyable.

High alcohol intake

A regular high intake of alcohol causes hypertension and is associated with excess IHD. A moderate intake, particularly of red wine, is thought to protect against IHD.

Personality characteristics

The risk of IHD is thought by some researchers to be increased in association with a person displaying characteristics of the type A behavioural pattern, including aggressiveness, competitive drive and a chronic sense of time urgency. However, a number of methodological difficulties in measuring these psychological characteristics has led to the results being viewed with caution. An extensive study in the UK failed to show any relationship between type A behaviour and the incidence and prevalence of IHD (Johnston et al 1987). Research studies to determine whether reduction in type A behaviour reduces mortality and morbidity rates from IHD are being conducted. Interventions directed at group counselling have indicated that this may be an effective strategy in modifying type A behaviour.

Factors influencing high-risk behaviour

High-risk behaviours such as smoking, lack of exercise, excessive alcohol consumption and unhealthy diet are often seen as voluntary elements of lifestyle. There is, however, some debate as to the extent to which this is so. Diet may be determined at least in part by income and the availability of different foods. Smoking and alcohol consumption, in particular, may be regarded as being determined by social and peer pressures. Certain individuals or

Diabetes
See chapter 2.6

groups of individuals may not have the time, money or necessary transport to enable them to engage in leisure or sporting activities.

The environmental, political, economic and social forces that act on individuals and groups to influence behaviour need to be understood before change interventions can be identified and implemented.

Cardiovascular disorders and nursing

Ways in which nurses can contribute to the reduction in mortality rate and personal suffering caused by cardiovascular disorders include (Ashworth 1992):

- providing physical treatment and monitoring for pathophysiological problems

- modifying activities of living to balance demands on patients with their capacity to meet them

- modifying the nursing environment to achieve for each individual the optimum possible environment within available resources

- reassuring, supporting and comforting patients and their families

- facilitating lifestyle adjustment to enable each individual to attain and maintain a level of health compatible with the achievement of personally desired life goals.

Many nurses come into contact with individuals with cardiovascular disorders at the time of an acute illness episode; however, many patients have to come to terms with long-term chronic consequences of their disease process and their whole way of life will be affected far beyond the hospital experience. This has led to the broader involvement of nurses in nurse-led clinics and in the community to maintain the health of patients with cardiovascular disorder.

The person with a cardiovascular disorder

Assessment

Assessment of the individual's cardiovascular function provides data needed to identify actual and potential health problems, guide nursing intervention and evaluate care. A cardiovascular assessment includes:

- health history

- physical examination

- diagnostic procedures

- knowledge of manifestations of cardiovascular disorders.

The nurse collects and analyses the assessment data, formulates patient-centred problems and develops a goal-oriented plan of care with the patient and family, which is then implemented and evaluated. More recently, and particularly in cardiac care, integrated care pathways (ICPs) are being used (see p. 10) (Johnson 1997).

Health history

The health history will assist the nurse in defining the patient's health problems. The depth and manner in which this information is collected will depend on the patient's clinical status and availability of family or significant others.

If the patient is acutely ill, then brief, direct questions should be used to identify essential information during admission procedures. If the patient's status is stable, the nurse may conduct a formal interview using more open-ended questions. Other information can be obtained through less formal conversation throughout interaction with the patient. The nature of the nurse–patient relationship is important is establishing the significance of the problem for the patient and family.

The health history includes data concerning the patient's primary health problems, history of present illness, past health history, family history, and social and personal history.

Primary health problem The patient identifies the chief concern or reason for contact with the healthcare system. Common cardiovascular health problems include chest discomfort, dyspnoea, syncope, palpitations and intermittent claudication.

History of present illness This is a detailed investigation of the patient's primary health problem and previously prescribed treatment plan. It is important to use a systematic approach when gathering these data to ensure the information is comprehensive. One method of organizing this data collection is use of the PQRST mnemonic (Box 12.2).

Past health history Assessment includes the patient's general state of health, major health problems and treatment plans, hospital admissions, surgical procedures and

Box 12.2 PQRST mnemonic for symptom assessment		
Letter	Aspect	Sample questions
P	Provocation Palliation	What brings the pain on? What relieves the pain?
Q	Quality	What does it feel like?
R	Region Radiation	Point to where it hurts. Does it move anywhere?
S	Severity	On a scale of 0–10, how would you rate the pain?
T	Time	When did it start?

injuries. The patient's response to these events provides data concerning coping strategies. Allergies to food, medication and environmental agents are identified and allergic reactions described.

Family history Information concerning the patient's blood relatives may suggest a specific cardiac problem. The patient may be questioned about whether any family member has ever had hypertension, diabetes mellitus, ischaemic heart disease, vascular disease or hyperlipidaemia.

Social and personal history These data facilitate an understanding of the person's uniqueness as an individual and suggest needs for health teaching and discharge planning. Data are gathered in the following areas:

- *Personal characteristics*. These include patient's age, marital status, education, occupational experiences, socioeconomic status and religious beliefs.

- *Lifestyle*. Information concerning the individual's daily activities is collected, including dietary, bowel and sleep habits, and usual activities, and data concerning use of tobacco, alcohol, caffeine and social drugs. Identification of these factors can help to facilitate planning in the areas of health promotion and prevention of progression of disease.

- *Patient's perception of the illness and ability to cope*. What does this illness mean to the patient? This provides information as to the patient's level of understanding about the condition and the impact on his or her life. How the patient has coped with other problems may identify coping strategies that the nurse can facilitate when planning care with the individual.

- *Relationships with others*. The patient is questioned about the network of family and friends to assess social support systems available. The family and significant others' perceptions of the patient's condition and coping will provide information as to their level of understanding and their ability to handle the situation.

- *Home environment*. Who is living with the patient? Describing the physical characteristics of the home including stairs, location of bathroom (toilet facilities), etc. will help start discharge planning. This is particularly important for the individual with reduced activity resulting from cardiac dysfunction as daily routines will need to be modified to accommodate changes in function.

- *Knowledge of cardiovascular function*. The patient's understanding of the condition and the treatment plan is important for planning health education. Does the patient know the current medical diagnosis and what this means in terms of treatment and lifestyle? For example, does the patient who has had a myocardial infarction understand activity limitations and medication schedules?

- *Quality of life*. There is a wide individual variation in response to physical illness. Some individuals are able to continue to lead full and satisfying lives despite major symptoms and disability, whereas others with much less serious medical problems become gravely handicapped (Mayou and Bryant 1993). This issue needs to be explored so that a knowledge of the reality of illness for each individual can be used in subsequent care planning. Kleinman et al (1978) give the following questions designed to elicit important patient information:
  a. What brings you here?
  b. What do you think has caused your illness?
  c. Why do you think it started when it did?
  d. What do you think this illness does to you?
  e. How severe is your illness?
  f. What kind of treatment do you think you should receive?
  g. What are the most important results you hope to receive from treatment?
  h. What are the chief problems your illness has caused for you?
  i. What do you fear most about your illness?

Basic physical examination of the cardiovascular system

In this section, basic physical examination techniques for assessing the person's cardiovascular system are described. The more specialized techniques are beyond the scope of this text and the nurse is referred to advanced texts such as Walsh et al (1999). Certain of the techniques described are normally carried out by the doctor. However, increasingly, nurse practitioners are undertaking these skills as part of nurse-led practice. It is also necessary for nurses to understand the principles of these techniques in order to gain a wider appreciation of the patient's experience and to be equipped to explain the nature of the techniques to patients.

Basic physical examination is a cornerstone of the nurse's methods of data collection. Performing a physical examination facilitates gathering the objective data on the person's cardiovascular system, which is necessary to establish a baseline of the person's condition and to assess ongoing changes in health status.

General appearance

1. *Facial expressions*. Does the patient appear alert, anxious, distressed, exhausted? Grimacing, biting of lips are noted as they may be signs of pain.

2. *Posture*. Does the patient appear comfortable, restless, agitated? Is he or she sitting, lying supine?

3. *Skin and mucous membranes*:
   a. Colour: examine skin in symmetrical areas, noting any increase or loss of pigmentation, redness, pallor, cyanosis and jaundice. Ask the patient

whether there have been any recent changes in the colour of the skin. Observe for signs of bleeding such as petechiae, bruising or haematomas.

b. Moisture: inspect skin for dryness, oiliness or sweating (diaphoresis).

c. Hair pattern: note hair distribution on limbs, glossy, shiny appearance of skin surface.

Palpation

This method of examination is used to assess **skin** and peripheral pulses.

Skin

1. *Capillary refill*. This is noted by applying pressure to the nail-bed and releasing quickly. A normal response is for the nail-bed to blanch on pressure and quickly to reperfuse and become pink when pressure is released. An abnormal response is a delay of more than 2 s in the return to pink.

2. *Temperature*. The skin is palpated symmetrically to establish the temperature of the skin using the back of the hand and noting generalized warmth or coolness of any localized areas.

3. *Turgor*. A fold of skin is lifted and the speed with which it returns into place is noted.

4. *Oedema*. Assessment is made for oedema in symmetrical locations, including feet, ankles, lower arms and sacrum. Three fingers are pressed firmly over symmetrical bony surfaces for 5 s, and released. Pitting oedema, which is continued depression of the skin and underlying tissue after pressure is released, is noted.

Skin assessment
See chapter 6.1

Blood pressure measurement
See chapter 4.2

Peripheral arterial pulses

Arterial pulses are assessed for rate, rhythm and amplitude (volume) at symmetrical locations on the body. The carotid, brachial, radial, femoral, popliteal, dorsalis pedis and posterior tibial pulses can be included.

The heart rate can be assessed by counting the pulse rate. The radial or carotid pulse rate can be palpated and counted for 60 s to establish heart rate.

The heart rhythm can be initially assessed using the pulse. The radial or carotid pulse is palpated to identify whether the rhythm of pulses is regular. If it is irregular, any pattern present is noted.

The pulse amplitude may be graded and recorded as follows:

0   Not palpable

+1   Barely palpable, weak, thready

+2   Decreased, moderate impairment

+3   Full

+4   Bounding

Auscultation

Arterial blood pressure

Arterial **blood pressure** is an important predictor of morbidity and mortality, and is therefore one of the most important clinical observations. Recording a blood pressure appears simple, but it is a skill that must be performed carefully. There is clear evidence that care is not always taken to do this (Hatchett 2001). Importantly, treatment for high blood pressure (hypertension) will be initiated on the results of these readings, although, unless the reading is very high, several recordings will be taken over a short period of time to provide a more accurate assessment (Hatchett 2001).

Arterial blood pressure is most frequently measured in millimetres of mercury (mmHg). This is by means of a sphygmomanometer and a stethoscope, using the brachial artery. Increasingly, electronic digital devices are used which do not contain mercury, because this is known to be a toxic substance. Its use is slowly being banned worldwide in medical devices because of the dangers of accidental spillage. Not all non-mercury devices are electronic, but may use a dial and needle to note the pressure instead of the column of mercury. The general technique of recording a blood pressure is described here, but it should be noted that the mercury column is likely to be replaced by the digital display or dial. However, the technique is similar in many ways and should be followed to ensure an accurate reading. The rubber cuff of the blood pressure apparatus is applied to the upper arm just above the elbow and is inflated with air, which compresses the brachial artery. The pressure in the cuff is transmitted to the column of mercury of the manometer or to the electronics of the digital device. The stethoscope is applied over the brachial artery just below the cuff.

When the cuff pressure becomes greater than the blood pressure, no pulse is heard or sensed by the machine. The air in the cuff is slowly released and the height of the mercury on the manometer is noted when the pulse is first heard. This corresponds to the systolic blood pressure.

With further slow deflation of the cuff, the pulse gradually becomes softer. The level of the mercury is again noted just before the pulse becomes inaudible or when there is a pronounced change in the sound heard, known as muffling. This represents the diastolic blood pressure. Electronically, the device will note the changes in these sounds and provide a digital figure. If the blood pressure is recorded as 100 mmHg, this simply means that the pressure of the blood on the walls of the vessel is sufficient to raise a column of mercury to a height of 100 mm. The normal systolic pressure in a healthy young adult in a sitting position is 100–135 mmHg; the normal diastolic pressure is 60–80 mmHg.

When the person has a history of fainting or dizziness when changing position, or of hypertension or may be dehydrated, the blood pressure should be taken in three positions if possible: supine, sitting and standing. Under normal conditions, the systolic pressure will either drop slightly or stay the same when the person rises, while the diastolic pressure rises slightly.

For accurate readings the patient's arm should be at the same level as the heart. The arm should be supported to remove the effect of muscle tension and there should be no constriction around the upper arm, such as a rolled-up sleeve.

Heart sounds

Auscultation of the heart involves listening to the heart with a good stethoscope using a systematic approach. **Heart sounds** are assessed considering the following characteristics: frequency, intensity, duration and location.

Two loud sounds are produced in quick succession in each cardiac cycle and two other very soft sounds which only the experienced ear will normally detect. These are followed by a brief pause before being repeated in the next cycle. Through a stethoscope, the heart sounds will be heard as a lubb-dubb and are produced by closure of the heart valves.

The first heart sound, S_1, is a prolonged low-pitched sound (lubb). It is produced by the closing of both atrio-ventricular valves, the mitral and the tricuspid, just before ventricular systole. Although closure of the two valves occurs almost simultaneously, the mitral valve closes slightly before the tricuspid valve. Therefore, the mitral component is heard slightly before the tricuspid and is the main component of the first heart sound. S_1 is heard best over the apex (fifth left intercostal space) of the tricuspid and mitral areas using the diaphragm of the stethoscope.

The second sound, S_2, is briefer and higher pitched (dubb). It is produced by the closing of both semilunar valves, the aortic and the pulmonary, just before diastole. As the aortic valve closes slightly before the pulmonary valve, the aortic component of S_2 will be heard slightly before the pulmonary. The components of the second sound are normally affected by respiration. During inspiration, closure of the pulmonary valve is delayed because of the increased venous return to the right heart. The difference in the two components of S_2 is therefore more apparent. This is referred to as *physiological splitting* and disappears during expiration. S_2 is best heard in the second intercostal space, either side of the sternum using the diaphragm of the stethoscope.

The remaining faint sounds are known as S_3 and S_4, and are connected with atrial emptying. They follow S_2.

Clinical characteristics of impaired cardiac function

Any impairment in circulation due to an abnormal heart condition is reflected in signs and symptoms, which are produced by various factors: (1) a reduced blood supply to the heart and tissues throughout the body, causing a reduced nutrient and oxygen supply and an accumulation of metabolic wastes; (2) malfunctioning of the conduction system; and (3) the inability of the heart to eject the blood it receives. The last factor results in an excessive volume in the venous system, creating congestion and increased pressure that interfere with the function of tissues and organs.

The signs and symptoms of cardiac conditions vary with the degree to which circulation is impaired and with the form and location of the heart condition. Those that are discussed here do not necessarily all occur in every patient, nor are they all inclusive; they are the more common problems presented by cardiac patients.

Abnormal pulse

The pulse rate may be abnormally fast or slow and the intervals between the heart beat may be unequal. The volume may vary. Some specific abnormalities of the arterial pulse are described below.

Pulsus alternans With pulsus alternans, the heart beats are regular but vary in amplitude. This condition is produced by changes in the left ventricular contractile force and is often precipitated by a premature ventricular beat. It is frequently associated with left ventricular failure resulting from hypertension, cardiomyopathy or aortic valve disease.

Pulsus bigeminus Premature contractions alternating with normal heart beats result in variation in the strength of the heart beats. This alteration in pulse volume from beat to beat is called the bigeminal pulse. It differs from pulsus alternans in that the weaker beat occurs regularly after a stronger, normally conducted, beat.

Pulsus paradoxus Normally, the strength of the arterial pulse falls during inspiration because of pooling of blood in the pulmonary vascular system. This occurs because of the more negative intrathoracic pressure and expansion of the lungs causing a reduced left ventricular stroke volume. If the blood pressure falls more than 10 mmHg (the normal fall during inspiration), the pulse is called pulsus paradoxus. Causes include cardiac tamponade, chronic constrictive pericarditis, emphysema and bronchial asthma.

Blood pressure

Arterial blood pressure is an important indicator of the patient's circulatory status. The systolic pressure depends on the cardiac output and, obviously, will fall with a reduced output by the left side of the heart. Venous pressure is frequently used to assess the ability of the heart to accept the inflow into the right side of the heart. A venous pressure in excess of the normal may indicate cardiac insufficiency or failure, or an excessive intravascular volume (i.e. there is more blood returning to the right side of the heart than it can cope with).

Heart sounds
See chapter 4.2

Dyspnoea

The patient may experience shortness of breath or laboured breathing only on exertion, or it may be present even at rest. This is due to pulmonary congestion. The left side of the heart may not be forwarding all the blood it receives, and the blood is dammed back in the pulmonary veins. The pulmonary congestion and hypertension resist alveolar expansion, increasing the work of breathing and decreasing the vital capacity. If the congestion is long standing, alveolar tissue changes occur: the elastic tissue is replaced with fibrous tissue and normal gas exchange is disturbed.

Dyspnoea that occurs when the patient is recumbent is referred to as *orthopnoea*. It may be relieved when the patient sits upright.

Cough

Fluid escapes into the alveoli from the capillaries in the congested pulmonary system and acts as a cough stimulus. This collection of transudate in the alveoli may be referred to as *pulmonary oedema*. The fluid may be expectorated as a frothy sputum and in severe heart failure may contain blood.

Hypoxia

Any impairment in circulation will create an oxygen deficiency in tissues. The cardiac output may be reduced, or a disturbance in pulmonary circulation may reduce the exchange of gases in the lung. Symptoms of an oxygen deficiency are many and varied, because the function of all structures is affected. The brain quickly reflects oxygen deprivation and reduced mental efficiency, restlessness, apathy and disorientation are manifested. If the deficiency is severe, consciousness is lost and, unless the supply to the brain is promptly re-established, there is likely to be permanent brain damage.

Severe pain (angina) occurs when muscle tissue, such as the myocardium, is deprived of adequate oxygen. Hypoxia may also cause cyanosis, a bluish colour, which is usually seen first in the lips and nail-beds.

Oedema

Excess fluid accumulates in the interstitial spaces of the tissues in cardiac disease when the heart cannot forward the blood it receives. The blood backs up in the veins and venules, raising the venous blood pressure. Normally, at the venous end of the capillaries, the colloidal osmotic pressure exceeds the hydrostatic pressure of the blood, and interstitial fluid moves into the capillary. However, if the hydrostatic pressure of the blood in the distal portion of the capillaries exceeds the blood protein osmotic pressure, interstitial fluid will not be moved into the capillaries.

The retention of sodium ions also contributes to the formation of oedema in the cardiac patient. The decreased sodium excretion is promoted by the reduced blood flow through the kidneys, which results from the impaired circulation. It is also suggested that some

Dyspnoea
See chapter 5.3

Hypoxia
See chapter 5.3

Oedema
See chapter 4.2

Pain
See chapter 2.3

Heart sounds
See chapter 4.2

mechanism may exist that causes an increased secretion of aldosterone by the adrenal cortices. This hormone promotes reabsorption of sodium in the kidney tubules.

Oedema is a very characteristic sign of some weakening in heart function. Considerable fluid accumulates before the oedema becomes apparent; a person may retain 4.5–7.0 kg of excess fluid before the oedema becomes evident. It appears first in the dependent parts of the body where gravity most hinders venous return. If the patient is ambulant, it becomes evident first in the ankles and feet but, if in bed, it appears initially in the sacral region.

Pain

Chest **pain** may result from a variety of conditions. Non-cardiac causes include musculoskeletal disorders such as cervical arthritis, gastrointestinal disorders such as reflux oesophagitis and gallbladder disease, pulmonary conditions such as pulmonary embolus, and psychological states such as severe anxiety.

Pain of non-cardiac origin may mimic that of cardiac origin. For example, the pain of oesophageal spasm is usually burning in nature, located substernally and may be relieved by glyceryl trinitrate (GTN). Non-cardiac disease is ruled out by a careful history, physical examination and specific diagnostic tests such as gastric or gallbladder investigations. The chest pain that cardiac patients experience is usually due to the deficiency of oxygen in the myocardium. It is important to determine the location, nature and precipitating or contributing factors of chest pain in order to distinguish the specific cause. The pain may be described as sharp, aching, squeezing, a feeling of heaviness or weight on the chest or a sensation of pressure within the chest. It may be mild or excruciating. It may be localized to one area or may radiate across the chest, and into the back, neck, jaw, shoulders and/or arms. It may be precipitated or aggravated by activity, breathing cold air or certain bodily positions, and may be relieved by resting or a change of position. Table 12.1 describes some causes of chest pain.

Palpitation

Change in heart function may cause the person to be conscious of heart beats. Palpitation may be due to the apex of the enlarged heart striking the chest wall with each contraction, or it may occur with an increased stroke volume in extrasystole, or ectopic beats (see p. 298).

General debilitation, loss of strength, and decreased mental and physical efficiency

Weakness, loss of appetite and weight, general apathy and reduced efficiency occur as the result of the reduced nutrient and oxygen supply, venous congestion and the accumulation of metabolic wastes.

Abnormal heart sounds

Cardiac murmurs are abnormal **heart sounds** caused by abnormalities within the heart. The most frequent causes

Table 12.1 Differential diagnosis: causes of chest pain

	Angina	Gastrointestinal	Musculoskeletal	Respiratory
Provocation	Exercise Emotional upset	Related to food consumption	Related to trauma, physical effort	Increases with inspiration or trunk movement
Palliation	Rest Glyceryl trinitrate	Antacids	Mild analgesics, heat, rest	Little relief
Quality	Tightness	Burning, discomfort, wind	Ache	Sharp, grabbing (pleurisy, pneumothorax or pulmonary embolism) or dull, aching in pneumonia
	Stops patient activity	Patient carries on activity	Patient carries on activity	Lower chest, sometimes bilateral
Region	Retrosternal	Epigastric /retrosternal	Intercostal	Pneumothorax on entire side of chest
Radiation	Arm, wrist, hand, jaw	Unlikely, but possibly through to back	Backache	Pneumothorax radiates to back
Severity	Moderate	Variable	Moderate, but variable	Moderate to severe
Timing	Recent specific onset	Vague onset, but may waken patient from sleep	Shortly after physical effort	Sudden onset and then continual pain

From Walsh et al (1999). Reprinted by permission of Butterworth–Heinemann.

of heart murmurs are stenosed and incompetent valves and openings between the right and left sides of the heart. Murmurs may also occur in an aneurysm – a localized saccular dilatation of an artery.

In determining the significance of a murmur, the doctor considers when it occurs in the cardiac cycle, its intensity, quality of sound, duration, factors that alter the sound (such as respiration and change of position) and the patient's history. Murmurs in some persons may have no great significance.

Occasionally the S_3 or S_4 heart sound becomes pronounced, producing a gallop rhythm. This may be associated with significant pathology such as hypertension, CHD or thyrotoxicosis, or may be heard in pregnancy.

Clinical diagnostic studies

The cardiac patient may require a number of diagnostic studies to evaluate disease processes and treatments. The nurse requires an understanding of these procedures and their implications to manage patient care effectively and to teach patients who wish to be more knowledgeable about their own care. Blood tests, non-invasive and invasive diagnostic procedures are discussed below.

Blood tests

A number of blood tests are conducted when investigating heart disease, including biochemical markers for myocardial damage (such as troponin levels), cardiac enzymes, blood cholesterol levels, and urea and electrolyte levels. These are discussed elsewhere in this book.

Non-invasive diagnostic procedures

Non-invasive diagnostic procedures include electrocardiography, echocardiography, nuclear magnetic resonance imaging and chest radiography.

Electrocardiography (ECG)

Electrocardiography is the study of the electrical activity associated with heart contractions. The **electrocardiogram**, which produces a graphic recording of heart activity, provides one of the most dependable aids in assessing heart function and in diagnosing heart disease. It is also non-invasive and painless to the patient.

Each heart contraction results from electrical currents that spread from the heart and can be monitored from the surface of the body. These currents are detected when electrodes are placed on the external surface of the body and make up the ECG recording.

The electrical complexes are recorded on graph paper (see Fig. 12.5). The horizontal axis of the graph paper represents time. Each small horizontal square indicates 0.04 s. Each large square is composed of five small squares and is therefore equal to 0.20 s.

The vertical axis of the graph indicates voltage. Each small vertical square represents 0.1 millivolt (mV), whereas a large square composed of five small squares equals 0.5 mV.

The electrical activity over each cycle is divided into the P, Q, R, S and T sections.

The baseline of the graph paper represents zero electrical potential. Deflections above the baseline are considered positive, and deflections below the baseline are considered

Electrocardiogram
See chapter 4.2

Figure 12.5 A normal electrocardiogram.

negative. When a wave form has both a positive and negative component, it is considered biphasic.

The *P wave* represents atrial depolarization. It begins when the electrical impulse leaves the SA node and initiates atrial depolarization. The P wave may be positive, negative or biphasic, depending on the monitoring lead, and should be no more than 2–3 mm high.

The *P–R interval* is the time interval from the beginning of the P wave to the beginning of the QRS complex. The normal P–R interval is 0.12–0.20 s. The P–R interval represents the time for an impulse to travel from the SA node to the ventricular Purkinje fibres.

The *QRS complex* represents ventricular depolarization. The Q wave is the initial downward (negative) deflection following the P wave, the R wave is the initial upward (positive) deflection following the Q wave, and the S wave is the downward deflection following the R wave. The QRS complex should not exceed 0.10 s in duration and the normal amplitude varies significantly depending on the monitoring lead.

The *ST segment* is an interval of zero potential, the period between completion of depolarization and the beginning of repolarization (recovery) of the ventricles. Usually it is isoelectric, but it may normally deviate 2.0 mm above or below the baseline.

The *T wave* represents the recovery phase after contraction or return of the ventricular muscular fibres to their resting state. Normally, the T wave is slightly rounded, asymmetrical and not more than 5–10 mm in height, depending on the lead.

A *standard 12-lead ECG* records electrical conduction events from 12 different angles or leads, six recordings from the limb leads, and six recordings from the chest leads. The ECG tracing is studied for deviations by understanding the tracing made by a normal heart, including the direction, contour and timing of the waves and segments. Information is obtained that is related to impulse formation and conduction, and to the condition and response of the myocardium. As the 12-lead ECG can provide a variety of angles of the conduction waveform, this enables a far easier diagnosis of an arrhythmia than can be offered by a bedside monitor alone. It also indicates whether any specific area of the heart is damaged, because each lead examines a particular area of the heart (Walsh and Kent 2001).

The patient should be given a brief explanation of the procedure and told that it takes approximately 5 minutes and that it is important to lie still during the procedure to produce a good tracing. The patient should be aware that the electrical recording will not cause any discomfort and there is no danger of electrocution.

In most coronary care units the nurse is responsible for obtaining the ECG. Nurses working in these specialty areas interpret ECG patterns and changes in the ECG tracings of patients connected to cardiac monitors. Nurses are becoming increasingly responsible for ECG interpretation and should always be aware of the results and their significance for the individual patient. However, nurses who are trained to administer thrombolytic (clot busting) agents will have to act upon ECG interpretation, as will nurses trained in the skills of advanced life support (ALS).

Bedside monitoring

While on a specialized cardiac unit, the patient's cardiac functioning may be monitored by bedside equipment. This equipment allows continued surveillance of the patient's ECG tracing, with rapid identification of abnormal or changing rhythms and prompt treatment.

Telemetry monitoring

A telemetry monitoring system can be used in hospital to monitor an ambulant patient's cardiac activity. This method incorporates a transmitter (a small battery-powered unit), which can fit into a pocket, and a receiver and monitor, which are commonly housed in the coronary care unit. The patient, attached to the transmitter by means of chest electrodes, can be in a ward in another part of the hospital as long as he or she is within the working radius of the transmitter and receiver. The cardiac rhythm can therefore be monitored in the coronary care unit by nurses who are able to recognize cardiac arrhythmias. This system is important because it allows patients to begin the process of appropriate mobilization without feeling imprisoned by the monitoring system.

Ambulatory electrocardiography

The Holter technique of electrocardiography is a means of studying, over a prolonged period of time, the electrical activity of the heart during a person's normal daily activities. The ECG is recorded continuously on a magnetic tape while the patient performs normal activity, usually for 24 hours. The patient keeps a diary of activities and symptoms over the recorded period. The tape is then analysed by computer for arrhythmias, which can be correlated with activities (such as sleep and exercise) and symptoms.

This technique can be used to detect and document suspected or known cardiac rhythm disturbances and to assess cardiac function during symptoms such as syncope, palpitations or chest pain.

The nurse should explain the procedure to the patient. As the machinery cannot be immersed in water, the patient will not be able to have a bath or shower during the test. It is very important that the patient maintains a normal level of activity during the test and records all symptoms and activities in the diary.

Exercise electrocardiography

An exercise ECG, also known as a stress test or graded exercise test, is used to detect and evaluate ischaemic heart disease while the individual exercises. Exercising increases myocardial oxygen demand and this test assesses the ability of the coronary arteries successfully to meet the increased demand. Thus it is useful in the evaluation of chest pain and the assessment of cardiac reserve or presence of IHD following myocardial infarction or cardiac surgery. Electrodes are attached to the patient, who is monitored continuously during the procedure. Periodically, recordings are printed.

The patient exercises on a treadmill or rides a bicycle at gradually increasing speeds against a regulated amount of resistance, according to an established protocol (often called a Bruce protocol). The exercise continues until the patient reaches a predetermined maximal heart rate according to age and sex. The test is discontinued earlier if the patient develops chest pain, hypotension, severe ventricular arrhythmias, marked ST depression, undue dyspnoea or fatigue. The exercise ECG is considered positive for ischaemia if the ECG shows an ST segment depression of 1 mm or more.

The nurse should be aware that the patient may have nitrates, calcium channel blockers and beta-blockers withheld 48 hours before the test.

On the day of the test, the patient should have a light meal and should not smoke for 2 hours before the procedure. The patient should come to the test prepared to exercise, wearing loose-fitting trousers or shorts and lace-up walking shoes, with socks to prevent blisters. It is important that the patient knows that she or he can stop the test at any time and that any symptoms, including chest discomfort, light-headedness, leg cramping and weakness, must be reported to the staff. After the test, the patient should be encouraged to rest and not to take a hot shower within 2 hours of completing the test.

Patients are likely to want to know the outcome of the test and any implications for their future. Many patients feel reassured as their performance on the test gives them some indication of their exercise capabilities, which they can then translate into activities of daily living.

Echocardiography

This is a non-invasive test used to detect ventricular dysfunction, valvular abnormalities, pericardial effusions, intracardiac masses and congenital defects.

High-frequency sound waves are aimed at the heart from a transducer held against the skin. Some sound waves reflect or 'echo' off thoracic structures, are picked up by the transducer, visualized on a screen, and recorded on videotape or on a strip chart recorder for analysis.

Doppler echocardiography

This is a valuable adjunct to the conventional echo examination. Using ultrasound, it provides information concerning blood flow patterns by assessing blood velocity at multiple locations of the heart or great vessels. Doppler colour flow mapping provides information concerning direction of blood flow. Doppler imaging is especially useful in evaluating valvular heart disease and the presence of septal defects.

Patients should be aware that they will need to lie quietly in a dimly lit room for 20–30 minutes while the technician performs the echocardiogram. They will also be asked to change position several times during the procedure.

Oesophageal echocardiography

Minute transducers mounted at the end of a gastroscope have been developed to image the heart anteriorly. This procedure is useful for visualizing the aortic and mitral valves, the aorta and the left ventricle. It is useful because it reduces the impedance of skin, muscle and bone in gaining a clear picture. The patient is asked to fast for 6 hours before the procedure and is likely to be given lidocaine (lignocaine) spray to anaesthetize the throat.

Nuclear magnetic resonance imaging

Magnetic resonance imaging (MRI) is a non-invasive diagnostic technique used to obtain high-resolution, tomographic, three-dimensional images of body structures. It allows visualization of cardiac chambers and blood vessels to determine structure, function and tissue characteristics.

Contraindications for MRI include the presence of pacemakers or implantable cardioverter defibrillators (ICDs) because the magnetic field can interfere with their operation. The presence of surgical clips and mechanical valves may produce considerable image artefact. The patient who suffers from claustrophobia or those who are acutely ill and unstable are not good candidates for this investigation.

Patients should be aware that they will be enclosed in the MRI scanner for about 30 minutes. No discomfort is felt during the procedure. The development of magnetic resonance contrast media to enhance images is creating a greater interest in this technique in cardiac patients. These require a much smaller injected volume and are less toxic than the more usual X-ray contrast media.

Chest radiography

A radiograph of the chest provides valuable information about the heart and lungs. Heart size may be assessed relatively accurately; the normal heart should be less than 50% of the width of the thoracic cavity and not exceed 16 cm. Cardiac enlargement is an early sign of cardiac failure, but an enlarged cardiac shadow may be seen in other conditions, such as valvular disease, cardiomyopathy, cardiac aneurysm and pericardial effusion. The location of invasive catheters, such as pacemaker or pulmonary artery catheters, can also be identified. There have been several advances in chest X-ray techniques in recent years. Of note are computed and digital radiography. Computed radiography uses a phosphor plate instead of conventional film. Following exposure the phosphor plate is scanned by a laser, the image digitized and stored electronically. In both computed and digital radiography, images can be manipulated electronically from one exposure, without increasing the radiation dose to the patient by taking a further radiograph (Halstead et al 2001).

A brief explanation by the nurse may help allay any apprehension on the part of the patient.

Invasive diagnostic procedures

Radionuclide imaging techniques

Nuclear cardiology includes a group of diagnostic tests in which tracer substances called radionuclides are injected into the bloodstream and their distribution in cardiac chambers is measured using a computer and a gamma camera. Tracer substances are composed of two components: the radionuclide and the substance to be tagged.

Tracers are characterized by their chemical behaviour, their physiological and biological half-life, and by the type of radiation emitted. For example, tracers that emit gamma radiation are used to make most of the measurements in nuclear cardiology.

Gamma rays emitted from the patient are detected with a gamma camera, and an image of the distribution of radioactive isotope in the area of interest is obtained. This information on isotope distribution and the relative amounts of isotope present can be obtained in fractions of a second and stored in a computer for subsequent analysis.

Nuclear cardiology techniques are relatively non-invasive, requiring only peripheral intravenous injections, and are considered safer than invasive techniques. Some measures are carried out while the patient is at rest and others during exercise.

Information provided varies with the test performed. Some tests estimate myocardial blood flow; others show cardiac haemodynamics such as cardiac output, stroke volume or ventricular performance. Radionuclide techniques

may be divided into two general types: (1) first-pass techniques, in which only the first transit of a radionuclide bolus through the circulation is analysed; and (2) equilibrium studies in which serial studies can be obtained over time.

Two nuclear myocardial imaging techniques will be described: the thallium and technetium scans.

Thallium myocardial imaging

Thallium-201 is an element with properties similar to potassium and is the radiopharmaceutical of choice for myocardial perfusion scintigraphy. Clearance from the blood is rapid and extraction by the myocardium is high.

Thallium-201 scanning provides an assessment of myocardial tissue perfusion. Normally, coronary blood perfusion is equal throughout the myocardium, and thallium-201 would be distributed evenly in the tissue. In areas of myocardial ischaemia or necrosis, little or no thallium would be picked up. These areas of no perfusion would be seen as dark or 'cold' spots on the composite computerized image. In some patients, myocardial perfusion may be normal at rest, even with severe coronary disease. With exercise, however, the blood supply in the area supplied by the diseased vessels will differ from that supplied by normal vessels. Thus thallium imaging may be paired with exercise stress testing to evaluate myocardial perfusion at rest and when stressed.

After the heart has been stressed, exercise-induced ischaemia or previous myocardial infarction with a non-viable scar will produce a perfusion defect or cold spot. A second myocardial scan (or reperfusion image) is usually done 3 hours later. During the rest period, the exercise-induced ischaemic tissue will be reperfused and will no longer show as cold spots. This is called the redistribution pattern.

Technetium myocardial imaging

The radioactive substance in this procedure is ^{99m}Tc-labelled pyrophosphate. This test detects the size, location and approximate age of myocardial damage within 7–10 days of damage. The technetium-99m is absorbed by injured myocardial cells and images obtained of the heart will show these areas as 'hot' spots or bright areas. The scanning to obtain images takes approximately 30 minutes to perform.

Cardiopulmonary angiography

There are various techniques whereby the pulmonary and cardiac circulation can be assessed. The most widely used method involves the selective placement of a suitable catheter in the vessel or cardiac chamber proximal to the region being investigated. Injected radio-opaque contrast medium flows away from the catheter tip, and its path may be recorded and stored electronically on a compact disk (CD).

Cardiopulmonary angiography may be used to investigate and diagnose a number of abnormalities, including valvular lesions, such as stenosis or regurgitation, pulmonary emboli, cardiac tumours, myocardial dysfunction, coronary artery stenosis or occlusion.

Cardiac and pulmonary angiography is invasive and not without complications; these may include a haematoma at the catheter insertion site, an allergic reaction to the contrast media, and chest pain during the procedure. As with all investigations, the potential benefit from making a correct diagnosis must exceed the risk from the diagnostic procedure. The indications for the test must be clear and the patient fully informed of what to expect. It is the doctor's duty to discuss the procedure with the patient and to gain consent, but the nurse must have sufficient understanding to respond to additional questions and be reassuring, thereby reducing anxiety. High levels of anxiety may exist amongst patients before the procedure, particularly if invasive, because of a fear of the unknown (Halstead et al 2001). Peterson (1991) found that patients had concerns over a variety of issues, including the waiting time on the day of the procedure, the actual test, lying flat on a hard table, insertion of the catheter and possible complications. Teaching the patient relaxation techniques prior to the procedure reduces stress. Patients are likely to be less anxious if they are told what sensations to expect (Peterson 1991), although some respond better if they are not told in too much detail what the procedure is like.

It is the policy of most hospitals that informed, written consent be obtained before angiography. Food and fluids are withheld for the preceding 4 hours and opiate premedication is advisable. There are few contraindications to the administration of radio-opaque contrast media. Although most patients experience a sensation of warmth with the injection, major side-effects, which include respiratory distress, hypotension, urticaria, nausea and vomiting, are fortunately rare. Treatment will depend on the severity of the reaction, but intravenous fluids, antihistamines, steroids, adrenaline (epinephrine) and oxygen should be available. Full resuscitation equipment needs to be on hand in case of problems resulting from ischaemia.

Right heart and pulmonary catheterization

This investigation provides information about the right side of the heart and the pulmonary circulation. Under local anaesthesia and sterile technique, the common femoral vein (usually the right) is punctured using a stiletted needle. The stilette is withdrawn and, once venous backflow occurs, a guidewire is threaded through the needle into the vein as far as the inferior vena cava. The needle is removed and an appropriate catheter is passed over the wire until it is in a satisfactory position, as judged by fluoroscopy. A small injection of contrast medium will confirm the position of the catheter tip.

If a pulmonary angiogram is required for suspected pulmonary emboli, the catheter is guided through the

Table 12.2   Range of normal resting haemodynamic values

	Pressure (mmHg)		
	Mean	Systolic	End diastolic
Right atrium	0–8		
Right ventricle	9–16	15–30	0–8
Pulmonary artery		15–30	3–12
Pulmonary artery 'wedge' and left atrium	1–10		
Left ventricle		100–140	3–12
Systemic arteries	70–105	100–140	60–90

tricuspid and pulmonary valves. In the assessment of right ventricular function, valvular disease or congenital defects, the catheter will be placed in the appropriate cardiac chamber.

Left heart and coronary artery catheterization

The femoral or brachial artery is used for evaluation of the left heart and coronary arteries. The technique of catheter introduction is similar for arterial studies, but more care is required because the pressures are higher. The catheter is passed retrogradely up the aorta. Crossing the aortic valve usually causes very little disturbance to cardiac or valve function; however, arrhythmias may be induced, so continuous cardiac monitoring is mandatory.

Cardiac catheterization also allows haemodynamic measurements and other parameters, such as the degree of oxygenation of blood within the various chambers, to be recorded (Table 12.2). This may be valuable in the investigation of congenital heart disease. For example, with an atrial septal defect, increased oxygen tension may be found in the right side of the heart.

The role of the nurse

The nurse has a major role in preparing the patient for cardiopulmonary angiography. As indicated above, informed written consent is required. The patient is informed of the equipment that may be seen during the procedure, the sterile precautions that will be taken, and some of the physical sensations that will be experienced, such as a feeling of pressure when the catheter is introduced and the warm flush that immediately follows injection of the contrast medium. Although each step is usually explained during the procedure, the patient's anxiety is often decreased when given this information beforehand. Some institutions may provide leaflets describing the experience.

The patient's reaction must be observed closely during the procedure. The ECG is monitored constantly. Irritation of the myocardium by the catheter may rarely precipitate ventricular fibrillation, so a defibrillator is close at hand. The patient experiences little discomfort

Figure 12.6   Placement of catheters in electrophysiology studies. SVC, superior vena cava; IVC, inferior vena cava.

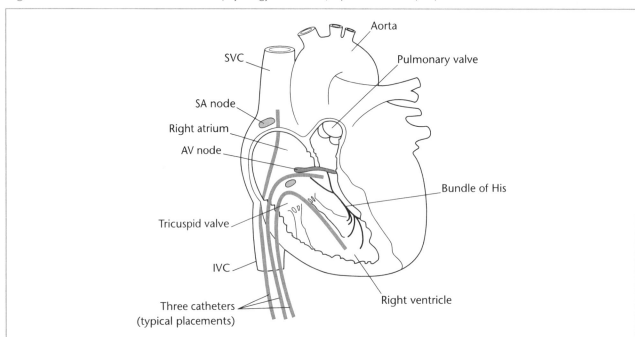

but may complain of a fluttering or irritation in the chest, especially during movement of the catheter. The patient is advised that this is a temporary sensation.

The sheaths, which introduced the catheter, are often removed by the doctor in the angiography laboratory. However, the nurse may perform this when the patient returns to the unit. Pressure is then applied over the groin area, which can be for a minimum of 10 minutes to stop bleeding from the artery. Special manual compression devices and collagen seals into the vessel have all been designed to reduce the length of time for which the nurse has to press on the groin. There has been controversy recently over how long the patient should then stay on bedrest to reduce damage to the artery and haematoma formation. It is likely that patients will lie flat for an hour and gradually be sat upright. The patient needs to be able to drink in order to clear the radio-opaque dye from the system. Searle and Hoff (2000) found that bedrest of 2–3 hours, followed by gentle mobilization, produced few side-effects such as haematoma formation. In addition, the pulse below the catheter insertion site is checked every 15 minutes for the first hour and then at gradually increased intervals if it remains normal. An irregular, rapid or weak pulse is promptly reported to the doctor. The wound is observed for redness and tenderness, which may indicate irritation or phlebitis.

Despite the above measures, there may still be an area of bruising and skin discoloration as a result of bleeding into the tissues around the puncture site. This will fade over a week or so. Patients discharged straight home need to be given advice and a contact telephone number in case of any problems. Patients frequently wish to discuss their feelings following the procedure. Although one probable reaction is relief that the procedure has been completed, anxiety about the findings and their implications is often evident.

Electrophysiology studies

An electrophysiology study (EPS) is an invasive procedure used to assess and facilitate management of recurrent symptomatic arrhythmias. The heart is deliberately provoked in an attempt to identify the existence, type and severity of the rhythm disturbance. The heart is stimulated using pacing catheters. The catheter electrodes are usually introduced via the right femoral vein (it is rare to use an artery), and are positioned with radiographic (fluoroscopic) guidance in the right side of the heart, which will receive the stimuli. Once the pacing catheter(s) are in place (Fig. 12.6), programmed stimulation is used to induce the rhythm disturbance. Figure 12.6 illustrates the three catheter positions, but a fourth may be placed in the coronary sinus, enabling recording and pacing from the left atrium (Bygrave 2001).

If the arrhythmia is induced, medications and various manoeuvres may be attempted to prevent or treat it. A long-term treatment regimen can thus be established.

Preparation and post-procedure management of the patient undergoing EPS by the percutaneous route are similar to those described for cardiopulmonary angiography. However, the patient will also have to be in a 'drug-free state' to prevent their usual medication suppressing the arrhythmias that are being induced. After the procedure it may be necessary to monitor the heart rhythm, depending on the diagnosis (Bygrave 2001).

The patient with significant arrhythmic disturbances may require ongoing evaluation using EPS.

Measurement of venous blood pressure

Venous **blood pressure** is an important parameter in the care of seriously ill patients. It reflects the intravascular volume and the ability of the heart to cope with the blood it receives via the venous system. Measurement of the venous pressure may be made in a peripheral vein, such as the median basilic, or in a large central vein, such as the superior vena cava.

Central venous pressure

Central venous pressure (CVP) is more reliable than the peripheral, and is being used clinically more often to assess the patient's condition. It may be used as a guide for fluid replacement in the dehydrated or postoperative patient, or for a critically ill patient.

An intravenous catheter is passed into the superior vena cava via the subclavian or internal jugular vein, or occasionally into the inferior vena cava via a femoral vein. The catheter is attached to a three-way stopcock which is also connected to a water manometer and intravenous infusion. An alternative, and more frequently used, method employs a pressure transducer in the CVP cannula and electronic monitoring of the CVP reading. In setting up the CVP line, the zero level of the manometer is positioned at the level of the right atrium, which is approximately in line with the mid-axillary and suprasternal notch. The most important factor is that the equipment is at the same level for each recording, so the initial level is usually marked on the patient's skin. In most instances the changes in the venous pressure or the trend of recordings are more significant than the actual level.

To take a CVP reading, patients should be lying on their back, although they can sit up; however, they must be in the same position for each recording. The pressure is generally recorded hourly. When the catheter is introduced, the stopcock is adjusted to allow fluid to flow to the patient. Then, to determine the venous pressure, the stopcock is turned to direct the fluid up into the manometer to a level of approximately 30–35 cm. The valve is then adjusted to close off the flow from the intravenous bag and to establish a flow between the manometer and the catheter. When the back pressure fluid from the venous system balances the downward pressure of the column fluid, the fluid level remains relatively stationary, rhythmically rising and falling 1–2 cm with respirations. The height of the fluid column above the base line is the CVP. After recording this, the stopcock is readjusted to allow the intravenous solution to flow to the patient.

The normal CVP is approximately 3–12 cmH$_2$O when recorded with a water manometer set on an infusion (drip) stand. When an electronic transducer is used to measure CVP, the normal range is recorded in millimetres of mercury, and is approximately 0–8 mmHg. This varies with the patient's size, position and state of hydration.

As the normal range is quite wide, it is important to note the recorded trends in CVP readings to detect changes in the patient's condition. The significance of CVP is determined in conjunction with the arterial blood pressure, the hourly output of urine, pulse rate and volume, and ECG. The nurse needs to know the levels at which the doctor is to be informed, and the type, volume and rate of flow of the infusion must be prescribed.

Other nursing responsibilities include observation for complications such as inflammation at the insertion site. This may be prevented by the use of aseptic technique during catheter insertion and during the application of dressings. Interference with flow may be minimized by periodic flushing with a solution of heparinized saline to prevent clotting, and loosely coiling the tubing to prevent it from kinking.

Measurement of pulmonary artery pressure (wedge pressure)

To obtain more specific information about the functioning of the left side of the heart, pulmonary artery and pulmonary capillary pressures are measured. This procedure is used for critically ill patients in whom early detection of left ventricular dysfunction is important.

A flow-directed pulmonary artery catheter (sometimes called a Swan–Ganz catheter) (Fig. 12.7) is inserted under sterile conditions into a central vein, such as the internal jugular or subclavian vein. A tiny balloon at the tip of the catheter is inflated and the catheter floats into the right atrium, right ventricle and pulmonary artery, at which time the pulmonary artery pressure may be measured. The catheter is then advanced into a branch of the pulmonary artery until it becomes wedged in a pulmonary capillary. The changing monitored pressure tracings allow the doctor to know where in the heart the catheter is as it is advanced. The balloon is inflated and 'wedged' in the pulmonary artery, hence the term 'wedge pressure'. It may then monitor pressure in the lungs and the left heart chambers. Thus, the catheter offers a reflection of the functioning of the left side of the heart, without directly entering these high-pressure chambers. The balloon must always be deflated until the next pressure reading, to allow blood to flow through to the lungs.

The nurse is responsible for monitoring pressures, reporting abnormalities and preventing complications. The normal pulmonary artery pressure is 25/10 mmHg, and the normal pulmonary capillary 'wedge' pressure is 4–12 mmHg. An increase in this latter reading can indicate left ventricular failure.

Nature of patients with a cardiac condition

Patients with cardiovascular problems are a diverse group. There are varying degrees of impairment and a wide range of psychological responses. Individuals will display different ways of coping with and adapting to

Blood pressure
measurement
See chapter 4.2

Central venous
pressure
See chapter 4.2

Wedge pressure
See chapter 4.2

Figure 12.7 Thermodilution pulmonary artery catheter.

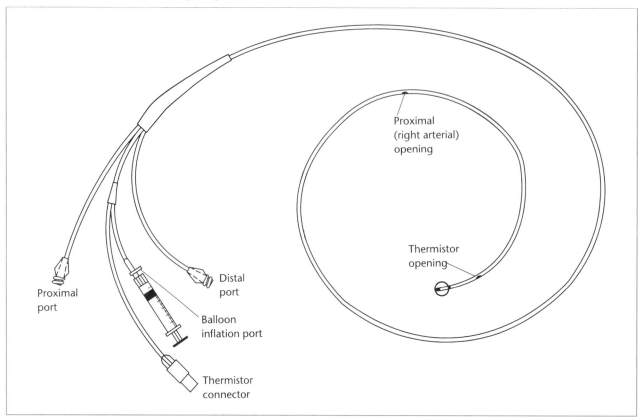

unique situations. The heart is frequently perceived as symbolizing life and health. Not being able to see the heart and related structures means that those with problems need to rely on information from healthcare professionals before they can conceptualize the extent of their disorder. Misconceptions and unfounded fears are common. Most people will know someone who has had a cardiac condition, and it is easy for information to become distorted. Significant others will also be greatly affected, as will the dynamics of family life. The ability to plan ahead and to retain a sense of control over the future may be lost.

Some individuals may have a slight physical abnormality or a condition that has been cured. The heart may carry some structural change or a scar (e.g. after myocardial infarction) but cardiac efficiency is such that no long-term restrictions on activities are necessary. Some such people may have unwarranted fears and, despite advice to the contrary, restrict their activities unnecessarily. There may be a fear of extending the damage or triggering off an old problem. Some people worry about dying. There is often a feeling that a first event, such as a myocardial infarction, is a warning and a subsequent second attack is inevitable and will be fatal. Alternatively people may experience benefits as a result of their diagnosis and continue to display activities associated with the sick role in order to guarantee themselves continuing attention and support from others. Families are

frequently uncertain how to respond to individuals with cardiac problems. They may have similar perceptions to the patient or their views may contrast significantly. A tightrope is often walked, balancing between overprotection and apparent indifference. Wives of coronary patients, for example, have been shown to engage in secret surveillance activities, monitoring their partner's every move, during the first few weeks at home (Thompson et al 1995). The role of the nurse with these patients is to try to dispel any unfounded fears and encourage an active and fulfilling lifestyle. Talking through unresolved fears and offering positive reassurance may be of benefit.

Some people are left with limited cardiac function, and some restrictions on activity are necessary. The disorder may have resulted in adaptive changes to the heart (dilation, hypertrophy and/or acceleration) in order to avoid heart failure. Energy expenditure needs to match functional capability and therefore limitations will be individual. Some may only have to give up strenuous competitive sports. Feelings of anger and a reduced sense of self-worth may accompany enforced changes in lifestyle. Frustration is a common response. Relationships may suffer as partners have to take on new roles and accept limitation in their own lives. Other relationships may be enhanced through caring and the increased openness that illness sometimes brings. The aim is to help each individual to live a useful and satisfying life within their own limitations. Individuals and their families may need support in accepting and adjusting to changes in lifestyle. Advice about appropriate activities – work, leisure, etc. and the importance of rest – may help in regaining a sense of direction and control. Ongoing medical treatment may be necessary to control symptoms. Compliance with such treatment is more likely if the individual understands the reasoning behind it and has a good relationship with the healthcare team. Realistic expectations are important.

Some patients may have a functional capacity that means they experience symptoms such as shortness of breath and chest pain on minimal exertion. They may be limited to self-care activities or be completely dependent on others. Such individuals are likely to be dependent on the care and support of their families, with resulting consequences for family dynamics. There may be a regression to child-like status with associated feelings of inadequacy, powerlessness and low self-esteem. Individuals may resent their situation and become angry and uncooperative in the eyes of their carers. They may become depressed and withdraw from life as they once knew it. Such individuals need to be helped to retain some sense of self-value and purposefulness. The family needs to be involved in care planning and decision making. Physical care can be demanding and demoralizing, and carers need a forum to express their feelings in confidence. Family members may suffer physical exhaustion and experience feelings of guilt at possible negative feelings towards their situation.

If the patient is at a terminal stage in their disease process, they need care geared towards supporting them and their families through this difficult time. Deciding when the condition has become terminal can be a problem for some healthcare professionals geared to preserving life. End-stage heart failure, although irreversible, has often not been given the same priority as other conditions such as cancer or acquired immune deficiency syndrome (AIDS). Respite care in hospital or hospice may be a way of relieving pressure on the family. The primary healthcare team may also have input at this stage.

Common problems related to cardiovascular function

Analysis of data gathered during assessment may identify a number of problems related to the individual's cardiovascular status, emotional response to disease and alterations in lifestyle. The most common problems occur as a result of:

■ decreased cardiac output

■ activity intolerance

■ chest discomfort

■ effects on family/carers

■ anxiety and other psychological responses

■ alterations in lifestyle and self-care.

See Table 12.3.

Decreased cardiac output

The individual may experience shortness of breath, lethargy, weakness, palpitations, swollen ankles, weight gain, changes in elimination pattern and/or changes in appetite. Management *goals* include:

1. reducing the workload of the heart

2. improving contractility of the heart

3. identifying and treating associated patient problems

4. monitoring effects of interventions.

Nursing intervention

Reducing the workload of the heart

Rest

Rest is important in the treatment of the patient with reduced cardiac output because it reduces the demand on the heart by reducing body requirements for oxygen. The decrease in muscular activity leads to a reduction in venous return. Filling pressure (preload) is decreased and there is greater efficiency of ventricular emptying at systole. Thus, the heart works more effectively and cardiac output increases. Renal blood flow increases as less blood is needed to supply the muscles. Recumbency-induced diuresis also decreases intravascular volume, increases urine volume and reduces oedema.

The benefits of rest need to be weighed against the severity of the problem and possible consequences of inactivity. The patient could be advised to be on *complete bedrest*, which tends to mean absolute minimal activity with help with most activities of living, or *bedrest*, which refers to the patient being able to participate in some degree of personal care. Care plans need to be specific in the amount of activity the patient is performing. The patient may react negatively to restrictions on activity and they need to know the rationale behind such restrictions and the length of time they are likely to last. Strategies need to be worked out with the patient which allow activity that induces minimal symptoms. The effect of any activity on or by the patient needs to be monitored. Intervention by the various health professionals needs to be coordinated to allow time for rest. Activity needs to be spaced out. Creating an environment conducive to rest is important.

Once an acute episode has passed, the patient is likely to be able gradually to increase activities. Intermittent rest periods throughout the day and after activities should be encouraged.

Positioning

The position that the patient with decreased cardiac output finds most comfortable in bed may be determined by

Table 12.3   Common problems related to cardiovascular disorders

Problem	Related factors	Defining characteristics
Decreased cardiac output	Cardiac arrhythmias Impaired contractility of myocardium Changes in preload Altered afterload Coronary vasospasm Changes in myocardial automaticity	Altered level of consciousness Changes in blood pressure Changes in cardiac output, pulmonary capillary wedge pressure Arrhythmias Jugular venous distension Decreased or absent peripheral pulses Increased bodyweight Altered rate and depth of respirations Crackles in lungs Changes in skin colour Decreased or absent urine output Fatigue

Activity intolerance	Immobility
	Imbalance between oxygen
	  supply and demand
	Generalized weakness
	Sedentary lifestyle
	Impaired myocardial contractility
	Impaired nutritional status
	Limited cardiac reserve
	Arrhythmias
	Lack of knowledge about energy conservation
		Statement of fatigue, weakness
		Inactivity
		Dyspnoea on exertion
		Chest pain on exertion
		Expression of decreased energy
		Significant changes in heart rate, blood
		  pressure on exertion

Chest discomfort	Decreased myocardial perfusion Increased myocardial oxygen requirements	Statement of chest pain Facial grimacing Clenched fist on chest Changes in rate and depth of respirations Altered blood pressure Changes in heart rate, rhythm Sweating

Effects on family	Disruption of family functioning due to
	  patient's illness, hospitalization, treatment
	Lack of knowledge of cardiovascular
	  disease process, management plan
	Altered sexual feelings and behaviour
		Decreased family involvement in social and
		  community affairs
		Failure to participate in usual family activities
		Lack of family participation in patient's care

Anxiety and other psychological responses	Prognosis Diagnosis Treatment plan	Complaints of anxiety, anger, denial, guilt, depression Sleeplessness Restlessness Abnormal rate or rhythm of pulse Abnormal rate of respirations Increased blood pressure Lethargy, withdrawal, hostility, non-compliance

his or her breathing. If the patient is experiencing a profound decrease in cardiac output and little dyspnoea, the supine position is preferable. This position facilitates venous return to the heart and reduces the heart's workload. The patient who is experiencing dyspnoea will be more comfortable with the head of the bed elevated, but the height of elevation should only be that at which the dyspnoea is minimal.

Patients may manifest orthopnoea, that is, less difficulty in breathing with the trunk in the upright position. This position increases the vital capacity and tends to reduce the volume of blood returned to the heart and to the pulmonary system. Pressure of abdominal viscera on the diaphragm is reduced. Some patients may be still more comfortable in a true sitting position – with the lower limbs down. A special cardiac bed on which the foot of the bed can be lowered to provide a chair-like support is available. Alternatively the patient may find comfort from sitting in a chair. The sitting position promotes the formation of peripheral oedema in the dependent parts but relieves the pulmonary congestion to some extent; peripheral oedema is much less serious than pulmonary oedema.

In the sitting position a pillow placed longitudinally at the patient's back may help provide some comfort. Pillows should be used at the sides to support the arms and relieve the fatiguing pull on the shoulders. A change may be effected by arranging a table and pillow over the bed, upon which the patient may rest the head and arms. Cot sides may be kept up on the bed to safeguard the patient when in the upright position, as the patient may become drowsy and fall to the side, or may experience cerebral hypoxia which causes disorientation. The sides are also useful when a change of position is made because they may be grasped by the patient and used for added support. Patients in the upright position are encouraged to assume the recumbent position for periods to help reduce circulatory stasis and oedema in the lower parts of the body. However, patients should not be forced to do this if they are suffering from severe dyspnoea.

In patients with heart conditions, as with all patients, the general principles of positioning apply. Good body alignment is respected to prevent contractures, hyperextension and circulatory stasis. *Even a slight change in position* every 1–2 hours is helpful. A footboard is used to prevent foot drop.

Constipation should be prevented and the patient cautioned against straining at stool because of the stress it places on the heart. A mild laxative or stool softener may be given as necessary.

Drug therapy

Nursing responsibilities towards patients receiving drug therapy include:

- administering the drug
- explaining its purpose
- monitoring the effect – changes in fluid balance, weight, oedema and breathing pattern
- observing for side-effects – dehydration, hypokalaemia, muscle weakness, arrhythmias, etc.

Vasodilator drugs reduce the workload of the heart by producing either venous dilatation (relaxing smooth muscle in the veins, thereby reducing venous return) or arterial dilatation (reducing myocardial work by decreasing peripheral vascular resistance). This lowers the heart's demand for oxygen, because less blood is returned to be pumped through the chambers due to the vessel dilatation. *Diuretics* reduce preload, blood volume and ventricular filling pressure, and resolve pulmonary and systemic congestion. *Angiotensin-converting enzyme (ACE) inhibitors* inhibit the conversion of angiotensin I to angiotensin II and are therefore very effective in lowering blood pressure. *Thrombolytics* are drugs that dissolve thrombi, which may be occluding a vessel. They are of major value when a patient is suffering a myocardial infarction (MI). *Beta-blockers* (beta-adrenergic blockers) block the β-adrenergic receptors in areas such as the heart. They can be used to treat the pain of angina by reducing the heart rate and thus the demand for oxygen. It is the mismatch between the supply and demand of oxygen by the myocardium that causes anginal pain.

Improving contractility of the heart

Myocardial contractility can be enhanced with the use of inotropes, which increase ventricular activity. They tend to be given by intravenous infusion and are commonly seen in the coronary and intensive care environment. Examples are *dobutamine* and *dopamine*. *Digoxin* is a mild oral inotrope. Unfortunately, inotropes can overstimulate the heart, leading to myocardial hypoxia with the possibility of ventricular arrhythmias.

Identifying and treating associated patient problems

Shortness of breath

Appropriate positioning of the patient, spacing out activities, encouraging rest and administering drug therapy may help ease **shortness of breath**. In addition, oxygen therapy may be beneficial because it helps correct the ventilation–perfusion imbalance that leads to hypoxia. Sometimes opiates in the form of diamorphine prove helpful as they reduce anxiety, leading to systemic vasodilatation, which improves cardiac efficiency.

Palpitations

The patient in hospital may require frequent ECGs or constant cardiac monitoring. Individuals, particularly those at home, need to be aware of the importance of reporting any abnormal heart sensations. Changes in heart rate and rhythm need to be assessed for their nature and frequency, and for the effect they have on the individual concerned.

Oedema and weight gain

The patient with fluid retention and **oedema** is at increased risk of pressure sore development and problems associated with reduced mobility. They may also have negative feelings about their body image and become depressed and withdrawn. Drug therapy needs to be given as prescribed and its effects monitored. Elevating swollen limbs may also help. Individuals need to have realistic expectations about the effects of treatment and to be aware of the importance of frequent pressure relief for affected areas.

Changes in elimination pattern

Prolonged immobility and gastrointestinal stasis may lead to constipation requiring a mild aperient.

Diuretic therapy is likely to lead to an increase in the volume and frequency of urine output. The timing of administration of these drugs should be planned around the patient's day to avoid disruption, particularly at night. Despite possibly feeling lethargic, it is usually easier to use the bedside commode than a bedpan.

Dyspnoea
See chapter 5.3

Oedema
See chapter 4.2

Changes in appetite

Gastrointestinal congestion, ascites and/or lethargy may lead to a reduction in appetite. An easily digestible diet should be available and encouraged. A high salt intake needs to be discouraged because it attracts excess water and has been linked to factors such as high blood pressure, which can lead to further complications (e.g. heart failure). Those who are overweight need to be advised of the benefits of weight reduction as this reduces myocardial workload and enables exercise to be taken more easily, thus improving cardiac function.

Monitoring effects of interventions

The effect of interventions designed to improve cardiac output can be evaluated through monitoring:

- fluid balance
- daily weight
- blood pressure, heart rate
- subjective feelings
- level of exercise tolerance
- associated clinical features.

Activity intolerance

Patient goals

1. The patient will be able to perform planned activities without increased dyspnoea and fatigue.

2. The patient will understand and participate in a planned physical activity programme.

Nursing intervention

Activity progression

An acute episode of cardiovascular dysfunction will often confine the patient to bed until symptoms abate. This means that the patient is dependent on the nurse to facilitate care. It is important to discuss this necessary dependence with the patient so that its purpose, importance and temporary nature are understood.

The patient is encouraged to perform mild activities such as cleaning teeth, washing face and hands, and feeding, as long as reaching is avoided. Exercising the lower limbs to prevent venous stasis is commenced. Most patients are helped to use a bedside commode, as this demands less energy than using a bedpan. Undisturbed rest periods are provided following short periods of activity, for instance after eating or bathing.

As the patient's condition improves, activities and ambulation are gradually increased. An important principle in gradual ambulation is pacing activities. Rest periods are alternated with activity, and certain activities may be avoided for a period of time. These may include pushing, pulling, lifting or straining.

When patients learn that they have a heart condition or are recovering from an acute cardiac illness, they are advised as to whether former activities may be resumed or whether it will be necessary to curtail some activities. On the basis of the functional capacity of the heart, some individuals may consider themselves doomed to complete invalidism and an early death. They may have an unjustified fear of another attack or of participating in any activity, creating unnecessary problems and hardships for themselves and their families or carers. Maximum independence should, however, be the ultimate goal. Some may find that a few simple adjustments in their pattern of living are necessary, while others are more restricted.

There are several ways of assessing the patient's capacity for activity and any limitations. The patient's response to a gradual increase in energy expenditure is a key indicator of progress. This will probably begin with self-care activities which are progressively extended to include more strenuous efforts. The assessment programme may go on over several weeks or months, and the patient may require considerable encouragement to persevere. An exercise tolerance test may give the patient positive encouragement as to how far they can push themselves.

The nurse may assist in the assessment of the patient by observing and recording responses to various activities. Any complaint of shortness of breath, palpitation, fatigue or an undue increase in the pulse rate are noted, and the effort is discontinued.

It is helpful to have patients list their regular pattern of activity. It may then be apparent what changes, if any, are necessary. This is useful in getting patients to think and talk about how much they will be able to do. It encourages patients to plan independently and to reach a compromise between activity and restriction. Ideally, patients should be given the information, advice and support, and encouraged to decide for themselves what they can or cannot do. Individuals need to have the confidence to listen to their own body's response to activity and exercise, and to interpret what they find and modify their activity levels accordingly. Those with cardiovascular disorders will be of a variety of ages and previous levels of fitness. They will have varying expectations of and needs for future activity levels. Standardized activity programmes are likely to be inhibitive for some and overambitious for others. Individually setting short- and long-term objectives will give a sense of direction and encourage motivation. Practical information regarding daily activities such as gardening is more useful than simply suggesting a gradual return to normal.

Once the patient is free of pain and other early symptoms and feels quite well, activities may still be restricted. Time may drag, so some effort should be made to provide suitable diversions in which the patient is interested. Reading or radio and television programmes may occupy the patient. Some hobby may be pursued without over-taxing the heart. Visitors are restricted at first, but later they help to relieve the patient's boredom. Visitor selection should be made by the family to avoid those who might excite or distress the patient. Visitors should be made aware of time limitations as it may be difficult for patients to ask them to leave if they become tired.

Planned physical activity programme

Physical activity refers to any body movement that uses energy, for example housework, gardening, etc. *Exercise* refers to structured body movement that is performed with the purpose of enhancing health and fitness.

Following an acute cardiac event, or the diagnostic label of some form of heart disorder, there is a temptation for many consciously to avoid physical activity and exercise. The symptoms brought on by exercise may mimic those of a cardiac problem (e.g. breathlessness and sweating), and therefore cause anxiety. Loss of confidence may prevent participation in the simplest of activities. A vicious circle ensues: the less active the individual becomes, the more likely they are to experience symptoms of breathlessness and fatigue.

The benefits of physical activity include:

- enhancement of physical working capacity, enabling individuals to work harder for longer with less effort
- improvement in the efficiency of the cardiovascular system
- improvement in posture
- helping in weight management, thus improving self-esteem
- improvement in sense of well-being and stress reduction
- reduction in the risk of disorders such as IHD, hypertension, diabetes and osteoarthritis.

The benefits of aerobic exercise for cardiac patients include:

- improvement of collateral circulation
- decreased resting heart rate
- increased maximal exercise capacity
- improved peripheral circulation and blood pressure reduction
- increased levels of high-density cholesterol.

Elderly individuals with heart disease have been shown to make significant improvements in functional capacity with a regular exercise programme (Hellman and Williams 1994). Structured exercise is now generally viewed as beneficial to the majority of patients with heart failure, to increase their functional capacity (Gould 2001).

Individuals who experience angina need gradually to increase their exercise levels. The threshold at which they experience pain is likely to increase. Following myocardial infarction or heart surgery, activity levels should again be built up gradually and regular exercises introduced as soon as surgical wounds have healed (4–6 weeks).

In hospital

Many hospitals have structured activity programmes beginning as soon as the acute stage is over. The more active the patient is in hospital, the more likely they are to have the confidence to build up activity at home. A typical plan of activity progression in hospital would involve the following:

1. Rest in bed, chair, carrying out own toilet/hygiene activities at the bedside. Perform gentle neck, arm and leg exercises.
2. Walk around the bed area, sit in the bathroom for wash at the sink, be wheeled to bathroom, gradually increase gentle exercises.
3. Walk around ward area, walk to bathroom and toilet, increase exercises.
4. Walk around more frequently. Use the shower, then rest.
5. Build on the above plus monitored use of the stairs.

First weeks at home

Day-to-day activities should be gradually increased over the first few weeks at home. The distance walked each day should gradually be increased to build up stamina. Small amounts of activity need to be followed by rest. Individuals should be encouraged to monitor their own body's response and recognize appropriate and inappropriate signs. Warming up before exercise is important to loosen the joints, as is cooling down once the activity is over.

Exercise should be avoided until at least 2 hours after a heavy meal as blood and hence oxygen is diverted to the gut to aid digestion. Extremes of temperature should also be avoided. If chest pain, nausea, excessive shortness of breath, faintness, palpitations and/or excessive sweating is experienced, the activity should be stopped.

Activity that is moderate, rhythmic, continuous and aerobic such as walking, cycling and swimming should be encouraged initially. Heavy lifting, pulling, pushing, impact activity or anything that involves a sudden burst of activity should be avoided at first.

Chest discomfort

Patient goals

Management goals include:

1. early recognition of chest discomfort
2. elimination of chest discomfort
3. prevention of further chest discomfort.

Nursing intervention

Early recognition of chest pain

This requires that: (1) the individual is able to acknowledge and report chest pain as appropriate; and (2) healthcare professionals are aware of chest pain.

Each patient needs to be taught the significance of chest pain and to be made aware of the importance of acknowledging the signs and symptoms, and of reporting them to others when appropriate. Some patients may not realize that the sensation they are experiencing is anything to do with the cardiovascular system. The pain can be similar to that of indigestion. Others may have been told that their pain is cardiac, but choose to ignore or deny it. People sometimes try to work through their pain, continuing with activity as a method of distraction. The response to pain is likely to depend on an individual's perception of the significance of the pain and other factors, such as health perception and the need to be seen by others as being well.

Some studies have shown that nurses' assessments of patients' pain are not always reliable (Drayer et al 1999, Watt-Watson et al 2000), although others have demonstrated that assessments are more accurate if nurses have been taught about the significance of symptoms (Thompson et al 1994). Nurses need to be aware of typical words used to describe cardiac pain, the site and radiation of such pain, and likely associated symptoms, bearing in mind that individual experiences can differ widely. In hospital there will be access to other means of assessment including ECG, cardiac monitoring, blood pressure recording and blood tests. Totally painless cardiac ischaemia is possible; nurses therefore need to be aware of changes in the ECG pattern associated with ischaemia.

Elimination of chest pain

Administration of nitrates

Nitrates act by relaxing vascular smooth muscle. This results in decreased peripheral vascular resistance and venous return, with a subsequent decrease in heart size, stroke volume and cardiac output. The net effect is a decrease in the oxygen consumption of the heart.

Glyceryl trinitrate (GTN) is a short-acting vasodilator administered in tablet, skin patch or spray form. The tablet is placed under the tongue where it is absorbed very quickly (sublingual). The patient may experience a tingling feeling on the tongue at first and should obtain relief in 1–2 minutes. Patients should not take multiple doses to obtain quick relief of pain. If relief is not apparent after three tablets taken at 5-minute intervals and the patient is outside the hospital, he or she should come to the hospital as soon as possible. If the patient is in hospital, the nurse will initiate therapy as ordered by the doctor or dictated by a predetermined protocol. The initial dosage of GTN should be 0.3 mg. This reduces the likelihood of severe headaches, which often occur in the initial

Oxygen therapy
See chapter 5.3

stage of treatment. People who suffer attacks of angina are advised to carry the drug at all times. It should be replaced periodically so that a fresh supply is available when required. Tablets should be kept in a dark glass container and those not being carried should be stored in a cool, dark place, because GTN is affected by both light and heat. The patient is advised that there may be a mild fullness, warmth or throbbing in the head, but fortunately with continued use these side-effects usually diminish.

In emergency situations GTN may be administered intravenously.

Administration of analgesics

An analgesic such as diamorphine is usually given to relieve severe pain not relieved by nitrates. The drug may be administered intravenously in small doses in pre-hospital care, the accident and emergency department and in the coronary care unit. Intramuscular injections raise creatine phosphokinase readings, as this enzyme is also present in skeletal muscle, and diagnosis of a myocardial infarction may be obscured. However, the majority of units are now using biochemical markers such as the troponins, with levels recorded a set number of hours apart to determine the presence of myocardial damage. The effect of diamorphine on the respirations should be noted, as depression of the respiratory centre may occur. This drug will reduce preload, afterload, sympathetic tone and the patient's anxiety.

Administration of oxygen

Oxygen is usually administered in order to increase arterial oxygen tension, which may help to relieve the myocardial pain caused by hypoxia and prevent extension of the infarction. Observations are made of the patient's response to oxygen. Its effectiveness will be indicated by reduced pulse rate, less dyspnoea, improvement in colour, less restlessness and improved oxygen saturation levels as monitored by pulse oximetry.

Prevention of further chest pain

Administration of nitrates

Long-acting nitrates, such as the buccal tablets that are placed in the buccal cavity (between upper lip and gum) and left to dissolve, can be used if regular attacks of angina are being experienced. Other nitrate tablets used to control angina include *isosorbide dinitrate* and *isosorbide mononitrate*. Modified-release preparations prolong the effects. In hospital, intravenous nitrate therapy may be prescribed. The dose is usually low initially and increased in response to pain. Some people may experience hypotension and feel light-headed on standing. A headache is common, and paracetamol may help. GTN tablets may be taken prophylactically before an activity known to produce angina, although there is a danger of psychological dependence and not being able to get an accurate picture of the level of activity needed to produce pain.

Reduction of workload on the heart

The reduction of workload on the heart is important so that there is sufficient oxygen available to the myocardium to meet the demands placed upon it. Pacing of activities to ensure adequate periods of rest between periods of activity can facilitate balanced supply and demand on the heart.

Anxiety reduction

Increased anxiety levels increase the likelihood of chest pain as the stress response stimulates the sympathetic nervous system. Biofeedback or relaxation techniques such as background music may help some. Distraction, such as watching the television, may help others. The nurse should ensure a calm relaxing environment for the patient at all times.

Anxiety and other psychological responses

Goals

Goals will be individual and centred around the response of each person concerned. They may include the person being able to talk about feelings of anxiety or to show signs of a reduction in anxiety.

Nursing intervention

People with heart disease are frequently anxious. Serial measurements of the anxiety levels of coronary patients have shown that anxiety is highest on admission to the coronary care unit and immediately after transfer to the ward, falling rapidly over the following week and rising just before discharge (Thompson et al 1987).

The common knowledge that the heart is a most vital organ and that heart disease is a frequent cause of death produces a great emotional reaction in the person advised of a diagnosis of a heart disorder. This response is likely to be very individual and depends on factors such as age, perception of the significance of the diagnosis, and expectations for the future. The complex range of emotions produced can be described in terms of response to loss: loss of health, loss of status, loss of income, loss of confidence, and loss of any notion of invincibility. The individual is likely to go through the stages described in models of mourning, including numbness, denial, disbelief, grief, guilt, anger, despair, depression and disorganization. Anxiety is the most common initial response, peaking again in the early recovery period (Thompson et al 1987). All the above responses are normal, although they may become prolonged and then lead to serious distress. There is no set pattern to coping, and responses will depend on individual personality and experience. Reorganization and acceptance are the final stages of adaptation, although not all will work through to this response.

The aim is to encourage individuals to accept the reality of their situation and adjust accordingly. The emotional energy invested in grief and anger needs to be reinvested in positive coping for the future. The individual needs to:

- accept the reality of the situation
- work through negative emotions
- adjust emotionally to changed circumstances
- make necessary changes in lifestyle, employment, etc. in order to move with confidence to an acceptable quality of life.

The nurse who understands the patient's condition, and who knows what to look for and what to do, usually displays calm and composure which contribute to the patient's confidence and security. Brief and precise explanations of all equipment, routines, tests and procedures usually prove helpful. A quiet, controlled atmosphere may do more toward allaying fear than verbal reassurance.

Patients may pose direct questions about their condition, such as: 'Is it serious?' or 'Will I recover?' Answers should be honest and supportive. Each patient must be helped to find a coping strategy appropriate to his or her personal situation and own strengths and weaknesses. This is done through effective communication with the patient. Effective communication includes listening to the patient and responding to any cues, introducing statements to which the patient might respond, and allowing the patient to discuss feelings. Considerable help and peace of mind may be derived from a priest or other religious leader.

If the patient is very upset, the nurse remains until the patient is less apprehensive, and confirms that someone is close by and will be in and out frequently. The presence of a close member of the family who will not disturb the patient may provide additional comfort. Occasionally, diazepam or another anti-anxiety drug may be prescribed.

There may be a problem at home that contributes to the patient's unrest, which should be discussed if appropriate or arrangements made for assistance from the social services or primary healthcare team.

Effects on family/carers

Patient's family or carer's goals

1. The family/carer(s) will express feelings of support and awareness of available resources.

2. The family/carer(s) will be able to participate in the patient's treatment as appropriate.

It is important to understand that the family may not necessarily be a close or blood relative of the patient. A detailed nursing assessment will ascertain who the patient regards as closest emotionally to them and who can offer support.

Nursing intervention

Members of the patient's family often experience shock and anxiety in response to the patient's diagnosis. Seeing someone close to us in pain and seriously ill is a very frightening experience. Relatives of patients have described their initial reaction as 'feeling numbed and dazed'. As reality sets in, anxiety about the patient's survival and future increases.

Good relationships between family members and healthcare professionals need to be fostered early on. Soon after admission the family needs to be advised about suspected diagnosis and initial treatment. Family members may be uncomfortable in approaching nursing staff to ask questions and so should be invited to discuss their feelings and concerns. Relatives as well as patients are reassured by simple explanations of equipment, procedures and routines. In talking to the family, the nurse may elicit information about the patient's habits, likes and dislikes, and emotional reactions, which are helpful in planning care.

Alleviating the anxieties of relatives and/or close family friends allows them to be more supportive of the patient. As with the patient, concern may prevent the members of the family from absorbing all that they are told. Explanations and instructions may have to be repeated. The family should be included in teaching programmes provided for the patient or in programmes specifically designed for them to ensure they understand the patient's condition. Visiting times need to be viewed as an important contribution to recovery. Open visiting is encouraged in many areas with thought to individual patient needs. Restricted visiting may distance the family from the patient's recovery (Fairburn 1994).

Dynamics within the family may take a while to re-establish themselves. They may never return to how they were before the event. Relationships may be perceived as stronger or weaker. The anxiety created from having cardiac disease can have a clear detrimental effect on resuming sexual activities (Friedman 2000). Unfortunately specific teaching, supporting and/or counselling interventions aimed at managing the effects of illness and treatment on sexual function are not usually provided by nurses (Gamel et al 1993). Couples are often open about discussing sexual matters once the subject has been mentioned, and nurses need to examine their own feelings towards the issue. Partners may have unresolved feelings of guilt at having contributed in some way to the problem. It is not always relevant for nurses to become involved in complex family issues but they need to be aware of the important part they play in recovery and offer support and advice as appropriate.

Patients in the community will need the support of their general practitioner and practice or district nurse. More practices are establishing support groups for individuals with similar problems. Self-help groups may help to foster positive attitudes and provide a means of social support (Hildingh et al 1994).

There is evidence that spouses experience significant distress when a partner is experiencing a cardiac disease (Kettunen et al 1999, O'Farrell et al 2000), yet professional support, particularly of the spouse, is often inappropriate or inadequate. The main need is to feel that there is hope (Norris and Grove 1986). A simple programme of in-hospital counselling for coronary patients and spouses has a number of benefits, including a reduction in anxiety and depression (Thompson 1990). Patients in early recovery from myocardial infarction or cardiac surgery have been found to want information on the side-effects of treatment and knowledge of their disorder (Jaarsma et al 1995).

Alterations in lifestyle and self-care

Patient goals

1. The patient will show knowledge of the disease process.

2. The patient will engage in lifestyle modification to reduce risk.

Nursing intervention

Patient's knowledge of the disease process

To make the best possible adjustment to illness and recovery, the patient must have some understanding of the illness and how he or she can assist in recovery. Provision of this information helps to give the patient realistic expectations and some control over the situation. Teaching programmes are adjusted to specific patient needs and capabilities, as learning capacity varies among individuals. Patients experiencing cardiovascular conditions often have many misconceptions of their condition and how it will affect their future. It is useful for the nurse to find out what the patient already knows and to obtain information about lifestyle. The nurse has many opportunities to reinforce and elaborate on explanations given by the doctor and to respond to further questions.

During the acute stage, the patient is often too anxious to absorb much information. *Simple* explanations of equipment being used and procedures common to coronary care units are usually adequate. Following transfer to the general ward, the patient is usually better able to participate in a planned programme. Written as well as verbal instruction may be provided. Visual aids such as heart models or diagrams help to enhance learning.

Short teaching sessions are necessary, as many patients with cardiovascular conditions tire easily. It is helpful if one of the family can be present during the teaching session. Acknowledgement is made of the feelings that the patient has in response to the illness. The patient may wish to express verbally the feelings being experienced, such as discouragement, fear, anger and/or depression; the nurse should provide opportunities for free expression and should be a willing listener.

Use should be made of the many useful pamphlets and booklets available from the British Heart Foundation. Many of these deal with rehabilitation, and appropriate copies may be given to the patient to read, backed up with individual information and advice.

Lifestyle modification

The harmful effects of smoking are so severe that the patient is advised to discontinue.

Clarification of the prescribed diet is made. Many patients are advised to continue with a low sodium (salt) intake and a limited number of calories. Foods allowed, those restricted and meal planning are discussed. The importance of keeping the weight normal and avoiding large meals is explained. Preferably, the discussion of the diet should be with the family as well as the patient. Directions and suggestions are given to the patient in writing, and an appropriate diet booklet can be obtained from the British Heart Foundation, the Health Education Authority or the dietetic department.

The medications that are to be continued are discussed, and written instructions are provided. Early signs of untoward reactions are cited; included with these are directions about what to do if they develop. For example, if an anticoagulant such as warfarin is to be continued, the patient and a family member are advised of the action of the drug and the necessary observations to recognize bleeding. They are told that bleeding from body orifices, discoloured areas of the skin (bruises and petechiae), bleeding gums, and persistent bleeding from minor cuts or injuries are to be reported immediately to the doctor or clinic. If there is dental work to be done, the patient should advise the dentist that he or she is receiving warfarin. The patient is given an identification card to carry which states that he or she is receiving warfarin. A weekly visit to a clinic for prothrombin time evaluation is usually requested by the doctor.

Many patients with heart conditions are required to take digoxin continuously and should understand that loss of appetite, nausea or diarrhoea may indicate the need for some adjustment in the dosage of the drug. If the patient is an elderly person who lives alone, it is advisable for a calendar to be kept available with the time that a medication is to be taken clearly marked. It is stressed that the patient should adopt the habit of marking off the medication as soon as it is taken.

Progressively increased activity is encouraged to condition the patient to the level of activity that corresponds to the heart's ability.

Changes may be necessary at home if the patient is not able to use stairs. It may be helpful to have a member of the primary healthcare team or an occupational therapist or social worker assess the home situation before the patient is discharged. For example, a bedroom and bathroom may have to be provided on the ground floor.

It should be pointed out to the patient and family that moderation in everything is a good rule for persons who have had a heart illness. Some work, exercise, rest and recreation are important for everyone. Situations that are likely to add undue strain should be anticipated and avoided. Enough time should be allowed to prevent rushing. For example, rather than having to run for a bus, the patient should plan to leave earlier. Climbing, walking against a strong wind, lifting, pushing and fatigue are to be avoided. Constipation, infections and emotional upsets also tend to increase the demands on the heart. Suitable recreational activities, which meet both interests and cardiac functional capacity, may be suggested. Exercise is beneficial and walking is a particularly good exercise. Regular hours of rest at night and, if necessary, a rest period during the day are recommended.

The doctor, a social worker or the nurse may discuss necessary adjustments in the person's work situation with the employer or occupational health nurse. Assistance might be given to find suitable employment or to obtain retraining if a change in occupation is indicated.

Some follow-up service is important. The patient and family are advised of the resources outside the hospital, and a referral may be made to the cardiac rehabilitation programme, general practitioner or district nurse. Home visits by a nurse can be very helpful; they provide an opportunity for the patient and family to ask questions and receive counselling on the various aspects of care. At the same time the patient's condition and progress are observed.

An individual may choose not to follow advice given but still gain support from the nurse–patient interaction. Understanding what has happened and what to expect during recovery may enable the patient and family to cope, without necessarily influencing subsequent behaviour patterns.

Causes and types of heart disorder

Heart disorders may be classified as *congenital* or *acquired*. Various subclassifications may be used in acquired heart disease. Some authors concentrate on structure, such as pericardium, myocardium and endocardium. Others highlight the causes of heart disease, such as trauma, infections, degenerative processes, and hypermetabolic and hypometabolic processes. This text classifies heart disorders as:

- congenital cardiovascular defects

- disorders of cardiac muscle

- disorders of myocardial blood supply

- disorders of electroconduction

- disorders of myocardial pumping capacity
- disorders of the vascular system.

Congenital cardiovascular defects

Congenital cardiovascular defect implies a structural abnormality that was present at birth in the heart or the large proximal blood vessels. It has been only within the past two or three decades that many of the congenital cardiovascular defects have been identified and successfully treated by surgery. Many are recognized shortly after birth if the infant survives. Others may go undiscovered for months or years because the heart maintains an adequate circulation by compensation. As in so many congenital deformities, the cause remains obscure.

An individual's response to a congenital condition is likely to alter with time. The significance of the problem may not become apparent until the person gets older and starts to want to plan ahead, for example starting a family. Uncertainty as to how symptoms of the disorder will increase with time may produce feelings of fear, uncertainty and loss of control. To meet such needs there has been an emergence in recent years of Grown Up

Congenital Heart Teams, known as GUCH teams. They aim to meet the needs of adolescents and young people with congenital cardiovascular defects who are making the transition to independent adulthood.

Many types of heart malformation occur. They may be classified into three main groups: (1) those that produce a left-to-right shunt of blood; (2) those that offer resistance to the blood flow; and (3) those that cause a right-to-left shunt (Fig. 12.8).

Anomalies that cause a left-to-right shunt

Several malformations occur that produce an abnormal pathway that permits a direct flow of blood from the left side of the heart or aorta to the right heart or pulmonary artery, creating a bypass of the systemic circulation and an overloading of the pulmonary circulation. These anomalies include patent ductus arteriosus and septal defects.

Atrial septal defect (ASD)

An opening between the two atria (Fig. 12.8c) may be due to failure of the foramen ovale to close after birth or

Congenital defects
See chapter 4.2

Figure 12.8   Congenital cardiac defects: (a) patent ductus arteriosus; (b) tetralogy of Fallot; (c) atrial septal defect; (d) coarctation of aorta.

to a gap in the septum, either above or below the foramen ovale. There are three types. The most common is termed an *ostium secundum* defect and is found in the middle of the atrial septum. The other two are *ostium primum* and *sinus venosus* (Farrelly 2000). Blood in the left atrium will flow through the opening into the right atrium, increasing the volume of blood in the pulmonary system. The right atrium, right ventricle and pulmonary artery enlarge. Pulmonary hypertension develops and causes dyspnoea, particularly on exertion. The reduced systemic circulatory volume retards physical and mental development and efficiency. The size of the opening may be so small that it goes undiscovered, and the patient may not experience any respiratory or circulatory difficulty.

Surgical repair of an atrial septal defect is usually accomplished by open heart surgery. Some defects may be closed simply by suturing, whereas others may require a patch of Teflon.

Ventricular septal defect

An opening in the ventricular septum results in a left-to-right shunt and produces problems similar to those cited in atrial septal defect: pulmonary hypertension, enlargement of the right ventricle and pulmonary arteries, and a deficient systemic circulation. If the defect is small and the patient is asymptomatic, surgery is not indicated. Moderate to severe defects may be closed by patching with either pericardial tissue or Teflon. Occasionally the defect closes spontaneously in the young child.

Patent ductus arteriosus

Normally, after birth, a gradual spontaneous constriction and atrophy of the ductus takes place. If it remains open, the blood in the aorta, under a pressure approximately five to six times that in the pulmonary artery, is shunted into the pulmonary artery (Fig. 12.8a). This increases the volume of blood entering the lungs, resulting in a high pulmonary blood pressure and dilatation of the pulmonary vessels. The patient experiences dyspnoea, particularly on exertion. There is a corresponding increase in the venous flow into the left atrium and left ventricle, causing dilatation and hypertrophy of the left side of the heart. The volume of blood in the systemic circulatory system is less than normal, and the resulting oxygen and nutritional deficiencies delay normal mental and physical development.

The patent ductus arteriosus is corrected by surgical division and suturing of the two ends of the vessel.

Anomalies that cause resistance to blood flow within the circulation

The severity of the problem is determined by the degree of constriction or stenosis found in the pulmonary artery or aorta.

Pulmonary stenosis

A stenosis of the pulmonary valve or artery offers resistance to the outflow of blood from the right side of the heart. The right ventricle enlarges and the pressure in both the right ventricle and atrium is above normal. Blood may be backed up in the venous system, while the blood volume entering the pulmonary system is below normal. The latter creates an oxygen deficiency throughout the body which is manifested by fatigue, shortness of breath and, less frequently, cyanosis. Symptoms may not be present for several years.

This malformation may be treated surgically by incision of the constricted ring.

Aortic stenosis

A defect comparable to pulmonary stenosis may occur in the aorta and offer resistance to left ventricular outflow. The left side of the heart enlarges and the pressure in both left chambers is greater than normal; this may be reflected in an increased pulmonary pressure if the restriction is severe. The cardiac output is lower and reduces arterial blood pressure and the systemic circulation as well as the blood supply into the coronary arteries. The defect may be treated by operation, using an extracorporeal pump oxygenator (cardiopulmonary bypass) during the procedure.

Coarctation of the aorta

Coarctation is a stricture in a segment of the aorta (Fig. 12.8d). *Postductal coarctation* occurs just beyond the obliterated ductus arteriosus and distal to the origin of the left subclavian artery. The second type, *preductal coarctation*, develops in the segment of aorta before the entrance of the ductus arteriosus. With this latter type the ductus usually remains patent.

Blood volume and pressure are increased behind the stricture, and the work of the left side of the heart is increased greatly. The blood volume and pressure are high in the upper extremities and head, but are abnormally low in the body parts that derive their blood supply from below the stricture. A difference in growth and development may be seen between the areas supplied from behind the stricture and those supplied from the aortic flow distal to the stricture. The patient may experience headaches, epistaxis, dyspnoea on exertion, leg cramps and fatigue.

Surgical treatment of the condition involves resection of the constricted area and an end-to-end anastomosis, or, in some instances, the area is excised and a graft of inert material introduced.

Anomalies that cause a right-to-left shunt

A shunting of blood from the right side of the heart to the left involves a combination of two or more anomalies. Normally, the pressure is much higher in the left side of the heart than in the right. A stenosis that offers resistance to flow from the right ventricle may increase the pressure in the right side to a level exceeding that in the left side. If a septal defect coexists with this increased pressure, blood is shunted from the right to the left side of the heart.

One of the most frequently seen combinations of anomalies that produces a right-to-left shunt is the *tetralogy of Fallot* (Fig. 12.8b). Tetralogy denotes a set of four conditions: pulmonary stenosis, ventricular septal defect, dextraposition of the aorta which causes it to override the septal defect, and right ventricular hypertrophy. The pulmonary stenosis produces an increased pressure in the right ventricle, causing a right-to-left shunt. The volume of blood flowing through the pulmonary system for oxygenation is reduced. Unoxygenated blood escapes into the aorta and a general systemic hypoxia occurs, manifested by cyanosis and dyspnoea, especially on physical exertion, and by clubbing of the fingers. Compensatory responses to the oxygen deficiency develop in the form of polycythaemia, high haemoglobin level, and increased pulse and respiratory rates.

Correction of these defects is possible by means of open heart surgery and the use of the cardiopulmonary bypass machine. The septal opening is patched, and the pulmonary stenosis is relieved. Occasionally the surgeon may decide not to perform corrective surgery but will proceed with a palliative surgical procedure, referred to as a 'shunt'. This consists of an anastomosis between the subclavian and pulmonary arteries (Blalock–Taussig shunt) to divert a larger volume of blood through the lungs for oxygenation.

Miscellaneous congenital cardiac anomalies

A wide variety of anomalies can occur; many are not yet amenable to treatment, and others may be so severe that the infant cannot survive. *Transposition of the great vessels* is relatively common and may be treated surgically. In this anomaly, the pulmonary artery originates from the left side of the heart and conducts the oxygenated blood back to the lungs, and the aorta rises from the right ventricle, carrying unoxygenated blood into the systemic circulation. *Valvular atresia* (absence of an opening) is another form of anomaly that occurs most frequently with the tricuspid valve, but may also develop with the aortic valve. Tricuspid atresia raises the pressure within the right atrium to a level exceeding that in the left atrium, and blood flows through the foramen ovale. This anomaly is frequently accompanied by a ventricular septal defect and is corrected surgically.

Disorders of cardiac muscle

In this section, discussion will focus on cardiomyopathies and inflammatory disorders of the heart, including rheumatic fever, infective endocarditis and pericarditis, as well as the nurse's role in caring for people with these disorders.

Cardiomyopathy

Cardiomyopathy is a term used to describe diseases that affect the myocardium and have no obvious cause.

Three types of cardiomyopathy have been identified, based on their pathophysiological abnormalities: (1) dilated cardiomyopathy, where enlargement of the cavity of the ventricle is seen; (2) hypertrophic cardiomyopathy, where there is a thickening of the ventricular wall, associated with a small cavity, and (3) restrictive cardiomyopathy, where the ventricle becomes stiff and resistant to filling (Oakley 1998).

Dilated cardiomyopathy (DCM)

This is the most common of the three types. It is characterized by dilated, usually thin-walled, ventricles which produce poor systolic function and low cardiac output. A variety of conditions has been associated with this disorder, including viral infections (poliovirus, coxsackie B virus), immunological disorders, systemic hypertension and exposure to toxic agents (particularly alcohol).

Symptoms of this disorder include congestive heart failure, particularly left-sided failure, fatigue, activity intolerance, chest pain and tachyarrhythmias. As a result of relative stagnation of blood in the ventricles, patients may experience systemic or pulmonary emboli.

The patient will be supported with a range of drugs, such as digoxin and furosemide (frusemide), for as long as possible. End-state dilated cardiomyopathy may be treated surgically with cardiac transplantation. More recently the use of mechanical left ventricular assist devices, such as the Jarvik 2000 Impeller Pump, have been used to reduce the workload of the ventricle and facilitate some improvement in cardiac function.

Hypertrophic cardiomyopathy

This is characterized by a hypertrophied left ventricle, particularly the septum, with no dilatation of the chamber. Thus the left ventricle has thickened walls but there is no enlargement of the chamber size.

Symptoms of hypertrophic cardiomyopathy include dyspnoea, palpitations, syncope, angina pectoris and activity intolerance. The first sign of this disorder may be sudden death.

Medical management of hypertrophic cardiomyopathy focuses on improving cardiac output by enhancing diastolic function, reducing contractility and preventing ventricular arrhythmias.

Surgical management may be indicated, with a septal myotomy being performed. This procedure involves the removal of a portion of the hypertrophied septum, thus widening the outflow track from the left ventricle to the aorta. However, the patient is usually very sick at this stage and the surgical risk is high. A specific form of cardiac pacing, which depolarizes the septum at a slightly earlier stage of the cardiac cycle, may be used to encourage a particular movement in the cardiac muscle to reduce the obstruction to the outflow of blood. An implantable cardioverter defibrillator (ICD) (see p. 306) may be used for those who have survived cardiopulmonary arrest.

Several medications are generally contraindicated in the treatment of hypertrophic cardiomyopathy, although they may be used with careful supervision. Digitalis is contraindicated because it increases contractility and increases outflow obstruction. Nitrates and diuretic therapy are avoided because they cause decreased venous return to the heart, increased contractility and increased outflow obstruction.

Restrictive cardiomyopathy

This is the least common of the three types of cardiomyopathy. It is characterized by rigid, hypertrophied ventricular walls and impaired diastolic filling, leading to decreased cardiac output. This loss of compliance may be a result of myocardial infiltration and/or fibrosis.

This disorder may manifest as pulmonary congestion, activity intolerance and chest pain. Atrial arrhythmias, particularly atrial fibrillation, are common.

Medical management of this disorder is also palliative in nature and involves managing the symptoms of heart failure by diuretic therapy, and fluid and sodium restriction.

Inflammatory disorders of the heart

The inflammatory process may result in destruction of normal functional tissue followed by its replacement with scar tissue, which is fibrous in nature and less specialized.

Diseases that produce inflammatory heart lesions and impaired function include rheumatic fever, infective endocarditis and pericarditis.

Rheumatic fever

Rheumatic fever causes inflammation of heart structures and can still be cited as a factor linked to valve replacement in later life. However, the incidence of the disease has declined significantly over the past 50 years in Western Europe and the USA. In industrialized countries the annual incidence is around 0.5 cases per 100 000 children of school age. In developing countries rheumatic fever remains an endemic disease, with an annual incidence ranging from 100 to 200 per 100 000 school-aged children (Olivier 2000). Although any or all parts may be affected by rheumatic fever, the valves and the myocardium are the most frequent sites and tend to sustain greater permanent damage. The disease is a complication of a group A streptococcal infection, which is usually respiratory. A period of 1–5 weeks may lapse between the infection and the onset of rheumatic fever, during which time the patient may have recovered completely from the infection.

The inflammatory response, which may occur in the joints as well as the heart, is thought to be due to a sensitivity of the affected individuals to the antibodies that were formed in response to the invading bacteria. This sensitivity is present only in certain individuals – not all those with streptococcal infection develop rheumatic fever. The symptoms of the acute stage vary in intensity and may be so mild that they go unrecognized. In some, joint involvement and fever may be predominant with no evident symptoms referable to the heart, and it is not until much later that it becomes known that cardiac tissue was involved and sustained permanent damage.

Rheumatic fever may cause acute myocarditis with subsequent scarred areas that reduce myocardial efficiency and impair the conduction system.

The valves are the most common area of the heart to be affected, and the mitral and aortic valves are the most susceptible. They frequently become scarred, distorted and functionally impaired. Both the valve ring at the opening and the valve cusps may be affected. Following the acute inflammation scarring occurs, the orifice is diminished and the edges of the cusps may fuse. These changes result in resistance to the forward movement of the blood, thus increasing the work of the heart chamber behind the obstruction. Damage of this type is referred to as a *stenosis*. Normally, the mitral opening in an adult is large enough to admit three fingers; in severe stenosis it can become so restricted that only one finger may be introduced.

In some instances, the scarring of the valvular cusps produces a thickening and loss of tissue which prevents them from coming together to close off the opening completely. This incomplete closure allows a regurgitation or backflow of blood through the valve, and is called *valvular incompetence* or *regurgitation*. An added strain is placed on the heart chamber behind the incompetent valve. Many patients with rheumatic heart disease have combined stenosis and incompetence in the affected valve. If the mitral valve is involved, the left atrium develops dilatation and hypertrophy to compensate for the resistance of stenosis and the backflow of valvular incompetence (i.e. the leaking of the blood back through the valve). In the case of aortic valvular damage, the left ventricle dilates and hypertrophies. Prolonged strain created by a damaged valve, increased demands on the already weakened heart, or further progress of the initial rheumatic disease process may result in decompensation or heart failure.

Treatment of rheumatic fever includes drug therapy (antimicrobial preparations, salicylates, corticosteroids), rest and possible surgery.

In the acute stage of rheumatic heart disease the patient may receive large doses of penicillin to destroy any haemolytic streptococci that may still be active in the body. Reactivation of the disease occurs very readily with any subsequent streptococcal infection. Patients with rheumatic fever, particularly children, continue on prophylactic doses of oral penicillin or on a monthly intramuscular injection of a large dose which is slowly absorbed. Anti-inflammatory drugs may be used to decrease inflammation.

Nursing management of patients with rheumatic fever may focus on:

■ lack of knowledge about prophylactic antibiotic use

■ activity intolerance related to fatigue

■ ineffective coping related to managing the disease process.

Infective endocarditis

Infective endocarditis is inflammation of the endocardium, primarily the heart valves. Factors predisposing to infective endocarditis include parenteral drug use (of note is prolonged intravenous drug abuse, with poor skin preparation), valvular abnormalities (either congenital or acquired in origin), rheumatic fever, minor infections, dental procedures and cardiac surgery. The term subacute bacterial endocarditis (SBE) is slightly dated now, as the disease can be caused by organisms that are not bacterial in origin (Mason 2001). Presentation can vary between patients, but tends to include fever, sweats, chills, anorexia, fatigue, weight loss, arthralgia (pain in the joints), myalgia (pain in the muscles) and back pain (Mason 2001). The fever is usually low grade unless an organism such as S*taphylococcus aureus* is involved. The onset of symptoms may be insidious and more commonly affects previously damaged heart valves.

In infective endocarditis, the organisms implant on areas of the endocardium, and clusters of vegetative structures form consisting of inflammatory exudate, fibrin, platelets and bacteria. As the infection subsides, the affected areas become scarred; if a valve was involved, incompetence is likely to develop, and the patient then has the same problems as mentioned in relation to rheumatic fever.

Symptoms may include signs of infection such as fever, malaise, chills, joint tenderness and petechiae. Valvular destruction usually produces a cardiac murmur, heard on auscultation, and signs of embolism, caused when fragments of vegetative lesions break away and lodge downstream in an artery. Diagnosis is confirmed by blood cultures which identify the causative organism. Echocardiography may be useful in visualizing vegetations on heart valves.

Treatment of infective endocarditis includes eradicating the infecting organism by long-term antimicrobial therapy. Surgical repair of damaged valves may be required.

Nursing management of the patient with infective endocarditis may focus on the following problems:

■ lack of knowledge about the disease process, need for antibiotic prophylaxis and treatment

■ activity intolerance related to fatigue

■ anxiety related to the disease process and length of the recovery period.

To assist in reducing issues related to the last point, some hospitals have been using home intravenous antibiotic therapy (HIVAT). This is generally used with patients who understand the illness and the importance of the antibiotic treatment, and is usually reserved for specific bacterial infections such as penicillin-sensitive streptococcal infections. Importantly, these tend to have a reduced risk of disease-related complications (Mason 2001).

Pericarditis

Pericarditis is an inflammation of the pericardium and is most commonly caused by bacterial and viral infections, cardiac injury or an autoimmune reaction. Fluid accumulates in the pericardium as part of the inflammatory response, causing a pericardial effusion. The pressure exerted on the heart by this fluid may prevent its normal filling, creating a condition referred to as *cardiac tamponade*. In some instances, extensive scarring of the visceral pericardium may prevent normal stretching and filling of the heart chambers.

Symptoms of pericarditis may include chest pain, which is exacerbated by movement, pyrexia and dyspnoea. A pericardial friction rub may be heard on auscultation. A paradoxical pulse may be present if cardiac tamponade has occurred. ECG changes characteristic of pericarditis include elevation of ST segments, followed several days later by T-wave inversions. Chest radiography and echocardiography may be used to identify a pericardial effusion.

Treatment goals for the patient with pericarditis include relieving pain, controlling the underlying cause and preventing complications. Explaining the cause of pain is important because there may be fears that it is due to a myocardial infarction.

Medical treatment includes non-steroidal anti-inflammatory agents, such as salicylates and indometacin, and occasionally corticosteroids to combat inflammation. Antibiotics are prescribed for bacterial pericarditis. The patient must be observed carefully for complications such as cardiac tamponade.

Nursing management of the patient with pericarditis may focus on the following problems:

■ chest pain related to pericardial inflammation

■ anxiety related to illness

■ lack of knowledge about the disease process and management.

Pericarditis
See chapter 4.2

Disorders of myocardial blood supply

Coronary atherosclerosis

A narrowing or obstruction in the coronary arteries reduces the blood supply to the myocardium, and causes what is called *ischaemic heart disease*. It results in a deficiency of oxygen and nutrients to the muscle. The reduced oxygen supply is most significant and is quickly reflected in reduced myocardial efficiency. The heart muscle can withstand only a very small oxygen debt, as it is much more susceptible to a reduced oxygen supply than skeletal muscle. In most instances the decreased blood supply to the myocardium is due to degenerative changes in the arteries that produce a narrowing of the lumen of the vessels. Fatty substances, which include cholesterol, are deposited within the intima of the arteries to cause *atherosclerosis*. These fatty plaques interfere with the nutrition of the cells in the intima, leading to necrosis, scarring and calcification, which leave the surface rough and the lumen reduced. These roughened constricted areas allow less blood through and predispose to thrombus formation and occlusion of the vessel.

Atherosclerosis usually develops gradually. While the blood supply through the artery is being reduced, a collateral circulation develops in an effort to increase the supply to the myocardium, but this supplementary circulation is rarely sufficient to provide enough oxygen to the heart muscle during strenuous physical exertion. *Acute coronary syndromes* (ACS) is a term use to define patients with ischaemic cardiac chest pain of recent origin, with one of the following: unstable angina, non-Q-wave myocardial infarction (no Q waves seen on the 12-lead ECG), acute myocardial infarction with ECG changes of ST segment elevation and Q-wave development (National Institute for Clinical Excellence 2001).

Angina pectoris

The term angina pectoris describes a clinical syndrome characterized by chest pain. 'Pectoris' indicates the general location (chest) and '**angina**' refers to the choking, suffocating nature of the pain. This condition arises because of an imbalance between the oxygen being supplied to the myocardium and the energy being expended. The pain, arising from heart muscle fibres that are deficient in oxygen, is usually precipitated by physical exertion or emotional stress, which increases the workload of the heart. There is a need for a greater blood supply than is being delivered by the coronary circulation. It is estimated that more than two million people in the UK suffer from angina, with 333 000 new cases being diagnosed each year (British Heart Foundation 2001).

Chest discomfort often develops suddenly and is retrosternal, and frequently may radiate to the left or both shoulders and arms, and occasionally up the neck to the jaw. The pain may, however, be atypical and arise only in the arms, jaw or neck, and not in the chest. It is usually relieved within a few minutes by resting and/or by glyceryl trinitrate (GTN) but may last as long as 30 minutes. The patient may become short of breath.

Angina may remain a stable condition brought about by predictable precipitating factors with no change in the severity or frequency of the attacks. *Stable angina* is usually associated with fixed obstructive coronary artery disease (Fig. 12.9a). It is then controlled by limiting those activities or situations known to cause pain and by medication. However, the pain may progress in frequency and intensity if the atherosclerotic process in the coronary arteries proceeds more rapidly than the development of collateral circulation. This condition is known as *unstable angina*. Activities may then need to be curtailed greatly. Pain may be experienced at rest.

Unstable angina is distinguished from stable angina by four characteristics:

1. The syndrome has developed within the previous month.

2. A pattern of stable, exertion-related angina pain becomes less predictable, more prolonged, frequent or severe.

3. The syndrome occurs at rest.

4. The pain is not relieved as promptly with GTN as it is with stable angina.

Unstable angina frequently precedes myocardial infarction and is the reason why it is treated promptly. The pathology of unstable angina involves varying amounts of fixed obstructive coronary disease and dynamic obstruction caused by platelet activation and thrombosis (Fig. 12.9c).

Prinzmetal angina refers to a type of unstable angina in which the pain occurs at rest and often at the same time each day. It is not precipitated by exertion. The underlying cause is spasm of the coronary arteries, and obstructive coronary artery disease may or may not be present.

Diagnosis of angina pectoris is made by means of a thorough history, resting electrocardiography, exercise stress test and/or radionuclide imaging. Cardiac angiography is used to assess the degree of narrowing and occlusion within the coronary arteries.

Medical management

Management of angina pectoris is focused on balancing myocardial oxygen supply and demand to ensure the supply is greater than or equal to the demand. Interventions focus on immediate care, reducing or eliminating risk factors, activity management, medications, percutaneous transluminal coronary angioplasty (PTCA) and the intra-aortic balloon pump.

Angina.
See chapter 4.2

Figure 12.9 Coronary artery obstruction by (a) plaque formation, (b) clot formation around plaque, (c) thrombi on top of fixed plaque formation and (d) vessel haemorrhage.

Immediate care

At the start of an angina attack, patients should be advised to stop whatever they are doing, sit down and take a sublingual glyceryl trinitrate (GTN) tablet or a squirt of their GTN spray. If this does not relieve the pain in 5 minutes, a further dose of GTN should be taken. Once the pain is resolved, any remaining tablet can be spat out or swallowed. Tablets can be bitten to increase the surface area and speed up the action of the drug if the pain is particularly severe.

In hospital, it is useful to monitor how often pain is occurring and to identify any precipitating factors. A 12-lead ECG recorded during pain can highlight the area of heart muscle involved and record any abnormal heart rate or rhythm associated with ischaemia.

Risk factor modification

Altering lifestyle to reduce the progression of coronary artery disease is highly desirable (see p. 279).

Activity management

The patient is advised that strenuous physical activity and emotional outbursts should be avoided. Moderate exercise below the point of producing pain is encouraged. Walking is excellent exercise and should be done on a regular basis. The individual should begin with short walks on level ground, gradually increasing the distance over a period of weeks. Regular, medically supervised, exercise programmes are recommended for some patients. Regular exercise improves muscle tone and general well-being and stimulates the development of collateral circulation in the myocardium. Normal weight is more easily maintained. The psychological benefit of exercise to the patient cannot be overestimated.

Medications

One of the cornerstones of the management of angina is pharmacological therapy. The medications commonly used are presented in Table 12.4.

Percutaneous transluminal coronary angioplasty (PTCA)

PTCA provides an alternative for some patients who might otherwise require coronary artery bypass surgery. It can also be used as an alternative to thrombolysis in acute myocardial infarction (MI). PTCA is a non-surgical method of dilating stenotic or occlusive lesions in the coronary arterial system. Thomas (1991) recommends that patients should be prepared as for cardiac catheterization. However, as approximately 2–3% of patients may require subsequent coronary graft surgery due to complications such as *acute coronary occlusion* (closure of the vessel during the procedure), PTCA is carried out

Table 12.4 Drugs used in the management of angina

Medication	Example	General action in angina
Nitrates		
Short-acting	Glyceryl trinitrate	Vasodilate vascular smooth muscle
		Decrease preload, decrease afterload
		Vasodilate coronary arteries
Long-acting	Isosorbide dinitrate GTN ointment	As above
Beta-blockers	Propranolol	Decrease heart rate, automaticity
	Atenolol	Decrease force of contraction
		Decrease myocardial oxygen consumption
Calcium channel blockers	Nifedipine	Dilate coronary and peripheral vessels
	Diltiazem	
Anticoagulant therapy	Aspirin	Decrease platelet aggregation
	Heparin	Decrease thrombosis formation
Potassium channel openers	Nicorandil	Sustained dilatation of arterial resistance and conduction vessels
		Little haemodynamic effect on heart rate, blood pressure or cardiac contractility

on sites with a cardiothoracic surgical capability or rapid accessibility.

Criteria for selection of patients include:

1. Acute MI, where:
   a. thrombolysis is inappropriate
   b. there is cardiogenic shock, or
   c. large anterior infarct – known as primary angioplasty – is present

2. Recent onset of angina pectoris

3. Angina resistant to medical treatment

4. Angina symptoms of sufficient severity to compromise the quality of life of the patient

5. Single-vessel disease, which technically makes the procedure easier, although those with multivessel disease will be treated. However, the risk of complications is higher

6. Anyone being considered for coronary artery bypass grafts.

Diagnostic testing before this procedure is similar to that for coronary bypass surgery and includes coronary angiography. Nursing care includes giving both physical and emotional support to the patient, as the procedure is often frightening. The patient should be given an explanation of ischaemic heart disease and of all the tests carried out before the procedure, the risks involved, the possible need for bypass surgery and the expected results of this treatment.

PTCA is performed using local anaesthesia in the cardiac catheterization laboratory. A guide catheter is introduced into the right or left femoral or brachial artery. This catheter is advanced under fluoroscopy to the affected coronary artery. Once through the stenotic narrowing in the coronary artery, a dilating catheter is slipped through the guide catheter. When positioned within the atherosclerotic lesion, the dilating balloon is inflated. The resultant stretching of the coronary arterial muscle wall widens the lumen of the artery, allowing blood to flow more freely.

Possible complications include bleeding or thrombosis of the affected artery due to injury of the vascular endothelium, acute coronary occlusion, coronary artery spasm and rupture of the artery, causing cardiac tamponade. These complications may result in acute myocardial infarction (1–2% of cases).

Medications such as nifedipine and beta-blockers may be given either before or during the procedure to prevent coronary artery spasm. Intravenous GTN may be administered to promote vasodilatation. Generally patients receive an anticoagulant such as heparin, which may be followed by treatment with warfarin or antiplatelet drugs (National Institute for Clinical Excellence 2000).

After the procedure the patient is returned to the acute cardiac unit. Cardiac monitoring is initiated and a 12-lead ECG is recorded to assess for signs of ischaemia or infarction related to the vessel that has been treated. Heparin will have been administered during the procedure. It is important for the nurse not to remove the introducer sheaths until the recorded activated clotting time (ACT) is reduced to the desired protocol range. This is normally between 130 and 175 s, and indicates that excessive bleeding will not occur on sheath removal. Pressure is applied to the groin during sheath removal to reduce the risk of bleeding. Biochemical markers such as troponin T are recorded to assess whether any myocardial damage has occurred because of the procedure. Time spent on bedrest following sheath removal varies, but will be at least 2–3 hours. It is likely that a *stent* (a tiny circular wire mesh used to hold open the coronary artery) will be inserted during the PTCA procedure to offer greater patency to the vessel wall. Some units perform a PTCA in the morning and discharge that evening, but many will stay in hospital for 24 hours. Patients will be discharged home on aspirin for long-term use, and with a short course of an oral antiplatelet drug such as *clopidogrel* or *ticlopidine* to prevent vessel occlusion.

Intra-aortic balloon pump

Occasionally counter-pulsation with the intra-aortic balloon pump is utilized for the patient with unstable angina prior to coronary artery surgery. The intra-aortic balloon is inserted into the aorta from one of the femoral arteries; it is inflated during diastole and deflated as the heart ejects its contents during systole. In this way it reduces afterload and myocardial oxygen demand, decreases myocardial ischaemia and relieves angina. The intra-aortic balloon pump is an invasive method of treatment; consequently, the patient and family require a great deal of support from nursing and medical staff. Further discussion of this intervention is beyond the scope of this text (Hatchett 1998).

Nursing management

The nursing management of a patient with angina focuses on the following health problems:

- lack of knowledge
- activity intolerance
- potential for chest discomfort
- anxiety and other psychological problems.

Myocardial
infarction
See chapter 4.2

Case Study 12.1

Ann Carter was a 70-year-old woman diagnosed with stable angina 6 months ago. She had been referred to the community nurse to be monitored for her ability to manage her angina. Mrs Carter lived with her daughter and son-in-law in a bungalow. When visited in her home, Mrs Carter expressed anxiety related to her inability to cope with chest pain when it occurred. She was concerned that she would not do the 'right things'.

Mrs Carter's primary health problem was identified as knowledge deficit related to her disease process and management. The *goals* of care for Mrs Carter were that she could:

1. recognize symptoms of myocardial ischaemia

2. undertake appropriate interventions to reduce and eliminate myocardial ischaemia if it occurred

3. engage in activities to prevent myocardial ischaemia.

Nursing intervention

- Mrs Carter was asked to describe the signs and symptoms of myocardial ischaemia which she had experienced. Descriptors that described myocardial ischaemia were reinforced and other possible symptoms were discussed.

- The patient was questioned as to her understanding of the cause of her angina. The concept of myocardial ischaemia was clarified. The heart's need for enough oxygen to meet its demands was emphasized and the impact of ischaemic heart disease was discussed. This was achieved using straightforward language, reinforced with diagrams.

- Mrs Carter was prompted to discuss what she did when she experienced chest pain. The use of rest and correct administration of glyceryl trinitrate were reinforced. She was encouraged to tell whomever she was with that she was experiencing chest discomfort, so that they could assist her as needed. If the chest pain was not relieved by rest and glyceryl trinitrate in the prescribed time, Mrs Carter was advised to ask to be taken to the nearest hospital where she could be assessed by healthcare professionals.

- Preventive strategies to avoid angina were also discussed. Mrs Carter indicated that she did not get overtired. The need to alternate activity and rest was reinforced. Use of glyceryl trinitrate prophylactically when Mrs Carter engaged in activities that caused angina was encouraged.

- An educational booklet was given to Mrs Carter to read. This provided her with a reference so she could review any concerns.

Evaluation

At the end of the visit, Mrs Carter could describe signs and symptoms of myocardial ischaemia, actions she would take if she developed chest pain, and how she planned to pace herself. On a follow-up visit, 2 weeks later, Mrs Carter described how she had successfully managed an episode of chest discomfort. She had also paced her activities, incorporating more quiet periods into her life. Mrs Carter expressed feelings of increased confidence in her ability to manage further episodes. She was also referred for assessment of further treatment that would reduce the symptoms of angina, such as PTCA or coronary artery bypass grafting.

Acute myocardial infarction

Acute **myocardial infarction** (MI) or 'heart attack' is the most serious and acute form of ischaemic heart disease. A coronary artery becomes blocked and the myocardial area which it supplies suffers oxygen deficiency and cell necrosis. The blockage may be due to the rupture of an atheromatous plaque, with associated thrombus formation as blood clots around the area. This can occur suddenly, and compensation through collateral channels is inadequate to maintain the myocardial cells. The resulting area of necrotic tissue is referred to as an *infarction*.

The extent of the infarction varies from patches of 1–2 cm in diameter to widespread areas of necrosis. One or more layers of the heart may be involved. The area of infarction becomes soft and then eventually fills in with firm, fibrous, scar tissue. Survival and the extent of subsequent restrictions depend upon the amount of myocardial damage and the area of the heart affected. Death may occur immediately or within a few hours. Obviously, the remaining viable heart tissue must compensate for the loss of functional tissue.

Occlusion may be preceded by some manifestations of coronary insufficiency such as angina, or it may occur suddenly without any previous warning. Although the condition can clearly be fatal, it is estimated that 1.3 million people have survived an MI in the UK, of whom 850 000 are men (British Heart Foundation 2001). Survival will depend critically on prompt diagnosis and instigation of appropriate treatments such as early thrombolysis (see below).

Types of myocardial infarction

It is difficult to delineate the precise area of the myocardium that is affected, but general areas can be identified from the 12-lead ECG. This is important to know because damage to each area can produce different complications. Although other areas of the heart may be involved, most infarctions occur in the left ventricle.

Anterior wall infarction

The anterior wall of the left ventricle is infarcted due to an occlusion of the left anterior descending artery. The interventricular septum may also be involved, in which case it is called an *anteroseptal* infarct.

Lateral wall infarction

An infarction in the lateral wall of the left ventricle is associated with an occlusion of the lateral branch of the left circumflex artery. Occasionally both the anterior descending and the left circumflex branches are obstructed, and the infarction is designated *anterolateral*.

Inferior wall infarction

This term implies an infarction of the part of the left ventricle, which rests on the diaphragm. It is usually due to occlusion of the right coronary artery.

Posterior wall infarction

This type is usually due to occlusion of the posterior branch of either the right coronary or left circumflex artery. It is sometimes called a true posterior infarction to distinguish it from an inferior infarction.

Right ventricular infarction

The right ventricle may infarct in conjunction with an inferior or posterior left ventricular infarction. It is usually caused by occlusion of the artery that perfuses the posterior ventricular wall, either the right coronary artery or, less commonly, the left circumflex artery.

Symptoms

Pain The most common presenting complaint of patients with myocardial infarction is severe chest pain. The pain may last for several hours or until relieved by analgesics. It should not persist for days; prolonged pain may be an indication of pericarditis or an extending infarction. Up to 25% of patients do not experience any pain (*silent MI*). Time of onset of pain has been shown to peak at around midnight and 6 am – times when individuals are likely to be awoken from sleep with pain rather than engaging in vigorous physical activity (Thompson et al 1991).

Dyspnoea Dyspnoea may be due to pulmonary congestion or pain. It may also occur as activity is increased. Relief of pain and congestion may relieve the dyspnoea. It is important to note whether shortness of breath is present at all times or, if intermittent, how it is precipitated and what measures relieve it.

Skin The skin may be cool and moist, and have a greyish colour in response to the decreased cardiac output.

Nausea and vomiting Nausea and vomiting may be experienced at the time of the attack, lasting from several hours to 2–3 days. Occasionally, nausea and vomiting occur in response to the opiates being administered.

Weakness and tiredness Extreme weakness may be experienced and may persist for many days. Many patients complain of tiredness for weeks after an infarction; the exact cause of this is not clearly defined. Some suggest it results from decreased oxygen perfusion of the tissues due to a lowered cardiac output. It has also been attributed to weakened skeletal muscles as a result of even a brief period of immobilization. The patient may have been in a state of physical exhaustion before the attack or may be emotionally exhausted from the experience.

Heart rate The pulse becomes rapid and weak, and may be imperceptible at the time of the attack. Initially, a few patients may exhibit bradycardia, followed by tachycardia.

Blood pressure Owing to the decreased pumping efficiency of the heart, the blood pressure can fall, but initially following a MI it may be raised due to an augmented sympathetic response.

Temperature Myocardial necrosis causes an increase in body temperature ranging from 37.7 to 39°C. The temperature usually rises within 24–48 hours and returns to normal by the sixth or seventh day. If the increased temperature persists for longer, it may be due to complications.

Psychological reactions A MI carries the threat of death or long-term disability of the patient. The sudden change in well-being may lead to feelings of vulnerability and helplessness. The patient is required to make very rapid adjustments to both the illness and change in environment.

Anxiety is the most common psychological response. It is manifested by various overt and covert behaviours, such as tenseness, restlessness, short attention span, inability to concentrate, crying, constant talking and expression of feelings of anxiety. The patient may appear generally relaxed but may exhibit more subtle manifestations of anxiety such as darting eye movements. There are various instruments available for measuring anxiety. Three of them, the Stait-Trait Anxiety Inventory (STAI), the Hospital Anxiety and Depression scale (HAD scale) and a linear analogue anxiety scale, have been shown to give effective measurements for coronary patients (Elliot 1993). Patients may also show denial, refusing to acknowledge the seriousness or even the presence of symptoms, and may be angry and/or depressed. These emotional responses may appear in varying degrees and at any time during hospitalization or may not become evident until after discharge from the hospital. The individual's interpretation of the experience and personal coping pattern influence responses.

Diagnosis

Medical diagnosis of an acute MI is made using the clinical history, changes in the 12-lead ECG, and via biochemical markers and serum enzymes.

Changes in the electrocardiogram

Theoretically, three types of changes are present in the myocardium when an infarction develops. These define three concentric areas, referred to clinically as the *area of infarction*, the *area of injury* and the *zone of ischaemia*, resulting in a distinctive ECG pattern. In the central infarcted area, irreversible structural changes occur with resulting necrosis of tissue. As electrical impulses cannot be conducted through this tissue, the normal ECG pattern is altered resulting in a pronounced pathological Q wave (see Fig. 12.10).

Surrounding the zone of infarction is an area of injury that suffers a decreased blood supply, but the damage is not permanent. Although specific abnormal ECG changes are produced, these may revert to normal if the blood supply is restored. Electrodes placed over the injured area will record an ST segment elevation due to leakage of positively charged ions from damaged cells.

The zone of ischaemia surrounds the area of injury and may also return to normal once the blood supply is restored. Inverted T waves indicate ischaemia.

ST elevations appear within several hours following an infarction and disappear in a few days. In the early stages T waves become taller and appear as an extension of the

Electrocardiogram
See chapter 4.2

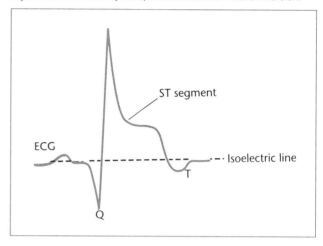

Figure 12.10 Electrocardiographic changes indicating acute myocardial infarction: Q wave, ST elevation and T-wave inversion.

elevated ST segment. They later become inverted. Q waves appear within 1–2 days and persist (Fig. 12.10). The area of infarction will be reflected in leads that view that portion of the heart. Thus, *inferior* infarctions can be identified in leads II, III and AVF, *anterior* infarctions can be identified in the anterior leads V_1 to V_4, and *lateral wall* infarction in leads I, AVL, V_5 and V_6. Under normal conditions no leads face the posterior wall of the heart, so diagnosis is based upon reciprocal changes in leads facing the opposite wall; that is, increased R waves in leads V_1 and V_2.

Changes in biochemical markers and serum enzyme levels

Certain intracellular biochemical markers and enzymes known to be persistent in myocardial cells are released into the blood when the cells are damaged or destroyed. Serial determinations of the serum concentrations of these enzymes can provide information concerning the presence and degree of cardiac damage. The normal values of serum enzymes vary depending on laboratory techniques and sampling methods.

In the coronary care unit, the most commonly ordered biochemical markers and enzyme level estimations are those for troponin T or I, creatine phosphokinase (CPK), aspartate aminotransferase (AST) and lactic dehydrogenase (LDH) (see Table 12.5). Diagnosis of a myocardial infarction can be confirmed by elevations of these biochemical and enzyme levels.

Creatine phosphokinase (CPK)

CPK is present in cardiac and skeletal muscle and in brain tissue. CPK levels begin to rise in the serum 4–8 hours following MI, peak at 12–24 hours, and return to normal in 3–4 days.

A rise in CPK levels may also be caused by pericarditis, severe congestive heart failure, electrical cardioversion and intramuscular injections. Thus, to determine the source of raised CPK levels, electrophoresis or radioimmunoassay can be used to separate CPK into three

Table 12.5 Increases in serum enzyme levels (units/litre) following myocardial infarction

Enzyme	Day of admission	Day 2	Day 3	Day 7
CPK	6	162	5	5
AST	14	177	201	23
LDH	151	513	789	419

A troponin T value should be less than 0.1 μg/L. There are several Troponin I assays available and values will vary depending on the system used to record the level. It is advisable to consult the manufacturer's literature. Myoglobin concentration should be less than 100 μg/L.

fractions or isoenzymes. The *MB isoenzyme* has been found predominantly in the myocardium. Studies have shown that CK-MB (or MB-CPK) is very sensitive and specific for the diagnosis of acute MI, provided that it is determined between 6 and 36 hours after the suspected infarction.

Thus, in assessing the presence of an acute MI by means of CPK levels, it is important to ensure that blood samples are drawn on admission and every 6–8 hours for 24 hours after the onset of chest pain.

Aspartate aminotransferase (AST)

The concentration of AST rises within 8–12 hours after a MI, reaching a peak at 18–36 hours and usually returning to normal within 3–4 days. Raised AST levels are also seen in patients with hepatic and skeletal muscle disease, pulmonary embolism and pericarditis. This is a problem for the diagnosis of MI because there are no cardiac-specific isoenzymes of AST. Thus, the routine use of AST in diagnosis of acute MI is debatable.

Lactic dehydrogenase (LDH)

LDH is present in most body organs including the heart, kidneys, lungs, liver and skeletal muscle. After an acute MI, the LDH level becomes raised in 8–24 hours, peaks at 3–6 days and returns to normal in 8–14 days.

A rise in total LDH concentration may also occur in patients with pulmonary embolism, neoplastic disorders, hepatic disease and shock. Thus, it is important to assess LDH isoenzyme levels to assess whether cardiac damage is causing increased enzyme levels. LDH has five isoenzymes and cardiac muscle contains primarily LDH_1. A rise in the proportion of LDH_1 exceeding 40% of the total LDH value and an increase in the ratio of $LDH_1 : LDH_2$ is considered a sensitive indicator of MI. Thus, when a patient has a suspected MI that occurred more than 2 days previously, LDH isoenzyme analysis can be more revealing than CPK analysis.

The troponins and myoglobin

The troponins are known to be highly sensitive markers of myocardial damage, and may ultimately supersede cardiac enzyme testing. The blood levels do take several hours to rise, and it is usual to record a troponin level on admission and again in approximately 8 hours, to rule out myocardial damage. The other advantage is that, together with another biochemical marker called myoglobin, their presence can be measured as a bedside test. Treatment for myocardial damage can therefore be given quickly with the assurance of a positive test result. Myoglobin rises at an earlier stage compared with other markers, owing to its small molecular size, allowing it to escape more easily from damaged myocardium into the bloodstream.

Other diagnostic procedures

Other procedures that may be used to assess the extent of MI include echocardiography, radionuclide imaging and thallium stress electrocardiography.

Medical management

Patients with acute MI are best managed on a coronary care unit, although some are cared for on medical wards and some at home. Coronary care units have essentially been designed to serve three purposes:

1. The provision of a separate area within the hospital for the care and monitoring of patients with acute MI or other cardiac disorders.

2. The provision of high-quality specialized care.

3. The provision of personnel and equipment immediately available for resuscitation.

Ideally, this service should be available for all, with no exclusion criteria such as advanced age.

The most important area of management must be the attempt to re-establish blood flow to the myocardium through the blocked coronary artery. Management will also focus on areas of control of symptoms, reducing the workload of the heart, and the recognition and treatment of complications. It is also important to have a strategy to identify patients at high risk, to reduce subsequent development of heart failure, and to have effective measures for secondary prevention to reduce the incidence of reinfarction as well as to promote rehabilitation.

Control of symptoms

Pain relief

See page 276.

Prevention of arrhythmias

During the convalescent phase of MI, ventricular extrasystoles and supraventricular and ventricular arrhythmias are associated with a poor prognosis. However, treatment with prophylactic antiarrhythmia drugs is no longer popular because of adverse side-effects.

Reducing myocardial workload

Reducing the myocardial oxygen demand may limit the size of the infarcted area. Beta-blocking agents are used to reduce heart rate, myocardial contractility, blood pressure and cardiac output. They are used with extreme caution or contraindicated in patients with hypotension, chronic airway disease or peripheral vascular disease.

Acute myocardial reperfusion

Thrombolytic therapy

Evidence that coronary thrombosis is a very early event in acute MI, recognition of the prognostic importance of infarction size, and evidence that infarction size might be reduced by early intervention have resulted in thrombolytic therapy becoming the most significant recent development in the management of the patient with acute MI. Several intravenous agents that lyse (break down) clots are currently being used in patients who have sustained an acute MI; these agents include streptokinase and tissue plasminogen activator (tPA). Research to evaluate the impact of these agents on morbidity and mortality, as well as to establish the most effective management protocols, is ongoing. However, the benefit of this form of treatment is clear, together with the need to initiate therapy as soon as the diagnosis has been confirmed. In addition, it has been known for some time that all patients who are experiencing an MI should be given 300 mg aspirin to chew as soon as possible (ISIS-2 1988). This is not for its analgesic effect, but its antiplatelet properties. Aspirin appears to augment the effects of thrombolysis and increase the chance of survival. Patients who are allergic to aspirin or who have a history of problematic bleeding, such as those with a peptic ulcer, are generally not offered aspirin.

Therapy needs to be initiated as soon as possible after the onset of MI to give maximum benefit. Thus, enabling patients who are experiencing chest pain to attend units that can promptly administer these agents has become increasingly important. Contraindications are related to issues of bleeding problems. These will vary between units but generally include active bleeding, CVA within the previous 3 months (in some units this may extend to periods of up to 1 year), severe systemic arterial hypertension, bleeding disorders, and major surgery or traumatic injury in the last 6 months.

Nurses need to be aware of the possible complications of bleeding, arrhythmias, allergic reaction, drop in blood pressure, as well as anxiety and lack of knowledge, which might accompany the administration of thrombolytics. There is evidence that individuals who have received streptokinase develop antibodies that reduce the effectiveness of subsequent administration of the drug. Those having this form of thrombolytic therapy need to be issued with a card detailing the date and dose of drug given so that an alternative can be offered if necessary. To speed the administration of thrombolytic agents, specially trained nurses are now instigating treatment to agreed protocols before the medical team has arrived (Quinn et al 2001).

Anticoagulants

Heparin therapy is used routinely by some cardiologists when there is evidence on ECG of left ventricular thrombus, active deep vein thrombosis or anterior wall MI. Heparin may also be used prophylactically for a patient with an inferior wall MI experiencing atrial arrhythmias, and also those having congestive heart failure. Heparin may also be administered after thrombolytic therapy. Low-dose heparin may be used for patients with a high risk of venous thromboembolism.

Antiplatelet drugs

Multiple trials with aspirin have shown that daily low-dose aspirin (75–150 mg) significantly reduces the risk of reinfarction and death following MI.

Percutaneous transluminal coronary angioplasty (PTCA) and coronary artery bypass surgery (CABG)

These procedures may be indicated for the acutely unstable individual who requires aggressive therapy to prevent death after coronary angiography is conducted. Discussion of PTCA can be found on page 286.

Stents

Some centres are increasingly using stents inserted during a procedure similar to angioplasty to increase and maintain myocardial perfusion.

There is much evidence that certain drugs and therapies when administered to the patient with angina, unstable angina and MI do improve survival and clinical outcome. The National Service Framework for Coronary Heart Disease (DoH 2000b) is a government-initiated document that has highlighted specific standards to achieve in the treatment of these and other cardiac conditions. These standards include, unless contraindicated, the use of thrombolytic agents, aspirin, beta-blockers, angiotensin-converting enzyme (ACE) inhibitors and lipid-lowering drugs such as the statins in the treatment of MI. Much work is in place and ongoing in the hospital and community to improve service delivery to meet such standards, and includes innovative practice between all members of the healthcare team.

Recognition of complications

Doctors and nurses share responsibility for assessing and recognizing complications of an acute MI. It is important for the nurse to have a sound understanding of the possible complications so that rapid identification and initiation of treatment, as required, is conducted. Complications following MI include arrhythmias, congestive heart failure, pericarditis, mitral regurgitation, myocardial rupture, aneurysm, and systemic or pulmonary emboli.

Arrhythmias

Arrhythmias usually occur early following a myocardial infarction. The most serious arrhythmia that may be seen is *ventricular fibrillation*; this is treated by cardiac defibrillation. *Bradyarrhythmias* are unusually slow heart rates (e.g. Wenckebach heart block), and are most often associated with inferior wall infarctions. As the SA node and the AV junctional tissue are most often supplied by the right coronary artery, occlusion of this vessel will lead to their decreased functioning. Anterior MIs are more likely to lead to failure and arrhythmias, such as *sinus tachycardia* and rapid *atrial arrhythmias*, and to interventricular conduction disturbances, such as *Mobitz type II block*. *Complete AV block* (third-degree or complete heart block) may follow either inferior or anterior wall infarction.

Heart failure

Mild congestive heart failure occurs in many patients due to the decreased efficiency with which the heart contracts. Gross left ventricular failure is more common following an anterior infarction. Heart failure is diagnosed by the presence of crackles on chest auscultation, complaints of shortness of breath and chest radiography.

Patients with left ventricular failure or asymptomatic left ventricular dysfunction are increasingly being prescribed angiotensin-converting enzyme (ACE) inhibitors.

Pericarditis

Pericarditis following a MI is thought to be due to an autoimmune reaction in which antigens originate from the injured myocardial tissue and cause inflammation of the pericardium. It is known as Dressler's syndrome, and may occur as early as 24 hours after the infarction. The pain that accompanies pericarditis is similar to that of MI, but is sometimes more excruciating. It is alarming to the patient, who may think that he or she is having another MI. A friction rub may be heard on auscultation, but is not always present in the early stages. The patient's temperature may remain raised for more than 1 week. Treatment is usually with non-steroidal anti-inflammatory drugs such as indometacin or soluble aspirin. A corticosteroid preparation may be used.

Mitral regurgitation

This complication may occur when a papillary muscle dysfunctions or ruptures, causing the valve to become incompetent. This is a grave complication which may be corrected by surgery. Less severe mitral insufficiency may be due to infarction of the papillary muscle.

Myocardial rupture

Myocardial rupture, when present, usually occurs within 7 days. It is more often seen in patients with transmural infarctions. Rupture of the interventricular septum usually occurs within the first 2 weeks and is a very grave prognostic sign. Instead of flowing normally from the left ventricle into the aorta, blood is re-routed to the right ventricle, increasing the demands on it and flooding the lungs.

Aneurysm

An aneurysm is a ballooning out of the infarcted myocardial tissue, causing the heart to contract in a disruptive fashion. If large, it seriously impedes the maintenance of normal cardiac output. The extent of the aneurysm may be determined by a myocardial scan, and in some instances may be corrected by surgery.

Emboli

Emboli occur because clots formed in the healing area of the myocardium break loose and escape into the circulation. Pulmonary emboli may arise in the leg veins due to circulatory stasis, and may be prevented by exercising the limbs. The treatment for emboli includes anticoagulant drugs.

Risk stratification

Assessment of left ventricular dysfunction, residual ischaemia and the tendency to arrhythmias is important for identifying patients at high risk of complications so that treatment can be targeted appropriately. Clinical features, ECG, chest radiography, echocardiography, exercise testing and radionuclide studies are important assessment tools.

Rehabilitation

Cardiac rehabilitation is the process by which patients with ischaemic heart disease (IHD) are enabled to achieve their optimal physical, emotional, social, vocational and economic state (World Health Organization 1993). Cardiac rehabilitation services for the patient and partner need to include the following (Stokes and Thompson 2001):

- a tailored exercise programme
- risk factor modification, including specific advice on activity, work, changes in lifestyle, relaxation and stress management
- attention to the psychological sequelae of IHD for both the patient and family, especially the partner.

Numerous studies have shown that comprehensive rehabilitation programmes can produce worthwhile improvements in quality of life and it is recommended that they be routinely offered to all patients with IHD (Thompson et al 1996, Department of Health 2000b). Ideally, programmes should be individually targeted and cater for groups such as the elderly, women and those from minority ethnic groups. Routine care needs to be accompanied by a means of identifying those who need additional support.

Rehabilitation can be seen as a process that begins in hospital from the time of admission and extends out into the community.

Community support needs to follow on as soon as possible from that provided in hospital. Ideally, the patient and partner should have some support during the first 2 weeks at home – even if this is only a telephone link with the hospital or practice nurse. Some programmes incorporate home visits in the first few days at home. Later support can involve individual and group sessions linked with exercise, either in hospital or a community-based setting. Home-based rehabilitation may be more appropriate for some individuals. The 'Heart Manual', a home-based programme, has been shown to increase confidence in recovery and produce a positive perception of progress (Linden 1995).

After 3 or 4 months, some programmes offer a long-term community-based support group which encourages self-help and peer support for long-term health maintenance.

Nursing management

The nursing management in the acute phase of a patient who has sustained a MI is illustrated using a clinical example (Case Study 11.2).

Case Study 12.2

Robert MacGregor was a 57-year-old man, married with two grown-up children. He was admitted to hospital via ambulance with the diagnosis of acute anterior wall myocardial infarction. On the day of admission, he awoke from sleep at 12.15 am with 'crushing' chest discomfort, which radiated down his left arm. He felt nauseated and sweaty, and was short of breath. He felt something was seriously wrong and woke his wife. She telephoned the ambulance service and Mr MacGregor arrived at the hospital approximately 1 hour after his chest pain started.

Mr MacGregor's past medical history did not include any cardiovascular disorders or bleeding problems. He had sustained several injuries to his left knee which had required surgical correction. Mr MacGregor had several risk factors for ischaemic heart disease, including his age, sex and habit of smoking a pack of cigarettes a day for 40 years. He did not know his cholesterol levels and did not have hypertension. Mr MacGregor considered his position as a taxi driver to be stressful. His father had died from a myocardial infarction in his seventies.

Care in the coronary care unit

Mr MacGregor's initial assessment indicated that he was medically stable. His vital signs were stable and he was in normal sinus rhythm. Interventions included:

- Oxygen via nasal cannulae at 4 litres per minute was commenced.

- An intravenous line was set up.

- A 12-lead electrocardiogram showing changes consistent with an anterior wall myocardial infarction was recorded.

- A troponin T level was obtained and again in 8 hours to assess for myocardial damage.

- Diamorphine hydrochloride 5 mg i.v. was given with good relief of chest pain.

- Aspirin 300 mg was administered, and thrombolytic therapy was commenced to reduce the size of the myocardial infarct, as there were no contraindications. Streptokinase was administered via intravenous infusion.

- The doctor and nurse met with Mrs MacGregor to discuss her husband's condition and to provide reassurance.

Mr MacGregor was somewhat restless and fully conscious. He indicated that he had no discomfort in his chest and that he was worried about his wife. Mr MacGregor knew that he had had a myocardial infarction. His respiratory rate was 14 breaths per minute and he remained on oxygen 4 litres per minute via nasal cannulae. His blood pressure was equal in both arms and was 120/60 mmHg. The cardiac monitor showed that Mr MacGregor remained in normal sinus rhythm, 72 beats per minute with ventricular ectopic beats (VEBs) approximately 5–10 per minute.

After 1 hour the streptokinase infusion was complete and a heparin infusion was started.

Four priority health problems were identified in the provision of nursing care for Mr MacGregor:

1. potential for chest pain
2. potential decrease in cardiac output
3. anxiety
4. potential for haemorrhage.

Potential for chest pain

Mr MacGregor was encouraged to report any episodes of chest pain. A visual analogue scale was used to quantify any pain experienced, a score of 10 meaning the worst possible pain and a score of 0 no pain. Diamorphine intravenously was given for pain during the acute period, a total of 12.5 mg being required over the first 12 hours. Glyceryl trinitrate was placed at the bedside on the second day so that Mr MacGregor could have control over his pain management and rapid pain relief. He kept nursing staff informed when he used this so that they could assess the effectiveness of pain management and the degree of ischaemic pain.

Evaluation

Mr MacGregor experienced only one episode of pain after the first day. He felt confident at using GTN tablets and in managing any episodes of pain experienced after discharge.

Potential decrease in cardiac output

This was related to damaged myocardium, as evidenced by 12-lead ECG changes, presence of ventricular arrhythmias, clinical history and biochemical markers/cardiac enzymes.

The *goals* in caring for Mr MacGregor were that:

1. Mr MacGregor would be pain free.

2. He would reduce the workload on his heart.

3. No further ventricular arrhythmias causing haemodynamic instability would be experienced.

4. Mr MacGregor would report any episodes of myocardial ischaemia (experienced through chest pain, and assessed by nursing staff via the 12-lead ECG).

Nursing intervention

- Mr MacGregor's vital signs were monitored every 4 hours for any changes in blood pressure. His heart rate and rhythm were monitored continuously for any changes. Close attention was paid to ventricular arrhythmias as the patient had had VEBs. Initial damaged ventricular muscle predisposed him to fatal ventricular arrhythmias.

- Mr MacGregor was initially advised to remain on bed/chair rest to limit cardiac workload. His activity level was gradually increased over several days to allow the heart time to recover and to facilitate assessment of his activity tolerance.

- The importance of avoiding straining and of performing isometric exercises was stressed. A laxative was given, as necessary, to avoid constipation.

- A quiet environment was provided to facilitate rest. Mr MacGregor was encouraged to rest for an hour after each meal to reduce myocardial workload.

- Supplemental oxygen via nasal cannulae was administered continuously for the first 24 hours and if he had chest pain. This ensured additional oxygen was available to improve myocardial oxygen supply if required.

Evaluation

Mr MacGregor experienced no further arrhythmias. He reduced his cardiac workload by resting quietly in bed and performing gentle exercises. He reported that he experienced no episodes of chest discomfort.

Anxiety

Anxiety was related to diagnosis and admission to hospital, as evidenced by inability to concentrate, apprehension and difficulty in sleeping.

The *goals* in treating this problem were that:

1. Early signs of anxiety would be detected.

2. Mr MacGregor would participate in activities that would reduce or eliminate his anxiety.

Nursing intervention

- Reassurance and comfort were provided for Mr MacGregor. The nurse stayed with him frequently, speaking calmly and providing competent, efficient care.

- A quiet environment was provided and sensory stimulation was reduced. The door was partly closed and the lights were dimmed during rest periods to facilitate sleep.

- Mr MacGregor was informed of the procedures and treatments he could expect. He was kept up to date, with the use of language he could understand. The patient was encouraged to ask questions about his environment and condition. Honest, concise information was provided to clarify his understanding of heart disease. As Mr MacGregor liked to read, he was given a pamphlet to reinforce information provided. He was informed that many patients find it difficult to concentrate while in hospital, so he should not be alarmed by his poor concentration span.

- Visitors were limited to the immediate family. Mrs MacGregor was encouraged to visit her husband and was kept informed of his condition. She was encouraged to attend the cardiac family support group to meet other partners and receive support from them.

- Mr MacGregor took a mild sedative in the evening to encourage sleep.

- Mr MacGregor was informed about the cardiac rehabilitation programme, and he and his wife were invited to attend.

Evaluation

Mr MacGregor indicated that he felt less anxious and more in control of his environment when he was well informed. He eagerly asked questions about his condition and prognosis. The booklet was helpful as he recorded questions he wanted to ask the doctor in it, so that he would not forget them. Mrs MacGregor enjoyed the family support group and found it helpful. Both Mr and Mrs MacGregor were keen to join the rehabilitation group which started 3 weeks after discharge. The rehabilitation coordinator would visit them at home during the first week to offer support, answer questions and assess their progress.

Potential for haemorrhage

There was a potential for haemorrhage related to thrombolytic agent and concurrent administration of anticoagulant.

The *goals* were that there would be:

1. Absence of all subjective and objective signs of gastrointestinal, vascular and soft tissue haemorrhage.

2. Early detection of bleeding, within 15 minutes of commencement.

Nursing intervention

- ■ Vascular punctures were kept to a minimum.

- ■ All intravenous and puncture sites were observed frequently for bleeding. Any bruising was outlined and assessed more frequently for increasing size.

- ■ All bodily excretions were inspected for signs of blood.

- ■ Mr MacGregor was informed of the risk of bleeding and was encouraged to report immediately any signs of bleeding to the nurse.

- ■ Mr MacGregor used his own electric razor and soft toothbrush.

Evaluation

Mr MacGregor showed no signs of haemorrhage during his stay in the coronary care unit.

When Mr MacGregor improved and was transferred from the coronary care unit to the general medical ward, several other health problems became more important. These included activity intolerance, potential for chest pain and alteration in lifestyle and self-care. The cardiologist requested further investigations of his cardiac functioning and the condition of his coronary circulation, to determine further care. Medical treatments such as beta-blocking therapy were commenced and the cardiac rehabilitation team became involved prior to an uneventful discharge.

*Arrhythmia.
See chapter 4.2*

Disorders of electroconduction

Normally, the rate and rhythm of heart contractions are established by impulses generated in the sinoatrial (SA) node at a rate between 60 and 100 beats per minute (Fig. 12.11). A disorder of rate or rhythm is referred to as a *cardiac arrhythmia*, and is due to some disturbance in the formation or conduction of impulses. The **arrhythmia** may be of short duration or persistent, and may be functional in origin, result from organic heart disease or be associated with an electrolyte imbalance, such as hypokalaemia.

An arrhythmia may have significant haemodynamic consequences. For example, an excessively slow or fast

Figure 12.11   Sinus rhythm.

heart rate may decrease the cardiac output and blood pressure, thus compromising the perfusion of vital organs such as the brain, kidneys, liver and the heart itself. Arrhythmias may also predispose the patient to thrombus formation. It is important for nurses to have a sound knowledge of arrhythmias and their management in order to plan and provide care for patients with these health problems. Arrhythmias can also act as a prewarning to further, more life-threatening, rhythm disturbances, and a knowledge of certain arrhythmias is imperative for the employment of skills where nurses are trained to provide prompt definitive treatment, such as in the use of defibrillation in cardiopulmonary arrest.

Common irregularities include tachycardia (fast heart rate), bradycardia (slow heart rate), ectopic beats (extrasystoles), flutter, fibrillation and heart block. The arrhythmia is further defined by the site of its origin: *sinus* arrhythmia originates in the SA node, *atrial* originates in an atrium, *junctional* originates in the AV junctional area, and *ventricular* originates in a ventricle. Importantly, tachycardia needs to be treated promptly to slow and steady the heart, producing a good cardiac output. Bradycardias are treated cautiously to avoid inadvertently stopping the heart altogether. Cardiac pacing may be used to speed up the rate in a longer-term bradycardic problem.

Tachycardias

Sinus tachycardia

In this rhythm the heart rate is greater than 100 beats per minute, and the impulse originates in the SA node. It is not always an abnormal rhythm, because it occurs during and after exercise and in response to emotional stress. It may be a normal response to an abnormal state, such as pain, severe anxiety, fever, anaemia, infection, hyperthyroidism, myocardial infarction and heart failure. It may also result from medications, for example atropine, adrenaline (epinephrine), isoprenaline hydrochloride and thyroid extract, or other drugs such as alcohol and nicotine (Fig. 12.12).

Tachycardia is significant for two reasons: coronary blood flow occurs predominantly during diastole. With tachycardia, the diastolic time is shortened, reducing the time for perfusion of the myocardium. Also, an increased heart rate increases the need of the myocardium for

Figure 12.12   Sinus tachycardia: rate over 100 per minute; P wave and QRS are normal in 1 : 1 relationship.

Figure 12.13   Paroxysmal atrial tachycardia.

Figure 12.14   Ventricular tachycardia.

oxygen. In someone with narrowed coronary arteries, tachycardia may precipitate myocardial ischaemia.

Primarily, treatment is directed at correcting the underlying cause, but it may be necessary to reduce the rate by giving a drug such as a digitalis preparation or a beta-blocker.

Paroxysmal atrial tachycardia (PAT)/narrow complex tachycardia

This is an abrupt onset of a very rapid heart rate, usually 150–250 beats per minute, initiated in the atria. It has several names and may be called a supra (meaning above) ventricular tachycardia (SVT). It may last a few seconds or longer. Such attacks cannot be explained in some persons; in others they may be related to organic heart disease or digitalis toxicity (Fig. 12.13). The narrow QRS complex indicates that the fast arrhythmia is originating in the atria, not in the ventricles, as this part of the ECG (the QRS segment) is normal.

A rapid heart rate of this type is serious if imposed on a diseased heart. When this arrhythmia occurs, the patient is advised to rest and the doctor is notified. If the patient is subject to recurring attacks, he or she is encouraged to recognize and avoid possible precipitating factors such as fatigue, emotional stress, or excessive smoking or coffee drinking. In some instances an attack may be relieved by measures that increase parasympathetic (vagal) innervation to the heart. Among those suggested is pressure on the carotid sinus. *Caution must be used in relation to the manoeuvre.* Carotid sinus massage applied injudiciously

may result in asystole. It should be performed only by a doctor. The Valsalva manoeuvre, which involves an inspiration followed by voluntary closure of the glottis and an effort to exhale, may prove helpful. This reduces the venous return from the extremities and head, thus reducing the volume of blood entering the heart, which in turn decreases the cardiac output and the arter-ial blood pressure. An antiarrhythmic agent such as adenosine (which blocks the electrical impulses reaching the ventricles for a few seconds, breaking the tachycardic cycle), verapamil, a beta-blocker or digoxin may be used. Disopyramide or amiodarone may be useful. Long-acting quinidine preparations are sometimes prescribed.

Ventricular tachycardia (VT)/broad complex tachycardia

The term ventricular tachycardia (VT) usually refers to a run of rapidly repeated ventricular beats, essentially regular in rhythm, at a rate of 100–210 per minute. The impulses actually occur in the ventricles themselves and dominate as the fast pacemaker of the heart. Any rate above 60 per minute that is initiated in the ventricles might be considered tachycardia because the ventricles normally do not initiate impulses at more than 25–40 beats per minute. However, rates between 60 and 100 per minute are usually distinguished from the faster rates. They are usually referred to as *accelerated idioventricular rhythms* but are also called *slow ventricular tachycardia* (Fig. 12.14). The broad QRS complex indicates that the abnormal impulse originates in the ventricles themselves.

Figure 12.15   Sinus bradycardia.

Ventricular tachycardia is a serious arrhythmia as there is always the danger that it will lead to ventricular fibrillation. It is usually due to ischaemic heart disease and is frequently present following myocardial infarction.

Treatment includes defibrillation, cardioversion (if a pulse is present) and/or antiarrhythmic drugs such as intravenous lidocaine (lignocaine). Other drugs that may be used include intravenous procainamide or bretylium tosylate.

Bradycardias

Sinus bradycardia

Sinus bradycardia is discharge of the SA node at a rate less than 60 beats per minute (Fig. 12.15).

Circulation may be adequately maintained by an increased stroke volume in a person with sinus bradycardia. With fewer contractions, more blood collects in the heart chambers to produce greater stretching of the myocardial fibres, resulting in a stronger contraction and increased output. Obviously this can occur only if the myocardium is in good condition. If the heart rate is less than 30–40 per minute, circulatory insufficiency is likely to occur, especially with physical activity.

The most common causes of sinus bradycardia are a decreased blood supply to the SA node or increased vagal tone. Circulatory reflexes may initiate a compensatory increase in the heart rate but, if the cause persists and becomes progressively severe, the heart muscle will gradually become weaker and less responsive, producing fewer contractions. Any disturbance that initiates an increase in the number of vagal nerve impulses to the heart will produce a decrease in the heart rate. An example of this would be bradycardia produced by carotid sinus massage or, in some people, by vomiting. Other examples of conditions in which slowing of the heart rate may be secondary are increased intracranial pressure (see p. 705) and myxoedema (a deficiency of thyroid secretion; see p. 588).

The pulse rate may normally be slower in those with well developed cardiac reserve, such as well trained athletes. In such people, the venous return is of greater strength, producing an increased stroke volume with each contraction.

Sinus bradycardia does not require treatment unless the individual is symptomatic. Atropine sulfate may be administered to decrease vagal tone. If the arrhythmia is due to the administration of medication, this should be withheld and re-evaluated.

Ectopic beats (extrasystoles)

When impulses that influence the heart rate and rhythm are generated elsewhere than in the SA node, the contractions are called *ectopic*, *premature beats* or *extrasystoles*. The beats tend to be individual, but may occur in a small sequence or increase in frequency. The ectopic or premature beat occurs when the myocardial fibres are in the relative refractory period following a normal contraction. The impulse from the SA node for the succeeding normal contraction is ineffective, because it arrives when the muscle fibres are in the absolute refractory period following the premature beat, and no contraction takes place. This causes a longer than normal pause before the next normal contraction, and the heart 'misses' a beat. The next normal contraction may be stronger because of the prolonged filling period. The time between the normal heart contraction, which precedes the extrasystole, and the one that follows is equal to two normal cardiac cycles. The subject usually describes the experience as the heart 'missing a beat'.

Ectopic, or premature beats, may be due to ischaemic areas or to inflammation in the heart muscle. The fibres may also become irritated and hypersensitive as a result of certain toxic conditions, such as may occur with the excessive use of tobacco, coffee, tea or alcohol. The ectopics may occur irregularly, with varying lengths of time between them. The incidence may be so rare as to have no clinical significance but they should be investigated if persistent, even though they occur irregularly and at relatively long intervals. Ectopic beats may arise regularly and at a rate in excess of that of the normal SA pacemaker, resulting in tachycardia.

Atrial ectopic beats

The ectopic focus is in the atria and the complex occurs earlier than expected. Atrial ectopic beats are significant because, if they occur during the vulnerable period of the atria, they may precipitate more serious atrial arrhythmias, such as atrial flutter or atrial fibrillation. They may or may not be conducted to the ventricles, depending upon the state of conduction through the AV node and the refractory period at which they occur. Treatment is not usually required unless they occur with great frequency or unless progression to more serious arrhythmias is feared, as may occur following myocardial infarction. If a precipitating cause is recognized, it should be eliminated (Fig. 12.16).

Figure 12.16 Atrial ectopic beat (arrowed).

Figure 12.17 Ventricular ectopic beat (arrowed).

Figure 12.18 Atrial flutter.

Ventricular ectopic beats (VEBs)

The ectopic focus is in the ventricle, and therefore there will be no related P wave on the ECG. Occasional ventricular ectopic beats may be innocuous, but they may also precipitate ventricular tachycardia and/or fibrillation. If they occur in a diseased heart, in groups of three or more, more frequently than 5 per minute, arise from more than one focus (multifocal) or are on the T wave of the preceding complex, they are considered serious and require treatment. The usual immediate treatment is lidocaine (lignocaine), given by bolus i.v. injection followed by a continuous i.v. drip. An oral drug such as disopyramide might be given when the lidocaine (lignocaine) infusion is gradually tapered

off; however, many patients do not require this (see Fig. 12.17).

Flutter

Atrial flutter

As with atrial tachycardia, atrial flutter is due to a rapidly firing ectopic focus in the atria. The atrial rate usually falls between 250 and 350 beats per minute and a characteristic sawtooth pattern is seen on the ECG. AV block is usually present, so that the ventricular response may vary from 150 to 175 beats per minute (Fig. 12.18). Atrial flutter may occur with mitral stenosis, ischaemic heart disease and chronic obstructive pulmonary disease. The

Figure 12.19 Atrial fibrillation with varying ventricular responses.

Figure 12.20   Ventricular fibrillation: chaotic ventricular activity.

usual treatment is electrical cardioversion (see below) when the patient is haemodynamically unstable. Digoxin is the drug of choice to slow the ventricular rate by blocking impulses at the AV node. It may convert the flutter to atrial fibrillation, which is easier to manage.

Fibrillation

This is an arrhythmia in which the normal rhythmic contractions of the myocardium of either the atria or ventricles are replaced by extremely rapid (250–500 per minute), ineffective contractions, irregular in force and rhythm. As a result the heart does not achieve the contraction and relaxation that permit normal emptying and filling of the chambers.

Atrial fibrillation (AF)

Atrial fibrillation is a fairly common arrhythmia in which electrical activity in the atria is totally disorganized. It is due to myocardial disease which may be the result of coronary insufficiency, valvular heart disease, congestive heart failure or acute infection. The atria are never completely empty, and normal filling cannot occur. Since little pressure is created by the atrial contractions themselves, the flow of blood into the ventricles is due mainly to drainage under the influence of gravity. This aspect may not adversely affect the cardiac output. Only a proportion of the impulses arising in the atria are conducted through the AV node to the ventricles. However, those that do pass through may far exceed the normal in frequency, and are irregular, although the QRS complex is normal (Fig. 12.19). Cardiovascular problems may therefore occur, owing to the high heart rate experienced. Cardiac output falls as a result of decreased ventricular diastolic filling time, and the pulse may be weak and irregular.

To control the ventricular response, digoxin, verapamil and beta-blockers such as propranolol may be used. To decrease atrial tissue irritability, quinidine can be used. Procainamide and amiodarone may be used in more resistant cases. Cardioversion may be used with the patient who is haemodynamically unstable.

A complication that may follow atrial fibrillation is embolism. The blood that was not forwarded into the ventricles during fibrillation may have formed a thrombus in an atrial chamber and then, when normal heart action is re-established, the thrombus may be moved out into the circulation. Therefore, for those who have been in atrial fibrillation for some time, anticoagulation will be given for several weeks with warfarin, in addition to a drug such as digoxin to slow the heart rate, before cardioversion is attempted. In the elderly, treatment may fail to revert them to sinus rhythm and a drug such as digoxin is used on a long-term basis to slow and steady the heart rate.

Ventricular fibrillation (VF)

In ventricular fibrillation very rapid, asynchronous quivering arises in the ventricular myocardium because the electrical activity occurs in a totally disorganized sequence (Fig. 12.20). The contractions are so ineffective in pumping that the condition very quickly proves fatal. The pulse and blood pressure become unobtainable within a few seconds, the patient quickly loses consciousness, pupils dilate, reflexes are lost and cyanosis is likely to develop. Prompt emergency treatment may re-establish circulation. If the patient is being monitored in a coronary care unit, the arrhythmia may be identified immediately at onset, and treatment would consist of immediate defibrillation. Defibrillation is an expanding part of the nurse's role but hospital policy on who may defibrillate should be followed at all times. An important guideline is that it must be initiated very quickly to increase the chance of survival.

Ventricular fibrillation may occur with irritation of the heart during heart catheterization, because of coronary occlusion by the catheter or when conditions such as myocardial infarction, hypothermia, hypoxia, hypokalaemia and electrical shock exist. Very frequently ventricular fibrillation is preceded by ventricular ectopic beats. Prompt administration of an antiarrhythmic drug may prevent serious ventricular tachycardia and fibrillation.

Heart block

This is a condition in which impulse formation is depressed or impulse conduction is blocked. Although conduction may be interrupted between the SA node and the atria, the term 'heart block' usually refers to a disorder of conduction at the junctional tissues, which are the AV node and the common bundle (bundle of His). The SA node or the conduction pathway may be damaged by

Figure 12.21   Sinoatrial block (the arrows indicate where a sinoatrial impulse (P wave) should have occurred).

Figure 12.22   First-degree heart block.

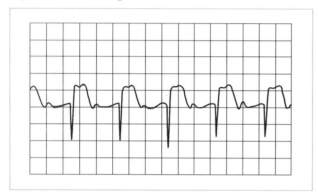

inflammatory disease such as rheumatic fever, coronary insufficiency, pressure from scarred or calcified tissue, or surgical trauma. In the latter, this is notably following cardiac valve surgery.

Sinoatrial block

In sinoatrial block, impulses either are not formed in the SA node, fail to be conducted from it, or emerge very slowly (Fig. 12.21). If sinoatrial impulses are not received by the atria, occasional beats may be dropped, cardiac standstill may occur, or the ventricles may respond to impulses arising from a lower pacemaker, such as the junctional tissue. In the latter instance a junctional rhythm will result .

The seriousness of a SA block depends on the extent to which the heart rate is slowed and cardiac output is decreased. A slow rate may precipitate other arrhythmias. Specific precipitating causes include drugs such as digoxin and some antiarrhythmic drugs, salicylates, ischaemic heart disease, myocardial infarction and increased vagal tone.

Treatment is directed at removing the cause, when possible, and improving conduction between the SA node and the atria by drugs such as atropine and isoprenaline. If drug therapy is not effective, artificial pacing may be required.

Heart block at junctional tissues occurs in varying degrees of severity and may be categorized as first degree, second degree (types I and II) and third degree, or complete AV block. Conduction may be impaired in the bundle branches, referred to as *right* or *left bundle branch block*.

First-degree atrioventricular block

First-degree heart block is usually due to delayed conduction through the AV node, and the interval between atrial and ventricular contractions is lengthened. This is exhibited on the ECG by a prolonged P–R interval (greater than 0.20 s) (Fig. 12.22). It may be caused by increased vagal tone, digoxin toxicity, inflammatory heart disease or coronary artery disease. First-degree AV block may progress to second- and third-degree block, but in the absence of evidence of disease requires no treatment. Digoxin may be discontinued or the dosage reduced.

Second-degree atrioventricular block

Second-degree or partial block refers to a more advanced disturbance in which some of the sinus impulses fail to get through and activate the ventricles. It may be divided into Mobitz type I or Wenckebach, and Mobitz type II.

In *Wenckebach block* the period of time between atrial and ventricular conduction becomes progressively longer, until finally an atrial impulse is completely blocked. The ECG shows progressively longer P–R intervals, until finally a P wave is not followed by a QRS complex. The P–R interval following this dropped ventricular beat is close to the normal range, but with each successive beat it lengthens and the cycle repeats itself. The patient may be conscious of a decreased ventricular rate if the change occurs suddenly, but may exhibit no physical symptoms (Fig. 12.23).

Type II second-degree block is more serious than type I. At specific intervals impulses are blocked at the AV node and an atrial beat fails to be followed by a ventricular beat. The ratio of atrial to ventricular beats may vary, for example 2:1, 3:1, 4:3, or 3:2. The P–R interval is constant. The patient may experience syncopal (fainting) attacks (Fig. 12.24).

Figure 12.23   Wenckebach block.

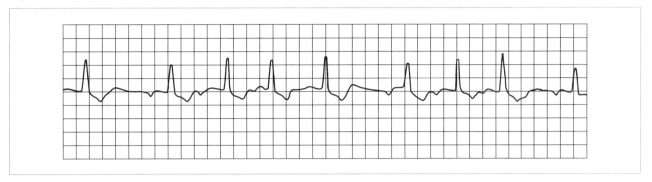

Figure 12.24   Type II second-degree block.

Figure 12.25   Complete heart block (the arrows indicate sinoatrial impulses (P waves) occurring regularly but independently of ventricular activity).

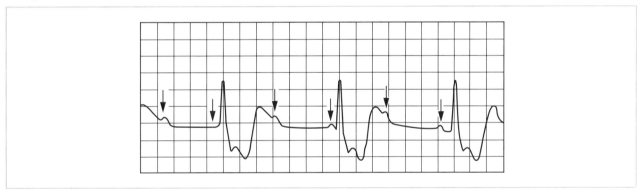

Both second-degree blocks may be due to inflammatory or fibrotic processes, ischaemic heart disease, infarction, or drugs such as digoxin, beta-blockers or verapamil. Atropine sulfate may be required to increase the heart rate, and temporary cardiac pacing may be needed if the ventricular rate is slow.

Complete atrioventricular block

In this arrhythmia conduction is so disturbed that no impulses reach the ventricles, and the atria and ventricles beat independently at their own inherent rhythms. The block may occur at the AV node, or the bundle of His. It is a more advanced block and may be caused by any of the disorders responsible for type II partial blocks. As atrial impulses are unable to penetrate the AV node, a lower pacemaker takes over and controls the ventricles. If this 'rescuing' pacemaker is initiated in the junctional tissue, the ECG will show a QRS complex that is normal in appearance and is not wide unless there is an associated bundle branch block. If the pacemaker is in the ventricles, the QRS complexes will be wide and abnormal in shape (Fig. 12.25).

This condition may be managed with an infusion of isoprenaline if the patient shows signs of a decreased cardiac output. A temporary cardiac pacemaker may be required and evaluation of the need for permanent cardiac pacing conducted to manage this arrhythmia. A permanent pacemaker is rarely used in the first instance, because the condition may be temporary, for example following cardiac surgery.

Treatment of cardiac arrhythmias

Treatment of heart arrhythmias includes the use of a pacemaker, implantable cardioverter defibrillator (ICD), medications and/or defibrillation.

Artificial cardiac pacemakers

In serious conduction defects, and sometimes in the treatment of tachyarrhythmias, electrical stimulation may be provided by an electronic battery-operated pacemaker to stimulate or control cardiac contractions.

An artificial pacemaker generates an electrical stimulus which is used to send a specific electrical current to the myocardium to control or maintain a minimum heart rate. Every pacemaker consists of a pulse generator, which emits and senses electrical impulses, and a wire catheter with one or more electrodes that conduct the impulses to the heart. This electrode or lead system may transmit impulses by contact with the endocardium established through the venous route into the right atrium and/or ventricle, or by contact with the epicardium established by thoracotomy (e.g. after cardiac surgery). Contact may also be made by the transthoracic approach when the pacing stimulus is delivered through electrodes applied on the external anterior and posterior chest wall in an emergency. This latter method is quite painful to the patient.

If the conduction defect is transient, a *temporary* pacemaker is used. A pacing electrode is introduced through the external jugular, subclavian, antecubital or femoral vein, and advanced into the right ventricle under fluoroscopy or via a special flotation catheter with a little balloon on the end. The electrode wire is connected to an external battery-operated pacemaker. The site of insertion of the electrode is secured with a sterile dressing.

When the conduction defect is irreversible, a *permanent* pacemaker is implanted within the body. The electrode is introduced transvenously, usually through the right cephalic or right external jugular vein, and the battery unit is implanted subcutaneously in a supermammary pouch on the chest wall. Alternatively, it is implanted beneath the muscle of the upper abdominal wall. This requires a small incision. Pacemaker functioning can be described based on: (1) the heart chamber paced, (2) the chamber in which the heart's intrinsic electrical impulse is sensed, (3) the mode of pacemaker response, (4) its programmable characteristics, and (5) the antitachy-arrhythmic features. Often, only the first three positions are used to describe a particular pacemaker's functioning (Table 12.6).

Essentially all pacing systems must have two wires to complete the electrical circuit. The *bipolar* system uses two wires placed against the myocardium (Fig. 12.26b). A temporary system will invariably use a bipolar system (with an external pacing box). If one of the wires is believed not to be working, perhaps because pacing spikes cannot be seen on the ECG with a good electrical output, either wire can be 'bypassed' by pushing a needle under the skin and connecting this to the temporary pacing box to complete the electrical circuit.

There are several modes of pacemaker, categorized according to their pattern of activity. The pacemaker may

Table 12.6   Positions describing pacemaker functioning

	Position		
	I	II	III
Category	Chamber(s) paced	Chamber(s) sensed	Mode of response
Letters used	V – ventricle A – atrium D – dual (atrium and ventricle)	V – ventricle A – atrium D – dual (atrium and ventricle) O – none	T – triggered I – inhibited D – dual O – none

Figure 12.26   VVI pacing systems.

(a) Unipolar pacing   (b) Bipolar pacing

From Barnett (2001), with permission.

be preset to discharge at a fixed rate, by demand or at a rate that corresponds to cardiac activity. *Fixed rate pacing* is asynchronous, meaning that it does not sense the heart's own impulses. The pacemaker therefore delivers a predetermined rate of impulses, even if the heart is generating its own spontaneous rhythm. A second mode of pacing is the *demand mode*. In this mode, the pacemaker is programmed to sense the heart's intrinsic electrical activity and to fire only when the intrinsic rhythm falls below a preset rate. This avoids dangerous competition between the heart and the pacemaker, as well as the risk of two differing messages being sent to the myocardium, for example a stimulus to depolarize during repolarization. This would run the risk of inducing a life-threatening cardiac arrhythmia.

Nurses caring for patients with cardiac pacemakers learn how to recognize that the device is working from the characteristic ECG patterns. Generally, when working, a small vertical horizontal *pacing spike* occurs before a P wave in atrial pacing and before a slightly abnormal QRS complex in ventricular pacing. In the latter, if the wire is quite high in the ventricle, the QRS complex may appear fairly normal. Also, P waves may be seen to wander through the rhythm strip, because atrial activity may still be functioning while the ventricle is paced, but there is no association between the two chambers. In dual-chamber pacing, a spike appears before the P wave *and* before the corresponding QRS complex. Pacing spikes with no complexes indicate a lack of electrical *capture*, or depolarization of the myocardium.

Nursing care of the patient with a pacemaker

Nursing care involves assisting in the preparation of the patient for implantation of the pacemaker. The patient may be apprehensive because of the symptoms of bradycardia such as dizziness and fainting, and may also be fearful of the procedure and being dependent on an electrical device for their heart beat. When explaining the need for a pacemaker, the doctor reviews the procedure with the patient. The nurse reinforces this explanation and answers any further questions before the patient signs the consent form. Explanations are also given to the family/carers.

Temporary pacemakers are usually implanted under local anaesthesia in the angiography department, in the radiology department or occasionally, in an emergency, at the bedside. Permanent pacemakers are inserted in the operating theatre or the angiography department.

Following the implantation of a permanent pacemaker, the patient is monitored continuously until it has been established that the pacemaker is functioning properly. Rest is indicated for the remainder of the day. If a temporary pacemaker has been inserted, mobility is restricted, depending upon the site of insertion as well as the patient's general condition. Cardiac monitoring may be continued as long as the temporary pacemaker is being used.

The nurse is responsible for monitoring and reporting the patient's rhythm, for checking the operation site and cleansing the wound as necessary, for assessing and reporting any complications, and for supporting the patient and providing any information needed.

Complications that could occur include malfunction of the pacemaker, perforation of the myocardial wall by an electrode, breakage or dislodgement of the electrodes, thrombus formation, and infection, such as phlebitis, endocarditis or septicaemia. Malfunction may occur because the pacemaker fails to fire, fires too rapidly, or fires erratically. Malfunctioning may be detected by cardiac monitoring or by ECG, as well as by the presence of signs and symptoms, such as decreased pulse rate, dizziness and/or fainting.

Following perforation of the myocardium, blood can seep into the pericardium, causing cardiac tamponade. The resulting compression of the heart causes low blood pressure, tachycardia, increased central venous pressure and distended neck veins. The electrode may also stimulate innervation to the upper abdominal or lower chest muscles, resulting in spasm. This is uncomfortable for the patient and more common with a large and thinned right ventricle. The doctor should reposition the wire in such cases. Breakage or dislodgement of the electrode will result in a change in the shape of the QRS complex and in the heart rate.

The nurse should be alert to electrical hazards in the environment. Electrical equipment must be properly earthed and the external pulse generator of temporary pacemakers must be kept dry. If epicardial wires are used, which emerge through the chest wall, following cardiac surgery, the ends should be wrapped in gauze or the fingers of rubber or latex gloves. This prevents static from clothes sending an electrical impulse along the wire to the heart.

Caution regarding electrical hazards includes avoiding close contact with large electrical motors; for example, in a machine shop the patient may develop arrhythmias as a result of the electrical interference (Sager 1987). Microwave ovens may cause similar interference with some pacemakers if the oven is faulty with an inadequate door seal. Small home appliances, if properly grounded, produce no untoward effects. Contact sports might be allowed on the doctor's advice. The patient's dentist should be advised that the patient is wearing a pacemaker before any electrical equipment is used. It is advisable for the patient to notifiy airport security of their cardiac pacemaker to avoid triggering the alarms.

The patient should carry an identification card indicating the type of pacemaker in place and the doctor to be notified in case of difficulty. Before travelling, the patient should obtain the name of a local doctor or hospital in case of an emergency.

The implantable cardioverter defibrillator (ICD)

This is a small internal device which looks rather like a pacemaker. It is designed to track the heart rhythm and deliver a series of small direct current (DC) shocks to the myocardium when a life-threatening arrhythmia is detected. This aims to terminate the arrhythmia. It is designed for patients who are known to be prone to this sort of event, perhaps due to cardiac disease, and where other treatments alone are not effective. Although the use of these devices has saved many lives, it has emerged that there is a need for psychological support for patients receiving the ICD (James 2001). This is because patients are often discharged home within a few days of implantation and may have concerns over a variety of issues. These include how the shock will feel (although many units now administer a test shock before discharge), whether they can be touched during the shock, whether an ambulance will need to be called after a shock is delivered, through to the dangers to partners during sexual activity. In fact, the shock is small enough not to affect those touching the patient. However, a structured programme for patients receiving the device is needed to allay fears in both the patient and loved ones, and to prevent the device from having an adverse effect on quality of life.

Drugs used to manage arrhythmias

Drugs commonly used to manage cardiac arrhythmias are described in Table 12.7.

Defibrillation and cardioversion

In *defibrillation* two electrodes ('paddles') are placed on the chest wall. The standard technique is to place one paddle to the right (the patient's right) of the upper part of the sternum, below the clavicle and the other paddle over the fifth left intercostal space in the mid-clavicular line. A strong electrical discharge is passed through the electrodes for a brief period. All the muscle fibres of the myocardium are thrown into contraction together and then enter a refractory period simultaneously. This quiescent period may give the normal pacemaker, the SA node, an opportunity to take over. It is important to make sure that no one is touching the bed or the patient during the electrical discharge to prevent them from receiving a shock. Shocks are delivered in a set sequence of usually three shocks: 200, 200 and 360 joules in adults, followed by a 1-minute pause, then 360 joules in sequences of three (Resuscitation Council 2000).

Cardioversion differs from defibrillation in only one important aspect. It is a synchronized procedure designed to deliver smaller amounts of electrical energy to the heart at a set time in the cardiac cycle. The same equipment is used to perform cardioversion as defibrillation but a synchronization circuit is activated to allow for timing of the cardiac cycle. After the machine is discharged, the shock is held until the next QRS complex is tracked and then it is discharged. This prevents the shock from being delivered during ventricular depolarization and causing ventricular fibrillation. Cardioversion is used

Table 12.7   Drugs commonly used to manage cardiac arrhythmias

Drug	General actions	Clinical uses
Cardiac glycosides e.g. Digoxin	Increase force of contraction without significantly increasing oxygen utilization Decrease conduction through AV node	Atrial arrhythmias, notably atrial fibrillation

Sodium channel suppressors
e.g. A. Quinidine sulfate
       Procainamide
 	
    B. Lidocaine (lignocaine)
	Depress automaticity
	Slow conduction
	Decrease myocardial contractility
	Depress ventricular ectopic foci
		Atrial arrhythmias
		Ventricular arrhythmias
		
		Ventricular arrhythmias, ventricular ectopic beats

β-Adrenergic blockers e.g. Sotalol	Decrease ventricular ectopy Decrease heart rate Increase PR interval Decrease myocardial contractility Decrease myocardial oxygen demand	Ventricular arrhythmias Supraventricular arrhythmias
Prolong repolarization e.g. Amiodarone	Decrease ventricular conduction Increase duration of the action potential	Atrial arrhythmias Recurrent ventricular tachycardia/fibrillation
Calcium channel blockers e.g. Verapamil	Prolong refractory period of AV node	Atrial arrhythmias

to treat ventricular tachycardia and rapid atrial arrhythmias, such as atrial **fibrillation** and flutter, when the patient is haemodynamically unstable.

Some patients are admitted for electrical cardioversion as day cases, such as those in atrial fibrillation. They will have been fully anticoagulated on warfarin to avoid the formation of any clots that might be forced into the circulation on restoration of normal sinus rhythm. Patients need to be advised not to eat or drink for at least 5 hours before the procedure as they will be having a general anaesthetic. Cardioversion is normally performed on a coronary care unit or a day-case ward. The procedure takes about 15 minutes. After-effects tend to be related to the anaesthetic, although the patient may have a sore chest requiring the application of a topical cream. Cardioversion is not always successful as it does nothing to remove the underlying cause of the arrhythmia. The outcome therefore needs to be fully explained.

Cardiopulmonary arrest

Cardiopulmonary arrest means the sudden cessation of effective ventricular contraction *and* respirations. **Cardiac arrest** essentially means the cessation of effective ventricular function, but the terms may be used interchangeably. The condition includes ventricular tachycardia (VT) when there is no pulse, ventricular fibrillation (VF) and asystole. Possible causes are myocardial ischaemia, respiratory insufficiency, heart block, electric shock, metabolic acidosis and adverse reactions to medications.

Cardiac arrest must be recognized as a critical emergency. This condition is diagnosed when the individual is assessed as unconscious, not breathing and having no carotid pulse. It is imperative that oxygen supply be re-established to the brain within 3–4 minutes of cardiac arrest to prevent irreversible anoxic brain damage.

Basic cardiopulmonary resuscitation (CPR) must be commenced as soon as cardiac arrest is diagnosed. The ABC steps are Airway, Breathing and Circulation (Fig. 12.27). It is every nurse's responsibility to be prepared and well versed in conducting basic life support. Regular practical updates, usually 6 monthly to yearly, allow the skill to be reassessed and competence maintained.

A: Airway

After unresponsiveness has been determined, help is summoned, the airway is opened using the head-tilt/chin-lift or jaw manoeuvre. A Guedal airway may be used to maintain patency of the airway until such time as endotracheal intubation occurs.

B: Breathing

After the airway is opened, assessment for respiration is conducted. Once absence of breathing is determined, definitive assistance such as an ambulance or the cardiac arrest team is called. Artificial respiration using the

Figure 12.27 Resuscitation in cardiac arrest.

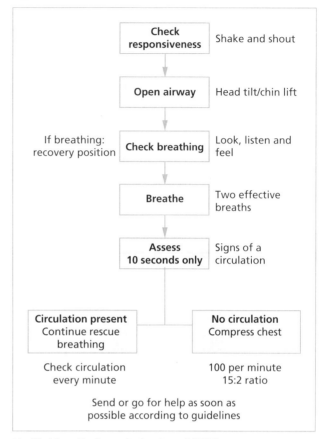

Modified from the Resuscitation Council (2000).

Fibrillation:
See chapter 4.2

Cardiac arrest:
See chapter 4.2

mouth-to-mouth method is started. The rescuer gives two initial breaths, ensuring the patient's nose is pinched closed. In a hospital or clinic, resuscitation should be performed using a pocket mask with oxygen attachment, or a self-refilling bag-mask device, again attached to an oxygen source. This offers a greater percentage of oxygen to the patient. The bag-mask device is hard to use by one person, as there is a need to keep the airway open, hold the mask in place and inflate the bag. It is much more effective if one person holds the mask over the face with two hands while tilting the chin, and another squeezes the bag to ventilate the lungs. Laryngeal mask airways (LMAs) are being used by nurses in hospital to offer an even higher oxygen percentage. These consist of a tube with a rubber flange on the end. This is inserted into the mouth and inflated over the larynx, then connected to the bag-valve device (Simons 1999). The use of these devices is known as basic life support with adjunct therapy.

C: Circulation

Circulation is checked by palpating the carotid pulse. If no pulse is found, external chest compression is started immediately. This consists of the regular application of vertical pressure at a point one-third up the sternum from its tip (xiphoid process). Both hands should be used, with the fingers interlocked, applying pressure with the heels of the hands and maintaining the elbows locked in an extended position so that the arms are straight. The increase in intrathoracic pressure produces a limited circulation of blood which, if it is to be effective, must force sufficient blood into the arteries to produce pulsation in the carotid and femoral arteries. The sternum should be depressed 4–5 cm in an adult. The thoracic cage is quite flexible in an unconscious person and the possibility of injury to the ribs is therefore reduced. This technique of resuscitation is simple, requires no special equipment, and may be done anywhere. Finding the carotid pulse can be difficult in a collapsed patient.

If one rescuer is present, compressions are interrupted at every 15th compression for the lungs to be ventilated twice. If two rescuers are present, the task is shared, with one performing chest compressions and the other ventilations in the ratio of 15:2 (Resuscitation Council 2000). The aim should be to deliver at least 12 respirations per minute.

Basic CPR is enhanced by the provision of advanced cardiac life support by trained personnel who are prepared to diagnose and provide definitive therapy. One member of the team attaches electrodes to the patient and continuous cardiac monitoring is begun to determine the underlying cardiac rhythm. Another member of the team inserts an intravenous line for the infusion of medications. If ventricular fibrillation or pulseless ventricular tachycardia has caused the arrest, a defibrillator is used to deliver an electric shock through electrodes into the chest wall. Emergency drugs are given as required. To be optimally effective, advanced life support follows a particular algorithm guideline from the Resuscitation Council (2000) (see Appendix 1).

Care following resuscitation

The patient who has been resuscitated requires constant observation of the vital signs. If possible, the patient is transferred to an intensive care unit and continuous monitoring of heart action is established. An intensive care unit will be used if mechanical ventilation is required. An X-ray is usually ordered to assess for any damage to the chest following CPR, the position of any central lines or an endotracheal tube if in place. A variety of blood tests will be taken to assess electrolyte and blood gas levels (e.g. oxygen and carbon dioxide levels). What has happened will be discussed with relatives and loved ones, and if there are any specific problems encountered such as cerebral oedema due to hypoxia of the brain these will be assessed and treated. Peripheral pulses are checked for volume, rhythm and rate, together with regular recordings of the blood pressure and oxygen saturation levels via a pulse oximetry probe. The defibrillator and mechanical ventilator are kept nearby and ready for immediate use.

The patient may be very apprehensive and should be advised of the improvement in condition and of the

---

> **Box 12.3**   The decision to withhold CPR
>
> Mrs Jones is an 86-year-old woman who has been admitted to hospital with increasing shortness of breath. Tests show that she has lung cancer that has metastasized throughout her chest. She has been an active woman until recently and agrees to a trial of radiotherapy to control the malignancy to a certain extent. After a week she starts to deteriorate.
>
> ■ If Mrs Jones has a cardiac arrest, should she be resuscitated? How should such a decision be made?

importance of rest and minimal emotional stress, and is assured that someone will either be present or close by so that treatment may be quickly instituted should it be needed.

Ethical issues: decisions to withhold cardiopulmonary resuscitation

Although decisions to withhold CPR have been debated extensively during the past two decades, such decisions remain a common and difficult ethical problem for most healthcare providers. The usual presumption in any instance of cardiac arrest is that CPR will be attempted. However, there are situations in which CPR does not appear to be appropriate. The main difficulties in trying to determine whether or not CPR is appropriate can be reduced to three: determining in *which* situations CPR should be withheld, determining *who* should make that kind of decision, and determining *how* the decision should be made and implemented. A typical situation is described in Box 12.3.

Background

Deciding not to resuscitate is, of course, a controversial issue. Like many technological advances, CPR raises ethical issues that previous generations of healthcare providers did not have to face. The imperative to extend life-sustaining technology to an ever wider range of patients brings eventually with it the need to set limits to the use of the technology. When CPR was introduced in 1960 its goal was to prevent sudden and unexpected death from cardiac arrest. Before long it was applied to almost anyone who suffered cardiac arrest (i.e. anyone who died). Now, in most hospital practice, and in most hospital policies, it is presumed that in the event of cardiac arrest CPR will be performed unless a specific decision not to resuscitate is made. In the 1960s, any decisions not to resuscitate were made by doctors verbally at the time of making rounds.

As practitioners were confronted with increasing and sometimes inappropriate use of CPR, and as nurses became more uncomfortable at being left with only verbal orders, attempts were made to establish guidelines for making decisions about CPR. The nurse has an obligation to determine whether there are such advance directives.

Although limitation of treatment decisions is usually couched in terms of the principle of autonomy, or 'patient wishes', other principles are involved in actually coming to the decision. A decision to forego CPR is usually guided by balancing the benefits and the burdens of the treatment for a patient. When the burdens of a treatment such as CPR appear to be disproportionate to the benefits that may be obtained, it is important for the caregivers to initiate a discussion of the appropriateness of CPR for the individual. In evaluating a decision, the benefits and the burdens are both considered from the point of view of the patient. At present, most policies require that decision making on this issue include the patient or relatives, and that decisions be made only after discussion with the patient or relative.

A further issue that might be considered is balancing the benefit to the patient with the burdens that the treatment will place on family members or society in general.

Certain types of underlying disease and other characteristics of the patient are associated with reduced survival, and for some associated complications (e.g. pneumonia) the chances are practically zero. It may be possible, with further study, to define the circumstances in which CPR would be definitely futile, and would therefore not even have to be offered. Until then, the patient or patient's family should be involved in the decision making. To aid decision making and the support of everyone involved in such a decision, the British Medical Association, the UK Resuscitation Council and the Royal College of Nursing have produced guidelines (BMA/RCN 2001). The term *do not attempt resuscitation* (DNAR) is used, and the overall responsibility lies with the consultant or general practitioner in charge of the patient's care. He or she should discuss the decision with other healthcare professionals involved in the patient's care. The decision must always be on an individual basis, be clearly documented in the medical and nursing notes, and should be conveyed to all those who need to know it. Unless the patient refuses, decisions on resuscitation should be communicated to those close to the patient, who should be a part of the decision-making process.

Since the early 1990s there has been an increased awareness of the need to allow relatives and loved ones to witness the resuscitation of the patient. Traditionally, staff have considered that loved ones would get in the way, or be unable to cope with seeing events. However, there is little evidence to support this and many are grateful to see all that was done, as opposed to sitting for prolonged periods in a waiting room. We do also need to question whether we have the right and whether it is ethically correct to stop a loved one being with the patient at what may be the end of their life. There is, however, a need for someone to stay with the person, explain proceedings and support them (Quinn and Hatchett 2001).

Communication

While there has been increased awareness of the ethical aspects of decisions regarding CPR, actual practice does not seem to have kept pace with our understanding. Thus, although it is common for institutions to have policies on the subject, the level of communication on this subject between patient and doctor is still disappointing. Decisions need to be communicated both verbally and in writing.

Although it is still considered to be the role of the doctor to carry out the discussions and make the decisions regarding CPR with patients and families, it is often the nurse who makes the initial assessment that the appropriateness of CPR should be questioned and who assumes the role of facilitator of the decision-making process. It is important, therefore, that the nurse has a clear understanding of the principles on which decisions regarding the withholding of CPR should be made.

Heart failure

Heart failure can be defined as an insufficient cardiac output to meet the metabolic demands or needs of the body. It may be acute or chronic. In the acute situation there is a sudden and severe failure of cardiac function, perhaps due to myocardial infarction or a condition such as cardiomyopathy. In the chronic situation, failure occurs over many months or years, primarily due to ischaemic heart disease, or a condition such as hypertension or a valvular disorder. In this case the body will implement a variety of compensatory mechanisms to maintain cardiac function, for example enlargement of the heart (hypertrophy). The person may be admitted to hospital many times with a worsening of their condition, when it is known as *decompensated* heart failure, i.e. they can no longer compensate for the deterioration in their heart's function. Chronic heart failure is a debilitating condition, with the person becoming increasingly breathless, tired and severely restricted in activities. The incidence in the UK is high at 0.3% per annum (McDonagh and Dargie 1998). More recent figures from the British Heart Foundation (2001) indicate that 760 000 people are living with chronic heart failure, with 63 000 new cases appearing each year.

Although the mortality rate from CHD is slowly declining, admissions for chronic heart failure appear to be rising (Sharpe and Doughty 1998). This is due to an ageing population, but also because treatments are allowing patients with the condition to survive for longer periods. It is now clear, however, that mortality figures for chronic heart failure are comparable to those for many malignant diseases. In fact, those with the condition often fair much worse (Millane et al 2000). This has led to the increased involvement of palliative care teams in managing this condition, as well as the use of specific treatments to improve the quality of life.

Heart failure
See chapter 4.2

Figure 12.28   Events leading to left ventricular failure.

Heart failure may involve either side of the heart. However, as both sides of the heart work in series, one side does not usually fail for long before the other is affected.

In *left-sided heart failure*, the left side of the heart cannot forward all of the blood it receives to the systemic circulation. As a result, blood backs up in the pulmonary circulation (Fig. 12.28). The pulmonary vessels become congested and the alveoli gradually fill with serous fluid.

A serious consequence of left-sided heart failure may be acute pulmonary oedema. This condition occurs when the alveoli fill up with serous fluid and the exchange of respiratory gases is impaired. A patient in acute pulmonary oedema will manifest symptoms of acute respiratory distress including dyspnoea and cough. Rapid treatment is necessary to prevent further deterioration of respiratory function. This will include the use of a diuretic, often intravenously, and nitrates. The diuretic reduces oedema and therefore helps breathing, while nitrates dilate the venous system to reduce blood returning to the heart (reducing the preload). To a lesser extent, nitrates also reduce the resistance in front of the heart (the afterload) through arterial dilatation. These actions reduce the workload on the heart and enable it to pump more effectively. Augmentation of contractility will be achieved with the use of a drug such as digoxin.

Right-sided heart failure may be secondary to failure of the left side, or it may occur independently. When the right side of the heart fails, it cannot effectively forward blood to the pulmonary arteries and lungs. As a result, increased pressure is placed on the venous system. This leads to venous congestion and oedema developing in tissues and organs (Fig. 12.29).

Symptoms of heart failure

Respirations Dyspnoea is the most common symptom of heart failure. Pulmonary oedema impairs gas exchange and may induce hypoxia. In mild or early failure, dyspnoea may be experienced only with exertion. With severe heart failure, it is present at rest. With acute pulmonary oedema, it is severe. The respirations are checked every ½–1 hour in acute failure and every 4 hours in moderate or mild failure. With breathlessness related to activity, the degree of exertion is noted.

Cough Due to congestion and fluid in the alveoli and bronchial tubes, cough may be present. The frequency, characteristics and amount of sputum are noted. Frothy, colourless sputum occurs in pulmonary oedema, and blood may appear from the rupture of capillaries and arterioles in severe congestion.

Pulse The pulse may be rapid, weak and irregular, as tachycardia frequently accompanies severe heart failure. The strength, rate and rhythm of the pulse are noted frequently and in relation to activities.

Blood pressure The blood pressure is checked frequently because it reflects the cardiac output.

Body temperature Many patients with cardiac insufficiency register a subnormal temperature as their heat production is reduced because of inadequate circulation, deficiency in oxygen and resulting decrease in metabolism.

Colour The colour of the lips, nail-beds and skin is observed, and any changes noted. The skin may show pallor due to generalized vasoconstriction. There may be cyanosis of lips and nail-beds.

Generalized oedema Failure of the right side of the heart causes fluid to accumulate in the systemic venous circulation. The reduced venous return to the heart leads to a reduction in left ventricular output, and compensatory mechanisms occur in an attempt to maintain adequate perfusion of vital organs. This causes further retention of fluid. Systemic venous and capillary pressures are raised due to back pressure from the failing heart. As a result of abnormal pressure gradients, fluid escapes from the vascular system into the interstitial tissues, resulting in oedema.

Oedema is usually found in the dependent areas of the body. If the person is mobile, swelling first appears in the feet and ankles, but if the person is confined to bed oedema may first become apparent in the back and sacral region. As it becomes more severe, all body tissues become affected and ascites may develop.

The most accurate method of observing the patient for oedema is by daily weighing, which should be at the same time each day wearing similar clothes. Up to 7 kg (7 litres) of water may be retained before oedema becomes visibly obvious.

Figure 12.29 Sequence of events leading to right heart failure.

Fluid balance An accurate record is kept of the patient's fluid intake and output. A positive balance is brought to the attention of the doctor, particularly if the urinary output is decreased to less than 0.5 mL per kg per hour. The amount of sweating is noted as a large amount of fluid may be lost in this manner. In the patient whose cardiac function is severely deteriorated, a urinary catheter allows an hourly assessment of urine output. Urinary output provides a useful guide to general tissue perfusion, because the kidneys are one of the last organs to be served with blood when there is disruption to cardiac function. If the person is passing at least 0.5 mL/kg of urine per hour, then the vital organs of heart, brain and lungs are receiving an adequate blood and oxygen supply.

Chest or abdominal pain Chest pain and any apparent precipitating causes are observed and reported immediately. Abdominal pain may be due to the congestion and poor perfusion of internal organs. Abdominal distension may be associated with reduced peristalsis as a result of congestion and reduced blood supply to the intestines.

Anorexia The patient may not eat because of lack of strength or because of dietary restrictions that make meals unpalatable. Congestion of internal organs due to oedema may contribute to loss of appetite. Anorexia may also result from drug toxicity (e.g. digoxin). The amount and type of food the patient eats should be observed at every meal.

Fatigue The degree of fatigue is noted at rest as well as in relationship to specific activities.

Orientation and level of consciousness When circulation and/or the oxygen content of the blood perfusing the brain are inadequate, the patient's cerebral functioning may decrease. Observations are made regarding the patient's level of consciousness; orientation to person, time and surroundings; and response to stimuli such as questioning.

Anxiety It is very important to observe the patient for fear and apprehension. Anxiety may initiate the release of adrenaline, which stimulates the heart at a time when the aim is to reduce cardiac workload. The patient's apprehension may indicate a need for information, explanations or sedation.

Diagnosis

Diagnosis of heart failure can be made using the history, physical examination, chest radiography, arterial blood gas levels and two-dimensional echocardiography. Haemodynamic monitoring may be initiated to assess the patient's preload, contractility and afterload.

Medical management

Management of a patient with heart failure focuses on two areas. The cause of heart failure must be determined and corrected if possible. Often the underlying cause is a myocardium that is so severely damaged after myocardial infarction(s) that it cannot function effectively and the condition cannot be cured without a heart transplant. The second focus of treatment is improving the functional ability of the heart. This is accomplished through the following interventions:

- *Decrease myocardial workload.* This focuses on facilitating the patient's physical and mental rest. This will decrease the resting heart rate, reduce myocardial oxygen consumption and improve myocardial oxygen supply.

- *Afterload and preload reduction.* Reduction of afterload can improve stroke volume, reduce myocardial workload and decrease oxygen consumption. The use of vasodilator medications can be very effective in managing heart failure. Arterial and venous dilators such as sodium nitroprusside and the angiotension-converting enzyme (ACE) inhibitors (e.g. captopril) may be used. Direct arteriolar dilators with no venous effects, such as hydralazine, may be beneficial. Nitrates that are good venous dilators and poor arteriolar dilators may be useful in reducing preload.

■ *Improve cardiac contractility*. Medications utilized to enhance myocardial contractility are positive inotropes. These include digoxin, which is the traditional medication for heart failure. Digoxin improves myocardial efficiency by improving contractility with only a moderate increase in oxygen consumption by the myocardium.

■ *Reduce fluid accumulation*. A diet restricted in sodium may be useful in decreasing fluid retention. Diuretics are essential in the treatment of heart failure. In severe heart failure a fluid restriction may be advocated of 1–1.5 litres in 24 hours. It is important to explain this to the patient and to devise an acceptable distribution of fluid intake over each 24-hour period.

Nursing management

Nursing management of the person with congestive heart failure focuses on several specific problems. These include:

1. decreased cardiac output
2. fluid volume excess
3. anxiety (see p. 277)
4. alteration in lifestyle and self-care (see p. 279).

Decreased cardiac output

Goals

1. The patient will demonstrate signs of improved cardiac contractility.
2. The patient will show signs of improved oxygenation.
3. The workload of the heart will be reduced.

Nursing intervention

Drugs commonly used to improve cardiac contractility are inotropic agents such as digoxin, dobutamine and dopamine. Nursing staff are responsible for their administration and monitoring for adverse reactions. Structured exercise programmes are now also advocated for patients with chronic heart failure to increase their functional capacity.

Oxygenation of the tissues

Oxygen may be administered by mask or nasal cannulae to increase arterial oxygen concentration. It will be effective only if delivery to the tissues is improved.

The nurse should explain the procedure to the patient briefly and remain until the patient is accustomed to the mask or nasal cannulae. Observations are made of the patient's response to the oxygen. Its effectiveness will be indicated by reduced pulse rate, less dyspnoea, improvement in colour and less restlessness.

In severe pulmonary oedema, oxygen may be given under positive pressure (i.e. greater than atmosphere pressure) to counteract the movement of fluid from the capillaries into the alveoli.

Reducing the workload of the heart

Administration of medication Drugs that reduce cardiac workload (including vasodilators) are used to treat heart failure (see Table 12.8). The nurse will monitor the effectiveness of these medications and needs to ensure that each patient understands their medication (Hagenhoff et al 1994).

ACE inhibitors and beta-blockers, when given in small doses and gradually increased over several weeks, have a beneficial effect on the morbidity and mortality of patients with chronic heart failure (Clark et al 2000). Spironolactone has also proved beneficial in this respect. The nurse may note that these drugs have been added to the patient's medication regimen.

Promotion of rest Rest is important in the treatment of the patient with heart failure because it reduces the demand on the heart by reducing body requirements for oxygen. For the patient in failure, rest in bed is necessary until the oedema has decreased.

Once the acute episode has passed, the patient is able to get out of bed for gradually increasing intervals. Intermittent rest periods during the day and after activities are arranged, and the patient rests before and after meals and between procedures.

Physical comfort will contribute to the patient's rest and may be promoted by change of position, bathing, warmth, etc. Anticipation of need and the planning and provision of undisturbed rest periods are important. Cooperation is sought from the laboratory, dietary and house-keeping staffs to minimize interruptions to rest periods.

Activity Rest has been emphasized as an important phase of the treatment of cardiac patients, but it is well known that there are certain disadvantages inherent in bedrest. The limbs should be put through passive movements to promote venous drainage and prevent phlebothrombosis. Gentle massage is also helpful. If the patient's condition permits, it may be suggested that he or she gradually commences foot, leg and arm exercises. The patient is also encouraged to take 5–10 deep breaths every

Table 12.8   Medications used in the treatment of heart failure

Medication	Example	General action related to heart failure
Reduce myocardial workload		
Vasodilators	Nitrates	Reduce preload and/or afterload
	Angiotensin inhibitors	Reduce systemic vascular resistance
		Improve cardiac output
Improve cardiac contractility		
Cardiac glycosides	Digoxin	Increase force of contraction
		Increase cardiac output
Sympathomimetic agents	Dobutamine	Increase force of contraction
		Systemic vasodilatation
		Reduce ventricular filling pressures
Phosphodiesterase inhibitors	Amrinone	Increase force of contraction
	Milrinone	Systemic vasodilatation
		Improve cardiac output
Reduce fluid accumulation		
Diuretics	Loop	Reduce venous return to heart
	Thiazide	Vasodilatation

1–2 hours to expand the lungs fully. As soon as possible, the patient is encouraged to get out of bed to use a commode, because the use of a bedpan for defaecation places considerable strain on the patient.

Observations are made of reactions to any activity so that undue stress on the heart may be avoided. These will also assist in defining the patient's future activities and the amount of rest and restriction that will be necessary.

Positioning   The patient should be positioned in such a way as to facilitate ease of breathing. The person who is experiencing dyspnoea will be more comfortable with the head of the bed elevated, but only by a sufficient amount to be effective.

Patients with congestive failure manifest orthopnoea, that is, less difficulty in breathing with the trunk in the upright position. A semi-upright or upright position increases the vital capacity and tends to reduce the volume of blood returned to the heart and the pulmonary system. Pressure of abdominal viscera on the diaphragm is reduced. Some patients may be still more comfortable in a true sitting position (i.e. with the lower limbs down). A special cardiac bed on which the foot of the bed can be lowered to provide a chair-like support is available. Alternatively the patient may find comfort from sitting in a chair. The sitting position promotes the formation of peripheral oedema in the dependent parts but relieves the pulmonary congestion to some extent; peripheral oedema is much less serious than pulmonary oedema.

In the sitting position, a pillow placed longitudinally at the patient's back may help to provide some comfort. Pillows should be used at the sides to support the arms and relieve the fatiguing pull on the shoulders. A change may be effected by arranging a table and pillow over the bed, upon which the head and arms may rest. Cot-sides may be kept up on the bed to safeguard the patient when in the upright position, as the patient may become drowsy and fall to the side, or may experience cerebral hypoxia which causes disorientation. The sides are also useful when a change of position is made because they may be grasped by the patient and used for added support. Patients in the upright position are encouraged to assume the recumbent position for brief periods to help reduce circulatory stasis and oedema in the lower parts of the body. However, patients should not be asked to do this if they are suffering from severe dyspnoea.

Good body alignment is essential to prevent contractures, hyperextension and circulatory stasis. *Even a slight change in position* every 1–2 hours is helpful. A footboard is used to prevent foot drop.

Elimination   Constipation and straining at defaecation are to be avoided because of the unduc strain placed on the heart. A mild laxative may have to be given to keep the stool soft. Abdominal distension is also to be avoided, because it raises the diaphragm and further inhibits the patient's breathing. Use of the bedpan requires more energy than getting out of bed and using a commode. Therefore it is preferable for the patient to use a bedside commode. When a patient receives a diuretic it will mean frequent use of the urinal, bedpan or commode, which can be very exhausting.

Fluid volume excess

Goals

1. The patient will demonstrate a decrease in weight.

2. The patient will reduce dietary sodium and fluid intake as appropriate.

Nursing intervention

Administer medications to produce diuresis as prescribed by the doctor (Table 12.8) and monitor the effectiveness of these.

Low-sodium diets may be prescribed to reduce oedema and prevent further accumulation of fluid in the tissues. Sodium restriction varies with patients, depending upon their cardiac function and amount of oedema. Normally the average daily salt intake is 10 g daily. This is approximately double what is recommended for any person's needs. If no salt is added to food either at the table or in cooking, and no salted foods are used, the intake may be reduced to approximately 3 g. With the advent of the newer and more potent diuretic drugs, severe dietary sodium restriction is not mandatory, as it was previously for most patients with heart failure. A great deal of salt is found in ready-made meals, processed meats, soups and snacks. Food may initially appear tasteless without adding salt, but taste receptors do adjust over a few weeks, so that salted food is then difficult to take. A sodium content of less than 0.2 g per 100 g of food label is generally recommended (Hatchett 2001). The nurse should explain the purpose of the diet and relate it to symptoms the patient is experiencing. There are many spices and foods allowed that help to make a low-sodium diet more palatable.

If the patient with heart failure is overweight, the calorie intake is reduced in an effort to reduce weight. The lower-calorie diet should contain less fat but enough of the other foods to meet nutritional requirements.

The person having cardiac surgery

Correction of acquired heart disease includes surgery for coronary artery disease and for stenosed or incompetent cardiac valves. The fact that the heart must function immediately after operation presents a problem different from that in many areas of the body. The heart must heal while continuing to maintain adequate circulation. This creates the need for greater support and for minimizing physiological demands.

Progress in this area was delayed until the introduction of the pump-oxygenator (bypass machine). This machine permits extracorporeal (outside the body) oxygenation of blood and maintenance of circulation while the heart is arrested and opened to provide a direct surgical approach. During operation the heart is exposed by median sternotomy; the aorta is clamped off and cardiopulmonary bypass maintained via cannulae in the atria and descending aorta. Circulation thus bypasses the heart and lungs. The body temperature is lowered to 32°C in order to reduce the metabolic activity of the heart so that the cells can survive the interruption of the coronary circulation. In addition, to reduce metabolic demand further, cardiac arrest is induced by a variety of methods. This may be the use of electric paddles, which causes the heart to fibrillate (the muscle twitches rather than contracts), or through the use of high doses of potassium in a solution known as *cardioplegia* injected around the heart. The blood is heparinized in order to prevent coagulation and thrombus formation. On completion of the cardiopulmonary bypass, the heparin is neutralized by the administration of protamine sulfate.

After the procedure, the aorta is unclamped, the patient rewarmed and normal cardiac rhythm restored by internal defibrillation. Cardiopulmonary bypass is stopped, the cannulae removed and the chest closed. As a general rule the whole operation takes 3–4 hours.

The bypass machine is not without complications and these have been noted for several years. Those of particular note include the potential for neurological, renal and pulmonary damage. Neurological damage is the most significant. This can range from temporary memory loss and changes in personality, through to disorientation, agitation and inappropriate behaviour. The latter is known as *post-pump psychosis* or *delirium*, and the exact cause is unknown. The nurse can assist by orienting the patient to time and place, reducing noise levels and sensory overload, such as maintaining night and day patterns, and the use of familiar people such as family and friends. Ultimately, sedation may be required until recovery occurs over the following few days. At worse the patient may suffer a cerebrovascular accident (CVA), perhaps through emboli entering the cerebral circulation. Because of these effects, *off-pump* cardiac surgery has emerged. This form of surgery is performed on the beating heart, and may use a variety of mechanical devices to stabilize the area of the heart that the surgeon is working upon (Glenville 1999, Openshaw and Durbridge 2001).

Surgery for ischaemic heart disease

Both direct and indirect methods are used to revascularize the myocardium. The indirect method involves implanting the internal mammary artery into the myocardium, but is rarely used because revascularization is not immediate.

The most popular procedure is the *aortocoronary bypass surgery*, in which one end of a resected saphenous vein is anastomosed to the aorta and the other to the coronary artery beyond the point of obstruction. The right or left internal mammary artery may also be used as a grafting vessel. The blood supply to the myocardium is immediately improved.

There were approximately 28 000 bypass operations carried out in the UK in 1997–1998 (Fisher et al 2001). This figure has gradually increased over recent years. The overall mortality rate is approximately 3–4%. A strategy of early operation significantly reduces the mortality rate (Yusuf et al 1994). Coronary artery bypass grafts do not last indefinitely, and may require replacement in approximately 10 years. The mortality rate is higher for patients having a repeat procedure.

General indications for bypass surgery include:

■ symptoms despite maximum medical therapy

■ triple coronary vessel disease

■ left mainstem coronary artery stenosis

■ unstable angina.

The overall physical and psychological condition of the patient is generally taken into account. Patients who show a positive attitude toward risk factor modification may be more likely to have their case viewed favourably. Nurses may find themselves drawn into debates over issues such as whether smokers should be offered surgery. Patients who feel they have been unfairly treated may need specific support and advice.

Angioplasty (PTCA) may also be used in coronary artery disease (see p. 286).

Surgery for diseased valves

The surgeon can significantly enlarge the size of the orifice of stenosed valves in some individuals by dilating the valve. Others, however, may require valve replacement.

Certain patients with regurgitation of the aortic, mitral and/or tricuspid valves, who no longer respond to medical treatment, require total replacement. This is accomplished with an artificial valve prosthesis or the use of tissue homografts. Artificial valves require anticoagulation for life with warfarin to prevent thrombus formation on the valve. Tissue valves do not require this, but do not last as long. Tissue valves are usually advocated for patients such as women of childbearing age, for whom taking warfarin would be dangerous to the fetus, or the elderly.

Preoperative nursing care

Most patients have tests such as cardiac catheterization carried out several weeks in advance and then return to the hospital 1–2 days before the operation. Time is needed before surgery to gather baseline information such as weight, fluid balance and vital signs. A range of blood tests including cross-matching and blood-clotting measurements will be necessary. Nurses are ideally placed to provide cardiac surgery patients with advice, information and support before surgery. Patients and their families need to be clear about the operation itself and likely effects for the future.

Informed written consent will need to be obtained and any worries or misconceptions addressed. Anxiety is a normal response to impending surgery. The individual needs to appreciate the risks of surgery balanced against the risks of continuing untreated. Some patients will need support to help them arrive at a decision regarding surgery. There is evidence of a positive association between the length of time patients have to wait for surgery and levels of anxiety, depression and disturbed family relationships irrespective of the severity of illness (Underwood et al 1993).

Postoperative nursing care

Nursing objectives for the patient include:

■ monitoring and maintaining adequate respiratory and haemodynamic function

■ pain relief

■ assistance with activities of living

■ psychological support

■ evaluation of the recovery process

■ preparation for discharge home.

Box 12.4 shows outcomes from an integrated care pathway for a patient in the first 24 hours after cardiac surgery.

Complications

Complications of bypass grafting include:

■ angina

■ pain at both chest incision and graft sites

■ leakage at the incision site producing discomfort and shock

■ hypertension as a result of increased sympathetic activity produced by lack of blood flow during operation

■ shortness of breath due to heart failure or chest infection

■ hyperglycaemia as a result of increased sympathetic response

■ confusion or disorientation due to the effects of the bypass machine, cerebral hypoxia, medication and/or sepsis.

The patient is mechanically ventilated until normal body temperature has been regained, the patient is conscious and haemodynamically within acceptable parameters. Prolonged ventilation increases the risk of complications such as chest infection and pulmonary damage. Therefore, in many units, nurse-led extubation occurs. The nurse will assess the patient and follow a set plan, integrated care pathway or algorithm. When the nurse considers that all parameters have been met, including satisfactory blood gases, respiratory pattern and body temperature, the endotracheal tube is removed and an oxygen mask is put in place. Arterial and central venous pressure (CVP) lines are used to monitor cardiac pressures for the first 18–24 hours. Any cardiac arrhythmia or change in heart rate is detected with a cardiac monitor. Blood pressure, pulse and respirations need to be monitored closely. Fluid input and output are recorded

Box 12.4   Outcomes from an integrated (critical) care pathway for postoperative day 1 following cardiac surgery

Respiratory and cardiac monitoring

- Respiratory data assessed and recorded 1–2 hourly
- Air entry assessed and audible to all lung zones. Wheezing checked
  Aim: good air entry and able to breath deeply
- Blood gases collected p.r.n. to check respiratory function and potassium
- Transducers zeroed p.r.n. with position change
- Vital signs recorded 1–2 hourly
  Aim: haemodynamic parameters within prescribed limits

Fluid balance

- I.v. lines labelled and maintained patent
- Chest drainage recorded hourly with no evidence of bleeding
- Crystalloid infusions titrated to oral intake
- Maintain MAP and CVP within set parameters with prescribed blood/colloid as per consultant protocol
- Urine output maintained at >0.5 mL/kg with fluids and drugs as per consultant protocol
- Inotropes and vasodilators weaned off and discontinued in consultation with consultant

Sedation and pain control

- Neurological assessment performed
  Aim: patient alert/oriented and moving all limbs
- Pain assessment performed and appropriate analgesia (oral/i.v.) administered. PCA used by patient appropriately
  Aim: pain well controlled and patient able to move/breath deeply

Wounds

- Chest and leg wounds assessed once per shift
  Aim: dry and intact dressings
- Pedal pulses checked once per shift
  Aim: good peripheral circulation
- Remove leg bandages (unless otherwise indicated). TEDS if appropriate (as per consultant protocol)

Hygiene/positioning

- Oral, dental, hair and body hygiene maintained
- Patient made comfortable with 2–4 hourly position changes
  Aim: pressure areas intact
  Waterlow score_____
- Perform urinary catheter care with soap and water

Diet and fluids

- Oral fluids taken as desired
- Antiemetics administered if necessary, as prescribed
  Aim: patient free of nausea
- Soft diet taken when tolerated

(Continued)

Box 12.4 *(Continued)*

Physiotherapy	■ Chest physiotherapy maintained prior to discharge to ward. Encourage deep breathing and coughing
	■ Leg mobilization exercises performed regularly
	■ Patient sat out of bed when clinically appropriate Aim: patient confident and mobilizing with assistance
Clinical procedures and tests	■ Consultant round completed
	■ Bloods taken as per consultant protocol
	■ ECG taken as per consultant protocol
	■ Chest drain removed when two consecutive zeros recorded or as per consultant protocol
	■ Post-drain-removal chest radiograph completed
	■ Serum potassium maintained at preset parameters with prescribed supplements
	■ Arterial line removed prior to discharge to ward. Haemostasis achieved
	■ Remove neck lines as per consultant protocol
Education and support	■ Patient and relatives supported throughout Aim: well informed and happy with care
Transfer to ward	■ Transfer to ward agreed with consultant and sister in charge of ward
	■ Patient and relatives informed of ward transfer
	■ Portering services ordered and bed exchange organized
	■ Transfer patient notes, chest radiographs, valuables, toiletries and oral medications to ward
	■ Ensure necessary equipment is available on the ward
	■ Accompany patient to ward. Complete transfer as per protocol
	■ Complete data transfer on computer

Abbreviations: CVP, central venous pressure; ECG, electrocardiography; i.v., intravenous; MAP, mean arterial pressure; PCA, patient-controlled analgesia; TEDS, thromboembolic deterrent stockings.

Reproduced with kind permission of The Heart Hospital, London.

to detect possible fluid retention. One of the major roles of the nurse is to administer intravenous fluids and possibly an inotrope (a drug that stimulates cardiac contractility) depending upon the patient's haemodynamic status.

Level of consciousness, orientation and restlessness need to be observed as they may be linked to a fall in cardiac output/blood pressure or occur as a result of hypoxia, as well as inadequate pain relief. Any weakness or loss of function, possibly a result of a thrombus or embolus, needs to be reported. The chest drainage system needs to be observed at regular intervals to check that it is functioning correctly and the drainage observed for possible bleeding around the heart. One of the dangers of cardiac

surgery is *cardiac tamponade* (bleeding below the pericardium). This is indicated by rising CVP, falling blood pressure and tachycardia. This is an emergency situation and the surgeon will have to reopen the chest, stop the bleeding and evacuate the accumulated blood.

Dressings on the chest and graft sites need to be checked regularly for excessive bleeding and haematoma formation. Compression stockings may be used to reduce venous stasis and the risk of thromboembolic complications. The patient will usually be able to eat a solid diet on the first or second postoperative day. Intravenous fluids will be given before this. Mouth care may ease the discomfort of a dry mouth and help to prevent infection. Activity is increased as tolerated over the first 2 days and early mobilization is encouraged. The patient's way of coping needs to be assessed so that appropriate support can be given. Patients are usually ready for discharge after about a week.

Pain and discomfort

Pain from median sternotomy may cause discomfort for a few weeks; there may also be discomfort from incision sites. Leg pain and swelling may still be present for up to 1 year after operation. Delayed wound healing may also be a problem. Activities such as sneezing, coughing, bending over, raising the hand above the head and twisting to the side may cause difficulty. Helping the patient to hug a cushion when coughing supports the sternum and aids more effective expectoration. Patients may need help with washing and dressing for the first few weeks. Angina is likely to return in about 25% of patients within 5 years of bypass surgery, although the symptoms are not necessarily as severe as before operation.

Information for recovery

The increasing trend for shorter hospital stays minimizes the time available for information giving and support for discharge. It is therefore important that the time available is used effectively to establish a relationship with the patient and family on which to build individualized care. Finally, staff members need support and guidance concerning the patient's likely recovery pattern (Knoll and Johnson 2000). Patients need realistic expectations. A positive outcome for surgery does not have to mean a complete reversion to a presymptomatic lifestyle. Alternative goals may be more appropriate. Knowing how each individual perceives their situation may assist in helping them to identify realistic outcomes. Many patients find their early progress disappointing. Exercise tolerance may be less than expected. Pain may be more severe than anticipated. Appropriately supervised and progressive exercise programmes can be helpful in identifying problems, increasing activity levels, boosting confidence and providing support. Outpatient support via telephone links has been found to be associated with positive feelings about recovery (Gortner and Jenkins, 1990). However, there is evidence that, although helpful, such support does not necessarily reduce levels of anxiety and depression in the early period following discharge (Roebuck 1999). Those who have been severely restricted by angina for many years may find the return to normality difficult to cope with. The potential for a change in lifestyle is not always welcome.

Families need to be aware of the possibility of mood swings and signs of anxiety and/or depression. Short-term memory loss and difficulties with concentration are not uncommon. Some individuals experience feelings of poor self-esteem and of anticlimax.

Hypertension
See chapter 4.2

Disorders of the vascular system

Disorders may involve arteries or veins. Arterial disorder commonly leads to a reduction in blood supply to peripheral tissue resulting in ischaemic pain and possibly gangrene. Alternatively the patient may experience continuously raised arterial blood pressure, known as hypertension. Venous problems lead to interference with the normal drainage of venous blood back to the heart causing congestion and oedema within the tissues. Vascular conditions may be chronic, developing slowly over a considerable period of time, or they may be sudden and acute.

Hypertension

Hypertension is a condition in which there is a sustained increase in arterial blood pressure. Defining hypertension is problematic, because the normal range does vary – creating a blurring between normotensive and hypertensive people. A blood pressure of 140/85 mmHg may be seen as acceptable, but the reading does increase with age. If the patient has a condition such as diabetes, drug treatment should be initiated to keep to blood pressure below 140/80 mmHg in order to prevent microvascular and macrovascular complications (British National Formulary 2001). Antihypertensive drug treatment is recommended for those with a sustained systolic blood pressure reading of 160 mmHg or greater, or a diastolic pressure of 100 mmHg or more (Ramsay et al 1999). Figure 12.30 illustrates that blood pressure alone is no longer the sole indicator for treatment.

Sustained hypertension is a serious condition and is sometimes termed 'the silent killer', because few if any symptoms may be encountered until organ damage has occurred. A sustained increase in blood pressure results in vascular disease. The changes in the arterial walls involve thickening and sclerosis, which alter the blood supply to tissues and ultimately may reduce their functional ability. The arterial wall may develop necrotic areas that may weaken or rupture under high pressure. The wall may also thicken and so narrow the lumen of the artery. Thrombosis is likely with such diseased arterial walls.

Four organs that are the most frequent targets for damage are the heart, kidneys, brain and eyes. The sustained increase in arterial blood pressure greatly increases the workload of the heart. The myocardium hypertrophies in response to the increased demands, but there is not an adequate increase in the coronary blood supply and eventually some pump failure develops. Hypertension is a major risk factor for developing coronary disease. Thickening and sclerosis of the coronary arteries may cause ischaemic heart disease, the patient may experience angina pectoris or suffer a myocardial infarction. Kidney function becomes impaired as the result of sclerosing haemorrhage or thrombosis of the

Figure 12.30 Thresholds for intervention in patients with hypertension.

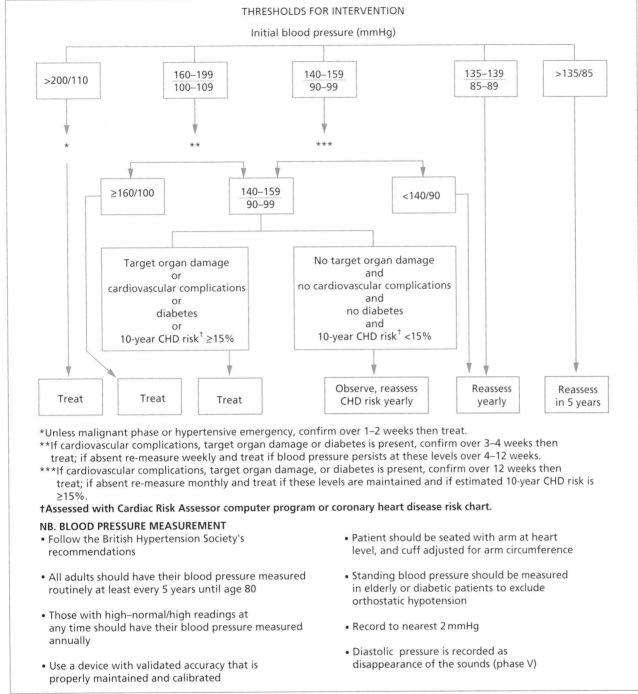

From the British Hypertensive Society (2000), with permission.

renal arteries, which destroys functional tissue. Retinal haemorrhages and oedema of the optic disc occur frequently, resulting in degenerative changes in the eyes.

Types of hypertension

Hypertension may be classified by aetiology as *primary* (essential) or *secondary*. Approximately 90% of people with hypertensive disease are said to have essential hypertension; the remaining 10% have secondary hypertension.

Primary or essential hypertension

Primary hypertension is most frequently referred to as *essential* or *idiopathic hypertension*. The cause of this type of hypertensive disease is not known; no initial disturbance in the areas commonly associated with secondary hypertension has been established. It may cause cardiac or kidney disease but is not preceded by either. Heredity is thought to be a factor, because most persons with the condition have a history of a parent or grandparent having had it.

Secondary hypertension

Secondary hypertension is distinguished from essential hypertension by having an identifiable cause. Common causes include renal disease, endocrine disorders and medications.

Renal disease

Any condition that reduces blood flow through the kidneys or destroys renal functional tissue causes hypertension. Examples of such conditions are sclerotic changes or stenosis of a renal artery, nephritis and polycystic disease. The ischaemic kidney reacts by secreting a proteolytic enzyme called renin. In the bloodstream, renin acts upon a plasma protein to produce angiotensin I, which is then converted to angiotensin II by another enzyme, primarily in the lining of the lungs. Angiotensin II causes widespread vasoconstriction of the arterioles and increased peripheral resistance, leading to an increase in arterial blood pressure. Angiotensin II also inhibits the secretion of aldosterone by the adrenal glands, which increases the blood pressure through its influence on sodium and water retention.

Endocrine disorders

A phaeochromocytoma is a tumour of the adrenal medulla. Tumours may be single or multiple. The tumour cells secrete adrenaline, in the same way as normal medullary cells; this produces vasoconstriction and an increased cardiac output with a corresponding increase in arterial blood pressure. Removal of the tumour restores a normal blood pressure.

An increased output of aldosterone by the cortex of the adrenal glands may also be responsible for hypertension. The increased secretion may be idiopathic or may be due to a tumour. Aldosterone increases the reabsorption of sodium by the kidney, leading to water retention and an expansion of the intravascular volume, increasing the arterial blood pressure. Aldosterone may also have a direct vasoconstricting effect. A general increase in the secretion of all of the adrenocorticoids causes Cushing's disease, which is also accompanied by hypertension.

Medications

Some women taking oral contraceptives may develop hypertension. It is thought that the oestrogen component of the pills may be responsible by stimulating hepatic synthesis of angiotensinogen, which leads to increased amounts of angiotensin. If the contraceptive agent is discontinued for 6 months, blood pressure usually returns to normal.

Symptoms

A person may have an abnormally high arterial blood pressure for a long period without symptoms. The condition is often discovered on a routine physical examination. Those who do experience symptoms may complain of a throbbing occipital headache or migraine. The headache may be accompanied by weakness, dizziness, visual disturbances, epistaxis, palpitations, angina pectoris and dyspnoea. Symptoms of emotional instability, memory lapses and personality changes may indicate cerebrovascular damage. Later, other manifestations appear as the heart, kidneys, brain or eyes become damaged by the persisting hypertension. The person who manifests even a slight increase above the normal in both systolic and diastolic blood pressures should undergo careful investigation to determine a possible primary cause. Several systems may be investigated in an attempt to identify the cause of hypertension. The renal and endocrine systems are the more important of these.

Medical treatment

If the hypertension is secondary, treatment is directed toward correcting the primary condition. In essential hypertension, treatment is directed at: (1) lowering the blood pressure in an effort to prevent serious complications; and (2) having the patient adjust life to reduce the demands on the cardiovascular system and kidneys. The treatment depends on the blood pressure and the signs and symptoms of impaired function in vulnerable organs (see Fig. 12.30). The patient with mild hypertension may simply be advised to reduce weight to normal, avoid overwork and overexcitement, and decrease salt intake to a prescribed level in order to prevent the development of hypertension.

People with more severe hypertension may receive drug therapy to lower the blood pressure (Table 12.9) and are likely to be more restricted in activities and diet.

Nursing care

Goals

1. The patient's blood pressure is within normal limits.
2. The patient can describe the disease process and the factors contributing to disease management.
3. The patient can describe health behaviours needed to manage the hypertension.
4. The patient actively participates in a disease management programme.

Nursing intervention

Diet

- Discuss with patient and family the need to achieve and maintain a normal bodyweight as this may facilitate lowering of blood pressure.

- Reduction of sodium intake is likely because excess sodium expands intravascular volume and aggravates hypertension. The degree of restriction depends on the severity of disease. A 'no added salt' diet may be recommended. If adequate sodium reduction is achieved by diet, drug therapy is likely to be reduced.

Table 12.9   Oral medications used in management of hypertension

Group	Example	General action
Diuretics		
Thiazides	Hydrochlorothiazide	Reduce interstitial fluid volume causing decreased vascular wall stiffness
Loop	Furosemide (frusemide)	
Potassium sparing	Spironolactone	
Angiotensin-converting enzyme (ACE) inhibitors	Captopril	Reduce peripheral arterial resistance
Vasodilators		
Predominantly arteriolar	Hydralazine	Relax arteriolar vascular smooth muscle
Drugs acting on central nervous system		
Centrally acting	Methyldopa	Displace noradrenaline from receptor sites, decreasing sympathetic nervous system activity
Post-ganglionic blockers	Guanethidine	Block release of noradrenaline from adrenergic nerve endings
Alpha-blockers	Prazosin	Peripheral arteriolar vasodilator
Beta-blockers	Propranolol	Block β-adrenergic receptors of sympathetic nervous system
Calcium channel blockers	Nifedipine	Potent arteriolar dilator

Patients should generally aim for foods with less than 0.2 g per 100 g, and be informed of those with a high sodium content (e.g. processed meats, soups, ready-made meals and certain snack foods).

■ Reduction of alcohol intake is recommended because alcohol increases the risk of obesity and may cause a rise in blood pressure. The recommended intake is 3–4 units of alcohol per day for men and 2–3 units for women. Binge drinking, for example saving up the daily units, is an unhealthy practice.

Exercise

Discuss with the patient a plan of regular exercise to be undertaken once the hypertension is under control. Regular physical activity is a beneficial strategy to achieve and maintain a satisfactory weight.

Stopping smoking

Great emphasis should be placed on encouraging patients to stop smoking as the coexistence of smoking as an additional risk factor in hypertensive patients confers a greatly increased risk of subsequent cardiovascular events.

Stress management

The relationship between stress and hypertension has not been clearly defined. However, stress reduction is advocated as a health promotion activity:

■ Encourage the person to express feelings of stress and to identify stressors in the environment that are both avoidable and unavoidable. Facilitate the patient's planning of strategies that can be used to reduce or eliminate the available stressors in a defined time.

■ Teach the patient relaxation techniques that can be used to reduce stress in a variety of settings. There are a number of resources available in the community to teach relaxation techniques, as well as books, cassette tapes and compact discs which can be purchased.

Medications

■ Medications required to control hypertension need to be taken regularly for long periods of time. This may be difficult for the patient to understand if they feel asymptomatic. Ensure that the patient and family have accurate perceptions of the use and need for these drugs and their possible side-effects.

■ Assist the patient in developing a simple, convenient schedule to take medications that is tailored to fit personal schedule and habits.

■ Discuss side-effects of the patient's medication and encourage the patient to seek advice from the practice nurse or doctor if side-effects occur.

Evaluation

Evaluate the effectiveness of care by assessing whether the patient:

1. has blood pressure within normal limits identified for him or her

2. can describe hypertension and the factors contributing to disease management

3. can discuss behaviours being followed to promote health.

Figure 12.31 Types of aneurysm: (a) fusiform; (b) saccular; (c) dissecting.

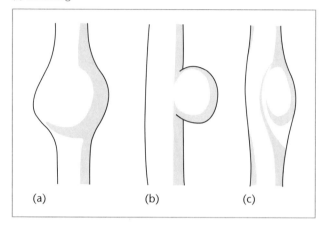

(a)   (b)   (c)

Arterial disorders

Aortic aneurysm

An aneurysm is a saccular dilatation of the wall of an artery and develops as a result of weakness in the wall of the vessel in that area. The weakness in the majority of cases is due to atherosclerosis but may also be caused by an infectious disease (e.g. syphilis), congenital defect, trauma or a condition of the connective tissue such as Marfan syndrome. The aorta and cerebral arteries are the most common sites of aneurysms.

The aneurysm that does not extend completely around the artery is referred to as a *saccular aneurysm*. If it involves the complete circumference, it is classified as a *fusiform aneurysm* (Fig. 12.31).

Separation of the layers of the aorta is referred to as a *dissecting* aortic aneurysm, even though no dilatation may be present. The tear is often in the intima and may be due to bleeding in the medial layer from the vasa vasorum. The dissection may extend lengthwise for a considerable distance and may involve branches of the aorta. The aortic aneurysm may also be classified according to the section of the artery in which the defect is located; for example, it may be designated as a thoracic or abdominal aortic aneurysm.

The Stanford classification identifies two types of dissecting aortic aneurysm: type A – involvement of the ascending aorta with or without extension into the descending aorta (De Bakey types I and II); type B: – involvement of the descending aorta without ascending aorta involvement (De Bakey type III). De Bakey is the older, although well known, classification system.

A serious threat to any patient with an aneurysm is rupture of the weakened vascular area: the rapid loss of blood almost always proves fatal.

Manifestations

Signs and symptoms may be absent until the aneurysm is large enough to compress adjacent structures. The majority of aortic aneurysms are abdominal. The patient may complain of mid-abdominal, lumbar or pelvic pain, often severe. Physical examination may reveal an expansile, abdominal mass. Femoral pulses may be reduced. The patient with a thoracic aneurysm may experience chest pain, dyspnoea, hoarseness due to vocal cord paralysis and/or congestion of the veins in the neck because of pressure on the superior vena cava. With an abdominal aneurysm, careful physical examination, radiography, echocardiography and/or aortography are means of confirming the diagnosis. Scanning techniques such as computed tomography, which may be performed with contrast dye to enhance results, and magnetic resonance imaging (MRI) are also used to provide images of the aneurysm.

Symptoms of a dissecting aortic aneurysm include pain, often described as ripping or tearing in nature, which may involve the chest, back and/or abdomen. There may be a discrepancy in pulses at various locations in the body. This is a serious situation with a need to control the pain, which may be severe, and to lower and stabilize the blood pressure with intravenous drugs such as a beta-blocker. This reduces the haemodynamic stress on the aortic wall. Controlling the blood pressure is very important to reduce the risk of the aneurysm rupturing. Occasionally hypotension may present, but hypertension is more common.

Treatment

In recent years, encouraging advances have been made in the surgical treatment of aneurysms. If a small blood vessel is affected, it may be tied off and the flow of blood diverted to another artery. In treating an aortic aneurysm, the area is resected and replaced with a graft of inert synthetic material such as Teflon or Dacron, which does not cause tissue reaction.

Acute arterial occlusion

Acute occlusion occurs suddenly as a result of external compression, thrombosis or embolism. It is serious because there is a lack of collateral circulation to the tissues supplied by this artery.

Arterial thrombosis occurs with the formation of an abnormal blood clot (*thrombus*) within an artery, usually as the result of narrowing of the lumen of the artery by atherosclerotic changes. The stasis in the blood flow predisposes to the formation of the clot, partially or completely blocking the vessel. If the vessel is not completely blocked, treatment is directed towards preventing the clot from enlarging to occlude the vessel and towards keeping it at the site of formation to prevent an embolism.

Arterial embolism is the blocking of an artery by a foreign mass that has been carried by the bloodstream until it reaches an artery too small for it to pass through. The foreign mass is referred to as an *embolus*.

Most frequently an embolus consists of a thrombus that breaks loose from its site of origin, but it may consist of air, fragments of vegetations from diseased cardiac valves, fat, atherosclerotic plaques or small masses of tissue or cancerous cells. The effects of an embolism are determined by the localization of the embolus. Obviously, if it is an end-artery, the tissue entirely dependent upon it becomes necrotic. An embolus originating in a vein or the right side of the heart is likely to cause a pulmonary embolism blocking the arterial supply to an area of lung tissue. One arising from the left side of the heart or a large systemic artery may produce a cerebral embolism or may plug a smaller artery. The site of arterial occlusion by an embolus may also be a lower extremity.

Chronic arterial occlusion

This most frequently develops as a result of gradual changes in the walls of the vessels, causing narrowing of the lumen. It may also be of functional origin due to hyperactivity of the sympathetic nervous system, causing excessive vasoconstriction. Gradual occlusion of an artery allows for collateral circulation to be established, which ensures a supply of oxygenated blood to peripheral tissue, for at least a while.

The most common causes of chronic occlusion are atherosclerosis and arteriosclerosis. The arteries in any area of the body may be affected, but the coronary, cerebral and renal arteries are frequent sites. The problems caused by their insufficiency are discussed under disorders of the relative structures. When the abdominal aorta and/or medium- and large-sized arteries are involved, the condition may be referred to as *arteriosclerosis obliterans*. The arteries of the extremities are also a relatively frequent site of chronic occlusion which may be referred to as *peripheral vascular disease*. In this condition there is progressive loss of the blood supply to the legs, leading to intermittent claudication and the appearance of necrotic tissue, usually on the toes and feet. Patients are typically of late middle age to elderly, have a history of smoking, and are often diabetic. Amputation may be necessary; this is discussed in detail in Chapter 24.

Two other forms of peripheral vascular disease are Raynaud's disease and thromboangiitis obliterans.

Raynaud's disease is a condition in which episodes of excessive vasoconstriction occur in the digits of the hands and/or feet. The cause is obscure, but the episodes are most frequently precipitated by cold or emotional stress. The disease is more common in women, usually develops before the age of 40–45 years and is bilateral.

Thromboangiitis obliterans (Buerger's disease) is a chronic occlusive disease in which there is an inflammation and thickening of the walls of limb arteries, predisposing to thrombosis. It has a higher incidence in young men and in Jewish people. The parts are very tender and painful, and necrotic areas develop in the distal portions of the digits.

The condition is seriously aggravated if the person smokes. The cause of this disease is unknown.

Signs and symptoms of arterial insufficiency in the extremities

Gradual reduction in the arterial blood supply to the extremities produces the following signs and symptoms.

Intermittent claudication This is leg pain that occurs with exercise and is relieved by rest. The blood supply is sufficient to meet the tissue needs when the part is at rest. However, with exercise, oxygen demands cannot be met and metabolic wastes are not readily removed from the muscle tissue. The result is ischaemic muscle pain. Rest allows increased supply of oxygen to tissues and removal of metabolic waste, thus relieving the discomfort. This symptom usually worsens progressively and increasingly limits the distance a patient may walk before the pain occurs.

Rest pain Muscle leg pain at rest indicates advanced peripheral vascular disease. This pain may be described as burning or numbing and may become more prominent at night.

Peripheral pulses Peripheral pulses may be absent or weakened. An oscillometer or Doppler flowmeter may be used to palpate the pulsation of arteries in an area where the vessels are deeper and cannot be palpated by the fingers. A comparison is made of the pulses in both legs and may reveal that one is weaker than the other, indicating partial occlusion in that leg. Complete occlusion would be indicated by an absence of the pulse.

Colour A difference in the colour of the two extremities or an abnormal change in both extremities, if both are involved, will probably be present. In caucasians the skin may become white and blanched, or it may become a dusky red or mottled, depending on the amount of blood in the capillaries and the amount of reduced haemoglobin in the blood. On being raised, the limb becomes even paler as the venous drainage increases but, on being lowered, it fails to increase its colour quickly as the normal limb would do with the rush of arterial blood into it. The superficial veins are slow in filling when the limb is lowered; normally, they fill in approximately 5 s.

Skin changes The skin temperature and moisture may be different in the two limbs. The affected one exhibits a coldness to the touch and may be unusually moist. Limb tissues may atrophy, causing the affected limb to become smaller than the other. The skin becomes dry and shiny, and loses its hair. Nails thicken and become brittle and ridged.

Necrosis Ulcerated or gangrenous areas may develop, denoting areas of tissue completely deprived of blood supply. Ulceration is a superficial area of devitalized tissue; gangrene is a more massive area of dead tissue.

Diagnosis

In most instances, a thorough history and an adequate vascular physical examination result in an accurate diagnosis of occlusive arterial disease. Various tests may be used to diagnose and assess vascular disease.

Exercise tolerance The patient is required to walk or perform some form of exercise until intermittent claudication occurs. The length of time from the start of activity until the occurrence of pain is noted.

Ankle brachial pressure index The systolic blood pressure in the legs should be equal to or slightly higher than the systolic pressure in the upper limbs. When arterial narrowing occurs, a reduction in pressure occurs distal to the lesion. The ankle brachial pressure index is calculated from the ratio of ankle to brachial systolic pressure (Donnelly et al 2000). It is a sensitive marker of arterial insufficiency.

A Doppler probe will assist in detecting blood flow at the ankle which occurs as the sphygmomanometer cuff is deflated, indicating the lower limb systolic pressure.

When the brachial systolic pressure is divided by ankle systolic pressure, the result should be greater than 1. A ratio of between 0.7 and 1.0 indicates significant arterial disease, and if the ratio is less than 0.4 severe ischaemia is present (Munro and Edward 1995).

Doppler ultrasonography Doppler ultrasonography is based on the principle that the frequency of reflected sound waves from moving objects (such as red blood cells) shifts in proportion to the velocity of the object and the direction of movement. Continuous-wave Doppler ultrasonographic equipment produces an audible signal when the probe is held over the artery, indicating movement of blood in the vessel (Donnelly et al 2000).

Duplex ultrasonography The combination of real-time ultrasonography and Doppler studies is being used increasingly in the evaluation of patients with arterial disease. A two-dimensional picture of the reflected ultrasound waves is provided. Characteristic changes can be seen near areas of stenosis. The great advantage is that it is non-invasive and in some parts of the body (e.g. carotid vessels) its accuracy in assessing the degree of stenosis is comparable to that of arteriography. Furthermore, the Doppler aspect of the study yields valuable information about the haemodynamic significance of any stenosis identified.

Angiography A radio-opaque contrast medium containing iodine is introduced into the arteries, and radiographs are taken. Arterial narrowing or obstruction may be located in this way, and some information regarding the amount of collateral circulation present may also be obtained.

Magnetic resonance angiography This technique has developed rapidly over recent years. It can image a moving column of blood, but does not require ionizing radiation or iodinated contrast dye (Donnelly et al 2000). It is limited by both cost issues and accessibility to the scanning equipment.

Medical management

Vasodilating and anticoagulant drugs have been used to treat patients with arterial occlusive disease.

Although many drugs are promoted as agents capable of increasing peripheral blood flow, many are universally ineffective. Any α-adrenergic blocking drug will increase the flow through the skin, but no drug can increase flow to muscles when the underlying disease is atherosclerosis of a major artery.

Anticoagulant drugs may be prescribed to prevent and treat thrombosis. The most widely used anticoagulants are heparin and warfarin. Aspirin may be used to prevent platelet aggregation. Heparin is given parenterally because it has no effect orally. It is thought to block the effect of thrombin on fibrinogen, thereby preventing clot formation. Heparin begins to be effective within minutes after administration and its action is prolonged for 3–4 hours. It may be given in a continuous i.v. infusion or at regularly spaced intervals. Heparin therapy is usually extended over several days and then gradually replaced by a warfarin preparation given orally. Warfarin takes effect in approximately 48 hours, so it is started before the heparin is withdrawn.

The dosage and frequency of warfarin administration is dependent upon the prothrombin time, which indicates the effectiveness of the extrinsic system in producing clotting. It is reported as the international normalized ratio (INR). The dosage of heparin is decided by the partial thromboplastin time (PTT), which is another measure of clotting time. A therapeutic level is generally considered to be 1.5 times to twice the normal values for PTT. The clotting time is determined when PTT cannot be measured.

Warfarin carries the risk of producing haemorrhage as a side-effect, especially as it is prone to interaction with other drugs that potentiate its effects. Broad-spectrum antibiotics, such as erythromycin and metronidazole, are one such groups of drugs. These drugs produce the risk of bleeding but their therapeutic value may be considered to outweigh this risk.

The nurse's responsibilities include close observation for signs of haemorrhage. The patient should be taught to monitor this potential problem for themselves before discharge. Profuse bleeding from minor cuts, bleeding gums, haematuria, haematemesis, blood in the stool, petechiae and abnormal vaginal bleeding indicate problems and should be reported promptly. In the event of bleeding, the drug is discontinued, and vitamin K (for those taking warfarin) and a blood transfusion may be given to counteract the reduced coagulation. Protamine sulfate, a heparin antagonist, is given if severe bleeding occurs as a result of heparin administration.

The prothrombin or partial thromboplastin time is determined before the anticoagulant drug is administered. Patients outside the hospital taking anticoagulants are usually required to report to the clinic, initially weekly, for an international normalized ratio (INR) (see p. 328) level check. More recently, drugs that prevent platelet aggregation, such as aspirin and sulfinpyrazone, are being used to prevent arterial thrombosis.

Surgical management of arterial disease

A direct surgical approach may be employed in which the surgeon chooses to perform an endarterectomy, bypass or graft. An endarterectomy is the removal of the thickened intima and atheromatous plaques from the artery, and is used when the disease is localized to a relatively small area. The establishment of a bypass channel in order to reduce the arterial insufficiency may be achieved by transplanting one end of another artery into the occluded artery below the site of obstruction or by an autogenous venous graft. The latter consists of the removal of a section of vein (usually the saphenous), reversing it (because of the valves) to ensure flow in the right direction and attaching it to the affected artery above and below the occlusion. The surgeon often elects to resect the affected segment of the artery and replace it with an inert synthetic (Teflon or Dacron) graft. This type of graft is relatively porous and is eventually incorporated into host tissues. An intima develops within it fairly quickly as cells proliferate through the interstices and from the host intima of the artery at each end of the graft. A layer of fibrous tissue also develops on the exterior surface, reinforcing the tube.

The most common site of major vascular surgery for occlusive disease is the aorta and the iliac and femoral arteries. Failure of surgical intervention may lead to amputation of the affected limb as ischaemic pain becomes continuous and gangrene may develop.

Nursing care

Arterial occlusive disease (peripheral vascular disease) is a chronic condition, and the patient will probably have to continue with the prescribed care and precautions indefinitely. This may create considerable hardship for the patient and family, depending on the severity of the disease and the limitations it imposes. Adjustments may have to be made in occupational and social life; the patient may become partially or completely dependent financially and for personal care, and will certainly find it difficult to accept the situation. The nurse must be alert to the possible implications for the patient and family/carers, and should provide the necessary assistance and guidance.

Impaired skin integrity related to ischaemia

Goals

1. The patient will have intact skin.
2. The patient will inspect the skin daily.

Nursing intervention

The patient is taught to inspect the skin daily for signs of irritation or injury. The presence of neuropathy may reduce the person's awareness or perception of pain, thus daily inspection may be the only reliable indicator of skin integrity.

Daily bathing in comfortably warm (not hot) water using a mild soap is recommended. Gentle and thorough drying is important, and special attention is given to the areas between the digits. If the skin is dry, the limbs may be gently massaged with lanolin or some light emollient. Nails are cut straight across but not right down to the soft tissue. Corns should be removed by a chiropodist; the patient should not undertake to 'pare' them with sharp instruments.

The patient is advised of the importance of well-fitting shoes and socks or stockings. Socks should be loose and are changed daily. The patient is instructed to avoid walking about in bare feet: a cut, abrasion or infection could be serious because resistance to infection is lowered and healing is poor as a result of the impaired blood supply. If injury does occur, even of a minor nature, it should receive prompt medical attention as the potential for sepsis and gangrene is great.

Good general nutrition is essential to promote tissue healing and prevent tissue breakdown.

Decreased tissue perfusion related to reduced blood flow

Goals

The patient will have:

1. extremities warmer to touch
2. improved colour of skin
3. reduced oedema of extremities.

Nursing intervention

Positioning The horizontal position is used when the patient rests. Occasionally, raising the head of the bed may be used to encourage the flow of blood into the lower limbs by gravity. Position should be changed at frequent intervals throughout the day, and long periods of standing must be avoided. The patient is advised not to cross the legs and, when sitting, pressure on the popliteal region should be avoided. If ambulatory, the patient sits or lies down every 2–3 hours and elevates the feet for 10–15 minutes.

Exercise Many authorities indicate the most effective treatment for intermittent claudication is physical exercise, especially walking. It is suggested that the patient should walk for 20–30 minutes each day at a slow to moderate pace on a level surface. The patient may do this by walking to the point of intermittent claudication, stopping until the discomfort disappears, and then continuing to walk until the distress develops again. The patient repeats this process for the prescribed period. The underlying theory is that exercise increases collateral circulation.

Passive and active exercises may also be prescribed: flexion and extension of the legs, feet and toes may be used for lower limbs, and similar exercises may be employed for the arms and fingers if these are the sites of the arterial insufficiency. Exercises promote emptying and filling of the vessels and stimulate the development of collateral circulation.

Protection from cold Exposure to cold with lowering of normal body temperature produces undesirable responses: peripheral vasoconstriction and increased metabolism. Special precautions are necessary in cold weather. Extra, warm clothing should be worn. If exposure to cold precipitates an episode, the patient is advised to take a warm drink and seek a warm environment. Local heat applications to the affected parts are discouraged because there is a reduced nerve sensitivity leading to the risk of localized tissue damage. The patient is advised to wear warm socks or to wrap the feet in a warm blanket rather than applying a hot-water bottle.

Smoking The use of tobacco is discontinued, because it promotes vasoconstriction and aggravates the disease.

Venous disorders

Reduction in venous return leads to congestion and oedema, which interfere with normal cell function and eventually prevent a normal arterial volume from reaching tissue cells. Common venous conditions are varicose veins, deep vein thrombosis (DVT), thrombophlebitis and phlebothrombosis.

Varicose veins

When venous blood meets with increased resistance to its forward flow, the walls of the veins become dilated and tortuous, the valves become damaged and incompetent, and the blood tends to pool and stagnate. The condition may be referred to as varicosities, or as varicose veins. Trunk varices are varicosities in the line of the long or short saphenous vein, or one of its branches in the legs. Reticular veins are dilated, tortuous subcutaneous veins, not belonging to the main branches of the long or short saphenous vein. Telangiectasia are intradermal and are often called thread or spider veins (London and Nash 2000). The superficial veins of the lower extremities are most susceptible. Because of our upright position, the venous pressure in the lower limbs is increased by gravity. Other common sites of varicosities are the veins of the anal canal (haemorrhoids), spermatic veins (varicocele), oesophageal veins (oesophageal varices) and the vulvar veins in pregnant women due to pressure from the enlarging uterus. Although resistance to the flow of blood is the main cause of varicosities, it is now believed that they are caused by inherently weak vein walls, which

leads to dilatation and separation of the valve cusps in the vein (London and Nash 2000). Long periods of standing, obesity and increasing age can all predispose to the development of varicose veins in the lower extremities.

Manifestations

Varicose veins cause local oedema of the tissues, crampy pains or aching, and a full, heavy feeling in the affected area. The congestion and oedema in the tissues interfere with the normal supply of oxygen and nutrients reaching the cells, leading to fibrosing of subcutaneous tissues and, in some instances, necrosis of superficial tissue, producing what is referred to as a varicose ulcer. The affected area appears swollen and discoloured, and the veins are seen as tortuous, bulbous protrusions. These veins readily become inflamed (phlebitis), and occasionally the vessel wall ruptures, causing haemorrhage.

Diagnosis

The test most frequently performed for varicosities in the lower limbs is the *Trendelenburg test*. While the patient is in the horizontal position, the leg is elevated above the level of the pelvis until the superficial veins appear to be empty. The patient then stands, and the veins are observed as they fill. Normally they fill relatively slowly from below; with varicosities, the incompetent valves allow them to fill from above as well. Hand-held Doppler or colour duplex scanning is used to asses the structure and functioning of the veins.

Conservative management

The patient is instructed to avoid situations and factors that tend to increase the resistance to venous flow, to provide support to the veins and tissues by elastic compression stockings, and to assist drainage by elevation of the limb at intervals.

If the varicosity is not extensive, the doctor may inject a sclerosing agent (sclerotherapy). This causes the veins to become inflamed and thrombosed. The use of this treatment has decreased in recent years owing to complications such as skin staining and ulceration, and because of the development of recurrent varicose veins in a proportion of patients (London and Nash 2000). It may be used to treat residual veins following surgery.

Surgical treatment

With more severe varicosities in the lower limbs, surgical treatment in the form of ligation and stripping of the veins may be employed, usually under general anaesthesia. The affected vein is ligated above the varicosity, its connecting branches are severed and tied, and the vein is removed. The venous blood then returns via the deep veins. The great saphenous vein is the one most frequently ligated and removed from the groin to the ankle. This necessitates several small horizontal incisions along the course of the vein. Compression bandages are applied from the foot to the groin after the operation, and the foot of the bed is elevated. The nurse observes the feet for colour and warmth to assess for an adequate circulation, and the incision sites are inspected for signs of bleeding. Mobilization is encouraged at an early stage, often on the day of operation if the patient is able, and certainly the next day. This facilitates good venous return. Standing is avoided. Compression stockings are provided for several weeks at home. The patient can return to work within 1–3 weeks depending on the occupation and its association with risk factors such as heavy lifting. Weight reduction is advised and support offered, straining at stool is discouraged, while regular walking is actively encouraged, increasing the distance each day.

Deep vein thrombosis

A **deep vein thrombosis** (DVT) is a blood clot occurring in the deep veins of the leg. It is usually due to venous stasis or slow flowing blood around the venous valve sinuses (Gorman et al 2000). Box 12.5 highlights the main factors predisposing to this condition.

Manifestations

Deep vein thrombosis may be asymptomatic and is notoriously difficult to diagnose by physical examination alone. It is confirmed in only one of every three cases suspected clinically (Gorman et al 2000). Further investigations are always required. Signs and symptoms may include pain in the calf area (particularly on walking) and localized tenderness. Swelling around the area of thrombosis may occur with pitting oedema, together with a raised skin temperature. It is important when performing a nursing assessment to consider whether the patient falls into one of the 'at risk' categories (Box 12.5), and to consider educating vulnerable patients with regard to identifying possible signs of DVT.

Diagnosis

A full medical history is always taken and a physical examination performed.

D-Dimer testing D-Dimer is a circulating degradation product of fibrin production. Fibrin is involved in the clotting process. D-Dimer concentrations are raised in conditions such as DVT and pulmonary embolism. Levels can be increased in other conditions, but this remains a valuable test, particularly if the patient presents out of normal working hours when other forms of investigation may not be available.

Contrast venography Contrast venography utilizes X-ray imaging with an injected contrast medium to see blockages in the vein. An alternative form is radionuclide (radioactive) venography, which uses the injection of radiopharmaceuticals to produce images of the occlusion. The latter is expensive and not the first line of investigation.

Box 12.5   Risk factors for the development of deep vein thrombosis (DVT)

- Varicose veins.
- Age above 40 years.
- Clinical history in the patient or family of DVT or pulmonary embolism.
- Immobility, for example as a result of prolonged bedrest, paralysis or stroke.
- Surgical procedures lasting for more than 30 minutes. These are notably orthopaedic, neurosurgical, urological or gynecological surgery (Gorman et al 2000). Surgery reduces venous return because of lack of mobility in the legs, preventing the muscles in the calves from squeezing blood back towards the heart. The clotting cascade is also be triggered by surgical intervention.
- Pregnancy. This can raise intra-abdominal pressure and hinder venous return of blood.
- Serious illnesses such as myocardial infarction, heart failure, sepsis; these can interfere with blood flow through the main and micro-circulation.
- Disorders that encourage abnormal blood clotting.
- Obesity. This may cause pressure and obstruction to the venous return.
- Underlying malignancy. This may affect both clotting and venous return.
- The term *thrombophilia* may be used, and refers to a tendency of the blood towards clotting.
- Recent controversy over the adverse effects of prolonged air travel has led to ongoing research into the so-called 'economy class syndrome' associated with the risk of DVT to passengers.

Deep vein thrombosis
See chapter 4.1

Compression ultrasonography This has emerged in recent years as a valuable diagnostic tool in DVT. Pressure is applied to the vein with an ultrasound probe. This compresses the walls of the vessel, but will not occur if a thrombus is present. The lack of vessel collapse can be visualized on a screen. As a technique it is known to be less effective in the veins of the calves.

Duplex scanning Colour duplex scanning utilizes ultrasound and may be used to image the venous system in certain areas, such as with more proximal DVTs.

Complications

Part or all of the DVT may break free and travel within the circulation. This may lead to emboli blocking the blood flow to organs, particularly in the lungs (pulmonary embolism). The patient becomes breathless and experiences chest pain. An area of lung may infarct – at worse, this may prove fatal.

Prophylaxis

Nursing staff should be aware of the factors predisposing to DVT. Patients should be encouraged to mobilize when able in order to encourage venous return. A good fluid intake is encouraged unless contraindicated, for example in severe heart failure. Subcutaneous heparin (an anti-coagulant) and graded compression stockings, which encourage venous return, may be necessary in high-risk groups.

Treatment

Nursing care should aim to reduce the presenting symptoms, prevent complications and reduce the size of the thrombus. The affected leg is elevated when resting. This will help to reduce swelling and compression around the area. Early mobilization is now seen as beneficial (Gorman et al 2000). Graded compression stocking will be prescribed. An accurate measurement of the limb is needed to ensure the correct size stockings are used. These should not be rolled down or have wrinkles in them. A spare pair is usually given to allow one pair to be washed. Anticoagulation is given as soon as a diagnosis has been made. This is usually a bolus dose of heparin (5000 units) and either a constant heparin infusion or subcutaneous low molecular weight heparin, such as dalteparin sodium (Fragmin). The dose of the latter form of heparin is weight related and is usually given once a day.

Monitoring the activated partial thromboplastin time (APTT) occurs at approximately 6-hour intervals to ensure that adequate anticoagulation has been achieved. A therapeutic range of 1.5–2 times the laboratory value of a normal PTT (the control) is usually recommended. Heparin will not break down the clot, but will prevent it from enlarging as it dissolves naturally. An oral anticoagulant, usually warfarin, is started immediately, but takes about 3 days to prolong the prothrombin time adequately, measured as the international normalized ratio (INR). The target range is approximately 2–3, or slightly higher for a recurrent DVT. Heparin is not available as an oral drug and is stopped when the INR has reached the target range for 24 hours with the oral anticoagulant.

The INR will be measured several times over the subsequent few days, then weekly as an outpatient assessment. The time is then lengthened as the INR target range stabilizes. Patients are advised of the risks of bleeding such as the occurrence of bruising or blood in the urine or stools. These should be reported to the healthcare team. A small booklet is kept by the patient with the result of the INR and the prescribed dose of warfarin, which alters depending on the result. Activities known to be a risk to bleeding, such as gardening, contact sports and handling pets that may scratch, should be avoided. The oral anticoagulant will be prescribed for a number of months. INR monitoring is now frequently undertaken in nurse-led clinics.

Approximately 35% of patients with a DVT are cared for in the community (Gorman et al 2000). Subcutaneous heparin is administered by the patient or community healthcare team. If the patient with a DVT is pregnant, heparin is administered by subcutaneous injection. It is stopped before delivery, then restarted following the birth for several weeks to approximately 3 months. Warfarin can damage the fetus.

Thrombophlebitis and phlebothrombosis

Phlebitis is an inflammation of the walls of a vein and may be caused by injury, prolonged pressure or infection. The endothelial lining is damaged and a thrombus develops at the site of inflammation, producing a secondary condition known as thrombophlebitis.

Phlebothrombosis is the formation of a blood clot within a vein with no associated inflammation, and for this reason may be referred to as a *bland* or *silent thrombosis*. It is nearly always due to slowness or stasis of the circulation, such as occurs with prolonged bedrest, inactivity or pressure causing resistance to the venous blood flow. The serious factor in both phlebothrombosis and thrombophlebitis is the blood clot, which becomes a potential embolus. The silent thrombus or that associated with inflammation may be carried along in the bloodstream and may eventually lodge in an artery to cause an embolism. Phlebitis and venous thrombosis may occur in any vein, but the most frequent site is the saphenous veins of the legs.

Manifestations

Thrombophlebitis in superficial veins produces local pain, tenderness and swelling. The pain may vary from moderate discomfort on touching the limb to severe cramping. If the leg is involved, there may be calf pain during dorsiflexion of the foot (Homans' sign). Systemic symptoms such as fever, headache and general malaise develop. If the vein is superficial, the overlying skin becomes red and hot. It may be taut and shiny.

With deep vein thrombosis, the process may be silent. No symptoms may be present until the thrombus is swept along and causes an embolism. In either phlebothrombosis or thrombophlebitis, the thrombus may become large enough to block the vein, causing severe congestion, oedema and pain.

Summary

Cardiovascular disease is one of the most important single causes of death in the UK and contributes to a significant level of morbidity. It is of multifactorial origin, so there is no one single preventive measure that would reduce its incidence dramatically. A combination of strategies is therefore needed to reduce the morbidity and mortality associated with cardiovascular disease. Nurses have a major role in preventing cardiovascular disorder and in improving the quality of life for patients, and their loved ones, living with heart disease. However, the government also has an important role in health promotion, and more recently considerable interest has been shown by the government in targeting heart disease through national standards, manifest in documents such as the National Service Framework for Coronary Heart Disease (Department of Health 2000b). This may go some way to addressing the issue of why Britain's mortality statistics from cardiovascular disease are amongst the worst in Europe.

Critical incident   Myocardial infarction

Bill Wright is a 65-year-old man with a known history of stable angina. Following his evening meal, he experienced chest pain which, although not intense, increased with discomfort throughout the evening. It was central, retrosternal, and radiated down his left arm. He took little notice, presuming it was indigestion from his rich evening meal. He awoke at 5 a.m., sweating, feeling nauseous and with an increased intensity of pain. His wife called the general practitioner, but he was at another call and, after eventually being contacted, arrived some 20 minutes later. The GP noted Mr Wright's ashen complexion and sweaty skin. He took the blood pressure, recorded as 110/70 mmHg, and assessed the presenting chest pain. He immediately called an ambulance and gave Mr Wright 2.5 mg diamorphine intravenously. In addition 300 mg aspirin was given. Oxygen was administered, together with a tablet of sublingual glyceryl trinitrate (GTN). Mr Wright was admitted via ambulance to hospital where a nurse-led thrombolysis programme was in operation. This allowed a rapid clinical assessment and the speedy administration of a thrombolytic agent.

Reflection
See Appendix 2 for guidelines on reflection.

References

Ashworth P (1992) Cardiovascular problems and nursing. In: Ashworth P, Clarke C, eds. Cardiovascular intensive care nursing, pp. 1–19. Edinburgh: Churchill Livingstone.

Balarajan R (1991) Ethnic differences in mortality from ischaemic heart disease and cerebrovascular disease in England and Wales. British Medical Journal 302: 560–564.

Barnett M (2001) Cardiac pacing. In: Hatchett R, Thompson DR, eds. Cardiac nursing: a comprehensive guide, pp. 391–425. Edinburgh: Churchill Livingstone.

British Heart Foundation (1999) Eating for your heart. London: BHF.

British Heart Foundation Statistics Database (2000) Coronary heart disease statistics. London: BHF.

British Heart Foundation (2001) Coronary heart disease statistics: morbidity supplement. London: BHF.

British Medical Association/Royal College of Nursing (2001) Decisions relating to cardiopulmonary resuscitation: a joint statement from the British Medical Association, the Resuscitation Council (UK) and the Royal College of Nursing. London: BMA/RCN.

British National Formulary (2001) British national formulary, Vol. 41. London: BMA/Royal Pharmaceutical Society of Great Britain.

British Hypertension Society (2000) Guidelines for the management of hypertension 2000. London: British Hypertension Society. Online. Available: http://www.hyp.ac.uk/bhs/gl2000.htm

Bygrave A (2001) Electrophysiology studies. In: Hatchett R, Thompson DR, eds. Cardiac nursing: a comprehensive guide, pp. 369–390. Edinburgh: Churchill Livingstone.

Clark J, Queener S, Burke V (2000) Pharmacological basis for nursing practice. St Louis: CV Mosby.

Department of Health (1999) Health survey for England. Cardiovascular disease 1998. London: DoH.

Department of Health (2000a) Saving lives: our healthier nation. London: DoH.

Department of Health (2000b) The national service framework for coronary heart disease. London: DoH.

Donnelly R, Hinwood D, London NJM (2000) ABC of arterial and vascular disease: non-invasive methods of arterial and venous assessment. British Medical Journal 320: 698–701.

Drayer RA, Henderson J, Reidenberg M (1999) Barriers to better pain control in hospitalized patients. Journal of Pain and Symptom Management 17(6): 434–440.

Elliot D (1993) Comparison of three instruments for measuring patient anxiety in a coronary care unit. Intensive and Critical Care Nursing 9: 193–200.

Fairburn K (1994) Nurses' attitudes to visiting in coronary care units. Intensive and Critical Care Nursing 10: 81–88.

Farrelly R (2000) Congenital heart disease 1. Nursing Times 96(24): 47–50.

Fisher S, Cross N, Walsh G (2001) Cardiac surgery. In: Hatchett R, Thompson DR, eds. Cardiac nursing: a comprehensive guide, pp. 426–461. Edinburgh: Churchill Livingstone.

Friedman S (2000) Cardiac disease, anxiety, and sexual functioning. American Journal of Cardiology 86(2A): 46–50F.

Gamel C, Davis BD, Hengeveld M (1993) Nurses' provision of teaching and counselling on sexuality: a review of the literature. Journal of Advanced Nursing 18: 1219–1227.

Glenville B (1999) Minimally invasive cardiac surgery. British Medical Journal 319: 135–136 (editorial).

Gorman WP, Davis KR, Donnelly R (2000) ABC of arterial and venous disease: swollen lower limb 1. General assessment and deep vein thrombosis. British Medical Journal 320: 1453–1456.

Gortner SR, Jenkins LS (1990) Self-efficacy and activity level following cardiac surgery. Journal of Advanced Nursing 15: 1132–1138.

Gould M (2001) Chronic heart failure. In: Hatchett R, Thompson DR, eds. Cardiac nursing: a comprehensive guide, pp. 187–217. Edinburgh: Churchill Livingstone.

Hagenhoff BD, Feutz C, Conn VS, Sagehorn KK, Moranville-Hunziker M (1994) Patient education needs as reported by congestive heart failure patients and their nurses. Journal of Advanced Nursing 19: 685–690.

Halstead F, Turner B, Wilson S (2001) Diagnostic procedures. In: Hatchett R, Thompson DR, eds. Cardiac nursing: a comprehensive guide, pp. 125–147. Edinburgh: Churchill Livingstone.

Hatchett R (2001) Clinical observation and monitoring devices. In: Hatchett R, Thompson DR, eds. Cardiac nursing: a comprehensive guide, pp. 69–95. Edinburgh: Churchill Livingstone.

Health Education Authority (1992) Allied Dunbar National Fitness Survey: a summary of the major findings. London: HEA.

Hellman EA, Williams MA (1994) Outpatient cardiac rehabilitation in elderly patients. Heart and Lung 23: 506–512.

Hildingh C, Segsten K, Bengtsson C, Fridlund B (1994) Experiences of social support among participants in self-help groups related to coronary heart disease. Journal of Clinical Nursing 3: 219–226.

ISIS-2 (Second International Study of Infarct Survival) Collaborative Group (1988) Randomised trial of intravenous streptokinase, oral aspirin, both, or neither among 17187 cases of suspected acute myocardial infarction: ISIS-2. Lancet ii: 349–360.

Jaarsma T, Kastermans M, Dassen T, Phipsen H (1995) Problems of cardiac patients in early recovery. Journal of Advanced Nursing 21: 21–27.

James J (2001) The management and support of patients with internal cardioverter defibrillators. In: Hatchett R, Thompson DR, eds. Cardiac nursing: a comprehensive guide, pp. 495–505. Edinburgh: Churchill Livingstone.

Johnson S (1997) Pathways of care. Oxford: Blackwell Science.

Johnston DW, Cook DG, Sharper AG (1987) Type A behaviour and ischaemic heart disease in middle aged British men. British Medical Journal 295: 86–89.

Kettunen S, Solovieva S, Laamanen R, Santavirta N (1999) Myocardial infarction, spouses' reactions and their need of support. Journal of Advanced Nursing 30(2): 479–488.

Khosla S, Laddu A, Ehrenpreis S, Somberg J (1994) Cardiovascular effects of nicotine: relation to deleterious effects of cigarette smoking. American Heart Journal 127: 1669–1672.

Kleinman A, Eisenberg L, Good B (1978) Culture, illness and care. Annals of Internal Medicine 88: 251–258.

Knoll SM, Johnson JL (2000) Uncertainty and expectations: taking care of a cardiac surgery patient at home. Journal of Cardiovascular Nursing 14(3): 64–75.

Law MR, Wald NJ, Thompson SG (1994) By how much and by how quickly does reduction in serum cholesterol concentration lower risk of ischaemic heart disease? British Medical Journal 308: 367–373.

Linden B (1995) Evaluation of a home based rehabilitation programme for patients recovering from acute myocardial infarction. Intensive and Critical Care Nursing 11: 10–19.

London NJM, Nash R (2000) ABC of arterial and venous disease: varicose veins. British Medical Journal 320: 1391–1394.

Macleod Clark J, Haverty S, Kendall S (1990) Helping people to stop smoking: a study of the nurse's role. Journal of Advanced Nursing 16: 357–363.

McDonagh TA, Dargie HJ (1998) Epidemiology and pathophysiology of heart failure. Medicine 26(1): 111–115.

Mason S (2001) Infective endocarditis. In: Hatchett R, Thompson DR, eds. Cardiac nursing: a comprehensive guide, pp. 287–298. Edinburgh: Churchill Livingstone.

Mayou R, Bryant B (1993) Quality of life in cardiovascular disease. British Heart Journal 69: 460–466.

Millane T, Jackson G, Gibbs CR, Lip GYH (2000) ABC of heart failure: acute and chronic management strategies. British Medical Journal 320: 559–562.

Munro J, Edwards C (1995) Macleod's clinical examination. Edinburgh: Churchill Livingstone.

National Institute for Clinical Excellence (2000) Appraisal guidance on technologies for specialist cardiac services. London: NICE.

Norris LO, Grove SK (1986) Investigation of selected psychosocial needs of family members of critically ill adult patients. Heart and Lung 15: 194–199.

Oakely C (1998) Heart muscle disease. Medicine 66(1): 129–133.

O'Farrell P, Murray J, Hotz SB (2000) Psychologic distress among spouses of patients undergoing cardiac rehabilitation. Heart and Lung 29(2): 97–104.

Olivier C (2000) Rheumatic fever: is it still a problem? Journal of Antimicrobial Chemotherapy 45: 13–21.

Openshaw A, Durbridge M (2001) Early extubation protocols, the emergence of high dependency units and the newer revascularisation techniques. In: Hatchett R, Thompson DR, eds. Cardiac nursing: a comprehensive guide, pp. 544–563. Edinburgh: Churchill Livingstone.

Oswald GA, Corcoran S, Yudkin JS (1984) Prevalence and risks of hyperglycaemia and undiagnosed diabetes in patients with acute myocardial infarction. Lancet i: 1265–1267.

Peterson M (1991) Patient anxiety before cardiac catheterisation. Heart and Lung 20: 643–647.

Quinn T, Hatchett R (2001) Cardiopulmonary resuscitation. In: Hatchett R, Thompson DR, eds. Cardiac nursing: a comprehensive guide, pp. 481–494. Edinburgh: Churchill Livingstone.

Quinn T, Webster R, Hatchett R (2001) Coronary artery disease: angina and unstable angina. In: Hatchett R, Thompson DR, eds. Cardiac nursing: a comprehensive guide, pp. 151–188. Edinburgh: Churchill Livingstone.

Ramsay LE, Williams B, Johnston GD et al (1999) Guidelines for management of hypertension: report of the third working party of the British Hypertension Society. Journal of Human Hypertension 13: 569–592.

Resuscitation Council UK (2000) Resuscitation guidelines 2000. London: Resuscitation Council.

Rice VH, Lepezyk M, Mullen M, Templin T (1994) A comparison of nursing interventions for smoking cessation in adults with cardiovascular health problems. Heart and Lung 23: 473–486.

Roebuck A (1999) Telephone support in the early post-discharge period following elective cardiac surgery: does it reduce anxiety and depression levels? Intensive and Critical Care Nursing 15(3): 142–146.

Sager D (1987) Current facts on pacemaker electromagnetic interference and their application to clinical care. Heart and Lung 16: 211–221.

Scandinavian Simvastatin Survival Study Group (1994) Randomised controlled trial of cholesterol lowering in 4444 patients with coronary heart disease: the Scandinavian Simvastsatin Survival Study. Lancet 344: 1383–1389.

Searle M, Hoff L (2000) Bedrest after elective cardiac catheterisation. Professional Nurse 15(9): 588–591.

Shaper AG (1987) Risk factors for ischaemic heart disease. Health Trends 19: 3–8.

Sharpe N, Doughty R (1998) Epidemiology of heart failure and ventricular dysfunction. Lancet 352(Suppl 1): S13–S17.

Simons R (1999) The airway at risk. In: Colquhoun MC, Handley AJ, Evans TR, eds. ABC of resuscitation, pp.19–24. London: BMJ Books.

Stokes H, Thompson DR (2001) Cardiac rehabilitation. In: Hatchett R, Thompson DR, eds. Cardiac nursing: a comprehensive guide, pp. 29–39. Edinburgh: Churchill Livingstone.

Thomas S (1991) Coronary angioplasty. Nursing Standard 5(42): 47–48.

Thompson DR (1990) Counselling the coronary patient and partner. London: Scutari.

Thompson DR, Webster RA, Cordle CJ et al (1987) Specific sources and patterns of anxiety in male patients with first myocardial infarction. British Journal of Medical Psychology 60: 343–348.

Thompson DR, Sutton TW, Jowett NI, Pohl JEF (1991) Circardian variation in the frequency of onset of chest pain in acute myocardial infarction. British Heart Journal 65: 177–178.

Thompson DR, Webster RA, Sutton TW (1994) Coronary care unit patients' and nurses' ratings of intensity of ischaemic chest pain. Intensive and Critical Care Nursing 10: 81–88.

Thompson DR, Ersser S, Webster RA (1995) The experiences of patients and their partners 1 month after a heart attack. Journal of Advanced Nursing 22: 707–714.

Thompson DR, Bowman GS, Kitson A et al (1996) Cardiac rehabilitation in the United Kingdom: guidelines and audit standards. Heart 75: 89–93.

Tortora G, Grabowski S (2000) Principles of anatomy and physiology, 9th edn. New York: John Wiley.

Underwood MJ, Firmin RK, Jehu D (1993) Aspects of psychological and social morbidity in patients awaiting coronary artery bypass grafting. British Heart Journal 69: 382–384.

Walsh M, Kent A (2001) A & E nursing, 4th edn. Oxford: Butterworth-Heinemann.

Walsh M, Crumbie A, Reveley S (1999) Nurse practitioners: clinical skills and professional issues. Oxford: Butterworth-Heinemann.

Watt-Watson J, Garfinkel P, Gallop R, Stevens B, Streiner D (2000) The impact of nurses' empathic responses on patients' pain management in acute care. Nursing Research 49(4): 191–200.

World Health Organization (1993) Needs and action priorities in cardiac rehabilitation and secondary prevention in patients with coronary heart disease. Copenhagen: WHO.

Yusuf S, Zucker D, Peduzzi P, Fisher LD (1994) Effect of coronary artery by-pass graft surgery on survival: overview of 10 year results from randomised trials by the Coronary Artery Bypass Graft Surgery Trialists Collaboration. Lancet 344: 563–570.

Further Reading

Cooke F, Metcalfe H (2000) Cardiac monitoring 1. Nursing Times 96(23): 45–46.

Cooke F, Metcalfe H (2000) Cardiac monitoring 2. Nursing Times 96(25): 45–46.

A well illustrated and brief guide to attaching a patient to bedside cardiac monitoring.

Farrelly R (2000) Congenital heart disease 1. Nursing Times 96(24): 47–50.

Farrelly R (2000) Congenital heart disease 2. Nursing Times 96(28): 43–46.

A well illustrated and briefly explained overview of the more common congenital heart defects in children, with a guide to current treatments.

Feather C (2001) Equipment for blood pressure measurement. Professional Nurse 16(11): 1458–1462.

A useful paper which provides information on the variety of blood pressure devices and the importance of choosing those that are known to be reliable, in recording this important haemodynamic parameter.

Hampton JR (1997) The ECG made easy, 5th edn. Edinburgh: Churchill Livingstone.

A popular and valuable handbook from the basics to the more advanced practice of ECG interpretation.

Hatchett R (1998) The principles of augmenting the cardiac output in adults. Intensive and Critical Care Nursing 14(5): 244–251.

A paper that uses a case study approach to allow the nurse to understand the various approaches to augmenting the patient's cardiac output and hence the oxygen tissue perfusion.

MacDermott AFN (2001) Approaches to improving outcomes in stable angina. Professional Nurse 16(8): 1302–1305.

An excellent overview paper of the management of stable angina, with an emphasis on the requirements of care outlined in the national service framework for coronary heart disease.

MacDermott AFN (2001) Reducing symptoms and improving outcomes in patients with angina. Professional Nurse 17(2): 103–106.

A further paper that reviews the initial treatment of stable angina and the secondary prevention of a cardiovascular event.

McGhie AI, ed. (2001) Handbook of non-invasive cardiac testing. London: Arnold.

There is an array of non-invasive cardiac investigations the patient may undergo from exercise electrocardiography, to echocardiography and nuclear cardiology tests. This useful handbook dedicates specific chapters to all of these tests, allowing the healthcare professional to allay fears and explain the procedures to patients and loved ones.

Riley J, Blue L (2001) Assessing and managing chronic heart failure. Professional Nurse 16(5): 1112–115.

A useful paper offering a general overview of the aetiology, presentation and assessment of a person with chronic heart failure. The body's more long-term compensatory mechanisms to this condition are presented briefly.

Stewart S, Blue L, eds (2001) Improving outcomes in chronic heart failure. London: BMJ Books.

A valuable research-based book for those involved in managing patients with chronic heart failure. It is aimed notably at nurse-led practice, where manipulation of medications to specific protocols, health promotion and psychological support is given. Its weakness is a lack of exploration of the education and support needed for nurses who are, or who wish to practise in, this area of increasing autonomy.

Swanton RH (1998) Cardiology, 4th edn. Oxford: Blackwell Science.

A very useful but detailed handbook, from the well respected cardiologist, which provides a quick reference to the many presenting cardiac conditions.

13

Caring for the patient with a respiratory disorder

Alyson Dickson and Graham Martindale

Introduction

Respiratory structures

Assessment

Specific disorders

Patients requiring respiratory assistance

Patients requiring mechanical ventilation

Localized airway obstruction

Summary

Introduction

Health problems affecting breathing and the respiratory system strike at the very root of human well-being and are common in a wide range of patients. Illness affecting the respiratory system ranges from acute life-threatening episodes (e.g. an acute asthmatic attack) to long-term debilitating conditions such as chronic bronchitis. Other systems of the body, particularly the cardiovascular system, are often involved. The consequences of such health problems are not only physical: severe psychological distress can also occur and be accompanied by major social disruption. After a brief overview of relevant anatomy and physiology, this chapter examines the assessment of patients with respiratory disorders before looking at some of the more specific issues relating to the care and treatment of patients with specific disorders.

Respiratory structures

The structures concerned with **ventilation** are the upper and lower respiratory tracts, respiratory muscles, thorax and portions of the nervous system (Fig. 13.1).

Upper respiratory tract

The upper airway is formed by the nose, mouth, pharynx and larynx. It serves as a passageway for air being inspired and expired; filters, warms and moistens the

inhaled air; and provides the protective reflexes of sneezing and the closing off of the larynx to prevent aspiration of fluid and solids. Irritation of the pharynx and larynx may also initiate the cough reflex.

Lower respiratory tract

The lower tract consists of the trachea, bronchi and two lungs. The trachea continues to warm and filter the inspired air. It divides into the two *primary bronchi* known as the right main bronchus and the left bronchus. The right bronchus is wider and shorter than the left and any foreign object that is inhaled tends to lodge in the right bronchus (Hinchliff et al 1996). The bronchi subdivide into the *bronchioles*, which in turn lead to the respiratory bronchioles. At the terminal end of each respiratory bronchiole is a thin-walled sac known as an *alveolus*. The alveoli are covered by networks of capillaries and it is in this part of the respiratory tract that gaseous exchange takes place.

Assessment

Nursing assessment of a patient with a respiratory disorder

When making an initial assessment of a patient, nurses need to use their skills of observation, measurement and

Ventilation of the lungs
See chapter 5.3

Figure 13.1 The respiratory system.

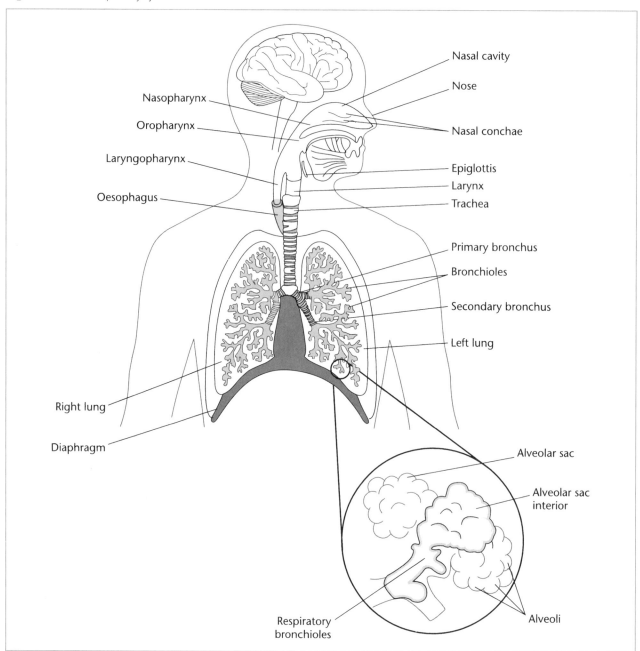

interpersonal communication. Information may be gathered from the patient, their relatives or significant others, and other members of the multidisciplinary team. Depending upon the patient's condition, the nurse will need to prioritize the information required to plan immediate care, adding to this at a later time when necessary and possible.

On first meeting the patient the nurse should take an overview of his or her general appearance in order to gain a feeling for the overall health status of the patient. The facial expression might give clues as to

mood; colouring should be noted to check for signs of a flushed, red appearance that might indicate pyrexia. Cyanosis (a bluish discoloration around the lips that is a late sign of severe respiratory failure) may be noted. The patient's posture should be observed to note whether it indicates a sense of ease and relaxation or anxiety and tenseness, associated perhaps with difficulty in breathing.

The nurse seeks to obtain information about the person's respiratory function, past history related to respiratory disorders and treatment programme, in order to identify factors that contribute to the promotion as well as any impairment of airway clearance. The information the nurse obtains from the patient and/or others should include:

- the symptoms that prompted the patient to seek health care
- a description of the precipitating events
- duration of the symptoms
- the person's perception of the causes and implications of the symptoms.

Possible symptoms manifested by the patient are described below.

Cough The presence, frequency and depth of the **cough** are noted as well as the nature and sound. The PQRST symptom analysis tool (see p. 258) should be used for an accurate description of the cough:

P *Provocation/palliation*: Does anything in particular bring on the cough (e.g. smoking) or relieve it (e.g. cough linctus from the chemists).

Q *Quality*: Is it hard and racking, croup-like, hacking, shallow, deep and rattling, or having a whooping sound? Does it produce sputum; if so, what colour is this?

R *Region/radiation*: Does coughing produce any sensations that are felt deep in the chest or localized to any particular area?

S *Severity*: Does the cough disrupt everyday life or prevent sleeping? Is it associated with pain? Is the cough getting worse or better?

T *Time*: How long have you had the cough? Is it worse at any particular time such as at night?

Sputum It is necessary to determine the consistency (mucoid, watery, purulent, tenacious, frothy or blood streaked), colour, smell and amount, and whether the amount has increased recently.

Breathlessness The patient may complain of breathlessness and the history should reveal whether it occurs with usual activity, increased effort or when at rest, and whether it interferes with daily activities and sleep pattern. It should be noted whether the patient's speech is audible, clear and effortless, or whether the responses are weak, short and jerky phrases with apparent effort. The patient is questioned as to what was done to prevent or modify the breathlessness and whether the suggested actions were effective in preventing or alleviating the breathlessness.

Fever/pyrexia The patient may have a **fever** and give a history of having night sweats. The recording of the patient's temperature should therefore form part of a baseline assessment against which changes can be monitored.

Pain and discomfort This may be associated with the chest, breathing activities or coughing; the nature of the **pain**, its severity, duration and precipitating factors should be noted alongside any strategies that the patient has found useful in relieving or lessening the discomfort.

The patient's understanding of the respiratory problems should be explored carefully. If the patient is severely distressed, questions should be kept to a minimum and if possible asked in such a way that they may be answered by a nod or shake of the head. More detailed discussions should be saved until the patient's breathing is easier.

Observation of whether the airway is patent, followed by assessment of respiratory rate, depth and rhythm, may identify serious problems immediately, and in all patients provides a vital basic record that can be used as a baseline to monitor subsequent progress. The tongue of an unconscious patient may, for example, block the airway. If the brain is deprived of oxygen, serious damage occurs within 3 minutes. Any obstruction to the upper airway is potentially fatal within minutes, hence the importance of always beginning an assessment by checking that the upper airway is clear.

Assessment of respiration

To avoid the patient being conscious of having the breathing monitored, which may affect the rate, it is suggested that the respiratory rate is taken immediately after the pulse, while still holding the patient's wrist. The healthy adult breathes 12–18 times per minute at rest, although this rate is much quicker in infants – 40 breaths per minute is typical of a newborn baby. A rapid respiratory rate (*tachypnoea*) in an adult may indicate anxiety, pain, pyrexia, metabolic disorders (e.g. acidosis) or may be the result of the body attempting to compensate for inadequate oxygenation due to a wide range of cardiovascular and respiratory disorders (e.g. heart failure or shock). Slower breathing rates are associated with sleep or with disorders and drugs that depress the respiratory centre (e.g. opioids).

Observation of the thorax should also be carried out to note its shape, size and symmetry, in addition to forming an impression about the amount of effort involved in breathing. Long-standing respiratory disease leads to a characteristic pigeon chest shape. Paradoxical chest movements (i.e. one part of the chest wall appears to move in the opposite direction from the rest of the chest wall) indicate ribs fractured in two places, known as a *flail segment*. This is potentially fatal as the ensuing lung collapse may make it impossible for the patient to achieve sufficient ventilation to be compatible with life.

Unequal participation of the two sides of the chest in respiratory movements may be evident, or unusual retraction or ballooning of the intercostal spaces may occur. For example, in patients with atelectasis or pneumothorax, in which a part or all of the lung is not being inflated, there is diminished movement of the chest wall on the affected side. Similarly, this may occur if a large section of alveoli is consolidated with fluid or secretions.

Coughing
See chapter 5.3

Fever
See chapter 6.1

Pain
See chapter 2.3

Excessive retraction or ballooning is associated with extreme difficulty in getting air in or out of the air passages.

Breathing pattern

Normal respirations are regular, effortless and quiet. Irregularities in breathing may relate to rate, volume, rhythm or the ease with which the person breathes. The following terms are used to indicate characteristic breathing patterns:

- *Eupnoea* is quiet, normal breathing at the rate of about 12–18 times per minute in the adult. Respirations are more rapid and shallow in the infant and preschool child, gradually reaching adult levels by the age of 10–12 years.

- *Tachypnoea* is rapid breathing, usually with reduced tidal volume.

- *Bradypnoea* is an abnormally slow rate of respiration.

- *Hyperpnoea* is an increase in the volume of air breathed per minute due to an increase in either the rate or depth of respirations, or to both.

- *Dyspnoea* refers to a subjective awareness of a disturbance in breathing. The patient experiences discomfort and/or the need for increased effort or work in ventilation. The individual's perception of difficult breathing or shortness of breath may be due to physiological or psychological stress. The experience of **dyspnoea** is anxiety provoking because the person knows that breathing is essential to life; the emotional reaction tends to aggravate and perpetuate the problem further. The individual may describe it as tightness in the chest, shortness of breath, unable to get enough air, or suffocating. The dyspnoeic patient frequently has a distressed appearance, is restless and may be perspiring. The difficulty may be present only on exertion and may be episodic. The frequency of the episodes and whether their occurrence is related to a particular time of day, activity or certain situations or factors are noted.

- *Orthopnoea* is dyspnoea which is present when the patient is lying down but is relieved to some extent by sitting up.

- *Cheyne–Stokes* respiration is characterized by a few seconds of apnoea followed by respirations that gradually increase in frequency and volume to a peak intensity and then gradually subside to a period of apnoea. This pattern is cyclical.

- *Biot's pattern* of breathing is characterized by a few respirations varying in volume, followed by a prolonged period of apnoea.

- *Kussmaul's* respirations are rapid and very deep.

Dyspnoea
See chapter 5.3

Other factors

When completing an initial assessment or as part of the ongoing assessment the nurse would also seek to gather information on the following factors.

Past history of respiratory disorders and treatment programme   The person is asked whether there has been any recent trauma or surgery to the chest or respiratory passages, or any respiratory infections. The existence of any associated health problems is also determined. Information is obtained about all prescription and non-prescription drugs the person has been taking regularly or intermittently. The name, dosage, frequency, purpose and perceived effectiveness of each drug is noted (if the patient is able to supply this information).

Health-promoting behaviours and risk factors   Assessment includes data about factors in the person's lifestyle and health habits that promote respiratory efficiency or increase the risk for problems. Exercise, diet, weight and utilization of the health service should be assessed. Information should be obtained about possible exposure to infectious agents; smoking habits including what is smoked, how often and for how long; the existence of any known allergies, the name of the agent and the nature of the reaction when exposed to it. Any risk factors or irritants to which the person is exposed at work, home or in the community should be noted.

The person's perceptions of altered respiratory status   The person's perception of their current health and attitude towards known risk factors such as smoking should be determined. It is important also to recognize which factors are beyond the control of the patient, such as working conditions, air pollution or poverty, and consider ways in which their effects may be reduced. Giving up work or moving away from a city may not be feasible or acceptable to the patient.

The nurse also assesses the individual's understanding of previously prescribed treatment. It is important to determine why the person sought health care and what his or her goals are for care. What does the individual state as the priority for care? Many respiratory problems are chronic in nature and it is therefore important that the person recognizes the long-term nature of the illness and the implications of this. Family support should be discussed to discover something of the social setting the patient has come from and will return to, as that setting may have significant influence over his or her health.

Pulse oximetry

Pulse oximetry is a non-invasive measurement of arterial oxygen saturation. Some 97% of the oxygen transported in the bloodstream is attached to haemoglobin (Hb) within red blood cells. The other 3% is dissolved in the plasma. When haemoglobin is carrying its maximum amount of oxygen (four molecules per Hb molecule) it is considered saturated; the extent to which this occurs is referred to as oxygen saturation or 'sats' for short.

To interpret oxygen saturation readings, Hb levels must be known. If the patient is anaemic (low Hb level), less oxygen is required to provide a high oxygen saturation. However, the total amount of oxygen in the bloodstream could be inadequate for metabolic requirements and the patient may be hypoxic despite an apparently satisfactory oxygen saturation reading on the pulse oximeter.

Pulse oximetry works by measuring the transmission of red and infrared light across a pulsatile arterial bed, such as a finger or earlobe. As these beams of light are transmitted, oxygenated haemoglobin absorbs more infrared light. Deoxygenated blood absorbs more red light. The pulse oximeter processor then determines how much of each type of light has been absorbed to calculate the saturated oxygen value.

Normal Hb levels and tissue perfusion are essential if oximetry readings are to provide an accurate picture of the amount of oxygen in the bloodstream. Abnormal Hb concentration, very low levels of normal Hb or severe tissue underperfusion (shock) can undermine the accuracy of oximetry readings. Temperature and blood pH also affect the relationship between saturation levels measured by oximetry and the actual amount of oxygen in the bloodstream as measured by the partial oxygen pressure (Po_2). Therefore, whilst the oxygen saturation is a useful measure of respiratory function, it should be combined with other measures of blood chemistry to obtain an accurate picture of patient progress.

Patient movement may cause interference with the oximeter reading, introducing inaccuracy. If blood pressure is being measured on the same arm, inflation of the cuff will affect saturation readings as arterial blood flow is temporarily impeded. Nail polish should be removed as this will interfere with the transmission of light through the nailbed and hence the oximeter reading, if the probe is attached to a finger. Finally, limb oedema may impede absorption of red and infrared light. If the patient has peripheral oedema, extra care should be taken not to cause pressure damage with the finger probe. When nursing the patient, the nurse should observe the probe site for pressure tissue damage. Frequently moving the probe to other digits will prevent this.

Peak flow rate measurement

One final method of assessment that the nurse may use is to measure peak flow rates for the patient. This is a test of the maximum rate of exhalation (**peak expiratory flow rate**) a patient can achieve (in litres per minute) by the patient blowing as hard as possible into a simple instrument. This assesses the degree of impairment in respiratory function due to airway narrowing in diseases such as asthma.

The nurse needs to instruct the patient on how to use the peak flow meter and should ensure that the patient adopts a position that is both comfortable and facilitates the greatest lung expansion (ideally the patient should stand). After taking a deep breath in, the patient should try to ensure that the mouth is closed around the mouthpiece, then exhale as deeply and rapidly as possible. It is usual practice to ask the patient to do this three times, with the best result being recorded. In addition to recording the result, the type of peak flow meter used should also be recorded as different instruments have been shown to give varying results (Sharp 1993). Peak flow meters have been available on prescription since 1990 and many patients now monitor their own respiratory function at home.

Medical assessment and related investigations

A range of techniques is employed to assess respiratory function. Although formerly the sole preserve of the medical profession, other health staff such as nurse practitioners and physiotherapists are now incorporating these techniques into their practice in order that they may expand their role. A fuller account of these techniques can be found in Walsh et al (1999).

Physical examination of the chest and breathing pattern

Inspection

Thorax

Normally, the thorax is symmetrical. It is important to note any difference on either side and any apparent abnormality in the shape or bony framework of the thorax. Scoliosis or kyphosis may interfere with normal breathing. If the chest is barrel shaped, this may indicate chronic airflow limitation. A funnel-shaped chest is characterized by depression of the sternum, whereas a pigeon chest involves an outward location of the sternum and inward depression of the first few ribs with minimal impairment of breathing.

Chest movements associated with respirations

The frequency, rhythm and depth of respirations are noted by observing the chest. The thorax is normally symmetrical. On inspiration, as the diaphragm descends, the lower rib cage moves slightly outward and upward. The upper rib cage simultaneously expands slightly. Expiration is a passive process of elastic recoil and of slightly longer duration than inspiration. A short pause occurs before the next inspiration

Accessory muscles

Rhythmic movement of the diaphragm is observed with normal respiration. Use of the accessory muscles indicates some degree of respiratory distress and is characterized by retraction of the supraclavicular and

Pulse oximetry
See chapter 5.3

PEFR
See chapter 5.3

suprasternal areas and elevation of the shoulders during inspiration. Enlargement of the accessory muscles, particularly the sternocleidomastoid muscles, occurs with chronic airflow limitation.

Palpation

This method of examination is used to assess chest excursion, symmetry, structural abnormalities and tenderness.

Chest excursion and symmetry

The chest excursion on inspiration reflects the extent of expansion and depth of respiration. It may be assessed by placing the hands on the chest with the fingers slightly outspread and the thumbs just meeting at the midline (Fig. 13.2). As the patient breathes in, the hands are normally separated by the chest expansion. Whether the range of the chest excursion is the same on both sides is also noted; if it is equal, the thumbs are moved an equal distance from the midline on each side. Normally the movements of the two sides are symmetrical.

Functional assessment

Functional assessment and investigations of the patient's effort tolerance are carried out to determine how energy expenditure in performing various activities may be reduced and how the environment may be modified to facilitate functioning:

1. The patient's level of daily activity should be assessed, especially the ability to:
   a. feed self
   b. dress, shave or shower without assistance
   c. climb stairs unaided
   d. perform household activities such as vacuuming, making beds, preparing food
   e. carry out strenuous activity at work.

Figure 13.2   Assessing the chest excursion on inspiration.

2. Factors that bring on breathlessness should be assessed:
   a. simple daily tasks such as shaving, dressing, tying shoelaces
   b. extra effort such as climbing stairs
   c. during the night
   d. getting up in the morning?

3. Steps that the person takes to relieve breathlessness should be noted such as using a bronchodilator before activity.

4. *Effort tolerance* may be assessed with the use of a treadmill. A chair should be available in case the patient needs to stop and rest. The resting heart rate is recorded as well as the pulse rate on completion of the test. An oximeter is used to determine changes in arterial oxygen saturation associated with the exercise. The test estimates the patient's horizontal walking capacity. This information assists in planning an acceptable daily routine and an exercise programme to increase effort tolerance.

5. Further data are obtained to identify how the patient perceives the respiratory dysfunction. Questions that could be asked include:
   a. What does it mean to the patient?
   b. What losses in functioning are most relevant to the patient?
   c. What losses is he or she able to accept?
   d. How does he or she feel about it?
   e. Is the attitude one of hopeless resignation or unrealistic denial?
   f. Is the patient motivated to pursue a self-care programme?

Breath sounds

The bell end of the stethoscope is best used to listen to breath sounds (auscultation). Normal respirations present characteristic sounds as air enters and leaves the lower respiratory tract. Absence of such sounds or the accompaniment of other sounds may indicate excessive secretions in an area or constriction or blockage of an airway in a section of the lung:

■ *Vesicular breath sounds* are heard in normal respirations. They are a soft, low-pitched sound and are heard over all the lung areas except over the main bronchi. The inspiratory phase of a vesicular sound is longer and louder than the expiratory phase. The differences may be attributed to the movement of inspiratory air into progressively smaller air passages (and vice versa in the case of the air being exhaled).

■ *Bronchial breath sounds* are associated with equal inspiratory and expiratory phases. The sounds are higher pitched and equally loud in both phases. They are abnormal and indicate consolidation of alveoli due to fibrosis or a disease process such as pneumonia.

■ *Adventitious sounds* are abnormal sounds superimposed on breath sounds as a result of a disease process within the tracheobronchial tree and/or lungs. These include crackles, wheezes and pleural friction rub:

— *Crackles* (*rales* or *crepitations*) are described as fizzing or popping sounds created by the equalization of airway pressures during the explosive reopening of previously collapsed airways closed on inspiration, or by air bubbling through pulmonary oedema

— *Wheezes* (rhonchi) are whistling, musical sounds associated with spasm of the bronchial walls and tend to occur on expiration

— *Stridor* is a distinctive sound heard on inspiration when there is partial airway obstruction; a totally obstructed airway is usually silent as there is no air movement to produce any sound

— *Pleural friction rub* is a characteristic rough, grating sound produced when inflamed roughened pleurae rub against each other on inspiration. It becomes audible during the latter part of the inspiratory phase.

Pulmonary function tests (Table 13.1)

Lung volumes may be determined by spirometry at the bedside, in the clinic, health centre or patient's home.

(Spirometry is the measurement of air taken into and expelled from the lungs.) Changes in lung volumes provide the best objective measurement of airflow limitation. Lung volume determinations are used to identify potential risks of respiratory complications in preoperative patients and to monitor changes in the postoperative period. Vital capacity (VC) and timed forced expiratory volume (FEV) are used most frequently at the bedside.

The normal values for the different lung volumes have been established from studies made on normal subjects. They vary with height, age and sex; tables of normal values are available.

■ *Vital capacity* (VC) is represented by the maximal volume of air exhaled following a maximal inspiration. To determine the VC, the individual breathes through a mouthpiece that is connected to a tube leading to a spirometer. The normal VC ranges from 3500 to 5000 mL. The VC provides information about compliance, which is the effort required to stretch the lung. Diseased lung requires more effort to achieve expansion and hence is said to have less compliance.

■ *Tidal volume* (V_T) is the volume of air exhaled following a normal breath. The normal is usually stated as being 450–500 mL with the individual at rest, but varies with individuals and their activities. *Minute ventilation* (or minute respiratory volume) is

Lung function tests
See chapter 5.3

Table 13.1 Summary of pulmonary function measurement

Test	Description	Comments
Vital capacity (VC)	The maximal volume of air exhaled following a maximal inspiration (normal: 3500–5000 mL)	Reduced in restrictive airway disease because of limited lung expansion. In obstructive airway disease, the total lung capacity is increased but VC may be reduced due to air trapping with increased residual volume
Tidal volume (V_T)	The volume of air exhaled following a normal breath (normal: 450–500 mL)	
Forced vital capacity (FVC)	The maximum volume of air that can be forcibly and rapidly exhaled following a maximal inspiration	Reduced in obstructive airway disease due to air trapping
Timed vital capacity (FEV_t)	The percentage of vital capacity that can be expelled in 1 s (FEV_1), 2 s (FEV_2) and 3 s (FEV_3) (normal ranges: FEV_1, 80%; FEV_2, 90%; FEV_3, 95%)	Reduced in obstructive airway disease because of increased airway resistance; usually normal in restrictive airway disease
Residual volume (RV)	The volume of gas remaining in the lungs at the end of a maximal expiration (normal: 25–40% of total lung capacity, e.g. 1500 mL)	Increased in obstructive airway disease
Functional residual capacity (FRC)	The volume of air remaining in the lung after a passive exhalation in normal breathing (normal: about 3000 mL)	Increased in obstructive airway disease

determined by multiplying the tidal volume by the number of respirations per minute.

- *Forced vital capacity* (FVC) is the maximum volume of air that can be forcibly and rapidly exhaled following a maximal inspiration.

- *Peak expiratory flow rate* (PEFR) measures the maximum rate at which air can be exhaled.

- *Timed forced expiratory volume* (FEV_t) records the percentage of vital capacity that can be expelled in 1 second (FEV_1). Normally about 80% of the vital capacity is expired in 1 second. FEV_t provides information about the resistance to expiratory airflow.

- *Residual volume* (RV) is the volume of gas remaining in the lungs at the end of a maximal expiration.

- *Functional residual capacity* (FRC) is the air remaining in the lung after passive exhalation in normal breathing; no forceful or increased effort is used.

Radiological examination

Chest radiography

Radiological studies of the chest may reveal a lesion in the respiratory tract or thoracic cavity, its location, the size of the area involved and something of the nature of the lesion. They also provide information about the mediastinum, the structure of the thorax, the size of the heart and aorta, and the level of the diaphragm.

The procedure is explained to the patient and clothing is removed to the waist to prevent the possibility of objects such as buttons obscuring the X-ray films. If the patient is wearing an identification tag or necklace, it is also removed; a gown is provided. The patient is advised to take a deep breath and hold it while the radiograph is being taken in order to ensure the lungs are fully expanded and there is no movement to blur the image formed on the film. The patient is then told to breathe normally.

Radiological investigation may include making a series of films of the lungs at different planes. This type of radiology is referred to as *plain film tomography*. In these films the lung tissue is visualized at different depths. They provide details that are not revealed in ordinary radiographs because of overlying structures. Tomograms are helpful in recognizing solid or calcified lesions and cavitations.

Computed tomography is a cross-sectional imaging modality that provides unique information about the lung fields and mediastinum. It is particularly useful in identifying small pulmonary nodules (e.g. early metastases), calcified foci and the degree of invasion of a malignant lesion (e.g. mediastinal involvement from a primary bronchial carcinoma). Such information may not be detected by other techniques.

Fluoroscopic examination (direct viewing by X-ray) of the chest may be done to view lung expansion and the respiratory excursion of the diaphragm.

Blood gases
See chapter 5.3

Pulmonary and bronchial angiography

Pulmonary arteriography may be performed via a catheter suitably placed in a large systemic vein (superior or inferior vena cava), the right side of the heart or the pulmonary artery. An injected radio-opaque contrast medium will depict the pulmonary circulation and confirm or exclude the presence of pulmonary emboli. The nature and extent of arteriovenous malformations can also be delineated.

The bronchial arteries arise from the thoracic aorta; they may be selectively catheterized and their circulation studied. The usual indication is to establish the site of bleeding from a chronic cavity. Once found, the radiologist has the facility to embolize the main feeding artery, occluding the vessel and thereby controlling the haemorrhage.

Perfusion lung scan

This provides images in multiple views of the distribution of blood flow to the lung. Small aggregates of albumin 1540 mm in size are labelled with technetium-99m and injected into a vein. These flow to and then stick in the first capillary bed they meet, which is the pulmonary capillary bed. Images of their distribution are made with a γ camera. This is the most sensitive non-invasive test of decreased blood flow to small regions of the lung.

Biochemical and haematological measurements

Blood gas analysis

Impairment of respiratory ventilation and gas exchange are reflected in changes in the levels of **blood gases**. Normal values are shown in Table 13.2. A blood specimen for gas analysis is withdrawn using an heparinized syringe, usually from the femoral artery, and any air is expelled from the syringe before it is covered with a cap to prevent atmospheric gas exchange (Szaflarski 1996). If the sample remains at room temperature it must be analysed within 10 minutes; otherwise the syringe is placed on ice in a special labelled container and sent promptly to the laboratory (samples stored on ice should be analysed within 1 hour) (Clutton-Brock 1997). Firm

Table 13.2   Normal values of blood gases

	Normal value
Pa_{O_2}	11–13.3 kPa (80–100 mmHg)
Pa_{CO_2}	4.8–6.0 kPa (35–45 mmHg)
pH	7.35–7.45
$[H^+]$	35–45 nmol/L
Plasma carbon dioxide level	20–32 mmol/L (20–32 mEq/L)
Arterial oxyhaemoglobin saturation	95–97%

pressure is applied to the arterial puncture site for at least 7 minutes, or until bleeding has ceased; it is then protected with a sterile covering.

Electrolyte concentrations

Determination of electrolyte values, particularly hydrogen carbonate ions (2428 mmol/L) is necessary to interpret changes in acid–base balance.

Erythrocyte count, haemoglobin and haematocrit determination

It is important to know whether the erythrocyte count is normal because erythrocytes contain the haemoglobin that carries the oxygen. Similarly, an assessment of the patient includes a determination of the haemoglobin concentration. Obviously, a deficiency of red blood cells or haemoglobin may produce an oxygen deficiency. The haematocrit represents the percentage of erythrocytes by volume. Normal values are shown in Table 13.3.

Leucocyte count

A total and differential count of the white blood cells may be ordered since this information may be useful in confirming infection and distinguishing between an acute disease, such as pneumonia, and a chronic one, such as tuberculosis (see p. 352).

Bacteriological and cytological studies

Specimens of sputum, throat secretions, pleural fluid or tissue may be examined for pathogenic organisms and/or malignant cells.

Sputum is examined microscopically in a smear or by culture for disease organisms, bronchial casts, eosinophils and cancer cells. Tests are also done to identify the antimicrobial drug(s) (usually antibiotics) to which the infecting organisms present in the sputum are sensitive. This denotes the drugs that will be effective for the patient. Ideally the sputum specimen should be collected first thing in the morning, because the secretions that accumulate during the night may have a higher

Table 13.3 Normal values for erythrocyte count, haemoglobin and haematocrit

	Normal value
Erythrocyte count	
Men	4.5–6.5 × 10^{12}/L
Women	3.8–5.8 × 10^{12}/L
Haemoglobin concentration	
Men	13–19 g/dL
Women	12–15 g/dL
Haematocrit	
Men	40–50%
Women	37–47%

concentration of organisms. The mouth should be clean and free of residual food particles. The patient is given a small sputum container and is instructed to cough deeply to raise the sputum from the lungs. When the specimen is obtained, the container is labelled and delivered to the laboratory. Sputum specimens may be collected during or after postural drainage. They may also be obtained by tracheal aspiration if the patient is unconscious or too weak to cough. The sputum specimen container is attached to the suction catheter, which allows the sputum to flow directly into the container.

Bacteriological studies may also be made of secretions from the *throat* and *pleura*.

Skin tests for tuberculosis

A tuberculin skin test is used in the diagnosis of tuberculosis and to identify those who have been exposed. The test involves an intradermal injection of tuberculin bacillus extract using a syringe and needle (Mantoux test) or a multiple puncture apparatus (Heaf, Tine or Mono-Vac). Tuberculin extract preparations include purified protein derivative (PPD) and old tuberculin (OT), which are available in several strengths. The forearm is the usual site of inoculation. Results are interpreted in 48–72 hours. A positive reaction is characterized by an area of induration of 10 mm or greater.

Histological examinations

When a malignancy is suspected a biopsy of the tumour is usually taken.

Bronchial biopsy Bronchial tissue can be examined visually by means of a bronchoscope, and samples of tissue and cells may be obtained by brushing or aspirating secretions from the involved areas.

Lung biopsy A lung biopsy may be necessary to confirm the diagnosis when radiological studies reveal pulmonary infiltration or lesions. Lung tissue can be obtained for examination by open thoracotomy, bronchoscopy or percutaneous needle biopsy. Transbronchial biopsy involves the introduction of a bronchoscope and the insertion of long flexible forceps into the involved area. Small samples of tissue may be obtained in this manner. Percutaneous needle biopsy involves the insertion of a needle into the diseased area to obtain a small sample of tissue. The procedure is useful when the lesion is localized, but other diseased areas may be missed.

Lymph node biopsy The scalene lymph nodes, which are situated in a pad of fat anterior to the scalenus anterior muscle in the neck, drain the lungs and mediastinum. The nodes are examined histologically to help determine the spread of bronchogenic carcinoma and the indications for surgical resection or the prognosis in diseases such as sarcoidosis, tuberculosis or lymphomas such as Hodgkin's disease.

Blood values
See chapter 4.1

Pleural biopsy Pleural fluid and tissue may be obtained during open thoracotomy but are usually obtained by thoracocentesis. A specially designed needle is inserted into the pleura and samples are taken. Tissue from several sites may be required to confirm a diagnosis of tuberculosis or a malignancy.

Specific disorders

Disorders of the lower respiratory tract

Pneumonia

Pneumonia is the term generally used to indicate infection and inflammation of lung tissue. Haslett et al (1999) define pneumonia as an acute respiratory illness with shadowing on the chest radiograph. It is an inflammatory condition of the lung in which the alveoli are usually filled with fluid and blood cells. Pneumonia is classified as community or hospital acquired due to the significance of potentially resistant bacterial strains in the treatment of the illness. This is a particular problem in hospital-acquired pneumonia. It is obviously imperative that the patient be treated with the correct antibiotic regimen to be effective against the causative organism. A further important category of patients who may develop pneumonia are immunocompromised persons, such as those with acquired immune deficiency syndrome (AIDS).

Pneumonia caused by pneumococci is a common type of pneumonia, but other bacteria or viruses may be the cause. Non-bacterial and non-viral causes include: aspiration of gastric secretions, food, fluids or lipoids (*aspiration pneumonia*), and retention of secretions, which occurs frequently in the immobilized elderly or debilitated individual (*hypostatic pneumonia*).

It should be remembered that the most common respiratory complication faced by individuals with human immunodeficiency virus (HIV) infection is *Pneumocystis carinii* pneumonia (PCP). The individual with PCP may be critically ill and is likely to present with a dry, non-productive cough, shortness of breath, high fever and night sweats. PCP may be difficult to diagnose as the individual may have a normal chest radiograph and breath sounds. Bilateral infiltrates are likely to be present in an abnormal chest radiograph. Diagnosis is usually made by cultures obtained by bronchoscopy.

PCP is readily treated with antibiotic regimens. Combinations of drugs such as trimethoprim–sulfamethoxazole (TMP/SMX) and dapsone or pentamidine may be used to treat the infection. These drugs must be used with caution because of their side-effects. For example, TMP/SMX may cause severe rash. Pentamidine given intravenously can cause nausea, orthostatic hypotension and hypoglycaemia.

Prophylactic regimens are also effective in preventing PCP. Prophylaxis is available to patients using a decreased amount of the above medications. Pentamidine when used for prophylaxis is given in aerosol form, generally with a hand-held nebulizer. Prophylactic regimens are usually initiated when the patient's T4 count drops below 200 000 cells/L. The patient is taught to assess for signs of infection and learns to monitor respiratory rate and function. Nursing care is similar to that for other patients experiencing respiratory impairment.

Manifestations

The onset, symptoms and course of disease vary with different types of pneumonia. Infection of the alveoli results in their filling with inflammatory exudate (plasma, blood cells, pathological organisms and cellular debris) that readily overflows into other alveoli, extending the infection. A whole lobe of lung tissue may become consolidated or the consolidation may be patchy; pulmonary ventilation and diffusion are impaired, and the oxygen tension of the blood is reduced to below normal. The P_{CO_2} level generally remains normal or may be decreased. The increased respiratory rate caused by the initial increase in the P_{CO_2} results in increased amounts of carbon dioxide being excreted by the normal areas of the lung. Within a few days the exudate becomes more liquid and may be gradually eliminated from the alveoli by expectoration and absorption. This process is referred to as *resolution*. The disease may clear up with dramatic rapidity when specific antibacterial drugs are administered. It may run a course of 5–10 days; untreated, it may rapidly prove fatal.

The onset of some infective pneumonias may be very sudden; they frequently begin with a chill, followed by fever (e.g. pneumococcal). Hypostatic, staphylococcal and atypical (viral) pneumonias have a gradual onset (less abrupt than the pneumococcal type). The last two may be associated at the onset with upper respiratory infection.

The pulse rate and respirations increase. The latter may be shallow and accompanied by an audible grunt characteristic of pleuritic pain. The nostrils flare on inspiration and the face may be flushed. Cyanosis of the lips, tongue and nailbeds may develop. The patient's cough may be hacking, painful and unproductive at first; later, it becomes less painful and is productive. In bronchopneumonia the sputum is tenacious, blood streaked and mucopurulent. In pneumococcal pneumonia, the sputum is usually rust coloured and becomes purulent as resolution takes place.

The patient experiences general malaise, weakness, headache and aching pains. The leucocyte count is raised in some types for pneumonia (e.g. pneumococcal, staphylococcal) and normal or below normal in others (e.g. atypical). Sputum examination and culture, blood culture and serology are used to identify the causative organism. Specific antimicrobial therapy is determined by culture and sensitivity tests.

Pneumonia
See chapter 5.3

An example of a clinical situation is described in Case Study 13.1.

Case Study 13.1

George Fleming was an emergency admission to the medical unit with a diagnosis of right lower lobe pneumonia. Upon admission, a thorough nursing history and assessment were completed. Further data were obtained from his daughter and from the results of diagnostic tests and additional assessments as they became available on his health record. Relevant findings included:

- *General appearance*. George was a well nourished man in his mid-seventies, with obvious respiratory distress and diaphoresis.

- *Vital signs*. Respirations were rapid at 32 per min; pulse was 110 per min; and oral temperature was raised to 38.2°C.

- *Respirations* were laboured with moderate retraction of the intercostal spaces. Crackles and wheezes were heard over the right middle and lower chest on auscultation. No abnormal breath sounds were heard over the left lung.

- *Cough* was dry and hacking, producing a small amount of blood-streaked sputum.

- *Pain and discomfort*. The patient experienced occasional episodes of stabbing chest pain that increased with respirations and travelled to his right shoulder.

- *Cognitive and perceptual status*. The patient was oriented to person but was confused as to time and place.

- *Chest radiography* demonstrated consolidation in the right lower lobe.

- *Sputum analysis* showed a positive Gram stain for bacterial pneumococci.

- *White blood cell count* was increased to 17 000 per mL.

- *Arterial blood gas* analysis showed a raised Pa_{CO_2} of 52 mmHg, a decreased Pa_{O_2} of 70 mmHg, and a decreased oxygen saturation level of 86%.

- *Psychosocial history*. George is retired. He lives alone in the home that he and his wife occupied until her death 3 years ago. His only daughter lives nearby.

The patient's daughter stated that her father was normally bright, alert and oriented. He was an active participant in planning and organizing events for the local pensioner's group. He had complained of a cold and flu-like symptoms a few weeks ago, but seemed to be improving. His present illness had come on suddenly.

Based upon an analysis of available data, the following major patient problems were identified:

1. The patient is unable to achieve normal lung ventilation due to the retention of respiratory secretions secondary to infection (i.e. ineffective airway clearance).

2. The patient is confused and disoriented in time and space, probably because of cerebral hypoxia as a result of problem 1.

3. The patient has severely limited activity owing to shortness of breath.

4. The patient is lacking in knowledge about how to improve airway clearance.

Box 13.1 illustrates the plan of care devised to deal with each of these problems. More than one goal may be devised and a time should be stated by when the goal is to be achieved. In this plan, where there are two goals for each problem, the interventions apply to both.

After 7 days the patient was able to feed, wash and dress himself, walk to the bathroom independently and describe plans for his discharge. He was alert and oriented. Owing to pressure on beds he was discharged a day earlier than planned; this caused considerable inconvenience for his daughter who had to take him home at very short notice. A community nurse visit was arranged as part of the follow-up but this was later than planned because of the premature discharge. Local social services promised that a home help would be able to visit once a week, but owing to staff shortages no-one came in the first week after discharge. Despite these problems, the patient recovered fully.

Chronic obstructive pulmonary disease and asthma

Disease of the airway may be broadly categorized as either reversible or irreversible, dependent upon whether the airways respond to treatment (Brewin 1997). The diagnosis of particular disorders is not, however, so simple as there is often overlap and what started as a reversible condition may over a period of time lead to irreversible damage to the airways.

Chronic obstructive pulmonary disease (COPD) has been defined by the British Thoracic Society (BTS) as 'A chronic slowly progressive disorder characterized by airways obstruction … which does not change markedly over several months. Most of the lung function impairment is fixed, although some reversibility can be produced by bronchodilator (or other) therapy' (BTS 1997b, p. 2). As airway obstruction gradually increases, breathing patterns change and become less efficient until eventually they are unable to meet the ventilatory needs of the body.

Chronic lung disease
See chapter 5.3

Box 13.1   Patient care plan for George Fleming, an elderly man with pneumonia

Goals	Nursing intervention	Rationale

Patient problem 1: Ineffective airway clearance related to retention of respiratory secretions secondary to inflammation of respiratory passages as a result of infection

Goals	Nursing intervention	Rationale
1. Respiratory rate will be 20–24 per minute within 3 days (date …)	Assess respiratory rate and depth, breathing pattern and breath sounds 2 hourly	Ongoing objective data provide a basis for planning further nursing interventions and identification of signs of respiratory failure
2. Breathing pattern will be regular, requiring minimal effort, and breath sounds normal within 3 days (date …)	Monitor body temperature 4 hourly	Provides objective data on disease progress and response to therapy
	Obtain a sputum specimen for culture and sensitivity as ordered	Antibiotic therapy alters sensitivity of organisms
	Administer i.v. antibiotics 6 hourly as prescribed	Treatment of infection
	Administer oxygen at 24% by mask as prescribed	To promote gas exchange and decrease respiratory effort
	Ensure patient is sitting upright	To facilitate lung expansion
	Demonstrate and supervise deep breathing and coughing techniques 2 hourly during day and when awake at night	To improve breathing pattern; promote removal of secretions
	Provide anti-inflammatory analgesic preparation 4 hourly as prescribed until temperature within normal range	To reduce body temperature and promote comfort to facilitate lung expansion
	Offer juice, warm tea or water 2 hourly or more often. Leave fluids within reach. Monitor fluid intake and maintain at 2 litres daily or greater	Adequate hydration facilitates movement of secretions
	Cleanse mouth with diluted mouthwash after coughing (2–4 hourly)	With increased expectoration of secretions, more frequent mouth care is required

Patient problem 2: Confusion and disorientation in time and space due to cerebral hypoxia

Goals	Nursing intervention	Rationale
1. Mr Fleming will be oriented to time and place as well as person within 4 days (date…)	Assess cognitive status 4 hourly	To evaluate changes in hypoxic state
	Call Mr Fleming by name and introduce yourself on each encounter	To promote orientation and decrease confusion and anxiety
2. Mr Fleming will participate in interactions with nurses, family and other visitors	Provide repeated explanations of all care activities before and during the procedures	
	Engage Mr Fleming in conversations during all activities	
	Encourage daughter to talk to him during visits	

Patient problem 3: Severely limited activity due to dyspnoea

Goals	Nursing intervention	Rationale
Mr Fleming will gradually resume self-care and other activities of daily living, becoming independent in 7 days (date …)	Plan care activities to allow for uninterrupted rest periods. Adjust assessment and care to be completed when he is awake	To promote maximum rest
	Assist Mr Fleming with all aspects of self-care initially. Increase his participation gradually as tolerated	To prevent exhaustion
	Assess daily for bowel function. Obtain order for stool softener if straining occurs	Constipation is a side-effect of analgesic medications and dehydration. Straining at stool increases energy expenditure
	Sit Mr Fleming upright	To depress diaphragm and decrease effort of breathing

Patient problem 4: Lack of knowledge concerning care after discharge

Goals	Nursing intervention	Rationale
Mr Fleming and his daughter will state a plan for home care and maintenance of respiratory function	To teach Mr Fleming and his daughter to observe for signs and symptoms of respiratory distress	Mr Fleming and his daughter will recognize complications quickly and seek help
	Assist them to develop a plan for Mr Fleming to obtain regular and adequate nutrition and fluids and adequate rest when he returns home	Mr Fleming and his daughter will be informed about his needs
	Make a referral to the community nurse for follow-up care	Resources should be available within the community to ensure continuity of care

COPD is a general term that covers many conditions (e.g. chronic bronchitis, emphysema and bronchiectasis) which share the same underlying lung conditions (Haughney 1998). COPD affects mainly older patients and most cases are linked to a history of tobacco smoking. Asthma may contribute to the development of COPD but is more usually characterized by variable and reversible airway obstruction, bronchial hyperreactivity and often persistent inflammation (Kilgarriff 2000).

The nursing care required by patients with COPD is discussed after an overview of the various disorders.

Chronic bronchitis

The disease is characterized by hyperactivity of the mucus-secreting glands of the bronchial mucosa in response to prolonged or frequently recurring irritation. As with all forms of COPD, tobacco smoke is the principal cause, although atmospheric pollutants such as dust, industrial fumes and smoke also contribute to the problem.

The bronchial mucosa undergoes a chronic inflammatory process, together with hypertrophy and an increase in the number of mucus-secreting glands. Airway obstruction results from the narrowing of the bronchial lumen as a result of hyperplasia of the mucus-secreting glands and the increased production of sputum. Initially the patient usually experiences a cough in the morning (often referred to as smoker's cough) but progressively becoming more frequent and accompanied by dyspnoea, cyanosis and the production of sputum. Although chronic bronchitis and emphysema are classified as separate disorders, they commonly coexist. A frequent complication of chronic bronchitis is chest infection as secretions are not expectorated and become infected. Individuals with chronic bronchitis are usually well aware of the further debilitation and lethargy that results from a chest infection and tend to be vigilant for the first signs in order to obtain prompt treatment (Williams 1993). Infective bronchitis is the most common cause of an acute exacerbation of chronic bronchitis, which may in turn lead to respiratory failure and death (Bloom, 1995).

Pulmonary emphysema

Pulmonary **emphysema** is a chronic disorder characterized by destruction of alveoli walls and a loss of lung surface area for gas exchange together with a loss of elasticity due to damage to the connective tissue (Springhouse Corporation 2000). Smoking is the principal cause. Destruction of the pulmonary lung units occurs with ageing in all lungs but is accelerated in some, leading to clinical emphysema. The damage is not uniform. It may affect only the central portion of the pulmonary lobules (centralobular emphysema) or it may result in destruction of most of the structures within a terminal unit, including the alveolar ducts and alveoli (panlobular emphysema). The onset is insidious but, once initiated, is progressive and non-reversible. The disease is more common in men than in women. The lung damage cannot be repaired but the patient may be helped to breathe more effectively and live with less disability.

Medical approaches to treatment of COPD

The British Thoracic Society categorizes COPD as mild, moderate or severe according to spirometry readings and provides treatment guidelines and recommendations for each group (BTS 1997b):

- *Mild* (FEV_1 60–79% predicted) – bronchodilator (short-acting β_2 agonist such as salbutamol or inhaled anticholinergic such as ipratropium) as required.

- *Moderate* (FEV_1 40–59% predicted) – bronchodilator p.r.n., but regular therapy may also be needed with one drug or combination. Consider corticosteroid trials in all patients.

- *Severe* (FEV_1 <40% predicted) – combination therapy regular β_2 agonists plus the addition of an anticholinergic agent consider steroid trial; assess for home nebulizer using BTS guidelines; oxygen.

Non-drug measures applicable to all groups include smoking cessation, exercise and vaccination against influenza.

Asthma

The prevalence of **asthma** in the UK has increased significantly in recent decades. It has been estimated by the Department of Health (1995) that approximately 3.4 million people within the UK suffer from asthma. The mortality rate for asthma rose steadily to peak at approximately 2000 deaths per year by the early 1990s but has since begun to decline slowly (Rees and Kananbar 2000). The increased incidence may partly reflect an increased awareness of, rather than a real increase in, the disease. Asthma can be described as a syndrome comprising of bronchial inflammation, airway hyperresponsivseness and usually reversible airway obstruction (Rees and Kanabar 2000).

Stimuli that may precipitate the asthmatic response include: allergens (especially the housedust mite), viral respiratory infections, irritating inhalants (chemicals, air pollutants), cold dry air, emotional stress and physical exercise. An asthma attack may also be triggered by a response to drugs such as acetylsalicylic acid (aspirin), beta-blockers and non-steroidal anti-inflammatory drugs. Asthma often begins in childhood but may develop at any age. Childhood asthma may gradually resolve with growth into adulthood, but adult-onset asthma tends to be a more permanent problem with which the person has to learn to live. Frequently there is a personal and/or family history of one or more allergies. Warning signs of increasing bronchial reactivity include frequent awakening at night,

Emphysema
See chapter 5.3

Asthma
See chapter 5.3

decreased physical effort tolerance, shortness of breath on getting up in the morning, and cough.

The reaction of the overresponsive airway to stimuli is oedema and thickening of the mucosa, hypersecretion by the mucous glands and spasmodic contraction of bronchial and bronchiolar muscle tissue. This causes diffuse narrowing of the tracheobronchial tree and obstruction to airflow. Inspiration is normal but expiration is impeded and the lungs become hyperinflated, resulting in severe dyspnoea and wheezing.

During an acute asthmatic attack the patient experiences tightness in the chest, wheezing and dyspnoea. The accessory muscles of respiration are used and expiration is prolonged. The patient usually appears distraught and may assume an upright sitting position. The sputum is scant and thick, and the pulse is rapid. Patients suffering a severe asthmatic attack may require intubation and artificial ventilation for a period if they do not respond to nebulized and intravenously administered bronchodilator therapy. Repeated peak flow measurements and arterial blood gas values are good guides to progress, together with vital sign monitoring. The importance of psychological support during acute episodes of respiratory distress cannot be overemphasized.

Medical approaches to the treatment of asthma

Most patients with asthma have their condition controlled and monitored by the primary healthcare team. There are, however, occasions when an individual's asthma may become so severe that hospital admission is required. Regardless of the location of care, the British Asthma Guidelines produced by the British Thoracic Society (1997a,b) provide comprehensive, multidisciplinary guidance on best practice. A key feature of the current approach to the treatment of asthma is the early use of preventive anti-inflammatory therapy, usually in the form of inhaled corticosteroids. The dose of inhaled corticosteroid should be titrated according to symptoms, peak flow recordings and other drug therapy with the goal of administering the lowest effective dose for long-term control and optimal quality of life (Lipworth 1999). The use of preventive corticosteroid reduces the need for symptomatic relief with short-acting inhaled bronchodilators (β_2 agonists). Currently there is controversy regarding the use of short-acting β_2 agonists as there is some evidence that regular use of this group of drugs may worsen the control of asthma (Lipworth 1999).

If β_2 agonists such as salbutamol are required to relieve shortness of breath more than once daily, the emphasis must be placed on prevention of attacks. Frequent use of these short-acting drugs in mild to moderate asthmatics is of no clinical benefit, although long-acting drugs such as salmeterol are of benefit (British National Formulary 2001).

The treatment of asthma is constantly under review and a new group of drugs known as leucotriene receptor agonists (LTRAs), which have an anti-inflammatory effect, have recently been introduced (e.g. montelukast). They are used as 'add on' drugs and may be prescribed for people with mild to moderate asthma if inhaled corticosteroids and an inhaled β stimulant are insufficient (British National Formulary 2001).

The main emphasis within asthma care is now prophylaxis – the prevention of an asthma attack or exacerbation. Prophylactic treatments such as inhaled steroids are, however, effective only when used correctly. For most patients with asthma medication needs to be taken on a daily basis even when asymptomatic (Ward and Reynolds 2000). From a review of the literature, Ward and Reynolds (2000) estimated that approximately half of all patients with asthma do not comply with their prescribed treatment regimen, emphasizing a very important role for nurses in improving patient cooperation.

The effects upon families or patients with asthma can be devastating, with the disease causing major practical and emotional problems for everyone, not just the sufferer. Nurses are ideally placed to help patients manage their asthma with the least disruption to their life. Patients should be taught that lack of response to a bronchodilator is a vital warning sign of an impending serious attack. This is a sign that is often missed. Patients can also be taught routine peak flow monitoring at home, in the same way that diabetic patients monitor blood sugar levels. Deterioration in peak flow is a warning sign that, if acted upon, could avert a major medical emergency.

The monitoring of peak expiratory flow rates (PEFRs) at home is becoming increasingly popular because it facilitates the early detection of decreased respiratory function and gives the individual with asthma the potential for greater control. Donaldson (1993), an asthma sufferer, describes the peak flow meter as a powerful aid that allows him to determine the mode of management for his asthma at any particular time. The protocol for the treatment of his asthma that Donaldson (1993) established with his physician is an example of the collaboration necessary for the effective treatment of asthma. A number of authors (Byrne et al 1993, Tettersall 1993) have highlighted the often poor compliance of asthmatics with prescribed treatments, despite these same individuals having adequate knowledge about asthma and its management. What these authors perhaps fail to acknowledge is that individuals with asthma may be better able to decide upon the most effective treatment regimen for themselves rather than purely complying with a doctor's prescription. More recent approaches to asthma care have included the use of self-management plans that involve patients in monitoring their respiratory function (usually by recording PEFR and noting any symptoms such as sleep disturbance, etc.) and providing them with guidelines on appropriate action to take based upon their observations (Partridge 1996).

For patients to take control of their asthma it is vital that they are able to identify the signs of an impending attack and understand what actions they should take. Patients also need to learn the skills of measuring (and recording) their PEFR and of taking their inhaled medication. Nurses need to be able to teach patients about their condition and provide correct instruction on the use of inhaler devices and peak flow meters. A small study by Howell (1996), involving 28 staff (17 qualified nurses, 11 auxiliaries) indicated that only a small proportion of those surveyed were competent to give advice and instruction on the full range of inhaler devices in use within the clinical setting. Although this survey is small and the results should not be generalized, it does give some indication of the need for clinical staff to develop and maintain their own skills and knowledge before attempting to teach patients. Ross-Plummer (2000) provides a useful checklist for nurses to use when planning a patient's discharge following hospitalization with asthma.

Management of a severe asthmatic attack

As the onset of an asthmatic attack may be sudden and without warning, treatment has to be immediate and appropriate to the severity of the attack. This can be categorized into four types: mild, moderate, severe and life threatening (see Box 13.2).

Key factors in the history that should be ascertained at assessment include whether the patient:

■ is a known asthmatic and what medication he or she takes

■ has any known allergies and may have been exposed to allergens

■ has a cough and whether it is productive

■ has any nocturnal symptoms

■ is wheezing

■ is a smoker.

The flow charts depicted in Figures 13.3 and 13.4 summarize treatment and care for a serious attack in hospital and in the community respectively.

If the patient has been admitted, the nurse should ensure before discharge that:

1. The basic pathophysiology of asthma has been explained to the patient and is supported by leaflets.

2. The patient knows about all his or her asthma medicines and their actions.

3. The patient's PEFR has been monitored throughout his or her hospital stay, not just during the acute exacerbation; it must be greater than 70% of the patient's predicted or best recent value.

> **Box 13.2** Characteristics of various types of asthma attack
>
> *Mild or moderate*
> The speech is normal
> Pulse < 110 per min
> Respiratory rate ≤ 25 per min
> Peak expiratory flow rate (PEFR) greater than 50% of the normal for that person
>
> *Severe*
> Unable to complete sentences
> Pulse > 110 per min
> Respiratory rate > 25 per min
> PEFR less than 50% of the normal for that person
>
> *Life threatening*
> The patient is unable to speak
> Bradycardia and hypotension
> Signs of exhaustion
> PEFR less than 33% of the normal for that person
> Silent chest on auscultation
> The patient is cyanosed

4. Inhaled corticosteroid therapy has been maintained throughout the admission and the patient is taking both inhaled and oral corticosteroids.

5. The patient has adequate inhaler technique and has been taking inhaled drugs for at least 24 hours.

6. In conjunction with the patient, the identification of trigger factors has begun and avoidance strategies are being considered.

7. Follow-up appointment arrangements have been made.

8. The patient has been instructed on how to monitor PEFR and supplied with a PEFR meter and diary card.

9. A detailed written discharge summary has been prepared for the general practice.

10. The patient knows what to do if his or her condition deteriorates soon after discharge.

It is clear that nurses and other health professionals need to work in partnership with patients to ensure optimum control of asthma and least disruption to daily life.

Problems common to patients with COPD

Altered breathing pattern

The most frequent symptom of COPD is a prolonged expiratory phase, as demonstrated by an increase in the forced expiratory time. Other characteristics of the breathing pattern of a person with COPD are rapid shallow respirations and use of the intercostal and accessory muscles.

Figure 13.3   Treatment of acute severe asthma in hospital.

Shortness of breath is experienced by many, but not all patients, despite severe airflow limitation. Dyspnoea varies daily with changes in activity, increased effort and during sleep.

Poor activity tolerance

Respiratory muscle fatigue develops in persons with COPD in response to the increased airway resistance, which in turn increases the work of breathing. The inspiratory muscles have to generate greater pressures to ventilate the lungs. Muscle fatigue occurs when the inspiratory muscles are no longer able to maintain the force required for ventilation.

Activity intolerance increases with exercise and stress and impairs the individual's ability to perform usual activities. Eventually, the effort of breathing consumes all the individual's energy.

Interestingly Williams (1993) comments on a study he conducted which found that poor lung function measurements (spirometry) were linked only weakly to dyspnoea and disability. He suggests that this finding indicates that psychological factors such as mood, beliefs and attitudes may have an equally strong role to play in the extent to which individuals with COPD can tolerate exercise. These findings endorse those of an earlier study (Morgan et al 1983) and emphasize the complex nature of disability.

Inadequate nutrition

Weight loss and muscle wasting are recognized problems in persons with chronic lung disease. An increased caloric intake is needed because of the increased energy expended with breathing. Associated problems include a loss of appetite and decreased senses of taste and smell. Dyspnoea

Figure 13.4   Treatment of acute severe asthma in primary care.

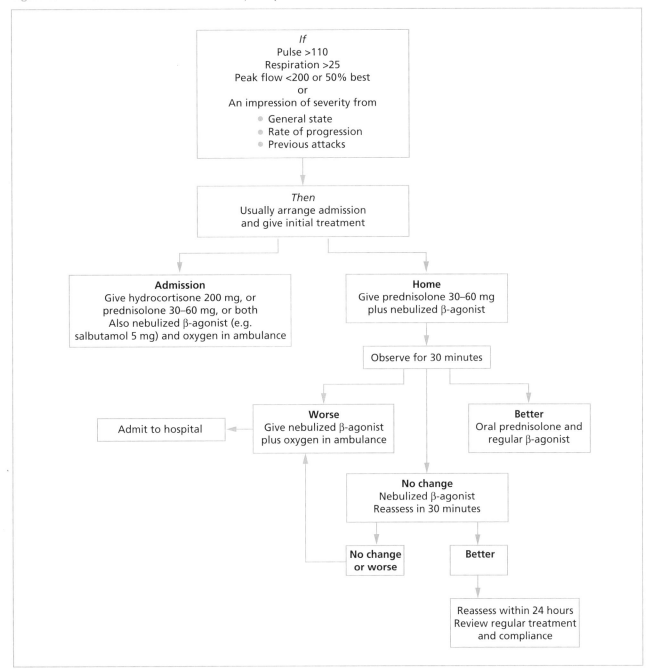

increases with eating because of the competition between eating and breathing.

Inadequate knowledge

Long-term management of COPD requires the patient to be an active participant in the care process. The individual requires knowledge of the disorder; an understanding of the use, actions, administration and side-effects of the medications; the ability to perform breathing retraining techniques; information on factors influencing respiratory function; and information about community resources.

Nursing intervention

Although COPD is irreversible, patient care has improved sufficiently over the past few decades to enable patients to live useful and satisfying lives. The patient's *goal* is to achieve an effective breathing pattern so that greater levels of activity can be tolerated. This can be shown by the patient being able to:

1. demonstrate a decreased respiratory rate and increased depth of respirations

2. demonstrate increased lung volumes

3. report decreased episodes and severity of dyspnoea

4. tolerate increased levels of activity.

Breathing

Assessment of the individual's respiratory status is ongoing and focuses on the relationship of the deterioration in respiratory function to the person's ability to function in daily living activities. Interventions to improve dyspnoea are limited. The person's home and work environments are assessed for possible respiratory irritants and the individual is directed to appropriate resources for help in altering the environment where this is possible.

The nurse can assist the individual to gain control over the respiratory pattern. During an acute episode, the nurse can provide emotional support and at the same time teach the person to relax and control breathing. The nurse should stay with the person and may place his or her hands on the patient's shoulder and abdomen while quietly repeating instructions and encouragement to breathe slowly and deeply, gradually altering the breathing pattern and decreasing fear. Patients are taught the techniques of breathing retraining and relaxation. The use of an anticholinergic bronchodilator such as ipratropium bromide has been found to be an effective treatment for people with COPD and can be taken via inhaler or nebulizer. Nurses need to educate patients about their medication and ensure that the patients are able to administer it correctly themselves.

During an acute episode of breathlessness the patient should be discouraged from talking unnecessarily and helped to find a comfortable position (usually sitting up with arms supported). The nurse works in collaboration with the patient, general practitioner, physiotherapist, occupational therapist and pharmacist to teach the patient and family to monitor and manage the respiratory care programme.

Activity

Once respiratory muscles become fatigued, they must be rested. Interventions are directed toward decreasing the work of breathing and increasing the individual's tolerance. Inhaled medications are administered to dilate the bronchial airways and to decrease inflammation, thus decreasing the effort of breathing. Postural changes such as sitting in the forward leaning position may also facilitate breathing. The use of general body exercises and respiratory muscle training shows promise in improving respiratory muscle strength and developing a more effective breathing pattern, but the evidence is not yet adequate to recommend routine application of these interventions.

Patients are helped to plan their daily activities to include periods of rest before and after activity, and to learn more effective ways of performing daily living activities.

In his study of people with COPD, Williams (1993) made extensive use of extracts from interviews conducted with sufferers. These graphically illustrate the tremendous difficulties that some people have to manage in order to continue with some semblance of everyday life. For example, one woman within the study described how it would take her more than 2 hours to vacuum her living room because of the need to take frequent rests. The study also highlights the extent to which some people go to disguise their reduced exercise tolerance, perhaps by pretending to be waiting for someone when they need a rest when walking. Nurses need to discover how an individual already copes in order to give effective advice and help.

Nutrition

Although no randomized controlled longitudinal studies have been carried out to date to show that nutritional support alters the outcome for persons with chronic respiratory disease, malnutrition is a recognized patient health problem.

A nutritional assessment should be carried out on all patients with COPD and, if necessary, a referral made to the dietician. Nurses can help by carefully timing the administration of nebulizers so that they are not administered immediately before meals, unless the patient requires the medication in order to have sufficient breath to eat. Oxygen can be administered via nasal cannulae (see Fig. 13.5) to enable the patient to benefit from the oxygen whilst eating. The presentation of small appetizing meals interspersed with nutritious snacks can be very helpful as many patients with respiratory problems feel unable to eat a large quantity of food at any one time. Fresh chilled water should always be available and the patient should be encouraged to take frequent small sips to counteract the drying effect of tachypnoea (and oxygen

Figure 13.5 Plastic cannulae or prongs inserted into the nostrils to deliver oxygen.

therapy). Regular mouth care can also enhance a patient's appetite and make the mouth feel more pleasant.

Teaching

Self-monitoring and self-care are essential components of the management programme. The patient needs to learn to cope with the limitations imposed by the disease, prevent complications and comply with the negotiated treatment plan if a satisfactory lifestyle is to be achieved. As with any chronic disorder, the individual ultimately has to learn to live with the disease process and to manage his or her daily routine accordingly. In recent years the use of guided self-management of asthma has gained in popularity and emphasizes the need for partnership between the patient and health practitioner. In simple terms, self-management involves the patient keeping well and adjusting treatment according to a treatment plan developed in advance with the doctor or appropriate health professional (Partridge 1996). Changes in treatment are usually in response to changes in peak flow recordings and other symptoms. Patients therefore need to be educated about how to measure and record peak flow and how to use the treatment plan to adjust their medication.

Drugs to promote ventilation and improve airflow

Patient teaching related to drug therapy

As there are no cures for many chronic respiratory disorders, treatment programmes and drug therapy are planned for each individual according to personal goals, lifestyle situation, respiratory status, response to drugs and other therapeutic measures. The patient usually assumes responsibility for self-management of the therapeutic regimen and therefore requires the knowledge and skill necessary not only to administer the drugs but also to make decisions regarding the plan. The individual learns to monitor responses to medications, determine when adjustments are desirable and when to seek further professional assistance.

The teaching plan should include:

- Information about the action, duration of effect, method of administration and side-effects of prescribed medications

- Instruction and practice in the proper use of metered-dose inhalers for optimal delivery of the medication into the bronchial tree. For individuals who have difficulty manipulating the metered-dose inhaler, a spacer device may be used which reduces the need for the patient to coordinate inhalation with the activation of the metered-dose inhaler, (Fig. 13.6)

- Participation in the development of the medication schedule to meet the individual's needs.

Bronchodilators such as salbutamol (β_2 agonist) or ipratropium (anticholinergic) may be taken up to 4 times per day (British National Formulary 2001). Administration may be planned to coincide with the beginning of specific activities to promote optimal functioning. The dose of corticosteroid preparations is adjusted so that the smallest dose necessary to maintain improvement in airflow is administered. Inhalation preparations are used to minimize systemic effects; also, a smaller dose is required.

The effectiveness of nurses teaching patients with chronic respiratory disease has been demonstrated by two studies in particular. Howard (1987) showed that a structured teaching programme had the effect of reducing hospital admissions and the lengths of such admissions when necessary, in a sample of 115 patients (predominantly white males). The effect was a reduction of between 15% and 25% in the number of days this group would have been expected to spend in hospital. Nursing time spent on such activities is cost effective when consideration is given to the substantial savings that could be made by hospitals, and clearly the improvement in health that occurred is very beneficial to the patients.

A community-based approach to patient teaching and support was used successfully by Heslop and Bagnall (1988), who studied the benefits patients might derive from monthly home visits by nurses. The major problems that were identified were patients' lack of knowledge and the great deal of fear and anxiety generated by breathless attacks, which severely restricted the patients' activity. Patients were encouraged to set their own goals and met with a great deal of success in achieving them. However, psychosocial problems proved very resistant to change

Figure 13.6 Using a metered-dose inhaler. (1) Shake the inhaler. (2) Exhale fully. (3) Spray once into wide open mouth as you inhale fully. (4) Hold breath for 5 seconds before exhaling. (5) Repeat for each puff ordered.

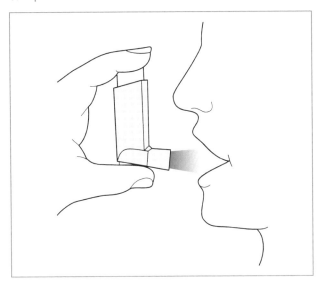

and caused major difficulties for many of the patients in this study.

Pulmonary tuberculosis

Tuberculosis is an infectious disease caused by the tubercle bacillus. The organism may attack other tissues in the body, but in Europe and North America the lungs are most frequently the primary site of invasion – although most organs in the body can be attacked. Infection is usually by inhalation of droplets bearing tubercle bacilli. The droplets have been expelled into the air by the sneezing or coughing of a person with active disease.

Tuberculosis is a disease of poverty, readily taking advantage of those with weakened resistance due to poor nutrition and general health. Social conditions therefore play a large part in determining susceptibility to the disease. Homeless persons and the elderly, together with members of ethnic communities originating from the Indian subcontinent, are perhaps most at risk in the UK. Children and adolescents are at greater risk than adults. The incidence of tuberculosis has increased in recent years from 5778 new cases in the UK in 1988 to 6564 new cases in 1993 (Central Statistical Office 1995).

Disease process

Small rounded nodules, with a tendency toward central necrosis, develop at the site of tissue invasion by the bacilli. These are referred to as *tubercles* and are composed of lung tissue cells, leucocytes, other phagocytic cells, fibroblasts and tubercle bacilli. If the body defences are strong enough to destroy the organisms, the lesion heals and may calcify.

In some instances, the reproduction of the tubercle bacilli may be minimal; a few continue to survive within the tubercle but remain confined and dormant. This person, having been infected and still harbouring live bacilli, will show a positive tuberculin test in approximately 2–10 weeks after the initial infection; defensive cells have become sensitized and tend to inhibit or slow up the growth of tubercle bacilli. At a later date, if resistance is lowered, the reproduction of the tubercle bacilli may be accelerated and active disease develops. When the bacilli continue to multiply, the tubercle necroses centrally, producing soft caseous material that may eventually be discharged from the tubercle, leaving a cavity. This caseous discharge is highly infective.

The initial infection does not affect pulmonary function. The later stages of tuberculosis, which are becoming again more common in Britain and Europe, produce systemic and local symptoms. The constitutional symptoms are vague and non-specific; they include lassitude, fatigue, malaise, loss of appetite and weight, fever (usually low grade) in the latter part of the day, tachycardia and night sweats. Symptoms produced by the local disease process at the site of the lesion in the lungs are cough, sputum, haemoptysis, dyspnoea and chest pain if the pleura is involved.

Diagnostic investigation

The investigation of a patient for pulmonary tuberculosis involves tuberculin testing, chest radiography and bacteriological examination of sputum.

Treatment

Patients remain at home and continue to work and live normal and useful lives during the course of their treatment. The principal factors in the plan of patient care are prolonged chemotherapy, rest, and patient and family education.

The administration of specific antimicrobial drugs over a long period of time has proved very successful in the prevention and treatment of tuberculosis. Preventive therapy for susceptible contacts involves the administration of isoniazid 300 mg daily for 6 months (Haslett et al 1999). The recommended treatment for infected patients commences with an initial phase of 2 months' treatment with isoniazid, rifampicin and pyrazinamide together to kill as many bacteria as possible, as quickly as possible (British National Formulary 2001). After 2 months of treatment this may be decreased to isoniazid and rifampicin only for a further 4 months. Longer periods of treatment or other drugs may be needed if there is evidence of resistance to these antibiotics. The nurse should be familiar with the treatment plan and with the actions and possible side-effects of the drugs so that adverse reactions can be recognized early and the patient can be taught what to look for and what to do if side-effects occur. The following drugs are used.

Isoniazid This is taken orally. This drug is usually well tolerated. Liver function should be checked before use as the drug can be toxic to the liver. Peripheral neuropathy is the main side-effect, and is usually associated with pre-existing risk factors such as malnourishment, alcoholism or diabetes.

Ethambutol This is used if resistance to first-choice drugs is likely. Patients receiving ethambutol should be assessed for visual acuity before treatment and monitored for changes, as the main side-effect is loss of visual acuity and colour blindness.

Rifampicin This is taken orally 1 hour before or 2 hours after the ingestion of food to promote maximum absorption. Adverse gastrointestinal effects such as heartburn, epigastric distress, nausea and diarrhoea may occur and can be minimized by administering the drug with food. Patients should be helped to establish a routine that best suits their responses. Patients should be aware that rifampicin may impart a red–orange colour to the urine, faeces, sputum, sweat and tears. Soft contact lenses may become permanently discoloured. The patient's liver function is monitored regularly.

Streptomycin This antibiotic is rarely used and only if resistance is a problem. It is given intramuscularly and serious side-effects are damage of the auditory nerves and consequent loss of hearing.

Pyrazinamide This drug is often added during the first 2 months of therapy. It occasionally causes hepatitis, hyperuricaemia, gastrointestinal disturbances or arthralgia.

In view of the lengthy courses of chemotherapy required to treat tuberculosis, there is a significant risk of patients failing to take their medication correctly or simply stopping altogether. This contributes to the problem of emerging resistance to current medication. Close supervision and reinforcement of teaching about the importance of completing the full course are therefore required in the community care setting.

Lung cancer

Lung cancer is the most common cancer in men and the primary cause of cancer deaths in both men and women. The incidence of lung cancer has been rising over the last 50 years; in England and Wales it now accounts for 17% of all new cases of cancer and 25% of all cancer deaths (Mera 1997). Cigarette smoking is a major risk factor for the development of lung cancer, with more than 85% of lung cancers being directly attributable to smoking (Mera 1997). Most patients present with symptoms late in the course of the disease and it has been estimated that approximately 70% of patients presenting with symptoms already have metastases (Mera 1997). In view of the high mortality rate for the disease and the strong links to smoking, the most important issue in relation to lung cancer is prevention and the use of health promotion strategies aimed at a reduction in smoking.

Characteristics of cancer of the lung

Early symptoms are usually absent or vague. The person may have a persistent non-productive cough. Later, the sputum may be blood streaked. Dyspnoea, localized chest pain and wheezing may develop. General symptoms include fever, chills, sweating (especially night sweats), anorexia, weakness, fatigue and weight loss. Symptoms are often insidious. Confirmation of the presence of lung cancer requires further diagnostic investigations.

Treatment of lung cancer

Treatment of lung cancer usually involves a combination of chemotherapy, radiation and surgical resection. Small cell lung cancers, which are characterized by rapid cell growth and metastases, are usually sensitive to chemotherapy and radiation. The non-small-cell variety are usually removed surgically. Most patients show some response to treatment but the 5-year survival rate remains poor.

Chemotherapy

Combinations of various chemotherapeutic agents may be prescribed for patients who have metastatic disease on diagnosis and for those with recurrent disease. No effective drug regimen for cancer of the lung has been proven; the use of chemotherapy is therefore limited primarily to individuals with small cell lung tumours.

Radiotherapy

Radiation is used as a primary treatment, in combination with surgery, or for palliation. The total dose of and the schedule for radiation depends on the treatment goal.

Surgical treatment

Surgical resection is the treatment of choice for persons with non-small-cell lung cancer with no evidence of extrathoracic metastases. Surgical treatment consists of a thoracotomy and resection of the involved lung tissue and regional lymph nodes.

Pneumonectomy, in which an entire lung is removed, involves the ligation of a large pulmonary artery, two large pulmonary veins and a bronchus. The phrenic nerve on the operative side is crushed or severed to permit the diaphragm to rise to reduce the size of the cavity that remains. Pneumonectomy is used when extensive tissue must be excised.

A *lobectomy* is the removal of a lobe of a lung and is used when the disease is confined to that particular lobe.

Segmental resection is used when the person's disease is localized to a segment of a lung, making it possible to conserve functional tissue and lessen the degree of overdistension in the other lung by removing only the affected segment.

Wedge resection is used when the disease is localized and small, or when conservative treatment is indicated because of a poor prognosis.

Nursing care of the person having chest surgery

Preoperative nursing care Before operation the patient and family may be anxious and frightened. They may be denying the diagnosis of lung cancer and the severity of the prognosis, while at the same time be struggling to make decisions regarding treatment.

The patient is usually fatigued and restless, and may appear thin and emaciated from recent weight loss and poor appetite. Chest pain and discomfort may not develop in the early stages. Respiratory function is usually impaired as a result of a history of heavy smoking and resulting chronic airflow disease as well as the lung cancer. The patient may experience a persistent non-productive cough and shortness of breath.

The patient's day is occupied with numerous diagnostic studies, including chest radiography, cytological studies of sputum, bronchoscopy and pulmonary function studies.

The goals for nursing intervention during the preoperative period are: (1) to improve respiratory function before surgery; (2) to alleviate the anxiety of the patient and family by providing support during the decision-making process and in coping with the diagnosis and prognosis; and (3) to provide information about the operative procedure and expectations for the patient and family before and after the operation.

Postoperative nursing care   The arterial blood pressure, pulse and respirations are noted every 15 minutes for the first 2–3 hours and then the interval is increased to 1/2–1 hour for the succeeding 8–10 hours if the vital signs are stabilized.

The rise and fall of both sides of the chest in respiration should be noted. Dyspnoea, decreased movement of one side of the chest on inspiration (except in pneumonectomy), cyanosis or chest pain may manifest a pneumothorax and should be reported promptly to the doctor. This may develop as a result of air or fluid collecting in the pleural cavity and compressing the lung. It must be treated quickly by chest aspiration (thoracocentesis), or the patient may die from respiratory insufficiency. Respirations are also observed for audible moist sounds. Portable chest radiography may be done daily for 2–3 days to determine lung expansion and detect the presence of fluid and air in the pleural cavity.

The wound area and chest drainage are examined frequently for any indications of bleeding. The sealed drainage system is checked frequently for functioning and the tubing connections are examined for security. The volume of drainage is measured at regular intervals. The intake and output are recorded and the fluid balance is estimated.

Arterial blood specimens may be necessary for blood gas determinations which indicate possible respiratory insufficiency and the need for mechanical assistance and/or increased oxygen inhalation.

In the case of a pneumonectomy, turning is from the back to the affected side only. With partial resection, the patient usually may be turned from back to left side, to back to right side, and so on. If a sternum-splitting incision is used, the patient is generally most comfortable on the back, but is encouraged to assume a lateral position for at least brief periods.

Disorders of the pleurae

Pleural effusion

Pleural effusion is an accumulation of an abnormal quantity of fluid in the interpleural space and is a symptom associated with a variety of conditions. The fluid may be a transudate or an exudate. A transudate may collect in the pleural space as a result of increased venous pressure incurred by congestive heart failure or an intrathoracic tumour which interferes with venous drainage in the area. Cirrhosis of the liver may cause a pleural effusion, as

Pneumothorax
See chapter 5.3

well as ascites. An accumulation of exudate in the pleural space indicates irritation and inflammation of the pleura associated with infection.

The patient with an effusion may experience some pleuritic pain, which is stabbing and is worse on inspiration before the excess fluid collects. The condition may develop insidiously and may go unrecognized until the increasing volume of fluid compresses the lung, causing dyspnoea and impaired pulmonary ventilation.

A chest aspiration (thoracocentesis) is done to relieve the pressure on the lung and to obtain a specimen of fluid for examination. Treatment is directed toward the disease causing the effusion. A culture is made of the aspirated fluid for identification of the causative organisms and their antibiotic sensitivity. The patient receives antibiotics parenterally or orally, and the drug may also be injected into the thoracic cavity following aspiration. Surgical drainage may be necessary, especially if the pus is thick. A collection of pus in the pleural cavity is known as *empyema*. Early breathing exercises to promote re-expansion of the lung are important, because the visceral pleura tends to become thick, fibrous and resistant to stretching, reducing lung compliance and the vital capacity.

Pneumothorax

Pneumothorax is a term used to describe a situation where a rupture in the visceral and/or parietal pleura allows air to accumulate in the pleural space, leading to collapse of part of the lung. This may occur after trauma or spontaneously. In *tension pneumothorax* the rupture acts as a one-way valve so that air enters the pleural space on each respiration but cannot escape. This leads to a progressive build-up of air in the pleural space, collapse of the whole lung and displacement of the trachea away from the affected side. Major blood vessels become kinked and blood flow to the brain may be seriously impaired. Unlike a *simple pneumothorax*, which often resolves itself with the air in the pleural space being gradually reabsorbed, a tension pneumothorax is a life-threatening emergency. An accumulation of blood acts in the same way to compress the lung and is known as a *haemothorax*.

In order to expand the collapsed lung it is necessary to remove any blood or air from the pleura. This is done by introducing a drainage tube which is sutured in place and secured via an underwater seal drain to prevent air re-entering the pleural space. If the patient has a pneumothorax, the chest drain is inserted high in the lateral chest wall, while to drain fluid and blood a site low down the lateral chest wall is selected. Drains may be inserted in both sites if blood and air need to be drained from the pleura (*haemopneumothorax*).

Assessment

Nursing assessment focuses on the person's respiratory status and breathing pattern. The breathing pattern of an individual with decreased lung expansion resulting from a pleural effusion or pneumothorax is characterized by decreased lung volumes, dyspnoea, use of the accessory muscles of respiration, and rapid shallow breathing. In non-emergency situations the nurse should ascertain the effect of the respiratory impairment on the patient's lifestyle and ability to carry out usual daily activities. Physiological measurements of pulmonary function are obtained, when possible, and the results used to validate the analysis of the nursing history and physical examination completed by the nurse. Additional data are collected from the patient, family and the health record to identify the factors contributing to the disorder.

The patient's *goal* is to achieve a functionally effective breathing pattern with adequate gas exchange. The patient should demonstrate:

1. slower and deeper respirations

2. increased lung volumes

3. blood gases within normal range.

Measures to restore normal intrathoracic pressure

The intrathoracic space is that between the visceral and parietal pleurae; the membranes are normally separated only by a thin film of fluid. Disruption of the pleura by disease, trauma or chest surgery results in air or fluid entering this space; the normal negative intrapleural pressure is lost. The increased pressure restricts lung expansion on inspiration and may cause collapse of the lung. Closed chest drainage is usually established. A thoracocentesis (pleural aspiration) may be performed to remove fluid from the pleural cavity, as well as for diagnostic tests.

Closed chest drainage

A closed or water-seal drainage system is established to allow the escape of air and fluid from the pleural cavity and re-establish the normal negative pressure, while preventing any reflux.

Methods

Various methods are used to achieve closed drainage, but the principle is the same with all: to allow air and fluid to pass in one direction only. The difference in the methods is generally in the number of compartments or containers used, whether or not suction is applied, and whether or not a flutter valve is introduced into the system. The compartments of the disposable chest drainage systems are comparable to the bottles or containers described in Figure 13.7.

Water-seal drainage may be established with one container fitted with a two-holed stopper through which two glass or plastic tubes pass (Fig. 13.7a). The chest tubes are connected to a fairly long tube leading to the drainage container. This drainage tube is connected to a tube that has its distal end submerged at all times in sterile water or sterile normal saline to a designated depth. The depth of tube submersion determines the pressure exerted by the water – hence the term water-seal drainage. A small, short tube, serving as an air vent, passes through the second hole of the tight-fitting two-holed stopper. The water level must be marked clearly on the container (or recorded in the care plan) so that the amount of drainage can be determined accurately.

With each expiration, the respiratory muscles relax, the intrapleural space is diminished and the pressure within the space is increased; this pressure exceeds that exerted by the water at the end of the tube, so fluid and air are forced from the cavity into the water in the container. The air may be seen bubbling through the water, from which it passes, escaping from the container through the vent. With inspiration the pleural space enlarges and the pressure within it decreases, causing water to rise several centimetres in the distal end of the tube. The evacuation of fluid and air from the intrapleural space results in greater space and less pressure. As a result, lung expansion is increased.

The alternating changes in pressure in the pleural cavity result in repeated fluctuations in the water level in the distal end of the drainage tube; these fluctuations correspond to the patient's breathing in and out, and indicate a patent system. If the water level does not oscillate, the tube may be blocked by a blood clot or fibrin. If this occurs the doctor should be notified at once as blocked tubing may cause a tension pneumothorax or surgical emphysema. The tube should not be milked by hand or by using mechanical rollers in an effort to relieve the blockage as even a small amount of negative pressure may result in lung tissue being sucked into the drainage system (Welch 1993). Fluctuation of the fluid level in the tube ceases when the lung has fully re-expanded. The doctor confirms this by chest radiography before removal of the drainage tube.

Coughing and deep abdominal breathing alter the intrapleural space and pressure to a greater degree than normal respirations and, as a result, are important in promoting drainage of the cavity, removal of air and fluid, and the re-expansion of remaining lung tissue.

To prevent water from being sucked into the chest, the drainage container must be kept well below the level of the patient (0.5–1 metre below the patient's chest). The negative chest pressure is equivalent to 10–20 cmH_2O and sucks the water up into the tube only to that level. If the container is lifted or moved, caution is observed to prevent traction on the tube, which might result in its dislodgement.

A safer method for preventing the possibility of water accidentally entering the chest cavity, and which also keeps the drainage separated from the water, is to use two containers. The second one contains the water, leaving the drainage container dry (Fig. 13.7b). When only one

Figure 13.7 Underwater-seal chest drainage system using (a) one bottle, (b) two bottles, and (c) two bottles and suction.

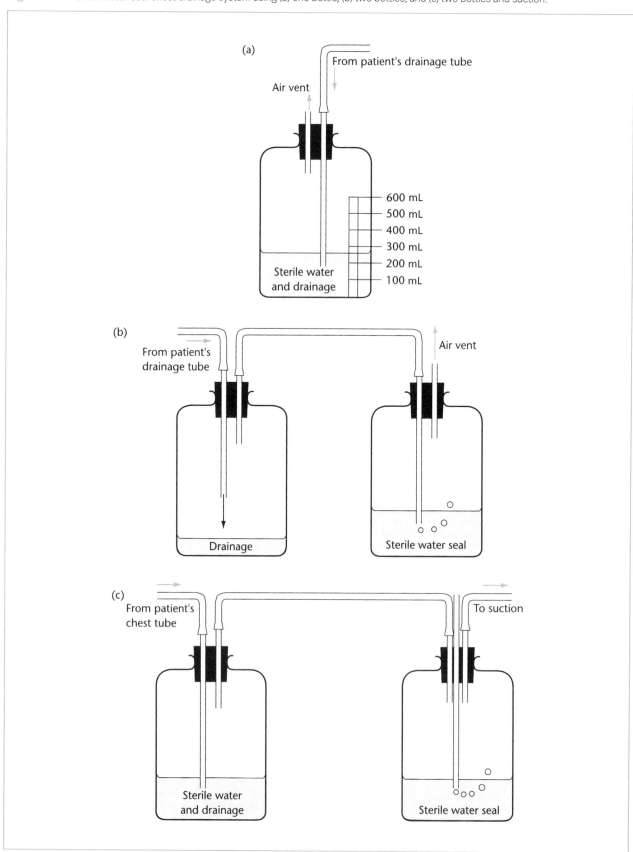

container is used, fluid drainage from the chest raises the level of the fluid, increasing the pressure at the distal end of the tube. More pressure is then required to force the fluid down on expiration and allow the escape of air and fluid. Blood and serum are more likely to collect and clot in the tube. In the two-container system, the first container is sealed and does not contain water. The arrangement is shown in Figure 13.7b. The second tube in container 2 is short and acts as an air vent. A disadvantage of the two-container system is its bulk, which makes it difficult for the patient to mobilize without assistance.

If there is a considerable amount of air leaking into the pleural cavity from the intrapulmonary space, or if the patient's cough and respirations are not sufficiently strong to facilitate the clearance of fluid and air from the chest cavity, *continuous gentle suction* may be applied. This necessitates a two-container system; the first container serves as a drainage container and water seal. The short air-vent tube in container 1 is connected to the second container, which has a three-holed stopper through which two short tubes and one longer tube pass (see Fig. 13.7c). The lower end of the longer tube is submerged in water to a designated depth. The upper end is open to the air. This tube controls the degree of suction applied to the pleural cavity. One short tube is connected to container 1; the second short tube is connected to a suction apparatus. The usual suction machine creates too strong a negative pressure to be applied directly to the pleural cavity. This may be reduced by a valve and meter (such as is used in wall suction) inserted between the suction and the water-seal container. If the portable suction machine is used, the negative pressure is controlled by the depth of submersion of the lower end of the open glass tube in container 2. A continuous bubbling in the control container (container 2) indicates that the suction is being maintained.

Disposable closed drainage receptacles with two compartments comparable to the two-container system are available. The receptacle is attached to suction and is suspended from the side of the bed, eliminating the danger of containers being knocked over and broken.

The water-seal system is cumbersome and also restricts patient mobility. The nurse and patient are continuously apprehensive of such things as tubes becoming disconnected and containers being broken. As a safety measure and to permit greater freedom in turning and earlier ambulation, some surgeons prefer to introduce a plastic flutter valve into the system. It is placed between the chest drainage tube and the drainage container. Suction may still be applied. The system may be placed on a small cart or pole with wheels to allow the patient to move around the unit.

Responsibilities and precautions

When any method of water-seal drainage is used, it is important that the nurse understands the purpose and operating principles of the system. The nurse must be familiar with the precautions to be observed to prevent air and fluid from entering the chest cavity, as this could cause a collapse of the lung and life-threatening respiratory insufficiency.

If the container system is used, the container should be calibrated so that the volume of water used is known and the drainage may be measured.

The system must be checked at frequent intervals for patency. This is determined by noting the oscillating water level in the submerged tube; this rises with inspiration and falls with expiration. When suction is employed, fluctuations of the water level do not occur because the continuous suction holds the water level in the tube at a fixed level. The suction may be interrupted briefly and the column of water observed for fluctuations. If the water level does not fluctuate in a closed system, the tube should be examined for possible kinks or compression caused by the patient lying on it. If the system remains non-functional, the doctor is informed at once.

As a precaution, connections may be taped with adhesive to prevent their separation and to keep air from entering the system. The taping of connections is controversial (Godden and Hiley 1998), but there is currently no firm evidence to support either taping or not taping and it is therefore up to the practitioner to decide on the most appropriate approach in a given situation. The containers may be placed in a rack to prevent accidental moving or knocking over. Visitors and ward personnel are warned not to disturb them.

To prevent dragging, the chest drain tubing may be loosely fastened to the patient's clothing using tape and a safety pin. This is better than securing it to the bedding as it allows the patient greater mobility, although care must be taken by the patient and staff to remember its presence when clothing is changed.

The characteristics and volume of the drainage are noted and recorded frequently, especially during the first 24–48 hours. The drainage may be coloured by blood at first, but gradually clears and decreases in amount.

The drainage container must be changed only by someone who fully understands closed drainage. Each drainage tube is clamped close to the chest wall with two chest drain clamps, and the container is quickly replaced by a clean, calibrated, sterile container.

If an interruption or break in the closed system should occur as a result of the disconnection of a tube or a broken container, a closed drainage system should be re-established as soon as possible. There has been debate as to whether or not clamps should be applied in this situation (Williams 1992), as the application of clamps could lead to the development of a tension pneumothorax and possibly death. In view of the potentially serious consequences resulting from clamping the drain for more than a few moments, it is safer to leave the drain open to the air as this will result in no more than a simple pneumothorax. As a precaution, an extra set of sterile containers and connections should always be available. As soon as the underwater-seal drainage system has been re-established, the doctor should be informed of the incident and the patient closely observed for signs of impaired breathing or other distress. It is important to remain calm and inform the patient of what you are doing, and why, as they will be understandably anxious.

Regular frequent staged coughing and deep breathing are important because they increase the intrapulmonary and intrapleural pressures, forcing air and fluid out of the cavity and promoting lung expansion. The patient should be ambulatory as soon as possible.

Patients should be instructed to inform the nurse if they experience any pain so that analgesia can be given or the prescription reviewed if it is ineffective. A patient experiencing pain will be reluctant to move about, cough or breathe deeply and this in turn will hamper lung expansion (Avery 2000).

When turning the patient, or when giving any care, precautions are taken not to dislodge or disconnect the drainage tubes. A final check is made to make sure the patient is not lying on a portion of the tube and that there are no loops or kinks present to interfere with drainage.

Even if the system appears to be functioning satisfactorily, any patient complaint of pressure or pain in the chest, dyspnoea, cyanosis or a rapid, weak pulse is reported promptly.

When the lung is fully expanded and no fluid remains in the pleural cavity, the tubes are removed. The water in the closed drainage container will have stopped fluctuating, and the lung expansion is confirmed by the doctor by percussion, auscultation and chest radiography.

When the tube is withdrawn from the chest cavity, the wound is covered with a dry, secure dressing. In most cases a purse-string suture has been inserted around the tube and this is tightened off when the tube is removed and covered with a dry, secure dressing. A chest radiograph should be taken following removal of the drain, and the respiratory rate recorded. The patient continues to be observed closely for the next 24 hours for possible leakage of air into the chest and ensuing pneumothorax.

Evaluation

If the person's breathing is more effective and dyspnoea, hypoxaemia and hypercapnia are absent or sufficiently modified to permit optimal daily functioning, care may be judged successful. Respiration should be regular, with symmetrical chest expansion, and of normal rate and depth for that individual. There should be evidence that the causative and contributing factors are modified: if pain was present, the person will state absence of pain; injuries to the chest will demonstrate healing; and repair and expansion of any impaired lung tissue will be shown by radiography.

Clamping of underwater-seal drainage systems

As mentioned above, some confusion exists among nurses and other healthcare workers regarding the indications for clamping underwater-seal drains. Following a review of the relevant literature, Williams (1992) identified only three valid reasons for clamping:

1. Following a pneumonectomy to maintain the central position of the mediastinum and its contents

2. When changing the drainage bottles

3. In patients with spontaneous pneumothorax, when re-inflation of the affected lung is confirmed by chest radiography, thus allowing observation for recurrent pneumothorax before the intercostal drain is removed.

When clamps are applied they should both be placed on the drain itself (i.e. above the first connection), not on the tubing connecting the drain to the drainage bottle.

Thoracocentesis (pleural aspiration)

A thoracocentesis is the withdrawal of fluid or air from the pleural cavity. Normally pleural fluid serves to lubricate the pleura. Excessive fluid and air interfere with lung expansion. Chest expansion will be asymmetrical, with distension and decreased movement present on the affected side. A thoracocentesis is performed to remove excessive pleural fluid to facilitate lung expansion, for diagnostic purposes or to instil medication into the pleural cavity. After preparation of the skin and injection of a local anaesthetic, the doctor inserts a needle through an intercostal space into the pleural cavity. A three-way adaptor (stopcock) is attached to the needle to enable withdrawal of fluid through attached tubing or a syringe, and closing of the system when fluid is not being aspirated. Care must be taken to maintain a closed system and prevent air from entering the pleural space.

Nursing interventions for the patient having a thoracocentesis are summarized in Box 13.3.

Restricted lung expansion

Ventilation may be restricted if bony structure is abnormal or there is rigidity of the wall. *Scoliosis* (a deformity in which the spine is S shaped with one shoulder higher than the other) causes stiffness of the chest wall, as well as limiting the size. Surgical removal of ribs (*thoracoplasty*) results primarily in a reduction in the size of the thoracic cavity. Restriction to thoracic expansion may also occur following chest surgery when the patient tends to immobilize the chest and take shallow respirations to minimize the pain.

Blunt trauma to the chest wall may produce fractures of one or more ribs. The pain caused by such an injury may be severe and, as a result, the patient is reluctant to breathe deeply. When ribs are fractured in two places (a flail segment), that section of the chest wall becomes

Box 13.3   Nursing intervention in the management of the patient having a thoracocentesis

Goals	Nursing intervention	Rationale
Patient problem: Ineffective breathing due to excess fluid in the pleural space		
1. The patient will state he or she understands the procedure and what to expect during the procedure	The patient is informed of the procedure, and what to expect during the procedure	Knowledge of what to expect can reduce anxiety and opportunity is provided to answer the patients concerns
2. The patient's breathing will be regular, rhythmical and not laboured	The nurse checks that the consent form has been signed following the doctor's explanation to the patient of the purpose of the test and expected and other possible outcomes, and that chest radiography has been carried out	Radiographs provide information as to the exact anatomical location of the fluid and air in the pleural cativity
3. Chest expansion will be symmetrical, with a usual degree of excursion		
	The prescribed sedation is administered prior to the start of the procedure	Sedation may be required to promote relaxation and decrease discomfort and anticipatory pain
	The patient is placed in a sitting position, leaning forward, with head and arms resting on a table or several pillows	Fluid is dependent and therefore accumulates in the lower portions of the pleural cavity when the patient is upright, making it easier to remove
	During the procedure the nurse provides physical support for the patient and instructs him or her to remain still while the needle is being inserted and while it is in place	To prevent spontaneous movement by the patient which may result in trauma to the pleura and lung
	During the procedure the nurse provides ongoing explanations as to what is occurring. As the antiseptic solution is applied, the patient is told to expect a feeling of cold; injection of the local anaesthetic will be felt and a pressure will be experienced as the thoracocentesis needle is inserted	Patient cooperation increases and anxiety is decreased when he or she is aware of what is happening
	A sterile transparent dressing or a gauze dressing sealed with tape is applied as the doctor withdraws the thoracocentesis needle	To prevent air from entering the pleural cavity To protect the site from micro-organisms
	The patient is assisted to a comfortable position in bed and assessed at least every 15 minutes for the first 2 hours. Observations include respiratory rate, depth and rhythm, pulse rate, presence of blood, frothy sputum, uncontrolled cough, dyspnoea, cyanosis, chest pain or tightness, and feelings of dizziness or faintness. The site is inspected and the surrounding tissue palpated for puffiness or crackling	If a large amount of fluid is removed, lung expansion occurs suddenly and pulmonary and cardiac distress may occur. Spontaneous pneumothorax and subcutaneous emphysema may occur following thoracocentesis. A portable chest radiograph is usually ordered to verify that a pneumothorax is not present
	The volume, colour and consistency of the pleural fluid is determined and recorded. The specimen containers are labelled and sent promptly to the laboratory	Accurate, prompt documentation is a legal requirement. Prompt labelling and discharge of specimens ensures identification of the specimen and that contamination of the specimen does not occur

unstable and, when negative pressure is created within the thoracic cavity for inhalation to occur, collapse of the chest wall inwards occurs (Fig. 13.8). This is known as *paradoxical respiration*. The result is that the lung is not adequately ventilated and life-threatening respiratory failure may ensue, particularly if the injury is associated with a haemopneumothorax. Early death after chest trauma is usually due to hypoxia or hypovolaemia. Such injuries often require urgent positive pressure artificial ventilation, for which the patient needs intubation.

Figure 13.8   A flail segment. Expansion of the chest wall leads to the pressure inside the chest being lower than atmospheric pressure. Therefore the flail segment collapses in on the lung, preventing proper expansion and ventilation.

Double fractures

Respiratory failure
See chapter 5.3

Restricted lung expansion may be the result of impaired nerve supply to the respiratory muscles, as occurs in the Guillain–Barré syndrome and poliomyelitis, or it may be due to muscular weakness incurred by a chemical deficit at the myoneural junction (myasthenia gravis). The impaired muscle contraction causes dyspnoea and, if severe enough, respiratory failure. Involvement of the diaphragm increases symptoms and assisted ventilation is usually necessary. Severe obesity alters the mechanics of breathing by decreasing lung inflation, chest wall compliance and lung volumes.

Respiratory failure

Respiratory failure is a disorder of respiratory function that is present when a person is unable to maintain adequate arterial blood levels of oxygen and carbon dioxide. A Pao_2 of less than 8.0 kPa (60 mmHg) or a $Paco_2$ of more than 6.2 kPa (45 mmHg) is the parameter used to define respiratory failure.

Causes

Respiratory failure may be encountered in any clinical area and may be associated with a variety of disorders, including:

- trauma or surgery that lead to shock

- intrapulmonary disorders, such as acute and chronic airway obstruction, resistive disorders and pulmonary vascular disorders

- central nervous system disorders, such as drug overdose, brain tumour, cerebral injury or haemorrhage

- neuromuscular disease that involves respiratory muscle innovation (e.g. myasthenia gravis and Guillain–Barré syndrome)

- sepsis, especially if the organisms are Gram negative.

- obstructive and central sleep apnoea.

Patients with a history of chronic obstructive pulmonary disease (asthma, chronic bronchitis) and cardiac or kidney disease, and those who are obese or debilitated, are predisposed to develop respiratory failure.

Respiratory failure may be the result of alveolar hypoventilation, inadequate oxygenation of the blood (as occurs in ventilation perfusion imbalance) or right-to-left shunt. In some instances more than one problem is present. Ventilation perfusion inequality is the most frequent cause and is largely responsible for the low Po_2 in respiratory failure that results as a complication of obstructive and restrictive diseases and adult respiratory distress syndrome (ARDS). Alveolar hypoventilation is characterized by the retention of an excessive volume of carbon dioxide (hypercarbia), accompanied by hypoxaemia. The patient develops respiratory acidosis because of the raised $Paco_2$. It is frequently associated with general hypoventilation due to neuromuscular disturbances and chest wall injury. When diffusion is impaired the carbon dioxide retention is initially slight and hypoxia is usually minimal.

Failure to oxygenate the blood adequately may be due to abnormal distribution of the inspired gas, ventilation perfusion inequality or shunting of the blood through unventilated areas of the lung. The alveoli may be filled with fluid, or the alveoli are not ventilated because of an airway obstruction or atelectasis. As a result, the blood may flow through the capillaries around the alveoli without gas exchange taking place. When blood enters the arterial system without going through ventilated areas of the lung, it is referred to as a shunt, such as occurs with a heart defect when the blood moves directly from the right side of the heart to the left. In other instances the alveoli may be ventilated but the respective capillaries do not receive an adequate blood supply or are occluded (*ventilation perfusion mismatching*).

When respiratory failure is severe, pulmonary capillary epithelium is damaged, which leads to haemorrhage and interstitial oedema. The oedema decreases diffusion because fluid lies between the alveoli and capillaries. Fluid infiltrates the alveoli; surfactant is destroyed by proteins that leak through the permeable capillaries; and functional terminal respiratory units collapse. The capillaries dilate, the alveolar walls hypertrophy and the lungs become fibrotic. Defective gas diffusion becomes extensive and very serious. This severe form of acute respiratory failure may be referred to as *adult respiratory distress syndrome* (ARDS) or *shock lung*. There is increased resistance to air entry in the airways and alveoli.

Characteristics

The person may manifest the effects of hypoxaemia or hypercarbia, or both. Dyspnoea or tachypnoea may be present, or in ventilatory failure respirations may be depressed and are slow, irregular and shallow. The pulse rate increases and arrhythmias may develop. The patient may be restless and complain of headache or dizziness. Disorientation, apathy and slow responses develop as a result of the cerebral hypoxia, and may progress to unconsciousness. Periodic sustained contraction of a group of skeletal muscles (asterixis), slurred speech and mood fluctuations may occur if there is marked retention of carbon dioxide. The tidal and minute volumes are usually reduced.

Respiratory failure may develop quickly in a few hours after the initial insult, or the onset may be insidious over a few days or weeks. Serial monitoring of the patient's blood gases and tidal volume, and close observation of the characteristics of the respirations in circumstances where respiratory insufficiency may occur, are important in early recognition of the problem.

Treatment

The underlying disorder that initiated the respiratory failure is treated and therapy is immediately directed toward improving ventilation and oxygenation of the blood. Airway obstruction is alleviated by removing retained secretions, through coughing, postural drainage and suctioning. A bronchodilator (e.g. salbutamol) is administered and respiratory stimulants may be given. Respiratory depressants are avoided. Corticosteroids are useful for some patients to improve their airflow.

Infections are treated promptly as they may produce respiratory failure in patients with chronic airflow limitation.

The aspiration of acid from the stomach into the lungs (acid reflux) occurs in many people with chronic respiratory failure, particularly when they are lying down. Measures to correct or modify the problem are developed in collaboration with the patient. Dietary measures include the avoidance of caffeine and eliminating evening snacks. The head of the bed is elevated on blocks. Antacid medications and histamine (H_2) antagonists such as ranitidine may be used to minimize the effects of the stomach acid.

Figure 13.9 Venturi mask (entrainment mask).

Diuretics are prescribed to decrease fluid overload in persons with cardiac complications. Changes in bodyweight are monitored and the person's ankles are observed for swelling.

Oxygen may be administered by Venturi mask (see Fig. 13.9) at a concentration of 24–28%. The administration of uncontrolled oxygen via nasal prongs or a simple mask may depress respiration and increase respiratory failure in individuals whose main respiratory stimulus is hypoxaemia. The number of hours of oxygen therapy per day is individually prescribed and will vary at different times for the same patient as the requirements fluctuate. A person who requires home oxygen for 14 hours a day when well may require continuous oxygen therapy during a respiratory infection that has increased the respiratory failure.

Additional nursing measures include exercise programmes to strengthen respiratory muscles and the use of breathing techniques. Patients with chronic respiratory failure are encouraged to remain active, eat a well balanced diet, maintain their desired body weight and get adequate rest and sleep. Individuals and their families are taught to monitor their respiratory status, to adjust the therapeutic regimen to prevent complications, and to treat them early when they do occur.

Patients requiring respiratory assistance

Care of the patient with an artificial airway

When there is an actual or potential obstruction of the upper airway, intervention is needed to secure efficient and reliable ventilation of the lungs.

Endotracheal Intubation

An oropharyngeal airway is useful in emergency and following anaesthesia to safeguard the airway against blockage by the tongue, should the patient be unconscious and have therefore lost the gag reflex and the ability to cough. The airway should be introduced inverted and then rotated into the correct position over the back of the tongue. Once in situ, it should be left until the patient recovers consciousness sufficiently for the gag reflex to return; at this stage the patient will cough the airway out spontaneously.

The site of the obstruction may be lower than the oropharynx; there may be severe facial trauma threatening the airway; or the patient may require artificial ventilation. In cases such as these a different solution is required and the patient will either have an endotracheal tube introduced as a temporary measure, or a tracheostomy may be performed, which could be temporary or permanent.

Common clinical situations in which an endotracheal tube is passed include emergency airway management (e.g. trauma, cardiac arrest), before operation to facilitate artificial ventilation and anaesthesia, and to allow efficient airway management for artificially ventilated patients in intensive care units.

The tube is usually passed (this is called *intubation*) through the mouth into the trachea, although the nasal route may also be used. If the patient is conscious, a quick-acting anaesthetic drug and a muscle relaxant (e.g. suxamethonium) are usually administered intravenously to permit intubation. The patient's airway is totally dependent upon the endotracheal tube thereafter; if muscle relaxant drugs have been used, the patient will be unable to breathe spontaneously as all muscles in the body will be paralysed. Maintaining ventilation, and hence the life of the patient, is therefore totally in the hands of the medical and nursing staff.

The endotracheal tube bypasses the upper airway where warming, humidification and filtration occurs; it also bypasses the vocal chords, so the patient cannot speak. If the tube is to be in situ for any length of time, it is important that the artificial ventilation system in use permits air to be warmed and humidified. The patient cannot drink, which means regular oral toilet is needed, otherwise the patient's mouth will become dry and *Candida* infection is possible.

If the patient is conscious, communication will be a major problem and aids such as a pencil and paper are vital. Ashworth (1980), in a now classical piece of nursing research, showed that nurses failed to communicate with intensive care patients if they could not talk back. Every effort should therefore be made to communicate with ventilated or unconscious patients. If possible patients should be informed beforehand that they will not be able to speak after intubation, and the temporary nature of the condition explained.

For intubation, any dentures should be removed and the patient should be positioned on the back, with the head extended and slightly supported to ensure correct alignment of the mouth, pharynx and larnyx. Using a laryngoscope the endotracheal tube is introduced and the proximal portion is secured to the patient's face. The tube, made from soft plastic, is more pliable and less traumatic to tissue than a rubber tube (Fig. 13.10). The tube is equipped with an inflatable cuff a short distance above the distal end. The cuff remains soft when inflated, thereby exerting only a low pressure on the tracheal walls and thus minimizing the risk of tissue damage through trauma or ischaemia. When inflated, the tube prevents the aspiration of vomitus and oral secretions. It also permits

Figure 13.10   An endotracheal tube with inflatable cuff which provides a seal between the trachea and tube. After the tube is inserted, the cuff is inflated by introducing a specified volume of air through the fine attached tube, which is then clamped.

more effective ventilation by preventing the escape of gases being delivered under pressure.

When the tube is in position, the cuff is inflated with air if the patient is to receive mechanical ventilatory assistance. Near the proximal end of the fine tube leading to the cuff, and through which the air is introduced, there is a small balloon-like dilatation that remains inflated when the tube is clamped. This dilatation is observed frequently and, as long as it remains inflated, the cuff is also inflated.

Immediately after insertion of the tube, and then at regular intervals, the chest is auscultated to determine whether air is entering both lungs. If the tube is too low, the inflated cuff could completely block off a bronchus and cause atelectasis of the respective lung. A radiograph may be taken to check the position of the tube.

The endotracheal tube is distressing and a source of discomfort to the conscious patient. Prolonged use may cause damage to the vocal chords and ulceration in the trachea. If an artificial airway is necessary for a prolonged period, a tracheostomy is done and the endotracheal tube removed.

Periodic deflation of the cuff should not be necessary if a large-volume low-pressure cuff is used. The inspired gas is humidified before entering the endotracheal tube to liquefy secretions and prevent encrusting within the tract and tube. Frequent deep suction through the endotracheal tube is necessary.

Suctioning may deplete the amount of oxygen reaching the alveoli. The patient may be given oxygen prior to suction, and again following suction. The patient's pulse is monitored for possible cardiac dysfunction and arrhythmias (due to hypoxia) during and after the suctioning. If any irregularity occurs, suctioning is immediately discontinued and oxygen is administered with the self-inflating bag and mask.

Using sterile gloves, the nurse passes a sterile catheter through the tube into the trachea. Suction is not applied while the catheter is being introduced. When in position, suction is applied intermittently and the catheter is rotated and withdrawn. If the airway is not clear of secretions, the catheter is not allowed to become contaminated and may be reintroduced into the trachea. It will probably be necessary to ventilate the patient with the self-inflating bag before passing the catheter again. If the secretions are tenacious, 5–10 mL of a sterile saline solution may be introduced into the tube, followed by immediate suction. After suction the patient is hyperoxygenated.

Frequent mouth care is necessary, and suctioning of the oropharyngeal area at frequent intervals is done to remove the secretions that may form in response to the presence of the tube. When the patient is to be *extubated*, the emergency (resuscitation) trolley should be accessible so the patient can be quickly reintubated if necessary.

Before the cuff is deflated and the doctor removes the tube, secretions are suctioned from the oropharynx to prevent aspiration. After removal of the tube, the patient is observed for respiratory distress and insufficiency. A nurse remains in attendance, constantly monitoring the patient's respirations, pulse and colour. The patient is usually apprehensive and needs the nurse's presence and reassurance.

Tracheostomy

Tracheostomy tubes are similar to endotracheal tubes but are inserted through an incision in the neck, directly into the trachea; they are therefore much shorter. The artificial airway bypasses the larynx and air passages above.

Indications for a tracheostomy include:

1. An upper airway obstruction (e.g. laryngeal tumour).

2. Prolonged, mechanically assisted, ventilation where a seal is necessary to prevent loss of ventilatory gas that is under pressure.

3. The need for more efficient access to retained pulmonary secretions which, unless removed, may cause serious respiratory problems such as atelectasis and pneumonia.

4. The prevention of recurrent aspiration of oral secretions and vomitus.

Since endotracheal intubation has been more commonly used and may be performed very quickly, tracheostomy is rarely used in an emergency situation. The procedure is generally elective, and is performed with an endotracheal tube in position and under aseptic conditions in an operating room. It may be necessary as an emergency measure if the patient cannot be intubated because of facial injuries or burns, laryngeal oedema or severe upper airway infection. If the tracheostomy is associated with laryngectomy, it becomes permanent.

The operative procedure is undertaken with the patient in the dorsal position, head and neck hyperextended. A pillow or folded sheet is placed under the shoulders. A vertical or horizontal incision is made about 2 cm above the suprasternal notch to expose the upper part of the trachea. This is then opened, usually at the level of the second and third cartilaginous rings, and a tracheostomy tube is introduced. The tube is held in position by laterally attached tapes which are tied securely around the neck.

Tracheostomy tubes are available in various sizes. The diameter and length of the tube selected depends upon the size of the trachea, and is slightly smaller in diameter than the trachea. The tubes may be made from plastic, silver or nylon, and may be single or consist of two parts – an inner and outer cannula (Fig. 13.11). When a double-lumen tube is used, the outer cannula is fitted with an obturator that extends beyond the distal end of the tube.

Tracheostomy
See chapter 5.3

Figure 13.11   Tracheostomy tubes. (a) Outer part of metal tracheostomy tube. (b) Inner part of metal tracheostomy tube. (c) Obturator used during insertion of the outer metal tube. (d) Polyethylene cuffed tube.

Its end is blunt and smooth, which facilitates the introduction of the tube. As soon as the tube is in position, the obturator is removed and the inner tube is inserted and secured.

The tube with an inner cannula provides a more efficient means of clearing the airway of secretions, because the inner tube can be removed and readily cleansed without the risk of compromising the airway. The single tube (without an inner cannula) must be changed about every 3 days or more often if secretions accumulate within the tube. The tube with an inner cannula may be left for a longer period.

Most synthetic tubes now in use have a high-volume low-pressure cuff which encircles the lower part of the outer tube. After the tube is in position, the cuff is inflated by introducing a small amount of air via a fine tube that leads into it. The cuff creates a seal between the trachea and the tube, and prevents air from entering or escaping around the tube, in addition to preventing the aspiration of secretions or fluid into the tract below. This type of tube is used most frequently for patients who require mechanical assistance in breathing.

The amount of air required to produce a seal without unnecessary pressure on tracheal tissue varies from 2 to 10 mL. While introducing the air, the nurse listens and tests for the escape of air from around the tube. The tracheostomy tube may be blocked off momentarily while testing for leakage around the tube. When the inflation is completed, the end of the fine tube is clamped. The amount of air used in inflating the cuff is recorded each time; any significant change observed from one time to another is reported. A decreased amount of air used may indicate swelling and oedema in the air passage tissues.

Near the proximal end of the fine inflating tube is a small balloon-like dilatation. This is inflated and, because it is visible, may be checked frequently to determine whether the tube and the cuff below remain inflated. Obviously, if the small pilot balloon becomes deflated, a leak in the system is indicated and the cuff will be deflated, thus losing the intratracheal seal.

A variety of tubes are available that facilitate upper respiratory breathing or speaking and are used when weaning patients from mechanical ventilation.

Tracheostomy care

The nurse should appreciate that the patient is dependent upon the patency of the tracheostomy tube for breathing. Constant attention and meticulous care are necessary to prevent serious complications and to reduce the patient's fear of choking. Sensitivity to the patient's fears and needs is important, because the patient cannot communicate verbally.

Preparation for tracheostomy

The doctor explains the procedure to the patient and family and informed consent is obtained. The nurse assesses the patient's understanding of the procedure. The patient is assured that someone will be in constant, close attendance and that provision will be made for communication by writing. A similar explanation is given to the family. Opportunities are provided for the patient and family members to ask questions and to receive further clarification.

Preparation to receive the patient

This includes assembling sterile suction equipment, ventilator if indicated, adaptor to fit the tracheostomy tube, oxygen administration equipment and a tray with various

Figure 13.12 Ambu resuscitator: a self-inflating hand-compressible breathing bag and mask.

sizes of sterile tracheostomy tubes in case the one inserted becomes dislodged. Sterile tape for securing the tube in place, gauze squares, tracheal dilator, artery forceps and a sterile syringe to inflate the cuff are required. A catheter mount, which can be used to connect an Ambu bag (see Fig. 13.12) to the tracheostomy tube should emergency resuscitation be required, is essential. A humidifier should also be switched on and ready for use; the type will depend on whether the patient is to receive mechanical ventilatory assistance; if not, a nebulizer may be available that fits over the opening of the tube. Equipment for frequent mouth cleansing should be available, and a pencil and slate or pad.

Position

The head of the bed is usually elevated to approximately a 45° angle if the patient is conscious and the blood pressure and pulse are stable.

Assessment

Frequent monitoring of blood pressure, respiratory rate and sounds, pulse and colour is necessary. An increase in the respiratory rate, crackles and wheezes, and an increased pulse rate may indicate the need for suction. The patient may still experience respiratory insufficiency due to obstruction in the tract below the tracheostomy. This could be evidenced by marked respiratory effort, unequal movement of the sides of the chest and retraction of the soft tissues in the intercostal and supraclavicular

spaces. Cyanosis and distress not relieved by suctioning are reported promptly. Increasing restlessness, especially if accompanied by a rapid pulse rate, may indicate hypoxia or bleeding.

The neck and area around the incision are inspected for possible interstitial emphysema due to air leaking into the subcutaneous tissue. The wound is observed for bleeding in the immediate postoperative period and then checked daily for signs of infection and sloughing.

The tube is checked frequently for patency and the characteristics (consistency, colour, amount) of the tracheobronchial secretions are noted. Increased secretion occurs in response to the tracheal trauma and is usually coloured by blood at first, but the blood content should gradually diminish and disappear.

Suction

Frequency of suctioning is determined by assessment of the patient's breathing and the rate of production of secretions. It is possible that an apparent decrease in secretions actually means they have just become thicker and more readily retained. Sterile saline may be instilled into the tube and followed immediately by suctioning to help loosen tenacious secretions.

If the patient is receiving mechanical ventilatory assistance or oxygen, he or she may be hyperoxygenated before suction (100% oxygen for 35 minutes). Suctioning removes air and oxygen from the respiratory tract, as well as removing secretions, and may cause hypoxaemia and ensuing cardiac arrhythmia. The development of hypoxaemia is related to the duration of suctioning and the frequency of passing the suction catheter.

The trachea is suctioned using a sterile glove and a sterile suction catheter moistened in sterile water or normal saline. The negative pressure is not applied during the insertion of the catheter but is applied when it is in position and during withdrawal. Suctioning must be brief, not longer than 10–15 seconds. If it must be repeated, the patient is allowed several breaths or is given oxygen again.

Secretions and suction may initiate coughing. Secretions escaping from the tracheostomy tube are gently wiped away with sterile unfrayed gauze (free of lint and absorbent). The mucus and exudate must be cleaned away quickly before being drawn back into the tube with a breath.

Tube and wound care

The wound and surrounding skin are kept as free of secretions as possible. The wound and area under the tube are protected with a dressing; a number of dressings are now available that have been developed for this specific purpose, many of which contain foam, thus increasing their absorbency and patient comfort. If the tapes securing the tube become soiled, they are replaced with fresh sterile tapes. It is advisable to have two nurses (or the help of a relative) when changing the tapes so that one person can gently but firmly hold the tracheostomy tube in place while the other changes the tapes. This reduces the risk of the tube becoming displaced during the procedure (e.g. as a result of the patient coughing). The tapes should always be tied in a double bow or knot as a single bow can easily become undone if the tapes are inadvertently caught on something.

The inner cannula of the tracheostomy tube is carefully removed and cleansed as often as necessary (perhaps even hourly). Hydrogen peroxide or sodium bicarbonate solution may be used to soak the tube to loosen crusts of mucus, and the cannula is then cleansed using a small tube brush or applicator. It is then rinsed in water and sterilized. The outer cannula is suctioned if necessary before the inner cannula is reinserted. Precautions must be taken not to displace the outer tube; the tapes that secure it are checked frequently.

Single tubes are usually changed by the surgeon or an experienced trained nurse, as often as necessary to ensure patency. The tube with an inner cannula may be changed weekly. A tray with sterile replacement tubes and the necessary equipment is kept at the bedside.

Should the tube come out of the trachea because of vigorous coughing or carelessly tied tapes, the tracheal opening closes and the patient is threatened with asphyxia. Prompt action is necessary. The tracheal wound may be quickly reopened with the sterile tracheal dilator or artery forceps, which are always kept at the bedside in the event of such an emergency. The opening is held open until the doctor (or experienced nurse) arrives and inserts the sterile tracheostomy tube.

An alternative course of action if you witness the displacement of a tracheostomy tube would be quickly to open one of the sterile tracheostomy tubes which should be by the patient and insert this into the stoma. This may be less traumatic than the use of tracheal dilators, particularly if the surgical wound is fresh.

Humidification

Humidification of the inspired gas is very important to prevent encrustations forming within the trachea and the tube, as these will increase airway resistance.

Fluids and nutrition

A minimum fluid intake of 3000 mL is recommended to help liquefy pulmonary secretions, unless contraindicated by cardiac insufficiency and oedema. An accurate record is kept of the intake and output. The patient is not usually permitted any fluids or food by mouth; they are administered intravenously. Some patients are fed via a nasogastric tube.

If the tracheostomy is to be permanent, or the patient is not on a ventilator, oral fluids are introduced gradually; if tolerated, a soft diet is given and increased gradually to a regular diet. The nurse remains with the patient until sufficient confidence is gained.

Mouth care

Oral hygiene is important for comfort and to reduce the risk of infection. The mouth is cleansed and rinsed every 2 hours until the patient is taking normal meals, at which time regular cleansing of the teeth and rinsing of the mouth after each meal and at bedtime suffice.

Communication

The patient is likely to be fearful of choking and concerned about his or her inability to cough up the secretions and to communicate. When the nurse leaves the bedside, the patient is advised of the errand and how long it will take. A call-bell is given to the patient, who will be more secure knowing that someone can be called if necessary.

The nurse talks to the patient, informing him or her of progress and what is to happen next. It is very helpful to try to anticipate information the patient might want but cannot ask for. A pad and pencil are kept readily within reach, and the patient is encouraged to communicate feelings and needs. Hand signals are developed to enable the patient to communicate yes or no, or to make routine requests by raising one or more fingers. Family members are encouraged to talk to the patient.

Extubation

If the patient has been receiving mechanical ventilatory assistance, removal of the tracheostomy tube is not considered until he or she is breathing successfully without the ventilator. When the tracheostomy is a temporary measure, the patient is gradually returned to breathing through the upper tract. In order to lessen tracheal injury and scarring, the tube is removed as soon as possible, but without compromising adequate ventilation. The protective reflexes should be responsive; the epiglottis and glottis should be closed to prevent aspiration, the gag reflex should be present and the patient should be able to swallow fluids and food without risk of aspiration.

If a cuffed tube has been used, the cuff may be deflated for 24–48 hours before the tube is removed and the patient's ability to keep upper tract secretions out of the lower tract is observed. A sterile tracheostomy tray with tubes of several sizes is kept at the bedside in case a tube has to be reinserted after extubation. Sterile suction equipment should also be available.

When the tracheostomy tube is removed, the wound is cleansed, the wound edges are approximated and taped, and a firm dressing is applied. Healing occurs spontaneously; sutures are not considered necessary. The patient is advised to place a hand over the area and exert some pressure when coughing. He or she may be fearful of not being able to breathe when the tube is removed, so is assured beforehand that breathing is adequate via the normal route. A nurse remains following removal to be certain that no difficulty is experienced. After discharge, the patient needs to be monitored to check for possible scarring and tracheal stricture resulting from irritation and trauma.

Home tracheostomy care

If the tracheostomy is permanent, the patient is instructed about the care of the tube and the stoma. This is done as soon as the patient is well enough to undertake the care in the hospital, so confidence will be developed. If possible, and with the patient's consent, a member of the family also receives instructions about the necessary care and precautions.

The patient and family are referred to the district nurse who is able to obtain the necessary suction equipment and dressing supplies, and also give instruction in the use and care of the equipment. The patient and family are advised how to conceal the site of the tracheostomy using collared shirts, a scarf or high-necked garments.

An explanation is made of the danger of aspirating water through the tracheostomy tube. In the past, a person with a tracheostomy was not allowed to swim, but there are now several devices available that make swimming a safe form of recreation. These devices need to be fitted professionally and care must be taken when first entering the water. Precautions must also be used when taking a shower.

The patient is advised to return to the outpatient department or to the general practitioner at regular intervals, as directed, for changing the tube and examination of the stoma. Eventually, when the stoma is firmly healed and the tracheal opening remains patent, the patient or a member of the family may be taught to change the outer cannula, or the tube may be removed permanently (if a laryngectomy has been performed). Precautions should be used to avoid close contact with those in the environment with respiratory infection.

Patients requiring mechanical ventilation

Mechanical ventilation supports respiration automatically by delivering air with an enhanced concentration of oxygen and in the process fully expanding the lungs. It is indicated when respiratory failure occurs and the patient is unable to maintain their own adequate arterial blood gases. However, only those patients who can benefit from respiratory support and have a realistic chance of survival should be established on ventilatory support.

Indications of the need for mechanical ventilation

The decision to ventilate a patient mechanically is usually taken by an anaesthetist. However, when appropriate, this may be discussed with the patient and family.

Mechanical ventilation may be indicated in a number of different circumstances including:

- post-surgery (e.g. following elective or emergency major abdominal, gastric, cardiac or neurological surgery)

- post-trauma (e.g. for a flail chest, multiple fractures, massive blood loss or spinal injury)

- acute ventilatory or respiratory failure (e.g. respiratory arrest, adult respiratory distress syndrome, infection or sepsis, or cerebral haemorrhage, multiple organ failure)

- impending acute respiratory failure (e.g. respiratory muscle weakness due to Guillain–Barré syndrome, self-poisoning)

- chronic conditions (e.g. chronic pulmonary disease).

Clinical investigations that may help to identify the need for mechanical ventilation include blood gas analysis, chest radiography and lung function tests. Mechanical ventilation is usually carried out via a positive-pressure ventilator which actively administers gas into the patient's lungs via a series of tubes and an artificial airway (commonly an endotracheal or tracheostomy tube). These ventilators are either volume or pressure controlled, reflecting the mechanism that terminates the inspiratory phase.

Volume-controlled ventilators

The inspiratory phase ends after a pre-set tidal volume or minute volume has been delivered. The machine will deliver this volume to the patient. However, lung compliance is reduced in most patients who require ventilation. This means that, to deliver a satisfactory volume to the patient, the pressure in the lungs may be high. This high airway pressure may cause further damage to the lungs. To prevent this, pressure-controlled ventilation may be used.

Pressure-controlled ventilators

This mode of ventilation delivers the inspiratory gas until a pre-set pressure is reached. This then determines the volume of gas the patient receives. The greater the compliance of the lungs, the lower the inflation pressures required to obtain a satisfactory minute and tidal volume. By controlling the airway pressure in this way, further lung damage may be avoided (*barotrauma*). Pressure-controlled ventilation also provides a greater distribution of gas around the lung.

Positive-pressure ventilation, regardless of the type of ventilator used, may be divided into controlled or assisted ventilation. In *controlled* ventilation the patient is making no respiratory effort and respiration is entirely dependent on the ventilator. An *assisted* ventilation mode may be used when patients are capable of making some respiratory effort themselves: the ventilator is literally assisting the patient to breathe. Recent advances in positive-pressure ventilator therapy have included development of the biphasic intermittent positive airway pressure (BIPAP) mode. In this mode, pressure alternates between two adjustable pressure levels. These levels are positive end-expiratory pressure (PEEP) and inspired pressure. Between these two pressures the patient can be ventilated manually or allowed to breathe spontaneously. This mode benefits the patient as it allows one mode to be used from the instigation of ventilation all the way through the ventilation episode. It allows much greater patient comfort whilst reducing the need for sedation. By having the airway pressure controlled, the patient is at much less risk of barotrauma. The extent of the assistance provided by the ventilator is variable and is determined by the mode selected by the anaesthetist.

The use of positive-pressure ventilators is largely limited to intensive care settings where nurses and other staff are skilled in the care of ventilated patients and the staffing levels allow close observation. Patients in intensive care environments who are mechanically ventilated are frequently sedated and in some instances will receive muscle relaxant drugs to enable them to tolerate the artificial airway and mechanical ventilation. These patients are totally reliant upon nursing staff for their personal safety and the fulfilment of their needs.

Localized airway obstruction

Localized obstruction of airflow is less common than chronic airflow limitation and causes less residual impairment.

Obstruction of the nasal passages

The narrow nasal passages are particularly susceptible to obstruction. Obstruction may be the result of:

- trauma causing deviation of the septum and nasal fractures
- foreign bodies in the nose, which are common in childhood
- growths and polyps
- inflammation of the nasal mucosa as a result of irritation from pollution, allergies, smoking or infection.

Signs and symptoms include asymmetry of the nose from trauma, bleeding, and thin to thick purulent drainage. The person breathes through one nostril or the mouth when obstruction is present.

Obstruction of the pharynx

Inflammation and enlargement of the adenoids in the nasopharynx and of the tonsils in the oropharynx interfere with breathing and swallowing. Foreign bodies that are of sufficient size to lodge in the oropharynx are usually relatively easy to remove. Smaller objects that pass on to the larynx and bronchi pose a greater hazard.

Obstruction of the larynx

Oedema, laryngeal spasm or aspiration of a foreign body may cause obstruction in the larynx. Any constriction or obstruction in the larynx is manifested quickly by hoarseness, dyspnoea, stridor, cyanosis, and increased but ineffective inspiratory effort, evidenced by the retraction of the intercostal spaces. Prompt emergency measures are necessary or death may ensue as a result of asphyxia.

Obstruction of the trachea

Aspiration of a foreign body, scarring following trauma or surgery, or pressure from an aortic aneurysm or neoplasm of a neighbouring structure may narrow the trachea and

Figure 13.13 The Heimlich method of dislodging a foreign body from the larynx or trachea. If patient has collapsed or is unable to stand, crossed hands can be placed just below the ribcage and a firm upward thrust exerted (a). Alternatively, if the patient can stand, the thrust may be performed by someone standing behind the patient and clasping their hands below the ribcage (b).

(a)   (b)

offer resistance to the flow of air. Inspiratory and expiratory stridor result and hypoventilation leads to hypercapnoea and hypoxaemia.

Obstruction of the airway by an aspirated foreign body presents an acute emergency. The patient should be slapped vigorously between the scapulae. Alternatively, someone standing behind the individual places the arms around the victim's trunk just below the diaphragm, clasping the hands in front. Pressure is applied with the arms and hands (Fig. 13.13). The compression (*Heimlich hug or manoeuvre*) forces air under pressure through the airway and may dislodge the aspirated mass. If this procedure does not dislodge the object, a laryngoscope may be quickly introduced through which the offending object may be retrieved. If the patient's breathing is completely obstructed, an emergency tracheostomy may have to be performed to establish an airway before the foreign body can be removed .

For *oedema* or *spasm*, intubation may be performed in which a tube is passed beyond the obstruction into the trachea to establish an airway, or the doctor may do a tracheostomy. If oedema of the larynx is due to an allergic response, the patient is given adrenaline 1 : 1000 subcutaneously. An adrenal corticosteroid preparation such as prednisolone may be prescribed for a brief period to reduce tissue sensitivity. Local applications of ice to the neck may also be suggested.

Obstruction of a bronchus

If a foreign body is inhaled, it may pass into either bronchus, but most often the right bronchus is blocked. Localized obstruction may also be caused by enlarged lymph nodes surrounding the bronchus. Complete obstruction leads to atelectasis (collapse of the lung) beyond the obstruction.

Summary

The constant exchange of oxygen and carbon dioxide between an individual and the environment is essential to life. Impairment of respiratory function threatens the individual's survival and either temporarily or permanently disrupts health and the quality of life. Respiratory disorders are common and familiar occurrences. Each of us has experienced the difficulties with airway clearance that result from acute respiratory infections. We can relate to the fear and apprehension demonstrated by persons with acute respiratory distress. It is much more difficult to appreciate fully the enormous personal impact that chronic respiratory disorders have on the patient and family, their daily functioning and lifestyles. Medical advances have been made in the management of acute and chronic respiratory disorders, but medical cures do not exist for most respiratory diseases. Patients and their families must learn to live with the resulting health problems.

The nursing care of people with respiratory problems includes the negotiation of long-term patient goals and outcomes as well as goals and outcomes for the current clinical situation. Nurses are assuming an increased role in helping patients with respiratory conditions and their families to acquire self-management skills and to achieve productive lives. Advances in nursing research related to respiratory function are providing scientific rationales for the selection of specific nursing strategies and are helping nurses to evaluate the effectiveness of therapeutic measures. Nurses are becoming better prepared and able to assume greater responsibility for providing nursing solutions to patients' respiratory health problems. Nurses need to be working collaboratively with other health professionals, patients and carers to optimize respiratory function and quality of life for those with respiratory disorders.

References

Ashworth P (1980) Care to communicate. London: Royal College of Nursing.

Avery S (2000) Insertion and management of chest drains. NT Plus – Respiratory Care 3–6, published with Nursing Times 96(37).

Bloom SR, ed. (1995) Tooheys medicine, 15th edn. Edinburgh: Churchill Livingstone.

Brewin A (1997) Comparing asthma and chronic obstructive airways disease (COPD). Nursing Standard 12(4): 49–53.

British National Formulary (2001) British National Formulary, Edition 41. London: British Medical Association/Royal Pharmaceutical Society of Great Britain.

British Thoracic Society (1997a) British guidelines on asthma management: 1995 review and position statement. Thorax 52: S1–24.

British Thoracic Society (1997b) Guidelines for the management of chronic obstructive pulmonary disease. Thorax 52(5): S1–S32.

Byrne DM, Drury J, Mackay RC et al (1993) Evaluation of the efficacy of an instructional programme in the self management of patients with asthma. Journal of Advanced Nursing 18: 637–646.

Central Statistical Office (1995) Annual abstract of statistics. London: HMSO.

Clutton-Brock TH (1997) The assessment and monitoring of respiratory function. In: Goldhill DR, Withington PS, eds. Textbook of intensive care, pp. 345–355. London: Chapman and Hall.

Department of Health (1995) Identifying R&D priorities for the NHS on asthma management: report to the NHS central research and development committee. London: DoH.

Donaldson J (1993) Asthma: the insider's view. Nursing Times 89(3): 64.

Godden J, Hiley C (1998) Managing the patient with a chest drain, a review. Nursing Standard 12(32): 35–39.

Haslett C, Chivers E, Hunter J, Boon N (1999) Davidson's principles and practice of medicine, 18th edn. Edinburgh: Churchill Livingstone.

Haughney J (1998) The role of inhaled steroids in COPD: the search for evidence. Asthma in General Practice 6(1): 5–7.

Heslop A, Bagnall P (1988) A study to evaluate the intervention of a nurse visiting patients with disabling chest diseases in the community. Journal of Advanced Nursing 13(1): 71–77.

Hinchliff SM, Montagne SE, Watson R (1996) Physiology for nursing practice, 2nd edn. London: Baillière Tindall.

Howard J (1987) Respiratory teaching of patients, how effective is it? Journal of Advanced Nursing 12(2): 207–214.

Howell M (1996) Staff knowledge of inhaler technique improved by survey. Nursing Times 92(13): 30–32.

Kilgarriff J (2000) A practical guide to treating asthma. Nursing Times 96(31): 43–44.

Lipworth BJ (1999) Modern drug treatment of chronic asthma. British Medical Journal 318: 380–384.

Mera S (1997) Understanding disease: pathology and prevention. Cheltenham: Stanley Thornes.

Morgan AD, Peck DF, Buchanan DR, McHardy GJR (1983) Effect of attitudes and beliefs on exercise tolerance in chronic bronchitis. British Medical Journal 286: 171–173.

Partridge MR (1996) Self-management plans: uses and limitations. British Journal of Hospital Medicine 55(3): 120–121.

Rees J, Kananbar D (2000) ABC of asthma, 4th edn. London: BMJ, Publishing.

Ross-Plummer B (2000) Preparing patients with asthma for discharge. Nursing Times Plus 96(24): 13–15.

Sharp J (1993) Which peak flow meter? Nursing Times 89(3): 61–63.

Springhouse Corporation (2000) Handbook of pathophysiology. Springhouse, PA Springhouse Corporation.

Szaflarski NL (1996) Preanalytic error associated with blood gas/pH measurement. Critical Care Nurse 16(3): 89–100.

Tettersall MJ (1993) Asthma patients' knowledge in relation to compliance with drug therapy. Journal of Advanced Nursing 18: 103–113.

Walsh M, Crumbie A, Reveley S (1999) Nurse practitioners; clinical skills and professional issues. Oxford: Butterworth Heinemann.

Ward M, Reynolds C (2000) Patient empowerment: the key to compliance in asthma. Nursing Times Plus 96(37): 8–9.

Welch J (1993) Chest drains and pleural drainage. Surgical Nurse 6(5): 7–12.

Williams S (1993) Chronic respiratory illness. (Experience of illness series.) London: Routledge.

Williams T (1992) To clamp or not to clamp? Nursing Times 88(18): 33.

Further Reading

Anderson P (1997) New British guidelines on managing asthma. Community Nurse 3(1): 8–9.

In this useful special news report, Pat Anderson reviews the most recent British Thoracic Society asthma guidelines. These are now known as the British Guidelines on Asthma Management.

Williams S (1993) Chronic respiratory illness (Experience of Illness series). London: Routledge.

This book provides a useful insight into the real life experiences of people living with a respiratory illness, and the problems they experience.

NT Plus (2000) Respiratory care (produced in conjunction with the Association of Respiratory Nurse Specialists). Published with Nursing Times 96(37).

This supplement to *Nursing Times* contains a number of useful articles relating to the care of patients with respiratory problems. The articles include: insertion and management of chest drains; patient empowerment: the key of compliance in asthma; asthma and women; identifying and treatment *Pneumocystis carinii* pneumonia.

Wooddrow P (2000) Intensive care nursing – a framework for practice. London: Routledge.

This British book on intensive care nursing contains sections throughout on the respiratory problems encountered by critically ill patients and related nursing care. As well as being a resource for nurses in intensive care units, the book is also a useful source of information for nurses caring for highly dependent patients outside specialist units.

14 Caring for the patient with a haematological disorder

Miriam Rowswell and Audrey Yandle

Introduction

Physiology

Blood disorders

Health assessment

Erythrocyte disorders

Leucocyte disorders

Lymphatic disorders

Haemorrhagic disorders

Transfusion practice

Summary

Introduction

Blood has been recognized as an important symbol of life throughout history. Folklore and religion have contributed to beliefs that blood has many attributes. These include not only its physiological functions but also its sacred and fantastic properties. Titmuss (1970) in his book *The Gift Relationship*, suggested that attitudes to blood and values associated with its possession, inheritance and loss are a distinctive feature of many different cultures. Bathing in blood, anointing with blood and drinking blood have been – and still are – practised either in reality or symbolically since ancient times. Historically, blood was identified as one of the four chief fluids or humours of the body along with phlegm, yellow bile (choler) and black bile (melancholy), the balance of which was believed to determine a person's physical and mental attributes. The sanguine temperament described the person in whom the blood predominates over other humours, giving rise to a person with a ruddy complexion, and a courageous, hopeful and amorous disposition. Blood-letting was practised as a treatment for many ailments in the belief that it would help to restore the balance of the body's humours.

Fears about blood also abound, and it is often the unexpected loss of blood that prompts individuals to seek medical advice without delay. Thus blood may simultaneously be perceived as a life-giving substance and a symbol of disease and death. Beliefs about so-called 'bad blood' have resurfaced in recent years, initially in connection with fears related to infection with the human immunodeficiency virus. More recently concerns have focused on risks related to transmission of the hepatitis C virus and Creutzfeldt–Jakob disease as a result of blood transfusion. Anxieties about blood transfusion are not new. Solzhenitsyn (1968) described the blood transfusion procedure and wrote of the fears and suspicions of the recipient of a transfusion in a Russian cancer unit in the 1950s. Issues relating to the transfusion of blood and blood products are considered later in this chapter.

Blood is one of the most familiar tissues of the body because it is frequently seen as a result of minor injuries. It is also easily sampled and examination of its constituents provides information about the function of other body tissues and organs. A specimen of blood is frequently taken and analysed as an aid to the diagnosis of a wide variety of conditions and to monitor the effects of treatment.

Blood
See chapter 4.1

Physiology

■ The haematological system consists of the blood and the sites of blood production including the bone marrow and lymph nodes.

Plasma
See chapter 4.1

Proteins
See chapter 4.1

- The average 70-kg adult male has a blood volume of about 5 litres. Blood constitutes 6–8% of bodyweight, the proportion being slightly lower for women and for the obese person (adipose tissue contains little blood), and greater for children.

- Blood is a red fluid connective tissue that is pumped throughout the vascular system by the heart.

- Blood is a medium for the transportation and distribution of cellular requirements and metabolic products between cells in different parts of the body and the external environment.

- Blood is vital to the maintenance of homeostasis. Continuous exchange of constituents across capillary walls between the blood and the fluid surrounding the cells (interstitial fluid) keeps the cellular environment relatively constant.

- Blood plays an important role in defending the body against infection and injury.

- Blood regulates body temperature and heat loss by distributing heat energy produced by metabolic reactions throughout the body and between the body and the external environment. This helps to keep the body's core temperature within narrow limits.

- Blood consists of a straw-coloured fluid called **plasma**, which is composed of water and a wide variety of solutes, and the formed elements (blood cells and platelets), which are suspended in the plasma (Fig. 14.1). Water and solutes are continually being added and removed. Temporary variations in solute concentrations occur but, in health, compensatory mechanisms act quickly to maintain plasma concentration within a normal range. An example of the operation of such a mechanism occurs following a meal when blood sugar levels are increased. Within 1–2 hours blood glucose levels are returned to a normal concentration of 3.9–6.1 mmol/L. Conversely if blood glucose falls, glucose is released into the blood to maintain a normal plasma concentration.

The plasma proteins

Serum albumin, serum globulin and serum fibrinogen comprise the majority of the solutes of the plasma. Their large molecular size prevents these **proteins** from diffusing easily through the capillary walls. The resulting

Figure 14.1 Composition of blood.

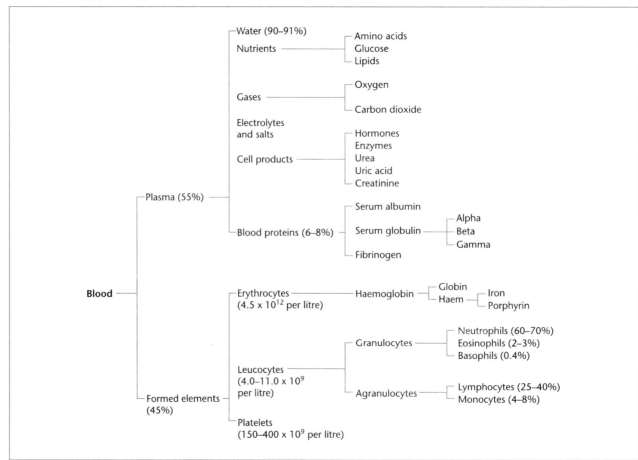

concentration of these relatively non-diffusible substances within the capillaries is responsible for what is referred to as the colloid osmotic pressure or oncotic pressure of the plasma (about 25–28 mmHg or 3.3–3.7 kPa). Reduction in the oncotic pressure may be due to excessive loss or diminished production, especially of albumin, and results in the accumulation of fluid in the tissues, known as oedema. The proteins also contribute to the viscosity (or thickness) of blood, which is 3–5 times that of water.

Serum albumin, fibrinogen and α- and β-globulins are formed in the liver from amino acids derived from ingested foods. In situations of protein starvation they can be synthesized from tissue protein. γ-Globulins are produced by plasma cells derived from B lymphocytes.

The functions of the plasma proteins may be summarized as follows.

Albumin

- Albumin exerts an intravascular oncotic pressure that influences fluid exchange between the interstitial and intravascular compartments.

- Albumin increases blood viscosity.

γ-Globulin

- γ-Globulin contributes to the immune response. It is the antibody fraction of the blood that binds to antigenic material and inactivates microbial agents and toxins.

Fibrinogen

- Fibrinogen plays a role in blood coagulation, which protects the individual from excessive loss of blood.

- At the site of inflammation or injury, fibrinogen forms an insoluble mesh in which the various tissues can grow and repair themselves.

General functions

- Plasma proteins combine with both alkalis and acids, and can act as a buffer to maintain a normal blood pH between 7.35 and 7.45.

- The proteins bind substances such as hormones, enzymes, lipids, fat-soluble vitamins and essential ions during their transport in the blood. This prevents too rapid an escape of these substances by filtration in the renal glomeruli.

- Many exogenous substances are also bound to plasma proteins. Drugs bound in this way (e.g. warfarin) may be biologically inactive until the protein reservoir is saturated or until they are displaced by a more strongly bound substance.

- Among the plasma proteins is a group known collectively as the complement system. These proteins enhance the inflammatory and immune responses.

Formed elements of the blood

The formed elements are the **red blood cells** (erythrocytes), the **white blood cells** (leucocytes) and the **platelets** (thrombocytes).

Blood cell production (haematopoiesis) starts at an early stage of fetal development, and by 6–7 months of fetal life the production of new blood cells is located in the bone marrow. After birth and during childhood most of the bones contain red bone marrow and participate in haematopoiesis. When growth is complete, only the red bone marrow in the cancellous (spongy) tissue of the skull bones, vertebrae, sternum, pelvis and proximal ends of the femur and humerus continue to produce blood cells.

The formed elements of the blood all develop from common pluripotent stem cells. When stimulated, these stem cells may differentiate into two types of committed stem cell: the lymphoid stem cell and the myeloid progenitor cell. The precursor cells respond to various haematopoietic growth factors which increase the production of one or other cell line as and when the need arises. Figure 14.2 summarizes how the different blood cells develop.

Erythrocytes

The normal red blood cell is a flexible, elastic, biconcave disc. During the process of maturation, the cell looses its nucleus and so the circulating **erythrocyte** has no nucleus and is incapable of division and repair.

The function of the red blood cells is the transportation of oxygen and carbon dioxide between the tissue cells and the lungs. The major constituent of the cell is haemoglobin, a complex protein made up of the protein globin and an iron-containing pigment, haem. Each red cell contains about 640 million haemoglobin molecules. Oxygen has an affinity for this compound: four molecules of oxygen combine with one molecule of haemoglobin to form oxyhaemoglobin. This combination is loose and reversible, so when there is little or no free oxygen in the red cell environment (plasma) oxygen is freed from the red blood cell and diffuses into the plasma.

It is the red pigment in the haemoglobin of red blood cells that gives blood its colour. The colour varies according to the amount of oxygen combined with the haemoglobin. A high concentration of oxygen produces a brighter red coloration.

Some of the carbon dioxide carried in the blood (approximately 27%) is transported in the red blood cells in the form of carbaminohaemoglobin. When the haemoglobin takes on oxygen in the lungs, the carbon dioxide is released into the plasma and then diffuses into the alveoli.

Erythropoiesis

In **erythropoiesis** a committed myeloid stem cell is stimulated to begin a series of cell divisions. During these cell divisions changes occur that result in the appearance

Cellular components
See chapter 4.1

Erythrocytes
See chapter 4.1

Erythropoiesis
See chapter 4.1

Figure 14.2   Development of blood cells. Sites of action of some haematological growth factors are indicated.

of haemoglobin in the cell: the loss of the nucleus, a reduction in cell size, and finally loss of the reticular network. The mature red blood cell is almost completely filled with haemoglobin and the whole process normally takes about 7 days.

In health, the rate of production and maturation of the red blood cells normally approximates to the rate at which old cells are removed from the circulation and destroyed. This results in the red cell count and the amount of haemoglobin remaining relatively constant.

Tissue hypoxia is the essential factor in the regulation of erythropoiesis. The red bone marrow does not respond directly to hypoxaemia (lowered concentration of oxygen in the blood) but the resulting tissue hypoxia stimulates

production of a hormone, erythropoietin, mainly by the kidneys. Erythropoietin acts by increasing the rate of production of red cells from stem cells and shortening the period of maturation. As more red cells are released, delivery of oxygen to the tissues increases and erythropoietin production declines. This negative feedback mechanism acts when the rate of red cell destruction is increased – if there is a loss of red cells as a result of haemorrhage and at high altitudes where the oxygen tension of the air is low.

Essential for an adequate production of normal erythrocytes by the bone marrow is a supply of protein, iron, vitamin B$_{12}$, folic acid and vitamin C. Iron is essential for the formation of haemoglobin. Only limited amounts are

Figure 14.3 Life cycle of erythrocytes.

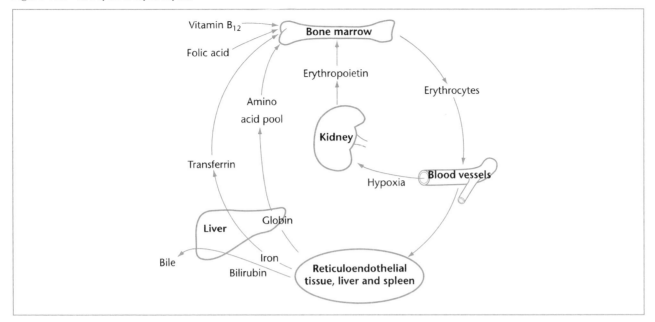

absorbed from the small intestine; this is then loosely bound with transferrin to be transported in the plasma. Excess iron is stored in the liver and other cells as ferritin and haemosiderin, and can be released as iron when needed by the bone marrow. The majority of iron used in the formation of haemoglobin is derived from breakdown of worn-out erythrocytes. Only a small amount of dietary iron is required under normal circumstances and its absorption from the small intestine is inhibited when transferrin and ferritin are saturated. Extra dietary iron and medicinal iron preparations are not absorbed but simply eliminated in the faeces. If erythropoiesis is increased, as it is in pregnancy, or in conditions causing hypoxia, the iron stores are utilized and intestinal absorption increases accordingly.

Vitamin B_{12} and folic acid are required for production of nucleic acids in all cells, and erythrocytes with their rapid rate of turnover are no exception. Vitamin B_{12} can be absorbed only in the presence of a glycoprotein known as intrinsic factor, which is secreted by the parietal glands in the gastric mucosa. Together they form a complex, which is absorbed in the distal ileum. The vitamin B_{12} is released into the portal circulation to be carried to the liver, where it is stored to be released as required. Stores are usually sufficient to last for up to 3 years even if the ability to absorb the vitamin is lost. Folic acid is absorbed in the small intestine and also stored in the liver, but stores are normally sufficient to last for only 3–4 months if intake ceases.

Vitamin C promotes iron absorption and also helps to preserve folic acid, which is very quickly destroyed during food preparation. It is also an important factor for red blood cell production.

Red blood cells survive in the circulation for approximately 120 days. The cell membrane becomes fragile and less flexible as the cell ages, and eventually it ruptures as it is squeezed through small capillaries. The phagocytic macrophages destroy damaged cells and haemoglobin is broken down. Iron is reutilized along with the constituent amino acids of globin, and the remainder of the haem molecule is eventually excreted in the bile. This cycle is illustrated in Figure 14.3.

Leucocytes

White blood cells are less numerous, larger than erythrocytes and have nuclei. Healthy people have at least five types of white cells or **leucocytes** in the circulating blood (see Fig. 14.2):

- **Granulocytes** are formed in the red bone marrow. Three types are recognizable by the staining characteristic of their cytoplasm: *neutrophils* (stain with a neutral dye), *eosinophils* (stain with and acid dye) and *basophils* (stain with basic dyes).

- **Lymphocytes** are smaller cells than granulocytes. They also are formed in the bone marrow. Some immature lymphocytes migrate to the thymus gland where they are processed and activated to become *T lymphocytes*. Several subsets of T cells exist, including *memory, helper* and *suppressor* cells. *Natural killer cells* also exist, and appear to be a further subset of T lymphocytes, although there is some uncertainty about their exact origin (Pallister 1994). Other lymphocytes, appear to be activated mainly in the red bone marrow and become *B lymphocytes*. These eventually develop into *plasma cells* and *memory B cells*. Mature lymphocytes circulate in the blood and

Leucocytes
See chapter 4.1

Granulocytes
See chapter 4.1

Lymphocytes
See chapter 4.1

Figure 14.4   Formation of white blood cells (leucopoiesis).

between the blood and the lymphatic tissues, where they spend most of their life.

■ **Monocytes** are the largest white blood cells. After their formation in the red bone marrow they circulate in the blood for only a short time (10–20 hours) before migrating into the tissues where they become *macrophages*. These cells form the reticuloendothelial system in bone marrow, liver spleen and lymph nodes.

Leucopoiesis

Stem cells in the blood-forming organs are stimulated to produce precursors of the white cells, *myeloblasts, monoblasts* and *lymphoblasts* (Fig. 14.4). The physiological stimuli responsible are not fully understood, but increased leucopoiesis is associated with infection, haemorrhage and tissue destruction, whereas drugs such as sulfon-amides, gold and most cytotoxic drugs result in a reduced white cell count. Numerous haematopoietic growth factors are involved in the process of differentiation and proliferation of the leucocytes. Some of these are normally found in plasma, others are detected only when there is an inflammatory response or in response to a stimulus such as an antigen or endotoxin. They include interleukins and colony-forming factors. Figure 14.2 illustrates the site of action of some of these growth factors.

Functions of the leucocytes

The leucocytes serve as an important body defence, destroying many injurious substances such as micro-organisms and the products of degenerating tissues. Neutrophils and monocytes are chemically attracted to areas of bacterial invasion and tissue damage. This process is known as chemotaxis. Neutrophils then ingest and digest foreign particles by a process known as phagocyto-sis and, when worn out, are themselves phagocytosed by

macrophages. Monocytes and macrophages respond more slowly but have a greater capacity for ingesting foreign particles and debris. Macrophages have a number of other functions concerned with the inflammatory and immune responses.

Eosinophils participate in allergic reactions, in defence against parasitic invasion and in the resolution of the inflammatory response. Basophils contain heparin and histamine, and are very similar to tissue mast cells. They are involved in hypersensitivity, anaphylactic and inflam-matory reactions.

T lymphocytes are responsible for cell-mediated immun-ity, and B lymphocytes for humoral immunity involving the production of antibodies (see Ch. 8).

The lifespan of the white blood cells varies enormously depending on the type of cell and the body's need for protection. A neutrophil may survive for only a few hours in the presence of an infection, whereas lymphocytes can survive for years in the spleen and lymph nodes. Leucocytes that are destroyed or die are disposed of by phagocytosis by the macrophages of the reticuloendo-thelial tissues.

Blood platelets

Platelets are the smallest of the formed elements of the blood. They are oval, non-nucleated, granular structures containing important substances, including calcium, potassium, several clotting factors, serotonin, adrenaline, adenosine diphosphate (ADP) and enzymes.

Stem cells in the red bone marrow develop into giant cells called *megakaryocytes* under the influence of a humoral growth agent called thrombopoietin. The megakaryocytes disintegrate, releasing platelets; each megakaryocyte is capable of producing about 4000 platelets. Platelets have a

Monocytes
See chapter 4.1

Platelets
See chapter 4.1

lifespan of 8–12 days and production is increased following tissue trauma and destruction and in hypoxaemia. At any one time about one-third of the platelets are to be found in the spleen, which acts as a reservoir.

The major function of platelets relates to haemostasis (arrest of bleeding) following injury to a blood vessel. This is achieved through:

1. Adhesion – platelets stick to the injured area, especially if collagen is exposed

2. Release of cytoplasmic contents as a result of cellular deformation

3. Aggregation – an increase in platelet stickiness caused by the release of cellular contents results in nearby platelets adhering to the original clump. This produces a platelet plug that prevents further blood loss.

Haemostasis and blood coagulation

The formation of a haemostatic plug by the clumping together of platelets is one of the mechanisms for restricting blood loss following the rupture of a blood vessel. The others are:

■ *Local vasoconstriction* – chemicals released by platelets stimulate a contraction of smooth muscle in the wall of the injured blood vessel which lasts for about 20 minutes.

■ *Clot formation* – this process involves the formation of a jelly-like mass in the blood by the conversion of the soluble plasma protein fibrinogen to an insoluble mesh of thin threads called fibrin in which are entangled blood cells forming the mass or clot. Clot formation is triggered either by contact of the blood with a foreign surface or by the release of tissue factor (thromboplastin) from damaged cells, and results in a chain of reactions between a series of clotting factors (see Table 14.1). The intrinsic and extrinsic pathways are now known to interact and complement each other. Figure 14.5 illustrates the

Table 14.1 Blood clotting factors

Factor number	Name
I	Fibrinogen
II	Prothrombin
III	Tissue factor (thromboplastin)
V	Labile factor
VII	Proconvertin
VIII	Antihaemophilic factor
IX	Christmas factor
X	Stuart–Prower factor
XI	Plasma thromboplastin antecedent
XII	Hageman factor
XIII	Fibrin stabilizing factor
Pre-K	Prekallikrein
HMWK	High molecular weight kininogen

The sequence of roman numerals indicates the order in which the clotting factors were identified and is not related to the sequence of their participation in the clotting process.

Figure 14.5 The process of blood coagulation.

Modified from Hoffbrand and Pettit (1993).

Table 14.2   The ABO blood group system

Phenotype (blood group)	Genotype	Red cell antigens present (agglutinogens)	Naturally occurring plasma antibodies (agglutinins)	Plasma agglutinates red blood cells of blood type
A	AA or AO	A	Anti-B	B and AB
B	BB or BO	B	Anti-A	A and AB
AB	AB	A and B	None	None
O	OO	None	Anti-A and anti-B	A, AB and B

Subgroups of the A antigen exist but are of little clinical importance.

clotting cascade. Clot formation takes about 3–6 minutes. The clot then shrinks in size as a result of contraction of contractile proteins, and serum (plasma minus the clotting factors and fibrinogen) is extruded. The fibrin mesh pulls together the edges of the break and further checks the loss of blood.

■ *Fibrinolysis* – as the healing process begins, fibroblasts proliferate, filling the area with fibrous tissue. Fibrin is degraded into waste debris by the action of the enzyme plasmin (an active product of the plasma protein plasminogen) and the debris is cleared by the macrophages.

These mechanisms operate during normal day-to-day activities when minute blood vessels sustain injury and in minor trauma. If a major blood vessel, especially an artery, is interrupted these physiological responses may not be adequate to control blood loss and pressure; ligation or cautery may be required.

Uncontrolled systemic coagulation is potentially dangerous, as is uncontrolled fibrinolysis. The body therefore produces various inhibitory substances such as anticoagulants and fibrinolytic inhibitors to counteract these processes.

Blood groups

In 1900 Karl Landstiener discovered that **human blood** differs from one individual to another. This difference arises from the presence or absence of specific antigens (agglutinogens) on the surface of red blood cells and on the presence or absence of specific antibodies (agglutinins) in plasma. This explains why blood cannot be taken at random from one person and transfused into another. The blood, when of a different type to that of the recipient, may cause a serious reaction and death. Many different blood group systems are now known, but the ABO and Rhesus systems are of most clinical importance.

The ABO blood group

Blood type is determined genetically, with the genes for A and B agglutinogens being co-dominant. An individual's

blood is typed as A, B or AB if it has those agglutinogens present on the red blood cells. If no agglutinogens are present, then the blood is termed type O.

The blood plasma does not contain agglutinins that will agglutinate the red cells; therefore, plasma of an individual with blood type AB will contain no antibody whereas plasma of an individual with blood type O will contain both. An individual whose red cells express either A or B agglutinogens will have plasma containing anti-B or anti-A antibodies respectively (Table 14.2).

Blood is grouped by adding specially prepared serum containing either anti-A or anti-B serum to a sample of the blood to be typed and observing for clumping of the red cells. The relative incidence of blood group antigens varies from race to race but, worldwide, types O and A are more common than B and AB.

The Rhesus (Rh) blood group

Several antigens (agglutinogens) are involved in this system but the D factor is of greatest clinical significance:

■ Approximately 85% of caucasians possess the D factor and are classified as being Rh positive. Those without the D factor are said to be Rh negative.

■ The gene for the D agglutinogen is always dominant, so an Rh(D)-positive individual may have inherited the gene from only one or from both parents (Fig. 14.6).

■ Antibodies against the D factor do not occur naturally: they develop in the plasma of Rh(D)-negative blood when the D factor is introduced on red blood cells of Rh(D)-positive blood. Anti-D antibodies develop slowly and, after an initial exposure, do not usually reach a sufficient concentration to cause a reaction before the red blood cells are destroyed naturally.

■ A second exposure to Rh(D)-positive blood will, however, result in a reaction causing agglutination of the donor cells.

When an Rh-positive fetus develops within an Rh-negative mother, some of the fetal red blood cells or

Blood groups
See chapter 4.1

ABO
See chapter 4.1

Rhesus
See chapter 4.1

Figure 14.6 Inheritance patterns of Rh blood group factors. The gene for agglutinogen D is always dominant. If the mother is Rh negative and her baby is Rh positive, the mother will form anti-Rh antibodies.

D antigen released by worn-out erythrocytes may pass through the placenta into the maternal circulation. This usually occurs at delivery. The mother then forms antibodies that diffuse into the fetal circulation in subsequent pregnancies causing agglutination of the fetal erythrocytes. This causes *erythroblastosis fetalis*, a severe haemolytic disease of the newborn. It is rare for this to occur in a first pregnancy. There is a chance that maternal sensitization may occur following spontaneous or induced abortion, amniocentesis, chorionic villus sampling, ectopic pregnancy, antepartum haemorrhage and abdominal trauma. This can be prevented by administering anti-D immunoglobulin to agglutinate Rh-positive antigen before the mother can produce her own antibodies. It is usual practice to administer anti-D after any of the potentially sensitizing episodes detailed above, at 28 and 34 weeks of pregnancy, and within 72 hours of delivery in order to protect any subsequent child from being affected.

When the fetus is Rh negative and the mother is Rh positive there is no problem, because there is no agglutinogen to stimulate antibody production.

Blood disorders

Blood disorders (dyscrasias) may affect erythrocytes, leucocytes, platelets or the coagulation process. The problem may be due to a defect originating in the blood-forming red bone marrow, or it may involve the lymphoid and reticuloendothelial tissues. Disorders may be inherited or acquired; they may represent a primary condition or occur secondary to some other pathological process or its treatment. A haematological malignancy such as leukaemia, an inherited haemoglobinopathy such as thalassaemia, and infection with the malaria parasite are examples of primary disorders. A condition such as renal failure that produces a secondary anaemia, and cytotoxic chemotherapy given for a non-haematological malignancy that causes bone marrow depression with anaemia, neutropenia and thrombocytopenia, are examples of problems caused by other disease states or by treatment. Deficiency of an essential requirement may also

result in a blood disorder. Blood cells that are defective, whatever the cause, are likely to function abnormally and may be rendered susceptible to premature or excessive destruction.

Blood disorders may develop at any point during a person's lifespan, although the incidence of some blood disorders predominates at the extremes of life. Women of reproductive age are subject to the particular demands of menstruation and pregnancy, and as such experience a greater risk of anaemia.

Like disorders affecting other body systems, disorders of the blood may be acute or chronic. Whatever the cause, dysfunction has an effect on many other body systems because of the numerous and essential functions of blood. The physical manifestations of blood disorders are therefore many, varied and frequently non-specific.

Health assessment

Assessment of an individual's normal and altered haematological status involves knowledge of the person's health history, physical examination and observation, medical diagnostic procedures and knowledge of the haematological system. Collection and analysis of these data form the basis for the identification of an individual's problems and the development of a care plan with specific nursing interventions.

History

In taking a patient history, information that may be of significance includes any family history of haematological disorders, a drug history (any cytotoxic drug, immunosuppressive drugs including antibiotics, and drugs affecting blood coagulation are of particular interest), an occupational history (providing clues about any exposure to toxic chemicals) and a nutritional history.

Common presenting symptoms are often non-specific and include fatigue, lethargy, weakness, breathlessness, and pain and weight loss. People with blood disorders also frequently report fevers, night sweats and repeated infections, and may have indications of unusual bleeding such as a tendency to bruise easily or prolonged or excessive bleeding from a cut. These factors should all be explored when taking a health history.

Physical assessment

Physical assessment should include observation of the person's general appearance and behaviour. Pallor and lethargy may suggest a decrease in the number of red blood cells and oxygen-carrying capacity. The colour of the mucous membranes is inspected, and may be abnormally pale in the case of the conjunctiva, or the tongue may be a beefy red with glossitis. Other unusual features such as stomatitis should be noted. On examination, the skin may be pale and dry; with some conditions jaundice may be present. This can result in itching and excoriation of the skin from scratching. The presence or absence of bruises and petechiae are noted when examining the skin, as this may indicate that the person has an increased tendency to bleed.

Blood pressure and pulse rate and volume are recorded and compared, if possible, to normal values for the particular patient. Respiratory rate and rhythm are also assessed at rest and after exercise, as a reduction in the ability of the blood to transport oxygen places a greater demand on the respiratory and cardiovascular systems which will be more obvious after activity. The patient's mental status should also be assessed for evidence of hypoxia, such as confusion.

Investigations

A variety of tests is used to assist in the diagnosis of blood disorders. Some of these are described in Tables 14.3–14.5. Microscopic examination of a stained blood film is used to assess the shape, size and appearance of blood cells and to detect abnormal cells and parasites such as that causing malaria. A variety of radiological investigations may also be helpful in determining the cause and extent of the haematological disorder, including radiography, ultrasonography, computed tomography, magnetic resonance imaging and nuclear medicine studies.

Bone marrow examination

This is a useful test for establishing haematological function. It involves examining a small sample of the bone marrow obtained from inside the bone (bone marrow aspiration) and a small piece of the bone itself (bone marrow trephine biopsy). Blood smears are made of the aspirated bone marrow and the bone specimen is cut into thin sections. Microscopic examination of these specimens provides information about the structure of the bone marrow cavity, the number and different types of cells and their stages of development and maturity. It may also show the presence of cells foreign to the bone marrow, as in secondary carcinoma.

Anaemia
See chapter 4.1

The site chosen requires red bone marrow to be easily accessible; in adults, the posterior iliac crest is usually preferred. An alternative site is the anterior iliac crest, and if only an aspirate is required the sternum may occasionally be used. In children, bone marrow may be sampled from the tibia and a general anaesthetic is given.

The individual is positioned prone or on their side when aspirating from the iliac crests; supine for a sternal aspiration. The skin is cleansed and the area infiltrated with local anaesthetic. When the anaesthetic has taken effect, the specialized aspiration needle is inserted. The individual should be warned that discomfort occurs from the pressure needed to pass the needle through the cortex of the bone into the marrow and from the aspiration of the marrow fluid. On removal of the needle, pressure is applied until bleeding stops and the site is covered with a plaster or dry dressing and should be kept dry for 24 hours. If an outpatient, the individual is observed for at least an hour to ensure bleeding has ceased.

Erythrocyte disorders

A deficiency or excess may occur in the number of circulating red blood cells, or the red blood cells may function abnormally. Variations in the size, shape and haemoglobin content may be present. Certain descriptive terms are used to denote some of the characteristics that are noted when blood is examined microscopically:

■ Macrocytes are erythrocytes that are larger than normal.

■ Microcytes are erythrocytes that are smaller than normal.

■ Normochromic describes cells that possess a normal amount of haemoglobin.

■ Hypochromic describes cells that are deficient in haemoglobin.

■ Hyperchromic describes cells with a haemoglobin content that is greater than normal.

■ Poikilocytic cells are cells with an abnormal shape.

Anaemia (erythrocyte and haemoglobin deficiency)

The term **anaemia** implies a reduction in the oxygen-carrying capacity of the blood. This occurs as a result of fewer circulating erythrocytes than is normal or a decrease in the concentration of haemoglobin. Anaemia is normally defined as a haemoglobin level in the blood of less than 13.5 g/dL in men and 11.5 g/dL in women. It is sometimes classified according to the size and amount of haemoglobin in the erythrocytes. For example, iron deficiency causes an anaemia where the cells are hypochromic and microcytic, and the disease may be referred to as a hypochromic microcytic anaemia.

Table 14.3 Laboratory tests for assessing erythrocytes (normal values vary slightly between laboratories)

Test	Normal values	Description
Red blood cell count (RCC)	Males: $4.5–6.3 \times 10^{12}$/L Females: $4.2–5.5 \times 10^{12}$/L	The normal red cell blood count varies with sex, age, altitude and exercise. It increases with hypovolaemia and decreases with hypervolaemia
Haemoglobin concentration (Hb)	Males: 14–18 g/dL (8.1–11.2 mmol/L) Females: 12–16 g/dL (7.4–9.9 mmol/L) Children (3 months to puberty): 10–14 g/dL	The normal values for haemoglobin vary with age, sex, altitude and exercise. Hypovolaemia leads to increased levels and hypervolaemia to decreased levels
Packed cell volume (PCV) or haematocrit	Males: 40–50% Females: 37–47%	The volume of red blood cells in blood is expressed as a percentage of the total blood volume
Erythrocyte indices		
Mean corpuscular volume (MCV)	76–96 fL (femolitres)	This is the average size of individual red cells (normocytic). A raised MCV indicates a macrocytic anaemia. A lower MCV indicates a microcytic anaemia
Mean corpuscular haemoglobin (MCH)	27–32 pg (picograms)	This is the average amount of haemoglobin per red cell (normochromic)
Mean corpuscular haemoglobin concentration (MCHC)	30–35 g/dL	This is the average weight in grams of haemoglobin in 1 decilitre of red blood cells
Reticulocyte count	0.5–1.5%	The percentage of circulating non-mature, non-nucleated red blood cells. Results are indicative of bone marrow activity
Serum vitamin B_{12}	160–925 ng/L	B_{12} is necessary for red blood cell production. It requires intrinsic factor for its absorption from the gastrointestinal tract. Its level is determined to diagnose macrocytic anaemia
Serum folate	3.0–15 µg/L	Folic acid is required for the normal production of red and white blood cells and DNA. Its absorption depends on a normally functioning intestinal mucosa. Its level is determined to diagnose macrocytic anaemia
Serum ferritin	10–250 µg/L	Indicates the total body iron stores
Red cell mass (RCM)	Males: 20–33 mL/kg Females: 20–27 mL/kg	Determined by labelling the red blood cells with chromium-51 (^{51}Cr). This is used in the diagnosis of polycythaemia
Erythrocyte sedimentation rate (ESR)	Up to 12 mm/h	Measures how rapidly red blood cells settle out of unclotted blood. Alteration in the blood proteins results in aggregation of the red cells and they fall faster. This is a non-specific test, but raised values are indicative of active inflammatory processes
Sickle-cell test	Negative	Demonstrates the presence of haemoglobin S. A reducing agent is used to deoxygenate the erythrocytes and the cells are examined microscopically for evidence of sickling. Red blood cells that contain haemoglobin S are distorted and sickle or crescent shaped when deprived of oxygen
Haemoglobin electrophoresis	Adult: (% of total) HbA 95–98% HbA_2 1.5–3.5% HbF_1 < 2% HbC 0% HbS 0% Newborn: HbF 40–70% Infant: HbF 2–10% Child (over 6 months) HbF 1–3%	Used to identify the different types of haemoglobin present in the red blood cells when investigating haemoglobinopathies and thalassaemia. Haemoglobin S is the most common of the abnormal haemoglobins
Coombs' test		
Direct	Negative (no agglutination)	Erythrocytes are mixed with Coombs' reagent to test for agglutinins that lead to clumping and haemolysis. The direct test detects antibody
Indirect	Negative (no agglutination)	or complement bound to the red cells as found in immune haemolytic anaemias. The indirect test is used in routine cross-matching before transfusion and during pregnancy. It detects antibody in the serum

Table 14.4 Laboratory tests for assessing leucocytes (normal values may vary slightly between laboratories)

Test	Normal value	Description
White blood cell count (WCC)	$3.7–11.0 \times 10^9$/L	
Differential count		In certain disease conditions the percentages of the various
Neutrophils	$1.7–7.5 \times 10^9$/L (40–75%)	types of leucocyte are increased relative to others
Eosinophils	$0.03–0.44 \times 10^9$/L (1–6%)	
Basophils	$0.015–0.1 \times 10^9$/L (<1%)	
Monocytes	$0.2–0.8 \times 10^9$/L (2–10%)	
Lymphocytes	$1.5–3.5 \times 10^9$/L (20–50%)	

Normal values may be lower for people of West Indian, African or Middle Eastern descent.

Table 14.5 Laboratory tests for assessing platelets and clotting functions of the blood

Test	Normal value	Description
Blood platelet (thrombocyte) count	$150–400 \times 10^9$/L	
Bleeding time	2–5 min (varies with method used)	This is the time it takes bleeding to stop naturally, i.e. the period of time for which blood continues to escape from an 'open' area
Prothrombin (PT) or International normalized ratio (INR)	11–15 s / 2–4	This is the time it takes for coagulation following addition of thromboplastin and calcium to the specimen. The INR is designed to produce consistent results in all laboratories regardless of reagents used; it is the ratio of the PT of the patient to that of a person not taking anticoagulants
Partial thromboplastin time (PTT)	40–100 s	PTT is a general test of coagulation used for screening and to monitor anticoagulant therapy.
Activated partial thromboplastin time (APTT)	30–45 s	Clotting deficiencies other than factor VII, XIII and platelets can be detected. APTT involves the addition of activators to the regular test reagent to shorten the clotting time
Plasma fibrinogen	2–4 g/L	This indicates the fibrinogen concentration

Causes

Anaemia may be caused by decreased production of red blood cells (erythropoiesis) or by excessive destruction or loss. Anaemia that is due to decreased erythropoiesis may result from a deficiency of factors essential for normal production or by depressed bone marrow activity. It may also occur secondary to some other disorder such as renal disease, and because of this the patient may undergo extensive investigation to determine the cause. Excessive destruction of red blood cells leading to anaemia may be caused by intracorpuscular defects or result from extra-corpusular factors.

General effects and characteristics

Whatever the cause or type of anaemia, it presents a common problem: a decrease in the capacity of the blood to transport oxygen. This is manifested in a variety of signs and symptoms attributable to tissue and organ hypoxia and the ensuing reduced metabolism. These are shown in Figure 14.7.

The occurrence and severity of these manifestations depend on three factors:

1. *Speed of onset* – a gradually developing anaemia may be tolerated without any significant incapacity, whereas a relatively small but rapid blood loss may produce marked symptoms.

2. *Severity* – mild anaemia often causes no problems, and even severe anaemia may result in relatively few symptoms in a young and otherwise healthy person.

3. *Age* – anaemia tends to be tolerated less well by the elderly because cardiac compensatory mechanisms may also be impaired.

Anaemia due to abnormalities of erythropoiesis

Anaemia may result from a lack of an essential nutrient in the diet – defective absorption or an increased demand – which cannot be met by the normal supply of factors essential for red cell production. The nutritional deficiency anaemias seen most often are those resulting from a lack of iron, vitamin B_{12} or folic acid. A healthy diet is very important in preventing such deficiencies occurring.

Nurses should be proactive in the primary prevention of such problems by promoting healthy eating guidelines at every opportunity as a normal varied diet supplies essential nutrients in excess of the body's usual requirements. A wide variety of community, workplace and institutional settings offer opportunities for nurses to interact with individuals, either on a one to one basis or in groups, to promote healthy eating. Those who should be particularly targeted include pregnant women, mothers with babies and toddlers, schoolchildren and adolescents, the elderly, and those in hospital or residential care. It is obviously important to take into account each individual's dietary preferences and circumstances, such as the special needs of vegetarians and vegans, and to be sensitive to cultural influences in diets and food preparation.

Dietary sources of iron are liver, red meat, some green vegetables, fish and cereals (which are often supplemented with iron during processing). Vitamin B_{12} is found in liver, red meat, eggs, shellfish and dairy produce. Sources of food rich in folate includes liver, eggs, vegetables such as broccoli, peas, spinach, brussel sprouts and potatoes, cereals and yeast, but cooking may reduce the folate content of food by up to 95%.

The ability of a person to afford or to access a healthy diet takes the problem to a different level. It is society's responsibility to ensure that its members can afford and obtain foodstuffs that will prevent any individual from developing diseases such as deficiency anaemias. This is a professional responsibility that may involve nurses in campaigning for client groups at risk, such as for healthier and affordable school meals, to prevent cuts in community care for the elderly and the closure of local food stores, or for rights of refugees and asylum seekers. The elderly form an especially vulnerable group because, even if they are able to afford a healthy diet, they often have physical disabilities and other health problems that make acquiring, preparing and eating food difficult.

Iron deficiency anaemia

This is the commonest type of anaemia worldwide (Gillespie et al 1991). It is characterized by small red blood cells with less than the normal content of haemoglobin (microcytic hypochromic). There is usually a slight reduction in the total number of red blood cells. Iron deficiency may be due to chronic blood loss, an insufficient intake, impaired intestinal absorption or an increased requirement. Pregnant and lactating women and preschool children are those most at risk of iron deficiency because of an increased need for iron to meet the needs of the fetus and for growth during infancy. In adults

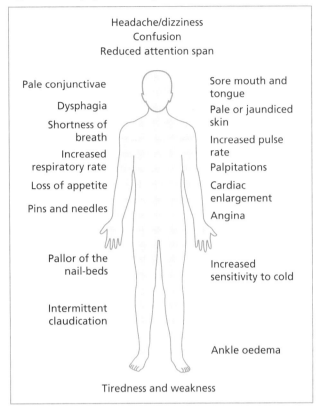

Figure 14.7 Symptoms and signs of anaemia.

Headache/dizziness
Confusion
Reduced attention span

Pale conjunctivae

Dysphagia

Shortness of breath

Increased respiratory rate

Loss of appetite

Pins and needles

Sore mouth and tongue

Pale or jaundiced skin

Increased pulse rate

Palpitations

Cardiac enlargement

Angina

Pallor of the nail-beds

Increased sensitivity to cold

Intermittent claudication

Ankle oedema

Tiredness and weakness

the most common cause is chronic blood loss, especially from the gastrointestinal tract or genitourinary tract. Women of reproductive age are at risk because of menstrual blood loss, increased demands during pregnancy and lactation, and blood loss at delivery. Iron deficiency anaemia is uncommon in men unless there has been a loss of blood, development of hypochlorhydria secondary to gastric disease, atrophy of the gastric mucosa or gastrectomy.

Causes of blood loss include cancer, peptic ulcers and haemorrhoids, and in tropical climates infestation with hookworms may be responsible for chronic blood loss. It has been estimated that it could take as long as 8 years for a normal adult male to develop iron deficiency anaemia solely due to poor diet or malabsorption.

In addition to the general symptoms of anaemia identified in Figure 14.7, the person with iron deficiency anaemia may experience soreness and inflammation of the mouth and tongue. The tongue may be very red and may have a smooth, glazed appearance due to atrophy of the papillae. Rarely the patient with a severe anaemia complains of dysphagia (difficulty in swallowing). The combination of dysphagia, stomatitis (inflammation of the mouth) and atrophic glossitis (inflammation of the tongue with atrophy of papillae) in anaemia may be referred to as the Plummer–Vinson syndrome. Changes in the fingernails are common in those with prolonged iron deficiency. The nails become brittle and concave or spoon shaped.

Investigations

Serum ferritin concentration is the most reliable guide to iron deficiency; it is likely to be less than $12\,\mu g/L$. When gastrointestinal bleeding is suspected as a cause of chronic blood loss, other investigations such as faecal occult bloods and endoscopy may be required.

Treatment

If a source of blood loss (such as a peptic ulcer, colonic cancer or uterine fibroids) is identified as the cause of the anaemia, steps should be taken to treat this and stop the blood loss. When iron supplementation is required, medicinal iron is usually given in the form of an oral ferrous salt such as ferrous sulfate 200 mg taken three times a day, or ferrous gluconate 600 mg three times daily. Both preparations are normally continued for at least 4 months in order to raise the haemoglobin to normal levels and replenish the iron stores. Gastrointestinal irritation and constipation or diarrhoea are not uncommon side-effects of iron therapy and may be reduced by taking iron preparations after food. Stools are discoloured by iron, and older patients in particular may find that iron has a constipating effect. Parenteral iron is rarely indicated.

Preventive strategies at an individual level include promoting dietary changes that will increase intake of haem iron (iron from animal products); increased intake of vitamin C and other acidic or fermented foods that promote iron absorption; and reduced intake of iron absorption inhibitors such as coffee, tea and some cereals. Other foodstuffs may be fortified, for example cereals and weaning foods and follow-on baby milks. Control of parasites such as hookworms and malaria are important strategies in some parts of the world for reducing iron deficiency. Iron supplementation is recommended for pregnant and lactating women in areas where iron deficiency anaemia is prevalent (Gillespie et al 1991).

Vitamin B_{12} deficiency (pernicious anaemia)

When there is a deficiency of vitamin B_{12}, red blood cells are produced that are larger than normal but fewer in number. The cells show considerable variation in both shape and size. Although the red cells have a haemoglobin content that is greater than normal, the deficiency in the total number of erythrocytes results in the oxygen-carrying capacity of the blood being inadequate. The condition is sometimes referred to as megaloblastic anaemia.

The cause of vitamin B_{12} deficiency is usually non-absorption of the vitamin. Inadequate dietary intake is rare and associated with starvation or in individuals who are vegans (eat no animal or dairy products). Malabsorption of the vitamin is the most common cause of deficiency and results from failure of the gastric parietal cells to produce intrinsic factor, the glycoprotein that binds vitamin B_{12} and facilitates its transfer across the intestinal wall. This condition, characterized by atrophy of the parietal cells, is known as pernicious anaemia. It is an autoimmune disorder that has a tendency to occur in families and is associated with those whose blood is group A. It is more common in females, and has an insidious onset and a peak occurrence around the age of 60 years.

Malabsorption of vitamin B_{12} may also occur as a result of partial or total gastrectomy, which removes the source of intrinsic factor. Any gastrointestinal condition or operation that results in the formation of blind or stagnant loops of small intestine (e.g. diverticular disease, Crohn's disease, ileal resection) may predispose to vitamin B_{12} deficiency because bacterial growth proliferates in conditions of stasis, using up available B_{12} before it can be absorbed.

Clinical characteristics

In addition to the general symptoms of anaemia, the patient may experience gastrointestinal and nervous system changes. The tongue is often sore and smooth, and a beefy red colour. There is loss of appetite but the person does not necessarily lose weight. The lack of vitamin B_{12} may cause degeneration of myelin and nerve fibres in the spinal cord and peripheral nerves. The patient may present with neurological symptoms such as a symmetrical tingling or 'pins and needles', or coldness and numbness in the extremities. Unless the deficiency is corrected, serious motor disturbances may develop in the form of muscular weakness, ataxia (loss of coordination and staggering) and paralysis. If the deficiency is prolonged and severe, degeneration of the optic nerves may occur, causing serious impairment of vision. When degenerative changes occur in the spinal cord, the condition is known as subacute combined degeneration of the cord. In severe pernicious anaemia the skin may show some jaundice – a result of increased haemolysis or erythrocyte breakdown.

Investigations

Laboratory examination of the blood reveals a deficiency in the number of erythrocytes and macrocytic hyperchromic cells. Bone marrow examination shows hyperplasia of the bone marrow but a failure in erythropoiesis, as evidenced by a large proportion of immature cells. A lack of intrinsic factor is often associated with a lack of gastric acid (achlorhydria), which is also produced by the parietal cells, and thus in investigation of pernicious anaemia there may be an attempt to test and stimulate gastric acid secretion after administering histamine or pentagastrin. The Schilling test or a variant of it may also used to evaluate the absorption of vitamin B_{12}. This involves measuring the concentration of radioactively labelled B_{12} excreted in a 24-hour collection of urine. The radioactive dose is administered orally and is followed by a dose of unlabelled B_{12} administered subcutaneously, which flushes the radioactive vitamin, which has been absorbed, out into the urine.

Treatment

Vitamin B_{12} deficiency is treated by intramuscular injection of hydroxocobalamin to overcome the problem of malabsorption. Up to 1 mg of hydroxocobalamin is administered on alternate days for 1–2 weeks or until the blood count is in the normal range. Thereafter an injection of the drug is required at 2–3-month intervals for life to maintain normal haemoglobin and erythrocyte levels.

The haematological response to treatment is rapid and may result in temporary depletion of iron stores and insufficient haemoglobin production. For this reason ferrous sulfate is sometimes administered concurrently when treatment is initiated. Potassium levels should also be monitored to detect potential hypokalaemia. Neurological symptoms improve only slowly and may never disappear completely.

In contrast to pernicious anaemia, the anaemia associated with a dietary deficiency of vitamin B_{12} or intestinal disease does not manifest as hypochlorhydria or lead to degenerative changes in the nervous system. Individuals who are strict vegans may take oral vitamin B_{12}. When the anaemia is secondary to intestinal disease and malabsorption has been demonstrated, parenteral vitamin B_{12} is given. Following total or partial gastrectomy or ileal resection, vitamin B_{12} should be given prophylactically.

Folic acid deficiency anaemia

Like vitamin B_{12}, folic acid (folate) is an essential requirement for DNA synthesis. Its lack results in a form of anaemia very similar to that of vitamin B_{12} deficiency. The cause of folate deficiency may be:

- an inadequate diet (alcoholics and those with anorexia are at particular risk)
- malabsorption (such as in coeliac disease, Crohn's disease and tropical sprue)
- increased requirements, particularly during pregnancy
- drug induced (e.g. by the cytotoxic drug methotrexate or anticonvulsants such as phenytoin).

Investigations

Haematological changes are the same as those found with vitamin B_{12} deficiency (macrocytic hyperchromic cells are seen microscopically); however, the person does not manifest achlorhydria, decreased vitamin B_{12} absorption or have nervous system involvement.

Treatment

Folic acid 5 mg orally daily for 4 months is usually sufficient to restore normal haematological findings and to replenish body stores. In malabsorption states a higher dose may be needed. A person with severe megloblastic anaemia needing urgent treatment should not be given folic acid alone until vitamin B_{12} deficiency has been definitely excluded. This is because there is a risk of precipitating neurological symptoms in a person with B_{12} deficiency. Until the underlying cause of the anaemia has been determined, it is therefore necessary to give vitamin B_{12} concurrently.

Folic acid is sometimes given prophylactically to women during pregnancy and to patients with severe haemolytic anaemias. It is recommended that all women who are planning to get pregnant take folic acid supplements at a dose of $400\,\mu g$ daily before conception and for the first 12 weeks of pregnancy. This has been shown to reduce the incidence of babies born with neural tube defects and also helps to prevent maternal anaemia (Department of Health 1992).

Vitamin C deficiency

This results in scurvy and is associated with a diet lacking in fresh fruit, potatoes and green vegetables. People eating a very restricted diet such as infants and the elderly sometimes develop anaemia and are deficient in vitamin C as well as iron and folate. Vitamin C improves iron absorption by reducing ferric iron to ferrous iron, which is more readily absorbed. It also enhances the catalytic action of folic acid in erythropoiesis.

Other anaemias due to abnormalities of erythrocyte production

A number of chronic inflammatory or malignant disorders result in abnormal red cell production, causing anaemias of varying severity. Erthyropoiesis appears to be suppressed to some degree by growth inhibitors such as interleukin in a number of the chronic disorders. If anaemia is severe, blood transfusions or therapy with erythropoietin may be needed to restore normal haematological values. A number of types of myelodysplastic syndrome result from changes in the red blood cell precursors in the bone marrow and are related to, or may eventually develop into, leukaemia. Sideroblastic anaemias are a varied group of conditions that all result in the toxic accumulation of iron in red cell precursors in the bone marrow and ineffective erythropoiesis. If associated with alcohol or antituberculous drug therapy, the condition is reversible on withdrawal of the agent. Other forms of the condition respond to pyridoxine (vitamin B_6) in doses of 100–400 mg per day. Blood transfusion may be required in individuals who fail to respond.

Aplastic anaemia is condition characterized by a failure of the bone marrow to produce all types of blood cells. This disorder is discussed later in the chapter.

Anaemia secondary to blood loss

Blood loss may be either acute or chronic. Common causes for chronic blood loss include gastrointestinal lesions and menorrhagia. In chronic blood loss, the result is often iron deficiency anaemia, which was discussed above. Acute blood loss may be the result of trauma, surgery, haematemesis, haemoptysis or obstetric haemorrhage.

The sudden loss of blood removes erythrocytes from the circulation, reducing the oxygen-carrying capacity of the blood. Initially the blood count may remain within normal parameters as there is an equivalent loss of plasma during a bleeding episode. As the plasma volume generally returns to normal within 1–3 days after the initial blood loss, the remaining pool of red cells is then dispersed into this increased circulatory volume. It is at this time that the severity of anaemia can be more accurately measured.

Under normal circumstances the bone marrow responds quickly to increased tissue hypoxia and the red cell count returns to normal within 4–5 weeks. As a considerable amount of iron may be lost as a result of the bleeding episode, haemoglobin production may be impaired, necessitating the administration of iron supplements to replenish iron stores and increase the level of haemoglobin production.

If the blood loss is 20% or more of the total blood volume, or if bleeding cannot be arrested quickly, rapid replacement by means of a blood transfusion may be necessary. This will help to prevent renal failure and minimize the normal physiological responses to acute blood loss that may lead to cardiac, renal, respiratory or gastrointestinal problems. Rapid transfusion quickly increases the total circulating volume as well as the number of red cells available to carry oxygen. In severe blood loss, the replacement of plasma, platelets and clotting factors may also be required. Specific protocols for the management of massive blood loss and transfusion exist as this represents a medical emergency associated with a high morbidity and mortality rate. Management of severe blood loss includes the surgical control of bleeding, management of the circulatory volume and maintenance of adequate blood oxygen-carrying capacity (McLelland 1996).

Anaemia due to abnormal red cell destruction (haemolytic anaemias)

A reduced red cell lifespan with abnormal or increased destruction is characteristic of the haemolytic anaemias. This abnormality may be either inherited or acquired. Destruction related to a defective red cell reflects the inherited haemolytic anaemias, whereas, for the most part, the acquired haemolytic anaemias are due to increased destruction of normal red cells. One exception to this is paroxysmal nocturnal haemoglobinurea, where an acquired red cell defect is the primary cause of the haemolysis. Destruction of the red cell may take place within the bloodstream (intravascular haemolysis) or in the spleen and liver (extravascular haemolysis).

Acquired haemolytic anaemias

Autoimmune haemolytic anaemia (AIHA) is caused by the production of an antibody that is targeted against one or more red cell surface antigens. AIHA is divided into warm or cold types, depending on the temperature at which there is maximum antibody activity (37°C or 4°C). Both types may either be primary or secondary to another disorder such as a lymphoproliferative disease or infection. Warm AIHA can be treated with immunosuppressive therapy such as steroid treatment or other immunosuppressive drugs, and a splenectomy may be considered if steroid treatment fails. Management of cold AIHA includes keeping the patient warm and immunosuppression.

Alloimmune haemolytic anaemia is caused by the reaction between the antibodies of one individual and the red cells of another. This may occur as a result of a mismatched blood transfusion, following transplantation or in haemolytic disease of the newborn, where a Rhesus-negative mother with Rh antibodies reacts to a Rhesus-positive fetus causing intravascular haemolysis in the child. Alloimmune haemolytic anaemia is a potentially life-threatening condition. *Transfusion-related haemolytic anaemia* is discussed in a subsequent section of this chapter.

Other extrinsic causes for abnormal haemolysis include drug-induced haemolytic anaemia and infections through either direct damage, toxins or autoantibody formation. Microangiopathic haemolytic anaemia may occur in disseminated intravascular coagulation, in patients with artificial heart valves, in thrombotic thrombocytopenic purpura (TTP), malignant hypertension, pre-eclampsia and meningococcal septicaemia (Mehta and Hoffbrand 2000). In these haemolytic anaemias, treatment of the underlying cause of the red cell destruction is a clinical priority, as well as managing the haemolysis itself.

Inherited haemolytic anaemias

Defects of the red cell can be related to:

■ an abnormality of the cell membrane

■ abnormal metabolism

■ abnormal haemoglobin.

Much of the pathology associated with these chronic anaemias can be described in terms of the process of red cell destruction. The anaemia itself may, in some disorders, be relatively mild and is often reasonably well tolerated. However, at times of stress, such as during a period of infection or extra need, the anaemia may become more pronounced. In these anaemias folate deficiency is fairly common; therefore folic acid supplements may be needed. The increased bilirubin concentration may predispose individuals to gallstones, particularly those with relatively high rates of haemolysis. There is also increased urobilinogen in the urine and faeces, making both darker in colour. Itching, either persistent or intermittent, may also be present. Splenomegaly may feature in disorders where the spleen is the major site of destruction.

Hereditary spherocytosis and hereditary elliptocytosis

Haemolytic anaemias resulting from an abnormal red cell membrane include *hereditary spherocytosis* and *hereditary elliptocytosis.* The haemolytic anaemia is classified according to the shape of the abnormal red cell, as the names imply. Most are inherited, although there is some evidence of spontaneous mutations in individuals with spherocytosis. In general the anaemia tends to be mild to moderate, depending on the rate of haemolysis. Folate deficiency is common, and infection (particularly some viral infections) can cause an acute haemolysis. A palpable spleen is relatively common. Nevertheless, many individuals remain only mildly symptomatic. For those whose symptoms are not easily tolerated, splenectomy may be helpful.

Glucose-6-phosphate dehydrogenase (G6PD) deficiency

An important example of haemolysis resulting from abnormal metabolism of the red cell is glucose-6-phosphate dehydrogenase (G6PD) deficiency. The genetic deficiency is on an X-linked gene, which means that by and large it affects males. The majority of women are only carriers, but a small population of women is affected, although usually only mildly. The incidence varies greatly throughout the world, from very rarely amongst northern Europeans to over 20% in southern Europe, parts of Africa and Asia. The highest frequency appears to be in southeast Asia and parts of the Middle East (Luzzatto and Gordon-Smith 1999).

In most, the haemolysis is acute and manifests itself only in the presence of a specific trigger. Certain drugs, fava beans and infections are known triggers. Care should be taken to avoid these as far as possible. For healthcare workers, this is particularly relevant in relation to specific drugs that may unknowingly be prescribed and administered to susceptible individuals. In acute attacks the intravascular haemolysis can greatly vary in severity, as can the symptoms. Renal failure is associated with G6PD haemolysis.

Treatment includes supportive care, treatment of any underlying infection and the immediate removal of any other specific trigger. In a few individuals the haemolysis may be chronic.

Haemoglobinopathies

The complex haemoglobin (Hb) molecule occurs normally in three forms. The type is determined by slight variations in the globin portions of the four subunits. HbA is the principal haemoglobin of adults, HbA_2 is approximately 2% of adult haemoglobin and HbF (fetal haemoglobin) is usally less than 1% Hb in adults (Arif and Mufti 1998). Adult haemoglobin contains two α and two β globin chains with a haem pocket within each chain.

The term haemoglobinopathy indicates the presence of red blood cells containing an inherited abnormality of haemoglobin, the result of a genetic mutation that causes a disorder in synthesis of the haemoglobin molecule. This may result in a structural variation in one or more of the globin chains causing a decreased production of structurally normal haemoglobin and premature haemolysis of the erythrocyte. The most common haemoglobinopathies are thalassaemia and sickle-cell disease.

Thalassaemia

The thalassaemias are a group of autosomal recessive inherited disorders affecting the synthesis of the globin part of the haemoglobin molecule in the red cell. Either the α or the β chain of the globin molecule can be affected, leading to an imbalance in the production of α and β chains and a fundamental instability of the globin molecule. This leads to a range of syndromes, the clinical characteristics of which are related to the degree of α- and β-chain imbalance (Howard and Hamilton 1997).

The thalassaemias occur predominantly in the Mediterranean, parts of Africa, the Middle East, the Indian subcontinent and south-east Asia (Weatherall 1999). They are among the most common inherited disorders (Howard and Hamilton 1997) and are thought to have evolved because they can confer partial resistance to the malaria parasite. The thalassaemias are classified according to their severity. Thalassaemia major is a severe transfusion-dependent form; thalassaemia minor is a carrier state with few, if any, clinical implications. Thalassaemia intermedia is a less severe form, with a degree of anaemia and splenomegaly (Weatherall 1999).

β-Thalassaemia major is a severe form of the disease, with red cell destruction both within the bone marrow and in the spleen. Children born with this disorder have severe anaemia, fail to thrive and have a myriad of problems. The spleen and liver enlarge and the chronic anaemia causes extramedullary haemopoiesis, causing bony deformities. These children are transfusion dependent: without treatment they seldom survive into adolescence. The need for frequent transfusions creates its own problems, including iron overload and organ damage.

Apart from regular transfusions, regular iron chelation therapy, such as subcutaneous desferrioxamine, is required to reduce iron overload. A splenectomy may be required to reduce transfusion requirements. Bone marrow transplantation may be an option for some individuals. Long-term cardiac, liver and endocrine problems require management as they arise.

Thalassaemia intermedia is less severe: individuals exhibit a moderate anaemia, sometimes requiring transfusion support. Many of the clinical symptoms of β-thalassaemia major are absent.

β-Thalassaemia minor (or trait) is least severe, with mild anaemia. Individuals often remain completely asymptomatic except perhaps at times of stress, such as in pregnancy (Weatherall 1999).

In α-thalassaemia, the clinical picture is related to the number of functioning α genes present. The complete absence of α-globin production is incompatible with life and results in intrauterine or neonatal death and the syndrome *hydrops fetalis*. Haemoglobin H disease is a consequence of only one functioning gene and results in anaemia and splenomegaly. One or two α-gene deletions result in thalassaemia trait. This is often asymptomatic, although some individuals may have mild anaemia.

Genetic counselling should be offered to those individuals found to be carriers. Partners of carriers should also be tested. Appropriate and unbiased information and support should be offered to couples who are both carriers, alongside the option of antenatal testing so that informed choices can be made about pregnancy.

Sickle-cell disease

Sickle-cell disease
See chapter 4.1

This is a group of hereditary recessive blood disorders characterized by red cells that contain an abnormal form of haemoglobin called HbS. The globin chain structure is changed by the substitution of one amino acid and this effectively changes the behaviour of the whole molecule. As this is a recessive disorder, individuals who inherit HbS from only one parent have what is termed as sickle-cell trait (HbAS), whereas individuals who inherit HbS from both parents have sickle-cell disease (HbSS) (see Fig. 14.8 for examples of inheritance of HbS). Other variants of sickle-cell disease include HbSC and HbSβ-thal. It is predominantly a disease of the African–Caribbean population, but also affects individuals with Mediterranean, Middle Eastern and Asian Indian ancestry. Sickle-cell trait seems to offer some protection from a common type of malaria, falciparum malaria, so there is a higher incidence of HbS inheritance in regions where malaria is prevalent. Diagnosis is often made within the first 2 years of life; young babies are often protected from symptoms of the disease because of the high levels of HbF produced in early life.

The exact mechanisms by which changes in the properties of deoxygenated haemoglobin molecules cause the red cells to sickle is not fully understood. It is thought that the red cells deform as they release oxygen molecules in the capillaries. These red cells undergo repeated cycles of sickling and desickling until they are no longer able to return to their normal shape. These distorted crescent-shaped red cells become trapped in the microcirculation, causing blockages and producing the range of clinical manifestations of sickle-cell disease. Another consequence of this sickling process is that the red cell lifespan is shortened from a normal 120 days to as little as 25–35 days, causing a haemolytic anaemia.

The course of sickle-cell anaemia is very variable. Some affected individuals are able to live almost normal lives, whereas others experience repeated crises and great incapacity. The reason for this variation is not known. The clinical manifestations of sickle-cell disease are varied but include:

- severe episodes of acute pain (referred to as a sickle-cell crisis)
- acute chest syndrome
- splenic sequestration crisis

Figure 14.8   Examples of inheritance of sickle-cell disease. S, gene for Hbs; A, gene for normal haemoglobin.

- avascular necrosis of bone and joints

- osteomyelitis

- chronic skin ulceration – frequently on lower limbs

- renal dysfunction

- stroke

- retinopathy

- priapism

- infections

- cardiomegaly

- bone marrow necrosis

- aplastic crisis

- anaemia.

Exacerbation of this sickling process, with vascular occlusion and severe pain, is termed a sickle-cell crisis. Precipitating factors of a painful crisis include physiological stresses such as exposure to cold or heat, dehydration, infection, physical exertion or any situation where the person experiences hypoxia as well as psychological stress. Often, it is a combination of factors that induces a crisis. At times there are warning signs, but often the crisis is unpredictable and quite sudden.

Pain is a key feature of a sickle-cell crisis, often requiring strong opiate analgesics to control it. Although some mild sickle-cell crises can be managed effectively at home with oral analgesics, often the person is unwell and requires hospital admission for management and pain control. Initially patients require large doses of strong analgesics to control the pain. This can be given as intramuscular injections, subcutaneous infusion or intravenous infusion, including patient-controlled analgesia (PCA) systems, depending on the clinical situation. Prompt, effective pain relief is imperative as pain is a potent physiological and psychological stressor, and may contribute to an increasing cycle of red cell sickling and to other serious complications – as well as being distressing to the person. Often the pain is intense, engendering fear and anxiety and rendering the patient immobile. Hydration is essential, orally if tolerated or as an intravenous infusion.

If the precipitating cause is a suspected infection, antibiotics are prescribed. This is important as a large proportion of patients with sickle-cell disease are functionally asplenic from an early age – a consequence of splenic infarctions from repeated crises. In the initial stages, rest and careful monitoring are also essential. Oxygen therapy is given to prevent any further hypoxia and the oxygen saturation levels are carefully monitored. Falling saturations may indicate a chest crisis or be a side-effect of the opiate analgesia. A chest crisis is a serious complication of sickle-cell disease and effective medical management should be instituted promptly. Another serious complication is splenic sequestration;

a rapidly falling haemoglobin level and abdominal discomfort or pain and distension are indicators of possible sequestration. Again, prompt medical intervention is essential. Transfusions of red cells or red cell exchange procedures may be required to reduce the proportion of sickle cells in the circulation and help to stabilize the seriously ill patient.

Once the person's condition has been stabilized and the pain is satisfactorily under control, gentle mobilization and rehabilitation can begin. This may be a rapid or slow process, depending on many factors. Regaining independence and a sense of control is a priority for patients. Pain relief can be titrated according to need, but a sudden increase in pain may signal the onset of another crisis and should be monitored carefully. A sample critical pathway that highlights some of the care interventions can be found in Box 14.1.

Chronic pain is often a consequence of bone and joint necrosis, and may be difficult to control effectively. Joint damage may reduce mobility, as can chronic skin ulcers. Strokes can occur at any age but are more frequent in childhood and can be devastating, leaving the person seriously disabled. Priapism (a persistent erection in the male) is another serious complication that may be difficult to treat and may induce impotence. The chronic anaemia and red cell breakdown may result in cardiomegaly and the development of gallstones. Patients with sickle-cell disease are often slightly jaundiced, a result of the continual red cell turnover. Renal damage to the renal capillaries may cause individuals to pass large amounts of dilute urine, predisposing them to dehydration. Repeated transfusions may lead to iron overload.

Prevention of crises and complications includes:

- good nutrition and hydration (3 litres of fluid per day)

- managing changes in the weather by keeping warm or cool as appropriate

- good housing with effective heating

- managing stress

- prophylactic antibiotics in the form of daily penicillin tablets

- folic acid supplements

- a home analgesia strategy including anti-inflammatory drugs and opiates

- access to effective medical and nursing care both in the community and in the acute sector.

Coordinated services with specialist medical and nursing teams as well as access to general practitioner services and sickle-cell specialist community nurses are important features of good care.

Sickle-cell disease: nursing management issues

Sickle-cell disease presents a challenge for nurses working in both hospital and community settings. The

Box 14.1   Critical pathway for sickle-cell crisis

ON ARRIVAL	DAYS 1–3	DAYS 4–10
ASSESSMENT	**ASSESSMENT**	**ASSESSMENT**

ON ARRIVAL

ASSESSMENT

- Pain assessment
- Baseline:
  — oxygen saturations
  — vital signs
  — level of consciousness
- Clinical examination including abdomen, chest and CNS
- Full blood count, U&E, blood cultures, group and save
- Chest radiography
- Assess need for vascular access

INTERVENTION

- *Analgesia*
  — institute promptly and at a dosage that relieves pain effectively
  — repeat regularly and titrate to pain levels
  — maintain a regular analgesia schedule
- *Oxygenation*
  — maintain oxygen saturations > 90%
  — oxygen via humidified mask
  — mechanical ventilation, if required
- *Monitor hourly*
  — pain levels
  — oxygen saturations
  — vital signs
  — level of consciousness/CNS
  — renal function
- *Hydration*
  — oral/i.v. – maintain input of 3 L in 24 hours unless contraindicated
- Intravenous antibiotics if infection is suspected
- Vascular access, if required

DAYS 1–3

ASSESSMENT

- Pain assessment (quantitative and qualitative, regular and consistent)
- Clinical examination including abdomen, chest and CNS
- Anaemia
- Respiratory function
- Level of consciousness
- Hydration
- Renal function
- Self-caring activities
- Psychological status/mood
- Support needs

INTERVENTION

- *Analgesia*
  — titrate to pain levels
  — maintain a regular analgesia schedule
  — institute an appropriate drug-delivery system (e.g. patient-controlled analgesia (PCA) device)
  — implement analgesia strategy to meet needs
- *Oxygenation*
  — maintain oxygen saturations > 90%
  — oxygen via humidified mask
  — mechanical ventilation, if required
- Monitor hourly initially – increase or reduce according to assessment findings (see above):
  — pain
  — vital signs and oxygen saturations
  — level of consciousness
  — nausea and vomiting
  — fluid input and output
- FBC, U&E if there are signs of anaemia, liver or renal dysfunction
- *Hydration*
  — oral/i.v. – maintain input of 3 L in 24 hours unless contraindicated
- Start or continue i.v. antibiotics in the presence of fever

DAYS 4–10

ASSESSMENT

- Pain assessment (quantitative and qualitative, regular and consistent)
- Clinical examination including abdomen, chest and CNS
- Anaemia
- Respiratory function
- Level of consciousness
- Hydration
- Renal function
- Self-caring activities
- Psychological status/mood
- Support needs
- Preliminary discharge assessment

INTERVENTION

- *Analgesia*
  — titrate to pain levels
  — maintain a regular analgesia schedule
  — discuss changing needs with the patient
  — review and maintain an analgesia strategy to meet needs
- *Oxygenation*
  — maintain oxygen saturations > 90%
  — oxygen via humidified mask if required
- Monitor 2–4 hourly – increase or reduce according to assessment findings (see above):
  — pain
  — vital signs and oxygen saturations
  — level of consciousness
  — fluid input and output
- FBC, U&E if there are signs of anaemia, liver or renal dysfunction
- *Hydration*
  — oral/i.v. – maintain input of 3 L in 24 hours unless contraindicated
  — consider an oral hydration schedule, if tolerated
- Start, continue or change i.v. antibiotics in the presence of fever
- Start a rehabilitation/mobilization programme titrated to energy levels and pain levels
- Review venous access – consider oral therapy in place of i.v. if client is stable
- Formulate a preliminary discharge strategy but only when client is physically and psychologically ready to start dialogue with the clinical team

(Continued)

Box 14.1 *(Continued)*

ON ARRIVAL	DAYS 1–3	DAYS 4–10
NOTES	**NOTES**	**NOTES**
■ Prioritize prompt and effective analgesia and assessment	■ Prioritize regular or continuous, effective analgesia and assessment	■ Prioritize regular or continuous, effective analgesia and assessment
■ Ensure adequate pain relief is maintained to minimize physiological stress and further sickling of red cells and deoxygenation	■ Consider possible complications: — chest crisis — splenic sequestration — cerebrovascular accident or other CNS involvement — sepsis	■ Consider possible complications: — chest crisis — splenic sequestration — cerebrovascular accident or other CNS involvement — sepsis
■ Keep client warm and comfortable		
■ Consider possible complications: — chest crisis — splenic sequestration — cerebral vascular accident or others CNS involvement — sepsis	■ At this early stage avoid reducing analgesia unless warranted by the clinical situation, i.e. respirations < 10–12/min or impaired level of consciousness	■ Avoid early withdrawal of analgesia ■ Remain alert for increasing levels of pain that may signal the onset of complications or a new crisis
■ Monitor client closely		

U&E, urea and electrolytes; FBC, full blood count.

---

establishment of sickle-cell centres has greatly enhanced knowledge, promoted understanding of the condition and promoted a multidisciplinary and culturally sensitive approach to care. This is important because the disorder affects ethnic and racial groups that may have been disadvantaged in relation to health care.

Although most individuals with sickle-cell disease have infrequent hospital admissions, a proportion will have repeated severe painful crises requiring regular admission to hospital. Unfortunately, because of their frequent and regular presentation in accident and emergency departments, many of these patients become labelled as manipulative and addiction prone, and analgesia is restricted at the very time it is most needed. In a small sample of patients admitted to hospital for management of a painful crisis, Alleyne and Thomas (1994) found evidence to support findings from other areas of nursing that nurses lack an understanding of the individual nature of pain and its management. These patients were treated as a stigmatized group labelled as 'sicklers'. A need for greater understanding of this disorder and its sequelae is therefore apparent. The impact of a poor client–carer relationship that arises from a lack of communication, lack of mutual understanding and a clinical situation that offers the potential for conflict is an important issue in the care of patients with sickle-cell disease (Oni 1998).

Physical care during a crisis is only part of the nurse's role. The ability of the nurse to help individuals and families to adjust their lifestyle and develop strategies for overcoming health difficulties is as important. Like other chronic illnesses, sickle-cell disease has many psychological and practical implications. Genetic counselling and support should be offered to individuals and couples when considering pregnancy and parenthood so that they are better able to make informed decisions. This counselling should provide an honest appraisal of risk but be unbiased so that couples can feel free to make personal informed decisions about their future and that of their children (Atkin et al 1998).

Social support has been identified as being extremely important to the well-being of families (Midence and Shand 1992, Midence et al 1993); local parent support groups and the Sickle Cell Society are helpful in meeting this need. The financial implications of raising a child with sickle-cell disease also need to be addressed, because maintaining an optimal environment may be very expensive in terms of heating, bills, etc. Teachers also need to be briefed on how the condition may interfere with a child's daily routines and school performance, as it is very easy for a cycle of disadvantage to be set up. Adolescents with sickle-cell disease, like those with any chronic illness, are a particular challenge to families and carers. In adult life individuals may be disadvantaged in terms of employment as a result of their need for a relatively constant environment, and as a consequence of the chronic manifestations of the disease, such as leg ulcers, the need for hip replacement following bone necrosis and visual loss from retinal damage. This complex disease and its many manifestations requires a multidisciplinary approach to care and nurses are ideally placed to coordinate care and resources so that the disabling effects on individuals and their families is minimized.

Nursing management of the person with anaemia

Anaemia is a symptom of an underlying disorder and the care required by an anaemic patient varies with the cause and the severity of the anaemia. Many individuals with anaemia are treated as outpatients, especially if the anaemia is chronic as in pernicious anaemia. Others may need continuous supervision, intermittent treatment and may need substantially to modify their way of life, as in the example of sickle cell anaemia. For some people anaemia may be cured entirely by treatment of the underlying cause, such as a bleeding ulcer. Depending on the underlying cause, there may be other symptoms and problems in addition to those attributable to anaemia. An example would be the problem of jaundice in haemolytic anaemia, or vascular occulsion in sickle-cell disease. Whatever the cause of the anaemia, the patients have one common difficulty: a decreased capacity of the blood to transport oxygen.

Assessment

History

It is important to begin by establishing to what degree the patient is incapacitated by the anaemia. This will vary from very mild to extensive disruption of their normal daily activities. Knowledge of the clinical characteristics of anaemia should lead the nurse to be alert to any indication of their presence from the history given by the patient. The patient is also asked about gradual or sudden changes in daily activities, changes experienced with exertion, and any increased need for rest and sleep.

The history should include information about the sequence of events leading up to the present situation, such as recent surgery or trauma or unusual bleeding. Occupational and social circumstances should be determined together with past health history and medication history. It may also be relevant to enquire about any history of anaemia in other family members. For women of reproductive age it is important to enquire about any menstrual problems, such as heavy, prolonged or frequent periods.

It may be relevant to obtain a nutritional history assessing the intake of essential nutrients and focusing especially on the adequacy of iron and vitamin B_{12} intake.

Taking a health history also provides an opportunity to assess the patient's knowledge and understanding of their anaemia, its cause and any prescribed therapeutic measures.

Physical examination

This begins with general observation of the person's appearance and behaviour, noting indications of anaemia such as pallor and signs of fatigue or pain. The skin and mucous membranes, especially the conjunctivae, are examined for pallor and in the case of haemolytic anaemia for initial or increasing jaundice. The tongue is inspected as vitamin B_{12} deficiency produces a red, smooth, sore tongue. Nails are observed for brittleness and any abnormalities of shape such as spooning or clubbing which can occur with anaemia. Respiratory and heart rates are recorded and any changes on exertion noted.

The person diagnosed or suspected of having pernicious anaemia may demonstrate signs of degenerative changes in the nervous system. Any complaint of tingling, numbness and paraesthesia (pins and needles) in the extremities, loss of fine movement, difficulty in holding small objects, limb weakness, ataxia or impaired vision should be noted.

If the person has sickle-cell disease, they are regularly observed for swollen, tender and painful areas, changes in body function or their mental and physical abilities that may be indicative of areas of vascular occlusion.

Laboratory test results should be consulted and nursing measures adapted according to abnormalities and changes. For example, a fall in the haemoglobin level, packed cell volume or erythrocyte count may suggest that the patient's activity level should be restricted to reduce oxygen requirements until treatment takes effect.

Patient problems related to anaemia

The reduced capacity of the blood to carry oxygen may give rise to some or all of the following problems:

- inability to sustain the usual level of activity
- potential risk of tissue damage and injury
- pain due to tissue ischaemia or hyperplasia of the bone marrow
- impaired thought processes.

The person may also experience problems such as:

- inability to maintain an adequate dietary intake of nutrients essential for red blood cell production
- lack of knowledge concerning the disease process, treatment and measures to promote health.

Nursing interventions

The goals of intervention for the person with anaemia are that:

1. The person will achieve an acceptable level of activity while maintaining vital signs within the normal range.
2. The person's skin and mucosal tissues will remain intact and no accidental injury will be experienced.
3. The person will state that he or she is pain free.
4. The person and their family will report improvement in thought processes.
5. The person will be able to select appropriate foodstuffs and maintain an adequate dietary intake, as indicated by improvement in laboratory blood results.
6. The person will be able to describe the cause and characteristics of the anaemia, the treatment plan, and discuss plans to modify lifestyle and minimize risk of complications.

Activity

Individuals are assisted to modify their level of activity in order to decrease the demand for oxygen, and nursing care is planned to achieve this. An explanation of the basis of the fatigue and weakness experienced, and emphasis on the importance of balancing rest and activity, may help the person to understand what is happening and to accept limitations on activity. Activity is encouraged but the importance of resting before becoming fatigued and breathless is explained. Assistance may be required to enable the person to perform essential activities, such as maintaining personal hygiene and dressing, with the minimum of effort.

Severe anaemia may cause shortness of breath or dyspnoea, even at rest, and the person may be less distressed with the head of the bed raised or in a sitting position, and with good ventilation. Oxygen administration may be necessary during the acute period. Prolonged use is inadvisable as increasing the concentration of oxygen in the blood suppresses erythropoiesis. A blood transfusion of packed cells may be administered. Individuals may have questions about the safety of blood transfusions and wish to explore problems associated with this treatment, especially if they are required regularly on a long-term basis.

In the long term, if the person is active and employed it may be necessary to encourage adjustments to their normal lifestyle. The nurse should help the individual and family to evaluate the usual daily routines and identify activities that are priorities so that a plan may be developed that aims at avoiding sudden strenuous activity and schedules rest periods. The person's activity tolerance is reviewed regularly and, taking the clinical condition into account, activity is increased or decreased accordingly.

Skin and mucosal tissues

The reduced oxygen supply to the tissues increases the risk of pressure sore development, especially if activity is limited. The person with anaemia should be carefully assessed, using a risk assessment scale such as that of Norton or Waterlow, and the appropriate precautionary measures instituted. This may range from 2-hourly changes of position to the use of special pressure-relieving systems. People with haemolytic anaemia who are jaundiced often experience *pruritus* (itching). Warm or tepid water is used for bathing and use of soap is avoided. Calamine lotion may be applied to relieve itching; the fingernails should be kept short and clean to prevent excoriation and infection, should the person scratch the irritated areas. Skin creams and emollients are useful in keeping skin hydrated and supple, and in preventing dry, cracked skin.

In pernicious and iron deficiency anaemias ulcerative lesions of the oral mucosa and a sore raw tongue may occur. Regular cool, mild mouthwashes may be soothing. A soft toothbrush is advised for cleaning the teeth. Hot spicy foods are best avoided and the mouth should be cleaned after taking nourishment.

The person who is very weak and dizzy as a result of anaemia may be at risk from falls. It is important to assess this risk and remove from the patient's immediate environment any object that might cause injury. The person who has sensory loss as a result of anaemia may demonstrate poor coordination and be at risk of injury from dropping objects. They will also be less sensitive to heat and may therefore be susceptible to burns.

If the person with anaemia is also susceptible to infection, additional safety precautions may be required. These are discussed later.

Pain

The person with anaemia may experience angina-like pain, headache, **pain** due to marrow hyperplasia or pain due to vascular occlusion and ischaemia as a result of a sickle-cell crisis. Whatever the cause, the pain should be fully assessed, using a pain chart, and analgesia administered as required to achieve pain relief. The person in a sickle-cell crisis may require regular 4-hourly opioid analgesia or patient-controlled analgesia, but non-invasive measures such as rest of the affected part, local heat application, use of a bed cradle and relaxation techniques may also be valuable.

Thought processes

The person with anaemia should be observed for signs of confusion and slow intellectual responses. The individual should be reassured that mental disturbance and a reduced concentration span are associated with the condition and should improve. This is because treatment, generally aimed at increasing the oxygen-carrying capacity of the blood, will also improve cerebral oxygenation.

Diet

When nutrition has been identified as a problem the nurse and dietician should discuss with the person and family the importance of diet. Food preferences are identified and help given to plan menus that will provide the necessary nutrients in an acceptable form. Foods should be light, easily digested and provide protein, iron, vitamins B_{12} and C, and folic acid. Dietary sources of iron include red meats, liver, eggs, fish, green leafy vegetables, enriched whole-grain cereals, and bread and dried fruits. The absorption of iron is reduced by the presence of tea, coffee, milk and antacids but is promoted in the presence of vitamin C. Sources of vitamin B_{12} include red meats, liver, eggs and dairy produce. Folic acid is present in meat (especially liver), whole-grain cereals, leafy vegetables, beans, brewer's yeast and dairy products. Citrus fruits, and other fruits and vegetables, are good sources of vitamin C. These vitamins are heat soluble and therefore destroyed by prolonged cooking.

Anorexia may be an accompanying problem and may be exacerbated if the person has a sore mouth. Small,

Skin assessment
See chapter 6.1

Pain
See chapter 2.3

frequent meals and avoidance of certain foods may help. Mouth care is important and food should be presented attractively. Help with feeding and social contact at mealtimes should be provided as necessary. Elderly people at home may require a carer or meals-on-wheels, arranged through their community care manager. Voluntary agencies such as Age Concern and local authorities provide day care and luncheon clubs, which provide a nutritious meal and social contacts.

Extra fluids are very important for the person with a haemolytic anaemia, especially sickle-cell anaemia. The person who is hospitalized during a sickle-cell crisis should have fluid intake recorded and may require intravenous hydration if unable to maintain a good oral intake (2–3 litres per 24 hours for an adult). Dietary intake may be supplemented by prescription of iron and vitamins.

Knowledge and lifestyle

A full explanation of the nature of the disorder and reasons for symptoms experienced should be made to the individual and family members. The person is advised of changes that might indicate a recurrence of the disorder and the need to seek medical help.

Information should be provided about the prescribed treatment and plan of care, and the person's understanding evaluated by having him or her carry out procedures such as medication administration and the planning and preparation of diet. Explanations should be provided about any prescribed drugs and possible adverse effects. For example, the person prescribed iron should be warned to expect dark stools and possible gastrointestinal irritation. Long-term iron therapy has a tendency to cause constipation and thus the importance of a high-fibre diet should be stressed. The necessity of getting regular maintenance doses of vitamin B_{12} should be stressed to the person with pernicious anaemia, and a district nurse referral made to facilitate this if attendance at the clinic for the injections is not possible.

In the case of sickle-cell anaemia, parents should receive an explanation of the disease and factors that predispose to crises. Children and parents can be advised of the importance of prophylactic care during remission. This involves living as normally as possible but avoiding chilling, contact with people with infections, high altitudes, overfatigue and stressful situations. A well balanced diet, plenty of fluids and adequate rest are important. Proper dental care and immunization against infectious diseases are stressed, as well as attendance at clinics for regular physical and haematological assessment.

Individuals with hereditary forms of anaemia may wish to be advised of genetic counselling opportunities for themselves. It is important that they feel able to make informed choices about their chances of having affected children (see Case Study 14.1).

Case Study 14.1

Claudia is a 19-year-old girl whose parents are Ghanaian. She came to a family planning clinic for advice regarding contraception. She and her boyfriend were having regular sex and she wanted a reliable method of contraception in addition to using sheaths to protect herself from sexually transmitted infection.

In taking a history it emerged that Claudia had sickle-cell disease and had experienced numerous crises throughout her childhood. She was currently well. She was well informed about her condition, as was her boyfriend, and very aware of the implications of pregnancy for her health.

Claudia's contraceptive choices were limited by her condition, as an intrauterine device would be unsuitable because of the risk of exacerbating anaemia and increased risk of infection, and the combined oral contraceptive pill is unsuitable because of the potential risk of thromboembolism. This left a progestogen-only form of contraception as her main option. Claudia was willing to try the progestogen-only pill; the possibility of irregular periods did not concern her as these were already irregular. She was in the habit of taking folic acid supplements and prophylactic antibiotics and therefore felt quite confident of her ability to take the pill on time. Following consultation with the doctor, Claudia left the clinic with 3 months' supply of Micronor to start on the first day of her next period, and condoms.

Persons with haemolytic spherocytosis who have had a splenectomy, and those with sickle-cell anaemia or thalassaemia who have impairment of splenic function, require teaching regarding the potential for post-splenectomy sepsis. Pneumococcal vaccine may be administered as a preventive measure.

Evaluation

Objective measurement of the effectiveness of nursing intervention for the person with anaemia is provided by ongoing laboratory results which show that the haemoglobin, red blood cell counts, haematocrit, vitamin B_{12} and folate levels are within the normal range for the individual. The person will report a decrease or absence of the clinical symptoms previously identified.

Evaluation of patient and family teaching is based on assessment of their knowledge of dietary and treatment measures and their verbalization of strategies to control symptoms and resume usual daily activities. Questions regarding the therapeutic plan should be answered and the person should be aware of community resources for ongoing health care.

Polycythaemia (erythrocyte excess)

Polycythaemia refers to a condition in which there is an excessive number of erythrocytes and a corresponding increase in the haemoglobin concentration. The red cell count may be $7\text{--}10 \times 10^{12}$ per litre (7–10 million per μL) with a haemoglobin concentration of 18–25 g/dL.

Secondary polycythaemia occurs when there is a physiological compensatory increase in the number of erythrocytes by the red bone marrow in response to a low concentration of oxygen in the blood and an increase in erythropoietin. It normally occurs at high altitudes where the atmospheric oxygen tension is low, and in pathological conditions in which there is tissue hypoxia. Examples of the latter are chronic obstructive pulmonary disease and certain congenital malformations of the heart. It can occur in individuals who are heavy smokers, and in people with renal disease when there is inappropriate secretion of erythropoietin. A relative polycythaemia also occurs as a result of excessive plasma loss, for example following extensive burns or excessive vomiting and diarrhoea.

Primary polycythaemia is also known as *polycythaemia rubra vera* (PRV). It is a rare, malignant, myeloproliferative disorder of the red bone marrow in which there is uncontrolled production of an excessive number of red blood cells. It may be accompanied by some overproduction of granulocytes and platelets. The cause of this malignant disorder is unknown, although it would appear to result from some mutation in a pluripotent stem cell which gives it a proliferative advantage in comparison to normal stem cells. Onset usually occurs in later life and its incidence is similar in men and women (Howard and Hamilton 1997).

Clinical characteristics

Primary polycythaemia increases the total red cell volume and viscosity of the blood. The blood pressure is raised and the workload of the heart is increased. Heart failure may develop insidiously as a result of increased cardiac demands. The rate of flow through the blood vessels is reduced, which, together with the increased number of erythrocytes and blood viscosity, predisposes to the development of thrombi. Occlusion of arterial or venous vessels may occur, causing a cerebrovascular accident, transient ischaemic attacks, coronary thrombosis, intermittent claudication, deep vein thrombosis, etc. The spleen enlarges in many cases because of the increase in red cell destruction.

Symptoms vary greatly: an individual may not experience any discomfort and be unaware of any problem until the condition is discovered during a routine blood test; others may experience symptoms such as headache, dizziness, blurred vision, or complain of a full feeling in the head. Pruritus (itching), especially after a hot bath, is an unpleasant although not dangerous symptom associated with this condition, as is gout due to uric acid derived from the increased breakdown of red blood cells.

A person with primary polycythaemia often appears plethoric (with a very ruddy complexion), whilst the distal parts of limbs, especially the lower limbs, may be cyanotic owing to the sluggish circulation. Peptic ulceration occurs in up to 10% of patients and is apparently attributable to an increase in gastric acid secretion (Hoffbrand and Pettit 1993).

The person with a secondary polycythaemia is usually cyanosed due to the underlying cardiac or respiratory disease. Diagnosis is based on a number of blood tests including increased haematocrit and red cell mass, and a bone marrow aspiration. Exclusion of respiratory and renal disease is indicative of PRV.

Treatment and care

The aim of treatment is to reduce the risk of thrombosis and alleviate the symptoms. How this is achieved varies and depends on the duration and severity of the condition and on the age of the patient. A phlebotomy (venesection) is the simplest way of producing a temporary reduction in symptoms.

Initially up to 500 mL of blood may be removed once or twice a week until the packed cell volume (PCV) is down to about 45%. Red cell and platelet apheresis is a rapid way of achieving this (see Box 14.2). Repeating this at regular intervals may be the only treatment needed, although iron and folate supplements may be prescribed to prevent deficiencies occurring. In patients with PRV, if phlebotomy is required very frequently or the platelet count is too high, the risk of thrombosis is high and treatment with a myelosuppressive drug such as hydroxyurea may be used to suppress erythropoiesis. Radioactive phosphorus (^{32}P) is of value in treating older patients with severe disease. These agents are avoided in younger persons, if possible, because of concerns about their carcinogenic potential. Allopurinol is prescribed to lower the excessive serum uric acid concentration and relieve the inflammation and pain of gout in joints. The value of other drugs such as recombinant interferon-α therapy and aspirin to inhibit platelet aggregation is still under evaluation.

Unless a complication such as thrombosis, peptic ulcer or cardiac insufficiency occurs, a person with polycythaemia is not usually treated as an inpatient. Pain should be alleviated and a reasonable amount of activity encouraged with the aim of preventing circulatory stasis. When pruritus is a significant problem, medication with antihistamines may be helpful in alleviating the itch. Close supervision by the haematology team and the patient's general practitioner is important, and the patient and family are alerted to early indications of potential complications such as thrombosis and advised of the importance of prompt action. Frequently PRV can be managed for long periods with relatively little disturbance to the individual's daily life. In the long term (10–15 years) about 20% of patients go on to develop acute leukaemia or myelofibrosis.

Polycythaemia
See chapter 4.1

Box 14.2   Apheresis

The term apheresis is derived from a Greek word meaning to take away or withdraw, and describes the process of removing one circulating blood component, usually through the use of automated blood cell separators, while returning the other components to a donor or patient. This procedure can be used for therapeutic purposes or as a method of collecting blood components for transfusion. Either cells (cytapheresis) or plasma solutes (apheresis) may be withdrawn.

The process involves the use of a closed system whereby an amount of blood is drawn from the person and mixed with anticoagulant to prevent clotting. It is then processed through a centrifuge or filter to remove the desired component. The remaining components are recombined and returned to the patient or donor. If required, the component being removed can also be replaced.

For example:

■ In polycythaemia, red cells and platelets can be removed from a symptomatic patient.

■ In sickle-cell disease, a large volume of abnormal red cells can be removed and these are then replaced through a simultaneous blood transfusion in order to maintain the patient's red cell count within normal limits (this is called red cell exchange).

■ In myeloma, plasma containing large amounts of abnormal paraproteins can be removed to reduce the symptoms of hyperviscosity, and normal plasma can then be transfused.

■ In acute leukaemia, large numbers of white cells can be removed from the circulation to relieve the symptoms of a high white cell count or to reduce the tumour load prior to chemotherapy.

■ In stem cell transplantation, stem cells can be collected from the donor using cytapheresis.

■ In transfusion practice, platelets can be collected from volunteer donors at specific blood donor sessions.

Therapeutic apheresis can be used for a range of indications other than those cited above; these have simply been selected as examples.

Leucocyte disorders

Alterations in the number of leucocytes may involve increased or decreased production of cells as a result of a variety of benign and malignant processes.

Leucocytosis

The number of leucocytes in the circulation increases to a level in excess of the normal ($4.0–11.0 \times 10^9$/L) in a variety of situations. These include infection, inflammatory diseases, pregnancy, after trauma or surgery, in malignancy, after acute haemorrhage or as a side-effect of drugs (Howard and Hamilton 1997). This increase is referred to as a leucocytosis and is usually predominant in one type of white cell.

Leucopenia

Leucopenia may be defined as a reduction in the number of leucocytes below the normal lower limit of 4.0×10^9/L. This may be due to a decreased production or an increased destruction of white cells. The deficiency is most commonly seen in the granulocyte cell line, particularly the neutrophils. Lymphopenia, a deficiency of lymphocytes is relatively uncommon but may be a consequence of corticosteroid therapy, trauma or surgery, Hodgkin lymphoma, systemic lupus erythematosus (SLE) and acquired immune deficiency syndrome (Arif and Mufti 1998).

Neutropenia

The primary function of neutrophils is as one essential part of the body's defence against infection. This requires the ability to migrate to the site of infection or injury and to destroy bacteria. A normal neutrophil count is generally between 2.5 and 7.5×10^9/L, although a lower threshold of 1.5×10^9/L is normal for some groups. Neutropenia may be defined as a peripheral count below 1.5×10^9/L. However, serious infections are not generally seen until the neutrophil count is less than 0.5×10^9/L (Howard and Hamilton 1997).

Neutropenia may be the result of a reduced production of neutrophils, as in bone marrow failure, increased destruction, as in immune neutropenia, or pooling into the spleen. *Benign idiopathic neutropenia* is a familial disorder that is not associated with an increased risk of infection. The production of neutrophils is normal but there is an increased proportion of neutrophils out of the circulation, with a resulting lower number in the peripheral blood. *Cyclical neutropenia* is a genetic disorder where the neutrophil count falls every 14–21 days and is associated with an increased risk of infection. Certain chemicals, drugs and infections may produce an *immune neutropenia* through a direct toxic effect to the bone marrow or through an immune process. Bone marrow infiltration with carcinoma, cytotoxic chemotherapy, irradiation, hypersplenism and some autoimmune disorders can also cause neutropenia, some with an associated pancytopenia.

Management and care

The cause of neutropenia should be identified and, if possible, eliminated. Infections should be treated promptly with broad-spectrum antibiotics, as septicaemia is a serious and potentially fatal complication of neutropenia. Prophylactic antibiotics may have a role to play in some patients, as does the use of haemopoietic growth factors. In a small group of patients with immune neutropenia, splenectomy may be considered (Roberts et al 1999). Nursing care of the patient with neutropenia includes a careful assessment of the current infection status and the risk of infection (including the client's environment, personal hygiene and dietary infection risk) and client education and support in the management of risk, and in identifying the early warning signs of infection or sepsis. A more detailed discussion of these issues can be found in the section on management of patients with white cell disorders.

Leukaemia

Leukaemia is a heterogeneous group of malignant disorders characterized by the uncontrolled proliferation of immature haematopoietic cells. It is thought that these malignancies arise from a single, mutated, early progenitor or stem cell. The malignant cells are characterized by uncontrolled cell growth, arrested development and resistance to normal cell death, and they also lack the expected mature cell functions. The cells rapidly overwhelm the bone marrow, preventing the production of normal red cells, white cells and platelets; they eventually spill over into the peripheral blood and may invade other organs such as the spleen.

Classification

Classification is important because it has a bearing on disease course, treatment choice and outcomes. The classification of leukaemia is, in the first instance, according to the general course of the disease, and is termed either acute or chronic. In general, acute leukaemias involve the more immature cells (blasts) whereas chronic leukaemias tend to involve more mature cells. The next classification is according to the originating cell line, either myeloid or lymphoid. These broad categories can then be further subdivided into subtypes based on other morphological or cytogenetic characteristics. So, for example, AML M3 refers to (A) acute (M) myeloid (L) leukaemia and M3 describes the cell as having stopped at the promyelocytic stage of development. CML Ph+ refers to (C) chronic (M) myeloid (L) leukaemia that is positive for the Philadelphia chromosome, denoting a particular genetic translocation.

Incidence and aetiology

Leukaemia is one of the less common types of cancer. Although leukaemia occurs in all age groups, it has a higher incidence in the older age groups and, overall, there is a higher incidence in males. There also are geographical variations in the incidence of particular types of leukaemia; for example, chronic lymphocytic leukaemia is common in countries such as the USA, Canada and the UK but much less so in Japan, India or South America (Cartwright 1998).

Certain predisposing factors have been linked to the leukaemias. A particular genetic predisposition, such as in Down syndrome, Fanconi anaemia, Bloom's syndrome and ataxia telangiectasia, is associated with leukaemia. There are also slightly higher rates of leukaemia in certain families, which also points to the possibility of a genetic predisposition. Pre-existing bone marrow dysfunction, such as in aplastic anaemia or myelodysplasia, is also associated with leukaemia.

Environmental factors associated with leukaemia include ionizing radiation, chemicals such as benzene, exposure to agrochemicals and previous treatment with particular cytotoxic agents (Cartwright 1998). The relationship between ionizing radiation and leukaemia was initially demonstrated by the high incidence of leukaemia in survivors of the atomic bombs and, subsequently, in follow-up studies with workers on atomic test sites. Long-term low-dose exposure, such as in the early days of the development of X-ray technology, also demonstrates an increased rate of haematological malignances, including leukaemia. Treatment with cytotoxic chemotherapy, particularly alkylating agents, can lead to the subsequent development of leukaemia, termed secondary leukaemia. There is also a reported increase in the risk of secondary leukaemia in solid organ transplant recipients as well as bone marrow transplant recipients, particularly those who received total body irradiation.

Despite a continued search for possible infective agents, only one to date has been strongly associated with the development of leukaemia. The human T-lymphocytic virus (HTLV-I) has been demonstrated to induce a T-cell leukaemia in susceptible individuals. This virus, although uncommon in Europe, is a common infective agent in the Caribbean, where its relationship with leukaemia has been demonstrated. Although there is some indirect evidence that infection may be one possible factor in childhood leukaemia, no clear evidence has yet come to light.

Occupational exposure to benzene and agrochemicals has been associated with leukaemia. Although there are reports of other possible occupational links with haematological malignancy, these are always difficult to demonstrate clearly owing to the inherent difficulties of epidemiological studies. One other possible associated factor is cigarette smoking, which is also associated with a myriad of other chronic conditions and diseases.

In the majority of *de novo* cases of leukaemia, however, the answer to the question of 'Why me?' must remain unanswered. The development of a malignancy is a complex, multistep process involving factors in the person, in

Leukaemia
See chapter 4.1

the environment and at a cellular level. For the individual facing an unwelcome diagnosis, this may seem a rather unsatisfactory response to an important question. One of the roles of the healthcare worker is to help the client look forward and to adjust to their situation, while also trying to make sense of what has happened.

Acute leukaemia

Acute leukaemia may be either myeloid or lymphoblastic. Acute myeloid leukaemia (AML) is most commonly seen in adults, whereas acute lymhoblastic leukaemia (ALL) is predominantly, although not exclusively, a disease of childhood. Presenting features vary from general non-specific symptoms at diagnosis to the disease manifesting itself as an acute illness. The presenting problems are, in the main, associated with ineffective bone marrow function. With the expanding pool of leukaemic cells in the bone marrow, the production of normal red cells, white cells and platelets decreases rapidly, resulting in signs and symptoms of anaemia, neutropenia and thrombocytopenia. The client often complains of feeling more tired than usual and may be short of breath on exertion or at rest. They may have an infection, such as a sore throat or chest infection, that they are unable to rid themselves of. More seriously, the patient may present with an overt septicaemia and be acutely ill. Often there is evidence of increased bruising or the client may describe a history of nose-bleeds or abnormal gum bleeding. Women may complain of heavy menstrual loss. The more acute presentations of thrombocytopenia include retinal haemorrhage resulting in loss of vision, gastro-intestinal bleeding or cerebral haemorrhage. Symptoms associated with a high peripheral white cell count include blurred vision and speech, memory changes and a fluctuating level of consciousness.

Diagnosis is made from examination of a bone marrow aspirate and trephine. Cytochemistry, immunopheno-typing and cytogenetic tests permit identification of the leukaemia type, help to identify some important prognostic factors and aid in deciding the optimal treatment strategies. Other tests include baseline blood counts to determine the degree of anaemia and thrombocytopenia, a clotting screen to detect abnormal clotting, biochemical investigations to assess renal, cardiac and liver function, microbiological cultures, chest radiography and physical assessment. A lumbar puncture to assess any central nervous system (CNS) involvement will be performed if ALL is suspected because CNS involvement is a feature of this condition. Other tests will be requested according to clinical need.

Priority of care at the time of presentation includes supportive treatment in the form of appropriate blood product administration, antibiotic treatment if required, and appropriate venous access, often through the insertion of a central venous catheter. Prevention of infection and haemorrhage are two important goals of care. Any clotting abnormalities require prompt treatment. If the white cell count is raised and the patient is symptomatic leucapheresis, a procedure involving the selective removal of the white cells from the client's circulation, may be considered.

Rapid confirmation of diagnosis is imperative to allow for the prompt institution of treatment. As fertility is an important issue in the care of patients with acute leukaemia, it may be possible to consider sperm banking before starting chemotherapy. For women, collecting eggs is not currently possible at diagnosis because of the time factor and technical difficulties. Even for men, the option of sperm banking depends on their clinical status at the time of diagnosis and on the services available. However, every effort should be made to address this important need, if possible.

The initial aim of treatment for acute leukaemia is to induce a rapid remission of the disease. This requires the use of an intensive schedule of combination cytotoxic agents appropriate to the type of leukaemia. These combinations are different for AML and ALL. Other factors, such as the patient's age and some specific prognostic factors, may alter the regimen chosen. The aim of combination chemotherapy is to increase cell death by combining drugs with different modes of action or ones that work synergistically. Box 14.3 lists common cytotoxic drugs used in the treatment of acute myeloid leukaemia and examples of combination chemotherapy for AML.

After treatment the patient will develop profound bone marrow failure with neutropenia and be at high risk of developing life-threatening infections. Careful monitoring of the patient's condition is fundamental to effective clinical care. A prompt response to any sign of infection is important. Any pyrexia should be investigated and the appropriate blood cultures and microbiological specimens sent. Patients will be started immediately on broad-spectrum intravenous antibiotics. Most units have specific protocols that provide clinical guidance on antibiotic use in neutropenic patients. As the risk of infection-related morbidity and mortality is high in this population of patients, the systematic use of appropriate antibiotic therapy is a cornerstone of good practice. Infection control measures such as effective handwashing by all members of the clinical team, a clean environment, the systematic use of aseptic technique when managing the central venous catheter and during any invasive procedure, and ensuring the patient's personal hygiene are important elements in a strategy to minimize the infection risk for the patient. The provision of a low microbial diet and the use of prophylactic antibiotics and antifungal agents may also be used to protect neutropenic patients from infection. Finally, minimizing the microbial load of the patient's immediate environment through the use of single rooms, controlled air-delivery systems and limiting visitors may also be used as part of the infection control strategy.

Blood product support at this time will be required to manage the anaemia and thrombocytopenia that follows intensive chemotherapy. The patient's haemoglobin level

BOX 14.3 Some cytotoxic drugs commonly used in the treatment of acute myeloid leukaemia

Antimetabolites	Alkylating agents	Anthracycline antibiotics/ DNA binding agents	Mitotic inhibitors	Miscellaneous
Cytosine arabinoside (Ara-c, cytarabine)	Cyclophosphamide	Daunorubicin Doxorubicin	Vincristine Etoposide	Amsacrine
Tioguanine (thioguanine)		Idarubicin Mitoxantrone (mitozantrone)		

Sample induction chemotherapy for AML

ADE: Cytarabine (Ara-c)	MAE: Mitoxantrone (mitozantrone)	DAT: Daunorubicin		
Daunorubicin	Cytarabine (Ara-c)	Cytarabine (Ara-c)		
Etoposide (VP16)	Etoposide (VP16)	Tioguanine (thioguanine)		

Sample consolidation chemotherapy for AML

MACE: Amsacrine (amsa)	MiDAC: Mitoxantrone (mitozantrone)	ICE: Idarubicin		
Cytarabine (Ara-c)	Cytarabine (Ara-c)	Cytarabine		
Etoposide (VP16)		Etoposide (VP16)		

Source: Dearnaley et al (1995).

will be maintained with the use of packed red cells. Often patients require a blood transfusion every 3 days. The need for more frequent transfusions should alert the team to the possibility of internal bleeding. Platelet transfusions will be required every 2–3 days, sometimes more frequently if there is evidence of bleeding or infection. The safe management of transfusion is an important feature in the care of haematology patients. This important aspect of care is discussed in a subsequent section.

Nutritional and fluid support may also be required at this time. Mucositis and its associated pain, oral candida infection, nausea and vomiting, and anorexia may all prevent the patient from eating and drinking sufficiently. Nutritional deficiencies, weight loss and muscle loss are all frequent features of this rigorous treatment. Ensuring a fluid and nutritional intake that maintains renal function and meets the body's increased metabolic requirements may require intravenous hydration and total parenteral nutrition at this time. A nutritious diet with supplements is important for those who are still able to eat and drink. A multidisciplinary approach to nutrition, including the expert support of a dietician and regular nutritional assessments, will prove valuable in preventing excessive weight loss and nutritional deficiencies.

Minimizing the inevitable consequences of chemotherapy invariably proves a challenge for the clinical team. Nausea and vomiting, diarrhoea, mucositis, pain, anorexia, pyrexia will all require prompt assessment and treatment. Renal failure as well as cardiac and liver problems may complicate the clinical picture. The patient will need intensive support for up to 25–30 days. Once bone marrow function is restored, the risk of infection and bleeding decreases markedly and the patient generally feels better. Problems with other organs, such as the kidneys, may persist in particular individuals. Loss of appetite and weight loss may also prove to be long-standing problems for some patients.

Remission induction chemotherapy usually comprises one or two cycles of treatment. Remission is defined as a specific reduction in the number of leukaemic cells or the absence of detectable disease, rather than the complete absence of disease. For this reason, consolidation and intensification chemotherapy are given as a prolonged attack on the leukaemia cells that are known to be present, even though they may be undetectable. In the case of ALL, CNS therapy will be added to treatment, as in this disease the CNS provides a particular sanctuary site for malignant cells. Consolidation chemotherapy involves giving repeated courses of the same drugs at similar doses as were given to induce remission, whereas intensification involves giving higher doses or different drug combinations (Lachant 1995). The specific drugs used for consolidation or intensification cycles may vary to some extent, but the treatment-related problems remain the same.

After the appropriate cycles of consolidation–intensification chemotherapy, patients with ALL will start a maintenance programme of chemotherapy. Maintenance chemotherapy usually involves lower doses of drugs and is given on an outpatient basis (Lachant 1995). At this point, also, particular subgroups of patients will be considered for other treatment strategies such as allogeneic bone marrow transplantation or autologous stem cell transplantation.

It is important to remember that with each cycle of treatment the patient may have accumulating problems such as weight loss and anorexia. The body's ability to heal itself will be seriously tested. The patient's own personal and psychological resources will also have been greatly challenged. Loss of weight and hair loss may engender issues of altered body image. The treatment-induced fatigue and loss of physical strength may be difficult for patients, particularly for those who had previously led active lives. The possible loss of fertility may need to be addressed sensitively. Extended periods of hospitalization may often lead to a feeling of loss and isolation from family life, friends and work. There may be concerns over financial matters or loss of income, affecting both the patient and their family. Changes in family members' roles may require personal adjustment. Fear and anxiety is a natural response to the threat of a serious illness and treatment; effective personal coping strategies and an effective support system will be helpful for the client at this time.

A therapeutic relationship between the clinical team and the patient and their families is a key aspect of care. Clients need to feel free to raise their concerns and personal worries; therefore the development of trust and confidence between staff and client is vital. This element of trust needs to be in relation to the quality of clinical care offered and the personal and team approach to the client. The individual's response to illness, its meaning for them and the worries they may have all need to be acknowledged, respected and explored in a sustained effort by the clinical team to support the person at this critical time in their lives (see Case Study 14.2).

Case Study 14.2

Helen, a 26-year-old woman, attended her GP surgery complaining of a persistently sore throat and a productive cough following a bout of flu. On examination Helen appeared rather pale and slightly short of breath. A blood sample was sent to ascertain Helen's full blood count. That same day, the GP rang Helen at home, requesting that she and her husband come to the evening surgery for the results. The doctor confirmed that Helen was anaemic, with a haemoglobin level of 9.1 g/dL, but also mentioned a low platelet count (25×10^9/L) and high white cell count (30×10^9/L) that were suggestive of leukaemia.

Helen was referred to her local hospital for immediate admission. That evening Helen had a bone marrow aspiration and trephine performed to confirm the preliminary diagnosis, and a central venous catheter inserted. She was started on intravenous antibiotics to treat the chest infection and was given a 2-unit blood transfusion. The diagnosis of acute myeloid leukaemia was confirmed by the haematologist later that evening. Helen was told that treatment would have to start as soon as possible, probably the next day.

Initial treatment included a combination regimen of cytarabine, doxorubicin and etoposide that lasted for 8 days. Helen was placed in a single room and remained in protective isolation until her white cell count returned to 0.5×10^9/L – in Helen's case, this took 24 days. Her main problems during this induction cycle of chemotherapy were mucositis, which prevented her from eating, and weight loss (3 kg in total). She did have one episode of fever and remained on intravenous antibiotics throughout most of this initial admission. Once her bone marrow function had returned, Helen was allowed home for a few days. After a week at home, Helen returned for a second course of chemotherapy, identical to the first. Again, mucositis and weight loss were two important problems and again she required intravenous antibiotics.

Following recovery of her bone marrow function, Helen had a bone marrow biopsy to determine her remission status. After another week at home Helen returned to the good news that she was in complete remission. The third course of chemotherapy included mitozantrone, cytarabine and etoposide. This resulted in a prolonged stay in hospital for Helen as the return of her bone marrow function was delayed following this cycle of chemotherapy. By this time, Helen was becoming rather withdrawn and had lost a considerable amount of weight, so it was agreed that a longer stay at home with the aim of putting on weight and spending time with her family and friends would be beneficial.

Some 2 weeks later Helen returned feeling generally better in herself and ready to face her final course of chemotherapy. At this point the possibility of a bone marrow transplant was addressed with Helen and her husband, as Helen had a sister who was an identical match. After careful consideration of the risks and benefits, Helen opted not to have a transplant as she did not want to face permanent infertility at this time in her life. She described her sister's bone marrow as her insurance policy for the future in case of relapse. Her final course of chemotherapy went reasonably well, and Helen went home after 27 days in hospital. Helen is still in remission after 18 months and attends the outpatient clinic regularly for check-ups.

Chronic leukaemias

Chronic myeloid leukaemia (CML)

This is a haematological malignancy characterized by the overproduction of neutrophils and their precursors. It is thought to arise from a genetic change in a pluripotent stem cell. The vast majority of patients have a specific translocation between chromosome 9 and 22. This is termed the Philadelphia (Ph) chromosome. The cause of CML is unknown, although there is an association with ionizing radiation (Cartwright 1998). The median age for its development is 40 years, and men and women are affected equally.

The disease appears to have two or three distinct phases; most patients present in the first phase, a relatively stable and chronic phase. After a period of months or, often, years, the disease frequently progresses to an accelerated phase, where the signs and symptoms of increasing bone marrow failure are in evidence. The final phase is one of transformation to acute leukaemia.

Presenting symptoms vary and the disease is sometimes found on routine blood testing. The patient may complain of left hypochondrial pain and may give a history of weight loss and night sweats. The spleen is often enlarged and there may be associated anaemia, with its accompanying fatigue, exercise intolerance and shortness of breath. The patient may occasionally have signs of hyperviscosity from the high white cell count and the often accompanying raised platelet count. These include disturbed vision, headaches and, rarely, priapism. High uric acid levels may predispose the occasional individual to gout. The presenting clinical picture is often related to the stage at which the disease is discovered. A relatively normal spleen and no anaemia probably indicates early disease. As the disease advances, an increasing proportion of blast (early precursors) cells can be seen in the bone marrow and peripheral blood. There are often increased signs of bone marrow failure leading to anaemia and a deterioration in general health. The final stage of the disease usually presents as acute leukaemia. The prognosis at this stage is often poor.

The choice of treatment for CML depends on a number of factors including the age of the patient at diagnosis and the availability of a suitable human lymphocyte antigen (HLA)-matched donor for allogeneic transplant. Although volunteer unrelated donors may be considered, sibling donors are preferred as the outcome is much more favourable with a sibling transplant. Although transplantation is the treatment of choice in CML, only a minority of patients will have this as an option. Alternative treatment choices include hydroxyurea and interferon-α. These may be given singly or in combination and can extend the chronic phase of the disease by months or years. Both of these treatments have side-effects, and interferon-α in particular may not easily be tolerated by all patients. It is only after careful consideration of all of the patient-related factors that the most suitable treatment regimen can be selected. Patients in blast crisis can be treated with the combination cytotoxic regimens available for the treatment of acute leukaemia with the aim of inducing an often short-lived remission.

Chronic lymphocytic leukaemia is a B-cell malignancy and is considered a disease of the elderly; it is rare before the age of 50 years. It is also the most common type of leukaemia in Europe and North America. Its cause is unknown. Many cases are discovered following routine blood tests. Symptoms, if present, may include those related to anaemia, weight loss and night sweats. An enlarged spleen is common and the patient may complain of a feeling of fullness after a light meal. Some 10–20% of patients develop an immune haemolytic anaemia (Hamblin and Oscier 1998). There may be urinary symptoms from kidney or prostatic involvement. Enlarged lymph nodes are present and are useful for disease staging. The presence of an enlarged spleen, liver and anaemia are other staging markers (Mehta and Hoffbrand 2000). The disease may remain stable for a period of years or may progress to more aggressive disease. A major cause of death in patients with CLL is infection (Hamblin and Oscier 1998).

Treatment is not necessary for a proportion of patients. For those whose disease or symptoms require treatment, chlorambucil, an alkylating agent, is a drug of choice. Corticosteroids, usually prednisolone, may be given if there is an associated haemolytic anaemia. For more advanced disease fludarabine may be considered. Splenic irradiation may also be useful for some patients (Catovsky 1999). Combination chemotherapy is another possible approach for patients with progressive disease. Good quality of life is an important objective in patients with CLL. Supportive measures, such as the prompt treatment of infection and minimizing possible treatment-related side-effects, are therefore important.

Aplastic anaemia

Partial or complete failure of bone marrow activity is an anticipated result of the toxic action of certain drugs or chemicals such as cytotoxics, excessive exposure to radiation, or invasion of the bone marrow by malignant cells. However, in susceptible individuals, an idiosyncratic response to particular pharmacological agents (e.g. chloramphenicol, gold salts), industrial chemicals (e.g. benzene) or certain viral infections (e.g. viral hepatitis) are thought to be capable of inducing bone marrow failure (Young 1991). Others may have an inherited predisposition such as in Fanconi anaemia, where a progressive deterioration of bone marrow function may be observed in affected individuals. However, the majority cases of bone marrow failure are idiopathic and the cause remains unknown.

Aplastic anaemia is an uncommon disease, affecting all age groups with an approximately equal male to female ratio. There is a greater incidence of aplastic anaemia in the Far East; this has led to suggestions of possible environmental factors in some cases. It is generally thought to be a consequence of multiple underlying factors including a reduced or damaged stem cell population, a damaged marrow microenvironment, and a complex and poorly understood immune process, resulting in either a sudden or insidious reduction in bone marrow production and eventual pancytopenia.

Presenting clinical features will be commensurate with the degree of marrow failure present. Many patients will manifest signs and symptoms of anaemia, neutropenia and thrombocytopenia. Infection, including life-threatening bacterial infections, bleeding and general weakness and lethargy with minimal exercise tolerance are common presenting features. Diagnosis is one of exclusion and is made from examination of the patient's bone marrow, peripheral blood count and a careful history. It is important to rule out other possible causes of bone marrow failure, such as malignancy or an inherited disorder, as this would have a great bearing on the appropriate choice of treatment. Initial treatment includes supportive care in the form of red cell and platelet transfusions and prophylactic or therapeutic antibiotics until the diagnosis is confirmed. Subsequent choice of treatment will be dependent on the severity of the bone marrow failure, any predisposing factors such as drug-induced aplasia, and the presence of a matched sibling donor for possible transplantation. Other factors involved in the decision-making process include the age of the patient, their general state of health and any concomitant health problems.

The current treatment of choice for patients under 55 years with severe bone marrow failure is allogeneic stem cell transplantation with a suitable matched donor (Marsh 1997). Currently this is the only potentially curative treatment for aplastic anaemia. Immunosuppression with antilymphocyte globulin (ALG) or antithymocyte globulin (ATG) is an alternative treatment, offering overall success rates of about 50–70% (Mehta and Hoffbrand 2000). With immunosuppressive therapy, treatment success is often defined as transfusion independence rather than a return to a normally functioning bone marrow. Treatment with ALG or ATG may be supplemented by the administration of cytokines or ciclosporin. For some patients with non-severe aplastic anaemia, immunosuppression with ciclosporin alone or support with transfusions may also be options. Patients treated with immunosuppression may well relapse after months or years, and can subsequently be offered further immunosuppressive treatment. For those individuals where treatment fails, supportive care in the form of transfusions and measures to prevent infection can be offered. Skilled nursing care in the management of the side-effects and complications of the disease and treatments is vital to the success of therapy. A therapeutic environment where supportive care, information giving and education facilitate the development of effective coping skills for living with a chronic and life-threatening illness is also paramount. A more detailed discussion of some of the nursing care issues can be found later in the chapter.

Stem cell transplantation

Stem cell transplantation (SCT) has become an increasingly useful treatment for a range of haematological conditions. The main purpose of SCT is to eradicate the patient's own faulty stem cell population and replace it with healthy haemopoietic stem cells. These healthy stem cells can be from another person (*allogeneic transplant*) or they can be the patient's own cells, which have been previously collected and stored (*autologous transplant*). SCT can also be used to replace or manipulate an abnormal immune system, as in autoimmune disease or immunodeficiency syndromes, for example.

Autologous transplant

The term transplant in the context of autologous transplantation is commonly used but can be a little misleading, as the cells returned to patients are their own. Another term for this is stem cell rescue, which reflects an important aspect of autologous SCT: one main objective of autologous SCT is to repopulate the patient's marrow after high-dose chemotherapy and/or radiotherapy. The bone marrow is very sensitive to the effects of cytotoxic chemotherapy and radiotherapy, and this has been an important dose-limiting factor in their therapeutic use. By collecting and storing the patient's stem cells before treatment with chemotherapy and/or radiotherapy, these therapies can now be used at a much higher dose. The stem cells are then returned to the patient and these repopulate the bone marrow, effectively rescuing the patient from treatment-related bone marrow failure. This technique is commonly used in the treatment of haematological malignancies when a donor is not available, or in older patients where allogeneic transplant would pose too great a risk. It is now also being used as part of the treatment strategy for some solid cancers, such as high-risk breast cancer. It may also have a place in the treatment of autoimmune diseases; all these strategies are currently being evaluated for their effectiveness.

Allogeneic transplant

Allogeneic transplantation requires a donor whose own genetic make-up closely resembles that of the patient. This type of 'matching' relates to the human lymphocyte antigen (HLA) complex that allows the immune system to recognize self and non-self. It is important that the donor and recipient's HLA complex closely match so that the donor stem cells are accepted and then tolerated by the recipient's immune system. Successful matching most often involves siblings as they have the best chance of inheriting similar antigen combinations from their parents. A volunteer unrelated donor transplant from either national or international donor registries is possible, but the chances of finding a match is often small and the immune problems associated with this type of donor transplant make it a less favourable option. A third type of allogeneic transplant is from an identical twin and is referred to as a syngeneic transplant.

The transplant process

Stem cells can either be collected directly from the bone marrow using a general anaesthetic, or can be obtained from peripheral blood (PBSCs). For a bone marrow collection no specific preparation is required, whereas PBSCs have to be coaxed out of the bone marrow with the use of growth factors, chemotherapy or both. There are benefits and limitations with each method of collection so that the choice of method depends, in part, on the clinical circumstances. Broadly speaking, PBSC collection is now the preferred method for autologous transplantations and a bone marrow collection is still often the method used for allogeneic transplants. One important benefit of the PBSC method is that the recipient's bone marrow function is restored more quickly compared with a transplant procedure using a bone marrow harvest. However, the use of growth factors in healthy donors prior to a PBSC collection may pose as yet unknown risks to the donor (Gluckman 1998), whereas the risks of anaesthesia are now well established.

SCT involves three distinct stages. The first stage is referred to as *conditioning* and involves high-dose cytotoxic chemotherapy and may also include total body irradiation. The exact type of conditioning used will depend on many factors including the nature of the disease and the degree of immunosuppression needed for a successful transplant. Once conditioning is complete the transplant stem cells are re-infused into the patient; this process is not unlike a blood transfusion.

Bone marrow failure is a feature of the next stage of transplant. This may last anywhere from 14 to 25 days or longer, depending on the type of stem cells and the conditioning used. As mentioned above, autologous stem cells and those collected from a peripheral stem cell harvest tend to recover more speedily than those from a donor or those collected directly from the bone marrow. At this time the patient is very vulnerable to infection, bleeding and anaemia, and requires intensive support.

The final stage of transplant is again variable in length and involves the reconstitution of the patient's *immune system*. The patient remains susceptible to bacterial, viral and fungal infections and may still require support including antibiotics and transfusions at this time. For allogeneic transplant recipients, this final stage is generally longer than in autologous transplantation as suppression of the immune system is greater and longer lasting, to allow the graft to establish itself. At this time, some of the long-term complications of conditioning and transplantation may begin to manifest themselves.

The list of possible complications associated with stem cell transplantation is extensive. Many complications arise as a consequence of the high-dose chemotherapy and radiotherapy used, the bone marrow failure, the immune dysfunction and the metabolic problems related to the prophylactic and therapeutic treatments needed during the acute transplant phase. Allogeneic transplant recipients are also at risk of graft-versus-host disease and graft rejection, and often require extended immunosuppressive therapy. Other transplant-related complications include pulmonary, endocrine and neurological problems or may involve other organs such as the kidneys or liver. Endocrine problems often include premature menopause for women. Infertility in both men and women is often a very distressing but inevitable side-effect of the treatment.

Undergoing such an arduous procedure and coping and living with its complications and side-effects is a challenge for patients and their families. A degree of psychological distress and anxiety is an inevitable consequence of the stress of transplantation and the subsequent disruption to normal life. Healthcare workers involved in caring for these patients require many skills to be able to minimize the physiological and psychological effects of the procedure effectively. Knowledgeable nurses with the skills to encourage and support patients are vital to the success of transplantation. As transplantation involves a number of complex events and processes, and these cannot be discussed in detail in a brief overview, further reading has been suggested at the end of the chapter.

Lymphatic disorders

Infectious mononucleosis (glandular fever)

This is a benign infectious disease involving the lymphatic system and is seen most commonly in adolescents and young adults. The causative organism is the Epstein–Barr virus (EBV). The disease is not highly contagious but is transmitted by the oropharyngeal route, via saliva, often through kissing. It has an incubation period of 4–6 weeks (Shaffer 1996).

Clinical characteristics

Symptoms vary from one person to another and are often non-specific. Common complaints include sore throat, headache, neck stiffness, fatigue, anorexia and general malaise. The person has a fever, which may be intermittent, and there is usually enlargement and tenderness of the superficial lymph nodes (cervical, axillary and inguinal). The spleen is often enlarged and tender, and palpation may also reveal abdominal tenderness due to involvement of the mesenteric lymph nodes. An erythematous or maculopapular rash is developed by some individuals with glandular fever and occasionally the person is jaundiced.

Investigations

The total leucocyte count is raised and may range from 10 to 20×10^9/L. A differential count reveals an increase in lymphocytes and monocytes, and many of the lymphocytes are atypical. The number of granulocytes may be below normal. A mild to moderate anaemia may exist together with thrombocytopenia. Diagnosis is confirmed by a positive Paul–Bunnell test. Heterophile antibodies appear in the serum of patients with infectious mononucleosis: these antibodies cause the agglutination of sheep red blood cells, which is the basis of the Paul–Bunnell test. The Paul–Bunnell reaction does not become positive until the second week of infection because it depends on production of immunoglobulin M (IgM). A rapid slide test (the Monospot test) using horse red blood cells is easier to carry out and considered to be more specific.

Treatment and care

The disease usually runs a self-limited course of 2–4 weeks and is managed at home with symptomatic care. Goals for the person with infectious mononucleosis are to:

- obtain adequate rest until the temperature returns to normal

- obtain a satisfactory degree of relief from distressing symptoms

- avoid spread of the disease to others

- avoid secondary infections.

Paracetamol or co-proxamol may be prescribed to relieve the headache, fever and general body discomfort. Warm saline gargles may help to soothe a sore throat. Rest is advisable until the temperature returns to normal.

Convalescence may take some weeks and occasionally a relapse can occur. The prolonged fatigue experienced may result in the person feeling discouraged and depressed. Nurses can convey understanding and reassurance that these reactions are normal and that fatigue will resolve over time. It may be helpful to set realistic goals for the resumption of normal activities whilst stressing the importance of adequate rest. When the spleen is enlarged the individual should be advised to avoid contact sports because there is a danger that an abdominal injury could lead to rupture of the spleen.

Malignant lymphomas

This term is applied to a group of neoplastic diseases that primarily affect lymphoid tissue rather than bone marrow. They are characterized by painless, progressive enlargement of the lymph nodes and the spleen. In some conditions the proliferating cells invade extralymphatic tissues and organs. This group of diseases is divided into Hodgkin's disease (HD), which is the most common form of lymphoma, and non-Hodgkin's lymphomas (NHL) (Souhami and Tobias 1995).

Hodgkin's disease

Hodgkin's disease is a disease of unknown aetiology. Although there is some evidence of a viral connection,

with traces of Epstein–Barr virus being detected in 30–50% of cases, it is not likely to be the sole cause. Hodgkin's disease may develop at any age but incidence peaks between the age of 20–30 years and after 50 years of age. There is a higher incidence of the disorder in males. The 5-year survival rate has improved dramatically, from only 20% in the 1960s, and is currently approaching 90%. This is mainly due to the introduction of interdisciplinary care and advances in chemotherapy and radiotherapy techniques.

Hodgkin's disease is classified histologically into four subtypes. This is known as the Rye classification:

1. lymphocytic predominant

2. nodular sclerosing

3. mixed cellularity

4. lymphocyte depleted.

Large atypical cells known as Reed–Sternberg cells seen in the affected lymph nodes are characteristic of Hodgkin's disease and are present in different numbers in the various subtypes. The lymphocyte-predominant form of the disease tends to be associated with a more favourable prognosis than the other subtypes.

Clinical characteristics

The disease often has an insidious onset and most patients present with a painless enlargement of one group of lymph nodes. In two-thirds of patients it is the cervical nodes that enlarge. The disease spreads progressively to other lymphoid and non-lymphoid tissue throughout the body, producing a variety of symptoms. The enlarging nodes may cause pressure on nerves, resulting in pain, or may impose on neighbouring organs causing dysfunction. Enlarged axillary and inguinal nodes frequently interfere with venous and lymphatic drainage, leading to oedema in the arms or legs. Enlarged mediastinal nodes may cause a distressing cough, dyspnoea or difficulty swallowing (dysphagia). The spleen becomes enlarged causing abdominal discomfort.

Constitutional problems do not usually present until the later stages. The patient gradually develops fatigue, weakness, fever, anorexia, loss of weight and pruritus. Drenching night sweats and alcohol-induced pain are sometimes reported.

Diagnosis is made by histological examination of an affected lymph node and observation of the Reed–Sternberg cell.

Non-Hodgkin's lymphomas

Non-Hodgkin's lymphomas (NHLs) are proliferative disorders primarily of B and T lymphocytes, with about 80% being of B-cell origin. The NHLs usually originate in the peripheral lymphoid tissues and are often widespread at diagnosis. They are less predictable in terms of pattern of spread than Hodgkin's disease and have a very variable prognosis. Some of the NHLs are relatively benign, whereas others are aggressive and rapidly fatal. The diverse nature of these disorders makes their classification very complex and various classification systems exist.

Although the cause is unknown, NHLs are associated with a variety of factors, including damage to the immune system caused by radiation, immunosuppresive drugs and environmental chemical hazards. Viral infections are also believed to contribute to the complex aetiological process and there is an increased incidence of NHL in individuals with AIDS. As a group, NHLs are the commonest form of haematological malignancy, with an incidence of around 1 in 10 000. Although forms of NHL affect all ages, the incidence increases with increasing age and men tend to be affected more often than women.

Clinical characteristics

Painless enlargement of peripheral lymph nodes may be the first indication of a problem, although generalized disease is not uncommon. Sometimes large masses are detected in the chest and abdomen, and the gastrointestinal tract is the most commonly involved extranodal site after the bone marrow because it contains a lot of lymphoid tissue. Many other tissues may be involved including tonsils, bone, skin, testicles, central nervous system, liver and spleen, giving rise to a wide variety of symptoms, including respiratory difficulty, superior vena cava obstruction, abdominal swelling and ascites, lower limb oedema and intestinal obstruction. Recurrent fever, night sweats, weight loss and fatigue are other general symptoms that may occur. Diagnosis is confirmed by histological examination of an excised lymph node or tumour biopsy.

Investigation and staging of malignant lymphomas

When a diagnosis of Hodgkin's disease or NHL has been confirmed, a series of investigations is organized to determine the extent of the disease. These include: a full blood count, bone marrow aspiration and biopsy, blood chemistry, liver function tests, chest radiography and immunoglobulin estimations. Computed tomography, magnetic resonance imaging, lymphangiography (occasionally), isotope scans, ultrasonography and lumbar puncture may also be indicated. For the person with Hodgkin's disease, accurate staging is crucial in determining the best treatment option. Surgical assessment with a staging laparotomy, liver biopsy and splenectomy used to be routine, but advances in radiological techniques have virtually eliminated need for such surgery with all its inherent risks.

Malignant lymphomas are staged according to the spread of the disease using the Ann Arbor classification, revised in 1989 to take account of specific nodal involvement in stage III and the importance of tumour bulk as a prognostic indicator (Fig. 14.9). NHLs are also classified according to histological appearance and immunological tests into different subtypes using the Revised European American Lymphoma (REAL) system. Knowledge of the particular histological subtype of lymphoma assists the doctors in making treatment decisions based on whether the tumour is indolent or aggressive, or likely to disseminate in the CNS, and is of greater clinical importance than the stage of the disease.

Treatment and nursing care

Treatment may consist of radiation therapy, chemotherapy or a combination of both. Care is aimed at helping the person with a malignant lymphoma to understand the disease and the side-effects of treatment and to cope with both the physical and psychological sequalae of diagnosis and treatment.

Treatment of Hodgkin's disease

Radiotherapy

Radiotherapy is used to treat early-stage disease, either alone or in combination with chemotherapy. Involved nodes and those in adjacent areas are irradiated in very early cases. When treating all lymph node groups above the diaphragm an extended 'mantle' field is irradiated. The equivalent field used to treat lymph nodes below the diaphragm is known as an 'inverted Y' field (see Fig. 14.10). A combination of the two given 3–4 weeks apart may be used for stage III disease and involves total nodal irradiation. Localized radiotherapy is also used to treat bulky or painful tumour masses in patients with advanced disease who are receiving chemotherapy as the primary treatment. Side-effects of the radiotherapy vary according to the field of treatment and all patients need information and opportunities to discuss treatment, potential side-effects and how these may be minimized.

A person having mantle irradiation may experience a dry mouth, altered taste, dysphagia, vocal changes, skin soreness and hair loss in the treatment area. These effects are temporary and usually completely reversible. A person having inverted Y irradiation is likely to experience gastrointestinal disturbances, colic, flatulence and diarrhoea, and will need dietary advice to control these problems. Young women who wish to remain fertile can be offered oophoropexy (repositioning of the ovaries) via laparoscopy to allow the ovaries to be shielded during treatment. Men normally have their testes shielded to protect testicular function. Blood counts and haemoglobin concentrations are determined frequently as bone marrow depression may occur. The general effects of radiotherapy are discussed in Chapter 11.

Chemotherapy

Chemotherapy with or without radiotherapy is used to treat stage III or IV disease, and anyone with adverse prognostic factors such as weight loss greater than 10% in 6 months, fever and night sweats (referred to as

Figure 14.9   Staging of malignant lymphomas: Ann Arbor classification. Each stage is further subdivided according to the absence (A) or presence (B) of any of the following symptoms: weight loss greater than 10% of bodyweight in 6 months; fever greater than 38°C; night sweats. Suffix E indicates localized extranodal involvement in stages I, II and III. Suffix S indicates involvement of the spleen in stage III.

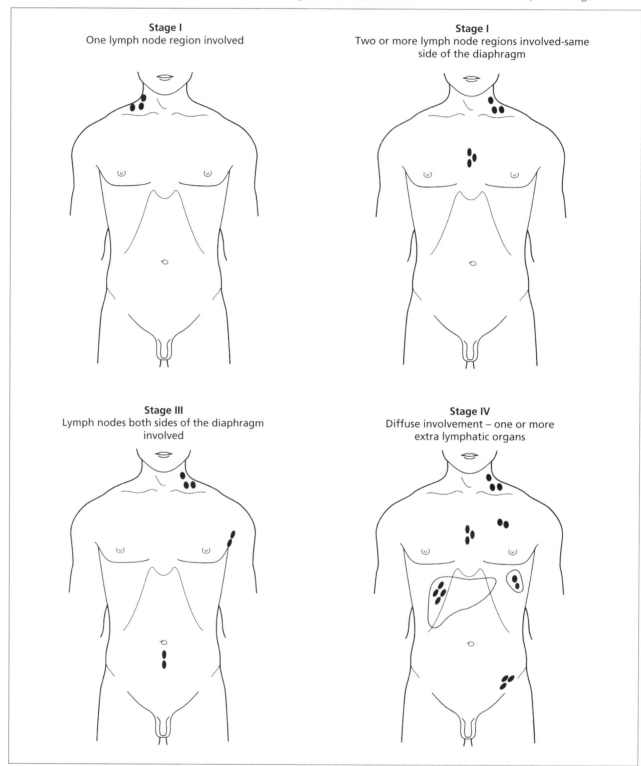

B symptoms), multiple sites and/or bulky disease. A variety of cytotoxic drugs is used, including chlormethine (mustine), vincristine, vinblastine, prednisolone, procarbazine, cyclophosphamide, chlorambucil, dacarbazine and bleomycin. These are usually given in combinations such as MOPP (chlormethine (mustine), vincristine, procarbazine and prednisolone) or ABVD (Adriamycin (doxorubicin), bleomycin, vinblastine, dacarbazine) given at 4-week intervals for up to 6 cycles. Some combinations (those containing alkylating agents) are more

Figure 14.10 Mantle and inverted-Y radiotherapy fields for Hodgkin's disease. Shaded areas are irradiated with 35–40 Gy given over 4–5 weeks.

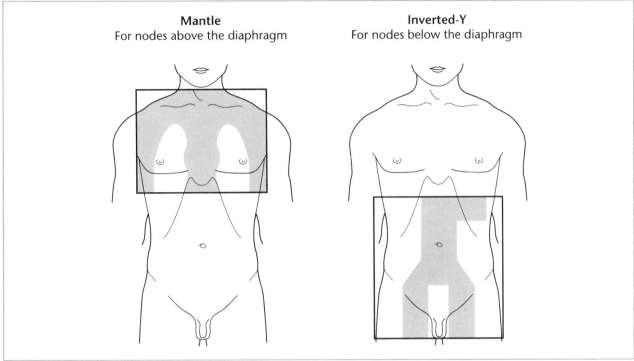

likely than others to cause infertility, which is an important consideration for many patients when selecting a treatment plan. They are also associated with an increased risk of developing a secondary malignancy at some later date. Six to eight cycles of chemotherapy are normally administered. See Case Study 14.3.

Chemotherapy is also used for patients whose disease relapses, and developments in the use of growth factors and stem cell rescue have offered opportunities for administering high doses of chemotherapy to this group and to younger patients with poor prognostic factors as primary treatment.

Case Study 14.3

Paul is 26 years of age. He has been married to Jane for 4 years and they have no children. Paul works in the computer department of a large bank. Two years ago he noticed a swollen gland on the right of his neck. His general practitioner treated this as an infected lymph gland for several weeks before referring Paul for a biopsy, which revealed that he had Hodgkin's disease. He was diagnosed as having stage Ia disease and a course of local radiotherapy was given to the neck and axillary area.

As the course of radiotherapy progressed, Paul started to complain of low back pain which got progressively worse. Shooting leg pains inhibited walking and the pain woke him at night. Various analgesics were prescribed but failed to control the pain adequately. Paul was reassured that the pain was unrelated to the Hodgkin's disease because investigations over several months failed to reveal a cause for the pain. Eventually Paul alerted medical staff to the fact that his back pain became much worse after drinking beer. A MRI scan was then performed and a shadow was detected on the lumbar vertebrae. Biopsy of the vertebra confirmed Hodgkin's disease and a bone marrow biopsy revealed extensive infiltration of the marrow.

At this point chemotherapy was planned and an opportunity to discuss sperm banking was offered. Paul was advised that only healthy sperm could be preserved successfully. As his disease was widespread and involved the bone marrow, it was felt that the quality of his sperm would be too poor to preserve and Paul and his wife decided not to proceed with sperm banking.

Paul then commenced 8 months of chemotherapy on a monthly alternating schedule of LOPP (chlorambucil, vincristine, procarbazine and prednisolone) and EVAP (etoposide, vinblastine, Adriamycin (doxorubicin) and prednisolone) chemotherapy. The first course of treatment was accompanied by severe nausea and vomiting but in subsequent treatments this was controlled with ondansetron. Although Paul was able to have his chemotherapy as a day patient, he experienced severe neutropenia and thrombocytopenia between courses of treatment and had to be admitted between cycles for intravenous antibiotics. Deep mouth ulcers causing severe facial swelling, pain and an inability to eat were the side-effects of treatment that Paul identifies as causing him the most distress. Eventually Paul had his wisdom teeth removed as it was believed that these were the source of the infection. Paul also recalls the repeated venepunctures by different members of staff as being the 'ultimate torture for someone with a bit of a needle phobia'.

After completion of the chemotherapy Paul returned to work and has been promoted. His response to treatment has been followed by 3-monthly bone marrow biopsies in outpatients, and these have remained clear to date.

Treatment for non-Hodgkin's lymphoma

The treatment chosen depends on the person's medical history and the classification and characteristics of the disease. Radiation therapy and chemotherapy are used singly or in combination. For low-grade tumours, radiotherapy alone or single-agent chemotherapy may be adequate treatment. For persons with intermediate-grade disease, combination chemotherapy with or without local radiotherapy is used to produce remission rates of up to 75% and a significant improvement in survival rates. Aggressive high-grade NHLs are managed with intensive combination chemotherapy.

A typical chemotherapy combination used is called CHOP, which is a combination of cyclophosphamide, Adriamycin (doxorubicin), vincristine and prednisolone. Response is often rapid but there is a high relapse rate. Intrathecal methotrexate may be given to prevent CNS relapse. High-dose chemotherapy and autologous bone marrow or peripheral stem cell transplantation may be recommended for patients who relapse. The role of interferon-α and other biological response-modifying agents are also being evaluated in the management of NHL.

Nursing intervention

The potential patient problems, goals and nursing interventions for the patient with a malignant lymphoma are similar to those for patients with leukaemia. Following the investigational procedures, initial therapy aimed at achieving remission may be given as an inpatient or on an outpatient basis depending on the drugs and doses used. During this period the patient will need careful surveillance and may need supportive measures such as blood transfusion and intravenous antibiotics and symptomatic care, for example analgesia for pain relief. Following remission the patient can usually return to a normal lifestyle.

Nurses should be closely involved with the patient and family members in discussions about treatment plans, care, and prevention of side-effects (especially infection). The need for rest, information about medication and follow-up are important, as is support in coping with the therapy and its side-effects such as fatigue and nausea.

Risks of future infertility should be explained. Opportunities for sperm banking exist and it may soon be possible to freeze and store eggs or ovarian tissue for future use (Donnez and Bassil 1998). Women treated with chemotherapy are less likely to become sterile than men, but periods usually become irregular or stop during chemotherapy. The re-establishment of menstruation after chemotherapy tends to be age related. Contraceptive advice therefore needs to be available and women who experience an early menopause may need hormone replacement therapy to control their symptoms.

With much treatment being given to outpatients, it is essential that patients have an out-of-hours contact number should problems arise at home and that details of most recent blood counts are easily available. Information for patients is available from a number of sources including The Hodgkin's Disease Association, Leukaemia Research Fund, Cancer BACUP and the Royal Marsden Hospital, and may be accessed via telephone helpline, information booklets or the internet.

Multiple myeloma

Multiple myeloma is a malignant disease characterized by a proliferation of abnormal plasma cells in the bone marrow. Plasma cells develop from B lymphocytes after they have been stimulated by an antigen, and they secrete antigen-specific immunoglobulins. These plasma cells exist in lymphoid and connective tissue throughout the body. In multiple myeloma a malignant clone (a group of identical cells derived from a single cell) of plasma cells produces one of the immunoglobulins in excess and in a form that is not capable of maintaining normal humoral immunity. The abnormal protein produced is known as paraprotein and may be found in the plasma and urine. It is a malignancy that accounts for about 1% of all malignant disease but remains an incurable condition affecting mainly those in late middle to old age.

Clinical characteristics

The disease tends to have an insidious onset, with early symptoms being pain and general malaise. Multiple, diffuse areas of bone destruction develop; these areas are seen as well circumscribed or 'punched out' lytic bone lesions on radiography and typically affect the skull, ribs and axial skeleton. The breakdown in bone structure frequently results in pathological fractures, especially in weight-bearing bones such as the vertebrae. Changes in posture and stature may be evident. The patient often experiences pain in the area of the bone lesions, which worsens with movement, jarring and pressure. As the disease progresses, the patient experiences more and more pain and may become increasingly incapacitated. The vertebrae are a common site of involvement and pressure on the nerve roots by the tumours and/or collapsing vertebrae causes severe back and/or lower limb pain. In extreme cases this may progress to spinal cord compression and, if treatment is delayed, interruption of nerve impulses may result in paraplegia.

The excessive production of abnormal paraprotein occurs at the expense of normal immunoglobulin synthesis. This reduction in the synthesis of normal antibodies predisposes the patient to infections, which are usually respiratory in origin, although bladder infections and skin lesions are not uncommon. Abnormal quantities of immunoglobulins in the blood occasionally cause a hyperviscosity syndrome which may result in bleeding problems, visual disturbance, neurological problems and heart failure.

As the bone marrow becomes crowded with plasma cells, red cell production falls and the person with multiple myeloma is frequently anaemic. In advanced disease white blood cell and platelet production are also reduced, further predisposing the individual to infection and a bleeding tendency.

Breakdown of bone tissue gives rise to the release of calcium, and hypercalcaemia (normal calcium level 2.33–2.6 mmol/L) develops in about 30% of patients. Excretion of the increased serum calcium by the kidneys entails an increased loss of water. If the fluid intake is not correspondingly increased, the patient becomes dehydrated, the serum calcium is retained and urinary output falls. Nausea, thirst, loss of appetite, cardiac dysrhythmias, constipation, and disorientation and confusion may all be symptoms of hypercalcaemia.

Urinalysis may record proteinuria, and electrophoresis of urine may demonstrate the presence of an abnormal protein known as Bence Jones protein, which is excreted by the kidneys. In high concentration this protein may be precipitated in the renal tubules, forming casts that damage the tubules and may cause renal insufficiency. A combination of factors such as proteinuria, hypercalcaemia and raised serum urate caused by rapid breakdown of cells contributes to the high incidence of renal impairment with this condition.

Investigations

These include blood tests, which may reveal an increased erythrocyte sedimentation rate, erythrocyte, leucocyte and platelet counts below normal, and raised serum calcium and urea levels. Examination of a specimen of bone marrow shows the presence of large numbers of plasma cells, often with abnormal forms. Serum electrophoresis and urine electrophoresis demonstrate the presence of an abnormal paraprotein in the serum, urine or both.

Treatment

Care of the patient with malignant myeloma involves the administration of chemotherapy, radiotherapy and supportive care to relieve symptoms. Often the person with multiple myeloma remains stable and symptom free for several years, but overall the prognosis of patients with this malignancy remains poor.

Palliative chemotherapy is given when the patient is symptomatic or has progressive disease, but is stopped when the patient's condition has improved or stabilized. Alkylating agents such as melphalan or cyclophosphamide are given in combination with prednisolone. High-dose chemotherapy using melphalan, allogenic or autologous bone marrow transplantation with peripheral stem cell support are used to prolong remissions. Combination chemotherapy is also sometimes used and interferon-α may be given as a second-line treatment. The toxicity of all these treatments has to be monitored carefully, especially the bone marrow depression they induce. Unfortunately current treatments do not offer a clear survival benefit and options must be considered carefully in terms of the potential benefits and inevitable side-effects of intensive treatment. Supportive care is crucial. Allopurinol may be prescribed to decrease uric acid production and prevent impaired renal function. Patients with hypercalcaemia are hydrated with intravenous fluids and given a diuretic and steroids to reduce serum calcium levels. Administration of a bisphosphonate drug such as pamidronate is an effective way of both reducing hypercalcaemia and managing bone pain. Analgesics are likely to be needed to control the pain of bone lesions until chemotherapy or radiotherapy produces a response.

Radiotherapy is very useful in the treatment of bony deposits as it alleviates pain and reduces the likelihood of pathological fractures or spinal cord compression. Multiple bone lesions may be treated effectively with hemi-body irradiation. Plasmapheresis is used to treat hyperviscosity syndrome. This involves the removal of plasma containing the paraproteins and replacement with plasma protein fraction. Surgery may be required to treat pathological fractures. Blood transfusion and platelets may be needed to manage anaemia and thrombocytopenia.

Nursing care

The person with multiple myeloma should be assessed frequently as significant changes can occur in a short space of time (e.g. vertebral collapse leading to spinal cord compression). Posture, the degree and difficulty of movement, and amount of incapacity and pain are evaluated. Laboratory data relating to blood counts and blood chemistry need to be evaluated to indicate whether the patient's condition is improving or worsening. For example, rising serum calcium levels or increasing uraemia may indicate the need for hydration and detailed fluid balance recording.

Specific goals for the patient with multiple myeloma include:

- achieving adequate pain control
- maintaining mobility to prevent further demineralization of bone

- preventing injury related to pathological fractures and/or vertebral collapse (any numbness or increasing loss of sensation; weakness and loss of movement; urine retention and constipation; and back pain of increasing severity should be reported urgently to the doctor).

Involvement of a multidisciplinary palliative care team is vital at an early stage to ensure good symptom control, preserve independence and provide ongoing emotional support for the individual with a myeloma.

Nursing management of the person with a leucocyte or lymphatic disorder

White blood cells (WBCs) or leucocytes are composed of populations of granulocytes (neutrophils, eosinophils and basophils), lymphocytes (T and B cells) and monocytes. Their primary function is the protection of the body against foreign invasion. When there is either a quantitative or qualitative (i.e. numerical or functional) decrease in leucocytes, the body's natural defences are impaired, the person becomes immunocompromised and is susceptible to infection from bacteria, fungi or viruses. Bacterial infections are often caused by the spread of commensal bacteria to a new and previously sterile site; for example, intestinal flora may enter the bloodstream. Infection may arise from either Gram-positive or Gram-negative bac-teria and quickly develop into sepsis; in the immuno-compromised individual life-threatening sepsis is a common problem. Virus infections are often a result of reactivation of a latent organism but may also be a new infection. Fungi such as candida or aspergillus can be a major threat to an immunocompromised patient. Candida is frequently found in small numbers in healthy individuals; simple colonization can quickly turn into a life-threatening systemic infection in the immunocompromised person. Aspergillus is a common airborne spore that can invade the lungs of a susceptible individual, with serious consequences.

Susceptibility to particular infections is related both to the degree of immunosuppression and to the predominant type of white cell dysfunction. Frequently, however, immunosuppression is complicated by a variety of other factors such as the nature of the disease, treatment, overall bone marrow function, reduced mucosal barriers (as with the use of central venous catheters) and the person's overall state of health.

Assessment

Systematic and continuous assessment of the person with a white cell disorder is important during the acute phases of illness and treatment. Changes in health status that may be indicative of infection need to be identified promptly, as infection may rapidly become generalized and life threatening.

Health history

During the initial assessment it is important to establish the possible factors that may have contributed to the person's current situation. Particularly in circumstances where the cause of the white cell disorder is unknown and malignancy is not suspected, previous or recent exposure to chemicals, radiation, toxins or drugs may cast some light on the possible causes of the disorder. The previous medical history may also provide some clues to the origin of the problem.

Specific questions aimed at identifying possible signs of infection may provide useful assessment information. These may include the presence or absence of:

- redness, swelling, warmth, abnormal discharge
- fever, chills, shivering, unexplained sweating
- general malaise or weakness
- sore mouth, throat, eyes or ears
- skin lesions or rashes
- pain and discomfort in the abdomen, joints, rectal or perineal areas
- changes in the character or colour of stools, diarrhoea
- nausea or vomiting.

Another major component of the health history is identification of the person's and their family's response to the illness, diagnosis and treatment. This is particularly relevant when the diagnosis may be malignancy or another life-threatening illness such as bone marrow failure. Anxiety and fear are common reactions, as may be denial and anger. In many instances, the treatment regimens as well as the disease process itself places the patient at risk of infection. The infections and their debilitating side-effects are often very distressing to patients and their families and, even if expected, may engender fear and anxiety. It is not surprising that the emotional responses of the patient and the family are likely to fluctuate as the person's clinical situation and health status alter.

Physical assessments

1. Baseline observations of the person's blood pressure, pulse, temperature and respirations are taken.

2. Skin and all body sites with high potential for infection are examined. These include the skinfold areas (buttocks, axillae, perineum, breasts), insertion sites of intravenous cannulae or central venous catheters, and wound sites for signs of redness, warmth, swelling or discharge.

3. The mouth is inspected for candida infection or ulceration. Dental hygiene is assessed.

4. The person's respiratory status is assessed. The presence and nature of any cough and sputum is noted as well as any dyspnoea, pain or discomfort or alteration in breathing pattern.

5. Patterns of bowel elimination and the colour and consistency of stools are noted. Any history or presence of diarrhoea is established.

6. Urine is examined for any signs of infection such as cloudiness or odour. Any report of frequency or dysuria is noted.

7. The person's state of hydration is assessed and fluid intake and output are monitored.

Tests

The person's white cell count and differential are monitored regularly. Throat, wound, perineal or other swabs are sent for microbiological culture and sensitivity, as required. Urine, stool or sputum samples are also sent for culture and sensitivity testing, as required. Blood cultures are also sent, to be cultured for an infective agent, if the person has a raised temperature. Some may be sent to establish a baseline; subsequent samples may then be sent if infection is suspected.

Patient problems

A key health problem is the potential risk of local or systemic infection due to immunosuppression or bone marrow failure. Other problems may include:

- risk of bleeding from thrombocytopenia in the presence of bone marrow failure

- fatigue in the presence of infection or bone marrow failure-associated anaemia

- anxiety related to the diagnosis, treatment and potential outcomes; lack of knowledge of the disease process and treatment; fear of the unknown; loss of control over life events and uncertainty over the future

- pain due to the disease process, infection (e.g. oral candida) and treatment (e.g. stomatitis)

- nutritional deficiencies, weight loss and inadequate fluid intake from a multitude of factors including treatment side-effects, nausea, pain, infection, diarrhoea, anorexia and others

- body image issues associated with treatment side-effects such as hair loss, weight loss, long-term central venous catheters, pallor, loss of muscle mass

- lack of effective coping strategies related to altered roles and relationships, prolonged treatment and hospitalization, body image and loss of control.

In addition, treatment-related toxicity may frequently generate a range of specific problems.

Nursing interventions

Prevention of infection

Environment

The decision to isolate the person with a white cell disorder depends on the level of risk assessed, the facilities available, the anticipated length of isolation required, the anticipated degree and length of neutropenia, and other factors such as the potential risk presented by other patients. In general terms, however, scrupulous cleaning, staff education and supervision, and the removal of items likely to introduce infection into the client's immediate environment (e.g. flowers) will help to reduce the risk of **infection**.

While in hospital, the person who is severely neutropenic (a neutrophil count of 0.5×10^9/L or less) is often nursed in a single room or, if facilities are available, in a room designed with positive air pressure to facilitate the provision of a clean environment. Again, it is assessment of the client's associated risk factors (e.g. the use of intensive chemotherapy, radiation, immunosuppressive drug therapy, bone marrow transplantation, the overall degree of bone marrow failure and the client's general state of health) that will ensure the risk is minimized. Protective isolation can then be used effectively for those patients who are at high risk of infection while not necessarily restricting those at lower risk. An assessment process is also useful when facilities are limited. In this environment, limiting the number of individuals in the room at any one time, maintaining equipment and supplies for the client's sole use, and maintaining a high standard of cleaning services are other important measures.

Personal hygiene

An important nursing responsibility involves the promotion of meticulous personal hygiene in order to reduce the potential for infection. The person is encouraged to shower daily, establish an oral hygiene routine and practice good perineal care. Particular attention is given to the perineum, groin, axillae and skinfolds when showering or bathing. The person is taught to note any redness, tenderness, swelling, unusual skin lesions or discharge and report these to the clinical team. Antiperspirants are avoided as they can lead to blockage of the sweat glands and subsequent infection. Men should be advised to use an electric razor to decrease the potential for causing breaks in the skin while shaving. Women are also advised to take precautions if wishing to shave areas such as the legs.

Oral hygiene

Effective oral care is central to the prevention of infection, the maintenance of nutritional status and patient comfort and well-being. Treatment for haematological malignancies often causes significant destruction of the oral mucosa, may induce a severe reduction in salivary secretion and increase the risk of infection. Infection originating in the mouth can easily lead to a systemic

Infection
See chapter 6.1

infection with its associated risks. Appropriate oral care is, therefore, an important part of health-promoting care. Regular and consistent assessment of oral status with an appropriate tool can provide useful baseline data, monitor the response to nursing interventions and help to identify new problems as they arise. Assessment may include both the physical assessment of the status of the oral cavity and a functional assessment of the client's ability to swallow, speak, eat and drink. A pain assessment may also be useful when damage to the oral cavity is a possibility.

The prevention of trauma to the oral mucosa is necessary in the prevention of infection. Dentures should be checked to ensure that they fit properly and ill-fitting dentures should not be worn. Dentures should regularly be cleaned thoroughly and, if prophylactic mouthwashes or suspensions are prescribed, the dentures should be removed before using the treatment. Oral hygiene should be practised regularly using a soft toothbrush, taking care to avoid gum trauma or bleeding. If the mouth is painful, soft swabs can be used in place of the toothbrush. Mouthwashes can be used to remove debris or thick mucus. Dental floss should be avoided when the white cell count or platelet counts are low or when there is damage to the mucosa. A dental referral may be required if the patient has not been having regular checks or there is evidence of dental caries or gum disease. This is often required before intensive treatments that predispose the patient to mucositis and opportunistic infections. The person should also be warned that any dental treatment may need antibiotic cover and that this should be discussed with their doctor.

Bowel care

As infections originating from the intestinal tract are common in neutropenia, it is important that the patient understands the importance of avoiding constipation and rectal straining that may damage the rectal mucosa and provide entry for organisms found in the gastrointestinal tract. Maintenance of regular bowel habits is promoted and a bowel routine using stool softening or other mild non-irritating laxatives can be established and implemented with each patient when needed. Careful assessment of regular patterns and risk factors, such as the use of opioid analgesia, can encourage the implementation of preventive measures. Suppositories, enemas and rectal tubes should not be used as they may cause damage to the mucosa. If constipation or diarrhoea is a problem, the person's diet and fluids are reviewed accordingly. Women should also be advised to wipe from front to back when performing perineal cleansing after each bowel motion to reduce the risk of introducing infection. Careful handwashing is also encouraged. Abnormal pain, tenderness, discharge or itching should be promptly reported to the healthcare team.

Food and fluids

The patient may need support and encouragement to maintain a nutritionally balanced diet containing sufficient calories, protein and vitamins to meet physiological needs. The person at risk of infection may need to follow a low pathogen diet as it is recognized that food can be a major source of pathogenic bacteria. At a minimum, they may be advised to follow Ministry of Agiculture, Fisheries and Food guidelines (MAFF 1996) and to avoid high-risk foods such as soft ripened cheeses, lightly cooked eggs and pâtés as well as Department of Health advice to avoid unpasteurized milk and milk products, ice cream, ripened and blue cheeses, and foodstuffs containing raw egg, raw fish and meat products, and other high-risk foods such as salads. Soft fruits and bananas may also need to be avoided. Other diets may recommend cooked food only and, for those in sterile environments, food may even be irradiated before eating (Buschel and Whedon 1995). It is recommended that water should be boiled (Bouchier 1998). Ice cubes can be a source of bacteria, so are not recommended for use by at-risk patients.

A range of diets with a variety of different recommendations has been developed over the years by teams with the primary responsibility of providing care for immuno-compromised patients, and this continues to be a source of ambiguity in terms of best practice. However, it is important to note that, as in other aspects of care, a range of factors can affect the overall infection risk from food. For example, the individual who is neutropenic but living at home will not have the same level of risk as a client taking prophylactic antibiotics to sterilize the gastro-intestinal tract or the bone marrow transplant recipient. Assessment and effective teamwork, including the dietician and the infection control team as well as the nursing and medical team caring for the person, can help to overcome some of these inevitable ambiguities. Nevertheless, a more consistent research-based approach to this aspect of care would be welcome.

Patient and family teaching

The person with a white cell disorder often wishes to be kept informed of their blood counts and needs to be taught the normal ranges for white cell and neutrophil counts and the significance of variations from normal. An understanding of the functions of white cells and the causes for a decrease in counts can also help the patient to understand the significance of changes. Inclusion of the patient's family in these discussions, if appropriate, is important.

Meticulous handwashing is an essential infection control measure for staff, patients and visitors. Good handwashing technique can be demonstrated to the person and to families and visitors, and this is encouraged before any direct contact between the patient and others. The person and family are also advised to caution anyone with a recent infection, such as respiratory infections, shingles or chickenpox, not to visit the patient in hospital or at home while their count is low. Crowds, particularly in poorly ventilated environments, should also be avoided. Other work-related or recreational activities with a possible infection risk can be discussed by the client and the team on an individual basis.

The early identification of infection when at home is also important and patients and their families can be taught how to recognize early signs of infection. A raised temperature above 37.5°C or chills, even without a fever, should alert the family to contact the hospital team.

Delivery of nursing care

The nurse and other caregivers should take precautionary measures to prevent the transfer of infection from themselves to the patient. The need for regular and meticulous handwashing cannot be overstressed. Clean uniforms or clothing and the removal of outer garments such as white coats before entering the room is also important, as is the effective use of aprons and gloves. It is also best if the least number of caregivers is used to provide care. Similarly, if there is an indication that the caregiver has a potential or actual infection, a change of allocation should be provided. Strict aseptic technique should be maintained in the management of wounds and intravenous sites and lines. Equipment should be cleaned regularly and disposables such as infusion lines changed at regular intervals, usually every 24–48 hours.

The nurse has the overall responsibility to maintain a safe environment for the patient at risk; this includes the supervision of domestic staff and the provision of safe food as well as ensuring that all team members maintain consistent and high-quality infection control measures. Effective management of the clinical environment is an essential part of the nursing role in the care of this group of patients.

Early identification of infection

Specific assessment for infection takes place at least every 4 hours, but as often as the clinical situation warrants. A member of the medical team is alerted if:

- the oral temperature rises above 37.5°C

- the person experiences chills, rigor, tachycardia, cyanosis, cold clammy extremities, unexplained abdominal or rectal pain

- the person becomes irritable, restless, complains of a headache or shows an alteration in level of consciousness.

A blood sample is taken for aerobic and anaerobic cultures and a specimen of urine, sputum, stool, wound swabs, throat swabs or swabs from any lesion are sent for microbiological analysis and culture, as appropriate. Intravenous antibiotic therapy is then initiated as quickly as possible if there is any suspicion of infection. It is usually continued for at least 5 days, or for 48 hours after any fever has resolved, depending on clinical circumstances. Further antibiotic therapy may be prescribed. As mentioned previously, antibiotic protocols that have been designed specifically for the particular needs of neutropenic patients are usually in place.

Management of central venous access

Many patients, particularly those requiring intensive or prolonged cytotoxic chemotherapy regimens, long-term transfusion support, bone marrow transplantation or other procedures requiring frequent and reliable venous access will have a central venous catheter (CVC). Although a variety of CVC devices is commonly used in practice, for patients requiring intensive treatments a skin-tunnelled single- or multi-lumen catheter such as the Hickman catheter is a frequent choice (Fig. 14.11). This CVC is tunnelled under the skin before entering the vessel. A Dacron cuff located under the skin permits the tissue to seal tightly around the catheter. Once healed, this can provide a natural barrier to microbes, potentially reducing the risk of infection. The material used for the catheter is relatively inert, allowing the catheter to remain in place for extended periods of time – often months or even years. Other CVCs in common use include peripherally inserted central venous catheters (PICCS) which, as the name suggests, are inserted via the antecubital vein.

The benefits of long-term CVCs include:

- reduced need for repeated venepuncture for blood sampling, so preserving the integrity of veins

- multiple access allowing for simultaneous administration of multiple therapies including intravenous drugs, fluids or total parenteral nutrition

- the administration of large volumes or continuous therapies

- safer administration of cytotoxic drugs, reducing the risks of extravasation

- reliable access for the administration of blood and blood products

- rapid intravenous access in the event of an emergency.

Despite the many clear advantages of CVCs in the care and treatment of patients with haematological conditions, there are a number of potentially serious complications that healthcare professionals must manage effectively. Microbial contamination of the catheter lumen is a serious problem that can often lead to life-threatening infections and sepsis. Strict asepsis in the management of CVCs, particularly when accessing the catheter lumen, changing equipment such as giving sets or caps, or when changing the exit site dressings is imperative.

The risk of air embolus or serious blood loss from an open lumen (as well as the potential to introduce infection) can be minimized through the use of luer lock connections, the systematic use of the integral clamp on each lumen (see Fig. 14.11) and the use of closed system caps and access devices. Artery forceps or sharp-edged clamps should never be used as these may damage the catheter.

Patency of the catheter can be maintained by regular flushing with an appropriate solution at least once a week when the catheter is not in use or after each use. Local

Figure 14.11 Central venous catheter: placement and safety precautions to be observed.

Cephalic vein

Superior vena cava

Entrance site

Dacron cuff

Subcutaneous tunnel

Exit site

Check that:

cap is in place

cap

catheter is clamped

clamp

connection is taped

tape

clinical practices vary in relation to flushing, with regard to both frequency and the solutions used. The British Committee for Standards in Haematology guidelines for the management of central venous lines (BCSH 1997) include some catheter-flushing protocols that may support decision-making in this area.

Although clinical practices may well vary, this is nevertheless an important aspect of catheter care, as a thrombus within the lumen can reduce the lumen size, limiting flow and predisposing the patient to a catheter infection. It can also cause a catheter to break with the pressure exerted during flushing or bolus administration, may cause a clot to enter the circulation or may require the removal of the catheter if all patency is lost. Occasionally, a thrombus may develop external to the lumen, causing partial or complete obstruction of the vessel. A patient complaining of discomfort in the shoulder region should be investigated promptly for the possibility of infection, a catheter break or the presence of a thrombus.

The patient will need time and support to become familiar with and accept the catheter. The nurse should be sensitive to issues of body image and help the client to feel confident and skilful in catheter management, particularly before discharge. Education of both the client and family members in the effective management of long-term CVCs is an important nursing role; addressing anxieties and concerns is also important for the long-term success of this intervention. Some of the possible goals of a teaching programme to facilitate client independence in catheter management are outlined in the care plan shown in Box 14.4.

Evaluation

Review of care should demonstrate that assessment for signs of infection has been continuous and that the patient and family have been taught and understand measures for decreasing potential sources of infection, can identify signs of infection and know what to do if an infection develops. Persons with disorders of white cells should be supported in altering their behaviours sufficiently to decrease the risks of infection while still enjoying a balanced lifestyle and social activities.

Box 14.4   Care plan for central venous catheters

Goal	Intervention
■ The catheter will remain in place and intact for the duration of clinical need	1. The CVC will be stitched in place and stitches will remain until the tunnel and exit site are fully healed (approx. 21 days) (or until the catheter is removed if not intended as long-term vascular access) 2. Appropriate dressings and support are used to reduce the weight of the catheter on the exit site and the tail(s) are fixed to the chest 3. Strategies are developed to support and protect the CVC during normal activities such as sleeping, exercise and work 4. Strategies will be implemented to maintain patency and prevent thrombus formation, including a regular flushing schedule and the use of a lock technique when flushing
■ The catheter will remain infection free	5. Strict aseptic practice will be maintained at all times when handling or using the line 6. The number of individuals accessing the line is kept to a minimum 7. Strategies are developed to minimize line accessing (e.g. blood tests are timed with drug administration, etc.) 8. An occlusive dressing is used to protect the exit site when bathing, showering, etc. 9. The dead space is removed prior to using or flushing the CVC 10. The integrity of the CVC is maintained whenever possible 11. Microbiological cultures are sent whenever infection is suspected and antibiotic therapy is instigated at the earliest opportunity
■ The client and key individuals will demonstrate skilled, confident and knowledgeable practice in the care, maintenance and use of the catheter	12. An educational strategy is designed to facilitate the client or family members to: a. explain the purpose, use and care of the CVC b. demonstrate the ability to hand-wash to a high standard and to apply basic principles of asepsis to catheter management c. demonstrate the ability to prepare a syringe with a flushing solution, flush the catheter and dispose of the equipment safely d. change the cap on the catheter safely e. identify safety precautions and action to be taken in case of problems arising f. identify how they will obtain further supplies of equipment g. identify likely activities that may need to be curtailed or restricted and modified
■ The potentially negative impact of the catheter on the client's body image, sense of self-mastery and personal freedom will be minimized	13. Support will be offered to the client before and after catheter placement and their personal concerns will be identified 14. Partners and family are included in the preparation and education process, as appropriate 15. The client is facilitated to take responsibility for catheter management as quickly as is appropriate in the individual clinical and personal circumstances 16. Help and support in catheter management is offered until the client feels confident 17. Access to other clients with long-term catheters may be appropriate

Responses of individuals to malignant disorders of white blood cells

The diagnosis of a malignant disorder of white blood cells such as leukaemia or lymphoma has a dramatic impact on the person and his or her family. The emotional and psychological impact of the diagnosis is only the beginning of a long and very challenging road to acceptance and adjustment. Their lives are altered forever.

The dialogue in the Case Study 14.4, condensed from an actual nurse–patient interaction (the names have been altered), helps to highlight some of the issues from an individual perspective.

Case Study 14.4

James Adams is a 22-year-old man who was in his second year of college when he was diagnosed as having leukaemia. During the interview he recalled many of his experiences from the time of his diagnosis to this 2-year interview. He shared his perceptions of the impact his diagnosis had on himself, his parents and his younger brother, and how his family and health professionals had helped him to cope.

James: When I was first diagnosed I felt that I was the only one who had this disease. I thought once you had it, it was the end. Slowly I began to realize there was a chance that this thing could be beaten through chemotherapy. I went through the stages of anger, denial and acceptance. I let the stages take their course, but it was very hard to accept and took a long time. I remember people coming up to me and saying, 'You have cancer', and I would say, 'No, I don't, I have leukaemia. There is a difference'. That was just another way of denying it, even though cancer and leukaemia are the same thing. I could not believe it was happening to me. I was the healthiest person in the world.

Cheryl (nurse): You have told me about the support and encouragement you have received during this time. How have your family, friends and the healthcare workers helped you in coping and adapting to your diagnosis of leukaemia?

James: My family and friends were always very supportive. There were times when I was very irritable and told them that I did not want anything to do with them. They always managed to give me a 'sort of shake' and put things back into perspective. When I was at my lowest point, they would drag me out of the house, even though I did not want to go, and take me for a drive. They made me look at things in a different perspective – to open my eyes – and say, 'What am I doing sitting here feeling sorry for myself?'.

The nurses taught me how to deal with all the different things I was exposed to like needles, hospitals, and dealing with things mentally and emotionally. The nurses could provide more support if they had more time for each patient – the time they have sometimes is not quite enough.

The chaplain made me look at things in a different light. The doctor, of course, helps with the treatments and all the side-effects. I think it takes a very caring and special individual to work on a haematology ward because you develop close relationships with the patients. I have known some of the nurses for 2 years. The nurses are aware of everything the patients are going through and know what each patient likes and dislikes. When you spend as much time in hospital as I do, you like to have a sense of independence. That is something the nurses on haematology allow me to have. It does a lot for me psychologically.

Cheryl: How has your leukaemia altered your life?

James: There are many restrictions. At certain times I cannot drink alcohol. I have to be in hospital a lot. I am in for 1 week each month, and if there are complications I am in longer. Following treatments you do not feel well and therefore are not up to doing what you would like to do. I have a Hickman [central venous] catheter and therefore cannot be as athletic as I would like to be. I cannot play contact sports. If I was injured it would cause a lot of problems for me. But the goal is to get through therapy and hopefully get back to a normal lifestyle.

Cheryl: Do you have any comments you would like to make to a newly diagnosed leukaemic patient?

James:
1. Try to lead as normal a life as possible.
2. Your attitude is important. If you let it beat you mentally, then you have not got a hope.
3. It is good to talk to people – that has been my experience. I speak to the nurses, the chaplain, the doctors – as many people as possible. They help you put things in perspective when you are really upset and you cannot look at things logically.
4. Speak to someone who has gone through a similar experience. When I spoke with a volunteer from the Cancer Society, I thought, 'How come you are okay? People with this disease do not have a chance.' Seeing this young man and realizing that he had gone through some hard times and was okay now I thought, 'Well, if he can do it, I can do it too'. As a result of my experience, I appreciate little things more and take advantage of every minute. The time I spend with family, friends and nurses, I appreciate a lot more. I take things one day at a time.

Haemorrhagic disorders

Effective blood coagulation is the result of a complex interaction between vascular, platelet and plasma factors. A defect or abnormality in any of these may predispose an individual to excessive or prolonged bleeding. The cause may be primary, either inherited or acquired, or secondary to other diseases or pathological processes. Abnormal bleeding is commonly the result of a deficiency in clotting factors, excess anticoagulant, or may arise from a reduced number of platelets (thrombocytopenia) or, less commonly, dysfunctional platelets or vessel wall abnormalities. Secondary causes of abnormal coagulation include liver disease, malignancy, obstetric complications, trauma and burns. A bleeding disorder is often characterized by one or more of the following features: (1) prolonged bleeding following tissue damage, (2) spontaneous bleeding into mucous membranes, tissue, joints, skin and/or organs, and (3) bleeding in multiple sites.

Disorders of platelets

Thrombocytopenia

Thrombocytopenia can be very broadly defined as a platelet count below 150×10^9/L. In practice, however, clinical manifestations of thrombocytopenia often reflect a much lower platelet count, certainly below 100×10^9/L, although often the count may drop to double or even single digits. As a slight drop in the platelet count may have a straightforward explanation, mild thrombocytopenia may not necessarily be a cause for clinical concern.

Thrombocytopenia can, however, also be the result of a number of different pathological processes. These include failure of production, a reduced platelet lifespan, removal of platelets from the circulation or dilution of platelets in the circulation. Bone marrow failure in diseases such as leukaemia, myeloma or aplastic anaemia is a frequent cause of thrombocytopenia. It can also be the result of bone marrow toxicity following treatment with cytotoxic chemotherapy or radiotherapy. Other causes for a reduced production of platelets by the bone marrow include infections as well as drugs known selectively to suppress platelet production.

A reduced platelet lifespan may be the result of an immune process involving platelet antibodies, drugs or infections. Platelet destruction within the blood vessels is one result of disseminated intravascular coagulation. Sequestration by the spleen may reduce the platelet count through pooling into the spleen. A dilution effect may be a result of massive blood transfusion. It is also important to remember this dilution effect when transfusing an individual with a low platelet count.

Bleeding from the mucous membranes is characteristic of thrombocytopenia. Conjunctival haemorrhages, nose bleeds, bleeding gums as well as skin bruising are all common sites of bleeding. Heavy menstrual blood loss or gastrointestinal bleeding may also be a feature. Intracranial bleeding is a less common but very serious complication of a low platelet count.

Immune thrombocytopenia

Drugs (e.g. quinine, heparin), infections (e.g. malaria, Epstein–Barr virus), connective tissue diseases (e.g. systemic lupus erythematosus) and some malignancies (e.g. chronic lymphocytic leukaemia) are associated with immune thrombocytopenias (Howard and Hamilton 1997).

Idiopathic thrombocytopenia purpura (ITP), as the name implies, is a spontaneous event involving the systematic destruction of platelets by the reticuloendothelial system. These platelets have previously been coated with antibody through an autoimmune process. Acute ITP is predominantly a disease of childhood and often follows a viral illness. The platelet count often falls to below 20×10^9/L and may lead to spontaneous bleeding. The problem may resolve spontaneously or may require steroid therapy or intravenous immunoglobulin.

Chronic ITP is a disease of adulthood and is more insidious in nature. It rarely resolves spontaneously and may become a lifelong illness. The platelet count varies in chronic ITP, and very mild cases may not initially require treatment. For those whose platelet count puts them at risk of spontaneous bleeding or who have signs of active bleeding, therapy in the form of oral corticosteroids or intravenous immunoglobulin may be required. A splenectomy may be considered for patients who fail to maintain satisfactory platelet counts. Other treatments for those who remain refractory to conventional therapy include other immunosuppressant drugs such as cyclophosphamide, vincristine and dexamethasone.

Platelet function disorders

Defects of platelet function may either be hereditary or acquired. Aspirin therapy, for example, is a common cause of an acquired platelet function defect. Platelet function can be assessed in a variety of ways. A bleeding time is a direct assessment of the formation of a **platelet plug** in a wound. This is done by making a small incision in the patient's forearm and recording the time to the cessation of bleeding. Platelet aggregation studies can also be used to assess platelet response to the common agonists (e.g. adenosine diphosphate (ADP), collagen) involved in the formation of an effective platelet plug. More specialist tests may also be required to diagnose the more obscure causes of platelet dysfunction.

Impairment may result from a failure of any of the stages of platelet plug formation; however, the majority of the syndromes associated with these defects are relatively rare.

Plug formation
See chapter 4.1

Coagulation factor deficiencies

Deficiencies in blood **clotting** factors may be inherited or, less frequently, acquired. Failure of coagulation may be result of a deficiency in factor production, clotting factors that are either structurally or functionally abnormal, presence of antibodies to clotting factors, or excessive consumption of clotting factors. The next section describes the most common disorders of clotting factors, including haemophilia A and B and von Willebrand disease.

Haemophilia

Haemophilia is an X-linked recessive inherited disorder that leads to a deficiency in either factor VIII (haemophilia A) or factor IX (haemophilia B or Christmas disease). As the genetic defect is carried on an X chromosome, it is transmitted from mother to son. Men inherit an X chromosome from their mother and a Y chromosome from their father. Women inherit two X chromosomes, one from each parent. As this abnormality is carried on the X chromosome, men who inherit the abnormal gene are automatically affected as they have only one X chromosome. Women who inherit the abnormal gene also inherit a normal gene on the second X chromosome and therefore become carriers of the disease. For this reason, haemophilia is a disease that almost exclusively affects men (see Fig. 14.12). It is interesting to note, however, that occasionally women have been born with haemophilia. This could occur if a female carrier and a male haemophiliac were to have children. In practice this is a very rare occurrence but there have been documented cases (Tuddenham and Laffan 1999). It is also thought that a proportion of new cases of haemophilia, as in families with no known history of the disease, may be due to spontaneous mutations (Lawn 1991).

Clotting
See chapter 4.1

Clinical characteristics

Haemophilia is usually recognized in the first year of life, often once the child begins to crawl. Transplacental transfer of clotting factors from the mother to the fetus prevents excessive bleeding at birth but in some cases there may be persistent bleeding from the umbilical cord. Persistent bleeding when the infant is circumcised or injured can also lead to early diagnosis of the disorder. Some babies present with large bruises, leading to the suspicion of non-accidental injury. This may be a source of great stress and trauma for parents and families until an accurate diagnosis is made. A sensitive approach to assessment and diagnosis in these circumstances is vital.

The severity of bleeding is closely related to the individual's factor VIII level. Severe haemophiliacs (about 50% of cases) will have frequent spontaneous bleeding into joints, muscles and organs. Moderately severe haemophiliacs (about 30% of cases) will bleed after minor trauma and have some spontaneous bleeding episodes.

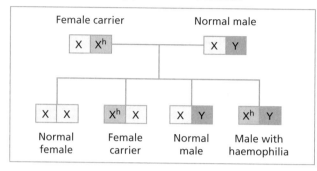

Figure 14.12   Inheritance of haemophilia. X^h, haemophilia gene; X, normal X chromosome; Y, normal Y chromosome.

Mild haemophilia (about 20% of cases) is characterized by severe bleeding after trauma or surgery (Tuddenham and Laffan 1999). The severity of the disease appears to be linked with the type of mutation found in the gene (Lawn 1991).

A key feature of the bleeding pattern is its persistence. Bleeding may be a continuous slow ooze or intermittent and continue for days. Joints, frequently but not exclusively the weight-bearing ones, are typical sites of bleeding. Some joints are more frequent 'targets' for bleeding; this leads to repeated irritation, inflammation and destruction of these target joints. Muscle bleeding is common and can cause pain and local neuropathy, as well as long-term ischaemic damage and contractures. Bleeding into soft tissues, such as the oropharynx, is less common but may cause problems such as obstruction. Gastrointestinal bleeding as in haematemesis or malaena requires investigation to exclude other possible causes for bleeding, such as malignancy. As blood is a potent irritant, repeated assaults on the integrity of joints and muscle tissue can lead to permanent and severe damage, resulting in a marked decrease in functional ability and long-term disability.

Treatment and care

The key to successful treatment of a bleeding episode is the prompt administration of clotting factors to limit the amount of blood leaking into joints, muscle or tissue. Clients frequently become adept at recognizing the onset of a bleeding episode, even before clinical signs appear. The availability of clotting factors in the home and skill in their self-administration offers the potential to minimize damage caused by frequent bleeding episodes. Although clotting factors are frequently administered as a response to bleeding, prophylactic administration of clotting factors is seen as the most effective strategy for minimizing the often crippling long-term damage of severe haemophilia.

Two limiting factors in the provision of prophylaxis have been availability of supply and cost. Increased plasma supplies and the development of recombinant factor VIII production have increased the overall availability of clotting factors, but cost continues to be a very real problem. In the long term, however, the cost implications need to be balanced against the benefits, including reduced need for orthopaedic surgery, hospital admissions and long-term disability as well as a myriad of other important quality-of-life issues.

Complications of treatment

A proportion of patients with severe haemophilia will develop antibodies to factor VIII. These are known as inhibitors. Inhibitors often develop in childhood but may occur at any point. The treatment options for a patient with inhibitors is dependent on the level of antibody and its response to factor VIII administration. In those whose antibody response is mild or whose antibody level is low, increased doses of factor VIII may be sufficient. In those whose response is high, porcine factor VIII may be an option. Others may require alternative factor infusions, in an attempt to bypass some of the clotting cascade. In refractory patients, the use of immunosuppression and immunoglobulin infusions and other complex therapies have been tried with varying degrees of success (Tuddenham and Laffan 1999).

A devastating complication of the use of factor concentrates has been the transmission of infections, of which two of the most important ones are hepatitis and human immunodeficiency virus (HIV). Screening for hepatitis B has been in place since the 1970s. Nevertheless, for years an unknown infective agent was causing liver disease in individuals with haemophilia. This is now known to be the hepatitis C virus (HCV). HIV infection in haemophilia was first documented in the early 1980s, and a proportion of patients now live with one or other, or both, of these viruses. The physical, psychological and emotional impact of chronic liver disease and HIV on clients and their fam-ilies cannot be underestimated. Care strategies that are able to meet the multiple and complex health needs of this client group pose many important challenges for healthcare providers. Careful screening of blood products and treatment with solvents has now eliminated new transmission of HIV, HCV and other known viral agents, but it must be remembered that as yet unknown infections may pose a health threat in the future to those dependent on blood product derivatives.

Care

Following a bleeding episode, local supportive measures can be instituted. An inflamed joint may require support and a period of rest, but activity and movement should be resumed as soon as possible to promote mobility. Appropriate pain relief measures must also be instituted at this time. Physiotherapy plays an important part in maintaining function and mobility in damaged joints or muscles and should be offered as part of a comprehensive care package.

The complex nature of this disease combined with the multiple problems associated with severe haemophilia have lcd to the development of a strategy for the provision of care and services to this client group. Designated haemophilia centres, where there is both expertise and access to a range of services, information and support, are considered key to the provision of quality care. Dedicated teams of doctors, nurses, physiotherapists and social workers combined with the availability of orthopaedic, dental, haematology, rehabilitation and other services within one locality can provide prompt, informed, appropriate services and a coordinated approach to care provision.

In the initial stages after diagnosis, one of the main functions of the nurse is to implement an effective teaching programme for the person and their family, enabling them to manage the disease and its consequences effectively. This can also promote a sense of personal control in the face of a lifelong condition with the very real risk of disability and ill-health. This programme may include information about the nature of the disorder and its possible consequences, management of home factor administration, risk assessment and essential precautions, management of a bleeding episode, effective self-care measures, and effective use of services available, including emergency access and long-term support. It is also important for parents of a child with haemophilia to be given the opportunity to reflect on the implications of the disease for the child during the various stages of development and to address their anxieties. This can help them develop a more realistic view of both limitations and possibilities. An important goal is to maintain as normal a home environment and lifestyle as possible and to minimize the risk of overprotection and the promotion of dependency. For this, parents may require personal support and encouragement, as well as practical support.

Managing the child at school can be a concern for parents, and problems may arise from a lack of knowledge and understanding on the part of the authorities. The expertise of haemophilia centres can be used successfully to facilitate this through the provision of information and education enabling children, their parents, teachers and the education authorities to develop effective strategies that meet the child's needs in the school environment.

Self-care measures such as the management of venous access, the management of childhood illness, the use of over-the-counter medications, dental hygiene and the home management of bleeding and rehabilitation can promote a sense of independence for the client and the family. As the child gets older, parents may need support in handing over the responsibility of health management to the child.

The adult with haemophilia will have gained considerable expertise in managing the condition but may still require support in areas such as employment and the management of increasing disability. The aim in any intervention should be the facilitation of independence and personal decision making. The Haemophilia Society, with its extensive support network, information, publications, events and campaigning, can be an effective resource for individuals with haemophilia, their families and professionals involved in their care.

Caring for the individual with haemophilia and HIV or HCV can be particularly challenging for the healthcare professional, who may share some of the great emotional strain experienced by the client, their partners and their family. Effective teamwork and a commitment to the provision of comprehensive care can help to support this particular client group.

Von Willebrand's disease (VWD)

Von Willebrand factor (VWF) is a protein synthesized by endothelial cells and megakaryocytes. Its primary purpose is to bind platelets to the endothelium and it also carries factor VIII in plasma. In VWD, the factor defect may be either quantitative or qualitative, so that either the factor is in short supply or there may be sufficient amounts but it functions ineffectively. The quantitative deficiency is by far the more common. A rarer type involves a defect of the actual platelet receptor sites for VWF, causing abnormal use of VWF.

Clinical symptoms vary depending on the severity of deficiency. A minority of patients have a severe form of the disease; this is characterized by a very limited production of VWF and a marked decrease in factor VIII levels. These patients are susceptible to spontaneous bleeding, which may at times be life threatening. This less common type more closely resembles the clinical picture of haemophilia A. Treatment of severe VWD involves the administration of factor VIII.

Milder forms of the disease reflect the reduced platelet function, with gum bleeding, epistaxis, prolonged bleeding after injury and increased bruising. Women may experience menorrhagia. Others may have noticeably increased bleeding only after surgical interventions, such as dental extractions or major surgery. Those with milder disease may require little or no intervention, except before operation. If bleeding is a problem and treatment is required, desmopressin (DDAVP) infusions can be used to stimulate the release of VWF from the body's stores. Some subtypes of VWD do not respond to DDAVP. Before a surgical intervention, DDAVP, cryoprecipitate or mixed purity factor VIII may be required. For those with a platelet receptor site defect, platelet concentrates would be a treatment option (Tuddenham and Laffan 1999).

Vascular purpura

An abnormality of blood vessels may be a cause of abnormal bleeding. A common cause for extensive bruising in older persons is senile purpura. This results from a loss of subcutaneous tissue and collagen, leading to inadequate support of the vessels and increased vessel rupture following mild trauma. Purpuric lesions may also follow

infections and certain types of septicaemia. Allergic purpura may be caused by inflammation of the vessel wall; this is precipitated by an allergic response to chemicals, toxins or other stimuli. Vitamin C deficiency (scurvy) may also cause bleeding from multiple sites. Vitamin C supplements quickly resolve the problem.

Long-term administration of steroid therapy may cause atrophy of collagen fibres, leading to a loss of support of blood vessels. Some rare collagen disorders may cause bleeding as a result of the failure of platelets to adhere to abnormal collagen after injury. Hereditary haemorrhagic telangiectasia is a rare disorder characterized by the development of angiomatous malformations in the nose, mouth, gastrointestinal tract, skin and urinary tract, which bleed easily with minor trauma. Iron deficiency anaemia is a common problem in persons with this rare condition.

Vitamin K deficiency

Vitamin K is essential in the production of prothrombin and factors VII, IX and X by the liver. Vitamin K is derived from vegetables in the diet and from intestinal flora. A deficiency may result from a dietary deficiency, impaired absorption or defective utilization of vitamin K. Dietary deficiency is most often seen in patients requiring intensive medical care and those on high or prolonged doses of antibiotics (Howard and Hamilton 1997) as these can seriously diminish the number of intestinal bacteria. Malabsorption may be the result of conditions such as coeliac disease or chronic biliary obstruction. Haemorrhagic disease of the newborn may be the result of lack of synthesis in an intestinal tract still free of organisms or low placental transfer of vitamin K, or even a low level of the vitamin in breast milk (Howard and Hamilton 1997). Liver disease may also result in reduced synthesis of clotting factors, including prothrombin. Vitamin K deficiency may be treated with parenteral or oral administration of vitamin K (phytomenadione). Haemorrhage or deficiency secondary to liver disease may also require the administration of fresh frozen plasma or clotting factors.

Excess of anticoagulant: heparin or warfarin toxicity

Excessive bleeding may be a result of anticoagulant drug therapy such as heparin and warfarin. **Anticoagulant drugs** are commonly used to treat acute venous thrombosis (e.g. deep vein thrombosis) and pulmonary embolus or as prophylaxis for individuals at risk of thrombosis. Patients with prosthetic valves, arterial grafts, transient ischaemic attacks and those with an inherited or acquired predisposition to thrombus formation are often on long-term or lifelong anticoagulant therapy. In all individuals on anticoagulant therapy, excessive bleeding following

*Anticoagulants
See chapter 4.1*

trauma or bleeding in the absence of vascular trauma may be an indication of an increased anticoagulant effect. This could be due to an excess of the drug or be the result of a drug interaction.

Unfractionated heparin disrupts the clotting process by potentiating the activity of antithrombin which, in turn, deactivates prothrombin Xa, IXa and XIa. In addition, it has an effect on thrombin and impairs platelet function. Low molecular weight heparin has a more specific activity, with a lesser effect on thrombin and platelets and a lower risk of bleeding (Mehta and Hoffbrand 2000). Warfarin inhibits vitamin K action on factors II, VII, IX and X, producing an overall decrease in these circulating factors over a period of 2–3 days. As warfarin does not offer an immediate anticoagulant effect, patients may commonly need alternative anticoagulant therapy such as heparin at the outset and will need to maintain multiple anticoagulant therapy until the optimum therapeutic level of warfarin-based anticoagulation has been achieved. The anticoagulant effect of continuous heparin infusion is monitored by measuring the activated partial thromboplastin time (APPT).

Warfarin requires regular monitoring for as long as the patient is on therapy. The prothrombin time is measured and expressed as an international normalized ratio, commonly referred to as the INR. Drug dosages can be altered to maintain the patient within a specified INR range to ensure maximum therapeutic effect and to minimize the risk of excessive anticoagulation with its increased risk of haemorrhage.

If bleeding does occur, or the INR is excessively raised, anticoagulant therapy is withheld and, if necessary, fresh frozen plasma or factor concentrates can be administered. Vitamin K may also be given but this results in a prolonged resistance to warfarin. Protamine sulfate inactivates heparin and may be used for serious bleeding but, as heparin has a short half-life, stopping the infusion or reducing the dose is often sufficient to correct an increased APTT.

Nursing responsibilities related to clients on anticoagulant therapy include assessment and education regarding:

- the aim of therapy and its possible side-effects and complications

- the importance of medication compliance and regular monitoring, including attendance at outpatient clinics

- the warning signs of possible over-coagulation requiring prompt intervention

- the importance of informing relevant individuals (e.g. dentists) of drug therapy

- the importance of maintaining adequate supplies of the drug to ensure continued therapeutic levels. This includes taking sufficient supplies on holiday, etc., and obtaining further supplies in good time to avoid running out of the drug

- the potential for drug interactions, including prescription and over-the-counter medications such as aspirin-based compounds, and alcohol

- the risk of injury and its immediate management.

Disseminated intravascular coagulation

Disseminated intravascular coagulation (DIC) is a potentially fatal condition that is a secondary development to a serious primary illness. It is characterized by inappropriate and excessive stimulation of the clotting mechanisms resulting in the simultaneous formation of multiple diffuse microemboli in the vascular system and haemorrhage resulting from the rapid depletion of clotting factors.

Common causes of DIC include:

- infection – septicaemia in particular

- shock associated with surgical trauma or burns

- malignancy – leukaemia and metastatic carcinoma

- obstetric emergencies such as septic abortion or eclampsia

- cardiac bypass surgery

- intravascular haemolysis associated with ABO-incompatible transfusion

- tissue rejection in transplantation

- liver disease such as cirrhosis.

DIC is the result of complex interactions involving an initial trigger such as damaged tissues, malignant cells or damaged endothelium. This trigger induces the activation of the coagulation cascade and platelet activation. Fibrin clots and strands form within the circulation and, in combination with activated platelets, cause partial blockage of the microcirculation, damaging red cells and inducing haemolysis. Localized clot formation in combination with this more generalized intravascular coagulation quickly leads to severe depletion of clotting factors. The liver is unable to compensate for this rapid depletion so that, as the circulating factors and platelets diminish and levels of fibrinogen degradation products (FDPs) increase, generalized bleeding ensues. There is then simultaneous bleeding and necrosis of the involved vessels and surrounding tissue.

Clinical characteristics

Diffuse bleeding may be evident as petechiae, haematuria, gastrointestinal bleeding, vaginal bleeding, epistaxis or persistent oozing from a surgical wound or needle puncture. The patient is often seriously ill and may be hypotensive and shocked. Pain may be experienced as a result of tissue ischaemia and bleeding. Organs such as the kidneys and lungs are particularly susceptible, and renal failure and acute respiratory distress are common features.

Management and nursing care

The diagnosis of DIC is made from the clinical picture and from a rapid laboratory evaluation of the patient's haemoglobin level and haematocrit (to establish possible haemolysis), platelet count, and the prothrombin and thrombin time as well as fibrinogen levels. Subsequent tests may include specific factor levels and FDP levels.

Prompt management of DIC is essential:

1. If at all possible, efforts should be made to eliminate the trigger factor.

2. Management of bleeding should be instituted to avoid hypotensive shock with red cell replacement. In the interim, plasma expanders or fluids may be required.

3. Coagulation replacement therapy in the form of fresh frozen plasma, cryoprecipitate and platelet infusion will be needed.

4. Intravenous antibiotics can be given if sepsis is suspected.

5. Central venous access should be considered to facilitate management.

6. Careful management of fluid replacement is important, particularly in the presence of renal insufficiency.

7. Respiratory management in the form of oxygen will be necessary; mechanical ventilation may be an option in some circumstances.

8. Cardiac function should be monitored and may also require support with inotropic agents.

9. Renal function should be closely monitored with careful measurement of output, and may also require support. In some instances, renal dialysis may be required.

10. Continuous monitoring of vital functions and regular assessment is an important nursing responsibility.

11. Pain management and comfort measures are also essential, as is the support of the critically ill patient and their family.

Nursing assessment of the person with a haemorrhagic disorder

Health history

It is important to ascertain at the outset the nature of the bleeding, the duration of bleeding, and any known or possible precipitating factors. The client may be asked to describe any abnormal bleeding such as rashes, bruising, swelling, tenderness or areas of discoloration on the skin or mucous membranes. Specific questions regarding changes that may have gone unnoticed for a period of time, such as nose bleeds, bleeding gums, increased menstrual bleeding, a bloodshot eye or a change in stool colour, may be helpful in establishing the possible history of the condition. A family history of bleeding may also help to elucidate the situation. For persons with known bleeding disorders, a history of recent episodes, expected severity of episodes, usual management strategies and commonly encountered problems may provide the healthcare team with valuable information for assessment and care strategies.

As bleeding is always a warning sign that something is wrong, the client may naturally feel anxious and concerned. Part of the health assessment may include assessment of the person's understanding and possible fears as well as support and relevant information giving to facilitate the client in coping with the situation.

Physical assessment

The person is examined for signs of bleeding. The clinical characteristics of bleeding that may be identified by inspection and palpation of the skin, mucous membranes and joints include:

■ *Haemorrhage.* The bleeding may be external or internal. The amount of blood lost will depend on the size of the blood vessel(s), whether an artery or vein is ruptured, and the effectiveness of the body's clotting mechanism. External bleeding can be assessed by direct observation; the amount of blood that has soaked into the person's clothing or pooled on or under the affected part may be estimated. Arterial blood is bright red and spurts; venous blood is dark red and flows steadily. A gastrointestinal haemorrhage may lead to *haematemesis* (the vomiting of blood) or *malaena* (faeces that are black and tarry as a result of containing digested blood).

■ *Petechiae.* These are small red spots about the size of the head of a pin and may be seen in groups over various parts of the body. They are the result of an increased permeability of blood vessels that enables blood to extravasate (leak) into the surrounding tissue. They are a common feature of thrombocytopenia.

■ *Purpura.* Purpuric spots are caused by the same mechanism as petechiae, but are larger in size.

■ *Ecchymosis or bruise.* This is an area of extravasated blood beneath the surface of the skin that produces a patch of blue or purplish discoloration. It often occurs as a result of trauma or in platelet disorders.

■ *Haematoma*. This is a large bruise caused by infiltration of blood into the subcutaneous or muscle tissue as a result of a coagulation defect, trauma in thrombocytopenia or an overdose of anticoagulant. It is characterized by discoloration of the skin, swelling, pain and deformity of the tissue.

■ *Haemarthrosis*. This is haemorrhage into a joint, usually caused by a severe coagulation disorder such as haemophilia. It is characterized by pain, tenderness and swelling of the affected joint.

It is important to note the sites and extent of bleeding. If the person has a haemostatic defect, bleeding may occur at multiple sites. Bleeding at individual sites may also be indicative of local factors such as trauma. Baseline measurement of pulse, blood pressure and respiration rates are an important part of the initial assessment, as are blood samples for the full blood count (particularly the haemoglobin, haematocrit and platelets counts) and a clotting screen. Subsequent monitoring may then yield useful information on trends, indicating possible increased or continued bleeding as well as patient status.

Specific nursing needs of patients with haemorrhagic disorders vary with each individual and with the cause, associated symptoms and severity of the disease. Some nursing care issues are discussed under the relevant sections and further information can be obtained from the relevant texts in the reference list. Some common problems and considerations are presented in the care plan for patients with a haemorrhagic disorder shown in Box 14.5.

Transfusion practice

Transfusion of blood and blood products

The safe and effective supply of blood products depends on the availability of healthy volunteer donors and an established blood transfusion service. Both the World Health Organization and the International Society of Blood Transfusion support the principle of blood donation and collection that is not motivated by financial profit (Contreras and Hewitt 1999). It has certainly been suggested that payment for blood may increase the risk of disease transmission and may also encourage concealment of relevant medical history or high-risk behaviours (Titmuss 1970, Hewitt and Wagstaff 1992). However, others suggest that there is no conclusive evidence that payment increases the risk of contamination provided there is thorough screening of donors and adequate regulation to ensure safe and non-exploitative practice (Rodriguez Del Pozo 1994).

Most countries in western Europe, including the UK, in so far as possible uphold the principle of non-profit provision of blood products, but in other parts of the world donors are paid for their blood donations. Worldwide, commercial companies are involved in the collection and supply of blood and, in particular, plasma products. One important factor is the relative scarcity of blood products combined with ever-increasing need. The social, political, scientific and practical issues involved in the provision of safe blood products are both a fascinating and complex subject, meriting careful consideration of the issues and debates.

The main indications for the transfusion of blood or blood products include:

■ replacement of blood lost during surgery, trauma or haemorrhage

■ the correction of anaemia, as in bone marrow failure, chronic diseases, and haemoglobinopathies

■ the correction of deficiencies in other blood and plasma components, such as platelets or clotting factors.

Donation

When blood is taken from the donor, it is collected into a sterile single-use collection pack containing a citrate-phosphate-dextrose-adenine (CPD-A) anticoagulant. Subsequent additions of plasma replacement solutions such as saline-adenine-glucose-mannitol (SAGM) permit the collection of large amounts of plasma from each donation and also increases the storage life of red cells to up to 35–42 days (Contreras and Hewitt 1999). It is important to remember the potential for interactions of these additives with drugs or other infusions. It is for this reason that safe practice guidelines dictate that no other solutions or additives be added to either the transfusion bag or giving set. Each unit of blood receives a unique identification number to enable it to be fully traced from donor to recipient. This is an important element of quality control in the event of a transfusion-related complication or an error in processing, storage or delivery. In the UK, as in many other countries, stringent quality standards are in place to ensure a safe blood transfusion service.

To minimize the risk of transfusion-related infections, donor blood is tested for human immunodeficiency virus (HIV), hepatitis B and C, and syphilis. Some donations are also screened for cytomegalovirus (CMV) to provide CMV-negative blood products for special recipient groups such as transplant recipients and neonates. All red cell and platelet products are currently also leucocyte depleted at source in view of the possibility of transmission of new variant Creutzfeldt–Jacob disease. Donors are also assessed at the time of donation for other potential problems such as a pre-existing illness or chronic condition and for possible exposure to infections such as malaria. The donor's haemoglobin (Hb) is also tested to rule out anaemia. Each donation is typed for blood group and Rhesus factor and for the presence of alloantibodies for common blood group antigens. Other tests may be carried out according to need.

Transfusion
See chapter 4.1

Box 14.5   Care plan: the person with a haemorrhagic disorder

Goal	Nursing intervention

Problem: Potential risk of bleeding due to a platelet disorder, deficiency of clotting factors, excess anticoagulant or a vascular defect

■ Bleeding will be limited due to prompt identification

1. Determine likely potential to bleed by checking current blood results (platelets, INR, etc.)
2. Inspect the skin regularly for appearance of petechiae and purpura
3. Record any change in size or new areas of petechiae and purpura
4. Observe open lesions, incisions, and intravenous and intramuscular injection sites for oozing or haematomas
5. Test urine and stools and examine vomit and sputum for blood
6. Examine joints for oedema, tenderness and limited movement
7. Assess symptoms of internal bleeding by recording changes in vital signs 4 hourly or as condition indicates
8. Observe for signs of cerebral dysfunction, confusion, disorientation or restlessness

■ Bleeding will stop with minimal blood loss and vital signs will be within normal range

9. Control overt bleeding with pressure and elevation of affected part if possible
10. Estimate and record blood loss in vomit, nasogastric drainage, stools, and on dressings and sanitary pads
11. Keep the person at rest in bed
12. Administer blood products and medications as prescribed, observing for potential reactions
13. Monitor and record vital signs regularly as indicated by person's condition
14. Maintain an accurate fluid balance record
15. Immobilize limbs or joints if bleeding is present in these areas

■ Patient will experience no further bleeding or long-term complications

16. Move the person gently to avoid causing tissue trauma
17. Remove objects that have the potential to cause injury from the immediate environment or ensure they are protected (e.g. cot sides may need to be padded)
18. If there is bleeding into joints, immobilize in the optimal alignment
19. Provide a bed cradle to keep the weight of bedding off the affected part
20. Begin range of motion exercises 48 hours after bleeding stops
21. Use pressure-relieving aids on beds and chairs
22. Avoid invasive procedures, injections, etc. and minimize number of venepunctures
23. Apply direct pressure to venepuncture sites for 10 minutes
24. Take blood pressure only when essential, and rotate sites

■ Patient will express decreased fear and anxiety and actively participate in the treatment plan

25. Administer analgesia to relieve pain
26. Encourage questions and expression of anxieties
27. Encourage participation in decisions concerning treatment and care

■ Patient will describe signs of bleeding, preventive measures and action to take if bleeding occurs

28. Inform the person about causes, signs and symptoms of bleeding disorders (epistaxis, bleeding gums, petechiae, bruising, haematuria)
29. Instruct patient and family to seek medical advice immediately if these occur
30. Discuss measures aimed at preventing tissue trauma, e.g. use of soft toothbrush, avoidance of constrictive clothing, use of electric razors for shaving, need to keep nails short and clean, need to prevent constipation and injury to rectal mucosa, need to avoid self-medication with any aspirin-containing drug
31. Review the safety of occupation and recreational interests and identify activities that are safe to continue and those to be avoided (e.g. contact sports)
32. Provide information on community support available, self-help and support groups, etc.
33. Instruct the person and family in first-aid procedures should bleeding occur
34. Advise the person to inform their dental practitioner of the bleeding problem before undergoing treatment
35. Inform patient of genetic counselling opportunities if appropriate
36. Suggest need to wear a Medic Alert identification in case of emergencies if condition is prolonged

Figure 14.13 ABO blood group compatibility. Note: plasma compatibility is the reverse.

Donor blood group	Recipient blood group			
	A	B	O	AB
A	✓	✗	✗	✓
B	✗	✓	✗	✓
O	✓	✓	✓	✓
AB	✗	✗	✗	✓

As another quality control measure, a standard label is used on each unit of blood. The ABO blood group and Rhesus factor, the date of collection and expiry, the additives used for collection and storage, and the unit's total volume as well as the unique identification number are clearly marked. Additional information specific to the unit such as CMV status, other blood groups such as Kell or Duffy, or leucodepletion will also be indicated, as required by the clinical situation. A label with the recipient details will be added at the time of cross-match to permit the correct identification of the unit and recipient in the clinical area.

To ensure compatibility between donor and recipient, a cross-match is performed. Initially the recipient's blood group and Rhesus status are determined and any antibodies to common blood group antigens identified. A number of units that appear suitable are then allocated. At this point plasma from the recipient is mixed with red cells from the donation and observed for clumping, indicating incompatibility. If no agglutination occurs, the donation is considered to be suitable for transfusion to that particular individual. An ABO compatibility chart is shown in Figure 14.13 to serve as a general guide for red cell and platelet transfusions. Please note that this chart should *not* be used as a compatibility guide for the administration of plasma.

Blood and blood product derivatives

Preparations used in transfusions (Table 14.6)

Whole blood

Whole blood is now seldom used but may be used to treat acute massive blood loss with hypovolaemia. The limiting factors in routinely using whole blood include the large volumes infused and the transfusion of potentially unnecessary blood products such as plasma, platelets and white cells with the risk they pose to the recipient, such as acute reactions or the development of alloantibodies. As donations of whole blood are routinely processed to provide a variety of other blood products, the frequent use of whole blood would also be an inefficient use of a scarce commodity.

Packed red cells

With the removal of a large volume of plasma from whole blood, a red cell concentrate can be obtained. This is commonly used to treat a variety of anaemias. One other advantage of packed red cells is that a greater number of cells can be transfused in a given volume as compared to whole blood, so that maximum benefit can be obtained from the transfusion with a lesser risk of circulatory overload.

Platelets

Platelets can be concentrated from individual units of whole blood or obtained directly from a donor using a cell separator. These are suspended in a small volume of plasma, and have maximum shelf-life of 5 days. Platelets require storage at room temperature and a steady supply of oxygen for survival. They are generally stored in a platelet agitator and, once removed, should be administered promptly to ensure maximum platelet survival. Platelets are used to prevent or control bleeding in patients with thrombocytopenia. ABO and Rhesus compatibility is strongly recommended, particularly for patients requiring multiple or long-term transfusions, as there is a risk of alloimmunization with subsequent platelet destruction as well as febrile transfusion reactions. However, this is not always absolutely essential and may depend on availability of platelets. If Rhesus-positive platelets are transfused to an Rh-negative recipient, anti-D immunoglobulin may be considered to prevent alloimmunization.

Granulocyte concentrates

White blood cells from an ABO-compatible donor can be collected using an apheresis procedure. Alternatively, white cells can be obtained from whole blood collections. Blood is separated into its various components and white cells and platelets are found in a 'buffy coat' at the interface between the red cells and the blood plasma. White cells are very fragile and must be transfused within hours of collection. Transfusion of white cells may occasionally be considered in profoundly neutropenic patients with life-threatening infections, but are used infrequently because there is little evidence for their therapeutic effect (Mehta and Hoffbrand 2000).

Plasma

Fresh frozen plasma (FFP) is separated from whole blood shortly after collection and rapidly frozen to ensure the viability of certain clotting factors, namely factors V and VIII. FFP contains all of the coagulation factors and plasma proteins and, once defrosted, must be transfused promptly.

Table 14.6   The administration of blood and blood products

Blood/blood product and composition	Administration	Common complications

RED CELLS
 	
Whole blood
Red blood cells, leucocytes, plasma, platelets, clotting factors (500 mL/unit)
 	
Packed red cells/concentrated red cells
Red blood cells, some leucocytes and platelets. Removal of some or most plasma gives a volume of 200–300 mL/unit
 	
Other red cell preparations available
 	
■ Red cells in optional additive solution (all the plasma removed)
 	
■ Leucocyte-depleted red cells (most leucocytes and platelets removed)
 	
■ Red cells buffy coat depleted (leucocytes, platelets and plasma removed)
 	
■ Frozen red cells (washed red cells are frozen and stored for up to 10 years)
	1. Allow blood to warm at room temperature for 20–30 min but administer within 30 min of removal from the blood fridge
	2. Check labels carefully according to hospital policy
	3. Use a blood administration set with a blood filter inside the drip chamber
	4. Use only normal saline (0.9% NaCl) solution for intravenous infusion before transfusion
	5. Fill the drip chamber to cover the filter with the blood
	6. Agitate the blood bag gently before and during administration
	7. Begin the transfusion at a slow flow rate of approximately 1 mL/kg per hour and observe patient constantly for the first 15 min. Adjust rate if there are no adverse reactions
	8. Record vital signs before each unit, every 15 min for 30 min then every hour until complete
	9. Discard any blood not transfused within 5 hours
		Cold blood may induce venous spasm and slow or stop the infusion
		Large volumes of cold blood may cause hypothermia
		
		Transfusion reactions include:
		  Fever
		  Back pain
		  Headache
		  Restlessness
		  Chills
		  Dyspnoea
		  Tachycardia
		  Palpitations
		  Thready pulse
		  Hypotension
		  Cold clammy skin
		  Altered level of consciousness
		  Risk of circulatory overload
		  Haemoglobinuria

PLATELETS Platelets and some plasma, leucocytes and red cells (single unit packs 40–60 mL/unit) (pooled donation approximately 150 mL)	1. A platelet set is preferable but a blood administration set may be used 2. Administer as rapidly as tolerated (20–30 min/unit) 3. Flush the line well with normal saline after infusion to ensure all the platelets are delivered	Chills, fever Alloimmunization producing rapid destruction of transfused platelets
PLASMA Fresh or fresh frozen – all plasma proteins and clotting factors (no RBC, WBC or platelets) 200 mL/unit)	1. Use a standard intravenous administration set 2. Administer as rapidly as necessary and tolerated for volume replacement 3. Administer fresh frozen plasma promptly after thawing to prevent deterioration of clotting factors 4. Requires ABO compatibility	Greater risk of allergic reactions than with whole blood Risk of fluid overload with rapid infusions Respiratory distress
GRANULOCYTES White blood cells and plasma with some red blood cells, platelets and other white blood cells (200–300 mL per suspension)	1. Use a standard blood administration infusion set 2. Administer first 50–75 mL slowly and observe for transfusion reaction 3. Administer over 1–2 hours 4. Use within 24 hours of collection	Chills, fever Allergic reactions (urticaria, wheezing) Hypotension, shock Respiratory distress

(Continued)

Table 14.6 *(Continued)*

Blood/blood product and composition	Administration	Common complications
ALBUMIN (PLASMA PROTEIN FRACTION) (PPF) Albumin with plasma and normal saline (isotonic 4.5% or 5% in 50–1000-mL bottles; concentrated 20% or 25% in 20–100-mL bottles) PPF (plasma protein) – at least 85% albumin and saline (100-, 250- and 500-mL bottles)	1. The rate of administration depends on the reason for administration. It is administered rapidly for volume expansion, but is usually given slowly 2. Use standard administration set with filtered air inlet	Fluid volume overload Allergic reactions Hypotension Chills, fever
CLOTTING FACTORS Cryoprecipitated antihaemolytic factors	1. Administer by standard intravenous drip set 2. Administer promptly on thawing 3. Multiple units are usually administered	Chills and fever
Factor VIII concentrate	1. Reconstitute freeze-dried powder with a small volume of sterile water for injection 2. Administer by syringe as an intravenous bolus through a butterfly needle 3. Use within 30 min of preparation	Short half-life of factor VIII means several administrations of the concentrate may be required to control bleeding Chills, fever Allergic reactions
Factor IX concentrate	As above	

Blood group-compatible FFP must be used. Single donor plasma is separated from whole blood up to 18 hours after collection and lacks the more fragile clotting factors.

Coagulation factors

Cryoprecipitate is prepared from plasma that has been frozen with subsequent controlled thawing, and contains fibrinogen and factor VIII. It can be used, for example, for patients with DIC or liver disease. Coagulation factor concentrates are available as high-purity freeze-dried powders. A variety of factors are available in this form, including factor VIII used in the treatment of haemophilia A and factor IX for haemophilia B. In many clinical situations, coagulation factor concentrates have superseded the use of cryoprecipitate.

Albumin

This is prepared from plasma and is available in different solutions. It is used to expand plasma volume rapidly in severe hypovolaemia, such as in burns or shock.

Nursing responsibilities

The safe administration of blood products is an important nursing responsibility. The nurse managing the transfusion should have sound knowledge of safe transfusion practice and the appropriate clinical skills to assist in the management any adverse transfusion-associated reactions. The nurse should also have effective skills in the education and psychological support of the patient, who may naturally be anxious about the procedure and its possible side-effects. Patients are often particularly concerned about the risks of infection transmission and should have their concerns addressed to their satisfaction. Appropriate information and support can help clients make an informed decision about the procedure. During any transfusion, it is important to consider the client's comfort, particularly as mobility may be restricted for long periods. It may, for example, be feasible for the transfusion to be interrupted at an appropriate juncture to enable the patient to have uninterrupted sleep. It is in circumstances such as these that appropriate knowledge and effective teamwork and communication can improve the overall care of the client.

Collection and storage of red cells

It is important always to follow the local policy for the collection of blood, as this provides some important safety measures. Once collected, blood should be stored only in designated refrigerators and each unit of blood should remain in storage at 4°C until required for use. Individual blood bags should not be kept out of the refrigerator for more than 30 minutes before transfusion.

Checks prior to transfusion

It is important to remember that the systematic use of appropriate checking procedures and vigilance ultimately offers the final protection to the patient. Becoming familiar with and following local guidelines for the checking of blood products before transfusion are key safety elements. It is important that all the information on the transfusion request form, on the compatibility label, on the unit of blood and on the patient's identification bracelet correspond. If any discrepancies are noted – no matter how trivial they may seem – these should be challenged and the transfusion postponed until the discrepancy has been clarified. All queries should be referred promptly to the relevant staff and/or to the prescribing medical officer.

Administration

It is always important use a standard blood-giving set with an integral filter to prevent the transfusion of small clots or lysed cells into the patient's circulation. Giving sets should be changed every 24 hours or when there are significant clots in the filter chamber. The minimum infusion time is a clinical decision and depends on a variety of factors, including the client's general health and the reason for transfusion. The maximum infusion time for a unit of blood is 5 hours because of the risk of bacterial contamination and the deterioration of red cells (McLelland 1996). No drugs or other infusion solutions should be added to the blood bag or the giving set during the transfusion, as there may be significant interactions or red cell lysis. Best practice dictates that other infusions should be given through a separate line. At the end of the transfusion it is important *not* to run normal saline through the giving set, as this can again introduce lysed red cells and small clots into the circulation.

Monitoring

Before the start of the transfusion, the patient's baseline pulse, temperature, respiration rate and blood pressure are recorded. At the start of each unit and at 15 and 30 minutes, the patient's pulse temperature and blood pressure are measured. Thereafter, hourly monitoring of pulse, temperature and blood pressure should be maintained (McLelland 1996). If the client is not in direct view, frequent checks of their general condition should be made. It is also important to monitor fluid balance during the transfusion and to be alert for signs of circulatory overload.

It is also vital to monitor for signs of incompatibility or other adverse reactions. These include chills, rigors, flushes, headache, loin pain, restlessness or feelings of dread, blood in the urine, itching, a rash, breathlessness or chest tightness. Although reactions frequently occur during the first 20–30 minutes of the transfusion, it is imperative to keep vigilant throughout. In the event of a transfusion reaction, it is important to store all of the used and/or partially used bags safely for return to the blood laboratory.

Documentation

Careful documentation of the checking process, the monitoring process, the patient's progress and the time element of the transfusion are all important aspects of safe practice. This is particularly relevant as some complications of transfusion are delayed and careful record-keeping can then provide vital information.

Disposal

Empty blood bags are normally stored locally for at least 72 hours in case of a delayed transfusion reaction. Safe disposal of blood products is an important health and safety issue.

Transfusion reactions

The transfusion of a blood product carries with it some inherent risks. Any blood product could potentially generate an immune response in the recipient. This immune response may take the form of an allergic reaction, a new attack to what the body perceives as a foreign protein, or an antibody response to an unwelcome antigen. Other complex mechanisms underlie some of the potential complications of transfusion. Blood products can also transmit infections from donor to recipient and may create problems such as circulatory overload in the suscep- tible individual. The transfusion reactions discussed below include immediate and delayed haemolytic, febrile non-haemolytic, allergic, infection, circulatory and transfusion-related lung injury.

Haemolytic reactions

Intravascular agglutination of donor cells and their subsequent destruction (haemolysis) are key features of acute haemolytic reactions associated with transfusion. The destruction of donor red cells by recipient antibodies are, in almost all cases, an avoidable consequence of human error in the transfusion process. Rarely, the antibodies fail to be detected in the compatibility tests (Contreras and Hewitt 1999). Usually, however, this is the result of a failure to follow strict protocol in the procurement or administration of blood products. Mistakes in sampling or failure to check the recipient and blood unit effectively are common reasons for this serious, and sometimes fatal, complication. A meticulous approach to procedure and systematic checks are imperative.

Occasionally, haemolysis may be a consequence of transfusing lysed cells from a unit of blood that has either been left to warm excessively for long periods or been incorrectly refrigerated and stored (Contreras and Hewitt 1999). The importance of following correct procedure cannot be overemphasized.

The severity of the ABO-incompatible haemolytic reaction will depend on a number of factors such as the amount of blood transfused, the strength of the antibody response in the recipient and whether destruction is intravascular or occurs in the reticuloendothelial system. Such reactions typically occur within 20 minutes to 1 hour after the start of the transfusion. The timing is, in part, dependent on the speed of transfusion. The patient will typically complain of pain at the infusion site, headache, back pain, flushing, nausea and breathlessness, and may experience a sense of dread. There will also be a rapid rise in the heart rate and drop in blood pressure with possible rigors and pyrexia. The patient may collapse. Acute renal failure and abnormal clotting are possible serious consequences of the acute haemolysis. In very severe cases disseminated intravascular coagulation may exacerbate the problem.

Management of acute haemolysis includes immediate termination of the transfusion, careful monitoring of vital functions and renal function, maintenance of a satisfactory blood pressure and urine output, and maintenance of vascular access. All urine should be saved for the first 24 hours and tested for the presence of haemoglobin. Blood samples should be sent and the unit of blood returned promptly to the laboratory for investigation and analysis. The event should be considered a medical emergency as it constitutes a major cause of serious transfusion-related morbidity and death. A list of actions to be taken in the event of an acute transfusion reaction can be found in Box 14.6.

Delayed transfusion reactions may occur as late as 7–10 days after transfusion. They are generally caused by a proliferation of a previously undetectable antibody to a red cell antigen in the transfused blood. Patients may often be at home by the time this develops, so appropriate information should be given to the client and family to alert them to the possible signs and symptoms. Fever, rapid anaemia, a degree of jaundice and general malaise are key features.

Febrile non-haemolytic reactions

These reactions are frequently a response to donor white cells; less frequently to donor platelets. They may occur at any point during the administration, but often at 30–90 minutes into the transfusion. Often, the patient will experiences chills with a rise in temperature. Occasionally, a prolonged rigor will ensue and this can be very frightening for the patient. Management includes slowing down or temporarily stopping the transfusion, administering antipyretics and reassurance.

Once other causes for the reaction have been ruled out and the diagnosis confirmed, the transfusion can be

---

> **Box 14.6** Management of a transfusion reaction
>
> - STOP THE TRANSFUSION
>
> - Maintain intravenous access with a slow infusion of normal saline
>
> - Contact medical staff for urgent assessment and management
>
> - Save remaining blood/blood product for prompt return to the blood bank for analysis
>
> - Check patient identity, blood product and documentation for possible error
>
> - Monitor patient continuously: pulse, blood pressure, temperature, oxygen saturations, urine output, evidence of bleeding
>
> - Save all urine passed. Send sample for haemoglobin determination, as required.

restarted and administered slowly, with appropriate monitoring. Sometimes hydrocortisone and an antihistamine may be prescribed for a prolonged rigor. This is more commonly seen as a reaction to platelet transfusions. Leuco-depleted blood may also be prescribed for patients with a history of transfusion reactions. With the onset of a pyrexia or chill, it is important to rule out the possibility of a haemolytic reaction or bacterial infection.

Allergic reactions

A severe anaphylactic reaction with breathlessness, wheezing and possible shock is a rare but serious complication. In this circumstance the transfusion is discontinued immediately and the patient should promptly receive medical treatment. Hydrocortisone, chlorphenamine (chlorpheniramine) and adrenaline (epinephrine) should be available; bronchodilators may also be helpful. Careful monitoring of the patient's blood pressure, oxygen saturation and renal function is important. A severe reaction is a medical emergency. Mild urticarial reactions can be treated with an antihistamine.

Infection

The risk of transmission of infection has already been discussed. Bacterial infections, due to a contaminated blood product or to poor asepsis in the management of the intravenous infusion, can lead to a febrile reaction or to sepsis and shock. Current processing and storage techniques minimize the potential for contamination, and effective aseptic technique should always be maintained in the management of blood product administration. The patient may develop pyrexia and feel unwell; often the response to the pathogen or toxins may be dramatic and as potentially serious as that of severe haemolytic reactions, or may even be fatal (Serious Hazards of Transfusion (SHOT) Group 2000). In this instance, aside from the supportive

Allergic reactions
See chapter 6.2

care described previously, the patient will require prompt administration of appropriate antibiotics.

Circulatory overload

A rapid transfusion rate and/or the administration of large volumes of blood or plasma, except in patients whose intravascular volume is depleted (such as those with active bleeding), puts the patient at risk of circulatory overload. Individuals with cardiac or renal insufficiency, pregnant women and the elderly are at particular risk. Careful monitoring of the transfusion rate, the administration of diuretics and careful monitoring of pulse, blood pressure and respiration rates can minimize the risk. Signs and symptoms include breathlessness, coughing, cyanosis and anxiety. Patients may expectorate pink frothy sputum.

Transfusion-related lung injury

Occasionally, pulmonary oedema may develop in the absence of compromised cardiac function. This transfusion-related acute lung injury (TRALI) is thought to be a consequence of sequestration of white cells in the lung microvasculature, leading to pulmonary oedema and respiratory distress. The underlying mechanisms are not fully understood but may in part be due to donor antibodies reacting to recipient white cells. Diagnosis is made from the clinical picture and the condition may initially be difficult to distinguish from circulatory overload. It can occur either during or after completion of the transfusion, and may even occur in the initial stages of the transfusion before any significant volume has been transfused. Treatment includes respiratory support and maintenance of haemodynamic status. This is an important but often difficult to diagnose complication of transfusion therapy with a high incidence of morbidity and death (SHOT Group 2000).

In 1996, the SHOT Group started a voluntary and confidential central reporting system for serious blood and blood product transfusion-related complications. This has led to an increased awareness of the frequency of transfusion-related complications and to some of the factors involved in their occurrence. To date, the most common incident remains the transfusion of an incorrect blood component (SHOT Group 2000), highlighting the need for systematic and careful procedures in the supply, issuing and checking of blood products before transfusion. A recently produced guideline from the British Committee for Standards in Haematology (BCSH 1999) aims to address some of the issues involved in the prevention of wrong blood incidents.

Patient refusal of transfusion

Although blood transfusion is a commonly used therapeutic procedure, it is important to bear in mind that blood is a potent symbol and that different cultures and religions may view the transfusion of blood or its derivatives very differently. Refusal of blood products on religious grounds is usually associated with the Jehovah's Witness community. The origins and functions of this doctrine are discussed by Singelenberg (1990), but it is based on certain biblical references. According to the Jehovah's Witness, the concern over blood products has been justified by what they perceive to be the lack of safety or clinical efficacy of blood transfusions and by the well documented transmission of infections such as HIV and hepatitis with the use of blood products. It is important to respect individual convictions, and most courts now recognize the right of adult Jehovah's witnesses to make this choice for themselves. It has, however, usually been judged that parents and guardians do not have the right to refuse life-saving treatment for children, so that application for court order to protect a child whose parents refuse to consent to a transfusion may be considered appropriate in particular clinical circumstances.

When it becomes apparent that an individual may refuse a transfusion on religious or personal grounds, the use of blood and blood products should be discussed with the person at an early stage. The clinical team should offer a clear explanation of the consequences of refusing treatment, and any possible alternatives to treatment with blood products should also be considered. It is advisable to document the discussion process carefully and to obtain a signed and witnessed statement if ultimately treatment is refused. It is important to remember that other persons may have either general or specific concerns about the safety of blood product therapy and these must also be addressed. In all possible circumstances appropriate informed consent must be sought prior to the use of blood products.

Autologous blood transfusion (ABT)

This technique involves collecting and transfusing the patient's own blood. In certain circumstances it may be an acceptable alternative for someone refusing transfusion. This technique has an important advantage in that it minimizes the risk of the complications of transfusion and, in particular, may reassure the individual who is particularly concerned about the transmission of infections such as hepatitis and HIV. It is also useful in elective surgery if there is a potential shortage of appropriate blood. Surgical procedures, such as major orthopaedic or vascular surgery, that have considerable requirements for blood are ones for which ABT may most commonly be considered. In total up to 2–4 units of blood may be collected over a period of time and stored for a maximum of 5 weeks. Alternatively, cryopreservation can offer long-term storage.

Although, in the right clinical circumstances, this technique can be useful, it is not without risk. First, the risks of bacterial contamination and errors in collection, storage and correct identification and administration are no less for this type of transfusion than for donor transfusions. Second, the patient needs to be fit for the removal of one or more units of blood in a finite time period. Third, there is no guarantee that the recipient will not require donor blood in addition to their own (McClelland 1996). Such procedures do require careful consideration of the risks versus benefits in the specific clinical context.

Two other techniques that allow the use of autologous blood are: (1) preoperative bleeding and isovolaemic haemodilution, and (2) blood salvage. The first method involves the withdrawal of blood from the patient between anaesthesia and the start of surgery with fluid replacement. The venesected blood can then be re-infused after the operation. Blood salvage involves the collection and processing of blood lost during operation. This is then filtered and returned to the patient. This technique is not recommended for patients with bacterial infections, bacterial contamination or malignancy.

Summary

The unique nature of blood – which is the body's only fluid tissue – and its functions, concerned with distribution, protection and maintenance of a constant internal environment, result in some aspect of the blood's composition and function being affected by almost any pathological process. As has been previously stated, blood tests are frequently the starting point for the investigation of a variety of health problems.

This chapter has focused on describing disorders that directly affect the haematological system, be it the blood cells themselves or constituents of the plasma. These disorders arise for a variety of reasons including deficiency in an essential nutrient, inherited genetic disorder, infection and malignant processes yet to be fully understood. They produce numerous acute and chronic symptoms resulting in disruption to the normal daily life of affected individuals. The problems commonly experienced by individuals include anaemia, a tendency to infection and bleeding. Care and management of the individual with these problems is discussed in detail, whilst other potential or associated problems are identified but discussed in less depth.

The nursing skills identified as essential to the nurse involved in caring for patients with haematological conditions specifically relate to:

- management of venous access
- management of the patient at risk of infection due to neutropenia
- management of the transfusion of blood and blood products.

Other non-specific skills of assessment, health promotion and patient education are as vital to the care of these patients as to all others. Symptom management and maintenance of independence are issues for many patients with blood disorders that are chronic in nature. In others, the course of the disease may be rapid and life threatening, as in the acute leukaemias and lymphomas. For these patients there may be ethical issues about when it is appropriate to treat aggressively, for how long, and when to focus on palliative interventions. Many nurses find difficulty in caring for patients with haematological malignancies because patients may be actively treated or experiencing the sequelae of this treatment up to the time of their death. This requires the nurse to take account of ethical principles of autonomy, beneficience, non-malificence and justice (Beauchamp and Childress 1983) and to engage in analysis of the burdens and benefits of treatment with the individual, family members and other members of the multidisciplinary team.

Nurses are pivotal professionals in the patient's pathway from presentation, through treatment, during follow-up and on return to independent living. For families with children with blood disorders, nurses are an essential source of support and encouragement. Thus, the challenges of caring for individuals with blood disorders are many and varied and offer great opportunities for the development of specialist practice.

Critical incident

Mr and Mrs Ng are a Vietnamese couple who settled in this country after escaping from Vietnam. They have a take-away food business. Mrs Ng has never learnt to read or write English and her spoken English is very limited. She always brings her husband to the hospital and he acts as her interpreter. They have one child who lives away from home and is studying at university. Mrs Ng was diagnosed as having a non-Hodgkin's lymphoma. She has been attending the oncology outpatient treatment suite for chemotherapy treatment and had her third course of CHOP chemotherapy just over 2 weeks ago. It is very difficult to establish how she is tolerating this treatment as she apparently insists that all is well.

The last course of treatment had to be postponed for 1 week as her blood count was too low. Mrs Ng was admitted to hospital on Saturday in a collapsed state with septicaemia. You learn that she had been feeling unwell on Friday – cold and shivery, but thought she had caught a chill. Mr Ng had phoned his GP and made an appointment for Monday morning. He had not indicated, and had not been asked, what problem his wife was

(Continued)

References

Alleyne J, Thomas VJ (1994) The management of sickle cell crisis pain as experienced by patients and their carers. Journal of Advanced Nursing 19: 72–75.

Arif S, Mufti A (1998) Immune, blood, and lymphatic systems. London: Mosby.

Atkin K, Ahmad WIU, Anionwu EN (1998) Screening and counselling for sickle cell disorders and thalassaemia: the experience of parents and health professionals. Social Science and Medicine 47(11): 1639–1651.

Beauchamp TL, Childress JF (1983) Principles of biomedical ethics. Oxford: Oxford University Press.

Bouchier I (1998) Third report of the expert group on cryptosporidium in water supplies. Department of the Environment, Transport and Regions. Online. Available: http:www.detr.gov.uk/dwi/pubs/bouchier/index.htm

British Committee for Standards in Haematology (1997) BCSH guidelines on the insertion and management of central venous lines. British Journal of Haematology 98: 1041–1047.

British Committee for Standards in Haematology (1999) The administration of blood and blood components and the management of transfused patients. British Committee for Standards in Haematology, Blood Transfusion Task Force, Royal College of Nursing and the Royal College of Surgeons of England. Transfusion Medicine 9(3): 227–238.

Buchsel PC, Whedon MB (1995) Bone marrow transplantation – administrative and clinical strategies. Boston: Jones and Bartlett.

Cartwright RA (1998) Epidemiology. In: Whittaker JA, Holmes JA, eds. Leukaemia, 3rd edn, pp. 1–21. Oxford: Blackwell Science.

Catovsky D (1999) Chronic lymphoid leukaemias. In: Hoffbrand AV, Lewis SM, Tuddenham EGD, eds. Postgraduate haematology, 4th edn, pp. 405–444. Oxford: Butterworth-Heinemann.

Contreras M, Hewitt P (1999) Clinical blood transfusion. In: Hoffbrand AV, Lewis SM, Tuddenham EGD, eds. Postgraduate haematology, 4th edn, pp. 215–234. Oxford: Butterworth-Heinemann.

Dearnaley DP, Judson I, Root T, eds (1995) Handbook of adult cancer chemotherapy schedules. Abingdon: The Medicine Group (Education) Ltd.

Department of Health (1992) Folic acid and the prevention of neural tube defects. London: DoH.

Donnez J, Bassil S (1998) Indications for cryopreservation of ovarian tissue. Human Reproduction Update 43(3): 248–259.

Gillespie G, Kevaney J, Mason J (1991) Controlling iron deficiency: nutrition policy discussion paper no. 9. Geneva: United Nations Administrative Committee on Coordination/Subcommittee on nutrition.

Gluckman E (1998) Sources of haemopoietic stem cells for allogeneic transplantation. In: Apperley J, Gluckman E, Gratwohl A, eds. Blood and marrow transplantation – the EBMT handbook, pp. 88–97. Paris: European Blood and Marrow Transplantation and European School of Haematology.

Hamblin TJ, Oscier DG (1998) Chronic lymphocytic leukaemias. In: Whittaker JA, Holmes JA, eds. Leukaemia, 3rd edn, pp. 105–135. Oxford: Blackwell Science.

Hewitt PE, Wagstaff W (1992) The blood donor and tests on donor blood. In: Contreras M, ed. ABC of transfusion, 2nd edn, pp. 1–4. London: British Medical Journal.

Hoffbrand AV, Pettit JE (1993) Essential haematology, 3rd edn. Oxford: Blackwell Scientific.

Howard MR, Hamilton PJ (1997) Haematology: an illustrated colour text. Edinburgh: Churchill Livingstone.

Howard RJ, Tuck SM (1993) Haematological disorders and reproductive health. British Journal of Family Planning 19: 147–150.

Lachant NA (1995) Acute leukaemias. In: Skeel R, Lachant N, eds. Handbook of cancer chemotherapy, 4th edn, pp. 395–424. Boston: Little Brown.

Lawn RM (1991) Molecular genetics of factor VIII deficiency. In: Hoffman R, Benz EJ, Shattil SJ, Furie B, Cohen HJ, eds. Hematology: basic principles and practice, pp. 1284–1289. New York: Churchill Livingstone.

Luzzatto L, Gordon-Smith EC (1999) Inherited haemolytic anaemias. In: Hoffbrand AV, Lewis SM, Tuddenham EGD, eds. Postgraduate haematology, 4th edn, pp. 120–143. Oxford: Butterworth-Heinemann.

Marsh J (1997) Management of aplasia. Hematology 2: 181–191.

McLelland B, ed. (1996) Handbook of transfusion medicine; blood transfusion services of the United Kingdom. London: HMSO.

Mehta A, Hoffbrand V (2000) Haematology at a glance. Oxford: Blackwell Science.

Midence K, Shand P (1992) Family and social issues in sickle cell disease. Health Visitor 65(12): 441–443.

Midence K, Fuggle P, Davies SC (1993) Psychosocial aspects of sickle cell disease (SCD) in childhood and adolescence: a review. British Journal of Clinical Psychology 32(Pt 3): 271–280.

Ministry of Agriculture, Fisheries and Food (1996) A guide from the Food Safety Directorate. Food Sense 1 'Food Safety'. London: MAFF.

Oni L (1998) Sickle cell disease and the carer–client relationship. Nursing Times 94(26): 64–65.

Pallister C (1994) Blood: physiology and pathophysiology. Oxford: Butterworth-Heinemann.

Roberts PJ, Linch DC, Webb DKH (1999) Phagocytes. In: Hoffbrand AV, Lewis SM, Tuddenham EGD, eds. Postgraduate haematology, 4th edn, pp. 235–266. Oxford: Butterworth-Heinemann.

Rodriguez Del Pozo P (1994) Paying donors and the ethics of blood supply. Journal of Medical Ethics 20: 31–35.

Shaffer S (1996) Benign lymphoproliferative disorders. Seminars in Oncology Nursing 12(1): 28–37.

SHOT (Serious Hazards of Transfusion) Group (2000) Serious Hazards of Transfusion. Summary of Final Report 1998–99. Manchester: SHOT.

Singelenberg R (1990) The blood transfusion taboo of Jehovah's witnesses: origin, development and function of a controversial doctrine. Social Science and Medicine 31(4): 515–523.

Solzhenitsyn A (1968) Cancer ward. Harmondsworth, UK: Penguin.

Souhami R, Tobias J (1995) Cancer and its management, 2nd edn. Oxford: Blackwell Scientific.

Titmuss RM (1970) The gift relationship: from human blood to social policy. London: George Allen & Unwin.

Tuddenham EGD, Laffan MA (1999) Inherited bleeding disorders. In: Hoffbrand AV, Lewis SM, Tuddenham EGD, eds. Postgraduate haematology, 4th edn, pp. 612–635. Oxford: Butterworth-Heinemann.

Weatherall DJ (1999) Genetic disorders of haemoglobin. In: Hoffbrand AV, Lewis SM, Tuddenham EGD, eds. Postgraduate haematology, 4th edn, pp. 91–119. Oxford: Butterworth-Heinemann.

Young NS (1991) The pathogenesis and pathophysiology of aplastic anaemia. In: Hoffman R, Benz EJ, Shattil SJ, Furie B, Cohen HJ, eds. Hematology: basic principles and practice, pp. 122–159. New York: Churchill Livingstone.

Further Reading

British Committee for Standards in Haematology, Blood Transfusion Task Force, Royal College of Nursing and the Royal College of Surgeons of England (1999) The administration of blood and blood components and the management of transfused patients. Transfusion Medicine 9(3): 227–238.

Important guidelines for anyone involved in blood transfusion.

Buchsel PC, Whedon MB (1995) Bone marrow transplantation: administrative and clinical strategies. Boston, MA: Jones and Bartlett.

This book offers an American perspective on ambulatory care settings, long-term problems and issues of quality assurance for bone marrow transplantation units. Useful for nurses working in this field.

Corner J, Bailey C (2001) Cancer nursing: care in context. Oxford: Blackwell Science.

This text provides a range of insights on cancer, its treatment and the management of cancer-related problems. Highly recommended for those interested in cancer care.

Grundy M, ed. (2000) Nursing in haematological oncology. Edinburgh: Baillière Tindall.

This book provides a good overview of haemato-oncology and associated nursing issues. It is a useful text for nurses new to the field as well as being a source book for those already involved in the care of patients with haematological cancers. The first section relates to diseases, the second examines treatment issues, and there is a final section on nursing care issues.

Hoffbrand AV, Lewis SM, Tuddenham EGD (1999) Postgraduate haematology, 4th edn. Oxford: Butterworth-Heinemann.

An excellent and comprehensive reference book.

Jenkins GC, Williams JD, eds (1994) Infection and haematology. Oxford: Butterworth-Heinemann.

A medical text that provides useful insights on aspects of infection in haematology including a chapter on infection in patients with sickle cell disease.

McLelland B, ed. (1996) Handbook of transfusion medicine; blood transfusion services of the United Kingdom. London: HMSO.

This handbook covers all aspects of blood and blood product transfusion, and is written in an accessible style. Recommended for all clinical areas involved in blood transfusion.

Thomas NT, ed. (1997) Pain: its nature and management. London: Baillière Tindall.

This book provides a comprehensive holistic approach to pain and its management. Of particular interest are the chapters on sickle-cell disease pain and cancer pain; however, the reader will also find other chapters in the book relevant, interesting and useful.

Whedon MB, Wujcik D (1997) Blood and marrow stem cell transplantation: principles, practice and nursing insights, 2nd edn. Boston, MA: Jones and Bartlett.

A book with an American nursing perspective that nurses with an interest in transplantation would find very valuable.

Caring for the patient with a disorder of the gastrointestinal system

Teresa Finlay

Introduction

Overview of the structure and function of the gastrointestinal tract

The person with a disorder of the gastrointestinal system

Health problems in the upper portion of the alimentary canal

Disorders of the stomach and duodenum

Intestinal disorders

The person with faecal diversion

Summary

Conclusion

Introduction

After a brief description of the normal structure and function of the gastrointestinal tract, this chapter considers the care of patients with disorders of the gut. The text considers the more commonly occurring diseases, syndromes and symptoms, both acute and chronic, and describes nursing, medical and surgical interventions for patients experiencing these distressing problems. Starting at the mouth, problems are considered in the anatomical direction of the tract.

To facilitate the conversion of knowledge into practice, some of the commonly encountered conditions are translated into specific aspects of prescribed nursing care including case studies, a care pathway and a care plan. The psychological impact of gastrointestinal disease and its treatment is demonstrated throughout the text and the significance of the professional's self-awareness in this aspect of nursing is highlighted in the critical incident at the end of the chapter.

Overview of the structure and function of the gastrointestinal tract

The alimentary canal

The alimentary canal, frequently referred to as the gastrointestinal tract, is divided into the mouth, pharynx, oesophagus, stomach and intestines. The primary function is to provide the body cells with a continual supply of nutrients, electrolytes and water in a form that is acceptable to the system. To do so, the **gastrointestinal** tract performs the functions of ingestion, digestion and absorption of food and fluid into the blood and elimination of residue and waste products. These functions are controlled by complex levels of integration.

Structural divisions of the gastrointestinal tract (Figure 15.1)

Mouth

The **mouth** or oral cavity, the first part of the tract, is lined by a mucous membrane that secretes mucus to mix with the food, facilitating its movement through the pharynx and oesophagus.

The tongue, teeth and salivary glands are contained within the mouth. The *tongue* is comprised of muscular tissue enclosed in mucous membrane.

There are three pairs of *salivary glands* whose ducts open on to the surface of the mouth. The parotid glands produce a thin, watery secretion which includes an important digestive enzyme, ptyalin. The sublingual glands secrete only mucus; the submaxillary glands produce both a watery and mucous secretion. The secretions of the salivary glands and the oral mucosa collectively form the saliva.

Gastrointestinal system
See chapter 5.1

Mouth
See chapter 5.1

Figure 15.1   Structural divisions of the alimentary canal.

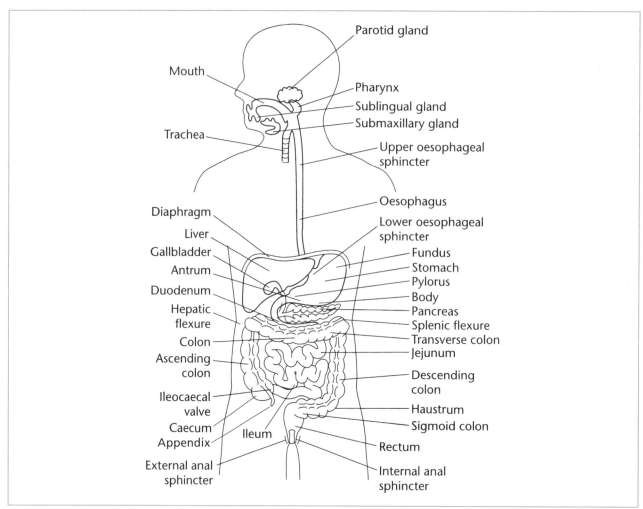

Pharynx

The pharynx serves as a common pathway for food and air. When its muscular tissue contracts, the band of striated muscle known as the cricopharyngeal or upper oesophageal sphincter relaxes; food and fluid are directed into the oesophagus, and the entrances to the larynx and the oral and nasal cavities are closed simultaneously.

Oesophagus

The **oesophagus** is a narrow muscular tube, approximately 25 cm long, that passes down behind the trachea and heart, through the mediastinum and diaphragm to the stomach. A thickened band of smooth muscle forms the lower oesophageal or cardiac sphincter, which opens when food is swallowed.

Stomach

The **stomach** is located just below the diaphragm and is divided into three segments: the fundus, body and pylorus.

The gastric walls have three layers of muscle tissue, one of which, the circular muscle layer, is thickened at the opening of the oesophagus into the stomach to form the *cardiac* or *lower oesophageal sphincter*. Similarly, the

opening into the small intestine is guarded by the *pyloric sphincter*.

The mucous membrane lining is thick and lies in folds to allow for distension as the stomach fills. It contains numerous minute glands made up of three types of secreting cells:

- zymogen cells secrete gastric enzymes
- parietal cells secrete hydrochloric acid
- mucous glands secrete mucus.

The glandular secretions are poured out into the stomach to form collectively the gastric juice.

Small intestine

The **small intestine** is the longest portion of the alimentary canal and is divided into the duodenum, jejunum and ileum. The *duodenum* is the short, proximal portion that originates with the gastric pylorus. It receives the bile and the pancreatic enzymes through a sphincter (sphincter of Oddi) at the junction of the common bile duct and the duodenum. The long *jejunum* and *ileum* lie in loops and fill the greater part of the abdominal cavity.

Oesophagus
See chapter 5.1

Stomach
See chapter 5.1

Small intestine
See chapter 5.1

Figure 15.2 Schematic diagram of two sectioned villi and a crypt to illustrate the histological organization of the small intestinal mucosa.

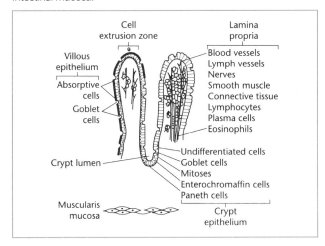

The mucosal surface of the small intestine is covered with many finger-like processes called villi (Fig. 15.2), each of which contains a central lymph channel, called a lacteal, and a network of capillaries. The villi with their microvilli serve to increase greatly the absorptive area of the gut. The small intestine contains many glands that secrete digestive enzymes and hormones on to the glycocalyx, which covers the microvilli. The molecules of digested food are absorbed into the blood in the capillaries and the lymph in the lacteals.

Large intestine

The **large intestine** has a greater diameter than the small intestine and is divided into the caecum, colon, rectum and anal canal. The ileum opens into a pouch-like structure, the *caecum*, in the right lower abdominal quadrant. The *appendix*, a slender blind tube, is attached to the caecum and is often a site of inflammation and infection (appendicitis). At the junction of the ileum and caecum, an *ileocaecal valve* functions to allow contents to pass in one direction only: from the ileum to the caecum.

The large intestine ascends the right side of the abdominal cavity from the caecum as the *ascending colon* and flexes at the undersurface of the liver to form the *transverse colon*. The *descending colon* passes down the left side of the abdomen and, because it takes an S-shaped course through the pelvis, becomes known as the *sigmoid colon*. The mucosa of the large intestine has no villi but has many *goblet cells* which secrete mucus.

The *rectum* is a continuation of the sigmoid along the anterior surface of the sacrum and coccyx. It is about 15–17 cm long.

The short terminal portion of the gastrointestinal tract, the anal canal, opens on to the body surface at the *anus*. The opening between the rectum and the anal canal is controlled by the *internal anal sphincter*, which is not under the control of the will. The anus is controlled by the *external anal sphincter* which, after infancy, is under voluntary control.

Peritoneum

The stomach and intestine are covered by an outer protective layer of serous membrane known as the *visceral peritoneum*. The abdominal cavity is lined with serous membrane called the *parietal peritoneum*. A fan-like expanse is reflected off the posterior abdominal wall and extends to the intestine, where it becomes continuous with the visceral peritoneum. This portion of serous membrane is known as the *mesentery*; it supports the intestine and transmits blood vessels, lymphatics and nerves.

Digestion

Digestion consists of mechanical and chemical processes. The mechanical processes involve the neuromuscular tissues of the alimentary tract and have as their purposes the movement of food through the tract, the mixing of it with digestive secretions, and the repeated breaking up of the food mass to bring more of it in contact with the absorptive surface. These processes include mastication, deglutition (swallowing), movements of the stomach and intestines, and defaecation. The chemical processes are chemical reactions catalysed by enzymes to reduce the food to simpler compounds.

The *digestive enzymes* are substances secreted by mucosal cells of the alimentary tract and by the associated digestive organs (pancreas and liver). They are classified according to the food they act upon. An enzyme that promotes the breakdown of protein is called a *proteolytic enzyme* or *peptidase*; one that acts upon starches is an *amylase*; and a fat-splitting enzyme is known as a *lipase*.

Digestion takes place within the lumen of the alimentary canal or the cells lining the tract. Most food undergoes several chemical reactions before it is reduced to a form that can be absorbed. The steps in the digestive breakdown of protein, carbohydrate and fat are as follows:

■ *Protein* → proteoses → peptones → polypeptides → amino acids

■ *Carbohydrate*
  Starch (polysaccharide) → maltose → glucose
  Disaccharides:
    maltose → glucose
    sucrose → glucose and fructose
    lactose → glucose and galactose

■ *Fat* → glycerol and fatty acids

The motility and secretions vary from one area of the digestive tract to another.

Large intestine
See chapter 5.1

Peritoneum
See chapter 5.1

Digestion in the mouth, pharynx and oesophagus

Motility

The mouth performs mastication (chewing) and the initial part of swallowing. The pharynx and oesophagus are concerned only with swallowing.

Deglutition

Deglutition is commonly referred to as swallowing and involves certain reflexes occurring in rapid succession. The most important action occurs when the larynx is raised, bringing its opening against the epiglottis and the base of the tongue, thus preventing the food from entering the respiratory tract.

The reflex responses of the pharynx to the entrance of food or fluid may be depressed by local anaesthetic. To prevent aspiration following anaesthetization of the pharynx, food and fluid are withheld until the swallowing reflexes have returned. This applies following laryngoscopy, bronchoscopy, oesophagoscopy, gastroscopy and surgery on the mouth or throat. Depression of the swallowing centre in the medulla occurs with general anaesthesia, alcohol and drug intoxication, and following some cerebrovascular accidents, and can lead to aspiration of food and fluid.

Swallowed food (bolus) is propelled through the oesophagus by coordinated waves of muscular contraction and relaxation in the oesophageal wall. This is called peristalsis.

Secretion and digestion

The amount of **saliva** secreted varies from approximately 1–1.5 litres per day. The saliva is swallowed and much of the fluid is reclaimed by absorption.

Saliva at rest has a pH of 6; with stimulation this increases to 7.8. The alkalinity helps to retain the calcium in the teeth. It consists of:

- water (97–99%)
- mucin
- sodium, potassium, bicarbonate, calcium and chloride
- enzyme: salivary amylase or α-amylase (formerly ptyalin)
- organisms
- epithelial cells from the mucosa
- antibacterial agents: lysozyme, which has an antiseptic action, and immunoglobulinA (IgA), which has a defensive action. These agents prevent dental caries and halitosis.

Functions of saliva

One of the **functions of saliva** is to moisten the food and lubricate the oral cavity in order to facilitate swallowing. In addition saliva has a cleansing effect, washing away food debris and maintaining oral hygiene. The sensation of thirst is linked to having a dry mouth owing to the absence of saliva. Saliva therefore plays a key role in fluid intake and fluid balance maintenance.

Regulation of salivary secretion

Control of the salivary glands is by the autonomic nervous system; each gland has both a parasympathetic and sympathetic nerve supply which deliver impulses from a salivary centre in the medulla of the brainstem.

Parasympathetic innervation results in an increased volume of a watery secretion containing the enzyme salivary amylase; sympathetic innervation causes a scanty flow of a thick, viscous saliva. The generalized sympathetic innervation associated with fright or nervousness and stress frequently produces a dry 'sticky' mouth.

Digestion in the stomach

Gastric motility

The stomach retains the food and churns it about for a period of time until it undergoes certain chemical and physical changes. The fundus acts as a storage vessel, whereas the body of the stomach contracts rhythmically about three times per minute to mix the food with enzymes, producing a mixture referred to as *chyme*. The gastric contraction is continuous from the antrum to the pylorus and through to the duodenum. Continued contraction of the pylorus prevents reflux from the duodenum after chyme has been expelled into the duodenum.

Approximately 3–5 hours after the last meal, strong contractions, which originate in the lower oesophagus and stomach, sweep the entire length of the small intestine at about 90-minute intervals. They expel undigested residue and seem to sweep debris along through the small intestines to the colon.

The presence of food in the stomach stimulates volume-sensitive nerve receptors as well as chemical receptors. Increasing volume stretches the stomach wall, which increases the force of contraction and secretion. The presence of proteins stimulates the release of gastrin and other polypeptide hormones that increase motility and enhance antral contractions, forcing more chyme through the pylorus. At the same time, acid and enzyme secretion is stimulated.

The duodenum, however, acts to slow down gastric motility and secretion, preventing overloading.

To summarize, gastric emptying is controlled by the volume and consistency of the stomach content, the effects of the hormone gastrin in stimulating motor and secretory functions, and by neural and hormonal feedback from the duodenum.

Gastric secretion and digestion

The gastric glands secrete a clear, colourless, slimy fluid of high acidity (pH 0.9–1.5) which contributes to

Saliva
See chapter 5.1

Saliva functions
See chapter 5.1

Saliva control
See chapter 5.1

Gastric motility
See chapter 5.1

chemical digestion and changes the food to a more fluid consistency.

The constituents of **gastric juice** are:

- water (97–99%)

- hydrochloric acid (0.2–0.5%)

- enzymes:
    pepsinogen (inactive pepsin)
    renin
    gastric lipase

- inorganic salts of sodium, potassium and magnesium

- haematopoietic or intrinsic factor (promotes absorption of vitamin B$_{12}$)

- mucus.

The hydrochloric acid and enzymes are the substances concerned with chemical digestion. Pepsinogen is activated to pepsin by the hydrochloric acid and the initial breakdown of proteins occurs. Pepsin reduces proteins to proteoses and peptones. The hydrochloric acid secreted by the parietal cells destroys many bacteria which are ingested with food.

Regulation of gastric secretion

The amount of gastric juice produced varies somewhat with the types of food taken, but with average meals it is about 2 litres per day. With fasting, and during the night, the volume is reduced.

Secretion is influenced by mechanical, nervous and hormonal factors, and it is customary to describe gastric secretion as occurring in three phases: the cephalic, gastric and intestinal phases. The *cephalic phase* of gastric secretion occurs before the food reaches the stomach. When food is anticipated, tasted and chewed, sensory impulses from the mouth enter the central nervous system and result in parasympathetic innervation via vagus nerve fibres, stimulating the gastric glands to pour out their secretions.

Food reaching the stomach further stimulates its secretion, producing what is known as the *gastric phase*. The food causes a direct mechanical stimulation of the gastric glands and initiates sensory nerve impulses that are delivered via vagus nerve fibres to the medulla, resulting in return impulses, via vagal motor fibres that increase the activity of the gastric glands. Chemical stimulation is by a hormone, gastrin, which is released by the gastric mucosa into the blood. A natural mucosal resistance prevents pepsinogen from digesting gastric tissue.

Histamine, which is produced, stored and released by enterochromaffin cells in the gastric mucosa, has been found to stimulate the parietal cells of the gastric glands, resulting in an increased output of hydrochloric acid. Two types of histamine receptors, H$_1$ and H$_2$ are present, and the H$_2$ receptors initiate the release of histamine which stimulates the secretion of hydrochloric acid.

The administration of H$_2$ antagonists (e.g. cimetidine, ranitidine) aids in the treatment of ulcerative gastric disease by inhibiting histamine-stimulated acid secretion. More effective inhibition of hydrochloric acid secretion is achieved with a group of drugs that inhibit the proton pump in the parietel cells (e.g. lansoprazole, omeprazole).

The *intestinal phase* of gastric secretion involves an increase in the concentration of various hormones which have a number of effects including stimulation of the parietal cells to produce gastric acid; enhanced contraction of the lower oesophageal sphincter, preventing reflux; and the secretion of insulin and glucagon by the pancreas.

Digestion in the small intestine

Motility

Food moves slowly through the **small intestine** so that digestion may be completed and the simpler molecules absorbed.

The small intestine terminates with the *ileocaecal valve*, which guards the opening into the caecum. The pressure in the small intestine forces open the valve and the fluid passes through into the large bowel.

Muscular and villous activity of the small intestine is regulated by both an intrinsic and an extrinsic mechanism. The intrinsic control is by receptors that are associated with the plexuses, and are sensitive to stretch or irritation of the mucosa. The reflex response is contraction of the muscle tissues which initiates segmentation, peristalsis and movements of the villi.

The extrinsic mechanism operates via parasympathetic impulses stimulating the muscle tissue and conversely sympathetic innervation slowing motility.

Secretion

The digestive juice in the small intestine includes external **pancreatic secretions** and **bile** as well as the secretions of the intestinal mucosal glands.

Pancreatic juice and bile

Approximately 700–1200 mL of pancreatic secretions enter the duodenum daily and consist of:

- water (97–98%)

- enzymes:
    amylase (amylolytic)
    amylopsin
    proteinases (proteolytic):
        trypsinogen (inactive trypsin)
        chymotrypsinogen (inactive chymotrypsin)
        procarboxypeptidase (inactive carboxypeptidase)
    lipase (lipolytic):
        steapsin

- salts: principal ones are sodium and potassium bicarbonate and sodium alkaline phosphate.

Gastric juice
See chapter 5.1

Control of secretion
See chapter 5.1

Small intestine
See chapter 5.1

Pancreas
See chapter 5.1

Bile
See chapter 5.1

Because of the salts, the pancreatic secretion is alkaline, with a pH of 7.5–8.4, and neutralizes the acid chyme. Bile does not contain a digestive enzyme, but the bile salts do facilitate the digestion of fat by the pancreatic lipase.

Regulation of pancreatic enzyme and bile secretion

Pancreatic secretion into the intestine is regulated mainly by hormones secreted by the intestinal mucosa. The entrance of the acid solution chyme into the duodenum causes the release of secretin (pro-secretin) into the blood. When secretin reaches the pancreas, it activates the cells to secrete a fluid high in sodium bicarbonate. Failure to produce this alkaline solution may result in damage to the duodenum by the chyme, which is strongly acid and contains pepsin. The duodenal mucosa is not as well protected by mucus as the gastric mucosa.

The liver cells secrete bile continuously, but the amount is increased when food is taken, especially fat and protein. It is thought that the hormone secretin, which excites the pancreas, may also cause an increased output of bile. The hormone cholecystokinin–pancreozymin, or CCK, causes the gallbladder to contract and bile flows into the common bile duct. It also causes relaxation of the sphincter of Oddi, and bile that has been stored in the gallbladder enters the intestine.

Intestinal juice (succus entericus)

The mucosa of the small intestine produces 2–3 litres of fluid per day. The solution, called succus entericus, is rich in bicarbonate, and the pH varies from 7.0 to 9.0, depending on the region of the intestine. Succus entericus contains:

- water
- salts
- mucin
- epithelial cells
- enzymes:
    entrokinase, which activates the trypsinogen and probably procarboxypeptidase.

Digestion

Most chemical **digestion** takes place in the small intestine.

Any polysaccharides that have not been reduced by salivary amylase to maltose are acted upon by the pancreatic enzyme amylase (amylopsin). Disaccharidases reduce disaccharides to monosaccharides by hydrolysis, producing the simple absorbable sugars, glucose, galactose and fructose. The intestinal enzyme maltase hydrolyses maltose, lactase splits lactose, and sucrase breaks down sucrose. These enzymes are secreted by the absorptive cells and are an integral part of the sticky layer, the glycocalyx. The final splitting of the disaccharides takes place at the microvillous level.

Protein digestion initiated in the stomach by pepsin is completed by several pancreatic and intestinal enzymes such as trypsinogen, which is activated in the intestine by enterokinase and is then known as trypsin. The proteolytic enzymes reduce proteins (polypeptides) to simpler forms of peptides. A considerable amount of ingested protein may be absorbed in the form of dipeptides and tripeptides rather than amino acids. The latter are more slowly absorbed than the peptides.

The breakdown of fats into glycerol and fatty acids is done mainly by the pancreatic lipase, steapsin. The intestinal lipase is less effective. Fat digestion is greatly facilitated by bile, which emulsifies the fat.

Digestion in the large intestine

Motility

Contractions of the muscular tissue in the **large intestine** mix and knead the content as well as move it through the large intestine toward the terminal portion.

Propulsion in the colon occurs as a mass movement three or four times a day, moving the content toward the rectum. When the content reaches the distal portion of the colon, it is then moved into the rectum. As the food proceeds through the mouth, stomach and small intestine, a large amount of water is added to it. Much of this water is reabsorbed in the colon, which changes the consistency of the remaining content. The latter becomes a soft, solid mass referred to as faeces.

Peristaltic **movements** in the large intestine are reflexly stimulated by the entrance of food into the stomach. This gastrocolic reflex results in the faeces being moved into the rectum, giving rise to the desire to defaecate.

Material such as fibre holds water in the faeces and facilitates the mass movements. Lack of mixing contractions and diminished absorption combined with strong frequent propulsive contractile activity result in diarrhoea.

Faecal matter consists of unabsorbed food residue, mucus, digestive secretions (gastric, intestinal, pancreatic and liver), water and microorganisms. The water content is progressively reduced by absorption as the faeces move through the large intestine so that, normally, on elimination the stool is a formed mass. If the faeces are moved rapidly through the large intestine, less water is absorbed and the stool is unformed and liquid. If movement of the faeces and elimination are delayed, an excessive amount of water is absorbed and the stool becomes hard and dry.

Secretion and digestion

The large intestine is a major site of electrolyte and water absorption. It secretes a large amount of viscous alkaline mucus that lubricates the faeces, facilitating their movement through the large bowel. The mucus also protects the mucosa from mechanical and chemical injury, and its alkalinity neutralizes acids formed by bacterial action, which is considerable in the **colon**.

Intestinal juice
See chapter 5.1

Digestion
See chapter 5.1

Large intestine
See chapter 5.1

Movements
See chapter 5.1

Colon
See chapter 5.1

Irritation of an area of the large intestine results in an increased output of mucus as well as an outpouring by the mucosa of large amounts of water and electrolytes in an effort to dilute and wash away the irritant. This causes the condition known as diarrhoea (frequent liquid stools). The loss of fluid and electrolytes may cause dehydration and an electrolyte imbalance.

Intestinal microorganisms

Many **microorganisms** inhabit the intestine, and colonic bacilli are present in large numbers. The tract is sterile at birth, but in a short time organisms that have been ingested with food are present in the intestine. These organisms are useful in that they synthesize vitamin K, which is essential to the production of prothrombin. A deficiency of vitamin K can result in uncontrollable haemorrhage. Intestinal bacteria also synthesize thiamine, riboflavin and folic acid. The organisms normally found in the intestine are non-pathogenic to the tract but may cause disease if they are carried into other tissues.

Absorption

Absorption is the movement of food, water or drugs from the alimentary canal into the blood to make them available to the cells throughout the body. It is performed passively by the physicochemical processes of diffusion and osmosis, and by active transport by the cells.

Like digestion, most absorption takes place in the small intestine. Its surface is especially adapted by the many circular folds in the mucous membrane to increase the surface area. The whole surface is also studded with millions of villi which contain epithelial mucosal cells that are specially adapted for both absorption and secretion. The network of capillaries and the central lymph channel of each villus take up much of the digested food.

Absorption in the stomach is negligible, although alcohol and some drugs are absorbed from the stomach.

Minerals, vitamins, water, drugs, amino acids, simple sugars, fatty acids and glycerol are freely absorbed from the small intestine. Large amounts of water are absorbed in the colon. Approximately 500 mL of fluid pass from the small intestine into the colon daily. About 400 mL of water are absorbed from this, leaving 100 mL to be excreted in the faeces.

The water-soluble vitamins, B complex and C, are generally readily absorbed from the small intestine. The exception is vitamin B_{12}. For absorption of B_{12}, a substance called intrinsic factor is necessary and is secreted by the mucosa of the stomach. A deficiency of the intrinsic factor or of vitamin B_{12} causes a deficiency in the production of mature red blood cells.

The fat-soluble vitamins, A, D, E and K, are absorbed from the small intestine if bile salts and pancreatic lipase are present.

The person with a disorder of the gastrointestinal system

Disorders of the digestive system are many and varied; they may interfere with the ingestion, digestion, absorption of food and fluids, elimination of residue and/or with the immunological defence mechanisms of the body. The clinical characteristics depend largely on the location of the disorder in the system as well as the nature of the aetiological factor. Different diseases may cause similar disorders of function; that is, several manifestations that develop are non-specific.

Modern health education places much emphasis on nutrition, and any interference with the ability to take and retain food creates anxiety in the individual. The common knowledge of the high incidence of malignant disease in the gastrointestinal tract may cause considerable concern in anyone with any digestive problem. Fortunately, the digestive system has considerable reserve; parts of it may be removed and the patient, with some necessary adjustments in diet and living habits, may continue to live a productive life.

Clinical characteristics

In reading the following section, which discusses some of the principal physical effects that gastrointestinal disorder has on the person, you should consider how patient assessment may be influenced and guided by these pathological effects. Not only is it important to discover whether any of these signs or symptoms are present, but it is also important to consider how they may affect the person's life and what fears and anxieties may be generated by these physical signs of disorder.

It is easy for the nurse to know that blood-stained stools are often associated with disorder of the rectum and anus, often without any malignant disease being involved; however, the patient may interpret this as a sign of cancer and understandably be very anxious and concerned. In addition there are powerful taboos and beliefs associated with the act of defaecation that inhibit discussion of what is a very personal and embarrassing bodily function for many people. You must therefore display tact and sensitivity in assessing the patient for evidence of any of the clinical manifestations discussed below and remember that how the patient feels about any sign is just as important as the sign or symptom itself.

Pain

Pain caused by a digestive disorder may be due to strong contractions of muscle tissue, stretching of viscera, chemical or mechanical irritation of the mucosa, inflammation of the peritoneum, or direct irritation or pressure on associated nerves. It may occur in any part of the abdomen, and in some instances the pain is referred to a site remote from its origin. For example, pain arising from a peptic

Bacteria
See chapter 5.1

Absorption
See chapter 5.1

Pain
See chapter 2.3

ulcer or from the biliary tract may be referred to an upper area of the back.

Heartburn is a form of pain that is described as a burning sensation felt behind the sternum. It is usually attributed to irritation of the oesophageal mucosa by reflux of gastric acid fluid into the oesophagus and may be accompanied by regurgitation of some stomach content into the mouth. It may contribute to altered gastrointestinal function.

A person may complain of a sense of fullness, especially after eating. Normally the stomach relaxes and distends to accommodate food without increasing the intragastric pressure. This accommodation may not occur if there is a disease, such as carcinoma, or if the patient is in an anxious state.

Significant characteristics of the pain must be noted and recorded. Meaningful clues include the duration, location, and the nature and onset of the pain as described by the patient. Aggravating factors such as activity, the taking of food or medicine, or some specific experience or emotional stress may exist. Nausea, vomiting, flatulence and defaecation associated with the pain are pertinent observations. The effect of pain on each individual varies and also the pain experience varies with the cause and nature of the pain. For example, the patient experiencing gallstone or kidney stone colic writhes in agony, whereas the patient with peritonitis or paralytic ileus tends to remain immobile.

Anorexia

Nausea and vomiting
See chapter 5.1

Anorexia is a loss of appetite for food and is a common complaint of patients with a digestive disorder, but is also associated with disorders in practically all parts of the body. It contributes to the general debilitation of patients. The individual may even express a revulsion to the odours of food. It may be functional in origin, resulting from an emotional upset.

Nausea and vomiting

Nausea is an unpleasant sensation producing a feeling of discomfort in the region of the stomach and the inclination to vomit. There may be nausea without vomiting, and vomiting may occasionally occur without being preceded by nausea. The involuntary muscular activity that precedes or accompanies vomiting is referred to as *retching*.

Nausea and vomiting are very common symptoms and are seen in a great variety of conditions. They may be manifestations of a digestive dysfunction, may represent hormonal changes such as occur in early pregnancy, or may accompany practically any acute illness or stressful situation.

The vomiting process is initiated by a *vomiting* or *emetic centre* in the medulla oblongata. This centre may be excited by sensory impulses originating in the stomach or intestines, by impulses of psychological origin when fright, unpleasant sights, odours or severe pain are experienced,

or by impulses from a group of neurones referred to as the *chemoreceptor trigger zone* in the floor of the fourth ventricle. The cells in the trigger zone are sensitive to certain chemicals in the blood and to impulses from the portion of the internal ear concerned with equilibrium. Vomiting in motion sickness, radiation therapy, toxaemia and as a side-effect of taking certain drugs (e.g. digoxin) results from impulses that arise from the chemoreceptor trigger zone. The sensitivity of the vomiting centre varies in different individuals; some vomit very readily and with little effort, whereas others are not affected even though the stimulus may be similar and of equal intensity.

The nurse should be alert to the possible effects of vomiting, regardless of its cause. Considerable muscular energy can be expended in frequent vomiting and may result in exhaustion.

Obviously, nausea and vomiting interfere with normal nutrition and, if prolonged, malnutrition and loss of weight and strength occur. The reduced intake and loss of fluid may rapidly lead to dehydration. Loss of gastric secretion may deplete the body electrolytes and cause acid–base imbalance. Acidosis may develop as the patient becomes dependent on body fat as a source of energy. Tooth enamel may be eroded by persistent vomiting, as in *bulimia nervosa*. The patient may complain of abdominal soreness from the retching and muscular effort, and may become increasingly anxious as a result of vomiting.

Regurgitation

Ejection of small amounts of chyme or gastric secretion through the oesophagus into the mouth without the vomiting mechanism being employed is referred to as regurgitation. It may occur as a result of incompetence of the lower oesophageal (cardiac) sphincter, as seen in infants or those with hiatus hernia, or it may be a symptom of organic disease.

Dysphagia

Dysphagia is defined as difficulty in swallowing. The patient may be able to swallow soft foods and liquids but may be unable to take firmer, more solid foods. Others may be able to swallow but complain of pain on doing so.

Dysphagia may be due to mechanical obstruction, dysfunction in the neuromuscular structures involved in swallowing such as motor neurone disease, or to diseases of the mouth, pharynx or larynx. Pain associated with swallowing frequently indicates an organic lesion such as an ulcer due to acid reflux from the stomach.

Loss of weight and strength

If food cannot be taken, digested or absorbed, body tissue cells are deprived of their requirements for normal functioning. Body stores and actual tissues are mobilized to meet the needs, but eventually these may be depleted. The person manifests loss of weight, strength and efficiency.

If the problem is related to a specific food, symptoms characteristic of a lack of that particular food will appear. For example, the effects of a protein deficiency include muscle wasting, weakness, hypoalbuminaemia, oedema, anaemia and, in the child, delayed growth and development. If there is a disturbance in the absorption of vitamin K due to a lack of bile salts in the intestine, the deficiency may be manifested by bleeding, because prothrombin, which is necessary for blood coagulation, will not be produced by the liver.

Changes in the mouth

Changes in the mouth may be of local origin or may be associated with digestive or general disorders. Disturbances may take the form of a coated or furry tongue, dryness, soreness, small ulcers and halitosis. Changes due to local conditions may be caused by inflammation, infection, neoplastic disease or injury of the tongue, buccal mucosa or lips.

Hiccup (hiccough, singultus)

Persisting hiccups or frequent attacks of hiccups may be associated with organic disease of the digestive system. They are caused by intermittent spasms of the diaphragm due to digestive distension, irritation of the phrenic nerve, or a metabolic disorder such as uraemia or toxaemia which affects the central nervous system. The frequency of the attacks and the effect of the hiccups on the patient should be noted. Dehydration, acid–base imbalance and malnutrition may develop, as hiccups may interfere with the taking of fluids and food. Disturbed rest and the expenditure of muscular energy may cause exhaustion. In many instances, the person becomes fearful because of the persistence of the condition.

A sedative or tranquillizer may be prescribed if the hiccups persist. Rarely, if they persist and are having serious effects on the person (exhaustion, dehydration, etc.), a phrenic nerve block or crush is done.

Flatulence

Flatulence is an excessive amount of **gas** in the gastrointestinal tract. The person may complain of a 'full, bloated feeling', pressure or actual pain. The abdomen may be distended and the person may pass gas from the stomach through the mouth or pass (flatus) from the bowel. Excessive gas in the stomach or bowel is frequently due to swallowed air.

Excessive gas in the intestine may result from the ingestion of excessive amounts of gas-forming foods (cabbage, turnips, onions, etc.) or from abnormal fermentation of the food due to bacterial action. Flatulence and distension occur with any obstruction in the gut and with paralysis of peristalsis. Another frequent cause is ingestion of milk in individuals who as adults do not possess the enzyme lactose. This may also occur in individuals who increase milk intake when they have been accustomed to very little.

Borborygmi is a term applied to the sounds made by the movement of a gas and fluid mixture in the intestines that are clearly audible. Borborygmi is an indication of bowel obstruction, although loud sounds do occur in the normal gut on occasion.

Abdominal rigidity

Rigidity of any area of the abdominal wall due to excessively tense muscle tone may be evident in patients with disease of the gastrointestinal tract. The muscle contraction is usually a response to irritation of an underlying structure.

Change in the normal pattern of bowel elimination

A disorder of the intestine may cause a retarded or accelerated movement of contents through the intestine. Delayed movement may cause *constipation*, whereas acceleration of the content causes *diarrhoea*.

Faecal incontinence

Involuntary defaecation is referred to as faecal incontinence. This form of incontinence is often preventable. Involuntary defaecation may be caused by underlying bowel disease, anal sphincter damage or neurogenic impairment.

Bleeding from the gastrointestinal tract

Bleeding in the alimentary canal may be manifested by the vomiting of blood (haematemesis), by melaena (the passage of a black, tarry stool containing blood pigments), or by the passage of frank blood from the bowel. Haematemesis and melaena occur as a result of bleeding in the upper digestive tract. Blood is a gastric irritant, and swallowed blood (e.g. in a nosebleed) will lead to vomiting. The characteristic black tarry appearance of melaena is due to the effect of the digestive enzymes on the blood. Frank blood in the stool usually originates with bleeding in the colon, rectum or anal canal.

It may be necessary in some instances to examine the blood that has been ejected through the mouth to determine whether it has been coughed up (haemoptysis) or vomited. Blood from the respiratory tract is a brighter red and frothy because of the contained air; that from the stomach is usually darker and may contain small clots and food particles. Melaena may be so slight that it goes unrecognized unless a stool specimen is examined for *occult blood*.

The most frequent cause of haematemesis and malaena is peptic ulcer, but oesophageal varices, carcinoma, injuries or a blood dyscrasia may account for the bleeding. Any evidence of bleeding should be promptly reported to a doctor. The patient who has haematemesis or tarry stool is put on bedrest; blood pressure, pulse, respirations, colour

Gas
See chapter 5.1

and general state (e.g. strength and consciousness) are checked frequently to detect signs of shock.

Frank bleeding from the lower part of the tract may be due to erosion of the mucosa, a congenital malformation of arterioles, carcinoma, ulcerative colitis, haemorrhoids or an anorectal fissure.

Health problems in the upper portion of the alimentary canal

Disorders of the mouth and contained structures are numerous and may be of local origin or secondary to disease elsewhere in the digestive system or in some other system. Primary lesions may be due to bacterial, viral or fungal infection, chemical irritation, congenital malformation, injury or neoplastic disease. General diseases frequently accompanied by a mouth disorder include vitamin B complex or vitamin C deficiency, blood dyscrasias, metallic medication intoxication, infectious disease and any condition that interferes with the normal fluid and food intake or salivary secretion.

Predisposing factors in mouth lesions are debilitation, poor dietary habits, poor oral and dental hygiene, dehydration, emotional stress and mouth breathing, and as a side-effect of chemotherapy.

Candida
See chapter 5.1

Disorders of the mouth

Toothache is the most dramatic common manifestation of a mouth disorder and should be distinguished from a dental abscess involving soft tissue. Bleeding of the gums or from a lesion may be present. An offensive breath may indicate sores or infection. Excessive salivation or dryness and/or disagreeable taste may be present. The individual may experience difficulty with clear speech or with swallowing.

Dental caries

Tooth decay is a major health problem caused by the action of organisms on ingested refined carbohydrates; acids are produced which eventually destroy the enamel surface of the teeth. Tooth decay, cavity formation, inflammation and eventual loss of teeth result if measures are not instituted to prevent progression of the process.

Periodontal disease

This disorder affects the tissues that support the teeth. Development of periodontal disease is influenced by the build-up of plaque on the teeth, poor nutrition, poor oral hygiene, malocclusion of the teeth and by some metabolic disorders. Symptoms include inflammation, bleeding and tenderness of the gums and loosening of the teeth. Formation of plaque is prevented by regular brushing especially with an electric toothbrush and use of dental floss and regular examination and care by a dentist.

Acute tooth infection

Infection of the dental pulp or development of an abscess at the 'root' of a tooth is very painful and may cause an increased temperature and general malaise. The person is advised to seek prompt treatment by a dentist.

Stomatitis

This is a term applied to inflammation of the oral mucosa. In some instances, it may involve the gums and the lips. The mucosa is very red and tender, and ulcerative areas may develop.

Thrush (moniliasis)

Thrush is caused by the fungus **Candida albicans** and may also be referred to as *candidiasis*. It may develop in the vagina as well as in the mouth. It occurs most frequently in infants and children and in the very old, but may also appear in debilitated persons. Areas of superficial ulceration occur in the oral mucosa or gums, and the membrane over the lesion becomes white and is easily detached. The condition is treated with nystatin, amphotericin or miconazole. Attention is directed to oral hygiene and also the person's diet in an effort to improve resistance and general condition.

Gingivitis

This is an inflammation of the gums (gingivae) followed by ulceration and necrosis. It is thought to be caused by proliferation of specific fusiform bacilli and spirochaetes which are present in only small numbers in healthy mouths.

The gums are swollen and painful and bleed readily. Excessive salivary secretion and an offensive breath are usually present. There is a loss of marginal gum tissue and of the interdental papillae by the ulceration and necrosis. Lesions may develop on the buccal and pharyngeal mucosa. A smear may be made from the affected area to confirm the diagnosis. Predisposing factors are poor oral and dental hygiene, malnutrition and debilitation. It may be associated with dietary deficiencies, infections, alcoholism or a blood dyscrasia.

Mouthwashes of warm saline are given frequently and normal oral hygiene measures are encouraged. The person is advised not to smoke, and a soft, nutritious diet of non-irritating foods is recommended. The patient will require treatment by a dentist as soon as the acute stage is over.

The condition is infectious and can be transmitted to other persons unless precautions are taken.

Leucoplakia

This condition is characterized by patchy, yellowish-white, firm, thickened areas of the oral mucous membrane or of the tongue. The lesion results from hyperplasia of surface epithelial tissue and keratinization.

The lesions are painless and are considered serious because they may be precancerous. They occur most frequently in men after the fourth decade of life. The lesions usually develop in response to chronic irritation that may be mechanical, chemical, thermal or infective in origin. The lesions may disappear with elimination of the irritation. In many instances, the cause is unknown.

Teeth are checked and defects corrected that may be causing irritation. Smoking should be discontinued and a high-vitamin diet is encouraged. If the area is fissured or ulcerated, a biopsy is done to determine whether cancer has developed. If malignant changes have taken place, surgical excision and radiation therapy are used.

Cancer of the mouth

Heavy smoking and alcohol consumption are the factors most associated with the causation of oral cancer. Poor oral hygiene and diet also contribute. The incidence rose in England and Wales until 1987, since when it has declined slightly, possibly due to less use of tobacco and alcohol, and improved nutrition. However, the incidence has risen slightly in women in the last decade (Munro 1995). Oral cancer has a higher incidence in Scotland. Evidence of the role played by social factors in explaining variations in health is apparent given the higher incidence of smoking and heavy drinking in this area.

The lesion usually appears as a small firm lump. Later the area breaks down, leaving a painful ulcer. If the condition goes untreated, swallowing and speech become difficult, hypersalivation develops, the mucosa becomes infected and the malignant growth metastasizes to the jaw and to the lymph nodes in the neck.

As with all malignant disease, early recognition and treatment are extremely important; *any sore that persists for 3 weeks should receive prompt medical investigation.*

Treatment involves surgical excision of the cancerous tissue, reconstruction using a skin flap and radiation therapy. Irradiation may be by interstitial implantation of needles or by external-beam radiation. When metastasis to lymph nodes is suspected, more radical surgery may be performed to include dissection of the cervical lymphatics, and chemotherapy may be employed. Extension of the malignant disease into the jaw may necessitate complete removal and reconstruction of the jaw. The specialized nature of the operation involved means that most patients are treated in regional units. Patients face major psychological problems in adjusting to the effects of the surgery and coming to terms with the life-threatening nature of the underlying disease. These may not become apparent until after discharge when multidisciplinary specialist skills are required to support patients. Adjustments in breathing, speech and nutritional intake may be needed as well as lifestyle changes in avoiding alcohol and tobacco use (Rhys Evans 1996).

Inflammation of the parotid gland

Inflammation of a parotid gland is the most common disturbance of the salivary glands and may be due to infection by the specific virus that causes **mumps**, or it may develop as a result of any non-specific bacterial invasion of the gland.

Preventive measures include frequent mouth care and keeping the mouth moist by ample fluid intake. The disorder is treated by the parenteral administration of antibiotics. If secretion of pus develops, surgical drainage is necessary. The fluid intake is increased and frequent mouth care is necessary.

Obstruction to the flow of saliva

Obstruction of any one of the salivary glands may be due to intrinsic or extrinsic causes. Disease *within* the gland or duct may be infection, neoplasm or a calculus. *Extrinsic* causes such as a tumour or infection in neighbouring structures may compress the duct, or scar tissue resulting from stomatitis may close off the duct orifice.

The obstruction is manifested by swelling of the affected gland. The swelling is most pronounced during meals because of the salivary stimulation and may subside between meals. Pain and tenderness may be due to the pressure or to the condition causing the obstruction. Fever and general malaise may accompany infection.

A *tumour in a salivary gland* causes a more gradual swelling unrelated to salivary stimulation. It is treated by prompt surgical excision of the gland, as malignant neoplasms of the salivary glands are radiation resistant. Carcinoma involves radical surgery. In the case of cancer of a parotid gland, removal of the mandible and dissection of the cervical lymphatics may be necessary. Surgical excision of the submaxillary gland for malignancy includes dissection of the cervical lymphatics and possible resection of the mandible. Following such disfiguring surgery as removal of the lower jaw, a prosthesis may be constructed from a synthetic material that is physically and chemically inert or from the patient's own bone, grafted from the pelvis or forearm. This is implanted in the area to restore a normal appearance. The psychological trauma of such surgery is a major factor in patient recovery and will need sensitive nursing care.

Following any operation on the parotid gland, the patient is observed for signs of facial paralysis because of the close proximity of the facial nerve to the operative site. In some instances the facial nerve may be involved by a malignant tumour and is removed with the gland, leaving the patient with some permanent facial paralysis.

Mumps
See chapter 5.1

Fracture of the jaw

Fracture of the jaw is a relatively common injury in motor accidents, some sports and assault.

Treatment and nursing intervention

If the fragments are displaced, they are approximated and the lower jaw is immobilized by wiring the lower jaw to the upper jaw or by attaching soft metal bars to the upper and lower teeth. These bars have hooks from which rubber bands extend between the upper and lower jaws, applying traction and fixation.

Following immobilization of the lower jaw, the patient is placed in a semiprone or lateral position to promote oral drainage and prevent aspiration of secretions during recovery from anaesthesia. A wire cutter is kept at the bedside; if the patient vomits, suction is applied and the wire or bands that immobilize the lower jaw must be released immediately so the mouth can be opened to prevent aspiration. A nasogastric tube may be passed and attached to low suction to remove gastric contents and reduce the risk of aspiration. Pharyngeal and oral suctioning with a small catheter may be necessary to remove secretions; trauma and resulting oedema of pharyngeal tissues may interfere with swallowing.

The patient receives a high-calorie fluid diet prescribed by a dietician. It may be given for a brief period via the nasogastric tube but as soon as possible it is taken orally through a straw.

The mouth is cleansed thoroughly every 2 hours and after each feeding. Normal saline or a mild antiseptic mouthwash, such as chlorhexidine gluconate (Corsodyl), may be used, and the teeth brushed as usual using a soft paediatric toothbrush if necessary (Turner 1996). The buccal mucosa and exposed area of the gums are examined twice daily for lesions and deposits of food, microorganisms and epithelial elements.

Early ambulation is encouraged and the patient may be discharged from the hospital as soon as he or she can care for themselves. You should teach the patient and/or a family member the importance of good oral hygiene and how to carry out the necessary cleansing and inspection. The diet, with suggestions for variation, and its preparation and digestion are discussed in detail in consultation with a dietician. When the wires are removed the patient is urged to see a dentist.

Health promotion relating to the mouth

A person's sense of well-being, comfort, ability to maintain good nutrition, and personal attractiveness are all enhanced by effective mouth care. The nurse can play an effective role in educating individuals and groups of all ages to develop health habits that encourage good oral hygiene and ensure the early identification and correction of problems. The aim is to promote healthy teeth, gums and oral mucosa.

Assessment

The following are key elements of the patient's health history:

- current oral hygiene
- any previous dental or oral disorders
- eating and drinking habits

- smoking or use of chewing tobacco
- general health status as related to oral health.

Physical examination

A tongue depressor and light are needed to inspect the oral cavity and tongue. In a normal, healthy mouth:

- the lips are moist and intact
- breath is free from odour
- teeth are white, intact, firm and free from caries, jaggedness or plaque
- the gums are moist, pink, intact and adhere to the teeth
- the mucosa is moist, pink, soft and intact
- the tongue is pink and moist with minute papillae on the superior surface.

Observation of the mouth may elicit significant information as to the person's state of hydration and nutrition as well as manifestations of systemic disease and local disorders. The tongue and mouth are the first sites to reflect dehydration; the mouth and tongue become dry and the latter may be furred. Dryness in some instances may be a side-effect of a drug that is being administered. Bleeding of the gums may indicate a deficiency of vitamin C or an infection. Excessive salivation (sialorrhoea) may be associated with a vitamin B deficiency or certain medications, or a neoplasm in the mouth or neighbouring structure.

The lips are scrutinized for lesions (e.g. lumps, cracks, blisters, ulcers), dryness and abnormal colour, and palpated if necessary to determine the presence and extent of a mass.

Goals

The individual will demonstrate:

1. Teeth that are white, intact and firm.

2. Pink, moist, intact gums, oral mucosa and tongue.

3. Understanding of the need for:
   a. daily oral hygiene
   b. dental check-ups every 6 months
   c. maintaining nutritional and fluid needs.

4. A plan to inspect mouth regularly for signs of irritation, inflammation and infection.

5. Properly fitting dentures and/or repair or reconstruction of teeth.

Nursing intervention

- Use of a toothbrush and toothpaste is the method of choice.

- A soft paediatric toothbrush or foam sticks can be used by individuals who are unable to tolerate toothbrushing. These will not remove debris from the surface or between the teeth but will cleanse the oral mucosa. The stick, after immersion in appropriate mouthwash solution, should be rotated gently over the mucosa, teeth, gums and tongue, ensuring that the whole surface is used.

- The choice of appropriate agent should be determined by assessing the person's needs and after assessment of the oral cavity. Turner (1996) points out that, although hydrogen peroxide is useful in dislodging debris, it has many disadvantages such as forming an excellent growth medium for candida, causing burns if not suitably diluted and causing tongue fissures. Saline solution has much to recommend it for safe effective mouth care. Petroleum jelly may be used sparingly on the lips to create an oil film, preventing loss of moisture.

- Provide artificial saliva and instruct the individual with a dry mouth or reduced saliva to use it to best effect.

- Frequency of mouth care will be dependent on the needs of the individual and factors which increase mouth dryness, debris accumulation and plaque formation, such as continuous oxygen therapy, intermittent suction, no oral intake, following anaesthesia.

Evaluation

Inspection of the person's mouth should show evidence of regular oral hygiene and dental care, and the individual should be able to describe measures taken on a regular basis to promote oral hygiene as appropriate.

Oral surgery

The major surgical procedures are performed most frequently for carcinoma (Box 15.1).

Disorders of the oesophagus

Manifestations of oesophageal disorders include dysphagia (difficulty in swallowing), regurgitation, heartburn, substernal pain and bleeding.

Causes

Interference with the transmission of food and fluid from the mouth to the stomach may be due to an abnormal condition within the **oesophagus** or to an extrinsic disorder. Swallowing may be impaired by a disturbance in innervation to the oesophageal muscle tissue, a decrease in or an obstruction of the lumen of the tube, or by mucosal irritation and inflammation.

> **Box 15.1**   Summary of the main oral surgical procedures
>
> - *Lip resection* is the excision of a portion of a lip. It is usually done to remove a benign or malignant tumour
>
> - *Glossectomy* is the removal of the tongue for the treatment of carcinoma
>
> - *Hemiglossectomy* is the excision of part of the tongue in either the oral or the pharyngeal area
>
> - *Mandibulectomy* is the removal of the lower jaw bone; it may be partial or complete
>
> - *Maxillectomy* is removal of the upper jaw bone and may be partial or complete
>
> - *Buccal resection* is the excision of a section of cheek (bucca)
>
> - *Radical neck dissection* (*en bloc* dissection) involves the extensive excision of cervical lymph nodes and non-vital tissues on the side of a primary malignant neoplasm of the salivary gland, tongue, mouth or pharynx.

Disease of neighbouring structures

As the mouth, tongue and pharynx are involved in directing food and fluid into the oesophagus, it is obvious that disease in any one of these structures may interfere with the initial phase of swallowing. This may be seen in severe stomatitis, pharyngitis, tonsillitis, cleft palate and neoplastic disease of the mouth or tongue. The condition may actually interfere with the swallowing process or cause so much pain that the patient avoids swallowing.

Compression of the oesophagus by enlargement or neoplasms of neighbouring structures occurs rarely. Examples are goitre (enlargement of the thyroid), thoracic aortic aneurysm and enlargement of the mediastinal lymph glands.

Neurological disorder

Dysphagia may result from a nervous system disorder that affects innervation to the central striated muscle tissue of the oesophagus. Damage to the swallowing centre in the medulla or to nerve fibres of the tenth cranial (vagus) nerve concerned with the swallowing mechanism may cause a partial or complete paralysis. Failure of the normal pharyngeal phase of swallowing may result in food passing into the trachea and the nasal cavities. The sphincter at the oesophageal opening may remain relaxed, allowing air to be drawn into the oesophagus during inspiration.

Conditions in which paralysis of swallowing is commonly seen include motor neurone disease (a progressive, degenerative disease of the central nervous system involving upper and lower motor neurones) and cerebrovascular accident (stroke).

Oesophagus
See chapter 5.1

Congenital abnormalities

A congenital abnormality may occasionally be the cause of impaired swallowing in the newborn infant. The most common malformations of the oesophagus include atresia, stenosis and tracheo-oesophageal fistula.

Reflux oesophagitis

The most common cause of oesophageal mucosal irritation is regurgitation of gastric content. Bacterial, viral or fungal infection may be imposed on the inflammation. Diagnosis is usually made on the basis of the patient's complaint of dysphagia, intolerance to hot, spicy foods, and substernal pain and heartburn. Endoscopy or barium studies may be performed to confirm the diagnosis. Biopsy and cytological examination of tissue of affected areas may be performed to exclude carcinoma.

In the case of chronic regurgitation of acid gastric content into the oesophagus, function studies are undertaken. The level of the lower oesophageal sphincter is measured and the pH of the oesophagus at 5 cm above the sphincter is recorded over 24 hours with a naso-oesophageal probe. If the lower oesophageal sphincter is incompetent, gastric contents reflux into the oesophagus, which leads to a burning sensation. The lower oesophageal sphincter is normally positioned within the abdomen (just below the diaphragm). When it is displaced into the thorax, as in a hiatus hernia, the lower oesophageal sphincter pressure is less than the intra-abdominal pressure, and reflux occurs. Sphincter incompetence also occurs in degenerative disorders of smooth muscle.

Treatment

This may include elevation of the head of the bed to reduce the reflux of acid gastric content during sleep; the administration of an antacid orally and inhibition of gastric secretion by a proton pump inhibitor such as lansoprazole (Zoton) or omeprazole (Losec). Rees and Williams (1995) also recommend the use of the reflux suppressant Gaviscon to protect the oesophageal mucosa. Smoking, alcohol, onions, tomatoes, spicy food and fatty meals should also be avoided.

The person is advised to remain upright for at least 2 hours after a meal and should avoid medication that could exacerbate the problem, such as salicylates, phenylbutazone and anticholinergics. Drinking milk is contraindicated because the high calcium content stimulates gastric acid secretion. A weight reduction programme in the obese may help to reduce symptoms. If the cause of persistent oesophagitis is an incompetent lower oesophageal sphincter, surgical repair to prevent reflux may be necessary. The operative procedure frequently used is a fundoplication, in which the fundus of the stomach is wrapped around the lower end of the oesophagus and sutured to it, or a modified form of this may be performed.

Chronic oesophagitis may incur progressive formation of scar tissue leading to stricture. This may be treated by intraluminal dilatation or may necessitate surgical correction. Also, chronic reflux can lead to altered cell histology, known as Barrett's oesophagus, in the lower oesophagus. This is asymptomatic but highly increases the likelihood of developing oesophageal cancer (Hamilton 1998).

Oesophageal achalasia

This is the term used to describe the inability of the lower oesophageal sphincter to open in response to swallowing, accompanied by a lack of tone in the musculature above the sphincter and loss of peristalsis in that area. The cause of achalasia is unknown. The oesophagus gradually dilates above the denervated sphincter. The result is an accumulation and stagnation of food and fluids in the dilated segment.

The symptoms of the disorder are a full, uncomfortable feeling in the substernal region, heartburn, inability to belch, dysphagia, regurgitation and eventually weight loss. The person may also experience coughing and dyspnoea due to pressure on the trachea by the distended oesophagus; a disturbance in normal cardiac functioning or pulmonary complications (aspiration pneumonia), due to inhalation of oesophageal contents, may be manifested.

Achalasia may be treated by repeated endoscopic dilation or by the surgical procedure oesophagomyotomy, which involves division of the muscle fibres at the lower end of the oesophagus. The food bolus then enters the stomach simply due to the effect of gravity. The patient then tends to develop reflux oesophagitis.

If dysphagia is accompanied by severe chest pain, the patient may undergo repeated cardiovascular examinations. A diagnosis of an oesophageal origin of the pain may reduce the anxiety and the dysphagia as emotional stress and anxiety tend to aggravate the disorder.

Trauma of the oesophagus

Dysphagia or aphagia may occur as a result of the ingestion of a caustic substance, foreign objects or too large a mass of food.

When a *caustic substance*, such as a strong acid (e.g. sulfuric or nitric acid) or base (e.g. household bleach) is swallowed, serious corrosive burning occurs in the oesophagus. The larynx may also be affected, as well as the lips, mouth and pharynx. The mucosa manifests acute inflammation, blisters, oedema and possible ulceration. If the chemical is not removed or neutralized promptly, burning and corrosion of deeper layers of tissue occurs. Later, with healing, scar tissue forms and the lumen of the oesophagus is constricted. Dysphagia progressively becomes more serious over several weeks as scar tissue is laid down.

There will be evident corrosive burns on the lips and in the mouth; the voice may be hoarse and the patient experiences dysphagia and probably dyspnoea, and difficulty with speech due to laryngeal irritation and oedema. Shock may develop quickly.

Management

Management of the person who has swallowed a caustic substance includes the following:

1. The chemical swallowed is immediately identified: the lips, mouth and clothing are examined if necessary for evidence. If a container of the chemical that was taken is available, the label is checked for suggestions as to an effective antidote. Milk may serve as a neutralizing agent.

2. Vital signs are assessed and treatment for respiratory insufficiency and shock commenced promptly.

3. An oesophagoscopy is done as soon as possible (within 12–24 hours) to determine the extent and depth of the burns.

4. An analgesic is prescribed for the relief of pain.

5. Oropharyngeal suctioning may be necessary to prevent aspiration of secretions.

6. Sips of water may be permitted. Gastric lavage and induced vomiting are contraindicated to prevent further damage to the oesophageal wall. An intravenous infusion is given to provide fluid and electrolytes.

7. A tracheostomy may be necessary if laryngeal oedema is indicated by respiratory distress and stridor. Blood gases are monitored.

8. A corticosteroid preparation is prescribed to reduce the inflammatory response and to lessen scar tissue formation and ensuing stricture. An antibiotic preparation is usually given to prevent serious infection.

9. A gastrostomy may be necessary in severe constriction in order to provide adequate food and fluids or the administration of parenteral feeding.

10. Stricture of the oesophagus is treated by bougienage; as soon as sufficient healing has taken place, bougies are placed into the oesophagus every day or two to dilate the lumen. The interval between treatments is gradually lengthened, but the dilatation may extend for over a period of a year or more.

11. If bougie therapy is not successful, surgical resection of the constricted area with an end-to-end anastomosis may be performed. When the area is extensive, surgical reconstruction of the oesophagus may be undertaken. A plastic tube or a section of intestine may be implanted to provide a patent passageway.

Nursing intervention

The oesophagus may be injured by a rough or sharp foreign body (e.g. a fishbone). The object may cause dysphagia or aphagia. The person experiences choking and becomes frightened and agitated. An oesophagoscopy is done and the foreign body located and removed. The person may complain of soreness and dysphagia for a few days.

Neoplasms of the oesophagus

Benign neoplasms

These occur rarely in the oesophagus. The most common of these are leiomyomas, which are tumours of non-striated muscle tissue. Those encountered less frequently are polyps, cysts, fibromas, adenomas and fibrolipomas. As the tumour imposes itself on the lumen of the oesophagus or interferes with normal muscle activity, dysphagia occurs. Usually the patient first experiences difficulty in swallowing the more solid foods, such as meat and bread.

Carcinoma

Cancer of the oesophagus tends to develop more often in the older age group. Its incidence is increasng and is more common in males aged 50–70 years, and the lower third of the oesophagus is the most common site. One in 5000 people die from oesophageal carcinoma per year in England and Wales (Finlay 1997). The majority of malignant tumours of the oesophagus are squamous cell cancer. Adenocarcinoma may occur, but is most frequently secondary to gastric carcinoma.

Clinical characteristics

The patient complains first of dysphagia with solid foods which gradually progresses to difficulty with liquids. Substernal discomfort and pain, regurgitation and loss of weight and strength are experienced with steadily increasing severity. In advanced states, bleeding may occur. Structures adjacent to the primary lesion may become involved: the disease may spread to the trachea, bronchi, stomach, diaphragm or associated lymph nodes, depending upon its location in the oesophagus.

Diagnosis is made by oesophagoscopy and/or barium swallow. A biopsy and a smear from the lesion are taken for cytological study during the endoscopic examination.

Treatment

Treatment may be by surgical resection and/or irradiation. Various surgical procedures may be employed, but many tumours are inoperable and only palliative treatment is possible. If surgical intervention is carried out, the affected part of the oesophagus is resected with a wide margin of normal tissue as well as the regional lymph nodes. If the lesion is in the lower part, the upper portion of the stomach is also removed (oesophago-gastrectomy). The remaining proximal portion of the oesophagus is anastomosed to the stomach, which is drawn up into the thoracic cavity (oesophagogastrostomy). A nasogastric tube is passed and remains in place until the anastomosis is well healed and peristalsis is established.

If the tumour is located in the middle or upper portions of the oesophagus, surgical treatment involves excision and radical reconstruction of the oesophagus, which is associated with significant risk; radiotherapy may be preferred.

Relief from dysphagia in individuals with extensive disease may be achieved by the palliative surgical approach of inserting a stent or a feeding tube through the constricted area.

The prognosis is very poor, with only a minority of patients likely to survive for more than 1 year whatever treatment regimen is employed.

Oesophageal varices

This serious condition is associated with cirrhosis of the liver and is discussed in Chapter 16.

Assessment of the patient with oesophageal disorder

The patient admitted to hospital will probably have had a period of increasing difficulty in swallowing, leading to undernourishment. It is important to discover what foodstuffs can still be swallowed in order that the patient be given an appropriate diet. Height and weight should be assessed and the patient asked whether they have lost weight recently. Serious undernourishment may be present, which can significantly reduce the patient's prospects of recovery; consequently dietary supplements may be necessary and the involvement of a dietician is important.

The person's mood and feelings about the illness should be explored. The inability to eat and subsequent loss of weight may lead to great anxiety and fear. The person may suspect cancer but not have been told the diagnosis; clearly it is important to discover how the person feels about the illness and what questions he or she has. The patient may also see a significant change in his or her body, which constitutes a serious challenge to self-concept. The nurse needs to know how successfully the person is coping with this challenge and what methods are being used to adapt in order to approach the patient sensitively and give support.

Oesophagoscopy

The oesophagus may be examined and a biopsy specimen obtained by oesophagoscopy if the patient has complained of dysphagia, gastric reflux or regurgitation, or haematemesis. Oesophagoscopy is useful in localizing bleeding and is also used to remove a foreign body or a bolus that has lodged in the oesophagus (oesophago-gastroduodenoscopy (OGD); see p. 454).

Nursing care of the person having surgery of the oesophagus

Preoperative care

Early involvement of other members of the health-care team, such as dieticians, medical social workers, occupational therapists and physiotherapists, are of the utmost importance. The nurse has an important role in coordinating the multidisciplinary team, ensuring continuity and encouraging the individual to participate in therapy.

Anticipatory grief and *anxiety* are real problems for both the person facing the operation and their family. The nurse must spend time assessing their understanding of the surgery and prognosis, provide information as indicated, identify their needs for emotional support, promote the development of coping strategies and help with the grieving process.

Preoperative preparation also includes emphasis on the promotion of *respiratory function* and teaching deep breathing and coughing techniques. Stopping smoking is essential for all patients who smoke.

The establishment of good *oral hygiene* and the alleviation of infections and potential causes of oral infections are important aspects of care. The person is referred for necessary dental repairs before operation.

Optimal *fluid and nutritional status* is an important goal, involving the administration of oral, nasogastric and/or parenteral nutrition as indicated. Fluid intake should be adequate and deficits corrected.

Postoperative care

Principal patient *goals* in the postoperative period are that respiratory complications will be avoided, the wound will heal without complications, and the patient will be free of pain, having a fluid intake of 2.5 litres per day, avoid weight loss and be able to discuss plans for discharge and self-care in a positive way.

Hiatus hernia

The openings of the diaphragm that accommodate the oesophagus and aorta are potential sites for the herniation of abdominal viscera into the thoracic cavity. The hiatus through which the oesophagus passes is the most vulnerable area; normally, when oesophageal content passes into the stomach it does not return to the oesophagus. If it does, it is referred to as reflux (a return flow).

Causes

The chief causes of the defect in the diaphragm are considered to be a congenital weakness and the ageing process. The former probably results from a defect in the fusion of tissues around the opening. The incidence of hiatal hernia is much greater in middle-aged and elderly persons, and is probably due to weakening of the diaphragmatic muscle. The weakness or gap that occurs results in imperfect closure of the hiatus around the oesophagus. Rarely, the hernia may be caused by trauma such as a fractured rib or perforating foreign object (e.g. bullet) or prolonged, extreme, intra-abdominal pressure as occurs in ascites or pregnancy.

Figure 15.3   (a) Sliding hiatus hernia. (b) Paraoesophageal hernia.

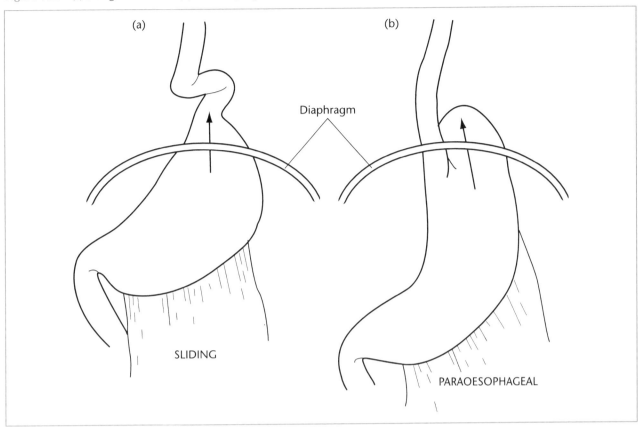

Classification

The hernia may be classified as sliding (oesophago-gastric) or rolling (paraoesophageal) (Fig. 15.3). A *sliding hiatal hernia* is one in which the oesophagogastric junction and a portion of the fundus of the stomach ride up into the thoracic cavity. In a sliding hernia, the lower oesophageal sphincter at the oesophagogastric opening (cardia) loses function, resulting in reflux of the gastric contents into the oesophagus. In a *rolling* or *paraoesophageal hernia*, a sac-like portion of the peritoneum and stomach herniates through into the thorax alongside the oesophagus. A section of omentum may also be extruded. The cardiac sphincter usually remains competent but the displaced portion of the stomach occupies space within the mediastinum and may cause respiratory distress or impaired cardiac function by direct pressure on the heart. Distension of the herniated segment or strangulation may develop, which demands emergency surgery.

Clinical characteristics

The symptoms depend upon the size of the hernia and the amount of displaced viscus. Intermittent mild digestive disturbances only may be experienced. The patient may complain of substernal burning pain or discomfort (heartburn), regurgitation of acid fluid, belching, a feeling of fullness and shortness of breath. The symptoms are frequently precipitated by stooping over, straining

associated with increased intra-abdominal pressure or a large meal. It may also be brought on when the patient is recumbent and may be relieved by sitting up.

Frequent reflux may cause oesophagitis, ulceration and bleeding. Scarring may develop that causes some constriction and probably dysphagia.

Diagnosis

This is made by the person's history and by an OGD or barium swallow. The pain of reflux oesophagitis associated with hiatal hernia is often similar to that associated with angina pectoris and myocardial infarction.

Therapeutic management

The principles of management are similar to those described for the treatment of reflux oesophagitis (see p. 448).

If a loop of the intestine or a portion of the stomach becomes confined in the thoracic cavity, surgical treatment is essential to return the viscus to the abdominal cavity. The surgical approach is usually made through the chest, but occasionally may be made via the abdominal cavity. Following replacement of the viscus, the hiatus hernia is repaired. A nasogastric tube is likely to be introduced, and mild suction is applied to prevent vomiting and intestinal distension. Fluids are administered by intravenous infusion for the first day or two, and then gradually introduced by mouth when the gastric suction is discontinued.

Case Study 15.1 describes the management of a patient with hiatus hernia and gastro-oesophageal reflux.

Case Study 15.1   *Hiatus hernia and gastro-oesophageal reflux*

Mrs Vines, a 60-year-old widow is admitted as a day case to the endoscopy unit. On arrival she explains that her husband died following a myocardial infarction a year ago. She has two adult children and three grandchildren, all of whom live some distance away. She has had symptoms of heartburn and 'indigestion' for over a year and attributes them to being upset about her husband's illness and death. She is particularly disappointed to miss out on the retirement they had planned.

Mrs Vines is scheduled to have an oesophagogastro-duodenoscopy (OGD) to diagnose or exclude peptic ulcer, gastric carcinoma, gastro-oesophageal reflux disease and oesophagitis. Mrs Vines describes the symptoms specifically as a central chest pain, which frightens her. This is associated with a burning sensation at the back of her throat before and after eating, and feeling full with only small amounts of food. She has lost weight (about 4 kg) over the last 6 months. She was referred for OGD by her GP when ranitidine 300 mg daily at night had no effect, and a serum *Helicobacter pylori* test had proved negative.

Mrs Vines is accompanied by a neighbour who will take her home later and ensure she recovers from the sedation. She has starved for 6 hours beforehand as advised, and has not taken ranitidine for 2 weeks prior to the OGD. Mrs Vines is naturally anxious about the procedure as the GP has briefly explained it to her. Having been assessed, she is seen by the person who will perform the OGD and signs a consent form after a thorough explanation of the procedure. In the endoscopy room she is seated on a trolley and the back of her throat is sprayed with lidocaine (lignocaine) to numb it. She is then asked to lie down and a mouthguard is inserted to prevent biting the endoscope. Sedation is given intravenously and oxygen administered via a face mask held by the nurse, who monitors her vital signs throughout the procedure. The OGD is completed without difficulty and reveals a sliding hiatus hernia of 3 cm, which could explain Mrs Vine's symptoms. Mild oesophagitis is noted from the reflux and biopsies are sent for histology to rule out Barrett's oesophagus. Her stomach and duodenum both appear healthy.

Mrs Vines is then wheeled to the recovery area where blood pressure, heart rate, respiratory rate, colour and

percentage oxygen saturation are measured regularly until the sedation begins to wear off. When she is awake, she is offered a cool drink. As Mrs Vines drinks this without pain or discomfort, she is given biscuits to eat. When able to move independently she is discharged home in the company of her friend. She is advised to rest for the day, and not to drive or sign any important documents for 48 hours. She is also asked to contact her GP in the event of sudden pain or fever in the next 24 hours, and to make an appointment after 2 weeks to discuss the findings of the procedure including the histology report. She may resume her medication that night.

The GP is advised of the diagnosis by the endoscopist and it is suggested that she be prescribed a proton pump inhibitor, such as lansoprazole 15–30 mg daily, and Gaviscon 15 mL as required up to four times daily after meals and last thing at night. Mrs Vines should avoid heavy physical work or lifting. She should eat regularly three times a day, not within 3 hours of going to bed and have her main meal in the middle of the day. Tomatoes, onions, spicy foods, caffeine and excessive amounts (> 2 units/day) of alcohol are to be avoided. If reflux continues to be a problem at night, she may consider raising the head of her bed 20–30 cm from the floor to facilitate stomach emptying and avoid reflux. Her symptoms will need to be monitored and a further OGD may be indicated to check for changes in the oesophageal mucosa. Mrs Vines may require surgery in future if lifestyle changes and the prescribed drug treatment are not effective.

Disorders of the stomach and duodenum

The gastric and duodenal disorders most frequently seen include gastritis, peptic ulcer and carcinoma.

Gastritis

The term gastritis implies inflammation of the stomach. The condition may be acute or chronic and the pathological process is usually limited to the mucosa.

Causes

The causes of acute inflammation may be the ingestion of large quantities of alcohol, contaminated foods or non-steroidal anti-inflammatory drugs (NSAIDs) (e.g. aspirin, ibuprofen). Infective gastritis is most frequently due to the ingestion of foods bearing staphylococci or salmonella organisms.

Clinical characteristics

The patient with acute gastritis becomes ill suddenly and suffers severe epigastric pain, nausea, vomiting and fever.

The treatment includes giving the patient nil by mouth, parenteral fluids and maintaining bedrest. Clear

Stomach
See chapter 5.1

Duodenum
See chapter 5.1

fluids are given when the symptoms subside and, if tolerated, a bland diet of soft foods is introduced and progressively increased until a normal diet is resumed.

Chronic gastritis occurs with prolonged and repeated irritation of the mucosa and results in atrophic changes in the **mucosa** and glands. The cause may be unclear, as the condition may be associated with other diseases such as pernicious anaemia, and with the degenerative changes of ageing. The condition may precede the development of gastric ulcer or gastric carcinoma. It is widely believed that the organism *Helicobacter pylori* is likely to be a significant factor in the development of chronic gastritis and peptic ulceration (Scheiman and Cutler 1999).

The symptoms of chronic gastritis are usually ill defined but may include anorexia, discomfort and a full feeling after meals, flatulence, heartburn, nausea and occasionally haematemesis. The patient may lose considerable weight as there is a tendency to restrict food intake to avoid the distress it may precipitate. Attention is directed toward improving the general nutritional status by encouraging a well balanced diet of non-irritating foods.

Peptic ulcer

A peptic ulcer is the erosion of a circumscribed area of tissue in the wall of the gastrointestinal tract that is accessible to gastric secretions. The actual erosion is caused by the digestive action of hydrochloric acid and pepsin. The most frequent sites of an ulcer are the stomach (*gastric ulcer*) and the proximal portion of the duodenum (*duodenal ulcer*), but the oesophagus or jejunum or any other part of the gastrointestinal mucosa may be susceptible if the surface comes in contact with gastric secretions.

The ulcer penetrates the mucosa and may invade the underlying submucosal and muscular tissues. Ulcers tend to recur; some heal promptly, whereas others become chronic.

Causes

There is no consensus as to the initiating cause of peptic ulcer, although the presence in the stomach of the bacterium *H. pylori* has recently emerged as a likely main causative factor. Normally, hydrochloric acid and pepsin are secreted but ulceration does not occur. This is attributed to the following defensive factors. The mucosa secretes sufficient mucus to dilute the secretions and provides a protective coating that prevents mucosal digestion by the acid–pepsin action. The duodenum has the additional protection of the strong alkalinity of the bile and pancreatic and intestinal secretions which neutralize the acidic chyme. Still another defence is a healthy resistant mucosa which has a good blood supply and is capable of continuous rapid generation of the mucosal epithelial cells.

A peptic ulcer may develop when the secretory output of hydrochloric acid and pepsin is in excess of the normal or when the protective mechanisms are inadequate in relation to the amount of acid and pepsin produced. An ulcer is therefore caused by an imbalance between pepsin secretion and the body's natural defences. Stress is also involved as it causes capillary shutdown, decreasing the blood flow to the area, and a reduction in bicarbonate production, which results in an acid–base imbalance.

The following are potential contributing factors in the development of an imbalance between the secretion of hydrochloric acid and pepsin and the defensive mechanisms of the mucosa:

- *Stress* – particularly associated with serious trauma and illness.

- *Inflammation*. Gastritis and trauma of the mucosa reduce the resistance of the membrane to digestion. Cell destruction is accelerated and cell reproduction, which normally renews the superficial layers quickly, may be retarded.

- *Heredity*. Genetic factors appear to have a role, as studies on incidence show there is a tendency for peptic disease to occur in families.

- *Certain drugs*. Some drugs, e.g. NSAIDs (aspirin, ibuprofen), corticosteroids (cortisone), indometacin and phenylbutazone.

- *Bile reflux*. The reflux of bile and pancreatic enzymes into the stomach due to an incompetent pyloric sphincter may lead to a gastric ulcer. The bile salts damage the gastric mucosa, predisposing it to ulceration.

- *Endocrine secretions*. Rarely, severe peptic ulceration is caused by marked gastric hypersecretion that occurs in response to an excessive gastrin concentration in the blood. The gastrin is produced by a tumour of the islets of the pancreas or the submucosa of the duodenum and stomach or regional lymph nodes (Zollinger–Ellison syndrome). Peptic ulceration also develops in hyperparathyroidism. The disturbance is attributed to the altered serum calcium level.

- *Histamine*. Histamine promotes stimulation of acid secretion; H_2-receptor antagonists, which inhibit histamine action, have been found in gastric parietal cells.

- *Cigarette smoking and high alcohol intake* (Butler 1997).

Clinical characteristics

The prominent symptom of peptic ulcer is epigastric *pain* with definite characteristics. It may radiate to the back. The pain is usually described by the patient as gnawing or burning and of being rhythmic in its development and

Mucosal structure
See chapter 5.1

Stress
See chapter 2.7

Inflammation
See chapter 6.1

relief in relation to the ingestion of food. The onset of pain may be immediate or up to 4 hours after a meal, depending upon the location of the ulcer, and is relieved by taking food or an antacid.

In the case of an *oesophageal ulcer*, the pain develops within a few minutes of the meal. It may be intermittent and the patient usually complains of heartburn and regurgitation. Pain associated with a *gastric ulcer* usually occurs ½–1 hour after the ingestion of food; that of a *duodenal ulcer* is delayed for approximately 2–4 hours.

The patient's rest is frequently disturbed by nocturnal pain, especially with a duodenal ulcer. Although the ingestion of food generally provides relief, in a few instances it may be the initiating factor of the ulcer pain, particularly if the food is coarse or highly seasoned. The association of eating with relief of pain ensures that the patient is not usually undernourished.

Vomiting is not a common incident in peptic ulcer but may occur if the ulcer pain is very severe or if the ulcer is in the pyloric region. In the case of the latter, inflammation and oedema of the surrounding tissues, pyloric spasm or contracted scar tissue resulting from ulceration may narrow the lumen of the pylorus. This may delay the emptying of the stomach and may cause vomiting.

Clinical diagnostic measurements

Investigation of the patient for peptic ulcer may include OGD or barium meal (see p. 480), serum gastrin assays, exfoliative cytology and stool examination for occult blood.

Endoscopy

This technique is now widely used for investigation of the upper gastrointestinal tract, for both chronic or acute disorders. The oesophagus is examined before passing the instrument through into the stomach where biopsy of any lesion and brushings for cytology may be carried out.

It is possible in some instances to arrest haemorrhage by the direct application of electrocautery or a haemostatic preparation to the bleeding site.

The endoscope is passed through the pylorus to examine the duodenum. The ampulla of Vater may be cannulated and viewed, and a radio-opaque dye injected to demonstrate the pancreatic and common bile ducts (cholangiopancreatography). Endoscopic examination may also be extended into the jejunum.

Nursing care in endoscopy

Preparation for this diagnostic procedure should begin with an explanation to the patient of what to expect. The doctor may have described the examination but the patient will probably still have questions, which the nurse should be able to answer.

Written consent for the procedure is required. The oesophagus and the stomach must be completely empty. No food or fluid is given for 4–6 hours before the procedure. In gastroscopy, the doctor may request a gastric lavage to be done several hours before the examination in patients in whom some pyloric obstruction is suspected. The dentures are removed and kept safe.

Intravenous sedation may be given to minimize patient discomfort.

The pharyngeal area may be sprayed with a local anaesthetic before the endoscopic instrument is introduced. The patient is unable to speak when the endoscope is in position and a mouthguard prevents them biting on the endoscope.

After the examination, the patient is allowed to rest. All food and fluids are withheld until the effect of the local anaesthetic has worn off and the gag reflex returns (usually 1–2 hours). Before giving any fluid, the reflex may be tested by gently touching the back of the throat with an applicator or spoon. The patient may complain of a sore throat or soreness in mid-chest. Warm fluids may be soothing and may provide some relief. Any expectoration or vomiting of blood or severe pain should be reported promptly to the doctor.

Assessment of the patient with peptic ulcer

The nurse will generally encounter patients admitted with peptic ulcer in one of three situations:

1. The person is undergoing investigation and diagnosis, increasingly as an outpatient.

2. The person is having an acute exacerbation with possible severe bleeding.

3. The person has been admitted for planned surgery as the ulcer is failing to respond to medical treatment.

Assessment will therefore tend to focus on different aspects of the patient in each of these situations.

The patient undergoing investigations may be very anxious and have fears of cancer being diagnosed. It is essential, therefore, that, in addition to the obvious physical parameters that are assessed, anxiety should be monitored and knowledge deficits explored. As health education about factors that predispose to ulceration will be a key part of the care plan, it is important to assess relevant areas of the person's lifestyle such as smoking and drinking habits, regularity and types of meals, and stress levels, all of which are amenable to health education. It is also important to discover the person's level of understanding and attitudes towards health education as this will have a major influence upon the approach used.

In an acute emergency situation, physical parameters such as blood pressure and pulse are a high priority because of the risks of hypovolaemic shock and a major bleed which may be fatal. Close assessment of stools for melaena or occult blood, and of vomit for the presence of fresh or altered blood, is required. Pain must be assessed carefully so that appropriate relief can be given as required. The nurse should not lose sight of the patient's psychological condition, however, and should carefully assess levels of both fear and understanding in what can be a very frightening situation.

The patient being admitted for surgery should be assessed along the lines discussed in the first scenario above. He or she may be optimistic as surgery is seen as a cure for a long-term and distressing complaint. However, lingering fears of cancer may be present along with all the fears that can be conjured up by the prospect of any operation. Such topics need careful exploration during assessment as it is also important to discover whether the patient has a realistic view of the benefits surgery may bring and is aware of the various measures that will be needed to cope with the side-effects of surgery in the long term. Successful health education before discharge will depend on discovering such information.

Management

Treatment of the patient is directed toward the relief of symptoms, healing of the ulcer and the prevention of complications and recurrence. A regimen of rest, non-irritating diet avoiding alcohol, stopping smoking (and the use of NSAIDs if applicable) is required. Medications designed to promote healing by reducing gastric secretory and motor activity, diluting the gastric juice and neutralizing much of the hydrochloric acid in order to promote healing are prescribed.

Hospitalization is not usually necessary.

Diet

Strict dietary control is not considered necessary. A regular, well balanced diet, free of foods that are upsetting to the individual, is recommended. Lengthy gaps between meals should be avoided. In the acute phase, small frequent meals will be more tolerable to the patient. These are gradually modified to the more customary three larger meals per day. In some instances five or six smaller meals may have to be continued.

Medications

Pain relief and healing of an ulcer are achieved by reducing the acidity at the ulcer site. However, it is important to diagnose infection with *H. pylori* in order to prevent a relapse when acid reduction is stopped. It is also important to avoid the use of NSAIDs. Current approaches to treatment for patients with peptic ulceration include antacids, antibiotics (if *H. pylori*-positive), proton pump inhibitors or H_2-receptor antagonists, and prostaglandin analogues.

Patients with *H. pylori* infection are given a 7–14-day course of 'triple therapy'. This consists of two of amoxicillin, clarithromycin or metronidazole, with either a proton pump inhibitor (lansoprazole or omeprazole) or an H_2-receptor antagonist (ranitidine or cimetidine). Maintenance therapy with a proton pump inhibitor or H_2-receptor antagonist may continue for some weeks thereafter.

The use of NSAIDs (prescribed for chronic arthritic conditions) inhibits the production of prostaglandin E, which results in loss of the mucous layer protecting the gastric lining. Prescription of misoprostol (a prostaglandin analogue) will help reduce the NSAID-related incidence of peptic ulcers (Trounce and Gould 2000).

Proton pump inhibitors are the most powerful gastric acid secretion inhibitors. They inhibit the adenosine triphosphate (ATP)-mediated pumping of potassium and hydrogen ions in parietal cells and have few side-effects. A single dose is usually given, before breakfast, on an empty stomach. Alternatively, they may be prescribed for both night and morning use. H_2-receptor antagonists block the histamine receptors in the parietal cells to prevent acid being secreted by parietal cells. They may be given either morning and night, or in a single dose at bedtime to have effect when acid secretion is greatest, at night.

Antacids are used to neutralize the acid in the stomach. To be effective they must be taken frequently throughout the day. Examples include aluminium hydroxide and magnesium hydroxide. Magnesium and aluminium salts are absorbed minimally and should not cause any disturbances in electrolyte levels. Hypermagnesaemia and hyperaluminaemia, however, can occur in patients with renal failure. Magnesium hydroxide can cause diarrhoea and aluminium hydroxide tends to cause constipation. Antacids may interfere with the absorption of certain drugs (e.g. ferrous sulfate, phenytoin, tetracycline) and it is usually recommended that the administration of antacids and other drugs be separated by at least 2 hours. Because of the availability of other drugs and the inconvenience of taking antacids so frequently, these drugs are used on a p.r.n basis rather than for long-term treatment.

Sucralfate is a sulfated polysaccharide that acts directly at the ulcer site. Sucralfate binds with the gastric mucosa and forms a barrier that inhibits the diffusion of hydrogen ions and the local action of pepsin. It is poorly absorbed and hence has few side-effects. Occasionally constipation may occur. Sucralfate should be taken 30 minutes before meals and at bedtime. If prescribed with antacids, administration should be separated by at least 1 hour.

Surgical treatment

If the symptoms persist and the ulcer becomes intractable, or if there has been bleeding or the ulcer has resulted in some obstruction in the gastric outlet, surgical treatment may be considered necessary. Various operative procedures are used in the surgical treatment of an uncomplicated ulcer in order to reduce the potential gastric acid secretion. Current operative approaches include the following procedures.

Gastric resection (subtotal gastrectomy) This is the removal of a portion of the stomach, including the ulcer-bearing area and part of the parietal cell mass. Resection is performed because of the risk of the ulcer becoming malignant in the future. An anastomosis is then made between the gastric stump and the duodenum (gastro-duodenostomy; Billroth I) or jejunum (gastrojejunostomy; Billroth II) to restore gastrointestinal continuity.

Gastric resection plus vagotomy Vagotomy is a resection of the vagus nerve to reduce the stimulation of gastric secretion. It also reduces the motility of the stomach and may interfere with gastric emptying. For this reason a highly selective vagotomy may be performed which leaves parts of the vagus nerve intact, particularly the sections that supply the antrum. Otherwise, vagotomy is combined with a gastric resection or with a gastroenterostomy to provide effective gastric emptying.

Vagotomy with pyloroplasty This involves a longitudinal incision made in the pylorus, which is then surgically closed transversely. This produces an enlarged outlet which compensates for the impaired gastric emptying resulting from vagotomy. In some instances a *gastroenterostomy* may be done instead of the pyloroplasty.

For nursing management of the patient who requires gastric surgery, see page 462.

Complications of peptic ulceration

The complications that commonly occur with peptic ulcer are serious and usually account for the deaths attributed to peptic ulcer. They are haemorrhage, perforation and pyloric obstruction.

Haemorrhage

Peptic ulceration is the most common cause of haematemesis and melaena. The loss of blood is due to erosion of a blood vessel at the ulcer site. Most of the patients who have a haemorrhage are known to have or to have had an ulcer, but in a few it may be the first symptom that prompts them to seek treatment.

Vomiting of blood and the passing of black tarry stools are the prominent indications of serious ulcer bleeding together with the development of hypovolaemic shock. The patient experiences weakness, apprehension, dizziness and faintness, together with the classical signs of shock. If a large vessel is eroded, the signs and symptoms appear rapidly and collapse occurs quickly.

Management

Management of the patient with haemorrhage may be conservative or include operation. The complication of haemorrhage is serious and demands prompt resuscitation and treatment of the site of bleeding.

Nursing assessment

Blood pressure, pulse and respirations are monitored frequently and the level of consciousness, colour and body temperature are noted. If a central venous catheter has been inserted, central venous pressure should be recorded from the same point, at regular intervals.

Blood typing and cross-matching are done immediately. The haematocrit and haemoglobin levels are determined, initially to determine the extent of the blood loss then later, at intervals, to assess the patient's response to treatment.

Accurate recording of the volume and characteristics of the emesis and drainage via the nasogastric tube is important. (Is the blood bright? Does the emesis contain clots?) An indwelling urethral catheter may be passed so that urinary output per hour can be monitored.

It is important to assess the person's reaction to the situation, because fear and anxiety aggravate the condition. The principal problem facing the patient is shock, and the main goals are that the patient's blood pressure and other vital signs will return to normal, indicating successful resuscitation.

Nursing intervention

Nursing intervention for a patient with haemorrhage includes the following:

- A plasma expander such as Haemaccel is given intravenously until compatible whole blood is available. The rate of flow is usually slowed as the patient's blood pressure increases; too rapid an increase in the blood pressure has the risk of increasing the bleeding. The blood pressure may need to be measured every 15–30 minutes.

- A central venous line may be inserted both to monitor central venous pressure and to provide wide, additional venous access for infusions.

- Rest should be promoted by reducing disturbances, keeping nursing interventions to a safe minimum. A sedative may be prescribed to promote relaxation and an analgesic for pain relief.

- The patient and significant others should be kept informed to allay anxiety. Information should be presented in short segments, without excessive use of medical terms, delivered in a calm manner, and regularly reinforced.

- A nasogastric tube may be passed to remove blood and gastric secretions. Gentle aspiration of stomach contents will remove acid and pepsin which could further irritate tissues. Aspiration of blood may prevent vomiting (haematemesis), allow estimation of loss, and reduce trauma and discomfort.

- OGD is usually performed to locate the bleeding site; injection of sclerosing agent (adrenaline/epinephrine), electrocautery or photocautery by laser, if available, may be used to control bleeding. If this is unsuccessful, emergency surgery may be necessary. If bleeding has ceased, close observation and fasting is usually continued until the person's overall condition is stable.

- If treated conservatively, and when bleeding ceases and the cardiovascular state is normalized, oral intake is permitted. Once small volumes of water are tolerated by the person, intake is gradually increased to include clear fluids, liquid diet, soft food, and eventually an ordinary diet. Being able to take food and fluid again improves the patient's morale and lessens anxiety. Iron may be prescribed to promote replacement of haemoglobin.

- Frequent mouth care is necessary because of the haematemesis, dehydration and the discomfort of extreme thirst.

Perforation

A peptic ulcer may progressively erode the submucosal muscularis and serous layers of the gastrointestinal wall. When the serous membranous layer is penetrated, some of the stomach or duodenal content escapes into the peritoneal cavity and causes a generalized peritonitis by chemical irritation and infection.

When perforation takes place, the patient immediately experiences sudden, incapacitating abdominal pain that begins in the epigastric region but spreads through the abdomen as more of the peritoneum becomes irritated by the intragastrointestinal content. Pallor, a cold clammy skin, rapid pulse, shallow grunting respirations and probably nausea and vomiting may be evident. The abdomen becomes rigid and board-like.

Perforation demands immediate treatment; emergency surgery may be performed to close the perforation or resect the affected area, or the patient's condition and history may be such that the perforation is treated by non-surgical conservative methods. The surgical procedure may consist of gastric resection or simple closure of the perforation by suturing the serous layer and reinforcing the area with a patch of omentum. The peritoneal cavity is cleared of the intragastrointestinal fluid that seeped through the perforation. In addition to the usual preoperative procedures for emergency surgery, preparation will include the insertion of a nasogastric tube and an intravenous infusion of electrolytes and fluids. An explanation of the need for operation and what it entails will be made by the surgeon and reinforced by the nurse.

Non-operative treatment usually includes parenteral administration of an analgesic such as morphine, aspiration of the stomach content using a large tube, followed by the insertion of a nasogastric tube and continuous gastric suctioning, intravenous electrolytes and fluids (fluids may include whole blood) and antibiotic therapy. If the patient's condition is satisfactory, continuous gastric suctioning is replaced by intermittent aspiration after 30–48 hours.

Pyloric obstruction

This may be caused by inflammation, oedema and spasm when the ulcer is in the acute stage, or by scar tissue that is formed as the ulcer heals. The ulcer may be gastric in the region of the pylorus, or it may be in the duodenum. The constriction causes gastric retention and dilatation.

The *symptoms* that the patient complains of include a 'full feeling' which causes greater discomfort toward the end of the day. Pain may be experienced after eating as gastric contractions increase in intensity in an effort to overcome the obstruction. The contractions gradually decline and the stomach becomes atonic and dilates. Severe anorexia develops and the patient vomits large amounts irregularly. The loss of nutrients, water and electrolytes leads to loss of weight, weakness, dehydration and acid–base imbalance (alkalosis).

If the obstruction is due to the active ulceration process, it is treated conservatively by gastric aspiration and intravenous fluids.

Obstruction due to contraction of fibrous scar tissue is treated by operation. A gastric resection with a gastro-enterostomy or pyloroplasty may be performed. For nursing care, see page 462.

Cancer of the stomach

Although cancer of the stomach still accounts for a large number of deaths each year, there has been a significant decline over the past three decades. The incidence is slightly higher in men and rises rapidly from the age of 40 years, with the highest number of deaths occurring in the 55–60 years age group.

Contributing factors

The cause of this cancer is unknown but certain conditions are considered predisposing. These include pernicious anaemia, achlorhydria, chronic gastritis, infection with *H. pylori* and benign gastric ulcer. It now seems likely that dietary carcinogens exist in some foods and contribute to the formation of gastric cancer.

Any region of the stomach may be involved, but the most frequent sites are the pylorus and antrum.

Clinical characteristics

The manifestations are vague and insidious. At first, the person may complain of some mild discomfort after eating but, as the disease advances, belching, regurgitation, nausea and vomiting may be experienced, and there is a progressive loss of appetite, weight and strength. Blood may appear in the vomitus and stool when there is ulceration at the tumour site. Pain is usually a late symptom. Unfortunately, because the early symptoms are mild and vague, the person tends to delay seeing a doctor, and the disease becomes well advanced before there is medical intervention. Nurses should be aware of this problem and, on learning that a person is experiencing even mild 'digestive' disturbances, should stress the importance of seeking medical advice.

Diagnosis

Investigation of the patient includes OGD and biopsy, barium meal radiography, cytological studies of gastric fluid, gastroscopy and biopsy, examination of the stool for blood, haemoglobin estimation and blood cell counts. Computed tomography of the chest and abdomen, and liver ultrasonography, may be performed to establish the extent of the tumour and infiltration or development of metastases in other organs.

Blood examinations will probably show some deficiency of haemoglobin and red blood cells, as anaemia is a characteristic of gastric cancer due to the chronic bleeding, reduced production of the intrinsic factor by the gastric mucosa, reduced absorption of iron because of the hypochlorhydria and nutritional deficits.

Metastases

Gastric carcinoma develops and metastasizes rapidly; all too often there has been a spread to some other structure(s) by the time of diagnosis. There may be direct extension to neighbouring organs (e.g. oesophagus, duodenum) or an indirect spread via the lymph and venous blood. The spleen, abdominal lymph nodes, peritoneum, liver, pancreas and lungs are frequent sites of metastases from gastric carcinoma. The left supraclavicular and axillary nodes may also be affected.

Dumping
See chapter 5.1

Treatment

Surgery is the treatment of choice but cure is possible only when the cancer is diagnosed in the early stages, i.e. before it has spread from the primary site or at least only to localized lymph glands. The surgical procedure used will depend on the site of the cancer and its extension or possible course of extension. A subtotal gastrectomy or, rarely, a total gastrectomy is performed and may include resection of the duodenum, excision of the areas of lymphatic spread (omentum, spleen), resection of the pancreas or resection of the lower oesophagus. In subtotal gastrectomy, the stomach is anastomosed to the duodenum (gastroduodenostomy) or to the jejunum (gastrojejunostomy) if the lower part of the stomach has been removed. With removal of the proximal portion of the stomach, the operation is completed by anastomosis of the oesophagus to the remaining stomach (oesophagoantrostomy). Total gastrectomy and resection of the oesophagus necessitate entrance into the thoracic cavity. Continuity of the alimentary tract is restored by an oesophagojejunostomy.

The preoperative and postoperative nursing care of the gastric surgical patient is presented on page 462. Care of the patient following complete gastrectomy includes the care necessary for any patient who has had chest surgery (see Ch. 13). The patient who has had partial gastrectomy requires small frequent meals of easily digested foods because of the development of dumping syndrome (see below) and vitamin B_{12} injections.

Radiotherapy and chemotherapy have unfortunately not made any significant impact in the treatment of gastric cancer.

Dumping syndrome

Normally, the gastric content is delivered in small amounts into the intestine by the pylorus. Following a gastric resection, vagotomy or gastroenterostomy, the normal pyloric control of the volume moving from the stomach into the small intestine is absent and a small proportion of patients develop the **dumping syndrome**. This is caused by the precipitous passage into the small intestine of a relatively large amount of gastric content that has not undergone the usual dilution by gastric secretions and digestive changes. This leads to a rapid absorption of a large amount of carbohydrate and a consequent increase in insulin release, leading to hypoglycaemia-like symptoms 1–2 hours later. The following factors are also implicated:

- The sudden distension of the proximal portion of the small intestine initiates sympathetic reflexes.

- The fluid that moved quickly out of the stomach is hypertonic, having a high concentration of sugar and/or electrolytes. The resulting hyperosmolarity on the intestine results in the movement of fluid from the intravascular spaces into the jejunum.

The effects on the patient are to produce faintness and palpitations immediately after meals, in addition to the symptoms referred to above 1–2 hours later. The person is advised to drink less at mealtimes and to eat fewer foods with high sugar or carbohydrate content to minimize these distressing symptoms.

Nursing care of the person with a disorder of the stomach and duodenum

Assessment

Health history

Gastrointestinal functioning and factors that influence it

- What is the usual diet of the individual?

- How has the diet changed in relation to symptoms?

- What strategies have been adopted to relieve symptoms?

- Does the person smoke or take alcohol or drugs such as aspirin or steroids?

- Has the individual experienced any particular stressful life events recently?

- What effects might the person's social circumstances have upon their diet?

Clinical symptoms

- Does the individual experience nausea, vomiting, epigastric fullness, discomfort or pain?

- Where is the pain located? Does it move to the back or shoulders?

- What factors appear to increase discomfort?

- What strategies has the individual adopted to relieve it?

- Is the pain or discomfort increased at night, when the stomach is empty or during any specific activities?

- How long have the symptoms been experienced? Have they changed?

General health status

- Has the person lost weight recently and how much?

- Have there been any other health problems such as breathlessness, reduced mobility or poor healing?

Patient problems common to those with disorders of the stomach and duodenum

- *Dehydration* due to nausea and vomiting

- *Malnutrition* due to increased gastric secretions, gastrointestinal discomfort, nausea, vomiting, and possibly surgical intervention

- *Fear and anxiety* that surgery may be necessary or that cancer may be present.

Goals

The person will demonstrate:

1. knowledge about the condition in terms of causes and treatment

2. absence or control of pain

3. absence or control of nausea and vomiting

4. awareness of dietary measures to relieve symptoms

5. an adequate nutritional intake, as shown by progressive increase in bodyweight towards normal

6. reduced anxiety levels and an ability to talk freely about the condition.

Nursing intervention

Alleviation of nausea and vomiting

Assessment

Assessment of the patient who is nauseous and is vomiting involves noting the following factors:

- Was the vomiting preceded by nausea?

- Was there retching or was the vomitus regurgitated without effort?

- Was pain associated with the vomiting?

- Was there any association with the ingestion of food or drugs?

- Do the nausea and vomiting occur at any time or are they more severe at a particular time of day?

- How frequent is the emesis?

- What is the quantity, consistency, colour and content of the vomitus?

- What are the effects (physical and emotional) on the patient?

Supportive measures

Sympathetic attention and understanding can mean a great deal to the patient. As stress and fear can perpetuate nausea and vomiting, the patient is encouraged to express any concerns. The plan of care and any diagnostic and therapeutic measures should be explained to the patient; knowing that something is being done or going to be done provides reassurance.

Support is also provided by remaining with the patient, supporting the head or painful site (e.g. incision), holding the basin, cleansing the mouth and lips, and making sincere efforts to relieve the discomfort.

Fluid and food

Oral intake is usually withheld for a period of time and is resumed gradually in small amounts. If vomiting is prolonged, an intravenous infusion of fluids may be necessary to prevent or correct dehydration and replace electrolytes. An accurate record is made of the fluid intake and output. The skin and oral mucous membrane are observed for dryness and skin turgor is assessed to identify dehydration.

Hygienic and comfort measures

The mouth is rinsed after each emesis and the basin emptied and disposed of promptly. Soiled bedding and clothing are changed and the room is ventilated. The odour or sight of vomitus may contribute to the patient's discomfort and may cause repetitive vomiting. The patient may be reassured by having tissues and a clean basin always within reach.

Rest, quiet and a minimum of disturbance may reduce the incidence of vomiting. Encouraging the patient to take several deep breaths may help to lessen nausea and offset vomiting. Nausea tends to increase with motion; any change of position should be made slowly. Positioning should facilitate drainage of the vomitus from the mouth to prevent possible aspiration. Subdued lighting may reduce external stimuli and be conducive to rest.

Relaxation techniques including muscular relaxation, meditation, guided imagery and deep breathing exercises may help to decrease stress and relieve the nausea and vomiting.

Some individuals find that food actually relieves nausea and prevents vomiting. Dry crackers or sips of soda water can be helpful.

Medication

An antiemetic or sedative may be prescribed. Diazepam may be administered orally or parenterally for sedation. Prochlorperazine or metoclopramide are examples of antiemetics that may be given, usually via the intramuscular or intravenous route depending on the drug.

The use of antiemetics or other drugs is restricted if there is any question of pregnancy, to prevent any effects on fetal development. Anticipatory nausea and vomiting are also controlled by preventive and regular doses of antiemetics. If the vomiting continues, gastric drainage by means of a nasogastric tube may be established.

Maintenance of adequate nutritional intake

Nutritional intake is maintained by decreasing stimulation of certain secretions, adapting the person's diet to relieve the problem or using alternative routes to administer nutrients.

Dietary measures

Measures to decrease stimulation of gastric secretions include withholding food for 24–28 hours to allow the stomach to rest. Fluids are given intravenously as even water taken by mouth will stimulate gastric acid secretion. Gastric intubation with aspiration may be used to remove gastric secretions to promote healing.

Recommended dietary modifications include the following:

- a nutritionally adequate diet
- substances that stimulate gastric secretion (e.g. coffee, strong tea, highly seasoned foods, especially those with pepper, citrus fruit and alcohol) are avoided
- meals are taken regularly at frequent intervals of about 3 hours to maintain the buffering action of food in the stomach
- meals should be small to avoid gastric distension, which stimulates gastric acid secretion
- foods that the person recognizes as actually precipitating symptoms are avoided
- the person should not smoke
- drugs such as NSAIDs (aspirin, ibuprofen) that are known to damage the gastrointestinal mucosa are avoided.

Alternative routes for the administration of nutrients

Oral intake of food is preferred, but when this is not possible nutrients can be administered intravenously or by nasogastric or percutaneous enteral routes.

Nasogastric tube feeding When a patient is unable to take fluid and foods by mouth, a fine-bore nasogastric tube may be passed, through which a specially prepared solution of essential nutrients is introduced directly into the stomach. This method of feeding a patient is known as *enteral feeding*.

Patients should always be nursed in an upright position whilst being tube fed to avoid the risks of reflux and aspiration.

Careful preparation of the patient before insertion will help in reducing discomfort and facilitate ease of insertion. The individual should have the procedure explained in full, including the sensations they will experience and how they can assist by swallowing when they feel the tube touching the back of the throat. Measures that can reduce the unpleasant sensations include: application of sterile, water-soluble, lubricating jelly to the tube, deep breathing, relaxation techniques and swallowing. Successful aspiration of gastric contents confirms the correct placement of the tube.

Nasogastric tubes can be secured by applying hypoallergenic tape to the individual's nostril or by an adhesive patch to the cheek.

Enteral feeding involves close cooperation between medical, dietetic and nursing staff, who have an important role in supervising the diet.

Commercially prepared feeds are commonly used because they have a known nutrient content, flow easily through the nasogastric tube, and are easy to prepare. They come sterilized and can be administered from a sterile reservoir through an administration tube attached to the nasogastric tube, reducing the potential for the introduction of contaminants.

The regimen is determined according to the individual's nutritional and fluid requirements, based upon their age, sex, bodyweight, medical condition and biochemistry. Continuous delivery of enteral feeding is the ideal as it minimizes side-effects, such as distension and nausea, and maximizes absorption. Intermittent feeding may be more convenient for some individuals, especially when at home.

When evaluating a feed, consideration is given to its osmolality, caloric value and protein, carbohydrate, fat, vitamin and mineral composition. Nutrients are present in simple form, are easily digested and absorbed, and leave minimal residue in the bowel. Patients with some malabsorption disorders may not tolerate some of the prepared feeds. Functioning of the patient's digestive tract and hydrational status are assessed before the preparation is selected.

For the initial feeding, an explanation of the procedure is given to the patient. The head of the bed is elevated to 35–40°.

A continuous infusion of the feed is given via a giving-set attached to the nasogastric tube. The fluid feed is given slowly, for example 500 mL over 6 hours, and the speed is regulated by a pressure regulator on the tubing or a peristaltic pump.

The feed is administered slowly and allowed to flow into the stomach by gravity. To avoid air entering the stomach, a collapsible plastic feeding container is used. When the feed is completed, the tube is flushed with up to 50 mL of water and clamped. If regurgitation or vomiting occurs, it may be that the prescribed volume is too great. A smaller amount given more frequently may be tolerated.

Frequent mouth care is necessary, as is the care of the nostril through which the tube passes.

The patient is encouraged to remain in a sitting position for at least 1 hour after each feed to decrease regurgitation and aspiration and to promote stomach emptying.

Gastrostomy This is the establishment of an opening into the stomach through the abdominal wall and the insertion of a tube through which fluids and liquefied food may be introduced directly into the stomach. General anaesthesia is not usually required. The stomach is visualized by an endoscope and the tube is inserted through the abdominal wall via a small stab wound. The tube is anchored with a flange in either side of the abdominal wall. This is often referred to as a *percutaneous endoscopic gastrostomy (PEG)*.

A gastrostomy may be a temporary procedure during a period of corrective surgery or it may be permanent, for example in conditions such as multiple sclerosis, motor neurone disease or brain injury (White 1998).

The patient generally finds it difficult to accept a gastrostomy because the natural process of eating and its associated pleasures such as taste and sociability have been removed. Personnel caring for the patient, the family and friends should acknowledge to the patient that they understand any negative feelings this leads to.

Regular feeds are given according to the patient's needs. The food preparations used in gastrostomy are similar to those cited above for gastric tube feedings or are the person's normal diet, liquidized. The required amount of feed is given through an administration bag attached to the gastric tube. The patient's head and shoulders are elevated and he or she remains in this position for half an hour after the feeding to prevent regurgitation into the oesophagus and leakage around the tube. The tube is cleansed following the feeding by flushing it with up to 50 mL of water and is then clamped.

A gauze or transparent (Opsite) dressing is applied to the wound following inspection of the skin for pressure necrosis from the flanges, or excoriation. The escape of even a small amount of gastric juice from around the tube may irritate the skin because of its acid pepsin content. The gauze dressing is changed whenever there is drainage, and the skin is cleansed thoroughly with water and dried. A protective coating of petroleum jelly or a prescribed ointment or powder may then be applied. Should excoriation occur, application of a hydrocolloid dressing or wafer

following cleansing of the skin may both promote healing and protect the skin from further damage. Evidence of necrosis should be communicated to medical/specialist staff as soon as possible.

The feeds may have to be adjusted from time to time. Too much fat or carbohydrate may cause diarrhoea. Complaints of a full feeling or abdominal discomfort may necessitate a decrease in the amount of feeds given. A record of the patient's weight is made, which also serves as a guide in adjusting the caloric value of the feed's formula. This should be recorded twice weekly at the same time of day.

The patient's mouth will require special attention. Frequent cleansing and rinsing are essential.

If the patient is to be fed by gastrostomy over a long period while various stages of treatment are carried out, or if the gastrostomy is permanent, teaching in the correct techniques is essential for both patient and family. Information should be provided regarding supplies of prescribed commercial feeding preparations and equipment. The nurse may direct the family to the appropriate community resources for the necessary assistance, or make the contact for them.

Although a life-preserving intervention, PEG has complications and risks. Peters and Westerby (1994) have listed the following as the main complications:

Stress
See chapter 2.7

- peritonitis
- pulmonary aspiration
- infection at site of tube entry
- gastrocolic fistula
- haemorrhage
- tube blockage.

Close attention to the entry site, tube patency, patient positioning and any complaints of abdominal discomfort are essential, therefore, to minimize the potential complications of PEG.

The problem of bacterial contamination of enteral tube feeds has been highlighted by Anderton (1995). She draws attention to poor hand hygiene, reuse of systems that should be disposable, poor cleaning of equipment, and storage at incorrect temperatures as frequent causes of enteral feeds being significantly contaminated.

Jejunostomy A jejunostomy tube may be inserted and used for feedings when it is necessary to bypass the stomach as a result of surgery or reflux.

Promotion of coping and control of stress

Emotional and physical **stress** affect gastric function, and ill-health of any type presents an additional stress to the individual. Whether stress is a contributing factor or a result of gastrointestinal disorder, the nurse can play a role in identifying both the causes of the stress and the person's responses to it, and help that individual to explore, test and evaluate various coping strategies. Nurses can facilitate the expression and exploration of feelings, provide information and teach patients self-management skills to alleviate the stresses imposed by the illness. The exploration of coping strategies that work for the individual and the development of relaxation and other stress management programmes with the patient and family fall within the role of the nurse. They can inform the individual and significant others about resources available to them in their community and work setting. They can also help patients to identify stressors in their daily lives, to develop strategies to alter their lifestyles to avoid these precipitating factors or to implement coping strategies when these situations occur.

Evaluation

When evaluating the care delivered it is important to remember that it is not just the individual's response to management of illness that is important but also their life situation and personal expectations.

Nursing care for the person requiring gastric surgery

Special considerations applicable to the patient experiencing gastric surgery are outlined below. The amount of gastric drainage obtained after operation and the extent of the potential nutritional deficit resulting from the surgical intervention vary according to the type and extent of gastric tissue excised during the surgical procedure. In clinical practice, the care plan is modified to meet the specific needs of the individual.

Preoperative care

The *goals* for the patient during the preoperative period are to:

1. improve fluid and nutritional status

2. learn and practise deep breathing and coughing techniques

3. reduce anxiety experienced by the individual and significant others.

If the patient's nutritional and fluid status is poor, enteral or parenteral nutrition may be administered. Intravenous solutions may be given to increase the person's fluid volume and to correct electrolyte imbalances.

The incision will be in the upper abdomen below the chest; it is important therefore that the patient is competent at performing deep breathing and coughing techniques, and understands the importance of performing these after operation. Introduction to the physiotherapist who will see the patient for chest physiotherapy after surgery is beneficial.

Explanations about the operation and hospital routines usually help to decrease anxiety in both the patient and family. The nurse should also take time to assess their learning needs and to determine their perceptions and expectations for the surgery and postsurgical outcomes.

Postoperative care

Health problems common to persons undergoing gastric surgery include:

- *altered fluid and electrolyte balance* due to gastric intubation and suction, and surgical fluid losses

- *malnutrition* due to preoperative nutritional deficits and decreased food intake after operation

- *pain* due to the surgical intervention

- *altered breathing pattern* due to incisional pain and the location of the incision

- *lack of knowledge* concerning postoperative care and skills required to achieve self-care.

Goals

The patient will have:

1. a patent gastric drainage system

2. fluid volume intake of at least 2.5 litres per day and output in balance

3. absence of pain

4. a clean, dry, intact incision

5. respirations, pulse and blood pressure within usual range

6. maintenance of nutritional status as shown by a weight loss of less than 2 kg

7. understanding of prescribed dietary regimen

8. understanding of plans for follow-up care.

Nursing intervention

Gastric drainage

The patient will return from theatre with a nasogastric, nasointestinal or gastrostomy tube in place.

The characteristics of the drainage fluid are noted and the total volume is recorded at regular intervals. Intermittent aspiration or free drainage will be ordered. It is important that the patency of the tube be maintained to avoid a build-up of secretions in the stomach. The drainage will probably be coloured by blood at first, but this usually clears in a few hours. The doctor is notified if large amounts of blood appear or if the drainage continues to be blood coloured. The volume is an important factor in determining the fluid and electrolyte replacement needed. Loss of gastric secretions incurs a loss of hydrogen ions (H^+) and chloride ions (Cl^-) that may result in alkalosis. Loss of intestinal fluid may result in a severe loss of hydrogen carbonate and potassium, and cause acidosis. The number of days for which the nasogastric tube is left in and oral fluids are withheld varies and depends partly on the patient's progress. The nasogastric tube is usually removed when normal bowel sounds return and drainage volumes reduce. Antiemetic drugs (metoclopramide, cyclizine) may be given regularly to avoid postoperative nausea and vomiting. Not only is nausea unpleasant for the patient, but vomiting poses undue strain on the anastomoses of the surgical areas.

Removal of the tube

Before removal, the tube may be clamped and left in place while oral fluid is introduced. If the fluid is tolerated, the tube may then be removed. It is withdrawn gently and quickly. The patient is instructed to hold the breath to avoid possible aspiration of fluid or mucus that may escape from the tube into the oropharynx during removal.

An intestinal tube is removed slowly, a few centimetres at a time. The lumen into the air-inflated balloon is opened, and the air is allowed to escape. When slight resistance is encountered owing to the intestinal peristalsis, the tube is left for a few minutes and then withdrawal is resumed. The doctor should be notified if resistance to removal persists; force should not be used. If the tube has a mercury-filled bag at its distal end, the latter is brought out through the mouth and the bag removed. The remainder of the tube may then be pulled through the nostril. As with the removal of the gastric tube, the patient is asked to hold the breath as the terminal portion of the tube is drawn from the oesophagus.

The mouth should be cleansed and rinsed immediately after removal of the tube. The patient may complain of soreness in the throat and nose, which usually subsides in a day or two.

Pain management

Considerable **pain** is experienced by the patient who has had gastric surgery. Analgesics such as pethidine are usually prescribed to relieve discomfort. Analgesia should be given regularly for the first few days and administered before activities that could increase discomfort, such as physiotherapy, turning and mobilization. Systems that allow self-administration of postoperative analgesia (patient-controlled analgesia; PCA) are increasingly used; these enhance patient control and increase participation in pain management. Continual assessment of pain levels is necessary in the postoperative period if the goal of a pain-free patient is to be achieved. Frequent regular change of position helps to relieve pain and discomfort.

Frequent cleansing and moistening of the mouth are necessary to lessen the patient's discomfort while the nasogastric tube is in place and oral fluids are restricted. The tube may cause irritation that results in mucus secretion which, if allowed to collect, might be aspirated.

The nostril through which the tube is passed is cleansed and moistened, and given a very light application of mineral oil or water-soluble lubricant to prevent the accumulation and crusting of secretions; adhesive tape securing the tube should be changed regularly.

Promotion of respiratory function

If a total gastrectomy was performed, the incision may involve the thorax, and chest drainage tubes will have been inserted. Remind the patient hourly to take five to ten deep breaths and to cough several times using the staged coughing technique to prevent undue tension on the suture line. Provide necessary encouragement and support by holding a small pillow lightly over the operative site and placing a hand on the patient's back during the coughing. Acknowledge the patient's distress but at the same time emphasize the importance of deep breathing and coughing in the prevention of other problems.

When vital signs are stable, the head of the bed may be gradually elevated to promote deeper breathing and gastric drainage. Change the patient's position at regular frequent intervals: side-to-side to back-to-side. Ambulation usually starts on the first postoperative day.

Fluid and nutritional intake

Parenteral fluids are used to sustain the patient over the first few days. Different procedures are used to introduce the first fluids into the gastrointestinal tract; the surgeon may have the nasogastric tube removed and small stated amounts of water given every half-hour or every hour. The amount is gradually increased if tolerated. The directive may be to introduce a specific amount of water at intervals through the nasogastric tube, which is then clamped.

If the patient tolerates the increased amounts of water without experiencing vomiting, pain or distension, liquids such as tea, fruit squash, soup and milk may be progressively introduced over 2–3 days, but only when normal bowel sounds are heard on auscultation.

With normal progress, the patient is usually receiving a soft diet by day 5–7. The volume given at any one time remains small because of the reduced capacity of the stomach. Foods high in calories and protein are selected and served frequently. The patient's weight is recorded regularly, and the doctor is advised if there is a loss or a failure to gain. Inability of the patient to take the prescribed diet, any regurgitation, vomiting, abdominal distension, or fever or complaint of pain is reported.

By the time the patient is ready to leave the hospital, a light diet of high calorie/protein foods divided into five meals is usually tolerated. Fluids may be omitted from the meals and taken in between so that their volume does not prevent the patient from taking sufficient solid food. The patient is advised gradually to increase the amount taken at regular meals and, if no discomfort is experienced, eventually to resume three or four meals with fluids taken between them.

Pain
See chapter 2.3

Fluid balance
See chapter 2.6

B complex vitamins and vitamin C and iron may be ordered, as the natural food sources of these will be restricted in the diet for a period of time.

Nutritional deficiency

Signs and symptoms of nutritional deficiencies include: the inability to maintain normal weight; insufficient food intake; and feelings of satiety and overfullness following a small amount of food.

The patient should be helped in developing a dietary plan that includes frequent high caloric intakes (small amounts at first and gradually increased as tolerated).

The patient's perception and responses to the necessary continuing dietary modifications after surgery should be assessed and discussed. The need for a period of time for the digestive system to adjust to the changes is discussed.

Anaemia

Monitoring of the patient's red blood cell count and haemoglobin is done regularly after gastric resection, and information is elicited as to energy, fatigue and food elements in the diet. The patient may develop an iron deficiency as a result of decreased iron absorption, which will be caused by measures that reduce acid secretion within the stomach. Normal absorption is facilitated by gastric hydrochloric acid which influences the change from ferric iron in the diet to ferrous iron, which is more easily dissolved and absorbed, mostly in the duodenum and jejunum. The bypassing of the duodenum by a gastrojejunostomy may therefore also reduce the amount of iron absorption. The deficiency may in some instances be due to a poor dietary intake of foods that provide iron (red meat, liver, leafy vegetables, whole milk, eggs and certain cereals). A supplemental preparation of iron is prescribed and the diet corrected to contain the necessary sources.

Anaemia frequently develops as a result of a deficiency in the secretion of the intrinsic factor (due to the loss of gastric mucosa by the gastric resection) which promotes the absorption of vitamin B_{12}. It may develop within a few months or not for 2–3 years after the gastrectomy. The patient may be given weekly vitamin B_{12} by subcutaneous or intramuscular injection until a normal erythrocyte count is established. A maintenance dose is then given monthly throughout the remainder of the patient's life.

Osteomalacia

This is characterized by decalcification of the bones and weakening of their structure, and is a rare complication following gastrectomy. It is attributed to decreased absorption of vitamin D and calcium. Associated symptoms include diarrhoea and steatorrhoea. Treatment involves the administration of vitamin D and calcium supplements.

Anaemia
See chapter 4.1

Osteomalacia
See chapter 3.2

Small intestine
See chapter 5.1

Patient and family teaching

The patient and family are helped to develop a plan to modify the diet and activity to accommodate temporary and long-term limitations imposed by the surgery. The importance of frequent small meals of non-irritating foods high in calories and protein is explained. The size of the meals may be gradually increased when comfortably tolerated, as the remaining portion of the stomach progressively adapts to larger quantities. After several months, the person may find that three regular meals can again be managed. Written dietary instructions and outlines should be provided to reinforce verbal information. Involvement of the dietician early in the patient's care will help in the dietary education process.

The patient is advised to weigh himself or herself regularly and to report to the clinic or doctor on scheduled dates. If pain, vomiting, progressive loss of weight or other distressing symptoms occur, the doctor is contacted promptly. Normal activities are resumed as tolerated and should not interfere with the regularity of meals.

If a total gastrectomy has been done or a large section of the stomach removed, the patient will require regular parenteral administration of a maintenance dose of hydroxycobalamin or cyanocobalamin (vitamin B_{12}). The importance of receiving this is stressed and arrangements are made for vitamin B_{12} administration at the scheduled times; it may be given by the community nurse. Alternatively, a family member may wish to be taught to administer the drug.

Information should be given to the patient and significant others concerning support available in the community. Early referral to the community nursing service will ensure continuity of care. Contact telephone numbers and addresses should be given to the patient.

Evaluation

Evaluation is based on the goals determined for each patient. On discharge from the surgical unit, the patient and significant others should be familiar with the immediate dietary needs and what to expect as he or she adapts to the changes and gradually tolerates increases in the amounts and types of foods and liquids. The patient and significant others should be familiar with measures to take to alleviate the symptoms of dumping syndrome. They should be aware of community resources for dietary assistance and any required wound care. Follow-up medical supervision is planned, scheduled appointments are given to the patient and transport arrangements discussed.

Intestinal disorders

Disorders of the **small intestine** may cause disturbances in the movement of the content along the gut leading to problems of digestion or absorption that may threaten the patient's nutritional status.

Disturbance in the function of the *large intestine* interferes with the excretion of bowel waste and, if the right half of the colon is involved, the normal absorption of water and salts may be reduced and cause dehydration.

A disorder in motility, secretion or absorption rarely occurs independently; a disturbance in one is usually accompanied by dysfunction in one or both of the other intestinal functions. For example, increased secretion may accelerate motility, decreased absorption causes dysfunction in motility and elimination, and inflammation usually causes a disturbance in all three functions.

Alteration in bowel elimination

Causative factors and defining characteristics for the assessment of problems relevant to elimination are listed in Box 15.2.

Diarrhoea

The term **diarrhoea** implies an accelerated movement of content through the intestine with a decrease in mixing and absorptive processes resulting in frequent liquid or unformed stools. The faeces pass through the colon before the normal amount of water is absorbed while fluids and electrolytes may be secreted into the gut also.

Diarrhoea is a symptom of many different disorders which may be within the bowel or extrinsic to the intestine. Changes characteristic of organic disease may occur in the intestine and result in diarrhoea, or the bowel may be structurally normal with the hypermotility being functional. The most common causes of diarrhoea are presented here as intrinsic or extrinsic, although there are many different aetiological classifications in medical literature.

Diarrhoea
See chapter 5.1

Box 15.2   Potential problems of patients with altered bowel elimination

Causes	Clinical characteristics
Diarrhoea	
Bacterial organisms and enterotoxins	Loose, watery stools
Intestinal neoplasms	Several bowel movements per day
Diet high in roughage, or spicy foods or alcohol	Dehydration: loss of skin turgor, weight loss, dry mouth
Allergy to ingested foods	Abdominal cramping and pain
Malabsorption syndrome	Weakness
Diverticulitis	Increased bowel sounds
Laxatives	Perineal excoriation
Antibiotics	
Inflammatory disorders of the intestinal tract	
Emotional stress	
Systemic diseases causing toxaemia (e.g. hyperthyroidism, uraemia, endocrine tumours)	
Radiotherapy to the abdomen and pelvis	
Chemotherapy (5-fluorouracil, cisplatin)	
Constipation	
Disease of the bowel	Abdominal pain
Decreased intestinal motility	Abdominal distension
Altered innervation to bowel and anal sphincter	Sensation of fullness and pressure in rectum
Megacolon	Loss of appetite
Inadequate fluid intake	Headache
Lack of fibre or cellulose in diet	Dry, hard, formed stools
Physical inactivity	Infrequent bowel movements (less than three times per week)
Medication (e.g. opiates)	Straining on defaecation
Weakness of abdominal muscles and diaphragm	
Irregular habits of defaecation	
Loss of bowel tone from excessive use of laxatives	
Haemorrhoids	
Hypercalcaemia	
Pregnancy	
Tumour mass in abdomen or pelvis	
Alteration in mental state	

(Continued)

Box 15.2 *(Continued)*

Causes	Clinical characteristics
Impaction	
Altered tone, motility and sensation in bowel as a result of ageing process	Cramping pain
	Oozing liquid stools
Immobility	Headache
Central nervous system disorders	Loss of appetite
	Abdominal distension
	Dry, hard formed stools
	Palpable hard rectal mass
	Straining at defaecation
	No bowel movement for more than 3 days
Incontinence	
Constipation	Involuntary defaecation
Faecal impaction	Constant soiling of clothing
Excessive use of laxatives and enemas	Faeces soft and semiformed, or loose
Drugs (e.g. iron, methyldopa)	Absence of sensation or urge to defaecate
Diabetes	Diminished propulsive contractions on rectogram
Diverticulitis	
Proctitis	
Carcinoma	
Rectal prolapse	
Regional enteritis (Crohn's disease)	
Malabsorption syndrome	
Ischaemic colitis	
Neurogenic disorders	
Sphincter damage	

Intrinsic causes

Normally the stimulus for peristalsis arises within the intestine. It may cause direct stimulation of the muscle tissue, or may initiate sensory nerve impulses that are transmitted into the central nervous system, resulting in parasympathetic nerve impulses being carried out to the intestine which then stimulate its motility. Disease or irritation within the bowel that may increase either direct stimulation or reflex hypermotility include the following.

Malabsorption Impaired absorption of foods may be due to incomplete digestion or to a defect in the absorptive process of the small intestine. Obviously, with reduced digestion and absorption, an increase in the bulk of the colonic content results and is a stimulus to intestinal motility. The stools are bulky, have an offensive odour and usually contain large amounts of fats, which are irritating to the bowel mucosa and initiate reflex peristalsis. The presence of unabsorbed osmotically active substances, such as glucose or a disaccharide that cannot be split, causes osmotic diarrhoea. The increased intraluminal osmotic pressure causes water to move into the intestine, producing diarrhoea. General malnutrition is also evident.

Inflammation Chronic inflammatory bowel diseases (Crohn's disease, ulcerative colitis and diverticulitis) all cause inflammatory processes in different parts of the gastrointestinal tract. Crohn's disease and ulcerative colitis, while progressive in nature, are characterized by periods of remission and exacerbation. The problems resulting from diverticulitis are constant.

Diverticulitis A pouch or sac may occur in the wall of the intestine and is known as a diverticulum. It may be congenital or may develop as a result of a weakening of an area of the muscle tissue in the wall. There may be several diverticula, or the defect may occur singly.

Diverticula of the large intestine are the most likely to give rise to trouble, as the more solid faecal content tends to collect and be retained in the sac, setting up an inflammation that causes increased reflex peristalsis and diarrhoea. In Western countries it is not uncommon in older people and is linked to a refined diet and associated high pressures in the colon. Diverticular disease arises most commonly in the sigmoid colon (Taylor 1997).

Laxatives Many laxatives act by direct irritation of the intestinal mucosa, resulting in the content being hurried through the colon before the normal amount of water has been absorbed.

Infection Food or fluid contaminated by salmonella, shigella or staphylococcal organisms is the most common cause of intestinal infection and may be referred to as bacterial food poisoning. Meat or milk contaminated with *Escherichia coli* 0157 has recently caused several serious community-based outbreaks of food poisoning.

Inflammation
See chapter 6.1

Infection
See chapter 6.1

A verocytotoxin produced by the bacterium causes haemorrhagic colitis and has profound systemic effects including renal failure.

The shigella bacterium causes bacillary dysentery, and the primary source is usually the excreta of an infected person. This disease is rare, except under crowded and poor sanitary conditions.

Salmonella bacilli may inhabit the intestine of humans, fowl and animals, and may be the source of infection to others. They may be transmitted by the meat of infected animals and by food or water contaminated by the excreta of infected humans or animals. Sporadic outbreaks occur and may be due to a human carrier employed in the handling of food. Ingested salmonella or shigella organisms multiply, causing irritation and inflammation of the intestine, resulting in diarrhoea accompanied by crampy abdominal pain, fever, nausea and vomiting.

Hypersecretory bacterial diarrhoea may be caused by toxin-producing organisms such as staphylococci, salmonella, shigella and *Vibrio cholerae*. The enterotoxins stimulate the release of excessive amounts of fluid and electrolytes by the small intestine.

Neoplasms   Diarrhoea may be a symptom of a malignant neoplasm of the colon and may be alternated with periods of constipation.

Dietary factors   An excessive amount of coarse foods or highly seasoned irritating food may produce hypermotility of the bowel. Occasionally, allergy to a certain food may account for diarrhoea; if the intestinal mucosa is sensitive to the food, it becomes hyperaemic and oedematous, and causes increased reflex hypermotility.

Antibiotics   Diarrhoea sometimes accompanies the administration of antibiotics. They may irritate the mucosa or alter the normal bacterial flora of the intestinal tract allowing infection by 'opportunistic' pathogens (e.g. *Clostridium difficile*). The most frequent offenders are the tetracycline and broad-spectrum antibiotics (e.g. Augmentin).

Idiopathic inflammation   Patients with ulcerative colitis or regional enteritis experience severe diarrhoea. No specific cause has been recognized for either condition.

Extrinsic causes

Diarrhoea accompanies a variety of disorders in which the stimulus that results in increased parasympathetic innervation to the bowel originates outside the intestine.

Emotional stress   Anxiety or underlying tension may be associated with diarrhoea, producing a condition that is referred to as the irritable bowel syndrome. On investigation, disturbances may be revealed that are secondary to the diarrhoea, but there is no organic disease in the intestine or elsewhere. Intestinal hypermobility and hypersecretion occur with both physical and mental **stress**. A study of the patient's total life situation may reveal a specific emotional conflict or ineffective coping that may account for the problem.

General or systemic disorders   Frequently, diarrhoea is associated with general diseases, particularly if they cause toxaemia. Examples of such conditions are acute infectious disease, hyperthryoidism and uraemia.

Assessment

It is important to obtain the following information:

- the patient's previous bowel habits
- the number of bowel movements each day
- the volume and consistency of the stools
- whether the stools contain blood or excessive mucus
- whether the patient experiences abdominal pain
- whether there is exacerbation with certain foods or activities
- whether the diarrhoea is worse during the day or the night. Functional diarrhoea tends to occur during the day, while that associated with organic disease is generally as disturbing at night as during the day
- the systemic effects on the person:
  — what is the hydrational status?
  — is the temperature increased?
  — is the person exhausted because of loss of sleep?
  — is the person losing weight?
- whether or not there are increased bowel sounds
- the individual's perception of, and reaction to, the diarrhoea
- the condition of the skin around the anus and over pressure areas
- fluid and electrolyte balances.

Stress
See chapter 2.7

Goals

The person will demonstrate:

1. formed stools
2. a return to the usual frequency of bowel elimination
3. fluid and electrolyte balance and absence of signs of dehydration
4. integrity of skin.

Nursing intervention

Measures to decrease peristalsis

Peristalsis of the small and large intestines may be slowed by the following measures:

1. Removal of the cause of the diarrhoea. This may involve the administration of prescribed antibiotics for intestinal infection, avoidance of specific foods for the patient with a malabsorption disorder or an

intestinal allergy, and avoidance of laxatives and treatment for systemic diseases such as hyperthroidism or uraemia.

2. Changing the diet to eliminate spicy foods, fruit juices, raw fruits and vegetables and gas-forming foods.

3. Use of drugs. Various medications may be used in the treatment of diarrhoea:

    a. Drugs to reduce intestinal spasm and motility may be ordered. Examples are diphenoxylate hydrochloride (Lomotil) and loperamide hydrochloride (Immodium).

    b. Opiates such as codeine phosphate are believed to increase absorption by acting on the opiate receptors.

    c. Drugs to provide a protective coating on the intestinal mucosa or to provide an adsorbent, which condenses and holds irritating substances, are used. Examples are kaolin, aluminium hydroxide gel and bismuth subcarbonate.

    d. An anti-infective drug may be ordered if the diarrhoea is persistent and of microbial origin. Sulfonamide preparations are poorly absorbed, have a local effect but are less frequently used orally; examples are calcium sulfaloxate, phthalylsulfathiazole and sulfaguanidine. Sulfasalazine (Salazopyrin) is indicated for the maintenance of remission in ulcerative colitis and Crohn's disease.

Infection
See chapter 6.1

Rest

The patient with diarrhoea feels weak and fatigued. Rest periods are provided and the person is encouraged to relax and pursue sedentary activities such as reading or watching television. If necessary, the patient is assisted to the bathroom, or a commode chair may be used at the bedside. The call-button should be answered promptly to avoid unnecessary effort or anxiety for the patient in attempting to reach the bathroom in time.

Some people are unable to relax and rest because of a constant fear of not getting to the bathroom in time; in such instances it may be helpful to make an exception and leave a covered commode at the bedside within the patient's reach.

Fluids and nutrition

Fluids and electrolytes are replaced by intravenous infusions. If oral fluids are tolerated, water or clear soup may be given but carbonated drinks, whole milk, fruit juice and iced fluids are best avoided.

The diet is expanded as soon as possible to reduce the possibility of nutritional deficiencies. A high-calorie, high-vitamin and high-protein diet is gradually introduced, and the patient is observed to determine the intestinal response. Roughage and gas-producing foods are restricted at first; whole-grain bread and cereals, raw fruits and vegetables and highly seasoned and fried foods

are not used. Concentrated sweets and fats are likely to be poorly tolerated Fibre-containing foods and roughage are introduced gradually, as tolerated. If the diarrhoea is due to malabsorption, a gluten-free diet may be ordered in which foods are avoided that contain any wheat, rye, and barley grains or flour.

The first few mouthfuls of a meal may initiate a mass peristaltic wave, and the meal is interrupted by defaecation. The patient may require some persuasion to continue the meal because of fear of provoking another attack of diarrhoea.

Hygienic factors

The patient who is mobile should be located as near to the toilet as possible on the ward and, if confined to bed, privacy should be provided so the patient is less embarrassed by frequent use of the commode.

The anal region should be left clean after each defaecation and, if the skin around the anus is irritated, it is washed and a protective cream applied. Soiled bedding or clothing is changed promptly. Provision is made for thorough washing of the patient's hands after each defaecation, and the nurse should also remember the importance of thorough handwashing. Commode or toilet facilities must be kept scrupulously clean. The patient may very well be embarrassed by the recurring episodes of diarrhoea. The nurse therefore should be sensitive and supportive, being aware of the demoralizing effects this problem may have on the patient. It may help to provide distractions for the patient, particularly if confined to a side ward as a precaution against the spread of infection.

Control of infection

Cases of acute diarrhoea are considered potentially **infectious** until indicated otherwise. Precautions are used to prevent the possible spread of infection to others. The hands are scrubbed with soap and running water after each contact. Contaminated waste such as soiled dressings or swabs are put into bags, which are sealed and labelled with a biohazard warning.

When performing any nursing care procedures requiring contact with the patient's faeces, disposable gloves are worn.

Acute infectious diarrhoea may readily spread throughout a family, school, hall of residence or neighbourhood because of a common source of infected food or water. The nurse may play an important role in the prevention of diarrhoea by alerting people to the hazards of exposed and unrefrigerated foods, particularly meat and those with cream filling or topping. Opportunities may arise to emphasize the hygienic handling of food and the importance of thorough handwashing after going to the toilet and the handling of soiled clothing.

Carers should be informed of precautions to take to prevent spread to others. Should other individuals who live with that person develop acute diarrhoea, the likely source of the problem needs to be investigated.

If a large number of cases is found in a school or community, the local health authorities should be notified so that a systematic investigation as to the possible source may be instituted. Occasionally, acute diarrhoea may spread through the patients on one ward. The primary source of such an outbreak should be sought. Personnel are urged to practise strict precautions, for infection may be carried from one patient to another or from a member of staff to patients through failure to wash the hands thoroughly between patients, after handling bedpans or linen, or after going to the toilet.

Evaluation

Evaluation of the goals and outcome criteria is based on examination of the person's stools, documented evidence of a decrease in the frequency of defaecation, and absence of fluid and electrolyte imbalances, as well as on the patient's reported perceptions that the diarrhoea is decreased or absent. For individuals with chronic bowel disease that causes diarrhoea, success of the interventions may be determined when they resume active participation in social and recreational activities.

Evaluation of the spread of infection may be determined on a particular nursing unit or by an infection control team. All incidences of infection are reported and recorded as part of the audit process.

Constipation

The majority of persons normally defaecate once every 24 hours but there is considerable variance in the frequency among healthy persons. Some persons have more than one bowel movement daily, whereas others may have an evacuation of a normal moist stool once every 2–3 days. Such variances in frequency of bowel elimination are compatible with health. An individual is considered to be constipated if bowel elimination is inexplicably delayed for several days or if the stool is so hard and dry that it is difficult to expel.

Constipation may be a delay in the passage of faeces through the colon, referred to as *colonic constipation*, or it may be a prolonged retention of the faeces in the rectum, designated as *rectal constipation* or *dyschezia*.

Causes

The causes of constipation are many and varied. It may be associated with organic disease, or may be a functional disturbance. It is frequently associated with a sedentary lifestyle or periods of prolonged bedrest.

Disease within the colon or rectum may narrow the lumen of the bowel and offer resistance to the forward movement of content. Common examples are:

- neoplasms of the intestine
- inflammation, which causes spasm, scarring and adhesions
- partial volvulus (twisting of the bowel).

Severe ascites (accumulation of fluid in the peritoneal cavity) or a tumour, such as an ovarian cyst or uterine fibroid, may compress the colon and delay the movement of intestinal content.

Failure of the normal propulsive movement may occur due to some disturbance or imbalance in the innervation of the intestine. The derangement may result in excessive tone and spasm in a segment of the bowel that retards the movement of the content. The spasm may be induced by a hypersensitivity of the colon or by anxiety. Constipation may be associated with injury or degeneration of the spinal cord or cauda equina, which affects the nerve supply to the colon and rectum.

Constipation may be associated with any illness in which there is diminished intake of food and fluid, or in cases where the diet is modified and lacks fibre, resulting less residue. The lesser amount of food does not provide sufficient bulk to stimulate peristalsis. Dehydration causes a small, dry, hard stool that may irritate the colon, causing spasm, or may fail to stimulate normal colonic motility.

Occasionally, drugs used in treatment may decrease intestinal motility and delay excretion. This increases mixing of the faeces and exposure to the absorptive surface, which dries out the faeces and produces constipation. Common examples of such drugs are opiates (e.g. codeine) and anticholinergic drugs (e.g. propantheline bromide).

Expulsion of the faeces is aided by increasing the intra-abdominal pressure to compress the colon and rectum. This involves contraction of the muscles of the abdominal wall and diaphragm. Weakness of these muscles due to disease, ageing, malnutrition or inactivity may contribute to constipation. Similarly, lack of tone in the intestinal musculature or weakness of the levator ani muscles may impair peristalsis and expulsive power.

Frequent causes of constipation in persons who are not ill are faulty defaecation habits, faulty diet and the habitual use of laxatives. If the urge to defaecate is ignored and evacuation delayed, the reflex becomes weak as the rectal mucosa adapts to the pressure of the content. Repeated failure to respond to the defaecation reflex may eventually result in the rectum becoming insensitive to the presence of a faecal mass and the reflex is not initiated. The person may delay response to the defaecation urge because it is inconvenient or because toilet facilities are not available.

A deficiency of foods with cellulose and fibrous content in the diet may be the cause of constipation. Refined foods and those that leave little residue after absorption fail to produce sufficient bulk to stimulate colonic motility.

Many persons have an inordinate concern about bowel elimination and think they must have a daily bowel movement or a frequent purge and resort to unnecessary, repeated use of a laxative. Loss of intestinal tone and reduced peristaltic response to normal food residue

Constipation.
See chapter 5.1

follow the use of a laxative, and then – too often – the laxative is repeated. The colon is not allowed to regain its natural rhythmic response to the normal faecal mass.

Constipation may cause considerable discomfort; the person may experience abdominal pain, a full feeling and abdominal distension. There is a loss of appetite accompanied by headache and eventually nausea and vomiting. The hard dry masses of faecal matter may damage the intestinal mucosa and lead to a fissure. Haemorrhoids are frequently the result of chronic constipation.

Assessment

The nursing history includes information about:

- the person's usual bowel elimination habits

- any unusual effort or stimulation used to promote defaecation including the use of laxatives or enemas

- the person's perceptions of what is normal bowel elimination

- the person's eating habits – types of foods taken and the volume of fluid taken daily

- the person's problem of constipation and potentially related factors:
    a. the duration and severity of the problem
    b. recent changes in usual eating habits, fluid intake and physical activity
    c. the person's perceptions of the problem
    d. pain, abdominal cramps, passing of gas associated with constipation
    e. history of disorders or medication therapy that may have altered food intake, digestion or absorption of foods, or bowel motility or sensation

- the person's living arrangements and the availability of toilet facilities

- the family's knowledge of foods that contain fibre and the value of fibre in promoting bowel function; the need to maintain an adequate fluid intake; the benefits of exercise and activity; and the action and untoward effects of various types of laxatives.

The person may be asked to keep a record over 2–4 days to determine the frequency and time of bowel elimination, the volume and characteristics of the faeces. Any warning signs of constipation experienced by the patient such as abdominal cramps or flatulence should be noted, along with the patient's own feelings about the problem.

Goals

The person will demonstrate:

1. understanding of the role of dietary fibre and fluid intake in stool formation and defaecation

2. awareness of the role of regular physical activity in the promotion of bowel elimination

---

> **Box 15.3** Steps to establish regular bowel elimination habits
>
> 1. Identify factors contributing to constipation
> 2. Discontinue the use of laxatives and enemas
> 3. Develop a diet plan to increase fibre and fluid intake
> 4. Develop a plan to increase daily physical activity
> 5. Establish a schedule for daily bowel elimination
> 6. Implement diet, exercise plans and elimination schedule daily
> 7. Evaluate the effectiveness of plan each day
> 8. Modify plan as necessary.

3. a plan to increase dietary fibre and fluid intake and to obtain regular physical activity

4. regular bowel elimination.

Nursing intervention

Box 15.3 lists the steps to be implemented in formulating a plan to develop regular bowel elimination habits for a patient.

Establishing a regular schedule

It is helpful to explain to the person in simple terms the physiological mechanism of defaecation so that the significance of responding to the initial urge for defaecation may be understood. The frequency of bowel elimination varies with the individual. It should be stressed to the patient that daily bowel elimination is not essential to health; defaecation every 2–3 days may be normal for some people.

Dietary modifications

The nurse and dietician work with the patient and family to evaluate current dietary habits and then help them to plan a diet that provides a liberal amount of fibre-containing foods, taking into consideration the person's food preferences, financial resources and daily routine. Emphasis is placed on whole-grain cereals and bread, fresh fruits and vegetables, and fruit juices. A daily fluid intake of 2000–2500 mL is recommended unless contraindicated by a cardiovascular or renal condition.

Peristalsis may be promoted by the drinking of a cup of hot water on rising in the morning (approximately half an hour before breakfast).

It has been demonstrated that regular bowel elimination can be achieved in the institutionalized elderly by adjusting the diet to increase fibre and fluid intake and increasing exercise (either active or passive). Reviewing medications and patients' toileting facilities are also

---

Box 15.4   Techniques to promote bowel elimination

1. Increase the amount of fibre in the diet

2. Increase daily fluid intake

3. Increase daily physical activity

4. Respond promptly to the urge for a bowel movement

5. Drink a cup of warm liquid half an hour before the usual time of defaecation

6. Go to the bathroom at the usual time for defaecation

7. Sit comfortably on the toilet in an environment that provides privacy, quiet and warmth

8. Use the following techniques to stimulate peristalsis:
   a. contract abdominal muscles, lean forward and bear down
   b. exert manual pressure downward on the abdomen

9. If the above techniques are not successful in producing a bowel movement, consider use of the following, in this order:
   a. glycerine suppository
   b. emollient laxative or stool softener
   c. bulk-forming laxative
   d. enema.

---

important in restoring regular bowel habit and reducing the use of laxatives (Nazarko 1996).

Techniques to promote defaecation

Box 15.4 lists various measures the person may use to promote regular bowel elimination; a scheduled time for **defaecation** is stressed as is the importance of prompt response to the urge to defaecate. Ensuring comfort and privacy during the defaecation attempt, contracting abdominal muscles, leaning forward and bearing down to increase abdominal pressure and application of manual pressure to the abdomen may be helpful.

The person is instructed to implement these techniques daily until defaecation occurs. If no bowel movement occurs in 2–3 days, glycerine suppositories may be used. If this is still not effective, a stool softener or bulk laxative may be administered. Once the person establishes a regular schedule, other laxatives or enemas should not be necessary.

Physical exercise

Some physical exercise is essential; walking is especially helpful and good tone in the abdominal muscles is important.

Laxatives and enemas

Laxatives, enemas and suppositories that the patient may be accustomed to using are discontinued. If increased dietary fibre, fluids and exercise are not sufficient at the beginning to establish normal bowel elimination, mild laxatives may be employed until the defaecation reflex is restored and bowel irritability and spasm are reduced. Glycerine suppositories placed in the rectum, and into stool if present, may be used half an hour before the usual time of defaecation to stimulate peristalsis and soften stool. The suppository may be repeated daily for several days. If this is not effective, a stool softener may be ordered to prevent severe straining at stool and injury to the rectal and anal tissues. The stool softeners in use are mineral oil and preparations of docusate sodium. These latter preparations act as wetting agents, allowing water to penetrate and mix with the faecal mass. Mineral oil should not be used for prolonged periods because it may prevent normal intestinal absorption, especially of fat-soluble vitamins.

Bulk-forming laxatives may also be recommended. These preparations swell when combined with fluid in the gastrointestinal tract and have a stimulating effect. Examples of bulk-forming laxatives are bran and ispaghula husk. Use of these laxatives should be assessed carefully in the elderly if dehydration is present. Osmotic laxatives such as lactulose syrup are disaccharides that are not absorbed in the small intestine. They are broken down by bacteria in the colon and acidify the colonic contents, which then stimulates peristalsis and serves as an effective laxative for the elderly. Magnesium hydroxide (Milk of Magnesia) is a cathartic that is not completely absorbed in the small intestine and causes retention of water in the intestinal lumen, stimulating peristalsis. It is contraindicated for those with any renal insufficiency.

Defaecation
See chapter 5.1

Evaluation

A programme of increased dietary fibre, increased fluid intake, regular physical activity and a schedule for defaecation can promote effective regular bowel elimination for most adults as well as for the frail elderly. The use of laxatives is usually not necessary if a comprehensive bowel elimination programme is followed. In hospital and long-term care settings, the documentation of bowel patterns and laxative use on the same assessment tool facilitates regular review of the effectiveness of nursing intervention. Information from chart audits on a nursing unit as well as data provided by a quality assurance programme help nurses to analyse their clinical practice and to identify strengths and areas for change in relation to common health problems such as constipation.

Faecal impaction

Occasionally, faeces accumulate in the rectum, producing a hard dry mass that forms a partial or complete obstruction. It occurs most often in older persons and in those with central nervous system disorders. These patients frequently suffer a loss of intestinal musculature motility and sensation. It may be associated with dehydration, lack of dietary fibre and volume, immobilization or narcotics. Manifestations include cramping pain, the passage of liquid stools without expulsion of the hard palpable faecal mass. The patient may complain of headache, fatigue, loss of appetite, and pressure and discomfort in the rectal and anal regions. Faecal impaction is identified by the presence of a palpable hard mass in the rectum, the oozing of liquid stools without passing the faecal mass and the absence of a bowel movement for over 3 days.

Goals

The patient will demonstrate:

1. regular bowel movements after relief of impaction
2. understanding of the role of dietary fibre and fluid intake in stool formation and defaecation
3. awareness of the role of physical activity in promoting bowel elimination
4. application of a programme to promote regular bowel elimination.

Nursing intervention

Relief of impaction

The faecal impaction is treated by the administration of an oil retention enema to soften the impacted stool and by oral administration of an emollient laxative such as docusate sodium, which also softens the stools. The enema is followed in a few hours by digital breaking up and removal of the faecal mass. The nurse lubricates a gloved finger and gently inserts it into the patient's rectum to loosen the impacted faeces. A cleansing enema of saline or tap water is then given. This process is usually both embarrassing and exhausting; following the enema the patient is made comfortable and allowed to rest. Psychological support is very important.

Promotion of regular bowel elimination habits

The patient experiencing faecal impaction should be assisted to develop a regular bowel elimination programme which includes dietary management, increased activity, a regular schedule and the use of techniques to stimulate peristalsis. Glycerine suppositories, stool softeners or bulk laxatives may be required initially. Impaction occurs most often in the elderly who do not eat adequate fibre and who have problems with mobility and experience difficulties in getting to the bathroom. The patient's living environment is assessed and the accessibility of the toilet taken into consideration. Assistance may be required from the district nurse, neighbours and friends to ensure the aged or incapacitated individual receives an adequate diet and necessary

physical assistance. If the patient is in a hospital or nursing home, a plan for bowel elimination is an integral part of the patient care plan. Excessive bedrest is avoided and physical activity encouraged.

Evaluation

Regular, spontaneous bowel movements will resume and further episodes of impaction will not occur.

Faecal incontinence

Assessment

The nursing history is reviewed to determine the patient's usual bowel elimination habits. The problem of incontinence is assessed by observing and recording the frequency of defaecation, the consistency of the stools, and warning signs experienced or expressed by the patient related to defaecation. It is important to note whether the patient experiences an urge to defaecate, manifests abdominal discomfort, massages the abdomen, or provides verbal clues that defaecation is occurring. Mental alertness is evaluated to determine the patient's ability to respond to the urge to defaecate and to follow a bowel elimination schedule.

Goals

The person will demonstrate:

1. controlled and regular bowel evacuation
2. absence or decrease in episodes of faecal incontinence.

Nursing intervention

Establishment of a regular bowel routine

Faecal continence can be established by developing regular bowel elimination habits, as discussed for the patient experiencing constipation, or by establishing a programme for regular bowel evacuation.

Programme to stimulate peristalsis

When the cause of the incontinence is constipation or faecal impaction, as commonly occurs in the elderly, a programme to adjust the diet and activity, maintain regularity and stimulate peristaltic activity is usually effective.

Prevention of reflex bowel emptying

When neuromuscular control is impaired, management of incontinence is directed to preventing reflex emptying of the bowel in response to rectal distension by faeces. If the patient has a predictable pattern of defaecation such as after breakfast each morning, a schedule can be developed to ensure that the patient is assisted to the bathroom or to a commode each morning after breakfast. If the patient's pattern of defaecation is irregular, attempts are made to establish a regular time for bowel evacuation. A daily routine is established, similar to that described for the patient who is constipated. The techniques described in Box 15.4 to stimulate peristalsis are employed. If no bowel movement occurs, the routine is repeated the next day. A glycerine suppository may be used on the second or third day to further stimulate defaecation. If the patient usually defaecates every 2 days, this measure would be introduced on the second day before the expected involuntary defaecation. A stool softener may also be used.

Patients with spinal cord injury or neurological disease are usually able to establish a regular defaecation pattern and avoid episodes of incontinence. Routine enemas and laxatives are avoided. Patient participation in developing and implementing a bowel-retraining programme is important if long-term results are to be achieved.

Personal hygiene

Until regular bowel evacuation is established, the incontinent patient is kept clean and dry, and skin irritation is avoided. Following faecal incontinence the skin is washed with soap, rinsed well and patted dry. Protective ointment may be applied to provide a coating over the skin. The clothing and bedding are changed as often as necessary to keep the patient clean. The nurse may reduce the patient's embarrassment and concern with reassurance that it is understood that the patient cannot control the bowel movements but that this can be achieved with a bowel-retraining programme. Episodes of incontinence may still occur if the patient develops diarrhoea or if the routine is changed, but most patients can achieve acceptable control if the programme is followed.

Irritable bowel syndrome

Irritable bowel syndrome (IBS) is a common but poorly understood syndrome characterized by multiple abdominal symptoms. It affects Western populations, and women are twice as likely to experience it as men. It is difficult to know how many people are affected as IBS does not appear on death certificates and general practitioners are likely to refer only about 20% of patients with IBS to a gastroenterologist (Thompson et al 2000).

IBS is used to describe a number of conditions with similar symptoms which have no organic cause. These include:

- cramping abdominal pain
- bloated abdomen
- altered and unpredictable bowel habit.

Abnormal colonic motility increases pressure in the large bowel. Spasmodic, non-propulsive contractions in the sensitive colonic muscularis result in cramp or spasm-like pain, but faeces may not be moved effectively through the colon. Consequently they become hard, dry and pellet-like. Alternatively, very loose stool may be passed with urgency, but also with associated pain and bloating.

Antispasmodics (e.g. mebeverine), osmotic laxatives and amitriptyline (to reduce gut motility) may help severe symptoms. However, many people prefer to try to adapt their diet and lifestyle, or use complementary therapies to manage their symptoms.

People with IBS often fear they have cancer. IBS is often diagnosed only when all other differential diagnoses have been excluded by means of extensive investigation. Thus the person can usually be reassured. Nursing support and encouragement to adapt lifestyle and manage symptoms is vital for these people, who often feel their symptoms are dismissed as unimportant by healthcare professionals (Taylor 1997).

Disorders of the small intestine

Malabsorption syndrome

Malabsorption involves failure to transport nutrients from the intestinal lumen to the vascular and lymphatic systems with loss of nutrients in the stool. It results from impairment of either the digestive or the absorptive process.

Nutrients are absorbed: (1) into the capillaries and from there are carried through the portal vein into the liver and then into the systemic circulation; or (2) through the lacteals into the thoracic lymphatic system and on into the systemic circulation. The absorptive cells of the intestinal villi are especially adapted for both absorption and secretion.

The causes of malabsorption may be:

- a lack of normal intraluminal digestion
- dysfunction of the absorptive cells of the intestinal mucosa
- impairment of the intestinal circulation or lymphatic system.

Clinical characteristics

The signs and symptoms of the malabsorption syndrome vary from severe to very mild; with the latter, the disorder may go undetected for years. The major manifestations are: weight loss; abnormal stools which are bulky, soft, light yellow to grey in colour and have a rancid odour; abdominal distension; anorexia; muscle wasting; peripheral oedema; weakness and skeletal disorders. Table 15.1 lists the signs and symptoms of malabsorption with their aetiological factors.

Digestive disturbances

Malabsorption due to digestive disturbances occurs with liver and biliary tract disease, following a gastrectomy and with bacterial overgrowth in the small bowel. With liver and biliary tract disease the primary symptom of inadequate digestion and absorption is the presence of

Table 15.1   Potential problems for the patient with systemic manifestations of malabsorption

Causes	Clinical characteristics
Nutrition less than body requirements	
Malabsorption of fat, carbohydrate or protein; calorie loss; and protein loss (albumin)	Muscle wasting, weight loss and oedema
Altered bowel elimination	
Impaired absorption or increased secretion of water and electrolytes	Diarrhoea, abdominal distension and flatulence, fatigue
Increased secretion of water and electrolytes with unabsorbed bile and fatty acids	Pale, bulky, odorous stools
Fluid and electrolyte load in excess of absorptive capacity of colon	Weight loss
Impaired carbohydrate absorption	
Impaired fat absorption and increased loss of fat	
Altered urinary elimination	
Delayed absorption of water; hypokalaemia	Nocturia and dehydration
Weakness and fatigue	
Impaired absorption of iron, vitamin B_{12}, folate; loss of electrolytes (potassium)	Anaemia and weakness
Increased potential for bleeding	
Impaired vitamin K absorption; increased prothrombin time	Bruising and haematuria
Altered muscle tone and sensation	
Impaired absorption of calcium and magnesium	Muscle cramps, tetany, and prickling and burning sensations
Impaired absorption of potassium	Muscle flaccidity, weakness, decreased tendon reflexes and cardiac arrhythmia
Increased potential for injury	
Impaired absorption of calcium and protein; demineralization of bone	Skeletal deformities and bone fractures
Altered sexuality patterns	
Impaired protein absorption; loss of calories	Amenorrhoea
	Decreased libido
Altered integrity of skin and oral mucosa	
Impaired absorption of iron, vitamin B_{12} and other vitamins	Dermatitis, glossitis and dry fissures of the lips
Altered visual acuity	
Impaired absorption of vitamin A	Night blindness

steatorrhoea or undigested fat in the stool. Decreased synthesis or excretion of bile salts results in impaired digestion of fat and interferes with the absorption of vitamin D and calcium. Following a gastric resection, emptying of the stomach occurs more rapidly; the duodenum may be bypassed, decreasing the stimulation of pancreatic enzymes; mixing of bile salts may be inadequate; stasis of intestinal contents may occur; and protein intake may be decreased.

Management includes the administration of pancreatic enzymes. Bacterial growth in the small bowel is controlled by normal peristalsis. When intestinal motility is impaired, bacterial proliferation occurs, resulting in changes in the action of the bile salts. Fat absorption is impaired and steatorrhoea is present. Vitamin B_{12} absorption is also decreased due to its utilization by the microorganisms. Treatment involves antibiotic therapy.

Dysfunction of absorbing cells

Malabsorption due to dysfunction or destruction of the absorbing cells may be due to an inadequate absorptive surface resulting from extensive resection of the small bowel, intestinal bypass or extensive inflammatory disease. Patient management includes a high-calorie diet: high in carbohydrates and protein and low in fat. Vitamin and mineral supplements are administered. Drugs such as belladonna alkaloids and codeine may be given to decrease intestinal motility. Ranitidine may be given to decrease gastric acid secretion. Long-term parenteral nutrition may be required in very extensive resection or total removal of the intestine, called short bowel syndrome.

Enzyme deficiencies

The malabsorption syndrome may be due to enzyme deficiencies in the intestinal mucosal cells. Adult lactase deficiency is a common disorder which causes an intolerance to lactose, the sugar found in milk. Hydrolysis of disaccharides takes place on the glycocalyx of the microvilli of the intestinal cells. When lactase is deficient, lactose is not hydrolysed to galactose, and glucose and is not absorbed; it remains in the intestinal lumen and draws water by osmosis into the lumen. Symptoms include abdominal cramps, distension, flatulence and diarrhoea following ingestion of dairy products. The diagnosis is made by taking a history and by a lactose tolerance test. The disorder is more common in African Caribbean and Asian people than in Caucasians. Treatment consists of a milk-free diet; cheese contains a minimal amount of lactose and is tolerated by most patients.

Gluten-sensitive enteropathy

Gluten-sensitive enteropathy (coeliac disease) is an immunological disorder characterized by a reaction of the intestinal mucosa, particularly in the jejunum, to gliadin (a component of the gluten of wheat). The mucosa is damaged, the villi atrophy and absorptive cells are infiltrated by lymphocytes and plasma cells. Other enzyme alterations may occur. Mucosal damage results in decreased stimulation of pancreatic hormones, impaired absorption of water and electrolytes, and the excretion of unabsorbed fats. Symptoms include weight loss, distension, diarrhoea and steatorrhoea.

A gluten-free diet is recommended; wheat, rye, barley and oats are avoided. Rice, corn, soybean and potato flours are used as substitutes in the diet.

Drugs

Certain drugs may also interfere with intestinal absorption. Examples of drugs that affect the absorption in the intestine include antacids, anticonvulsants, biguanides and folic acid.

Assessment

Health history

Data collected from the patient during the health history focus on the diet, bowel habits and the symptoms being experienced.

Problems commonly encountered by patients are listed in Table 15.1; these should be borne in mind during the assessment and form the basis for a patient interview. The patient's perspective is very important in considering these problems and the effects they may have on everyday life.

Physical examination

The nurse inspects the patient's skin for dryness, turgor and oedema. The specific characteristics of the patient's stools are observed and documented. The person's height and weight are recorded and their desirable body weight is determined. The perianal area should be examined discretely for soreness, excoriation, fissures and fistulae. Any episodes of faecal incontinence should be established, and how these were managed by the individual.

Goals

The person with malabsorption disorders will demonstrate:

1. achievement and maintenance of a desirable bodyweight
2. a decrease in diarrhoea
3. understanding of recommended dietary measures
4. integrity of skin and oral mucosa.

Nursing intervention

Health problems common to persons with malabsorption syndrome are listed in Table 15.1. As malabsorption syndromes are usually not curable, care for the patient is directed towards control of nutritional deficiencies and alleviation of symptoms.

Diet

Dietary measures include elimination of the specific inabsorbable nutrient from the diet and administration of the unabsorbed nutrients by other routes if necessary.

The person with gluten-sensitive enteropathy should eliminate wheat, rye, barley and oats from the diet and substitute cornmeal and potato, rice and soyabean flour. The dietician may provide recipes that substitute these products for the traditional wheat, rye and oat flours used in breads, pastries, cakes and pastas. The patient is also advised about health food stores and other outlets that carry gluten-free products.

The person with lactose intolerance should avoid dairy products, prepared foods and baked goods containing milk, butter and cheeses, instant coffee and chocolate. Some individuals with lactose intolerance are able to tolerate fermented dairy products such as yoghurt and cheese. Commercial products that are low in lactose or are lactose-free are available as substitutes for milk products in the diet or use as supplements.

Vitamins B_{12} and K are administered parenterally when deficiencies exist and persons with lactose intolerance may require calcium substitutes if dietary calcium is deficient.

Teaching

The nurse and dietician play a major role in patient and family teaching about the malabsorption disorder and dietary measures to manage the syndrome and associated symptoms. The person is taught to identify foods and food products containing the substances that cannot be tolerated and to avoid these in the diet. Skill and experience in reading product labels is emphasized. Individuals are also taught ways to alter the diet to incorporate substitute foods for the ones that are not tolerated. Patients also learn to identify their own symptoms and evaluate their diet to identify contributing factors and then to readjust their diet accordingly.

Evaluation

Symptoms associated with the malabsorption disorder should decrease as the person responds to the dietary changes that eliminate the responsible elements. Progress can be measured by changes in the stools and a decrease in diarrhoea, as well as by the establishment and maintenance of a desirable bodyweight.

Inflammatory disorders of the intestines

Inflammation may develop in any area of the small and large intestines and alter motility, secretion and/or absorption. The most prevalent inflammatory intestinal diseases include the acute condition of appendicitis and gastroenteritis, and the chronic disorders of Crohn's disease and ulcerative colitis.

Inflammation
See chapter 6.1

Appendicitis

The appendix, a narrow blind tube extending from the inferior part of the caecum, is a common site of inflammation, which may necessitate its surgical removal. The appendix has no essential function in the human and there is no change in body function when it has been removed.

Causes

The most common cause of appendicitis is obstruction of the lumen by a faecalith (a small, hard mass of accumulated faeces) or a solid foreign body, or by disease or scar tissue in the walls of the appendix. Secretion collects in the tube, causing distension that results in pressure on the intramural blood vessels. The mucosa becomes inflamed, ulcerates and readily becomes infected; the walls may become gangrenous because of the interference with the blood supply, and perforation is likely to occur. A ruptured appendix is serious; it allows the escape of organisms into the peritoneal cavity and may produce an abscess in the appendiceal region or a generalized peritonitis.

The disease may occur at any age but is more common in children over 4 years of age, adolescents and young adults. Early diagnosis and treatment of appendicitis is important to prevent serious complications.

Clinical characteristics

Manifestations of appendicitis are abdominal pain, nausea and vomiting, a moderate increase in temperature and a leucocytosis, with the increase being in the polymorphonuclear cells. At the onset, the pain may be diffuse or referred to the central portion of the abdomen or the lower epigastric region, and is described as crampy. As the inflammation involves the walls of the appendix, the pain becomes localized to the lower right quadrant or McBurney's point (the area about 5 cm from the anterior superior iliac spine on a line with the umbilicus, which corresponds to the normal position of the appendix). The area is tender on palpation, and rigidity gradually develops in the muscles (muscle guarding). Rebound tenderness may be present, and is determined by palpation of the left lower quadrant. With the sudden release of the pressure, the patient experiences pain or discomfort in the appendix region. The patient moves slowly and carefully to avoid jolting and movements that increase the pain, and tends to keep the right thigh flexed.

The omentum and adjacent bowel may become adherent to the inflamed appendix, walling off the area. If the appendix ruptures, an abscess will form in the walled-off cavity. If perforation occurs before the area is walled off, a generalized peritonitis develops; the patient complains of pain and tenderness over the whole abdomen, which becomes rigid and distended. The distension is due to inhibited bowel motility, and may be referred to as *paralytic ileus*.

Examination of the patient includes palpation of the abdomen and a differential leucocyte determination. The doctor may also conduct a rectal examination, and a vaginal pelvic examination may be done on the female.

The treatment of appendicitis is surgical excision of the appendix.

Nursing intervention

The person with abdominal pain should be urged to seek medical advice; self-treatment is discouraged, particularly the taking of a laxative or an enema which could be serious, because either could cause perforation of the appendix through stimulation of peristalsis. The patient is also advised not to take food or fluid until seen by the doctor. This is in case immediate surgery is necessary. In most instances, surgery is performed as soon as the diagnosis is established unless perforation is suspected. If the appendix was intact at the time of removal, the patient usually makes a rapid, uneventful recovery with a short period of hospitalization.

If an abscess is present, a drain is placed in the abscess cavity at the time of operation. The collecting bag attached to the drain allows observation of the discharge and accurate measurement of the volume of fluid draining. Antibiotics are prescribed and the patient should receive a minimum of 2.5 litres of fluids daily. An accurate record of the intake should be kept and, if the patient cannot take sufficient quantities by mouth, the administration of intravenous fluids may be necessary. Close observations are made for possible extension of the infection and generalized peritonitis, such as abdominal distension, nausea and vomiting, lack of bowel sounds, a raised temperature and rapid pulse; these are brought promptly to the surgeon's attention.

Box 15.5 gives a care plan for a patient having an uncomplicated appendicectomy.

Generally no follow-up is required for patients who have undergone straightforward appendicetomy.

Peritonitis

Peritonitis is a localized or generalized inflammation of the **peritoneum** and is most often a secondary condition. It is usually acute but may be chronic.

Causes

The inflammatory response may be due to bacterial invasion or chemical irritation caused by bile, pancreatic, gastric or intestinal secretions, urine or blood escaping into the peritoneal cavity. A common infectious agent is *Escherichia coli* that has escaped from the intestinal lumen.

Intestinal motility is depressed and the intestine becomes distended with gas and fluid. The peritoneal serous membrane becomes hyperaemic and oedematous, and there is an outpouring of fluid into the cavity that incurs serous fluid, electrolyte and protein imbalances.

Clinical characteristics

The patient experiences abdominal pain, nausea, vomiting and distension. The abdomen becomes rigid (muscle guarding) and progressively more distended. A leucocytosis and pyrexia may develop. The pulse becomes rapid and there is a decrease in blood volume due to loss of intravascular volume. The respirations may be shallow and rapid as a result of ventilatory interference by extreme abdominal distension. Unless quickly reversed, the patient shows signs of shock. Bowel sounds are absent as peristalsis ceases.

Treatment is directed toward the primary condition (e.g. an operation to close a perforated ulcer), relieving the distension and re-establishing peristalsis, combating infection and shock, and replacing fluids and electrolytes.

Gastric and intestinal intubation with continuous drainage are established. Nothing is given orally. An intravenous infusion is administered and the solutions used may be based upon laboratory determinations of serum electrolyte levels. A blood transfusion may be given to counteract shock and replace protein lost in the inflammatory exudate. An antibiotic is administered if organisms are the causative factor of the peritonitis.

Peritoneum.
See chapter 5.1

Box 15.5   Care plan for a patient undergoing appendicetomy

For a patient undergoing uncomplicated appendicetomy who does not live alone, the overall aim should be to be discharged home safely within 36 hours of operation. Such a patient's problems, the goals for care and the plan to achieve the goals are outlined below.

Problem	Goal	Action
Pain due to incision and resolving peritonitis	To be pain-free or at least to have a pain score of 1 or less (on a scale of 0 = no pain, 5 = worst pain imaginable). To be able to sleep, move and cough freely	Administer prescribed analgesia regularly. Do not wait for the pain to develop first. Assess effectiveness of prescription and consult about a change if indicated. Administer oral analgesia as soon as possible, also on a regular basis to avoid the development of pain. As pain subsides, advise a reduction in dose before reducing frequency. Ensure the patient moves in bed every hour and gets out of bed, and undertakes activities of daily living independently
Altered breathing due to discomfort and anaesthetic	Regular deep breathing; resting rate < 20 per min, > 10 per min. No smoking	Deep breathing exercises hourly. Encourage coughing and expectoration. Show the patient how to support the abdomen with a soft pad while doing so. Advise continuing these exercises at home for at least a week. If a smoker, discuss the habit with a view to encouraging cessation

(Continued)

Box 15.5 *(Continued)*

Problem	Goal	Action
Feeling weak after surgery	Blood pressure to be within the patient's normal limits as before operation. Heart rate <90 beats per min or as before surgery. Homeostatic fluid and electrolyte balance to be restored as soon as possible	Check vital signs regularly after operation for several hours until stable and goal attained. Check 6 hourly thereafter until discharge. Continue intravenous infusion (IVI) after operation until drinking and then discontinue. Check the patient has passed urine within 24 hours of operation and the volume is not more than 500 mL less than that taken in
Altered gastrointestinal function following surgery	Resume oral intake of light diet and 1500 mL fluid as soon as possible	Clear fluids orally as able. If tolerated, may drink as likes. Remove IVI. Administer prescribed antiemetic if nauseous. When drinks tolerated, offer soup and pudding or light breakfast as appropriate, and light diet thereafter. Advise three light meals and 1500 mL fluid intake at home, introducing larger, high-fibre meals gradually. Counsel about healthy eating as required. Re-establishing bowel habit may take a few days but provided the patient follows advice about healthy eating and drinking and takes daily gentle exercise, this should resolve. Advise to consult GP if not
Wound healing	Wound to heal by first intention within 2 weeks. Temperature to be <37.5°C	Check the wound regularly after surgery for oozing and inflammation. Monitor the patient's temperature 6 hourly until discharge. Change the dressing as indicated and before the patient goes home. Advise the patient that it is safe to get the wound wet and demonstrate how to apply clean gauze if desired. If sutures are not absorbed, arrange appointment for practice nurse to remove them at surgeon's instructions (usually 5–7 days). Advise the patient to see their GP if there is any oozing or inflammation in the wound, or fever >37.5°C for more than 12 hours

The patient is very ill and requires constant supportive nursing care and monitoring.

Chronic inflammatory bowel disease

Inflammatory bowel disease (IBD) is the term used to designate the two inflammatory gastrointestinal conditions of Crohn's disease and ulcerative colitis.

Crohn's disease is a chronic inflammatory disease that may affect any part of the gastrointestinal tract but most commonly involves the terminal ileum and proximal colon. Patches of granulomatous inflammation and ulceration develop in segments of the intestine and involve all layers of the wall. The bowel may perforate and form an internal or external fistula (an abnormal passage) into another loop of intestine or on to the skin. As the inflammation subsides, there is scarring and some stenosis, which may lead to a partial obstruction.

Ulcerative colitis is characterized by severe inflammation and ulceration of the mucosa of the rectum and of a part or all of the colon. The process begins in the rectosigmoid area and spreads up the descending colon. There is marked inflammation and oedema in the affected area, followed by ulceration. In affected areas there may be infection and a loss of fluid, electrolytes and blood.

Incidence

Crohn's disease and ulcerative colitis mainly affect young adults and are much more common in the industrialized West than elsewhere in the world.

Contributing factors

The cause of IBD is unknown. It is believed that Crohn's disease and ulcerative colitis are two distinct entities and not a progression of bowel disease, and that more than one mechanism contributes to the development of the disorders. There are many misconceptions about possible causes of IBD such as dietary and personality factors. For example, personality characteristics attributed to patients with the condition probably result from the disease and its pattern of exacerbations and remissions rather than contributing to its cause:

- *Immunological mechanisms* play a protective role in the gastrointestinal tract, which has its own immune system. To date, no specific immunological disorders have been identified as causes of either Crohn's disease or ulcerative colitis.

- *Genetic factors* are thought to be involved because of the familial incidence of the disease. There does appear to be a relationship in some families between ankylosing spondylitis, the HLA genes and IBD.

- *Infectious agents* have long been considered to be implicated in Crohn's disease. Investigators are currently studying the possible roles of anaerobic bacteria and viruses. No organisms have been found to cause IBD and there is no evidence of transmission from one person to another.

- *Environmental agents* have not been shown to cause IBD, despite numerous investigations and evidence of its worldwide distribution.

- *Emotional factors and stress* have not been shown to cause IBD, despite the demonstrated relationship between stress and bowel disorders.

Clinical characteristics

Ulcerative colitis

The major symptom of ulcerative colitis is diarrhoea, the severity and frequency of which depend on the extent of colon involvement. Stools are usually liquid, occur with tenesmus (painful, ineffective straining), and may contain blood, mucus and pus. The number of stools per day may vary from as few as 4 to as many as 24. Accompanying the diarrhoea is a sense of urgency and cramping abdominal pain. The pain is usually located in the lower left quadrant and is colicky in nature. After defaecation, pain may subside.

Ulcerative colitis varies in intensity and severity of presentation, ranging from mild to severe. As the disease becomes more severe, malaise and fatigue occur. Weight loss is common and individuals may limit food intake in order to decrease bowel movements. In the more severe cases, tenderness in the left lower quadrant, guarding and abdominal distension may occur, as well as anaemia, leucocytosis, tachycardia, fever and dehydration.

Crohn's disease

The patient with Crohn's disease may have occasional acute episodes of illness but more often has mild and intermittent symptoms. Acute inflammatory symptoms include pain in the lower right quadrant, cramping, tenderness, spasm, flatulence, nausea, fever and diarrhoea. Unlike ulcerative colitis, there is often no visible blood in the stools. Borborygmi and increased peristalsis may also be present. The most severe pain may mimic acute appendicitis or bowel perforation. The more typical picture is the chronic type, which has more persistent but less severe symptoms. When the terminal ileum is involved, the pain is in the periumbilical region. Jejunal pain is in the upper and left abdomen. Initially the ileal pain is intermittent; later it becomes more constant and may be noticed in the lower right quadrant.

Pain or discomfort accompanied by anorexia and malaise are the most common symptoms. The pain is usually peristaltic and intermittent. Cramps of regional enteritis are not closely associated with defaecation, and unlike cramps with colonic disease relief does not occur after passing stool or flatus. A constant aching, soreness or tenderness usually indicates advanced disease.

Diarrhoea is a consistent sign but is usually less severe than that associated with ulcerative colitis. The usual consistency of the stool is soft or semi-liquid. If steatorrhoea is also present, the stools will be quite foul smelling and fatty. A large amount of flatus is also likely to be a problem.

Abscess and fistula formation are common and may be characterized by a spiking fever and leucocytosis. Perianal disease, including fistulae and fissures, can occur. As Crohn's disease most often affects a portion of the small intestine, which then loses its ability to absorb nutritional matter, this can result in weight loss, malnutrition, cachexia, amenorrhoea in women and growth retardation in children.

Comparison of the two disorders shows differences as well as similarities. Crohn's disease may affect any part of the gastrointestinal tract. The lesions are patchy in distribution and transmural in nature, resulting in thickening of the wall, fistula formation and perforation of the bowel. Ulcerative colitis affects the large intestine, the lesions are continuous and as they progress the bowel thickens, narrows and shortens. There is an increased incidence of gastrointestinal cancer with both disorders. Both diseases may cause extracolonic manifestations, such as joint problems due to acute migratory polyarthritis, stiffness and pain in the back due to ankylosing spondylitis, jaundice and itching due to a chronic active hepatitis, and eye irritation due to episcleritis or uveitis.

Patients may suffer from weight loss, anaemia, debility, fatigue, nausea, vomiting, and fluid, electrolyte and metabolic disturbances. Ulcerative colitis and Crohn's disease are both characterized by remissions and exacerbations. Both are very disruptive to the lives of the patients and their families. They affect the person's ability to eat, participate in social and work activities, and personality.

Diagnostic investigations

The diagnostic process may be prolonged and cause considerable discomfort and inconvenience to the patient. The preparation for and the procedures themselves further aggravate the already troublesome bowel problems.

Stool cultures

Stool cultures may be carried out to identify the presence of several microorganisms that can mimic IBD.

Sigmoidoscopy

A direct examination of the anal canal, rectum and sigmoid colon may be made by means of a sigmoidoscope. A tissue specimen (biopsy) may also be obtained at the same time.

An explanation of the procedure is given to the patient, including advice about the position that will be required. The left lateral is the position commonly used. The lower bowel should be empty; cleansing enemas are usually given before the scheduled time.

Unnecessary exposure should be avoided by adequate drapes. In the left lateral position the lower limbs are flexed, with the right one being drawn up further than the left. Suction is made available to remove any secretion or fluid faeces that interfere with visualization of the bowel mucosa.

After the examination, the perianal region is cleaned and the patient encouraged to rest. The individual may experience discomfort during the examination as air is pumped into the bowel to distend the lumen.

Colonoscopy

The flexible fibreoptic colonoscope has made possible the visualization of the complete colon, the taking of a biopsy and pictures of a lesion, and the removal of polyps. Insufflation of air is used during the procedure to distend the bowel, permitting better visualization.

The patient should be advised of the purpose of the examination and what to expect, and is asked to sign a statement giving consent. The bowel must be absolutely clean. A low-residue or clear-fluids-only diet is usually given. Laxatives are given the day before the colonoscopy to ensure that the bowel is empty. The regimen is modified if the patient is suffering from acute colitis or rectal bleeding.

The patient is told that it will be helpful during the examination to take deep breaths with the mouth slightly open and to relax the abdominal muscles. Sedation (pethidine or midazolam) may be given before and during the scheduled colonoscopy. The patient is requested to indicate pain during the examination. The patient is usually placed in the recumbent position on the left side and the nurse remains at the patient's head, providing necessary psychological support.

Following the colonoscopy, the patient is allowed to rest and receives food and fluids. The patient is observed for signs of bleeding, pain, and abdominal tenderness and rigidity. The intake may be restricted to fluids for a period of time and then a low-residue diet is gradually introduced.

Radiological techniques and fluoroscopy

Introducing contrast medium into the lumen of the gastrointestinal tract allows it to be examined radiologically. Contrast medium may consist of a barium compound, an iodine solution, air or a combination of these. Barium sulfate is the most widely used and is very safe; however, its use is contraindicated when perforation is suspected. In such cases a water-soluble solution of iodine should be used. The aim of the examination is to outline the lumen with barium, utilizing its coating properties so that any mucosal destruction, distortion or deviation from the normal contour can be assessed. Lesions extending into the lumen are shown as filling defects or as an abnormal extension to the line of the mucosa. Failure of the barium to progress with dilatation suggests obstruction.

The passage of barium may be followed in 'real time' by X-ray fluoroscopy. This yields useful information about function (e.g. the swallowing mechanism) and also facilitates the optimal position of the patient for a 'spot' radiography. The fluoroscopic image can be recorded on video for later analysis.

Barium may be used to examine the oesophagus (barium swallow), stomach and duodenum (barium meal), small bowel (small bowel meal or enema) and colon (barium enema).

Patient preparation for the barium study will vary, depending on the part of the gastrointestinal tract being examined. Instructions are issued by the radiology department directly to patients in the case of outpatient investigations, and to the ward in the case of inpatients.

For barium swallows and meals the patient has nothing by mouth from the evening before, as residual food or fluid interferes with the technical quality of the examination and hinders interpretation. Mild to moderate laxatives are given before small bowel studies to clear small bowel contents and help empty stool from the caecum, which facilitates the visualization of the ileocaecal region. More aggressive measures are needed for colonic cleansing prior to a barium enema, as even small amounts of faecal material can mimic polypoid lesions. These measures vary from place to place, but usually include food restriction for 24–48 hours before the examination, and a purgative. Some centres also use colonic lavage or enemas. Frail, elderly patients may tolerate the bowel preparation poorly (e.g. they may become dehydrated and/or hypotensive). In these cases careful nursing supervision is required.

The majority of barium meals and barium enemas today are performed using double contrast – a combination of barium and gas. This achieves distension and a thin mucosal coating of barium, facilitating the identification of small mucosal lesions. Gas is given in the form of effervescent granules for barium meals; for barium enemas, gas is delivered directly through the rectal tube. It has recently been shown that carbon dioxide is more rapidly absorbed and causes less discomfort to the patient than air.

After any barium study the patient should be warned that the stools will be clay coloured until the barium has been eliminated. Fluids are encouraged as barium may become dry and thick, causing constipation. Should the patient suffer constipation or impaction of faeces following barium studies, an evacuation enema may be prescribed to relieve discomfort.

Treatment

The *goals* are that the patient with IBD will achieve an optimal nutritional state, physical and emotional rest, and a return to an active and desirable lifestyle.

Drug therapy

Anti-inflammatory agents, immunosuppressants and antibiotics are used alone or in combination to treat IBD. Other drugs may be prescribed for symptomatic treatment. These include antidiarrhoeal agents, including opiate preparations, such as codeine, which have a constipating effect.

- *Corticosteroid preparations* (e.g. hydrocortisone, prednisone, prednisolone). These are prescribed for their anti-inflammatory and immunosuppressant actions. Corticosteroids are often taken in the oral form or intravenously, and applied per rectum in retention enema. Observations are necessary for side-effects such as retention of sodium and water, hypokalaemia and hypertension.

- *Sulfasalazine*. This is an anti-infective and anti-inflammatory drug. When prescribed, it is important that the patient takes a minimum of 2500 mL of fluid daily, as with any sulfonamide preparation. This is to prevent possible crystallization of the sulfonamide in the renal tubules.

- *Antibiotics*. A fistula complicated by infection or a stagnant area or loop of intestine in which there is an overgrowth of bacteria may be treated with an antimicrobial agent, usually metronidazole.

Surgical intervention

Surgical intervention for persons with Crohn's disease is reserved for the patient with complications, as there is a high incidence of recurrence. Complications include the partial or complete obstruction of the intestine by the scar tissue, the formation of abscesses, perforation of the bowel and the formation of fistulae.

In patients with intractable ulcerative colitis, the diseased colon and rectum are removed and the ileum is brought through the abdominal wall to form an ileostomy. A portion of the ileum may be used to form an internal continent pouch (see p. 494) or the ileum may be anastomosed to the rectum. Strictureplasty (refashioning or release of narrowed areas) restores the lumen of the ileum without resection of small bowel, relieving obstruction. Surgery is usually effective but prognosis depends on the rate of development, severity and extent of the disease process.

Assessment of patient functioning

Assessment of a patient's quality of life provides insight into the problems that are most important for patients, allowing health workers to deal better with these problems. Obtaining such information, while important to understanding the patient's adjustment to IBD, may be difficult because of the embarrassment about discussing such topics as bowel movements and incontinence, and because of fear of the disease. It is important for nurses to consider their own feelings about those issues in order to anticipate patients' anxieties sensitively.

Quality of life

Inflammatory bowel disease can have a major adverse impact on patients' lives. Numerous descriptions of the problems affecting patients with IBD have documented limitations in work and social activities, home and married life, and emotional function. Patients tend to report symptoms that fall into five major categories: bowel symptoms, systemic symptoms, emotional function, social impairment, and functional impairment.

Bowel symptoms Problems most frequently cited by patients with IBD as having a significant impact on their lives include frequent bowel movements, loose bowel movements, abdominal cramps, pain in the abdomen, abdominal bloating, passing large amounts of gas, and rectal bleeding with bowel movements.

Systemic symptoms Systemic symptoms include fatigue, feeling unwell overall, tiring very easily, waking up during the night and feeling weak.

Emotional function Patients with IBD have sustained numerous losses, including loss of normal bowel habits, foods from the diet, body image, weight, relationships, work, valued leisure activities, familiar surroundings through hospitalization, income and self-esteem. They report feeling frustrated, depressed, discouraged, irritable, angry, anxious and impatient. They worry about not finding a toilet in time, about having to have surgery and about the next flare-up of symptoms.

Social impairment Loss of normal bowel habits resulting in bowel frequency, incontinence and embarrassment about sudden calls to the toilet can lead to a change in activities. Patients with IBD tend to avoid social events where toilets are not close to hand; social engagements may be cancelled if a flare-up occurs, and sporting activity may be severely curtailed.

Functional impairment Although some patients report an inability to attend work or school regularly, having to stop work or school, and difficulty doing housework, the majority of people with IBD lose little or no time from work over the long term. When symptoms are flaring, many patients have to get up earlier than usual in the morning because bowel actions delay departure for work.

Patients with Crohn's disease experience more systemic symptoms (most notably fatigue) than do those with ulcerative colitis. Problems in one area are likely to cause problems in another area. Overall, systemic symptoms are a major determinant of functional impairment, social dysfunction and emotional problems, whereas bowel symptoms predict emotional problems.

Serious disruption of personal relationships is a problem for only a few patients with IBD. The family may view the individual as a burden rather than as a capable, independent and functioning person who needs understanding and support during flare-ups. However, it is not uncommon for family members to be so attentive and wrapped up in the problems and needs of the individual with IBD that they tend to overlook their own personal needs. Such behaviour may result in increased family tension, fatigue, guilt feelings, resentment and a decreased ability to cope and offer support and reassurance over a long period of time.

In summary, symptoms of bowel disturbance such as frequent, loose bowel movements and abdominal cramps, as well as fatigue and malaise, have the most profound impact on the lives of patients with IBD. Disturbances of emotional function, including frustration and irritability, depression and discouragement, are common in patients with IBD. Impairment of social function is less frequent, with the majority of patients finding ways to cope with their job, social activities and family relationships.

Kelly (1992) describes the subjective experience of living with ulcerative colitis and, using autobiographical data, explains the personal strategies for coping with the disease. In his account he describes adjusting to ill-health using the processes of denial, normalization and accommodation, and proposes that these strategies can be both 'healthy' and problematic. He argues that some well-meaning counselling approaches that break down an individual's denial of their illness could promote adoption of the invalid or sick role, and cautions accordingly. His account also illustrates the miscommunication that can occur when the information given threatens the individual's personal construct of ill-health and the disease. This paper provides the healthcare professional, caring for the person with IBD, with insight into the experience of living with the condition and proposes approaches that can be adopted to encourage normal social development.

Nursing care

Patient problems

- *Malnutrition* due to the bowel inflammation, decreased absorption, diarrhoea, abdominal pain and lack of enjoyment of food
- *Dehydration* due to diarrhoea and inadequate fluid intake
- *Diarrhoea* due to the inflammatory process and disease complications
- *Stress and anxiety* related to the disease process, and the impact on quality of life and resulting personality changes
- Changes in *body image* and *self-concept*
- *Lack of knowledge* concerning disease, treatment and long-term management.

Goals

The person will demonstrate:

1. understanding of parenteral nutrition
2. gradual, consistent increase in bodyweight
3. understanding of measures to promote adequate nutritional and fluid intake
4. acceptable management of diarrhoea
5. awareness of emotional responses
6. recognition of positive coping strategies
7. communication and sharing of significant others' concerns, and changes in sexuality patterns
8. understanding of the disease process and its recurrent nature
9. understanding of the treatment regimen and disease management.

Nursing intervention

Nutrition

Nutritional deficits and weight loss are common to persons with IBD. When these are severe, all oral intake is withheld to decrease the mechanical, physical and chemical activities of the gastrointestinal tract.

Parenteral nutrition (PN) Parenteral nutrition is the infusion, into either a central vein or a large peripheral vein, of solutions of protein, glucose, electrolytes, trace amounts of essential minerals, vitamins and lipids (fat emulsions). This is carried out in sufficient concentrations to meet individual requirements for normal metabolism, tissue maintenance, repair and energy demands.

Parenteral nutrition is used with patients who have Crohn's disease or a bowel fistula that requires that the intestinal tract be rested.

The successful management of parenteral nutrition involves coordination of the efforts of all members of the multidisciplinary team. In some hospitals a special team – usually a specialist nurse, doctor, dietician and pharmacist – coordinate activities. Their responsibilities may include teaching and preparing the patient to manage the feeding regimen at home.

Strict surgical asepsis is mandatory throughout the insertion of the catheter, when handling the solutions and tubes, and when caring for the site of insertion. Infection causes a serious problem; the line serves as an excellent culture medium and, because it leads directly into the blood, bacterial colonization will cause septicaemia.

It is important to prepare the patient, especially if PN is to be prolonged or permanent, with a detailed explanation of the procedure, its purpose and subsequent care. The patient and family are encouraged to ask questions and time is taken to answer them. They may require assurance that the patient will be able to eat normally after a period of being fed this way, if this is the case.

A large vein is used for administration of the highly concentrated (hyperosmolar) solutions, as they are irritating to the veins and can cause phlebitis in smaller peripheral veins. The rapid flow of blood in the large vessels dilutes the PN solutions and lessens the risk of phlebitis.

The type of catheter inserted will vary from hospital to hospital and the patient's needs. When the PN is to be used over an extended period of time, and particularly when the patient is to go home with the catheter in place, a long-term central venous catheter (e.g. Hickman) is inserted and tunnelled under the skin on the chest wall to decrease the incidence of infection. Usually a multilumen catheter is inserted to provide flexibility of use. A peripherally inserted central catheter (PICC) may be used to give PN to patients in hospital. This avoids the higher risk of inserting a CV line but cannot be used indefinitely. Certain simple PN regimens can be given via a peripheral

vein for up to 1 week. A glyceryl trinitrate patch may be beneficial at the site to promote dilatation of the vessel.

The frequency with which the intravenous tubing and/or filter(s) are changed is indicated by hospital policy. If contamination occurs or is even suspected, a doctor is notified and the following investigations are performed:

- blood cultures from the catheter and a peripheral vein
- full blood count
- midstream specimen of urine for microscopy, culture and sensitivity
- chest radiography
- other tests to eliminate potential sources of infection, (e.g. wound swabs, throat swabs).

All tubing changes are made quickly while the catheter is clamped to prevent air entry and the risk of embolism. If the catheter cannot be clamped, the patient is instructed to bear down and hold the breath before tubing is disconnected and to breathe again once the connection has been made (Valsalva manoeuvre). The infusion line may contain one or two filters. Tubing connections are always luer locked to ensure maintenance of an intact line. PN solution consists of an amino-acid–dextrose solution, a fat emulsion solution and added vitamins, minerals and trace elements.

The rate of infusion is controlled by an automatic pump. This is essential because, if the infusion is too rapid, glucose is not metabolized rapidly enough to maintain a normal blood sugar level. The latter is likely to exceed the glucose renal threshold and glucose is excreted in the urine, taking with it essential water and electrolytes.

On dressing the site, strict aseptic technique is observed. Caution is necessary to avoid dislodging the catheter. The catheter site is inspected for redness, swelling or drainage; a swab is taken for culture if any irritation is observed. The skin is cleansed and re-dressed with an alcohol-based solution (chlorhexidine or iodine) and a sterile semi-occlusive dressing (e.g. Opsite) is then applied. The dressing of choice should be water- and bacteria-proof but permeable to air and water vapour. A transparent dressing permits frequent visualization of the area without disturbing the dressing, which can be left in place for 1 week as long as it provides a seal to a clean entry site.

Frequent mouth care is essential. Regular, frequent cleaning of the teeth followed by a mouthwash is very important. The lack of oral food and fluid intake causes discomfort and favours the growth of organisms present in the mouth, producing inflammation and tooth cavities. If the PN is prolonged or permanent, the patient may be permitted boiled sweets to suck, or a small amount of food which may be chewed and then expectorated. Some patients may be able to take small amounts of clear fluids or specified nutrients if their gastrointestinal tract is intact.

When assessing the patient the following observations are very important:

- The patient's blood pressure, pulse, respirations and colour are recorded frequently after the insertion of the catheter. Any complaint of pain or tightness in the chest or change in level of consciousness is reported promptly. Any such change may indicate air embolism, a pneumothorax or a haemothorax.

- The temperature, pulse and respirations are recorded one to four times daily, always in the evening. An increase in temperature and pulse rate may indicate infection.

- 24-hour collections of urine will be made several times a week to check urine biochemistry.

- Blood specimens are usually taken daily for estimation of urea, electrolytes and glucose. Hyperglycaemia may develop, necessitating the administration of regular insulin.

- Blood cultures are done and checked for fungi as well as bacteria.

- The patient's weight is recorded daily. The intake and output are recorded and the fluid balance noted.

Fluid
See chapter 2.6

- The site of insertion is examined carefully each time the dressing is changed and is inspected daily through the transparent dressing for inflammation, oedema, sloughing or purulent discharge.

Psychological support is necessary as the patient receiving PN for a prolonged period may report feeling 'very different'. Repeated explanations of the purpose and value of the feedings are necessary. As the procedure becomes more familiar and better understood, it becomes more acceptable to the patient. Activity is encouraged as exercise promotes protein synthesis as well as improving the patient's psychological well-being. Any weight gain should be reported to the patient as this may help morale; however, a failure to gain weight may have the opposite effect.

Bowel elimination decreases and the patient should be advised that, as nothing enters the tract, this is not surprising.

Oral intake is gradually increased when PN is to be discontinued. When the patient can take sufficient calories and protein orally, the infusion rate is reduced gradually over 48 hours. The catheter tip is sent to the laboratory for culture on removal.

Teaching must be given to the patient who requires long-term PN. Appetite decreases during parenteral feedings. This is attributed to the calorie intake, decreased gastric motility and underlying disease. Appetite remains suppressed when parenteral feedings are discontinued.

If this method of receiving nutrition is to be permanent or prolonged, carers and patient are prepared for discharge from the hospital. They are taught how to put up the solutions, the maintenance of asepsis, indications of problems (e.g. symptoms of infection), care of the site of catheter insertion, how often the tube is changed and by whom, and that the solution should not be frozen. They are advised of the necessary supplies and how they are stored and obtained. They should also have contact telephone numbers and addresses in case of emergency.

Referral to the community nursing services is important on discharge. This will ensure early identification of difficulties or problems, monitoring progress, provision of support, and assistance if necessary with aspects of care.

Most patients not only feel attached to the intravenous poles they have been pushing around for a period of time, whether as an inpatient, outpatient or on home care, they also feel protective of and dependent on their PN. They may require help in dealing with their ambivalent feelings of wanting to discontinue the feedings and anxieties over the loss. The patient needs positive reassurance to deal with the change in health status and what it will mean.

Oral intake When oral intake is resumed, the patient may be given nutritionally balanced elemental feedings. These preparations are bulk and residue free and low in fat, making them easier to digest in the upper gastrointestinal tract. Palatability is enhanced by providing the feed chilled and in different flavours.

Nutrition of the patient requires a great deal of attention. The patient may develop serious nutritional deficiencies. Anorexia presents a problem, and there are serious losses of essential nutrients, fluid and electrolytes in the frequent stools. In many instances, the nurse must work at getting the patient to take sufficient nourishment; it may be necessary to provide frequent small meals. An effort is made to serve foods the patient likes, to provide variety, and to have the tray arranged attractively. A discouraging factor commonly encountered is that, as soon as the patient starts to eat, peristalsis is stimulated and he or she must get to the toilet.

Fluid and electrolyte replacement

An excessive loss of **fluid** in diarrhoea and a probable reduced intake by the patient because of abdominal pain and 'feeling sick' may lead to dehydration. The daily intake and output are recorded and the fluid balance is noted. The patient is encouraged and, if necessary, given assistance to take adequate amounts of fluid. Intravenous infusion may be necessary to correct dehydration and maintain sufficient intake. If the patient has PN in progress, additional intravenous fluids and blood products should be given by a separate peripheral line to avoid contamination.

Serum electrolyte levels, especially potassium and sodium, are determined, as an abnormal amount may be lost in the stools or through fistula drainage. Replacement is made by intravenous fluids. A transfusion of packed red cells may be necessary to correct anaemia that has resulted from nutritional deficiencies. These develop due to insufficient food intake and/or impaired intestinal absorption.

Maintenance of skin integrity is an important role of the nurse when the patient is experiencing dehydration or malnutrition.

Bowel elimination: diarrhoea

The frequency, consistency, volume and colour of the patient's stools are recorded and the nurse and patient collaborate to identify foods, activities and emotional responses that increase or decrease the frequency and consistency of bowel movements.

Antidiarrhoeal medications may be given after each loose bowel movement. The rectal and perineal area are inspected for irritation and redness. Should moist excoriation develop, the area should be kept dry. Use of a hairdryer expelling cool air may help achieve this. Soreness may be relieved by the application of a local anaesthetic gel. A barrier cream can be used to protect the skin.

Individual coping

The nurse must appreciate that dependence and insecurity may be encountered in persons with IBD, and a great deal of tact and sensitivity is required in giving care.

Family coping

Family members, like professional caregivers, need help to understand the reasons for the person's changed behaviours and to appreciate the difficulties experienced in adjusting to a chronic illness that is probably progressive and definitely interferes with one's life. Awareness of the reasons for the behaviours and of the patient's needs provides a basis for understanding and the development of constructive coping strategies. The family may need assistance to identify and deal with their own needs as well as those of the patient.

Sexuality patterns

There is no evidence that IBD affects fertility, and pregnancy is possible. Sexual desire may be decreased by the disease and by the unpredictable bowel habits, odours and fatigue. The possibility of an ileostomy or colostomy raises additional worries about sex. The patient and partner may need support to discuss their concerns and to develop solutions to their particular situation.

Patient and family teaching

Assessment of patient and family learning needs is ongoing as needs change throughout the disease process.

The possibility of a recurrence is reduced if the patient understands the illness and follows the advice discussed in this section. The patient is encouraged to return to work and to live as normal and useful a life as possible. A balance between rest, work and recreation is advisable.

Referral to the medical social work department may be useful in resolving domestic or socioeconomic problems.

Some hospitals have a clinical psychologist or counsellor whose role is to assist the person with IBD and the family and significant others to explore the ramifications and meaning of the disease and develop positive coping strategies. Self-help groups can also be a useful resource to assist in adaptation, and have the added benefit of having members with similar experiences.

Emphasis is placed on the importance of a nourishing diet with the elimination of certain foods that are found to be irritating to the bowel.

Evaluation

Inflammatory bowel disease is characterized by remissions and exacerbation which, together with prolonged treatment, interfere with the person's life and impact on the family and caregivers. Disease management and coping strategies vary according to the status of the disease and the person's responses and ability to cope with the chronic progressive illness. Evaluation is ultimately based on the patient's perceptions, how well they are feeling, and how they perceive they are coping with the latest treatment, symptom, complication, remission or behavioural characteristics.

Intestinal obstruction

Obstruction to the passage of intestinal content may occur in the small or large bowel and is a serious, lifethreatening condition that demands prompt attention.

Causes

The cause of the obstruction may be within the wall or lumen of the intestine itself, or it may be extrinsic. It may be classified as mechanical, neurogenic or vascular and may be acquired or congenital (see Box 15.6).

Strangulated hernia, in which a loop of the intestine escapes from the peritoneal cavity through a defect in the abdominal wall, results in constriction of the lumen of the bowel and a blockage, as well as compression of the blood vessels. The constriction may lead to necrosis of the protruding segment of the intestine.

Obstruction may result from *intussusception*, a condition in which a segment of the intestine is invaginated into the segment immediately below. This telescoping results in compression of the attached mesentery between the layers of intestine in the intussusception and interference with the blood supply to the bowel. Intussusception occurs mainly in infants and young children.

Volvulus, which is a twisting of a loop of bowel on itself, interrupts the passage of intestinal contents and the blood supply to the involved segment. Older persons are more often affected, and the twisted section of bowel is usually the sigmoid colon.

Congenital malformations may be responsible for intestinal obstruction in the newborn. The anomaly may be a stenosis or atresia in an area of the small or large intestine,

Diarrhoea
See chapter 5.1

> **Box 15.6** Causes of intestinal obstruction
>
> *Mechanical*
>
> - Inflammation and oedema of the intestinal wall
> - Strictures or scarring (narrowing the intestinal lumen)
> - Adhesions (bands of fibrous scar tissue formed by the peritoneal tissue following inflammation and which may cause kinking and constriction of the intestine)
> - Neoplasms (intramural and extramural)
> - Foreign body
> - Incarcerated hernia
> - Volvulus
> - Intussusception
> - Congenital stenosis and atresia
>
> *Non-mechanical*
>
> - Neurogenic disturbances:
>   — paralytic or adynamic ileus
>   — dynamic ileus
> - Interrupted blood supply:
>   — mesenteric thrombosis
>   — strangulation of blood vessels secondary to:
>   incarcerated hernia
>   volvulus
>   intussusception

or it may be an imperforate anus. The infant fails to pass meconium.

In *neurogenic obstruction*, peristalsis is inhibited by a disturbance in the normal nerve supply to the intestine. Often this is an imbalance in the autonomic innervation which results in a cessation of peristalsis. It may develop with peritonitis, pancreatitis, severe toxaemia as in pneumonia and uraemia, shock, or spinal cord lesions, or after extensive abdominal surgery. An electrolyte imbalance in which the blood potassium level is below normal also predisposes to intestinal immobility. The inhibition of peristalsis due to impaired innervation causes the condition known as *paralytic* or *adynamic ileus*. Dynamic or spastic ileus occurs rarely in some toxic conditions and is associated with intestinal hyperactivity. The spasm of a segment is severe enough to obliterate the lumen.

Obstruction of vascular origin is due to interference with the blood supply to a segment of the intestine and may be secondary to mechanical obstruction, or it may be primary and itself cause failure of bowel activity. Thrombosis and occlusion of a mesenteric artery may occur, blocking the blood supply to a large portion of the bowel and arresting peristalsis. The interruption in the blood supply may be secondary to an initial mechanical cause, as occurs in strangulated hernia, volvulus and intussusception.

Clinical characteristics

The symptoms and effects of obstruction depend on whether it is in the small or large bowel and whether or not the blood supply to the intestine is maintained.

The first symptom of mechanical obstruction is colicky abdominal *pain* due to the bowel spasms. The crampy pains are accompanied by high-pitched bowel sounds. In paralytic ileus, the pain is steady and is due mainly to the distension. There is an absence of bowel sounds in this type of obstruction. No faecal matter or gas is passed after that which was below the obstruction is evacuated.

In small bowel obstruction, *vomiting* begins earlier and is frequent; the vomitus at first consists of stomach content and then of fluid containing bile. Eventually it becomes dark brown and faecal in character as the intestine becomes distended with excessive fluids and gas that overflow into the stomach.

The *abdomen becomes distended* because of the accumulation of gas and fluids in the bowel. Intestinal secretions are increased and the loss of fluid and electrolytes in vomiting leads to *severe dehydration* and *electrolyte imbalance*. Extravasation of plasma from the capillaries adds to the accumulation of fluid in the intestine as the veins are compressed by distension. This depletes the circulating blood volume and causes *shock*.

The patient's general condition may deteriorate rapidly. Unless the bowel is decompressed and fluid and electrolytes are replaced, a serious state of shock develops, manifested by restlessness, anxiety, a rapid weak pulse, low blood pressure, subnormal temperature, greyish pallor and cold clammy skin.

If decompression of the intestine is not established, the pressure created within the intestinal lumen may increase until it exceeds venous and capillary pressure. This causes congestion, oedema and necrosis of the mural tissue and may lead to perforation of the intestine.

The colicky pain becomes continuous as peristalsis diminishes, and the intestine loses its tone because of the marked distension and strangulation. Bowel sounds diminish and the vomiting changes character; it is no longer preceded by nausea and retching; the vomitus comes up without effort (regurgitated).

Peritonitis may develop as the weakened intestinal wall becomes permeable to organisms. *Generalized abdominal tenderness* and rigidity become evident.

Obstruction of the large intestine is less acute, and the symptoms develop over a longer period of time. Complete constipation (*obstipation*) and crampy abdominal pain are the patient's first complaints. Distension of the large bowel develops more slowly because fluid is absorbed, but eventually the distension may be very marked as the segment of the bowel is closed off by the obstruction at one end and the ileocaecal valve at the other. The ileocaecal valve will permit the entrance of content from the ileum, but not until the later stage does the content of the colon and caecum back up into the ileum. Vomiting and the attendant dehydration and electrolyte imbalance occur in this later stage.

Medical diagnosis

Diagnostic investigation in intestinal obstruction may include radiography of the abdomen in which the presence and levels of gas and fluid may be apparent without a contrast medium.

Treatment

Intestinal obstruction other than that due to paralytic ileus is treated surgically. In simple mechanical obstruction without strangulation, the operation may be delayed for a brief period in which medical treatment is used to improve the patient's general condition. This treatment includes nasogastric and intestinal intubation and suctioning to remove the accumulation of gas and fluid and to relieve the vomiting, pain and distension.

Fluid and electrolytes are given intravenously to replace the losses; as much as 5–6 litres may be administered daily. An accurate record of all fluid output and intake is necessary. The doctor bases the electrolyte replacement as well as the amount of intravenous fluid on the volume of intestinal fluid lost in vomiting and aspiration.

If there is evidence of interference with the blood supply to the obstructed intestine, emergency surgery is undertaken.

The surgical procedure used in intestinal obstruction depends on the cause of obstruction and the patient's general condition. If the obstruction is due to adhesions, they are severed. The operation may involve resection of the affected area of intestine and anastomosis to restore continuity of the tract or a bypass of the lesion by anastomosing a part above the obstruction to a lower part (usually the colon). In the case of an incarcerated hernia, volvulus or intussusception, the obstruction is relieved and the intestine examined for viability. If the blood supply has been interrupted for some time or is not re-established, a segment of the bowel may be gangrenous, necessitating resection and anastomosis. The operation may entail an ileostomy, or colostomy, which may be a temporary measure while an anastomosis heals or it may be done to establish drainage above the obstruction, making it possible to delay more extensive surgery until the patient's condition improves. In some instances, the stoma (colostomy or ileostomy) is permanent. (*Ileostomy* is an opening from the ileum on to the external surface of the abdomen. Intestinal content is eliminated through this opening. *Colostomy* is an opening through the abdominal wall from the colon. Faeces are diverted through this opening on to the external surface of the abdomen.)

For nursing care of the surgically treated patient, see Chapter 10.

Intestinal obstruction due to paralytic ileus is treated symptomatically. A nasogastric or intestinal tube is passed to drain gas and to fluid and to reduce distension. Fluid and electrolyte deficiencies are corrected; the serum potassium level receives special attention because hypokalaemia favours peristaltic dysfunction. Paralytic ileus is most frequently a secondary condition; as the primary disorder improves and decompression occurs, peristalsis is usually re-established gradually.

Cancer of the intestine

The most common site of carcinoma is the rectum; the sigmoid, caecum and ascending colon are next in order of frequency. Colorectal tumours are the second most common form of cancer in the UK and account for 1 in 500 deaths per year (Finlay 1997). These tumours are fairly equally distributed between the sexes. Small bowel cancers are uncommon and account for 2% of all gastrointestinal tumours. Cancer of the colon or rectum may occur at any age, but the incidence increases with age. The incidence is high in Western countries and low in less developed countries.

Contributing factors

The cause of colorectal cancer is believed to be multifactorial. Studies show a relationship between high-fat, low-fibre diets, lack of physical exercise and colorectal cancer. Specific substances in the mucous membrane lining the intestine may be the cause. The fat and fibre content of the diet, transit time of bowel contents and intestinal bacteria alter the microenvironment of the intestine.

A number of conditions carry an increased risk of developing large bowel and rectal cancer. These include prolonged history of inflammatory bowel disease and familial polyposis coli, which has a strong genetic element. Family screening using DNA probing should identify high-risk individuals who can then be followed closely with colonosopy (Finlay and Burns 1998).

Types

The malignant growth may be papillary, soft and friable, or a firm nodular mass projecting into the lumen; it may be a ring-shaped (annular) mass of firm fibrous tissue, causing a constriction of the bowel, or it may be ulcerative and necrotic, leading to bleeding and perforation.

Metastases

The malignant cells from bowel cancer spread by blood and lymph and by direct extension to neighbouring tissue and structures. Frequent sites of secondary growths are the liver, stomach, bones and peritoneal cavity. Direct extension may involve the bladder and reproductive organs.

Clinical characteristics

Manifestations vary with the location of the lesion in the intestine. If the neoplasm is in the *small intestine*, the symptoms develop insidiously and are vague and less noticeable. They include anorexia, nausea and vomiting, anaemia, loss of weight and strength, and occult blood in the stool. Obstructive symptoms appear gradually and the patient develops abdominal pain. If the tumour is in the duodenum, the manifestations may be similar to those of a peptic ulcer.

If the site of the neoplasm is in the *colon* or *rectum*, the most common early signs are a change in bowel habit and blood in the stool. Any person manifesting either of these signs is urged to seek prompt medical attention.

There may be increasing constipation or perhaps alternating bouts of constipation and diarrhoea. The stool may gradually become smaller and ribbon-like in form and may be streaked with blood, mucus and pus. A continuous defaecation urge and the feeling that evacuation is incomplete after passing a stool may be experienced. The patient presents a general picture of ill-health with loss of weight and progressive anaemia. Laboratory examination of the stool will probably reveal occult blood. In cancer of the large bowel, abdominal pain is usually a late symptom; at first the patient may have a vague discomfort, and later may experience a colicky pain which gradually becomes more severe. Unfortunately, if the cancer is in the caecum or ascending (right) colon, the early symptoms are more insidious and difficult to detect until the mass is large enough to be found by palpation. Occasionally, the first symptoms recognized are those associated with complications, such as obstruction or perforation of the bowel.

Screening and early detection

If the cancer is detected early, before lymph nodes become involved, the 5-year survival rate increases to 65–85%. However, if spread has occurred to the regional lymph nodes and beyond, the 5-year survival rate drops to less than 20% (Finlay 1997). This demonstrates the value of early detection of a malignant lesion before symptoms occur.

Screening for colorectal cancer at present is dependent upon occult blood estimation in stool samples. This test is estimated to produce a 25% false-positive result.

Flexible sigmoidoscopy or sigmoidoscopy are more specific but are concomitantly more expensive and risky. People with a positive faecal occult blood test result usually proceed to colonoscopy for diagnosis. Currently a screening programme for the UK population is being piloted. However, those at increased risk (IBD sufferers, those with a family history of familial polyposis coli or colonic cancer) are screened, usually with endoscopy. Others should be encouraged to discuss options with their general practitioner.

Diagnosis

A neoplasm in the *small intestine* may be recognized when barium sulfate is taken by mouth and the passage of the barium through the small intestine followed. Any delay at a given section may indicate narrowing of the lumen by a mass. The intraluminal contour of the small intestine is also recorded by radiography.

Investigation of the large intestine involves a colonoscopy, sigmoidoscopy or proctoscopy. A biopsy of the lesion, if it is located, is done at the time of the endoscopic examination. Radiography is done with a barium enema providing a contrast medium. The patient's haematocrit and haemoglobin level are checked for possible anaemia, and stool specimens are examined for blood, parasites and pus. Liver function tests may be done, to determine whether the malignancy has metastasized to the liver.

Treatment

Surgery is the first-line treatment and includes removal of the tumour, disease-free bowel on either side of it, and the surrounding tissue including lymph nodes. The remaining ends of the bowel are usually anastomosed (joined) using a stapling device. If the tumour is within a few centimetres of the anus, a permanent colostomy will be formed and the rectum and anus excised. If the anastomosis is low in the rectum or the bowel is inflamed, a temporary stoma may be formed to facilitate healing at the anastomotic site.

Depending on the site and stage of the cancer diagnosed, patients may have radiotherapy and/or chemotherapy before or after operation. Chemotherapy regimens of 5-fluorouracil and other cytotoxic drug (e.g. levamisole or leucovorin) have mild and reversible side-effects for patients with involved lymph nodes. Radiotherapy is indicated for patients with rectal cancer and is often given before the operation to shrink a tumour so that it can be excised more effectively. Radiotherapy is contraindicated in any area where the ileum is likely to be involved and so is used only for tumours in the pelvic area.

Case Study 15.2 describes the management of a patient with colorectal adenocarcinoma.

Case Study 15.2   *Colorectal adenocarcinoma*

Mr England, at time of diagnosis, is 57, divorced, has two grown daughters, lives with his woman friend whom his daughters dislike 'on principle', works as an insurance broker and describes himself as a workaholic. He takes little exercise, is slightly overweight and drinks in excess of 20 units of alcohol a week. In the preceding 6 months Mr England has been experiencing altered bowel habit: bloating, constipation and then loose stools, and more flatus than usual. The symptoms do not seem to be related to what he eats and after experiencing rectal bleeding on two occasions he visits his GP, partly at his partner's insistence. His parents are both dead, one from a stroke and the other from 'bowel cancer'.

Referral to the gastrointestinal (GI) outpatient clinic involves a flexible sigmoidoscopy which shows a mass at 8 cm from the anal margin, in the upper rectum. Having seen the GI clinic nurse and a consultant GI surgeon in the clinic, Mr England is referred for anorectal physiology measurement. Transrectal ultrasonography of the tumour shows invasion through the rectal wall, but Mr England's anal sphincter pressures are high and a low resection and anastomosis will be possible, avoiding a stoma, about which he is very relieved. Mr England is also seen by the colorectal cancer nurse specialist (colorectal CNS), who takes time to explore the implications of his diagnosis with him and to explain the treatment and possible outcomes. The nurse provides a contact number should Mr England or his family wish to discuss things further.

The plan for Mr England's treatment includes radiotherapy to shrink the tumour before surgical resection, and direct anastomosis. After recovery from the operation, a course of chemotherapy is planned in order to optimize his chance of remission from the cancer. Mr England is given external-beam radiation as an outpatient of the radiotherapy department, and the radiotherapy successfully reduces the size of the tumour.

Before admission for surgery, Mr England is seen in the surgical preadmission clinic by a nurse who takes his history and blood samples, performs an ECG and orders chest radiography. The nurse explains what to expect and that he will need a clean bowel for the operation. The bowel preparation prescription, dietary restrictions and high fluid intake are discussed.

Mr England is admitted for surgery and a low resection is undertaken as planned. The nurses on the surgical ward help him to recover and anticipate a healthy diet and normal daily bowel habit.

Histological reports of the resected cancer show an invasive rectal adenocarcinoma with local lymph node involvement.

Chemotherapy with 5-fluorouracil and levamisole is commenced 2 months after the operation (to allow healing of the anastomosis and suture lines) and is administered in the oncology day unit. During radiotherapy, surgery and chemotherapy events, the colorectal CNS sees Mr England and his partner to provide information and support, and ensure that the treatment is progressing according to plan.

When treatment is finally completed, Mr England has made a full recovery and continues to be seen regularly by both the colorectal surgery and oncology teams, with the colorectal CNS maintaining contact.

Some 12 months later, after feeling unwell for a few weeks, Mr England is found to have liver metastases, which are not surgically resectable. However, a further course of chemotherapy is organized to delay the growth of the tumour. Mr England sees the same staff in the oncology day unit and is also seen by the colorectal CNS. After the chemotherapy, the colorectal CNS suggests a consultation with the palliative care nurse specialist, emphasizing that this is for symptom management and to anticipate this need in the future. This point proves difficult for Mr England and his family to accept as it implies 'the end' to them. With careful counselling and support, the acceptance of symptom management as opposed to 'terminal care' is made clear and accepted by the family so that they are familiar with the team members in advance of becoming reliant on them.

Mr England's symptoms are managed successfully for more than a year after diagnosis of the metastases. With the help of the colorectal CNS and the palliative care team, who liaise with his GP and community nurses, Mr England and his partner and daughters learn to work together to maximize the quality of his remaining life. Mr England died at home, 4 years after his initial symptoms became apparent.

Critical pathway: colonic resection

Whilst it is important to individualize the care given to any patient, and the use of a pathway (see Table 15.2) does not preclude this, it is also useful to have a guideline for anticipated recovery from common illnesses and procedures. This can inform patients and new staff and facilitates the collection of data relating to complications or delays in recovery that may be helpful in improving care.

Depending on their state of health (nutrition, hydration, other pathology) patients admitted for colonic resection, without stoma formation, will usually stay in hospital for an average of 8 days in total and follow a predictable pathway of care and recovery. Admission before surgery will involve information giving about the plan for the patient's stay in hospital and subsequent recovery. This period spent in hospital is relatively short and intensive, and it is important that the patient and their family are prepared for this. It is important that plans for discharge are based on information about the patient's home circumstances and commenced as soon as possible in order to maximize the opportunity for convalescence. Advice to be included in preparing patients to go home is summarized below.

Discharge advice

■ Take analgesia regularly and increase the dose as prescribed if you anticipate doing anything that may cause more pain. You should expect to exercise and cough regularly. Do not try to avoid taking analgesia and then develop significant pain. It will be more difficult to control and could prevent you from sleeping or moving as easily as you should.

■ It is perfectly all right to wet the wound, although it should not be soaked. You should not require a dressing, but gauze could be taped over if the wound rubs or bothers you. If the wound still needs a special dressing when you go home, you will be shown what to do and/or the community nurse will be contacted to dress it for you. You should avoid direct sunlight to the scar, and should not rub any creams into it. It is normal for it to feel itchy or numb for some weeks

Table 15.2   Critical pathway for a patient undergoing colonic resection

Aspect of care	Preoperative	Day of operation	Day 1	Day 2	Day 3	Day 4	Day 5	Day 6
Respiratory	Assessment of baseline rate, O_2% saturation. Teach deep breathing and coughing. Refer to physiotherapist if indicated (smoker or chronic obstructive pulmonary disease)	Administer prescribed O_2. Respiratory rate > 12 per min. Saturation at or above baseline level. Check colour and perfusion. Deep breathing every hour	Wean O_2 to maintain O_2% saturation and respiratory rate. Deep breathing and coughing supporting the wound, every hour. Additional physiotherapy if required. Monitor regularly (2–4 hourly)	Deep breathing and coughing as previously. Monitor 4–6 hourly. Check any sputum produced. Report to doctors and culture if purulent	As previously	As previously. Monitor 8–12 hourly	As previously. Monitor 12–24 hourly	As previously. Should continue deep breathing and coughing at home until moving easily
Circulatory	Baseline assessment of BP, HR, history of problems and medication. Bloods for FBC baseline, cross-matching for 6 units of blood. ID with appropriate labels	Monitor BP and HR frequently and report deviation from preoperative baseline or parameters agreed with doctors. Check drainage from wound and wound drains frequently. If > 300 mL in one drain in 30–60 min, inform doctors immediately	Monitor BP and HR regularly. Check and record wound drainage for type and volume. FBC and check result	Monitor BP and HR regularly. Check and record wound drainage for type and volume. If still fresh blood, report to doctors. FBC and check result if significant loss from drains	As previously. If drains have drained < 30 mL in 24 h remove. FBC and check result	Check BP, HR 12 hourly. Remove remaining drain if < 30 mL in 24 h. FBC and check result	Check BP, HR 12–24 hourly. Remove remaining drain if < 30 mL in 24 h. FBC and check result	Check BP, HR 12–24 hourly. FBC only if previously < 10 g/L or transfused
Pain control	Explain measures for pain control and the importance of regular analgesia to enhance recovery. Assess ability to use PCA and teach technique	Monitor use of PCA; adjust prescription as indicated. Ensure other prescribed analgesia regularly administered. Monitor effectiveness using pain scale	As previously	As previously	As previously	As previously. Commence regular oral analgesia and wean PCA if able	As previously. Stop PCA if not already	As previously

(*Continued*)

Table 15.2 (*Continued*)

Aspect of care	Preoperative	Day of operation	Day 1	Day 2	Day 3	Day 4	Day 5	Day 6
Fluid balance	Assess current status (dehydration, use of diuretics, usual intake). Bloods for serum urea, creatinine and electrolyte (UCE) levels and check result. Ensure > 3-litre intake today (bowel preparation)	IVI to hydrate as prescribed (3 litres/24 h). Aim for urine output > 30 mL/h. Consider other losses (gut, drains, perioperative fluid losses). Assess balance 6 hourly and consult if > 500 mL positive or negative. Keep record of each 24-h balance and include in daily assessment	As previously. UCE and check result for appropriate IVI prescription	As previously. Assess balance 24 h. UCE as previously	As previously. Decrease IVI rate as oral intake increases. Assess balance 24 h. UCE as previously	Remove IVI when drinking freely. Assess balance 24 h. UCE as previously	Stop monitoring fluid balance	UCE if indicated
Nutrition	Assess nutritional status. Clear fluid only; supplement protein and calories with fortified drinks if indicated (cancer, recent weight loss, sepsis)	Nil orally from 6 h before surgery	Sips of water or ice by mouth only. Increase volume if bowel sound present	Increase volume of fluids by 30-mL increments hourly as tolerated	Free fluids by mouth including hot drinks as liked or tolerated when flatus passed. Use fortified drinks if indicated	Free fluids, soup and soft pudding as tolerated	Free fluids and a light diet	As previously
Excretion	Assess urinary function and screen urine with dipstick test. Assess usual bowel habit (before and since symptomatic). Explain and administer bowel preparation having familiarized patient with bathroom facilities. Give barrier cream if perineal irritation present or develops	Check urinary catheter patent and draining. Catheter care 12–24 hourly	As previously. Check for bowel sounds	As previously. Check for bowel sounds and whether flatus passed	As previously. Check for bowel sounds and whether flatus passed	Remove catheter; culture urine if indicated by dipstick test or fever. Check for resumption of urinary function; measure volumes and frequency. Check flatus passed and whether bowels opened	Check urinary function, volumes and frequency. Check flatus passed and bowels opened. Consider lactulose prescription if difficult	As previously

(*Continued*)

Table 15.2   (*Continued*)

Aspect of care	Preoperative	Day of operation	Day 1	Day 2	Day 3	Day 4	Day 5	Day 6
Activity and rest	Assess usual exercise pattern and limits, sleep pattern. Assess skin integrity and use pressure-relieving appliances as indicated. Start bowel preparation early to minimize sleep disturbance prior to surgery. Teach leg and ankle exercises for postoperative use and the importance of early resumption of activity and independence. Describe activity targets for postoperative period	Fit antiembolism stockings before surgery. Commence prescribed anticoagulant therapy	Help out of bed twice for as long as tolerated. Check calves for pain or inflammation. Hourly leg and ankle exercises. Prescribed anticoagulant therapy	As previously. Also take short walk around the bed twice. Clean stockings	As previously. Longer walk. Resume some independence in activities of daily living as able	As previously. Clean stockings	As previously	As previously. Remove stockings before discharge
Regulation (endocrine, temperature, immunity, healing)	Check temperature for baseline. Inform anaesthetist if febrile and consider cause. Assess history of endocrine disease (diabetes mellitus) and establish usual management. Consider implications for wound healing	Measure temperature 4 hourly after surgery. Consult with doctors if > 38.5°C. Check wound for oozing and inflammation frequently. Administer antibiotics as prescribed (three doses). Administer prescribed regimen and monitoring for diabetes if indicated	Measure temperature 4–6 hourly. Consult if > 38.5°C and culture wound, sputum and urine. Check wound for oozing and inflammation. Administer prescribed regimen and monitoring for diabetes if indicated	As previously. Dress the wound if indicated. Dress drain-sites daily when removed (more frequently if dressings wet). Change intravenous cannulae	As previously	As previously. Change intravenous cannulae if still required	As previously. Check temperature twice daily, always in the evening	As previously. If wounds still require dressing either show patient how to care or arrange for community nurse/practice nurse

(*Continued*)

Table 15.2 (Continued)

Aspect of care	Preoperative	Day of operation	Day 1	Day 2	Day 3	Day 4	Day 5	Day 6
Self-image	Assess feelings associated with diagnosis and impending operation. Provide information, explanation, support and reassurance as indicated. Check informed consent given for operation	Inform patient and family about outcome of operation as and when indicated depending on conscious level and need for further histology reports	As previously. Encourage the patient to look at the wound when able	As previously	As previously	As previously	As previously. Establish all parties are satisfied with current available knowledge and situation	As previously. Ensure appropriate referrals made and the patient and carer are fully aware of these
Interdependence and discharge plan	Assess current situation at home, who is there and their level of ability to support the patient. Assess patient's current level of ability and what help is or may be required. Discuss and initiate appropriate referrals	Provide information for the patient, family and friends as indicated and wanted. Pursue referrals for discharge plan and record progress	As previously	As previously	As previously. Outline discharge plan	As previously. Confirm discharge plan, arrange transport and appointments as required (GI surgical outpatients in 6 weeks)	As previously. Prescribe and order drugs to take home. Teach patient and family about convalescence using guidelines. Ensure clarity about drug regimens, appointments and when to seek help	As previously. Confirm discharge plan in operation with all relevant parties

BP, blood pressure; FBC, full blood count; GI, gastrointestinal; HR, heart rate; ID, identification; IVI, intravenous infusion; PCA, patient-controlled analgesia; UCE, urea, creatinine and electrolytes.

after the operation. If the wound becomes red or swollen, starts to drain fluid or you develop a fever (temperature >37.5°C) for more than 12 hours, you should contact your GP.

■ Initially you should continue to eat a light diet at home. Regular meals of food you like eating will help to restore your appetite. You will benefit from eating little and often, and eating low-fat foods but a higher protein and calorie intake will help your body to recover from surgery. Include natural yoghurt in your diet to help your bowel restore its normal environment and gradually increase your fibre intake in the form of cereals and fresh fruit and vegetables by one helping at a time. Aim to establish a three-meals-a-day pattern of a high-fibre (if you can tolerate it) low-fat diet within 4–6 weeks of going home.

■ You will have opened your bowels before you go home but a regular habit may not yet be established. This is not unusual. You may find you go infrequently or your stool is hard and difficult to pass. Ensure you establish a routine for meals and going to the toilet, and continue to take regular daily exercise. Drink at lease eight glasses of decaffeinated and non-alcoholic fluids per day. If the problem persists, consult your GP who may prescribe you some lactulose to soften the stool and make it easier to pass.

■ You should not drive, lift, undertake heavy exercise or do sit-ups for 6 weeks. When you first resume these activities (particularly driving) ensure you have someone with you and stop if you develop pain or get tired. However, exercise and rest are both important. You should not take to your bed, but get up and dress every day. You should aim to walk daily, going a little further each day; take someone with you if at all possible until you feel confident about going out on your own. When you feel tired, take a rest and lie down for a nap in the afternoon if you need to. Slowly resume your usual activities and try to include some strenuous exercise at least three times a week when you are fully recovered, if you have not done so previously. If you develop pain and swelling in your calf muscle, or sudden shortness of breath, contact your GP immediately.

■ Give advice about medications – when and how to take them, and why.

■ Give advice about stopping smoking where applicable.

Nursing intervention

Prevention

Evidence is accumulating in support of high dietary fibre as a protection against the development of colonic cancer. A low-fat diet is also recommended. The nurse's health education role can therefore make a substantial contribution to the long-term prevention of many cases of bowel cancer. By its very nature, such a contribution is not always apparent, however, and it requires long-term commitment by the individual for real benefits to accrue.

A major nursing issue is the promotion of colorectal cancer screening. The nurse is in a key position to teach individuals about the risk factors, to inform them about screening recommendations and to encourage participation in screening programmes. Nurses in primary health care, occupational settings and outpatient departments may have greater opportunities for initiating intensive health education programmes. An informed public recognizes the importance of early detection and treatment. Misconceptions exist that bowel cancer equates with a colostomy. The nurse can stress the positive outcomes of early detection and impress on patients that a colostomy may not be necessary. It depends on the location, extent and stage of the tumour.

The person with faecal diversion

Ileostomy and colostomy

The treatment of some intestinal disorders may necessitate surgery that establishes an opening into the bowel through which the intestinal content is discharged on to the surface of the abdomen. The opening may be temporary or permanent. A temporary diversion of the bowel content may be necessary while some abnormal condition below the level of the stoma is corrected or for quick decompression and drainage in obstruction. Later, the normal continuity of the tract is restored and the stoma reversed. If the opening is permanent, the portion of the bowel below is generally removed.

The operations performed are ileostomy or colostomy.

Ileum
See chapter 5.1

Colon
See chapter 5.1

Ileostomy

An ileostomy involves transection of the ileum, usually within the last 20 cm before the ileocaecal junction, and bringing the proximal end out to the abdominal surface to form a stoma. An ileal stoma usually protrudes 2–3 cm, which makes the management easier than with a stoma that is level with the abdominal surface. Because ileostomy effluent is liquid and corrosive to skin, if the stoma is flat, faecal fluid will leak under the appliance and cause excoriation. The removal of the distal severed portion of the bowel may be done at the same operation or may be postponed until the patient's condition is improved. If the lower part of the intestine is to be retained for a period of time, it is closed or, in some instances, the severed end may also be brought out to the abdominal surface. This second stoma is called a mucus fistula.

An ileostomy is most frequently performed for ulcerative colitis that does not respond to medical treatment and is incapacitating. It may also be necessary for patients with Crohn's disease, multiple polyposis of the colon or an intestinal obstruction in the upper portion of the colon. Major advances in surgery now offer new procedures that overcome many of the obvious disadvantages of the traditional ileostomy. The first such procedure was the Kock continent ileostomy which involved making a pouch or reservoir out of ileum (Fig. 15.4). This procedure is not performed on patients with regional enteritis (Crohn's disease) because the pouch may become affected.

The pouch serves as a reservoir for the intestinal content and is drained at regular intervals by the insertion of a catheter through the stoma. The capacity of the reservoir gradually increases, and may reach 400–600 mL over several months to a year. Continuous discharge and leakage of the fluid or semi-fluid between evacuations of the pouch is prevented by the formation of a valve-like structure at the internal end of the ileum which leads from the stoma to the ileal pouch.

More commonly an ileal pouch is formed and connected to the anus (Fig. 15.5), thereby eliminating the need for a stoma and restoring a normal means of passing faeces. The operation is performed in one or two stages, with bowel resection and construction of the ileoanal pouch. There may be a period when the patient has an ileostomy, but only on a temporary basis. The sphincter muscles around the anus are, however, conserved, permitting bowel evacuation in most patients via the anal route when the procedure is complete. At the second stage the ileostomy is closed and the pouch is activated to permit anal elimination.

The postoperative period for patients with a pouch ileostomy is longer than that for patients who have had a conventional ileostomy. It involves gastrointestinal drainage via a nasogastric tube, intravenous fluids and continuous catheter drainage of the pouch for several

Figure 15.4 (a) Pouch (continent) ileostomy. (b) Diagram showing the location of the ileostomy. Arrows show the direction of movement of bowel contents.

(a)

(b)

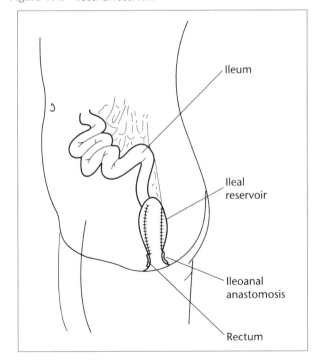

Figure 15.5 Ileoanal reservoir.

days while the pouch heals. There may be a problem with anal incontinence for several weeks after operation as the pouch tissue continues to secrete mucus. Diarrhoea and anal soreness can be serious problems until reservoir

adaptation has occurred, which may take 6–12 months. Eventually the patient will pass stool in a well controlled manner 4–8 times per day (Salter 1995). However, the advantages associated with an ileal pouch, such as the elimination of continuous drainage and the wearing of a bag, make the more involved procedure acceptable to the patient.

Young patients with familial polyposis may be offered a colectomy with ileorectal anastomosis and no pouch or reservoir. Salter (1995) points out that this is possible if it is considered that the patient has a strong enough anal sphincter to cope, but in later life there is the risk of cancer because the rectum is left intact. This may lead to further surgery and the formation of an ileorectal pouch after removal of the rectum.

Colostomy

A colostomy is an opening of the colon on to the surface of the abdomen. It may be in the ascending, transverse, descending or sigmoid colon. The types of stoma include:

- *Permanent colostomy* (usually called an end or terminal colostomy) carried out as a planned procedure with removal of all bowel beyond the stoma.

- *Temporary colostomies* divert faecal matter away from the distal colon while healing occurs. They are often carried out in emergency situations.

Various techniques can be used to fashion these types of stoma such as:

- *Loop colostomy*, where a section of the colon is brought out on to the abdomen, supported on the surface by a rod or bridge, opened longitudinally and the mucosal edges sutured to the skin.

- *Double-barrelled colostomy*, where the two ends of the colon are sutured together to make a spur and brought out on to the abdomen.

- *Divided colostomy*, where the proximal and distal ends of the stoma are brought out on to the abdomen to form two separate openings.

Nursing considerations in ileostomy and colostomy

Differences between ileostomy and colostomy

Certain differences exist between an ileostomy and colostomy that result in different problems and necessitate different types of care. For example, control of the discharge is determined by the location of the stoma; drainage from the ileum is of liquid consistency and is rich in enzymes that cause excoriation and erosion of the skin. Fluid from the ileum flows almost continuously, requiring the constant wearing of a receptive appliance unless an ileal pouch is constructed. There may be quiescent periods but they are not predictable and cannot be controlled. Complications are a more common occurrence with an ileostomy than with a colostomy, and odour presents a greater problem if there is continuous drainage. Irrigations are not used with the conventional ileostomy; the introduction of anything into the ileal stoma is discouraged for fear of injury to the intestine.

Colostomy drainage is usually more manageable and less irritating to the skin unless the opening is into the ascending colon; the drainage then is similar to that from an ileostomy. The colostomy is more often in the transverse or descending colon, and much of the fluid and electrolytes has been absorbed from the faecal content, leaving it semi-solid or solid by the time it reaches the stoma (Fig. 15.6). In some instances, the sigmoid colostomy may be so well controlled that it resembles normal bowel movement, and the patient does not have to wear an appliance continuously.

Intestinal activity in the individual with a colostomy or ileostomy may be influenced by diet, fluid intake and emotions – just as in the normal person.

Psychological preoperative preparation

When the doctor advises the patient before operation that a colostomy or ileostomy may or will be necessary, the patient may be emotionally disturbed. If the colostomy is a temporary measure it may be accepted more readily, but if it is likely to be permanent the patient may be more concerned about this than about the operation or the primary condition. Assumptions about the patient's

Figure 15.6 Colostomy sites and variation in faecal consistency within the colon.

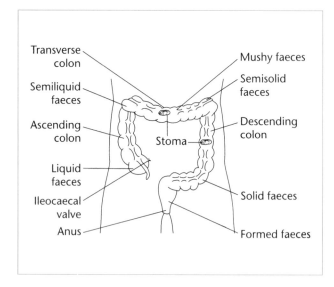

reactions can be misleading. The patient, for example, who is suffering much pain and disruption to their life from serious inflammatory bowel disease may be relieved at the prospect of surgery. However, a patient with only mild symptoms but a diagnosis of cancer may be devastated at the thought of surgery. The immediate response may be 'it would be better to die than have that'. The patient may become resentful or show marked depression, withdrawal and despair, perceiving this change to the body as making them unclean and unacceptable to society. There are fears because of odour and soiling. It is best to let the patient, family and partner express their feelings before attempting explanations. The nurse can help by being a willing listener, answering their questions and using every opportunity available to assure the patient that the 'ostomy' can be cared for without interfering with work and social life. When the patient recovers from the initial blow, discussions may then be held as to how to care for the ileostomy or colostomy. The patient should be actively involved in deciding the site of the stoma.

The stoma care nurse should be notified and meet with the patient and family before the operation. If no stoma care nurse is available, the nurse can encourage the patient and partner to handle the appliances, ask questions and look at literature or audiovisual resources on care and management of ostomies. It is important to reinforce that support and teaching will be available after surgery.

Some individuals, their families and significant others may welcome a visit from someone who has experienced a similar operation. Local branches of self-help groups such as the Ileostomy Association of Great Britain and Ireland or the British Colostomy Association have a list of suitable visitors. Some centres develop their own group of ex-patients who can fulfil this function.

> **Box 15.7**   Sites to be avoided when positioning a stoma
>
> - Areas affected by skin conditions
> - Bony prominences
> - Fatty bulges or skin folds or creases (present on lying, standing or sitting)
> - Groin creases
> - Old scars
> - Pubic area
> - Site of surgical incision
> - Site that cannot be seen by the patient
> - Umbilicus
> - Under large breasts
> - Waistline.

Physical preoperative preparation

Physical preparation for the formation of a stoma is important. This will include siting of the stoma and bowel preparation. Correct siting of the stoma will ensure ease of mastery of the techniques of management and ultimately speedier adaptation to altered bowel elimination. Although the site may be chosen by the stoma care nurse or surgeon, the nurse may be involved in assessing the patient and identifying physical disabilities (e.g. poor eyesight or poor dexterity) that will influence where the stoma is sited. Box 15.7 outlines the sites that should be avoided. The nurse may also be involved in applying test patches of appliances, skin protective wafers and adhesives to prevent later problems with skin sensitivity.

Bowel preparation should be carried out according to local policy as methods vary. Whatever method is used, the nurse should prepare the person by explaining the procedure and the reason why it is necessary. This will increase cooperation. Adequate privacy and hygiene needs should be provided, and monitoring of the patient for signs of dehydration, electrolyte disturbance, discomfort and exhaustion must be carried out. Bowel preparation can be psychologically traumatic, particularly if the individual experiences episodes of incontinence, as it may bring with it feelings of loss of control and realization of the impact of the planned surgery and future ramifications. The nurse should be supportive and encourage expression of anxieties about the future.

Nursing assessment

Initial and continuous assessment of the following is necessary:

- The patient's dexterity, eyesight and general ability to manage self-care of a stoma appliance

- The patient's perception of the ileostomy or colostomy
- The volume, colour, composition and consistency of the effluent (drainage)
- The patient's nutritional and hydrational status. The fluid intake and the quantity and composition of meals are noted. The patient's weight is recorded
- The condition of the stoma and surrounding skin surface
- The reaction to self-care
- The family's perception and reaction to the stoma
- The patient's ability to manage stoma care.

Patient problems

Health problems common to the person with a stoma during the postoperative and early rehabilitation periods include:

- *psychological distress* at the stoma
- *altered bowel elimination* due to the faecal diversion
- *potential for impairment of skin integrity* related to leakage of intestinal or bowel contents on peristomal skin
- *disturbances in body image* due to the abdominal stoma, the surgical incision, changes in faecal elimination and control of odours
- *altered sexuality pattern* related to altered self-image, stoma, ostomy appliance, altered sexual responses and lack of knowledge
- *lack of knowledge* concerning self-management of the stoma.

Goals

The patient will demonstrate:

1. a healthy stoma with clean, intact peristomal skin
2. ability to look at and touch the stoma
3. active participation in care
4. ability to empty, clean, change, prepare and dispose of appliances
5. absence of diarrhoea, constipation, excessive gas and abdominal distension
6. awareness of how diet and fluid intake affect bowel function
7. recognition of signs of complication and actions to take
8. ability to talk about feelings, concerns, questions and self-concept
9. awareness of community resources
10. understanding of how to obtain further supplies of appliances and accessories.

Nursing intervention

Physical management of the stoma

Postoperative assessment

The patient usually returns from the theatre with a clear pouch in place to allow for observation of the stoma. Initially the stoma is swollen and oedematous, pink to bright red in colour, and shiny in appearance. A purple or dusky colour and coolness to touch indicate ischaemia. The volume of drainage is small. The baseline assessment data include the colour, temperature, size, type and location of the stoma. It is important to note whether the stoma is flush, retracted or prolapsed and to document the condition of the skin. The stoma is assessed at least every 8 hours for the first 24 hours after operation, and at least daily during the remainder of the hospitalization. The peristomal skin is inspected each time the appliance is changed. If a loop ostomy has been created, note the type of support system (e.g. rod, bridge, drain). It is important to label the pouch to alert others to remove the pouch gently if a rod is in place.

Selection of the drainage appliance

Appliance selection is important for the person to be able to resume usual physical and social activities. The selected system should: (1) be odour-proof, (2) protect the peristomal skin, (3) stay secure, (4) be readily available in the community, (5) be acceptable to the patient, and (6) be invisible under ordinary clothing (Box 15.8). Drainage bags come as one- or two-piece systems. The one-piece appliances are used most commonly. The skin barrier is incorporated into the bag, eliminating the possibility of separation. Two-piece systems require that the drainage bag be snapped on over the solid skin barrier which is fitted around the stoma against the skin. The pressure of snapping the pouch in place can be uncomfortable against a newly operated area. There are two-piece systems available that avoid this pressure. After operation all ostomy patients require a system with a drainable bag. An ostomy belt may be attached to the appliance to hold it secure during activities and to prevent undue pull on the seal, but is usually unnecessary.

The skin barriers often come in precut sizes and the bags are available in different shapes and sizes, clear or opaque, odour-proof and drainable. Some can be cut to fit, decreasing the need for hospitals to stock all options.

The size of the stoma is determined by a stoma-measuring card and bags of corresponding size are used. Too large an opening in the adhesive that attaches the bag exposes the skin to irritating drainage; too small an opening may traumatize or constrict the stoma.

The disposable bag is emptied when it is one-third to one-half full (whether of gas or faeces); if allowed to fill it becomes too heavy and the pull on the bag may break the seal of the stoma and cause leakage. The lower end of the bag is opened and the contents are allowed to drain into

---

Box 15.8   Types of drainage appliance and indications for selection

One-piece closed pouch

- Suitable for solid effluent
- Discarded after use once emptied
- Changed once or twice daily
- Patient may need to use a peristomal wafer if skin sensitivity occurs
- Discrete appearance.

Two-piece system

- Skin sparing, because the baseplate or flange stays in place for several days
- Interchangeable sizes of pouch:
  — activity pouch
  — closed pouch
  — drainable pouch
- Can be used with a belt for extra security.

One-piece drainable pouch

- Suitable for liquid effluent
- Wear times of 3–5 days can be achieved
- Can be washed via emptying portal
- Clip or clamp used to empty device
- Can be used with a belt for extra security.

Colostomy plug (Bucharth et al 1986)

- Suitable for solid effluent, where stoma acts three or less times daily
- Stoma should be less than 45 mm in diameter
- Stoma should not protrude more than 6 mm from the skin
- Manufacturer suggests that a 12-day training period is necessary
- Patient may experience initial discomfort
- Patient needs to be motivated and dextrous
- Can be used with colostomy irrigation techniques
- Discrete appearance.

---

a receptacle. The volume and characteristics (colour, consistency and composition) of the drainage are noted and recorded. The appliance is changed as regularly as necessary but at least twice weekly to permit inspection and cleansing of the peristomal skin.

The stoma care nurse will help the individual choose the system most suited to the individual's needs and to make any adjustments required because of variations in the size, characteristics or placement of the stoma. Persons with a colostomy may not require skin barriers because the stool is usually formed. A small stoma pouch or cap can be worn by persons who have achieved continency of a sigmoid colostomy. Persons with an internal continent pouch usually require only a stoma cap or a gauze square with petroleum jelly over the stoma.

Colostomy irrigation

A colostomy can in some circumstances be controlled entirely by diet, especially if the colostomy is in the descending colon or sigmoid. Irrigation may be used to achieve control when the colostomy exudes solid faecal material. The technique can be time consuming and requires motivation and dexterity to master. The purposes of irrigating the colostomy are to remove faeces, gas and mucus from the intestine and to establish a regular time of emptying the large bowel so that spontaneous, irregular drainage is less likely to occur and interfere with the person's activities and usual lifestyle. The technique usually takes approximately 30–40 minutes to perform and is usually done every 24–48 hours. It involves lavaging the terminal colon with 1 litre of warm tapwater. The individual wears a long drainable pouch for the procedure but usually only wears a mini-pouch or cap to collect mucus or minimal faecal discharge at other times.

If the patient is constipated it may be necessary to irrigate the colostomy. An irrigation set can be used or alternatively a funnel is attached to one end of a catheter; the other end is lubricated and placed about 10 cm into the colon. Warm water is placed in the funnel, which is held above the level of the colostomy, and the water is allowed to run into the patient. The catheter is then removed and the outflow runs into the toilet. All the water that was instilled into the colostomy must be returned before the process is complete. When evacuation is complete, the patient cleans the skin and applies a new drainage bag.

The irrigation is most effective early in the morning, as this approximates the normal time of defaecation. If bowel regularity is maintained, irrigation should be unnecessary unless the person decides to use irrigation as a means of stoma control.

Care of a Kock continent ileostomy

Careful discussion before operation is essential to prepare the patient for surgery. The patient is returned from the operation with a catheter inserted through the stoma and valve into the pouch. The catheter is connected to a closed drainage system. It is important to maintain continuous drainage and prevent an accumulation of secretions, gas and faecal matter in the pouch in order to promote healing and prevent complications. Salter (1995) advises that the reservoir be flushed with 20–30 mL saline four times daily.

The colour of the drainage is checked frequently; it may be coloured by blood at first but the blood content progressively decreases over the first 2 days. The volume of the ileal discharge is also recorded. The faecal drainage eventually may become semi-liquid as the diet is increased and the capacity and retention of the pouch increase. Thicker pouch content may cause a drainage problem because 'solid' particles may obstruct the drainage tube, necessitating irrigation, increased fluid intake and adjustment in the diet.

A lightweight dressing with a slit for the catheter covers the stoma and surgical wound. This is changed daily and the stoma inspected for colour, swelling and oedema.

The nasogastric tube is attached to a drainage bag to prevent the possibility of gastric secretions and gas accumulating and distending the gastrointestinal tract. The catheter is left on open drainage for the first 10–12 days; thereafter it is clamped for progressively longer periods between drainage until it needs emptying only four times per day, utilizing the drainage catheter.

The capacity of the pouch gradually increases and in 6 months to 1 year a capacity of 400–600 mL is achieved.

Food tolerance tends to be an individual matter; the introduction of 'new' foods one at a time makes it possible to identify those that are troublesome. Gas-forming foods, raw fruits and vegetables, foods with a high cellulose or fibre content, corn, celery, lettuce, beans, peas and cabbage are frequently among those not tolerated.

Care of an ileoanal pouch

It is important that the patient understands this will not operate as a normal anal sphincter. Initial episodes of incontinence are common, with the mucus being discharged continuously from the pouch. The temporary stoma needs to be reversed in a second-stage operation; anal soreness can remain a problem and there is always the risk of the pouch becoming inflamed causing pain and frequent discharge.

Maintenance of skin integrity

Each time the appliance is changed, the **condition of the skin** and stoma are noted. The latter should be bright red and moist; if it is bluish or grey or dry the doctor is notified, as the change may indicate impaired circulation. The skin is examined carefully for possible excoriation or any break. Peristomal skin should be washed with warm water and gently patted dry. Skin irritation is treated promptly and a more effective protective barrier is provided. Fewer skin problems are encountered by the colostomy patient than the ileostomy patient.

Factors affecting the integrity of the peristomal skin include allergic responses, trauma, chemical irritants and infections. The individual may develop sensitivities to any of the products or appliances used to manage the ostomy. Known irritants are avoided and the method of use of each product is assessed and proper techniques taught. For example, skin barriers should be applied dry, not wet,

Skin assessment
See chapter 6.1

to avoid moisture under the pouch and against the skin. The use of adhesive tape should be kept to a minimum.

Mechanical trauma most often occurs as a result of frequent, repeated changes of the pouching system. The pouch should be changed every 3–7 days and whenever leakage occurs. If the person is changing it more frequently, the nurse should assess the technique being used and consult with the stoma care nurse regarding other actions the person might use to overcome the identified problem. Perhaps a different system would be more appropriate for the person and their particular activity pattern, or there may be another type of adhesive that will hold better.

The location of the stoma affects the composition, consistency and quantity of the faecal discharge. The drainage from an ileostomy contains more proteolytic digestive enzymes, which quickly erode the skin. Skin barriers are sized or cut to fit snugly around the stoma to protect the skin from faecal drainage but should not cut into the stoma itself as this will cause local trauma. The bag should be changed regularly and the underlying skin cleansed and inspected to guard against hidden leakage. Soaps are avoided on the peristomal skin as they leave a residue. If solvents are used, care must be taken to ensure that the skin is well cleaned. Adhesive preparations should be applied sparingly.

Infections of the intact peristomal skin are not common. *Candida albicans* (monilia) is the most common infection. It is usually treated with nystatin in the form of a powder. If infection is suspected, a swab is taken and sent to the laboratory and the surgeon is notified.

Alterations in nutrition

The ileostomy or colostomy patient usually starts out on a light, low-residue diet to which foods of a regular, normal diet are added gradually. Tolerance varies with patients but, by careful personal experimentation with foods, each person will recognize what can and cannot be taken. The foods that most often have to be excluded are those with a high-fibre or high-cellulose content. Nuts, prunes, celery, corn, pineapple, turnips, beans, cabbage and onions tend to be troublesome.

A well balanced diet is encouraged and the person's weight followed. Patients are advised to eat slowly and to chew their foods well, which reduces the risk of a faecal bolus blocking the stoma.

Considerable water and salts are lost in ileostomy drainage, especially during the first 2–3 months. Gradually, the small intestine adapts to the lack of colonic function and absorbs more water and salts. Until then extra water and food rich in sodium and potassium should be taken. The patient may erroneously think that limiting fluid intake will cause the intestinal drainage to be less fluid. Fluid intake should be more than 1.5 litres per day.

Coping with the change in body function

As soon as practicable after the operation, the nurse concentrates on helping the patient to accept the 'ostomy'

and on teaching the necessary care and management. Although there may have been considerable discussion of the modified method of elimination before operation, when the patient is actually faced with it, revulsion, discouragement and depression may occur. The patient with a temporary ostomy experiences the same feelings as the individual with a lifelong diversion. Allison and Stuchfield (1994) suggest it is common for stoma patients to experience intense feelings of loss as they lose control of such a fundamental body function as elimination. The patient has a constant reminder that they are now different from other people; the stoma stigmatizes the patient. The individual may show evidence of passing through stages of the grieving process as he or she mourns these losses (see Ch. 4).

The patient will probably be concerned about future social acceptance. Acceptance comes first from the nurse, who willingly makes every effort to keep the patient clean and comfortable without any hesitation or aversion. Personal contact by touch, when bathing the patient and positioning and cleansing around the stoma for example, in a perfectly natural and matter-of-fact manner helps the patient to feel that the stoma is acceptable. The nurse should encourage the patient and gradually introduce self-care with an understanding of the patient's reactions to the adjustments that are required (see the critical incident, p. 504). Competence in self-care of the ostomy promotes psychological adjustment. The patient may find it helpful to be visited by someone who has a stoma and is coping well. A visit by a stoma therapist should also be arranged well in advance of surgery.

Opportunities are created for the patient to interact and socialize with other patients on the ward. Return to normal activities and work are encouraged and may be achieved within 3 months.

Sexuality

The patient and partner are encouraged to ask questions about resuming normal sexual functioning, particularly as the partner may have more anxiety than the patient. Literature and pamphlets are available that may be given to the patient and partner regarding sex. Further opportunity for discussion should be arranged after they have read the information and formulated their personal questions and concerns.

Satisfactory sexual function improves the quality of life of the patient and promotes the closeness and sharing that the individual may perceive as lost or unattainable as a result of the alterations in body image and function. Identification of the patient's and partner's perceptions of the impact of the operation on their sexuality patterns and relationship should be assessed on an ongoing basis as they begin to cope with the realities of their situation. Box 15.9 lists the physical and psychological effects of ostomy surgery on sexual function. The patient and partner need help in understanding the meaning of these

Box 15.9   Sexual problems related to ostomy surgery

Direct effects

- Damage to sympathetic and parasympathetic nerves:
  — erectile difficulty
  — retrograde/no ejaculation
  — change in ejaculatory amount or force
  — orgasmic problems

- Penetration problems related to shortening or removal of vagina.

Indirect effects

- Altered expression related to:
  — altered body image
  — physical change
  — lack of knowledge

- Fears:
  — appearance of stoma or pouch
  — noise and odour
  — leakage
  — rejection
  — pain.

From Shipes (1987), with permission.

changes to their relationship. Misconceptions need to be identified, discussed and solutions explored. Responses to common misbeliefs about ostomy surgery and sexuality include:

- A stiff penis does not make a solid relationship, nor does a wet vagina.

- Absence of sensation does not mean absence of feeling.

- The presence of deformities does not mean absence of desire.

- Inability to perform does not mean inability to enjoy.

- Loss of genitals does not mean loss of sexuality.

The nurse plays an important role in helping the patient and partner adjust to the surgery and the effects of ongoing treatment and in the identification of problems related to altered sexuality patterns. If problems persist and interfere with the achievement of a satisfactory quality of life, the nurse should ensure that the patient and partner are referred appropriately and encouraged to utilize professional services.

As outlined in Box 15.8, a number of physical problems may occur following stoma surgery, especially when the rectum is excised. Impotence can be treated (see p. 786). Careful counselling of both partner and individual is important to ensure a satisfactory outcome. Impotence may resolve up to 2 years after operation. Women may experience dyspareunia, and careful assessment of the nature of the problem and appropriate advice may promote return to the desired level of sexual activity. Painful intercourse can be helped by strategies such as adopting different positions during intercourse, extended 'foreplay' to encourage relaxation, use of water-soluble lubricants or use of vaginal dilators. Some women respond to replacement oestrogen therapy.

Nurses can have a major role in encouraging discussion of issues related to sexuality and sexual functioning but it should be noted that it is an issue that is highly charged and requires sensitivity and understanding. Disclosure by the patient and the partner may threaten the attitudes and beliefs of the nurse, and, similarly, suggested strategies may frighten or disgust the individual's or partner's value system. If the nurse is unable to deal personally with this area, this should not be ignored. Encouragement to utilize other services (e.g. counselling) or to discuss problems with the stoma care nurse or general practitioner may be more advantageous in some circumstances in order to achieve a satisfactory outcome. In reviewing the literature, Allison and Stuchfield (1994) reported much evidence of positive adaptation between couples as well as acknowledgement of the major problems posed by stoma surgery. Some couples feel much closer as a result and others report such a dramatic improvement in the quality of life that sexuality has been enhanced.

Self-care

A plan of education is developed to prepare the patient for assuming care of the ileostomy or colostomy and for living a healthy, active life. During the first few days after the operation, the patient's experience with pain and discomfort generally precludes concern about the stoma and future care and activity. Gradually an awareness of the situation develops and the patient's reaction must be assessed. There may be a period of depression and withdrawal. Model (1990) emphasizes that this is all part of the patient's coping mechanism. Denial or suppression may be evident. The nurse should not challenge or confront the patient but rather work on building a supportive relationship so that eventually the patient can be helped to come to terms with their loss. In the meantime the patient is unlikely to be receptive to any formal teaching. The nurse encourages expression of concern by being a good listener and accepting the patient's reactions and anxiety.

It is suggested by Kelly and Henry (1993) that a useful strategy involves exploring the patient's usual coping strategies. Once the patient has explained how she or he usually copes with problems, the nurse can apply these approaches to the current problem. This is familiar territory, therefore, for the patient and if he or she can see that it is possible to apply familiar everyday solutions to the new challenge of a stoma, real progress with self-care can be made.

The preparation for the patient's discharge from the hospital should include a member of the family. Participation of a person with an ileostomy or colostomy who may have already visited the patient may be very helpful in reinforcing the information. Teaching includes explanations, discussions and demonstrations related to the following factors.

Management of the ileostomy and colostomy

Active patient participation in stoma and appliance care is introduced gradually but as early as possible. On discharge, the patient should be engaged in self-care and be confident in the fact that support and assistance are available in the hospital and at home.

At first, as the nurse cares for the ileostomy or colostomy, each step of the procedure is clearly described. Then, gradually, the patient participates in the care until eventually self-care is achieved. This progressive step-by-step approach takes time and patience but is less frustrating and discouraging for the patient. As self-care progresses, the community nurse should discuss any problems of self-care after discharge.

More formalized and detailed instruction includes directions for and demonstrations of the following.

Necessary equipment and supplies In addition to discussing and demonstrating the various parts of the appliance, a written list is provided and information given as to how and where the products may be obtained. Information regarding obtaining exemption from prescription charges, if not already exempt, should be provided.

Emptying the pouch, care of the stoma and changing of the appliance Planned discussions reinforce the learning that took place as the patient undertook, step by step, the daily care. It also gives the patient and the members of the family an opportunity to ask questions.

Additional directions for care and use usually accompany the appliance and should be read by the patient. Several useful booklets about ileostomy and colostomy care are usually available from the Colostomy Welfare Group or the Ileostomy Association of Great Britain and Ireland.

The hospital may also issue printed directions which serve as a guide for the patient. The importance of establishing a regular schedule for care is emphasized.

Irrigation of the colostomy (only if required by the patient). In addition to demonstrating and explaining the procedure and having the patient do it him or herself, written directions may be given. Assistance may be necessary in deciding how the irrigation can be fitted in with the daily routine.

Care of the skin The need for thorough but gentle cleansing of the skin is stressed, as is the use of a protective skin barrier because of the irritating effect of the enzyme-containing discharge. Inspection for redness and excoriation is described and advice given as to what should be done if either is present.

Emptying the bag The role of regular emptying, changing and thorough cleansing of the appliance in controlling odour is discussed.

Problems or complications Problems such as excessive drainage, blockage of the stoma, excoriation, burning sensation or itching of the skin are discussed with regard to possible causes, how they are recognized and the appropriate action.

Nutrition and fluids

The patient is advised that foods high in cellulose and fibre and some raw vegetables and fruits may be troublesome. A list of foods known to lead to a problem, and therefore to be avoided, is provided. The importance of a well balanced diet and the taking of additional amounts of sodium, potassium and water is explained. It is suggested that one new food be added at a time so those that cannot be tolerated may be identified.

Bathing

The patient may take a shower or bath with the appliance in place. Showering without the appliance is good for the skin and for cleansing the stoma. The patient must be sure that no soap is used on the peristomal skin. Bathing is usually done before applying a fresh appliance because the moisture is likely to loosen the adhesive disc.

Some people with stomas may have sufficient confidence to go swimming – the appliance is concealed by a bathing suit.

Activity

Activity for the stoma patient is normal except for heavy lifting, which predisposes to prolapse of the stoma and hernia, and body contact sports, which could result in injury to the stoma. The patient is encouraged to return to his or her occupation and recreational activities. Many people find that their general health is so much better than previously that they enjoy being able to participate in new activities.

The patient may be concerned about sexual relationships and is advised that the change in body image need not be a deterrent to satisfactory sex relations. If an abdominoperineal resection has been done, injury to parasympathetic nerves may very occasionally result in impotence. A woman may experience some discomfort during intercourse for a period of time because of the perineal wound. This matter of sexual relationships is something the individual may wish to discuss freely with the stoma therapist. Further help may be available from SPOD (Association to Promote the Sexual and Personal Relationships of People with Disabilities).

Medications

Laxatives or other drugs should not be taken unless prescribed. If a medicine is ordered by a doctor other than the gastroenterologist, the patient should remind the doctor about the stoma. Some preparations should be only in powder or liquid form to ensure absorption.

Sources of assistance

The patient is likely to be very apprehensive about leaving the protective hospital environment. A list of persons or associations from whom advice or assistance may be sought is provided, with telephone numbers. This list may include the stoma therapist, general practitioner or community nurse, and the relevant associations.

Differing models for support of the stoma patient in the community have emerged and there is no one correct approach. In some areas the hospital-based stoma nurse visits patients at home before they have the operation. Jefferies et al (1995) found in their survey that the stoma nurse was the most highly valued member of the care team, whatever model had evolved. They estimated that by discharge 65% of all stoma patients had achieved total independence in caring for their stomas, which still left a lot of community support work to be done. Three months after discharge Jefferies et al found that 89% of patients were independently caring for their stomas, even when away from home all day.

Complications

Potential complications of an ileostomy or colostomy include prolapse or retraction of the stoma, obstruction of the stoma, fluid and electrolyte imbalance, renal calculus and fistula.

In *prolapse of the stoma*, the mesentery of the remaining intestine is not secured sufficiently to the abdominal wall and/or the opening in the abdominal wall is too large. Increased intra-abdominal pressure results in a segment of the ileum or colon being forced out on to the abdomen. If several centimetres of the bowel are extruded, the patient should be placed in the dorsal recumbent position with the head and shoulders slightly raised and the knees flexed. A dressing moistened in sterile water or normal saline is placed over the area. The doctor may attempt manual replacement of the extruded segment or recommend surgical repair.

Retraction of the stoma occurs as the result of shrinking scar tissue in the supporting tissues of the abdominal wall. The opening becomes flush with the abdominal surface, making it difficult to protect the skin from the irritating effluent. Correction is by surgery.

Obstruction of the stoma may be caused by a faecal bolus formed as a result of insufficient mastication of food or the ingestion of fibrous or cellulose foods that are too bulky to pass through the stoma. The blockage may be relieved by an irrigation. An obstruction may also be caused by a volvulus of the ileum near the stoma. If there is no ileal or colostomy discharge, the doctor is notified. Unless the obstruction is relieved, the patient will develop nausea, vomiting, crampy pain and abdominal distension.

Ileostomy dysfunction sometimes occurs and is characterized by sporadic free liquid drainage with a very offensive odour. It is associated with peristomal scarring and stenosis which causes trapping of the intestinal contents until pressure and irritation result in the discharge. Dilatation of the stoma may be necessary.

Normally, much of the water and electrolytes contained in the small intestine content is reabsorbed in the colon. The person with an ileostomy loses considerable water, sodium and potassium in the ileal drainage and may develop *fluid and electrolyte imbalance*. The patient is encouraged to drink a minimum of 1500–2000 mL of fluid daily, to add salt to foods and to include potassium-containing foods (e.g. orange juice, banana, meat) in the diet. If the ileal drainage becomes excessive, fluids containing potassium and sodium, such as fruit juice, are increased to compensate for the loss. If the excessive drainage cannot be controlled, the doctor should be notified. An antidiarrhoeal drug may be prescribed, serum electrolyte levels determined and intravenous fluids administered to correct dehydration and electrolyte imbalance.

The ileostomy patient is predisposed to the formation of a *renal calculus* (kidney stone) because of the water and sodium loss in drainage. This further emphasizes the importance of a greater fluid and electrolyte intake for the person with an ileostomy or colostomy, especially if the latter is on the right-hand side.

Rarely, an ileostomy or colostomy is complicated by a *fistula*. An opening develops in the ileum and the drainage forms a tract to the surface. This may be the result of a poorly fitting appliance or the recurrence of the primary disease. The drainage causes tissue irritation and erosion. Surgical intervention may be used to resect the tract and may include reconstruction of the stoma. Healing may necessitate complete rest of the intestine; the patient may receive parenteral nutrition until the area is healed.

Herniation of the intestine due to a weakness of the muscular tissue at the site of the stoma may occur. It is recognized as a bulging area. Support may be provided by the ileostomy or colostomy appliance.

Evaluation

Physical management of the stoma is an important step in the person's adjustment to the change in body image and altered control of an important body function. Ostomy surgery impacts on the person's total well-being and family and social relationships. Adjustment is slow and requires support from the nurse, other healthcare providers and the patient's spouse and family.

A variety of products and appliances is available for ostomy care. The stoma therapist and/or nurse should assist the patient in selecting a drainage system most suited to his or her individual needs. Achievement of self-management and an acceptable quality of life are realistic goals for most persons following bowel diversion surgery.

Summary

Discussion in this chapter focuses on the person with disorders of the various functions and parts of the gastrointestinal system. Disorders of swallowing and absorption of foods are discussed. Diarrhoea and constipation are health problems that we all experience at some time in our lives. Constipation is a common, yet largely preventable, problem in the elderly. Inflammatory bowel disease may have devastating effects on the quality of life of those it affects, leading in many cases to stoma formation surgery. The creation of a surgical faecal diversion also has a tremendous impact on the quality of life of the patient and family. Adjustment is slow and requires teaching and support from nurses and other health professionals. Cancer of the gastrointestinal tract affects both men and women of all ages and carries a poor prognosis. Early diagnosis and treatment are important for a positive outcome. Preventive measures include the adoption of a diet high in fibre, fruits and vegetables, with adequate vitamins C and D, and low in fat, nitrate-preserved foods, salt and alcohol. The nurse's health promotion role may have a major long-term beneficial effect in reducing the incidence of bowel cancer.

Conclusion

The aim of this chapter was to give novice nurses, and nurses unfamiliar with the speciality, an insight into the effects of gastrointestinal disease and the syndromes that patients experience. With the imperative for evidence-based practice in mind, the text has sought to provide information about disorders and the current approaches to patients' care and treatment. More in-depth and specialist information for those wishing to explore the area further can be obtained from the further reading list and current papers in related nursing, medicine, surgery and pharmacology journals.

Critical incident

Sarah is a 23-year-old student who has had Crohn's disease for 10 years. After numerous episodes of remission and exacerbation, she has undergone surgery to have a colectomy and formation of an end-ileostomy. It is 6 days since her operation and she has made a good recovery, even stating that it is a relief to have the ileostomy. She has just started to learn to deal with it and is emptying the bag without supervision. She helps to change the bag but is not doing it herself yet. She has a boyfriend of a year's standing who has been visiting her regularly but, as far as you are aware, she has not discussed the details of her operation with him yet.

You are on night duty and busy settling patients for the night. Sarah seems comfortable; you have given her analgesia and ensured she has enough to drink during the night. You ask whether she has emptied the ileostomy and she says she has and there are no problems.

At 05:30 hours Sarah calls you. Her ileostomy bag has leaked; the odour and mess are obvious and Sarah is distressed to the point of not being able to move. You change the appliance for her and then help her to the bathroom. Whilst she is in the bath you clean and remake her bed and wash her nightclothes. You help her back to bed and quietly discuss what happened when she is ready.

Points for reflection and discussion

Why did it happen?

- The bag became overfull (more than half full of either gas or faecal fluid) and movement caused it to leak by lifting the adhesive flange off the skin.

- The bag was not well adhered and was beginning to lift off the skin anyway.

- Movement in bed when asleep may cause the bag to lift off if it is becoming full, particularly with gas.

- As Sarah is recovering she will have begun to eat solid food and this will result in more flatus forming, which she will not yet be used to.

How did it make Sarah feel?

- Disgusted by the mess?

- Appalled that this could happen to her?

- Reality shock – she had been doing well after the operation and this is the first pitfall she has encountered. She is not 'better' after all but has something else to deal with.

- She has possibly been in denial about the change in her body image as indicated by her not discussing the details of the operation with her boyfriend or showing him her stoma. This event will confront her with that reality. It may well cause her to feel unattractive and depressed.

- Angry – she did not realize this could happen.

How did it make you feel?

- Disgusted by the mess?

- Appalled that this could happen?

- Guilty?

- Disappointed that this episode has disrupted Sarah's apparently model recovery?

- Angry – you may be partly responsible for this happening.

What was bad about the situation?

- The mess?

- The distress it caused?

What was good about the situation?

- It gave Sarah the opportunity to overcome one of the practical and emotional aspects of her operation with your help and support.

- It gave you an opportunity to consider your feelings and action in the situation which you will be able to act on productively in future.

What was learnt from the situation?

- Leaking stoma appliances cause significant distress for the patient and those around them.

- Changes in dietary intake will affect the output of a stoma, particularly an ilestomy and need to be anticipated by the patient.

- Ilestomy appliances need to be emptied regularly, of flatus or faecal fluid, and adhesion of the appliance should be checked whenever this is done.

- New ostomists need guidance and reassurance every step of the way despite seeming to be 'in control'.

- Accidents happen to most ostomists sooner or later; learning to deal with them is an important part of the learning process and the adjustment to having a stoma.

- Discuss your practice and thoughts about such an incident with a stoma therapy nurse specialist.

What would you do differently in the future?

- Check new ostomists' appliances are empty and intact before going to sleep – do so with them as a teaching opportunity.

- Ensure new ostomists' learning and achievements are clearly documented so that all staff know what the patient is able to do independently, and where they need assistance, rather than making assumptions.

See Appendix 2 for guidelines on reflection.

References

Allison M, Stuchfield B (1994) Helping to adjust: an holistic approach to stoma care. RCN nursing update supplement. Nursing Standard 8(36).

Anderton A (1995) Reducing bacterial contamination in enteral tube feeds. British Journal of Nursing 4(7): 368–375.

Bucharth F et al (1986) The colostomy plug: a new disposable device for a continent colostomy. Lancet i: 1062–1063.

Butler M (1997) Gastrointestinal bleeding In: Bruce L, Finlay TMD, eds. Nursing in gastroenterology, pp. 119–139. Edinburgh: Churchill Livingstone.

Finlay TMD (1997) Malignancies of the gastrointestinal tract. In: Bruce L, Finlay TMD, eds. Nursing in gastroenterology, pp. 161–190. Edinburgh: Churchill Livingstone.

Finlay TMD, Burns SJ (1998) Digestive tract cancers. In: Garbett R, ed. Cancer nursing. Nursing Times PDNT Book 2, pp. 18–30. London: EMAP.

Hamilton SR (1998) Oesophagitis. In: Ming SC, Goldman H, eds. Pathology of the gastrointestinal tract, 2nd edn. London: Williams & Wilkins.

Jefferies A, Joels J, Wood J et al (1995) Service evaluation of stoma care nurses practice. Journal of Clinical Nursing 4: 235–242.

Kelly M (1992) Colitis. London: Routledge.

Kelly M, Henry T (1993) Discussion can lead to acceptance. Professional Nurse 9(2): 101–110.

Model G (1990) A new image to accept. Professional Nurse 5(6): 310–316.

Munro AJ (1995) Head and neck. In: Price P, Sikora K, eds. Treatment of cancer. London: Chapman Hall Medical.

Nazarko L (1996) Preventing constipation in older people. Professional Nurse 11(12): 816–818.

Peters R, Westaby D (1994) Percutaneous endoscopic gastrostomy: indications, timing and complications of the technique. British Journal of Intensive Care: 88–95.

Rees PJ, Williams DG (1995) Principles of clinical medicine. London: Edward Arnold.

Rhys Evans F (1996) Tumours of the head and neck. In: Tschudin V, ed. Nursing the patient with cancer. London: Prentice-Hall.

Salter M (1995) Advances in ileostomy care. Nursing Standard 9(49): 33–37.

Scheiman JM, Cutler AF (1999) *Helicobacter pylori* and gastric carcinoma. American Journal of Medicine 106(2): 222–226.

Shipes E (1987) Sexual functioning following ostomy surgery. Nursing Clinics of North America 22(2): 305.

Taylor C (1997) Diarrhoea and constipation. In: Bruce L, Finlay TMD, eds. Nursing in gastroenterology, pp. 27–54. Edinburgh: Churchill Livingstone.

Thompson WG, Heaton KW, Smyth GT, Smyth C (2000) Irritable bowel syndrome in general practice. Gut 46(1): 78–82.

Trounce J, Gould D (2000) Clinical pharmacology for nurses. Edinburgh: Churchill Livingstone.

Turner G (1996) Oral care. Nursing Standard 10(28): 51–56.

White S (1998) Percutaneous endoscopic gastrostomy (PEG). Nursing Standard 12(18): 41–45.

Further Reading

Bond S (1997) Eating manners. Newcastle-upon-Tyne: Centre for Health Services Research, University of Newcastle-upon-Tyne.

A vital, wide-ranging collection of information relating to nutrition for people and patients of every group. Includes self-test quizzes as well as numerous invaluable references on nutrition.

Bruce L, Finlay TMD, eds (1997) Nursing in gastroenterology. Edinburgh: Churchill Livingstone.

This text focuses on the wide range of difficulties that patients may encounter with gastrointestinal symptoms. Written by experienced nurses practising gastroenterology nursing, the patient-focused approach of the text gives valuable insight into how to care for people with gastrointestinal problems.

Burkitt HG, Quick CRG, Gatt D (1996) Essential surgery, 2nd edn. Edinburgh: Churchill Livingstone.

Chapters 6–18 give important information about surgical procedures and management relevant to the gastrointestinal tract. Clear diagrams clarify anatomical changes brought about by surgery.

Lennard Jones JE (1992) A positive approach to nutrition as treatment. London: King's Fund Centre.

A seminal paper about nutrition in hospital inpatients.

Pendlebury J (1997) Feeding by PEG. Community Nurse 3(4): 11–12.

Clear directive paper on PEG management.

Reilly H (1998) Parental nutrition: an overview of current practice. British Journal of Nursing 7(8): 461–467.

Recent publication on the use of parenteral nutrition and patient management.

Reilly H (1998) Enteral feeding: an overview of indications and techniques. British Journal of Nursing 7(9): 510–518.

Good background on the use and management of enteral feeding.

Smith L, Baker F, Stead I, Soulsby C (1999) Feeding via a nasogastric tube. Nursing Times 95(8 Suppl): 1–2.

Additional information about managing patients nasogastric tube feeding.

Travis SPL, Taylor RH, Misiewicz JJ (1998) Gastroenterology, 2nd edn. Oxford: Blackwell Science.

A medical text with comprehensive information about diseases of the gastrointestinal tract.

Caring for the patient with a liver, biliary tract or exocrine pancreas disorder

Sue Lee

Introduction

Assessment

The person at risk of a disorder of the liver and exocrine pancreas

Disorders of the liver

Disorders of the gallbladder and bile duct

Disorders of the pancreas

Summary

Introduction

Disorders of the biliary system account for many admissions to medical and surgical wards. Recent advances in surgical technique ('keyhole surgery') should reduce length of hospital stay for many patients with gallbladder disease, while recent studies indicate that treatment with interferon is effective in patients with hepatitis (Centre for Reviews and Dissemination (CRD) 2001a, b). Improvements have also been made in the care of patients with acute pancreatitis (McArdle 2000, Abou-Assi and O'Keefe 2001). For those patients suffering from chronic or malignant conditions of the biliary system and pancreas, the outlook may be bleak. However, organ transplantation, particularly of the liver and pancreas, is improving the morbidity and quality of life for many patients (Howard and Fahy 1997, Newton 1999). The anatomy and physiology of these structures will be reviewed briefly before entering into a discussion of the care and treatment required by such patients.

The liver

The **liver** is situated in the upper abdominal cavity immediately below the diaphragm. It is divided into four lobes and is highly vascular, receiving its blood supply from two sources. The *portal vein* carries blood from the stomach, intestines, spleen and pancreas into the liver. The *hepatic artery* delivers blood from the aorta. The blood from both sources leaves the liver by a common pathway, the hepatic vein, which joins the inferior vena cava.

The liver tissue is organized in functional units called lobules. The central veins from the lobules empty into sublobular collecting veins, which unite to form the hepatic vein. Minute ducts into which bile is discharged are also formed between the rows of hepatic cells within the lobules. The small lobular bile ducts unite to form larger ducts. Eventually, the bile from the lobules is transmitted in one main channel, the hepatic duct, which joins the bile duct from the gallbladder (cystic duct) to form the common bile duct (see Fig. 16.1).

Figure 16.1 The pancreas and associated anatomy.

The liver
See chapter 5.2

Functions of the liver

The liver performs a variety of very important complex **functions**. It is a vital organ, performing a major role in total body metabolism. The liver synthesizes, processes and/or stores many of the substances that are essential to normal body functioning. It also processes and excretes some substances that would be harmful if left in their original form or retained.

Bile production and excretion

The liver cells secrete 500–1000 mL of **bile** daily into the hepatic ducts. Bile is a yellow–green or brownish fluid that is strongly alkaline. The constituents of bile include water, bile pigments and bile salts:

- *Water (90–97%)*. The water content is reduced when the bile is stored in the gallbladder, where it is concentrated six to ten times.

- *Bile pigments*. The pigments resulting from the breakdown of red blood cells and from foods are excreted as the bile pigments, *bilirubin* and *biliverdin*. In the intestine, bile pigments are acted upon by bacteria and reduced to urobilinogen. Part of the urobilinogen is excreted in the faeces, giving them the normal brown colour. The remainder is reabsorbed through the intestinal mucosa into the blood. A small amount is excreted in the urine and the rest is returned to the liver, where it is reconverted to bilirubin and again is secreted in the bile.

- *Bile salts*. These are sodium and potassium salts of certain amino acids that function in digestion and absorption. The bile salts emulsify fats, increase the digestive action of the fat-splitting enzyme, and promote absorption of fats, fat-soluble vitamins and calcium salts. (Emulsification is the process whereby large fat droplets are dispersed into much smaller droplets.)

- *Other constituents*. Sodium and calcium salts, cholesterol, fatty acids and lecithin are other substances in bile.

Bile is discharged by the common bile duct into the **duodenum** through the sphincter of Oddi. The two main functions of bile are to promote the digestion and absorption of fats in the small intestine and, as it is alkaline, to neutralize the acidic chyme when it moves into the small intestine.

Metabolic functions

The liver has a role in the metabolism of carbohydrates, proteins and fats. Briefly, it converts glucose to glycogen (*glycogenesis*) and stores it, reconverting the glycogen to glucose, which is released into the blood when required to maintain an adequate blood sugar concentration. Glucose in excess of what can be converted to glycogen is converted to fat (*lipogenesis*) in the liver.

Functions
See chapter 5.2

Bile
See chapter 5.2

Duodenum
See chapter 5.1

Fats may be both synthesized and catabolized by the liver. Cholesterol, for example, may be formed by the liver. Fats are desaturated or may be broken down into ketone acids or acetate.

Protein may be deaminized, a process in which the amine radical is removed and the remaining elements are used to form glycogen or other compounds to meet tissue needs. The amine radical is converted to urea and released into the blood for elimination by the kidneys.

Storage

The liver stores glycogen, vitamins A, D, E, K and B_{12}, iron, phospholipids, cholesterol, and a small amount of protein and fat.

Formation of certain blood components

The liver stores vitamin B_{12} and releases it as necessary to promote the production of erythrocytes.

Heparin and the blood proteins serum albumin, fibrinogen and α- and β-globulins are formed by the hepatic cells. The liver also synthesizes most of the blood-clotting factors; it is the primary source of prothrombin, fibrinogen and factors V, VII, VIII, IX, XI and XII.

Destruction of erythrocytes

Worn-out erythrocytes are broken down by Kupffer cells in the liver. The haemoglobin is released, the iron and globin are split off, and bilirubin is formed from the waste products and excreted in bile. The iron is reclaimed, combined with a protein to form ferritin and stored until it is needed for the formation of haemoglobin.

Detoxification of harmful substances

Certain drugs and chemicals that could be harmful to tissue cells are changed by the liver and rendered harmless before being circulated and excreted by the kidneys.

The body itself produces certain chemicals (hormones) that, unless destroyed, would reach too high a concentration. Examples of physiological products that are destroyed in the liver are the antidiuretic hormone (ADH), progesterone and adrenocorticoid secretions. Some hormones, such as insulin and glucagon, undergo deamination in the liver, which renders them inactive.

The Kupffer cells also protect the body by destroying organisms that may have been absorbed from the intestine.

Heat production

The liver is second only to muscle tissue in the production of heat by its continuous cell activity. Under basal (resting) conditions, the liver is responsible for most of the body heat.

Gallbladder and bile ducts

The gallbladder is a sac on the undersurface of the liver with an average capacity of 40–50 mL. The cystic duct leading from the gallbladder merges with the hepatic duct to form the common bile duct. The latter unites with the pancreatic duct to form the ampulla of Vater, which opens into the duodenum. This opening is controlled by the sphincter of Oddi.

The functions of the gallbladder are to concentrate and store the bile. When the stomach and duodenum are empty of food, the sphincter of Oddi remains contracted. During this period, the bile that is continuously secreted accumulates in the gallbladder. Contraction of the sac to eject the bile is dependent upon hormonal stimulation. When food containing fat and partially digested protein enters the duodenum, a hormone called cholecystokinin-pancreozymin (CCK-PZ or CCK) is secreted by cells of the duodenal mucosa. It is carried in the blood and, on reaching the gallbladder, stimulates the smooth muscle tissue to contract and eject bile. CCK also produces relaxation of the sphincter of Oddi, which allows the flow of bile into the duodenum.

Pancreas

The **pancreas** is an oblong gland; a thicker portion, referred to as the head, lies in the curve of the duodenum, and the remainder extends to the left directly behind the stomach. It has two distinct types of essential functional cells. Groups of one type secrete into small ducts that drain into a main channel running the length of the gland. This collecting channel is called the *pancreatic duct*; it passes out of the head of the pancreas to unite with the common bile duct to form the ampulla of Vater. Because these (digestive) secretions flow through ducts they are classified as *external* or *exocrine secretions*.

The other type of parenchymal cell is scattered in insular groups, forming what are known as the *islets of Langerhans*. These cells produce secretions that are classified as *internal* or *endocrine secretions* because they are absorbed into the blood and are not secreted into ducts.

Exocrine functions

The external secretion passes through the ampulla of Vater and sphincter of Oddi into the duodenum. It is strongly alkaline, owing to a high bicarbonate content. Several important digestive enzymes involved in the breakdown of proteins, carbohydrates and fats are contained in the exocrine secretion. Regulation of the secretion of these enzymes and their role in digestion is discussed on page 437.

Endocrine functions

The endocrine functions of the pancreas are the production of insulin, glucagon and somatostatin. The effects of these hormones, particularly in relation to diabetes, is discussed on page 567.

Assessment

Disorders of the liver, biliary tract and pancreas affect overall body functioning. The body's energy balance is affected when the supply and storage of nutrients is altered, fluid and electrolyte balance is disrupted, bowel and bladder elimination are altered, blood-clotting mechanisms are affected, and heat production diminishes. Patient assessment includes the collection of data on lifestyle, behaviour patterns, dietary habits and changes in physiological functioning of most body systems. Also, the nurse should have some understanding of the various examinations and tests carried out in order to explain them fully to the patient and discuss the implications of the results.

The signs and symptoms of biliary tract disorder may be very distressing to the patient. It is not sufficient therefore, to note that a patient appears jaundiced. The alteration in skin colour may make the patient embarrassed or ashamed and be a cause of great concern to the family. The person may have heard 'old wives' tales' about jaundice, or associate the condition with a fatal outcome; consequently patient education is required to relieve a great deal of possible anxiety and fear. Jaundice represents a significant alteration in body image which requires the patient to adapt to this change. The nurse therefore needs to assess how effectively the patient is coping, as maladaptive behaviour, if present, suggests the need for nursing intervention.

It is important, therefore, that the nurse considers the effects of the various clinical manifestations of biliary, hepatic or pancreatic disease on the whole patient, besides the obvious physical changes that are present. This consideration should be borne in mind while studying the rest of this chapter. The question 'What does the patient make of this?' should therefore be to the forefront throughout the assessment stage.

Pancreas
See chapter 5.1

History

In taking a patient's history, the following areas should be looked at:

- *Activity and lifestyle.* Data are collected on the type and extent of daily activities, how the person feels after activity, how leisure time is used, and the usual pattern and amount of sleep received.

- *Nutritional history* includes identification of daily food intake, eating habits, and factors affecting eating. Daily food intake is analysed for adequacy of essential nutrients, vitamins, fluid volume and kilocalories. How the individual responds to food is elicited as well as symptoms that occur following ingestion of food. The presence of nausea, vomiting, anorexia, excessive thirst and changes in bodyweight are determined. Use of alcohol and drugs is carefully recorded.

- *Elimination.* The person's usual bowel habits are determined and questions related to the nature, formation, colour and odour of stools are asked. The presence of steatorrhoea, melaena or clay-coloured stools is noted. The volume and colour of urine and frequency of voiding are determined as well as the presence of nocturia.

- *Environmental and occupational history* includes the identification of factors in the person's work and home environment that might be toxic to the individual.

- *Pain and discomfort* are identified by questioning the patient about the location and duration of abdominal or epigastric pain or discomfort and factors which precipitate discomfort.

- *The patient's psychological and social status* should also be assessed, including the patient's own perceptions of his or her health.

Physical examination

Liver function tests
See chapter 5.2

In a physical examination the following points should be noted:

1. *General appearance.* Changes in posture or weight distribution as seen with abdominal ascites are observed, as well as the general colour of the skin and the sclera of the eyes.

2. *Height and weight* are measured and recorded. Changes in bodyweight are noted.

3. *Temperature, pulse, respirations and blood pressure* are recorded. Body temperature reflects both liver function and cellular metabolism. Advanced liver disease may lead to intrathoracic complications; dyspnoea (and hypoxaemia) may result and should be observed and recorded (Oh et al 2000).

4. *The skin* is inspected for signs of petechiae or bruises, open lesions that have not healed, and jaundice as evidenced by a yellowish colour to the skin and sclera and itching of the skin. Peripheral oedema is determined by pressing firmly for about 5 seconds with the thumb over a bony prominence such as the dorsum of the foot; on release of the pressure, the skin is observed and palpated for pitting or indentations and the rate at which it returns to normal.

5. *Abdominal ascites.* Inspection of the abdomen containing ascites will show distension, protrusion of the umbilicus and asymmetry when the patient shifts position.

Diagnostic tests

Laboratory tests for liver, biliary and pancreatic function

Blood tests

Serum bilirubin

This test gives an estimation of the concentration of bilirubin in the blood and indicates whether it is conjugated or unconjugated. Normally, the liver cells extract the pigment from the blood and convert it to a water-soluble compound (bilirubin diglucuronide) before excreting it in bile. In obstructive jaundice, the conjugate bilirubin level is increased (normal value: 2.0–8.0 μmol/L). In haemolytic jaundice, unconjugated bilirubin is the predominant pigment in the blood (normal: 0–12 μmol/L).

Serum alkaline phosphatase

Normally this enzyme is excreted in the bile by the hepatic cells. The blood concentration may be increased when there is liver disease or obstruction in the bile ducts (normal: 35–105 IU/L).

Serum enzymes (liver and pancreatic)

Liver enzyme tests   The liver cells contain the enzymes serum alanine aminotransferase (ALT; formerly referred to as serum glutamic–pyruvic transaminase (SGPT)) and serum aspartate aminotransferase (AST; previously called serum glutamic oxaloacetic transaminase (SGOT)). As these enzymes are released into the blood when the cells are damaged, their concentration may be used to estimate liver damage (normal values: ALT 1–12 IU/L, AST 0–40 IU/L). Opiates can cause a rise in ALT and AST levels. However, ALT measurements may also underestimate histological improvement occurring following treatment (particularly with interferon), so patients should still undergo liver biopsy (CRD 2001c).

The clinical value of serum lactate dehydrogenase measurement is still being assessed (CRD 2001d).

γ-Glutamyl transferase (GGT) is an enzyme found in greatest concentration in the liver and kidneys; it indicates liver cell dysfunction and alcohol-induced liver disease (normal: males 6–28 IU/L; females 4–18 IU/L).

Concentration of pancreatic enzymes   Some of the enzymes secreted by the pancreas are normally absorbed into the blood and eventually are excreted in the urine. An increase in the serum levels of amylase (>250 units/L) and lipase (>110 units/L) occurs when there is an obstruction of pancreatic ducts and necrosis of cells.

Serum globulin

This is produced in the liver and normally is of greater concentration than serum albumin. This situation is reversed in disease of the liver.

Prothrombin time

The liver is responsible for the synthesis of several clotting factors. The prothrombin time or activity reflects the effects of liver dysfunction on blood coagulation (normal: 11–15 seconds).

Blood lipids

The concentration of cholesterol and cholesterol esters in the blood falls in liver disease, when cell function is impaired, and rises in obstructive jaundice.

Blood ammonia

In severe impairment of liver function, the ammonia concentration in the blood is increased and may lead to hepatic coma.

Hepatitis tests

Viral hepatitis is caused by hepatitis viruses A, B, C, D or E. Serological tests on the plasma to identify known antigens and antibodies are available. The various tests for the hepatitis viruses are able to detect current infection and 'virus loading' (McCreaddie and Neilson 2001), long-term immunity or recent infection. However, they may have to be done in series, which can delay diagnosis (Shovein et al 2000).

Blood glucose concentration

Damage to the islets of Langerhans may cause a reduction in insulin secretion and hyperglycaemia.

Leucocyte count

The white blood count is raised in pancreatitis, with a marked increase in the polymorphonuclear leucocytes in necrotizing and haemorrhagic pancreatitis.

Carbohydrate-deficient transferrin test (CDT)

This new test is a very specific indicator of high levels of alcohol abuse affecting the liver. Transferrin molecules are responsible for iron transport; they occur in high concentrations in the liver and become deficient in carbohydrate as a result of alcohol abuse. Many employers now screen new staff for alcohol abuse and the CDT test, which requires only a small blood sample, is proving attractive to occupational health departments (Cooper 1995).

Urine tests

Urinary bilirubin

A urinalysis may be requested for bilirubin. Normally, this bile pigment is not present in urine. Conjugated, or direct, bilirubin is water soluble and is present in the urine in obstructive jaundice and hepatocellular jaundice but absent in haemolytic jaundice.

Urinary urobilinogen

Conjugated bilirubin is changed to urobilinogen by bacterial action when the bile reaches the small intestine. Most of the urobilinogen is then excreted in the faeces, and the remainder is absorbed. A small amount of the absorbed urobilinogen is excreted in the urine, but the larger portion is claimed by the liver to be excreted in the bile. If the liver cells are damaged they may not perform this latter function, and the amount of urobilinogen excreted by the kidneys is increased. The amount of the pigment in the urine may be decreased below the normal level in obstructive jaundice when bile is not reaching the intestine or when the bacterial content of the intestine is reduced, as it is in oral administration of antibiotics. If the individual is taking antibiotics this information should be noted on the laboratory form.

Stool test

Faecal fat test

Analysis of stool specimens made over a specified number of hours may be done to determine the fat content. Failure of the pancreatic lipase to reach the intestine results in undigested and unabsorbed fat.

Ultrasonographic examination

Ultrasonography is a quick, safe and non-invasive method of assessing the patient for gallstones, hepatic cysts or tumours and other biliary problems. It is less reliable in obese individuals and in those with an excess of bowel gas.

Computed tomography

Computed tomography (CT) detects most liver lesions; information about their density and enhancement characteristics often allows a specific diagnosis to be made (e.g. in haemangioma). Watanabe et al (2000) have also used CT to study spleen size: splenic index can indicate both the severity of oesophageal varices and hepatic functional reserve in patients with liver cirrhosis. As with all radiological examinations, the patient must remain still during the procedure. CT is often used with ultrasonography to investigate the patient thoroughly.

Endoscopic retrograde cholangiopancreatography (ERCP)

A fibreoptic endoscope is passed into the duodenum. A catheter can then be passed via the ampulla of Vater into both the bile and pancreatic ducts, and a contrast medium injected to facilitate radiographic investigation. Retrograde cholangiography is performed to determine the cause of biliary problems, to diagnose cholestatic jaundice, and to remove gallstones that are obstructing the common bile duct. Radiographic films are taken during the procedure. A catheter (stent) or T tube may be inserted endoscopically to bypass the obstructive lesion and relieve the jaundice in some patients with malignant biliary obstruction.

When gallstones are removed by ERCP and sphincterotomy the patient will need blood coagulation levels measured, and blood typed and cross-matched. An antibiotic and intravenous fluid are usually administered before the procedure. The major problems that may occur are haemorrhage and infection, and the patient is assessed for any signs of these following investigation.

Cholangiography may be used to aid diagnosis of the cause of jaundice, to determine the location of stones within the biliary tract, to diagnose cancer of the biliary system, and in the investigation of recurrent symptoms in individuals who have already had cholecystectomy.

Cholecystography

Radiography is also used in the diagnosis of gallbladder disease; the procedure may be referred to as cholecystography. A radio-opaque organic iodine compound that is eliminated in the bile is given orally or intravenously. The patient receives a fat-free evening meal which is followed by the administration of the contrast medium the night before the examination. Then the patient must not take anything by mouth until after the first radiograph has been taken. This procedure has increasingly been replaced by ERCP investigations.

Percutaneous liver biopsy

Jaundice
See chapter 5.2

A small specimen of liver tissue may be examined microscopically to assist in the diagnosis of liver disease. The specimen is obtained by aspiration with a special liver biopsy needle. Using a lateral approach, the needle is passed through the right eighth, ninth or tenth intercostal space, or may be introduced below the costal margin if the liver is enlarged.

Before the procedure, the patient's blood coagulation is evaluated by determining the partial thromboplastin time (PTT) and platelet count. Blood is typed and cross-matched so that blood is available for transfusion if required. An explanation is made to the patient of the purpose of the biopsy and what will happen during and after the procedure. Pulse, respirations and blood pressure are noted by the nurse as a baseline for comparison following the biopsy.

The patient is placed in the supine position close to the right side of the bed. The area is cleansed, and an antiseptic and sterile drape are applied. A local anaesthetic agent is then injected at the puncture site. The patient is instructed to take two or three deep breaths, and then to stop breathing following exhalation. The doctor should quickly introduce the biopsy needle, aspirate and withdraw, taking only a few seconds.

Following the biopsy, absolute bedrest is necessary until the next morning. The patient is required to lie on the right side with a small pillow under the costal margin. This position places pressure against the biopsy site, preventing the escape of blood and bile. Close observation is made of the patient for haemorrhage for 24 hours. The pulse, respirations, blood pressure, colour, puncture site and general condition are noted and recorded every 15 min for 2 hours, then every 30 min for 2 hours. The interval is

then gradually increased if there are no significant changes. Abdominal pain, tenderness and any rigidity are reported, because they may indicate irritation and inflammation of the peritoneum due to the leakage of bile from the liver. Severe pain and breathlessness are reported promptly as they may indicate that the lung or colon is perforated.

Transjugular liver biopsy

A biopsy of liver tissue may also be obtained via the transjugular route. This is particularly appropriate for patients who have significant abdominal ascites or have developed coagulopathy, when complications from the percutaneous approach are more likely to arise. The procedure is undertaken within a radiology setting; the procedure is generally regarded as safe, although some complications may occur such as arrhythmias or bleeding (Middlebrook et al 1999).

Radioisotope liver scan

The Kupffer cells of the liver phagocytose small particles in the blood such as technetium-99m sulfur colloid. When injected intravenously, this accumulates in the liver (and spleen). Any lesion in the liver does not take up the radiocolloid and appears as a cold area in the γ-camera image.

Clinical characteristics of disorders of the liver and biliary tract

Liver function is essential to life and, fortunately, this large organ has exceptional functional ability and regenerative capacity. If liver disease is limited and tissue damage is localized to one area of the organ, the body is not likely to suffer serious impairment of function. If there is diffuse disease and parenchymal damage, dysfunction is more marked. Liver disease may be acute or chronic, and disturbed function may be reversible or irreversible, depending on the amount of tissue involved and the nature of the cause.

Disorders of the gallbladder and bile ducts interfere with the flow of bile into the duodenum. They may be acute or chronic, and the intensity of the signs and symptoms parallels the severity of the condition. Like the liver, the pancreas has a large reserve capacity; a portion of the gland may be destroyed or become non-functional and the remainder will compensate sufficiently to maintain normal physiology.

Jaundice (icterus)

This is an indication of an excess of bilirubin in the blood, resulting in a yellowish staining of the tissues that may be seen in the sclerae, mucous membranes and skin. The cause may be intrahepatic or extrahepatic disease and, according to the cause, the **jaundice** may be classified as hepatocellular, obstructive or haemolytic (Table 16.1).

Table 16.1   Characteristics of different types of jaundice

	Urine			Faeces		Plasma	
	Colour	Urobilinogen	Bilirubin	Colour	Stercobilinogen	Unconjugated bilirubin	Conjugated bilirubin
Haemolytic							
Increased bilirubin load (e.g. hereditary spherocytosis)	Normal	Increased	Absent	Dark	Increased	Increased	Normal
Hepatocellular							
Deficiency of transferase (e.g. Gilbert's disease)	Normal	Variable	Absent	Normal	Normal	Increased	Decreased
Cellular damage (e.g. infective hepatitis)	Dark	Variable	Increased	Paler than normal	Low	Decreased	Increased
Obstructive							
Intrahepatic fibrous obstruction (e.g. biliary cirrhosis)	Dark	Absent	Increased	Pale	Absent	Increased	Increased
Extrahepatic obstruction (e.g. carcinoma of head of pancreas)	Dark	Absent	Increased	Pale	Absent	Increased	Increased

From Hinchliff et al (1996).

The *hepatocellular* type of jaundice is associated with intrinsic liver disease and is due to failure of the hepatic cells to take up the bilirubin resulting from the breakdown of red blood cells and excrete it as bile. Jaundice may not be present in chronic liver disease (e.g. cirrhosis), especially in the early stages, as regeneration of the hepatic cells may parallel the damage.

Obstructive jaundice is caused by an interference with the flow of bile in the extrahepatic ducts. It is most often due to the impaction of gallstones in the common bile duct, but may occur as the result of a stricture in the duct or neoplastic disease in neighbouring structures (e.g. pancreas) compressing the duct.

Haemolytic jaundice occurs when there is an inordinate destruction of red blood cells, resulting in excessive bilirubin formation.

The jaundiced patient's urine is likely to be dark because of the bilirubin or urobilinogen content. Urobilinogen is not present in obstructive jaundice, because it is formed in the intestine. The stools are pale grey in obstructive and severe hepatocellular jaundice.

Pruritus

The itching of the skin experienced by many patients with jaundice is attributed to irritation of the cutaneous sensory nerves by the retained bile salts.

General constitutional symptoms

The patient complains of a poor appetite, vague digestive discomfort and flatulence, and loses weight. McCollum (2000) reports a study in which appetite and nutritional intake in patients with chronic liver disease were assessed. No relationship was found between disease severity and nutritional intake. However, there was a strong association between liver disease and appetite suppression. Lassitude, weakness and muscle wasting develop as a result of the impaired storage of carbohydrates and protein metabolism. A low-grade fever may be present.

Pain

Dull, aching pain in the right upper abdominal quadrant is a common symptom, especially in acute liver disease. Tenderness is manifested on palpation.

The pain associated with gallbladder or biliary duct disease may be felt in the right upper abdomen or mid-epigastric region, or is referred to the right scapular area. It may be a persistent, dull ache, or very severe and disabling. The onset may follow a meal containing fatty foods. When it is very severe, causing the patient to writhe about, the pain is described as *biliary colic*. The pain of biliary colic or pancreatitis may be so severe as to cause reflex spasm of the chest wall and to interfere seriously with breathing (Pasero 1998).

Referred pain See chapter 2.3

Bleeding tendency

Inadequate production of prothrombin and other blood-clotting factors results in failure of the normal clotting process. Spontaneous bleeding may occur, manifested by purpura, epistaxis, bleeding of the oral mucous membrane and/or melaena.

Ascites and oedema

An accumulation of fluid in the peritoneal cavity develops with progressive liver disease, such as cirrhosis. The hepatic tissue damage, obliteration of blood vessels, and compression by the fibrous tissue (scar) replacement produce a resistance to the inflow and outflow of blood from the portal vein. The resulting increase in the blood pressure within the portal vein and its contributaries promotes the escape of fluid into the peritoneal cavity. The diseased liver produces less albumin and other plasma protein; therefore the person is unable to maintain the normal colloidal osmotic pressure of the blood. This increases fluid loss to the tissues from the circulation and may lead to a more generalized oedema developing (Woodrow 2000). Some blood protein is also lost in the transudate in ascites. Reduced liver activity results in increased concentrations of antidiuretic hormone and aldosterone (an adrenocorticoid secretion), further contributing to oedema. These secretions, normally destroyed by the liver, promote reabsorption of water and sodium by the kidneys.

Dilated veins and varicosities

The portal hypertension associated with liver disease is reflected in changes within the veins that drain into the portal vein. They become dilated and **varicosities** develop. The oesophageal and gastric veins are commonly affected and, because they are close to the surface, one may rupture, resulting in massive haemorrhage manifested by haematemesis or melaena or both. Haemorrhoids develop because of the pressure and resistance to blood flow within the rectal veins.

Ascites
See chapter 5.2

Varicosities
See chapter 5.2

Fever
See chapter 6.1

Alcohol
See chapter 5.2

Splenomegaly

The spleen enlarges because of the hyperplasia of the reticuloendothelial tissue and congestion, causing considerable discomfort for the patient.

Skin changes

In progressive chronic liver failure, several changes are likely to appear in the skin. 'Arterial spiders' (spider angiomas or naevi) may develop, in which a superficial arteriole gives rise to a series of fine, radiating branches readily visible on the surface. These lesions are seen predominantly on the face, neck, arms and chest, and are attributed to high oestrogen levels in the blood. Gynaecomastia and atrophy of the testicles may occur in males for the same reason. Normally, oestrogen is destroyed in the liver.

The palms of the hands are frequently mottled, bright red and warm because of capillary dilatation (palmar erythema). There is a loss of axillary and pubic hair in both sexes, and facial hair grows more slowly than usual in the male.

Neurological disturbances

Severe hepatic insufficiency leads to various mental changes. The patient may manifest irritability and behaviour not previously characteristic, such as becoming inactive, apathetic and forgetful. These symptoms may progress to confusion, lack of cooperation, stupor and eventually coma.

Twitching and a peculiar coarse tremor, referred to as *flapping tremor*, develop. Flapping tremor consists of a series of rapid, irregular alternating flexion and extension movements at the wrist and finger joints. The tremor may be referred to as *asterixis*. It occurs when the arms and hands are extended.

Ammonia toxicity is considered to be an important factor in producing the mental changes, coma and other abnormal central nervous system responses. The liver is unable to convert the ammonia that results from the breakdown of amino acids to urea.

Fetor hepaticus

In advanced liver disease, the breath has a faecal odour and the patient complains of a bad taste in the mouth. It is attributed to disturbed amino acid metabolism and abnormal bacterial action in the intestine.

Digestive disturbances

The patient with impaired bile transport may experience flatulence and an uncomfortable full feeling or nausea, especially after the ingestion of fatty or fried foods. Vomiting is usual if the patient has biliary colic or develops obstructive jaundice.

Fever

Chills and an increased temperature frequently accompany infection and inflammation within the gallbladder or bile ducts.

The person at risk of a disorder of the liver and exocrine pancreas

Alcohol and alcohol abuse

Box 16.1 outlines statistics on the consumption of alcohol in the UK in the late 1990s.

The UK guidelines for alcohol consumption were revised in 1995 to give weekly upper limits of 28 units per week for men and 20 units for women, where 1 unit is equal to half a pint of beer or a glass of wine. This upward revision by the Department of Health (DoH) has been criticized by many who consider that the old lower limits of 21 and 14 units respectively should have stayed in place. In 1997, the Government again revised the recommended alcohol intake, but in terms of daily units; this was believed to be more helpful and realistic for people, and to discourage binge-drinking (see Box 16.2 for details). Recent statistics indicate that alcohol intake has increased markedly in women and amongst the young. The highest prevalence of alcoholism occurs in those aged 16–29 years (DoH 1999a). The guidance issued by the

---

Box 16.1   Alcohol consumption in the UK

- In Great Britain in 1998, nearly two-fifths (39%) of men drank more than 4 units of alcohol on one day in the previous week; around one-fifth of women (21%) drank more than 3 units of alcohol on one day in the previous week.

- In 1996, mean weekly alcohol consumption in Great Britain was 16.0 units for men and 6.3 units for women.

- In 1996, 27% of men and 14% of women aged 16 years and over were drinking more than 21 and 14 units a week respectively. Drinking at these levels amongst men has remained stable at about 27% since 1986; that of women has risen from 10% to 14% in the same period.

- More than one-quarter (27%) of pupils aged 11–15 years drank in the previous week in 1996, in England, compared with one-fifth (20%) in 1988.

- It is estimated that the annual prevalence rate of alcohol dependence in private households is 75 per 1000 population among men aged 16–64 years and 21 per 1000 among women in the same age group.

- During 1997 in Great Britain there were 16 800 casualties in traffic accidents involving illegal alcohol levels – 5% of all traffic accident casualties.

From Department of Health (1999a), with permission.

Box 16.2   Recommended daily alcohol intake limits

Men: 3–4 units
Women: 2–3 units

Preventive benefit obtained:
Men > 40 years 1–2 units daily
Women (postmenopausal) 1–2 units daily

From DoH (1999a), with permission.

Box 16.3   The CAGE alcohol assessment

Cut down   Have you felt that you should cut down or stop drinking?

Annoyed   Have people annoyed you when they've told you that you should cut down or stop drinking?

Guilt   Have you ever felt guilty about how much you want to drink?

Eye-opener Do you wake up in the morning wanting to have an alcoholic eye-opener drink?

From Gorman (1997).

Government's chief medical officer merely recommends that: 'if you drink, do so in moderation' (DoH 1999b).

Nurses often hold negative attitudes towards individuals with drinking problems. This may be due to experiences of frequent A&E attendees, and inpatients with alcohol-related conditions who resume drinking despite advice to the contrary. As Helman (1990) has pointed out, a commonly held belief is that the responsibility for much illness rests with the person, especially in regard to alcohol use. The patient is therefore stigmatized and blamed for their ill-health. This can lead to a tendency for healthcare workers to stereotype the problem drinker as potentially violent, hopeless or unable to maintain relationships, employment or 'normal' social activity.

The reality in the UK is that regular, moderate drinking or occasional intoxication results in a range of alcohol-related health problems. Recurrent stomach disorders, hypertension and stroke, damage to brain, liver and heart, domestic, occupational and road traffic accidents and injury can result from quite light or moderate drinking (see Box 16.2). Alcohol is a major contributory factor to mortality and morbidity statistics in the UK (see Box 16.1). In 1995–96 there were 32 300 admissions with a primary diagnosis of 'mental and behavioural disorders due to alcohol'; of these there were 22 600 men and 9700

women (DoH 1999a). Estimates concerning the number of alcohol-related deaths in England and Wales vary from 5000 to 40 000 (DoH 1999a) annually.

Nursing assessment of alcohol intake

Early identification and education may be effective with 'at risk' drinkers in reducing serious health problems and dependence. Nurses, as the largest group of healthcare professionals with the greatest patient contact, may be ideally placed to re-educate and promote healthy drinking behaviour. Simple scare tactics, even with million pound government budgets behind them, do not produce any significant impact upon alcohol consumption (Naidoo 1994). Assessment of alcohol intake is therefore an essential part of any person's health history.

Gorman (1997) suggests that the most direct approach is the best. She recommends that all patients should have their alcohol intake assessed by simply asking the patient: 'How much alcohol do you drink daily? Weekly? When was your last drink?' She further describes the CAGE technique (see Box 16.3). If the patient answers 'yes' to two or more of the questions, then he or she may well have alcohol dependence. Unfortunately, some authors suggest that 'patient histories are often unreliable' and that nurses should multiply the patient's self-reported count by a factor of 3 (Crigger 1998). This author comments that patients may attempt to keep alcoholism secret, and that nurses should therefore take more account of physical findings and social history (family violence, multiple marriages, frequent job changes). The nurse has to take the patient's story at face value but should also seek evidence from other sources to build up an accurate picture of the patient's health status.

Alcohol abuse, like abuse of other substances, is a complex problem (see Ch. 26). Gorman (1996) details an approach that can help to educate and empower the patient to seek help (see Box 16.4). She reminds us that the underlying mechanisms at work in alcoholism include denial, low self-esteem and poor self-care.

The issue of denial frequently interferes with the identification of alcohol-related problems and the acceptance of treatment. It is difficult for people to accept both their alcohol dependency and a positive self-concept if they have held a negative stereotype of 'alcoholics'. People with alcohol problems who reject society's negative stereotype of 'alcoholics' are able to accept their own

---

Box 16.4   The empowering approach

This approach centres around respectful attitudes, empathy and patient education.

State your concern about the consequences of the patient's behaviour on health and quality of life:

- Don't assume the patient understands the link between poor health and drinking.

- Denial is common – you may have to point out the consequences several times in a respectful and open manner.

- Don't show your anger or frustration with the patient – it rarely helps.

- It is better to say: 'Coming into hospital must be scary and painful. Have you thought about getting help so this won't keep happening?' or 'Your GI bleeding is going to happen again unless you do something about your drinking. Would you be willing to talk to someone about it?'

- Don't threaten or isolate the patient.

Offer hope by assuring the patient that recovery is possible and they could feel better:

- For example, say: 'I realize that you might not know where to begin, given how seriously drinking has affected your life, but you can be sober and you can improve your health. It's not too late.'

- Or: 'Maybe giving up alcohol is the last thing you want to do, but if you're fed up with coming into hospital, I know that there is help available to you. You don't have to go through this on your own.'

Be prepared to refer the patient to the appropriate resources for help:

- Your own hospital resources – check them out.

- Community-based help and resources (e.g. Alcoholics Anonymous).

---

problems and still maintain a positive self-concept. Discussing the nature of alcohol dependency, and dispelling myths associated with the 'alcoholic' stereotype, can be an important nursing intervention in assisting the individual to accept the problem and the treatment for it.

It is important for nurses to examine their own feelings, beliefs and attitudes towards alcohol. Stereotypes not only make it difficult for the patient to accept their problem with alcohol but may also prevent the nurse from being supportive and emotionally available to assist the patient.

At times, the individual with alcohol or other substance abuse disorders will continue to deny the problem and/or refuse assistance. It is important to recognize that there is still likely to be a need for family support (e.g. Al-Anon treatment programme). Family members and significant others may require information about programmes and support even if the family member refuses treatment for their alcohol problem.

Nurses encounter persons with alcohol abuse problems in their daily practice, both in hospitals and the community. Unfortunately the person may be seriously intoxicated and displaying antisocial behaviour. As their behaviour deteriorates and becomes abusive and threatening, so too the possibility of meaningful communication disappears. The person has lost control of themselves and the nurse has lost control of the nurse–patient interaction.

In such difficult circumstances the following key points are essential for nursing care of an intoxicated patient:

- There should be no ambiguity between what the nurse says and does.

- There should be no difference between the nurse's verbal and non-verbal behaviour.

- Reduce any environmental stimuli to a minimum.

- Decide whether the planned therapeutic intervention warrants the risks involved.

- Keep communication simple.

Meaningful discussions can occur only when the patient is sober.

Case Study 16.1 presents an example of a clinical situation involving alcohol-related problems.

Case Study 16.1

Colin Bardsley is a 31-year-old salesperson who is married with two children. He was admitted via the emergency department with an acute case of pancreatitis. He appeared to smell of alcohol but explained that he had just come from a family celebration. Blood tests revealed his liver enzymes were generally at the high end of the normal range; his GGT results were raised by a factor of 4.

The nurse was aware that Mr Bardsley might have a drinking problem and that the nursing assessment would need to explore this possibility. The nurse therefore asked not only about alcohol consumption patterns, but also broad questions about legal, employment, social and family difficulties related to alcohol use. (For example: Have you ever had any difficulties at work related to the use of alcohol?) Mr Bardsley seemed annoyed with these questions. He explained he usually had a few drinks on a daily basis in order to entertain customers. 'I certainly can't ever get drunk or I'd lose customers. I'm very careful about how much I drink.' He denied any alcohol-related problems, except for two impaired driving charges. One charge was after an office Christmas party and the other after taking a client out to lunch to seal an important business transaction. Mr Bardsley explained he was just in the wrong place at the wrong time; such charges are an 'occupational hazard' for salespersons who are expected to do a lot of entertaining.

The nurse's awareness of a likely alcohol problem allowed anticipation of the potential problems of alcohol withdrawal. The symptoms of withdrawal include *nausea*, *vomiting*, *agitation* and *heavy perspiration*. As withdrawal progresses, symptoms such as *confusion*, *hallucinations* and *convulsions* may develop.

When Mr Bardsley became confused and appeared to be having visual and tactile hallucinations, the nurse recognized these as symptoms of alcohol withdrawal rather than a psychotic episode. Hallucinations and other psychotic symptoms (delusions, thought disorder) are frequently treated with antipsychotic medication. However, in the case of alcohol withdrawal this would not be done, because antipsychotics would generally further the seizure threshold further and therefore increase the risk of convulsions. Haloperidol may be used to treat hallucinations and diazepam to control convulsions.

In the period of detoxification and following detoxification, the fluid balance frequently needs monitoring. The patient is often prone to dehydration and therefore generally needs frequent fluids. In addition, from a behavioural point of view, the patient has become accustomed when drinking alcohol to consuming large quantities of fluid and may attempt to drink large quantities of other fluids to replace this loss. It is quite common for large quantities of coffee to be consumed as a readily available substitute. This may create difficulties because coffee can have a further diuretic effect, and the caffeine is also addictive. The patient could experience further withdrawal symptoms when later attempting to cut back coffee consumption.

The nurse was also aware of the potential for cross-addiction: many people with an addiction have more than one. Mr Bardsley was also a heavy smoker and frequently drank coffee. Mr Bardsley's emotional state was closely monitored for signs of anxiety, withdrawal and depression, all of which are associated with substance abuse.

Once the immediate physical problems related to withdrawal had passed, Mr Bardsley's nurse recognized his need to have specific treatment for his alcohol problem. Options include self-help groups such as Alcoholics Anonymous (AA) or more formal treatment programmes. Assessment and referral programmes may be community or hospital based. Similarly, treatment programmes may operate on an outpatient, day-patient or inpatient basis. It is therefore important to be aware of community resources.

In the case of Mr Bardsley, the nurse made a referral to a social worker who further assessed the drinking problem and then discussed treatment options. Mr Bardsley was able to take advantage of an employee assistance programme through his place of work to arrange for a short day-hospital programme, followed by a year of weekly outpatient follow-up.

Disorders of the liver

Viral hepatitis

This is an inflammation of the liver due to one of several viruses. Five viruses known as **hepatitis** A, B, C, D and E viruses are the most common causes, but other viruses such as the cytomegalovirus (CMV) or Epstein–Barr virus may also be implicated.

Hepatitis A

This type of hepatitis accounts for the greater number of cases. The disease may be epidemic and has a higher incidence in children and young adults. It has an incubation period of 3–5 weeks and is included in the list of *reportable diseases*. It is an acute, self-limiting disease which does not usually lead to chronic hepatitis or a carrier state.

Large amounts of the virus are eliminated in the faeces in the week preceding the onset of jaundice. The stools therefore constitute a low infection hazard once symptoms appear. Transmission is by the faecal–oral route and is therefore facilitated by poor hygiene. The virus, which is highly contagious, can also be spread by the ingestion of contaminated water or food (Shovein et al 2000). This disease may spread rapidly, especially in overcrowded and poor sanitary conditions.

Hepatitis B

Hepatitis B is caused by the type B virus (HBV), which consists of an inner **DNA** core enclosed in a protein coat. Both the inner core and the large surface mass contain distinctive antigens. The principal mode of transmission is by the injection of infected blood and blood products. Because of this, hepatitis B is a common problem among

Hepatitis
See chapter 5.3

DNA
See chapter 1.3

drug addicts who are sharing injection equipment. Needlestick injuries may result in transmission of the virus to healthcare workers. The same mechanism is also apparent in human immunodeficiency virus (HIV) infection. Hepatitis B can be transmitted like HIV, by intimate contact with carriers or those with acute disease. The virus can be found in saliva, semen and vaginal secretions, as well as blood. It may therefore be a sexually transmitted disease amongst homosexuals and heterosexuals. The incubation period for hepatitis B ranges from 6 weeks to 6 months. It is more common in adults than children, whereas hepatitis A tends to have a higher frequency in children and young adults. Hepatitis B has an insidious onset; it may persist or become chronic, or produce a carrier state in which the individual may be asymptomatic but harbour the virus.

Hepatitis C

Many cases of hepatitis associated with blood transfusions were known where there was no evidence of hepatitis B. These cases have now been shown to be due to a type C virus (HCV) which is transmitted via the blood, but has a low risk of sexual transmission. The illness is usually relatively mild in the acute phase, although up to 50% of patients go on to develop chronic liver disease (Kumar and Clark 1994). HCV is still more common in southern Europe and Japan than in the UK, although its true prevalence in the UK is difficult to assess as many patients are unaware that they have become carriers. The diagnosis, therefore, may not be made until they present with the symptoms of chronic liver disease.

Hepatitis D and E

Hepatitis D requires the presence of hepatitis B for transmission. It is very rare in northern Europe, as is hepatitis E, which is found mostly in Asia and is transmitted by the enteric route.

Prevention and screening

Prevention of the transmission of viral hepatitis focuses on two areas: education of carriers to prevent transmission to others, and protection of at-risk groups against contamination of the virus. Nurses have an important contribution to make in giving advice to carriers and their significant others to allay fears, reduce anxiety, provide education regarding potential routes of contamination, and abating misconceptions. However, this information should be relayed in such a way as to ensure reduction of risk to others but without promoting unnecessary restrictions or precautions that could cause distress. Nurses and other healthcare workers are also at risk of contracting hepatitis B and C – hence the importance of using universal precautions at all times when handling potentially infective material (De Palma 2000).

Education for drug users should focus on safe use and disposal of needles and syringes. Information regarding safe sexual practice, the use of condoms, etc. should be given and reinforced at every opportunity to homosexuals, prostitutes and drug users as these people are most likely to engage in high-risk behaviours. Leaflets and other educational material can be useful for spreading sound information, and may be easily displayed in many health settings to which the public have access. The parallels with the prevention of the spread of HIV are obvious.

Screening for hepatitis is usually targeted on the following:

- all admissions to renal dialysis and transplant units
- individuals who have recently travelled to countries with high levels of hepatitis
- drug users
- individuals who have received blood or blood products
- the acutely or recently jaundiced
- staff who have sustained a needlestick injury
- pregnant women.

It is extremely important to remember that anyone who is screened for any of the hepatitis viruses must give their informed consent, irrespective of the circumstances of diagnosis (McCreaddie and Neilson 2001).

Clinical characteristics

Whatever the virus responsible, the subsequent illness is very similar. The virus attacks the hepatic cells, and inflammation and necrosis follow. The swelling and congestion interfere with normal bile formation and flow, resulting in intrahepatic obstructive jaundice and raised blood bilirubin levels. Serum enzyme levels of alanine aminotransferase (ALT) and aspartate aminotransferase (AST) rise sharply because of the necrosis, and the serum albumin : globulin ratio may indicate a reduced formation of albumin and an increase in the γ-globulin. The latter points to the acute infectious nature of the disorder. Urinalysis reveals an excess of urobilinogen, especially in the initial stage. The blood is examined for the presence of hepatitis virus antigens and antibodies that have been identified.

Fortunately, in most cases complete regeneration of the liver cells occurs on recovery, with a minimal fibrous tissue formation and scarring. Very few persons experience residual impairment of liver function.

The signs and symptoms may vary in intensity from one individual to another. The onset is usually manifested by vague symptoms such as fatigue, loss of appetite, nausea, vomiting, headache, fleeting abdominal and joint pains, and fever. After several days, abdominal tenderness and pain in the right upper quadrant are more predominant, the urine becomes dark, either constipation or diarrhoea may be troublesome, the stools may be abnormally light in

Table 16.2 Assessment of the person with viral hepatitis

Pathophysiological alterations	Clinical characteristics
Liver structure and function	
Hepatomegaly	The liver is tender and enlarged on palpation Abdominal discomfort
Altered bile production, excretion and reabsorption	Pruritus Jaundice of skin and sclerae Urine, dark orange in colour Stools, clay-coloured Diarrhoea or constipation
Altered metabolism of carbohydrates, proteins and fats	Nausea and vomiting Anorexia Flatulence Malaise, weakness and fatigue Irritability Weight loss Muscle wasting Fever
Altered production and destruction of blood components	Spontaneous bleeding Purpura Melaena Haematuria
Extrahepatic	Skin rashes Arthralgia Headache Sore throat, cough, catarrh Depression

colour and jaundice becomes evident. Hepatitis B is usually more prolonged and debilitating. Table 16.2 lists the clinical characteristics of viral hepatitis.

Diagnostic tests

- ELISA (enzyme-linked immunosorbent assay): detects anti-HCV (presence of HCV shows current or previous infection).

- RIBA (recombinant immunoblot assay): confirmatory test, done after ELISA but being replaced by PCR.

- PCR (polymerase chain reaction): this test has two components that confirm HCV infection and also the 'viral load' circulating in the bloodstream.

- Liver function tests check for raised liver enzymes, e.g. alanine aminotransferase (ALT) and aspartate aminotransferase (AST).

- Liver biopsy to confirm liver damage – fibrosis and cirrhosis.

Treatment

There is currently no effective treatment for patients with hepatitis A, except for bedrest (the disease is debilitating), although children may be asymptomatic. There is some evidence to suggest that administration of interferon α is helpful for some patients with chronic hepatitis B (CRD 2001b). However, many patients respond only partially (i.e. the patient relapses following initial improvement) and some patients do not respond at all. Other research by Camma et al (1996) suggests that low-dose interferon is more helpful than no treatment for patients with hepatitis C. However, the research is still in a relatively early state and confirmatory studies are required. One of the problems is that ALT measurement may not be an accurate reflection of improvement (CRD 2001c).

In the USA and, more increasingly in the UK, liver transplantation is being offered to patients with chronic hepatitis who then go on to develop liver failure.

Assessment

Health history

The person is questioned with tact and sensitivity regarding exposure to hepatitis viruses from blood transfusions, the use of contaminated needles, sexual activity and possible contact with infected individuals, and personal hygiene. Emphasis is placed on identification of the clinical symptoms the person is experiencing. As the course of the disease varies from asymptomatic and mild to acute, fulminating and life-threatening, symptoms vary considerably as to frequency and severity. The patient is asked specific questions related to gastrointestinal disturbance and changes in the colour of the skin and mucous membranes, sclera, stools and urine. Changes in the tendency to bleed are also noted.

Physical examination

This includes the measurement of the person's temperature; observation of the skin, mucous membranes and sclera for changes in colour; observation of urine and faeces; observation of the skin and gums for signs of bruising and bleeding.

Nursing intervention

The *goals* of care are that the person will demonstrate:

1. alleviation of symptoms
2. fluid balance
3. maintenance of desired body weight
4. return of appetite
5. knowledge of self-management
6. resumption of usual daily activities.

It is also important that there should be no evidence of transmission to others.

Rest

The person is encouraged and helped to get adequate rest and relaxation. Both at home and in the hospital, plans should be developed to provide uninterrupted periods of rest throughout the day as well as at night. Activity is resumed slowly, and the person observed for reactions. Liver function is monitored by repeated tests to detect any adverse effects of increased activity.

Medications

Many drugs (such as oral contraceptives and morphine) that are normally inactivated by the liver are not pre-scribed. The patient is advised against taking any drug that has not been prescribed by the doctor during this illness. Alternative barrier methods of contraception and issues relating to safe sexual practices should be discussed.

Nutrition and fluids

In the acute stage it is difficult for the person to take suf-ficient fluids and food because of the nausea, vomiting and aversion to food. An increased daily fluid intake of at least 3000 mL is necessary because of the fever and to promote urinary elimination of the serum bilirubin. If the patient cannot tolerate fluids orally, intravenous fluids may be given. The patient is observed closely for signs of overhydration manifested by sudden weight gain, oedema and respiratory distress. Fluid intake and output are recorded. Parenteral administration of vitamin K may be recommended if blood coagulation is impaired as a result of impaired absorption of vitamin K when bile salts are decreased.

A high-calorie diet of 3000 kcal is recommended daily; nutritional deficiency retards the liver's ability to over-come the infection and regenerate functional tissue. As soon as the nausea and vomiting are controlled, the patient is offered small amounts of high-calorie foods fre-quently. These are gradually increased until the ultimate goal of 3000 kcal is achieved. The diet consists principally of protein and carbohydrate. The fat content may be restricted while there is jaundice but is increased, as tol-erated, by the addition of dairy products, which make the diet more palatable. Fried foods, fat meat and rich foods, such as pastries, are usually avoided for several weeks or months after recovery. The person is advised not to take alcohol for at least 6 months.

The individual's weight is checked at regular intervals because there may have been a considerable loss in the early phase of the disease.

Skin care

Frequent bathing and changes of linen during the period of fever are necessary. The use of soap is avoided; emol-lients may be added to the bathwater to relieve the itching associated with jaundice. Calamine lotion may be used and fingernails are cut short and kept clean. Most people with cirrhosis of the liver have abused alcohol, although many alcoholics do not develop cirrhosis. It is not clear why this is the case.

Prevention of the spread of infection

All patients with viral hepatitis are treated as potentially infectious. Universal and body substance precautions are used with all patients, therefore no additional measures are required. Needlestick injuries pose the greatest threat to healthcare workers as HBV is transmitted through the blood. As with all patients, needles should never be recapped and only disposable needles and syringes should be used for persons with hepatitis. Invasive proce-dures should be avoided whenever possible. Gowns and gloves should be worn whenever direct contact with blood or faeces is possible. Personnel caring for the patient are informed of the possible sources of the infec-tive particles (faeces, vomitus, urine and blood) and of the fact that they are usually resistant to heat, antisep-tics, and prolonged exposure to cold and freezing.

The hands are scrubbed under running water with liq-uid soap after each contact. Bed linen contaminated with faeces or blood is placed in a clean bag at the bedside, which is identified as an isolation bag. No special precau-tions are necessary regarding dishes or glasses. The use of disposable equipment for procedures involving penetration of the skin (e.g. needles and syringes) is recommended, and gloves should be worn by those handling them. Used needles and syringes are placed in a puncture-resistant container used for all such supplies. Blood, urine, faeces and sputum specimens should be clearly labelled 'bio-hazard' to protect laboratory personnel.

The person is advised of the importance of thorough handwashing after going to the toilet. Gloves are worn when handling the patient's bedpan; excreta should be flushed promptly down the toilet. If the patient is being cared for at home, the patient and family are taught sim-ple precautions and the importance of good handwashing.

Contacts

Known contacts of infectious hepatitis A are advised to consult a doctor as soon as possible. An intramuscular injection of human immune serum globulin may be given to provide protection. It is effective against the virus A organism. Hepatitis B immune globulin is available for contacts of HBV. Its use is usually reserved for individuals exposed to HBV through needlepricks or other accidental injection. The γ-globulin may not always provide immu-nity, but is found to lessen the severity of the disease should the person develop it.

Vaccines for active immunization against hepatitis are recommended for high-risk groups, especially health pro-fessionals at risk of contamination with patient's blood. Hepatitis B vaccine is available to nurses in the high-risk groups and to all who wish it through most employee occupational health services. Immunization involves three intramuscular injections, with the second and third doses being given at 1 and 6 months respectively.

Critical Incident: Needlestick injury

Student nurse Alice was caring for 27-year-old Allan who had hepatitis B. Allan had been an intravenous drug user for some years but had only recently contracted the disease after sharing needles with his new girlfriend. Unfortunately his condition was serious. Allan was tired, irritable and restless; he was experiencing extreme nausea and anorexia and had now developed coagulopathy. He was covered in bruises and had bleeding gums, and had been prescribed a vitamin K injection which Alice was giving under the supervision of staff nurse Joanne.

Allan appeared to be half asleep as Alice and Joanne approached him. Alice explained what she was about to do and asked him to turn over. Allan turned over but as Alice gave him the injection, he shouted loudly in pain and brushed her hand out of the way. Although Alice was wearing gloves, she felt the needle scratch her finger, which she had used to position the skin around the injection site.

The hospital policy was very clear. Although it was a barely perceptible scratch, Alice made the wound bleed and kept it under a running cold tap while Joanne completed the accident form. Alice then went down to the accident and emergency department for a blood test.

Both the initial ELISA and subsequent tests 3 months later showed that Alice had not developed anti-HBV. However, Alice has found this a very distressing and protracted experience; during this time, she split up with her boyfriend and found it very difficult to concentrate on her academic work.

Reflection

1. What could Alice and Joanne have done differently in relation to:
   a. Preparing Allan?
   b. Preparing Alice?

2. Is the hospital's policy for needlestick injury correct? Do you know what your placement's policy is?

3. What is the role of vaccination here?

4. What would the implications have been for Alice as a student nurse if she had developed HBV?

5. What would the implications be for Joanne had Alice developed HBV?

See Appendix 2 for guidelines on reflection.

Antibodies persist for at least 3 years. Booster doses are given at regular intervals. HBV vaccine is also available in the community for individuals who are at risk for contacting the infection. High-risk groups include those with illness-related factors requiring repeated transfusions of blood or blood products, and those with lifestyle-related factors such as homosexual practices, intravenous drug use and prostitution.

Follow-up

The person is encouraged to attend outpatient appointments; laboratory and physical examinations are carried out to detect possible progressive or residual impairment of liver function. Supervision is usually continued for 1 year. The intervals between visits to clinics or doctor are gradually increased if the findings are favourable.

Evaluation

Achievement of the established goals for the individual with hepatitis is determined by ongoing assessment showing alleviation of the person's symptoms. The individual's bodyweight should be maintained at a desirable level. The patient and family should be able to describe plans for meeting nutritional needs and needs for increased rest, as well as precautionary measures to prevent transmission of the virus to others. They should be familiar with plans for follow-up care.

Toxic hepatitis

Rarely, inflammation and degenerative changes in the liver occur as a result of a chemical. Carbon tetrachloride, phosphorus, sulfonamides, arsenical preparations and chloroform are examples of suggested offenders. The patient is treated by prompt withdrawal of the causative chemical, rest and supportive care.

Cirrhosis of the liver

The term **cirrhosis** denotes chronic diffuse degenerative tissue changes occurring in the liver. There is destruction of parenchymal cells and formation of excessive dense fibrous scar tissue. Blood, lymph and bile channels within the liver become distorted, compressed and effaced, with subsequent intrahepatic congestion, portal hypertension and impaired liver function. The fibrous tissue changes result in the liver becoming firmer. The surface is usually rough because of small projecting nodules of regenerated hepatic cells, and is frequently described as a 'hobnail surface'.

Causes

The mechanisms responsible for cirrhosis of the liver are not clearly defined, although the following factors are known to be associated with the condition.

Alcohol abuse Most people with cirrhosis of the liver have abused alcohol, although many alcoholics do not develop cirrhosis. It is not clear why this is the case. Ingestion of moderate to large quantities of alcohol over several years can produce fatty infiltration of the liver and liver dysfunction. The toxic effects on the liver develop more readily in the presence of malnutrition. Many

Cirrhosis
See chapter 5.7

persons show a marked improvement in the earlier stages of cirrhosis when alcohol ingestion is discontinued.

Hepatitis Severe type B viral hepatitis in which there has been extensive necrosis followed by considerable scarring may lead to cirrhosis.

Chronic cholestasis Degenerative changes characteristic of cirrhosis may also occur with prolonged cholestasis (obstruction to the flow of bile). The cause is usually partial obstruction by a stone or stricture within the extrahepatic bile ducts, but may be intrahepatic as a result of infection or inflammation and subsequent stricture of the small ducts within the liver.

Autoimmune processes Primary biliary cirrhosis is thought to be an autoimmune disease with progressive degenerative changes in the bile ducts within the liver, eventually resulting in liver failure. Mainly women are affected; it is thought that the incidence may be 670 people per 670 million adults (Fahey 1999).

Hepatic infiltration Fibrotic changes in the liver may be associated with the infiltration of certain substances. Examples include excessive glycogen which accumulates in the liver in the individual with von Gierke's disease; enlargement and fibrosis develop. Similarly, Gaucher's disease results from an abnormal reticuloendothelial cell content that incurs liver fibrosis and dysfunction.

Clinical characteristics

The liver has considerable reserve; early cirrhotic changes generally go unrecognized without apparent manifestations. With the characteristic insidious progress, signs and symptoms of impaired liver function appear gradually over a period of years. In the early stages the symptoms are vague digestive disturbances: the person experiences anorexia, flatulence, nausea and loss of weight. Intense pruritus is often the presenting symptom (Klainberg 1999). Later, jaundice, dependent oedema, spider angiomas, anaemia and increased abdominal girth due to ascites develop. Splenomegaly, neurological involvement (hepatic coma) and haemorrhage from oesophageal varices are characteristic of advanced cirrhosis and serious liver dysfunction.

The severity of liver dysfunction is determined by liver function tests as well as by history, symptoms and physical examination. Palpation of the liver and spleen provides significant information. The liver is enlarged and firm, and may have a rough surface; the spleen is enlarged owing to the resistance by the liver to flow of blood from the portal vein.

Treatment

The care required by the patient with cirrhosis depends upon the extent of the liver damage. There is no cure, as such, for cirrhosis. However, liver transplantation has been successful in patients with advanced disease (Klainberg 1999).

Medications

Methotrexate may improve liver function while urso-deoxycholic acid (UCDA) may actually slow the progression of the disease (Fahey 1999, Klainberg 1999).

Multivitamin preparations are prescribed. Parenteral vitamin K may be given if the prothrombin level is below normal and if a tendency to bleeding is manifested by petechiae, ecchymosis, epistaxis, melaena or haematemesis. Vitamin B_{12} injections may be necessary to correct anaemia.

Although the patient with cirrhosis usually develops oedema and ascites due to portal hypertension and decreased plasma oncotic pressure (because of reduced liver production of blood proteins), diuretics will be prescribed only with care. This is because of the risk of electrolyte imbalance, particularly excessive loss of potassium, as these patients often have low potassium levels initially. Fluid restriction is usual, depending on the level of serum sodium. Diuretics that are given initially are potassium-sparing diuretics (e.g. spironolactone), as hypokalaemia may precipitate hepatic encephalopathy. Cirrhotic ascites is often refractory and requires the use of a combination of diuretics. Rapidly acting diuretics waste potassium and necessitate frequent determinations of electrolyte and fluid balance.

Potentially toxic drugs normally inactivated by the liver are avoided. Examples of these are paracetamol, diazepam, oral contraceptives and opiates.

Abdominal paracentesis

An abdominal paracentesis may be necessary if the fluid in the peritoneal cavity reaches a volume that is causing respiratory distress, compression of abdominal viscera and blood vessels, and considerable pain and discomfort. The nurse explains the aspiration procedure to the patient and makes sure the bladder is empty. The head of the bed is elevated and the patient is supported with pillows. The doctor may wish to have the patient sitting on the side of the bed with a support for the back and feet. A blood pressure cuff is made ready on one arm so that the blood pressure may be monitored during and after the paracentesis. The necessary sterile equipment and fluid receptacle are brought to the bedside. Following the application of an antiseptic and sterile towels, the doctor injects the site with a local anaesthetic before introducing the trocar and cannula. A tube is attached to the cannula to drain the fluid into the receptacle.

During the procedure, the nurse checks the patient's pulse, colour and blood pressure, and provides necessary psychological support. The doctor should be alerted promptly if the pulse becomes rapid and weak, pallor is noted, or there is a fall in blood pressure. No more than 1 or 2 litres are withdrawn at one time. Removal of the fluid results in the loss of considerable plasma protein, especially serum albumin. Also, the sudden reduction of intra-abdominal pressure results in a dilatation of the abdominal blood vessels and a pooling of a large volume of blood, which may lead to circulatory collapse and shock.

A sterile dressing is applied to the site of the paracentesis when the cannula is withdrawn. The patient is returned to the dorsal recumbent position, and the head of the bed is lowered. The amount and character of the fluid are recorded and a specimen of the fluid is labelled and sent to the laboratory for examination. The abdominal site is kept clean and dry to prevent infection and discomfort. The pulse, colour and blood pressure are checked at frequent intervals for several hours. A plasma or whole blood infusion may follow the paracentesis to replace the lost protein. Increased diuresis may be observed with the decreased pressure on the renal blood vessels.

Peritoneovenous shunt

When ascites is persistent, a shunt may be placed between the peritoneal cavity and the superior vena cava. This draws ascitic fluid into the venous circulation and relieves the ascites.

Complications of cirrhosis and their management

Hepatic encephalopathy and coma, and oesophagogastric varices, are common complications.

Hepatic coma

Before the patient with cirrhosis of the liver develops coma, neurological disturbances are manifested. These include mental dullness, slow responses, forgetfulness and disorientation. Muscle reflexes are exaggerated, and muscular rigidity and asterixis (flapping tremor) are also present. The cause of the neurological involvement is failure of the liver to metabolize and detoxify nitrogenous substances; the toxic materials such as ammonia remain in the blood and are carried into the cerebral circulation. The failure may be due to hepatocellular necrosis or because portal blood bypasses the liver and reaches the central nervous system by being shunted directly into the systemic circulation.

Nursing measures used in the care of any unconscious person are applicable to the patient in hepatic coma. The condition is managed by reducing the level of nitrogenous substances. This is achieved by cleansing the gastrointestinal tract by administering lactulose orally and giving enemas (disposable magnesium sulfate). Sometimes a non-absorbable antibiotic (neomycin) is prescribed to suppress urea-splitting bacterial gut flora. Protein intake is restricted.

Portal hypertension

The flow of blood from the portal vein through the liver may meet with resistance due to disease and cirrhotic changes in the liver. Pressure rises within the portal venous system, causing **portal hypertension**. The increased pressure in the portal vein produces a back-up in the veins that normally empty into the portal system. Collateral circulatory channels develop between the portal vein and the systemic circulatory system to bypass the liver.

The veins most seriously affected by portal hypertension are those in the gastric cardia region and the lower part of the oesophagus. The veins become engorged and tortuous; the walls are weakened, predisposing them to rupture. These varicosed veins appear as large bulbous protrusions under the mucosa. The congestion in the mesenteric veins causes haemorrhoids and is also reflected in the apparent congested cutaneous veins around the umbilicus. In addition to varices, problems associated with portal hypertension include congestive splenomegaly and ascites.

The severity of portal hypertension may be assessed indirectly by evidence of oesophageal varices, which may be visualized using fibreoptic endoscopy or by liver scan.

Bleeding oesophagogastric varices

The oesophagogastric varices are frequently the site of rupture of the vascular wall and severe haemorrhage. The perforation and bleeding may be caused by mechanical trauma from 'rough' food passing over a varicosity, erosion and ulceration of the mucosa and venous wall by gastric acid secretion, or sudden increased intra-abdominal pressure associated with coughing, vomiting, straining at stool or physical exertion. Severe haematemesis occurs; some blood will enter the intestine and eventually the person passes tarry stools.

Prompt emergency treatment and care of bleeding oesophagogastric varices are necessary; the excessive loss of blood is life threatening.

Portal hypertension
See chapter 5.2

Control of bleeding

Various measures are used to control bleeding, including balloon tamponade, vasopressin infusion, sclerotherapy and surgical treatment.

Balloon tamponade A Sengstaken–Blakemore tube (a nasogastric tube with three or four lumens) may be inserted. One lumen ends in an elongated balloon that is inflated to exert pressure against the oesophageal wall; another ends in a small balloon that is positioned just within the stomach and, when inflated, compresses varices in the cardia and anchors the tube in place (Fig. 16.2); and the third lumen opens into the stomach, extending well beyond the balloon in the cardia. The third lumen permits drainage or aspiration of the gastric content; its proximal end may be attached to suction. Removal of gastric contents reduces the amount of blood entering the intestine. Digestion of blood in the intestine produces nitrogenous wastes that, when absorbed, predispose the patient to hepatic coma. Some Sengstaken–Blakemore tubes have a fourth lumen which permits suction above the oesophageal balloon.

Figure 16.2   Sengstaken–Blakemore tube which is used in the treatment of bleeding oesophageal varices. The tube has three lumens. One leads to the longer inflatable balloon that is positioned in the oesophagus to provide pressure. A second lumen ends in the smaller balloon that lies just within the stomach. The third lumen opens into the stomach to permit gastric aspiration.

Figure 16.3   A Sengstaken–Blakemore tube in position with the oesophageal and gastric balloons inflated.

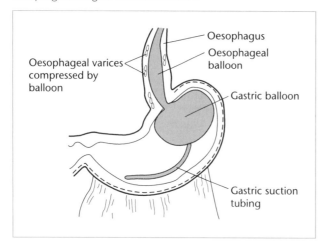

Continuous suction is applied so as to aspirate any blood or secretions above the oesophageal balloon. Before the tube is inserted, the tube and balloons are tested for leaks. Before insertion, the tube is usually chilled, which makes it firmer and easier to manipulate, and is lubricated to ease insertion. The nurse makes sure that the proximal end of each lumen is identified and clearly labelled to prevent possible error in inflation or deflation of tubes after insertion. The pressures to be maintained within the balloons are indicated by the doctor and are usually 25–30 mmHg; excessive pressure can cause tissue ulceration (Fig. 16.3). Inadequate inflation is ineffective in checking bleeding and may also permit shifting of the tube. The gastric drainage is checked frequently for blood content, which should progressively decrease following the insertion of the tube.

The patient is observed closely for any indication of respiratory distress. Saliva or blood escaping around the tube into the oropharynx may be aspirated. The patient is unable to swallow saliva, so provision is made for suction or for expectoration into tissues or a basin.

The tube is positioned within the nostrils to exert a minimum of pull and pressure, and then secured. Frequent moistening and a very light application of a lubricant to the nasal mucosa may reduce the irritation. Some doctors position the tube via the mouth.

Compression by the inflated balloons is not usually continued for longer than 48 hours. Pressure for a longer period could cause oedema, ulceration and perforation. The tube is left in position for continued gastric drainage and for the balloons to be reinflated readily if bleeding should resume. In some instances the doctor may order deflation of the balloons for 5 min at regular intervals to reduce the risk of tissue damage. Vomiting with the tube in place can lead to aspiration of the fluid – hence the extra fourth lumen which may be present.

Vasopressin infusion   Vasopressin (antidiuretic hormone; Pitressin) may be administered by an intravenous route. The vasopressin produces arterial vasoconstriction which reduces portal venous pressure by decreasing the volume of blood entering the portal system. The patient may experience crampy abdominal pain and be incontinent of faeces.

Sclerotherapy   This is the primary method of treatment. A coagulating substance is injected into the oesophageal varices. Visualization of the varices is achieved using fibreoptic endoscopy, and a coagulating substance is injected. The patient is closely monitored after the injection. The patient will be required to have this procedure repeated at regular intervals for 1–2 years.

Surgical treatment   If the measures cited above are not effective in checking the haemorrhage, emergency surgery may be performed. Different surgical procedures are used such as ligation of the submucosal veins that are involved in the haemorrhage by use of a stapling device. An incision is made for a gastrotomy and the target approached from below.

A transjugular intrahepatic portosystemic shunt (TIPS) may be more effective for patients with recurrent bleeding varices but should not be the first-choice treatment over endoscopic treatment (Papatheodoridis et al 1999).

Assessment

The patient with bleeding varices is seriously ill and requires continuous attention and ongoing assessment.

The blood pressure and pulse are recorded every 15–30 min until the bleeding is controlled. The intervals are gradually increased as the patient's condition shows improvement and stabilization. The patient's respirations, colour and responses are noted at similar intervals to monitor for signs of hypovolaemic shock.

The pressures in the balloons are checked at frequent intervals and corrected if necessary to the prescribed pressure (30–40 mmHg). The gastric drainage is observed for amount and blood content. Persisting bright blood in the drainage is brought to the doctor's attention as this indicates continued bleeding. The fluid intake and output are recorded, and the balance determined daily. Stools are examined for blood content.

Supportive measures

The patient with bleeding oesophagogastric varices is critically ill and needs physical and psychological support.

Blood transfusion Replacement of the blood lost is imperative. Fresh blood rather than stored is preferable in order to replace the thrombocytes lost.

Nutrition and fluids A large-bore intravenous line is maintained until the patient is able to take fluids by mouth.

Fluids may be introduced via the tube in the stomach before it is removed. When the tube is removed, small amounts of nutritious fluids are given. The diet is progressively increased to a light diet as tolerated. Roughage and raw fruits and vegetables are avoided. The patient is advised to chew food well, and in small amounts so that the bolus is small and less likely to cause trauma to a vulnerable area in the oesophagus or cardia of the stomach.

Rest and positioning The patient is kept absolutely at rest to avoid displacing the balloons. Passive movements of the lower limbs and deep breathing are usually carried out to prevent circulatory stasis and to promote airway clearance. The head of the bed is elevated, unless contraindicated by shock. This position may reduce the flow of blood into the portal system.

Psychological support The haematemesis, emergency measures and rapid loss of strength are very frightening to the patient. Fears and concerns should be acknowledged, and reassurance provided that everything possible is being done. Explanations are calmly made as to what is happening and what is going to be done. Sedation may be necessary to allay the patient's tension and anxiety, and provide rest. The patient may be less apprehensive and more relaxed if a family member is present. The family should be kept informed about the patient's progress and what is being done.

Mouth care The inability to swallow saliva and to receive anything by mouth necessitates special mouth care. Suction may be necessary to remove secretions. Tissues or a basin should be provided into which the patient may expectorate. The mouth is cleansed with moist applicators, and petroleum jelly or cold cream is applied to the lips to prevent irritation that may develop with the repeated use of tissues.

Nursing management (Box 16.5)

Assessment

Health history

The patient who is admitted with bleeding varices will be acutely ill and initial assessment should focus on the vital signs and the ABC of resuscitation. When the situation has been stabilized and the patient's condition improved, the person's perceptions of symptoms and cause of the illness are obtained. Data are collected about changes in bodyweight and the appearance of ascites; nausea and vomiting and any loss of appetite; skin colour and itching; changes in mental status; changes in bowel habits; changes in energy level and feelings of tiredness.

Ongoing assessment includes recording of the person's fluid intake and output, and accurate assessment of nutritional intake. A mental status examination is performed frequently if there is indication of confusion, lethargy or altered level of consciousness.

The person is weighed daily as short-term changes will reflect changes in body fluid. The abdomen is examined daily for signs of ascites, and the presence of oedema should be monitored. The skin is inspected for changes in colour associated with jaundice and for petechiae and bruising, which indicate bleeding.

Nursing intervention

The *goals* of care are that the person will demonstrate:

1. adequate nutritional intake
2. absence of pain and discomfort
3. regular, rhythmic respirations
4. loss of weight associated with a decrease in the ascites
5. absence of signs of infection
6. willingness to talk about feelings and concerns
7. understanding of and compliance with the treatment regimen.

Box 16.5   Care summary: Cirrhosis of the liver

Nurse

Admission assessment to include:

- Baseline observations of girth, vital signs, neurological status, home and social circumstances, alcohol intake
- Weigh patient daily
- Daily measurement of abdominal girth
- Daily recording of blood pressure, pulse, temperature and respirations
- Daily neurological assessment
- Assess, observe and record nutritional intake
- Assess, observe and record bowel function
- Apply anti-pruritic lotions/moisturisers and medications as prescribed (change bedding at least once daily)
- Observe for bleeding tendencies, e.g. melaena, bruising and jaundice
- Assist with investigations, e.g. paracentesis
- Administer medications as prescribed: vitamin B_{12}, methotrexate
- Patient/family education
- Assist with nutritional intake
- Maintain fluid balance chart
- Encourage patient to maintain sitting position.

Doctor

Medical history:

- Particularly alcohol intake, hepatitis, cholelithiasis
- Blood tests: check full blood count and coagulation studies, urea and electrolytes, liver function tests
- Prescribe medications: methotrexate, vitamin B_{12} injections, vitamin K
- Tests: abdominal paracentesis
- Patient/family education.

Dietician

- Nutritional assessment
- High carbohydrate, low sodium diet with vitamin supplements
- Liaise with medical/nursing staff regarding patient's protein requirements
- Potassium rich supplements
- Patient/family education.

Social worker

- Home social assessment
- Initiate home support measures.

Nutrition

As the progress of the disease is influenced by nutrition, a diet of 2500–3000 kcal per day, high in carbohydrates and vitamins is recommended. Protein content may be high (110–150 g), but can be restricted to 40 g, or eliminated according to the severity of the disease. Sufficient fat to make the diet palatable is added if the patient can tolerate it and is not jaundiced. Three small meals with in-between snacks will probably be more acceptable than three large meals. Sodium intake is restricted because of the tendency to develop oedema and ascites. Low-sodium protein concentrate and low-sodium milk are available and may be used to assist with the protein intake. Total abstinence from alcohol is very important.

If the liver insufficiency is serious and the patient is exhibiting neurological disturbances (e.g. depressed awareness, dulled mentation, confusion, asterixis and hyperreflexia) and has increased blood levels of ammonia, protein is eliminated from the diet. The patient is sustained with carbohydrates. The disturbance of the nervous system is attributed to failure of the liver to metabolize the nitrogenous wastes; the ammonia level rises because it is not deaminized to form urea. If coma develops, intravenous infusions are used to support the patient.

Control of pain and discomfort

The person's skin should be kept clean and dry. Soaps and perfumed skin products are avoided. The skin is inspected for areas of redness or breakdown. Moisturizers are used to treat dryness and antipruritic lotions may be applied to alleviate itching. The person's nails are kept short and they are encouraged not to scratch. Diversional therapy may be useful. The person will be more comfortable in a cool environment and should be cautioned to avoid heat and heavy clothing that will increase itching.

The person will probably be more comfortable in a sitting position to alleviate discomfort from abdominal distension due to the ascites. The sitting position also alleviates respiratory distress. The person's respirations are monitored regularly as indicated and the patient is encouraged to carry out deep breathing and coughing exercises if respirations are impaired.

Prevention of infection

Resistance to infection is lowered in the patient with cirrhosis of the liver. Precautions should therefore be taken to prevent possible exposure to any source of infection.

Patient and family teaching

Significant changes in lifestyle are required after discharge and these should be carefully discussed with the patient and family. Strict adherence to diet, total abstinence from alcohol, and the avoidance of infection and physical strain are stressed when interpreting the regimen to the patient and family. (If cirrhosis has been caused by alcohol abuse the nurse should encourage participation and commitment to therapy, and provide information and contact numbers and addresses of self-help groups such as Alcoholics Anonymous for the individual and significant others.)

The increased bleeding tendency associated with liver disorders makes it important to stress the need to avoid injuries and abrasions to the skin.

A referral to the primary healthcare team may be necessary so that consistent support and supervision is ensured.

The prognosis for patients with cirrhosis depends on the degree of liver insufficiency. If treatment is instituted in the early stages and the patient is sufficiently motivated to adhere to the suggested care, a normal lifespan is still possible. If portal hypertension has developed with resultant ascites and oesophageal varices, the prognosis is grave.

Evaluation

The person with cirrhosis of the liver is assessed on an ongoing basis for relief from symptoms and absence of discomfort. The skin is inspected for signs of irritation, scratches, breaks and signs of bleeding. The client and family should understand dietary and comfort measures and recognize when to seek professional help. The patient and family should be comfortable talking about their concerns and anxieties, and be aware of the prognosis for the patient. They should be aware of support groups and palliative care in the hospital and the community.

Accidental Injury to the liver

North American evidence indicates that in trauma patients, after the spleen, the liver is the second most commonly involved abdominal organ (Hudak and Gallo 1994). Any interruption of the capsule enclosing the hepatic tissue carries the risk of severe internal haemorrhage which may prove fatal before surgical intervention is possible. Urgent resuscitation is required together with surgical repair. Control of the bleeding is of prime importance. The area may be sutured or packed, or oxidized cellulose (Oxycel) gauze may be applied. The latter supplies fibres on which the clot may form more easily. In addition to the loss of blood incurred in injury, peritonitis may develop as a result of the chemical irritation caused by bile that may escape from the liver. Destruction of liver cells may also follow the injury, resulting in impaired liver function and serious clotting problems.

Neoplastic disease

Benign and primary malignant neoplasms in the liver are less common than the more frequent metastic growths. A primary tumour is usually associated with an already diseased liver (e.g. alcoholic cirrhosis). In the more frequent case where the growth is metastatic, the malignant cells will probably have been transported to the liver via the portal venous or hepatic arterial blood, or via the lymph. In many instances, secondaries in the liver are discovered before the primary source. The liver enlarges and signs of liver insufficiency develop. The patient experiences pain, food intolerance, anaemia, emaciation and ascites.

If a primary neoplasm is confined to one lobe of the liver, a hepatic lobectomy may be done. After the operation, the patient is observed closely for possible haemorrhage and biliary peritonitis. Chemotherapy may also be used. Mor et al (1998) conclude that liver transplantation for carcinoma has been effective in patients with advanced cirrhosis and small lesions. They also suggest that in the future the prevention of viral infection and genetic therapy should be studied.

Liver abscess

Infection with subsequent abscess formation occurs rarely and is most often associated with amoebic dysentery. The causative organisms (*Entamoeba histolytica*) are carried by the portal bloodstream from the bowel. The pyogenic infection may also be caused by staphylococcus, streptococcus or *Escherichia coli*. Along with manifestations of impaired liver function, the patient has chills and a high fever. There may be one or multiple small abscesses which frequently coalesce, forming one large cavity.

The patient is treated with antibiotics and also receives chloroquine or emetine hydrochloride (antiamoebic drugs) if the abscess is a complication of amoebiasis. The abscess is drained by aspiration followed by the injection of an antibiotic into the cavity. Open surgical drainage is avoided if possible because of the danger of dissemination of the infection within the peritoneal cavity and resultant peritonitis.

Liver transplantation

The number of liver transplants being performed is increasing each year, although the procedure remains limited to a few centres. Donor organs are generally matched to the recipient according to body size and blood type, as the liver is not as immunologically active as other organs. The recipient's immune system is suppressed usually with ciclosporin in combination with low-dose corticosteroids. Patients and families require a great deal of emotional support and therapeutic intervention to help them deal with the transplant and the implications for the patient's life and the quality of life that can be anticipated.

A number of recent studies have investigated the quality of patients' lives following liver transplantation. One of the key problems for researchers is the subjectivity of 'quality of life'. For some patients, this is related to returning to work (Newton 1999). Others, however, found that, although quality of life was improved, it was not the same as for the general population and that some patients had the same psychiatric morbidity as general medical patients (Collis et al 1995). In a qualitative study, Robertson (1999) found that patients felt that their independence was held back by their relatives/significant others, who continued to 'wrap them in cotton wool'. There is a clear need for more work to be undertaken in this area, as transplantation becomes more widely available.

Liver transplantation for end-stage alcoholic cirrhosis remains controversial: is it ethical for these patients to be offered an opportunity for transplantation, given the shortage of donor organs? Alcoholic liver disease is NOT medically contraindicated for transplantation and some studies report 'good' outcomes for former alcoholic patients. Howard and Fahy (1997) suggest that all transplant teams should include liaison psychiatrists to spot potential problems and initiate appropriate psychosocial interventions.

Disorders of the gallbladder and bile duct

Cholelithiasis

Gallstones
See chapter 5.2

Cholecystitis
See chapter 5.2

Cholelithiasis is the term used for stones in the gallbladder (Box 16.6). The stones vary in shape and size and consist mainly of cholesterol and bile pigments. There may be one stone or many and, although they may develop in both sexes, they occur more often in middle-aged women.

Clinical characteristics

Cholelithiasis may not give rise to any disturbance in many persons; in others, the stones cause signs and symptoms ranging from mild digestive disturbances following fat ingestion to the severe, disabling pain of biliary colic. **Gallstones** may cause acute or chronic inflammation of the gallbladder (*cholecystitis*), or *cholestasis* (stasis of the bile) within the liver leading to impaired function of that organ. Small stones tend to cause more acute problems, as they may escape into the ducts. They may pass into the duodenum or may lodge in the cystic or common bile duct or the ampulla of Vater. Impaction of a stone in the common bile duct leads to obstructive jaundice and biliary colic – an intense, incapacitating pain.

Treatment and nursing intervention

Cholelithiasis is treated surgically by removal of the gallbladder (*cholecystectomy*) and exploration of the common bile duct for a stone or stricture. Stones may be removed from the common bile duct by means of the ERCP technique. Percutaneous removal of gallstones is indicated in patients who are at high risk in terms of anaesthesia, but recurrence of gallstones is common (although this may be asymptomatic) (Courtois et al 1997).

Food and fluids by mouth are withheld, and the patient is given intravenous fluids. If vomiting and abdominal distension occur, a nasogastric tube is passed and regular aspiration is performed.

Box 16.6   Glossary of terms (extrahepatic biliary system)

■ *Cholelithiasis* – gallstones or calculi in the gallbladder

■ *Cholecystitis* – inflammation of the gallbladder

■ *Cholecystectomy* – surgical removal of the gallbladder

■ *Cholestasis* – stoppage or suppression of the flow of bile

■ *Cholecystostomy* – incision into the gallbladder and the insertion of a tube for drainage

■ *Choledocholithiasis* – gallstone(s) in the common bile duct

■ *Choledochitis* – inflammation of the common bile duct

■ *Choledocholithotomy* – surgical removal of stone from the common bile duct

■ *Choledochotomy* – incision and exploration of the common bile duct

■ *Choledochoduodenostomy* – anastomosis of the common bile duct to the duodenum.

After the acute episode and removal of the nasogastric tube, clear fluids are given and gradually increased to a light, low-fat diet as tolerated.

The patient is observed for signs of jaundice, and the colour of all stools is noted. The stools may be saved for examination for the presence of the stone, which may have passed from the biliary tract into the intestine.

If the patient is jaundiced and the stools are a pale grey, indicating an absence of bile in the intestine, a daily dose of vitamin K is given parenterally to maintain prothrombin formation and prevent bleeding.

Early surgical intervention has become much more common in recent years.

Cholecystitis

Inflammation of the gallbladder may be acute or chronic. Acute cholecystitis is most often associated with gallstones but may occur as a result of infection. The patient manifests pain and tenderness in the right upper abdominal quadrant or mid-epigastrium, fever, nausea and vomiting, and leucocytosis. The severity of the symptoms varies with the degree of inflammation. Jaundice may develop if the inflammation involves the biliary ducts.

Management

The treatment includes rest, intravenous fluids, analgesics and antibiotics. If the condition persists or worsens, it may indicate suppuration (empyema of the gallbladder), necessitating prompt surgery. A *cholecystostomy* (drainage of the gallbladder) or a *cholecystectomy* (removal of the gallbladder) may be done.

Chronic cholecystitis is characterized by a long history of vague digestive complaints. The person experiences abdominal discomfort and flatulence after a large rich meal or one high in fats. A dull, aching pain and nausea and vomiting may occur at times. The intensity and probably the frequency of the symptoms increase insidiously over months or years.

The chronic inflammation results in scarring and thickening of the wall of the gallbladder and cholestasis. If calculi are present, they progressively increase in size or number. The person may have subacute or acute exacerbations leading to nausea and vomiting, moderate fever and probably colic. The condition is usually treated surgically by removal of the gallbladder.

Bile duct disorders

Obstruction of the common bile duct may occur as a result of a gallstone that has escaped from the gallbladder (*choledocholithiasis*), inflammation (*choledochitis* or *cholangitis*), neoplasm or a stricture formed by scar tissue following trauma and inflammation. The duct above the obstruction dilates and obstructive jaundice develops.

In the case of an impacted stone, ERCP may be done and the gallstone removed during the cannulation of the common bile duct. Surgery may be undertaken to open the duct and remove the calculus. When a stricture is present and the area is sufficiently small, it is resected and an end-to-end anastomosis performed. If the obstruction is due to primary carcinoma, excision may be undertaken and the duct stump anastomosed to the duodenum (*choledochoduodenostomy*) or the jejunum (*choledochojejunostomy*).

Extrinsic pressure on the bile ducts obstructing the flow of bile may occur with cancer of the pancreas or duodenum.

When surgery involves an extrahepatic bile duct, a T tube is inserted at the site of entry into the duct to maintain bile drainage during recovery of the tissues (*choledochostomy*). The stem portion of the tube is brought out on the abdominal surface through a stab wound or the incision and is attached to a drainage receptable. Surgery on a bile duct is usually accompanied by a cholecystectomy, because the gallbladder is frequently the origin of the problem.

Nursing care of patients with extrahepatic disorders

The patient is kept at rest, and food is withheld as the patient is usually nauseous and vomiting. If there is vomiting, a nasogastric tube is passed and regular aspiration is performed. The temperature, pulse and respirations are recorded regularly. The patient should be checked for signs of obstructive jaundice and abdominal distension.

When the vomiting is controlled and the nasogastric tube removed, oral fluids are given and graduated, as tolerated, to a light, low-fat diet. Traditionally this conservative approach was followed by operation at a later date; however, early surgery is increasingly the favoured option.

Preoperative care

Preoperative preparation for surgery on the extrahepatic biliary system includes close observation for jaundice and the administration of vitamin K to raise the prothrombin level. Special attention is given to having the patient understand the importance of the frequent coughing and deep breathing that will be required after the operation. Because of the site of the operation, the patient tends to take very shallow breaths to prevent pain and discomfort, predisposing to respiratory complications as insufficient lung expansion occurs, which may lead to an accumulation of secretions and atelectasis. A nasogastric tube may be passed before the patient is taken to the operating theatre.

Postoperative care

The increasing use of laparoscopic techniques (so-called 'keyhole' surgery) should reduce the need for lengthy postoperative recovery periods as the incision is much smaller and much less tissue is involved. Close observation of vital signs and pain is essential to detect any postoperative complications that may arise, however.

Exploration of the common bile duct for stones will still necessitate a special drainage tube (T tube) being used. This is inserted in the common bile duct and generally clamped during the transfer from the operating room. After the patient has been transferred, it is immediately attached to a drainage receptacle. The tubing leading to the receptacle is secured to the dressing and lower bed linen, and should have sufficient slack to prevent traction and dislodgement. The patient is advised on how to turn to avoid a pull on the tube and of the need to be sure that the tube is not kinked or compressed. The drainage is observed frequently during the first 24 hours in case of haemorrhage. There may be a small amount of blood mixed with bile in the first few hours, but persistent bleeding is reported to the surgeon. The character and daily amount of bile drainage are recorded. If there is prolonged loss of bile, it may be given back to the patient through a nasogastric tube for the purpose of promoting more normal digestion and absorption in the intestine.

The dressing is checked frequently for possible bleeding or bile leakage. After a few days, the T tube is clamped for stated intervals and is removed when oedema of the common bile duct subsides. This is usually established by administration of a radio-opaque substance into the tube and the subsequent radiograph will show the outline of the biliary tract. Alternatively, the tube is clamped for

24 hours and, if the individual remains pain free, it is removed. After removal of the tube, the dressing is observed for bile seepage. If the dressing is soiled with bile, it is changed frequently; the skin and wound are cleansed. Should excoriation of the skin occur due to chemical irritation caused by strongly alkaline bile, a protective dressing such as a hydrocolloid wafer should be applied to the skin. If the drainage is heavy, application of a drainage bag may reduce soiling of clothing and reduce embarrassment or distress. The patient should be reassured that it will cease. The patient is also observed for signs of peritonitis, such as an increase in temperature, abdominal pain, distension and rigidity.

Until the procedures become less painful and the patient is less fearful, the nurse's assistance and support are required during the frequent, regular coughing, deep breathing and changes of position that are required.

Early ambulation is encouraged, and provision is made for a small drainage receptacle that may be attached to the patient's dressing gown if there is a T tube in the common bile duct.

The urine, stools, sclerae and skin are checked for any indication of obstructive jaundice.

The patient receives intravenous fluids until the nasogastric tube is removed and oral fluids and food are tolerated. The fat content of the diet is limited.

In preparation for discharge, the patient's diet is discussed. The individual can usually gradually include fat as tolerated in the diet but the health advantages of a low-fat diet should be discussed.

An alternative technique introduced recently is to dissolve the stones with bile acids. This non-operative approach is suitable only for certain patients, such as those with stones that do not contain calcium.

Disorders of the pancreas

Inflammation and neoplastic disease are the pathological conditions seen most frequently in the pancreas.

Pancreatitis

Inflammation of the pancreas may be acute or chronic with recurrent acute episodes.

Acute pancreatitis

Acute pancreatitis is a potentially serious and life-threatening disorder; the severity of the inflammation varies. In the mild form the pancreas becomes swollen and oedematous and, with treatment, the patient is likely to recover within a few days. If the process is severe and persists, necrosis and haemorrhage ensue. Necrosis results from intrapancreatic activation of the proteinases and lipase, initiating autodigestion of the pancreatic tissue and blood vessels. Enzymes and blood may escape into the surrounding tissue and peritoneal cavity; peritonitis, paralytic ileus or ascites may develop.

Cause

Pancreatitis is considered to be the result of some factor or change within the pancreas that effects activation of the proteinases and lipase of the exocrine secretion, with subsequent breakdown of the ducts, parenchymal tissue and blood vessels. The causative factor may be an obstruction to the flow of the pancreatic secretion within the ducts. The migration of a gallstone through the sphincter of Oddi is recognized as the most likely cause. It is suggested that such an obstruction causes a reflux of bile into the pancreas, promoting activation of the enzymes and ensuing autodigestion.

There are many other possible causes, amongst which an acute relapse of chronic pancreatitis secondary to an episode of heavy alcohol intake is a strong possibility.

Clinical characteristics

Acute pancreatitis has a sudden onset, being preceded usually by only mild, vague digestive disturbances. The principal signs and symptoms are pain, gastrointestinal disturbances, obstructive jaundice, shock and hyperglycaemia.

Pain

At first, constant severe incapacitating pain occurs in the upper abdomen, penetrating through to the back. It may be described as burning or boring. Later, with progression of the disease, the pain becomes more generalized in the abdomen.

Gastrointestinal disturbances

Nausea and vomiting occur and persist. Constipation may be a problem. Abdominal distension and rigidity appear as a result of the development of peritonitis. The latter is caused by chemical irritation of the viscera and peritoneum by the enzymes that escape from the pancreas. Peristalsis diminishes, and eventually paralytic ileus and intestinal obstruction may complicate the patient's condition further.

Shock

Shock is attributed to the severity of the constant pain, the exudation of plasma into the peritoneal cavity that occurs with the peritonitis, and the loss of blood resulting from the erosion of vessels within the pancreas associated with necrotizing and haemorrhagic pancreatitis.

Vital signs

The temperature may be raised in the early stage but may become subnormal if peritonitis and shock develop. The pulse is rapid and the **blood pressure** falls with the decrease in the intravascular volume. The patient is flushed at first, and then usually becomes pale. If peritonitis develops, a dusky or cyanotic colour is possible.

Referred pain
See chapter 2.3

Nausea and vomiting
See chapter 5.1

Shock
See chapter 4.2

Blood pressure
See chapter 4.2

Obstructive jaundice

If the head of the pancreas is involved, it may compress the common bile duct and cause **obstructive jaundice**.

Blood changes

With the escape of enzymes into the pancreatic parenchyma and peritoneal cavity, fatty tissue is broken down into glycerol and fatty acids. The latter combine with calcium to form insoluble calcium compounds. The serum calcium level falls and may be severe enough to produce tetany and affect heart action (prolonged diastole). The serum bilirubin level may be increased after 2–3 days.

Haemoconcentration develops as a result of the loss of plasma. The prothrombin level falls because of the lack of absorption of vitamin K. Serum amylase and lipase levels are raised.

Disturbance in glucose metabolism

A deficiency of insulin may develop when the islets of Langerhans are involved in the pathological process, and hyperglycaemia and glycosuria may be present.

Treatment

The patient with acute pancreatitis is critically ill. Care is directed toward the reduction of pancreatic secretion to a minimum, relief of pain, prevention of shock or correction if it has developed, prevention of electrolyte and fluid imbalances and prevention of infection.

Medications

Analgesia should be given regularly to relieve pain and discomfort and promote rest. Pethidine is usually prescribed as it depresses the central nervous system and relaxes smooth muscle. The patient may receive an anticholinergic drug such as propantheline bromide (Pro-Banthine) by intramuscular injection, which will inhibit vagal nerve stimulation of pancreatic enzymes and promote relaxation of the sphincter of Oddi. If an anticholinergic drug is prescribed, the patient will experience a very dry mouth, and close observations are made for the possible side-effects of urinary retention and paralytic ileus (see Case Study 16.2).

Parenteral administration of vitamin K may be necessary to maintain normal prothrombin production and prevent bleeding.

Case Study 16.2 *Pain management in pancreatitis*

55-year-old Paula is admitted to the medical admissions ward with acute pancreatitis. This is her first admission with this condition. Her social history shows that she has some problems related to alcoholism. Paula is in severe pain and calling out constantly for analgesia despite earlier

administration of intramuscular pethidine (she is postmenopausal). The nursing staff on duty are reluctant to administer any more analgesia because they suspect that Paula is 'crying wolf' because of her alcoholism. However, the nurse in charge makes an immediate referral to the acute pain team, who visit Paula within 15 minutes whilst the medical team is still present. The acute pain nurse explains that Paula's self-report of pain is valid and important; she initiates a pain assessment scoring system of 0–10; Paula says her pain is at 10 – 'worse than childbirth!'

The acute pain nurse is able to obtain a medical prescription for intravenous patient-controlled analgesia (PCA) with morphine. This is then commenced immediately. With this regimen, and under her control, Paula's pain susbsides to what she describes as 'manageable' – a pain score of 3. Often, pancreatic pain is resistant to opioid administration, however, and various combinations of analgesic drugs may be tried, along with anticholinergics. It is important to remember that this lack of response is about treatment failure, not drug-seeking behaviour.

Complications

If *paralytic ileus* and intestinal obstruction develop, a nasogastric tube may be passed into the stomach and decompression suction established. *Obstruction of the duodenum* may develop because of the swollen oedematous pancreas. Escaping pancreatic enzymes may digest an area of the gastric or duodenal wall, causing *severe haemorrhage* as well as perforation of the eroded organ.

Renal failure may develop within 24 hours of the onset of acute pancreatitis, necessitating dialysis.

Another complication that may develop in pancreatitis is the formation of one or more *pseudocysts*.

Accumulations of inflammatory exudate, liquefied necrotic tissue and secretions become walled off by a capsule of fibrous tissue. The cyst is atypical in that there is no epithelial lining characteristic of true cysts. This accounts for the term pseudocyst. The cyst may enlarge and impose on surrounding structures: the common bile duct may be blocked, the duodenum or stomach may be displaced, or the diaphragm may be elevated.

The symptoms depend on the size and location of the cyst(s). In some instances resolution takes place spontaneously, or the cysts may produce persisting pain, digestive disturbances, anorexia, loss of weight and mechanical interference with other organs. Percutaneous drainage of pseudocysts under ultrasonography or CT control is possible.

Surgical intervention

Surgery is not usually undertaken during an acute episode unless the patient is critically ill with extensive pancreatic necrosis. Surgery on the pancreas may involve the removal of calculi in the pancreatic duct, drainage of

Obstructive jaundice
See chapter 5.2

a pseudocyst, or partial or complete pancreatectomy. Rarely, in severe chronic pancreatitis, the sensory nerves (splanchnic nerves) that transmit pain impulses from the pancreas may be interrupted to relieve intractable pain.

Meticulous skin care and protection is essential to prevent excoriation. Use of skin-protective wafers or drainage bags with integral skin-saving adhesive plates may prevent problems. Early consultation with the stoma care nurse (if available) concerning skin care and appropriate appliances may prevent problems with skin integrity.

Nursing management

Assessment

The person's condition may change rapidly with progressive necrosis and resulting haemorrhage. The *vital signs* and the *general response and appearance of the patient* are observed frequently. A rapid weak pulse, a fall in blood pressure, pallor and increasing weakness may indicate haemorrhage or shock and are immediately brought to the doctor's attention. An accurate record is kept of the *fluid intake* and *output*. A catheter is necessary for accurate hourly measurements of urine output. A urinary output of less than 0.5 mL per kg per hour is indicative of impending circulatory collapse and must be reported to the medical staff immediately.

The *intensity and location of the pain* are noted, and the abdomen is examined for distension and rigidity. All *stools* are examined and, if they are bulky, greasy and foul-smelling or show other abnormalities, they may be saved for medical examination.

The *sclerae and skin* are observed for any yellow tinge that would indicate the development of jaundice.

Nursing intervention

The *goals* of care are that the person with acute pancreatitis will demonstrate:

1. fluid and electrolyte balance
2. blood glucose levels within normal range
3. absence of pain and discomfort
4. absence of respiratory complications
5. gradual increase in self-care activities
6. knowledge of prescribed dietary and lifestyle measures
7. plans for follow-up care.

Gastric drainage

A nasogastric tube is passed and regular aspiration is performed. This relieves vomiting and distension and prevents the acid gastric secretion from entering the duodenum, which would stimulate the release of the hormones secretin and cholecystokinin–pancreozymin. The colour, consistency and 24-hour volume of the drainage are recorded.

Fluids and nutrition

The patient receives nothing by mouth to avoid stimulating the secretion of the pancreatic enzymes. The restoration and maintenance of normal blood volume is very important to prevent or correct shock. Plasma or whole blood may be given intravenously, in addition to electrolyte and glucose solutions. A close check is kept on the blood chemistry, volume of gastrointestinal drainage, urinary output and amount of perspiration to determine the specific electrolyte and fluid needs. Total parenteral nutrition may be prescribed during the acute and convalescent phases of the illness. However, recent studies have indicated that enteral feeding via a nasojejunal tube is cheap, safe and effective (Abou-Assi and O'Keefe 2001). Frequent monitoring of capillary blood glucose is necessary. McArdle (2000) argues that glucose levels should be tested as frequently as the patient's condition requires, which could be hourly, rather than according to a fixed schedule. Insulin may be administered in line with blood glucose levels.

When oral intake is permitted, fluids are introduced in small amounts. The principal nutrient given at first is carbohydrate; protein is added gradually, according to the patient's tolerance. Fats are avoided. The diet is progressively increased to a high-protein, high-carbohydrate, low-fat, light diet. Four or five small meals are recommended daily. A preparation of extract of pancreas (pancreatin) may be prescribed orally with meals to assist in digestion. Large meals are avoided, and total abstinence from alcohol is stressed.

Mouth and nasal care

Frequent cleansing and rinsing of the mouth are necessary during the period in which oral intake is restricted because the antispasmodic, anticholinergic drug that the patient may be receiving suppresses salivary secretion. Oil, petroleum jelly or a cream is used on the lips to prevent cracking. The nostrils are cleansed with an applicator that has been slightly moistened with normal saline, and a light application of petroleum jelly or water-soluble lubricant is made to the nostril through which the tube passes to prevent irritation and excoriation.

Pulmonary care

The person with acute pancreatitis may develop respiratory difficulties due to acid–base abnormalities, distended abdomen preventing full expansion of the lungs, or experience of pain on respiration causing reduced effort. Anticholinergic drugs may reduce normal secretions of the respiratory tract. The person should be nursed in a semi-upright position to reduce pressure on the diaphragm and promote full lung expansion. Deep-breathing exercises and coughing should be taught and the patient should be encouraged to perform them regularly. Should oxygen therapy be prescribed, humidification may prevent further drying of the respiratory tract, and the use of nasal cannulae rather than a face mask may improve tolerance.

Psychological support

Support will be necessary throughout the illness as the experience is clearly very stressful for the patient and family. This will only be compounded by worries and anxieties over social factors such as loss of earnings, or even job, while a history of alcohol abuse brings with it a whole sequence of psychological and social problems.

Follow-up care

A long convalescence follows recovery from an acute episode of pancreatitis. The necessary care to avert an exacerbation is discussed with the patient and family. The importance of strict adherence to the prescribed diet, total abstinence from alcohol and the avoidance of large meals is explained. Verbal and written instructions are given about the content and preparation of the recommended low-fat, high-protein, high-carbohydrate diet.

Activities are gradually resumed and the individual may return to work in 1–3 months if the person's job has been kept available.

Evaluation

Evaluation of the outcomes of nursing intervention for the person with acute pancreatitis includes assessment of the person's symptoms and evidence that they have been alleviated; particularly important is the absence of pain. Vital signs and fluid and electrolyte balance should be returning to the person's usual levels. The patient should increasingly assume self-care activities. The patient and family should be able to describe the prescribed dietary measures, understand the need for rest, state plans to alter lifestyle factors such as alcohol consumption, and discuss plans for follow-up health care.

Chronic pancreatitis

Chronic pancreatitis may develop following an initial acute episode or may develop insidiously. It is frequently associated with alcohol abuse.

The chronic form of the disease is characterized by progressive fibrosing and calcification of areas in the pancreas following inflammation and necrosis. The degree of impaired function and the intensity of its signs and symptoms are proportionate to the amount of continuing inflammation or frequency of acute episodes and ensuing tissue damage.

Clinical characteristics

The person with chronic pancreatitis experiences recurrent attacks of pain in the epigastric region and right upper quadrant which progressively becomes persistent. Anorexia, nausea, flatulence and constipation are common problems. Episodes are frequently precipitated by the ingestion of alcohol or a large meal with considerable fatty content.

As more and more of the endocrine and exocrine cells become non-functional the effects on the patient become more severe. A deficiency of enzyme secretion occurs in the intestine. Less fat and protein is digested; the person's stools become bulky, greasy and offensive (steatorrhoea) and there is a progressive weight loss. A deficiency of insulin secretion may result in diabetes mellitus.

Treatment and nursing intervention

The key intervention is to secure total abstinence from alcohol. A low-fat diet will help to reduce the diarrhoea associated with steatorrhoea.

Impaired digestion due to insufficient quantities of enzymes in the intestine may be corrected by the administration of pancreatic enzyme supplements (preparation of pancreatic extract). Vitamin supplements, including vitamins A, D, K, folic acid and B_{12}, may be required.

Decreased insulin secretion may necessitate the giving of insulin to control glucose metabolism.

As the disease becomes more advanced, the pain experienced by the patient may indicate frequent doses of an analgesic. Not infrequently, this becomes complicated by the person's development of a tolerance for the drug, necessitating progressively larger doses or a change in the prescribed medication regimen.

Neoplasms of the pancreas

Carcinoma

Cancer of the pancreas usually arises from the ducts and, although it may occur in any part of the organ, it is most commonly seen in the head. It is usually fatal.

The patient experiences pain, progressive weakness and loss of weight. Obstructive jaundice develops if the neoplasm encroaches on the ampulla of Vater or common bile duct. The cancer may spread by direct invasion to adjacent structures or by metastasis to the liver.

Treatment

The condition is treated surgically if recognized sufficiently early and if it is the head of the pancreas that is involved. Neoplasms in the body and tail have usually metastasized by the time they are identified. Whipple's operation may be attempted in which the head of the pancreas is removed, along with the duodenum, with anastomosis between the common bile duct and jejunum, anastomosis between the pancreas and jejunum, and a gastrojejunostomy. Palliative operations may be carried out for inoperable tumours involving relief of jaundice by the placement of a stent to drain bile away to the small intestine, thereby relieving the obstruction caused by the tumour.

Preparation for surgery includes a high-calorie, low-fat diet if tolerated by the patient, intravenous rehydration, blood transfusions, and parenteral vitamin K if there is jaundice. Postoperative care includes gastrointestinal decompression to prevent distension of the jejunum and pressure on the sites of the anastomoses. The patient is supported by blood transfusions and intravenous fluids. Vitamin K administration may be continued.

Tumours of islet cells

A benign tumour may develop in non-β islet cells and may become malignant. The tumour cells secrete gastrin freely, causing the Zollinger–Ellison syndrome, which is characterized by gastric hypersecretion and persisting peptic ulceration. The treatment is surgical removal of the tumours or total gastrectomy.

Occasionally an adenoma develops from β cells of the islets of Langerhans, causing an excessive secretion of insulin (hyperinsulinism) and hypoglycaemia. The adenoma is usually benign but, rarely, may be adenocarcinoma.

The symptoms presented by the patient are mainly due to the effect of the abnormally low blood sugar on the brain cells. Brain cells are more sensitive to glucose deficiency than other body cells. The initial symptoms are hunger, restlessness and apprehension. These progress to weakness, loss of coordination, tremors, diaphoresis, disorientation, convulsions and coma. The manifestations appear during a fasting period (early morning) or after extreme exertion. Prompt administration of some form of glucose is necessary to raise the blood sugar level. If the hypoglycaemia remains untreated, the glucose deficiency may result in permanent brain cell damage or death. When early signs are recognized, the patient is given sugar or orange juice with sugar. In the more advanced stage of hypoglycaemia, 50% glucose is given intravenously.

Surgical treatment may consist of excision of the adenoma or subtotal or total pancreatectomy. Preparation for the operation includes a high-carbohydrate, high-protein diet and intravenous infusions of glucose solution to restore glycogen reserves. The glucose infusion is continued during the operation. Following surgery, close observation is made for a recurrence of hypoglycaemia. If a total pancreatectomy is performed, the patient will receive supplemental insulin and pancreatic extract for the remainder of his or her life.

Summary

This chapter provides an overview of the structures and functions of the liver, biliary tract and exocrine pancreas. The clinical characteristics and the nursing assessment of alterations in function demonstrated by the person with disorders of the liver, biliary tract and exocrine pancreas are discussed. Emphasis is placed on the role of the nurse in the early detection and treatment of persons with alcohol abuse problems and the potential for preventing serious disorders of the liver and pancreas.

The assessment and nursing management of persons with the more common acute and chronic disorders of the liver, biliary tract and exocrine pancreas are described. Discussion focuses on the occupational risk for hepatitis and measures to prevent the transmission of the various hepatitis viruses to nurses and the public.

References

Abou-Assi S, O'Keefe S (2001) Nutrition in acute pancreatitis. Journal of Clinical Gastroenterology 32(3): 203–209.

Camma A, Almasio P, Craxi A (1996) Interferon as treatment for acute hepatitis C: a meta-analysis. Digestive Diseases and Sciences 41(6): 1248–1255.

CRD (Centre for Reviews and Dissemination) (2001a) Interferon as treatment for acute hepatitis C: a meta-analysis. York: NHS Centre for Reviews and Dissemination, University of York.

CRD (Centre for Reviews and Dissemination) (2001b) The efficacy of interferon alfa in chronic hepatitis B – a review and meta-analysis, vol. 1. York: NHS Centre for Reviews and Dissemination, University of York.

CRD (Centre for Reviews and Dissemination) (2001c) Correlation of biochemical response to interferon alpha with histological improvement in hepatitis C: a meta-analysis of diagnostic test characteristics. Database of Abstracts of Reviews of Effectiveness. York: NHS Centre for Reviews and Dissemination, University of York.

CRD (Centre for Reviews and Dissemination) (2001d) The clinical value of lactate dehydrogenase in serum: a quantitative review. Database of Abstracts of Reviews of Effectiveness. York: NHS Centre for Reviews and Dissemination, University of York.

Collis I, Burroughs A, Rolles K, Lloyd G (1995) Psychiatric and social outcome of liver transplantation. British Journal of Psychiatry 166(4): 521–524.

Cooper D (1995) CDT screening for alcohol abuse. British Journal of Nursing 4(14): 804–808.

Courtois C, Picus D, Hicks M et al (1997) Percutaneous gallstone removal: long-term follow-up. Journal of Vascular and Interventional Radiology 7(2): 229–234.

Crigger N (1998) Defying denial: clues to detecting alcohol abuse. American Journal of Nursing 98(8): 20–21.

DePalma J (2000) HCV infection among nurses and surgeons: what are the odds? American Journal of Nursing 100(5): 28.

Department of Health (1999a) Statistics on alcohol: 1976 onwards. Online. Available: http://www.doh.gov.uk

Department of Health (1999b) Saving lives: our healthier nation. Online. Available: http://www.doh.gov.uk/ohn/popver.

Fahey S (1999) The experience of women with primary biliary cirrhosis: a literature review. Journal of Advanced Nursing 30(2): 506–512.

Gorman M (1996) Alcoholic patients: keeping hope alive. American Journal of Nursing 96(1): 20.

Gorman M (1997) Treating acute alcohol withdrawal. American Journal of Nursing 97(1): 22–23.

Helman C (1990) Culture, health and illness, 2nd edn. Oxford: Butterworth–Heinemann.

Hinchliff SM, Montague SE, Watson R (1996) Physiology for nursing practice. London: Baillière Tindall.

Howard L, Fahy T (1997) Liver transplantation for alcoholic liver disease. British Journal of Psychiatry 171(12): 497–500.

Hudak C, Gallo B (1994) Critical care nursing. Philadelphia: JB Lippincott.

Klainberg M (1999) Primary biliary cirrhosis. American Journal of Nursing 99(12): 38–39.

Kumar P, Clark M (1994) Clinical medicine, 3rd edn. London: Saunders.

McArdle J (2000) The biological and nursing implications of pancreatitis. Nursing Standard 14(48): 46–51.

McCollum J (2000) Appetite and nutritional intake in patients with chronic liver disease. Journal of Human Nutrition and Dietetics 13(5): 365–366.

McCreaddie M, Neilson M (2001) Hepatitis C: why all the fuss? Nursing Times 97(11): 34–41.

Middlebrook M, Cohen A, Wallace M, Clark J, Galati J (1999) Improved methods for transjugular liver biopsy. Journal of Vascular and Interventional Radiology 10(6): 807–809.

Mor E, Kaspa R, Sheiner P, Schwartz M (1998) Treatment of hepatocellular carcinoma associated with cirrhosis in the era of liver transplantation. Annals of Internal Medicine 129(8): 643–653.

Naidoo J (1994) Health promotion. London: Baillière Tindall.

Newton S (1999) Preliminary model of returning to work after liver transplantation. IMAGE – The Journal of Nursing Scholarship 31(1): 96.

Oh Y-W, Kang E-Y, Lo NJ, Suh W, Godwin J (2000) Thoracic manifestations associated with advanced liver disease. Journal of Computer Assisted Tomography 24(5): 699–705.

Papatheodoridis G, Goulis J, Leandro G, Patch D, Burroughs A (1999) Transjugular intrahepatic portosystemic shunt compared with endoscopic treatment for prevention of variceal rebleeding: a meta-analysis. Hepatology 30(3): 612–622.

Pasero C (1998) Assessing and treating the pain of pancreatitis. American Journal of Nursing 98(11): 14–16.

Robertson G (1999) Individuals' perception of their quality of life following a liver transplant: an exploratory study. Journal of Advanced Nursing 30(2): 497–505.

Shovein J, Damzo R, Hyams I (2000) Hepatitis A: how benign is it? American Journal of Nursing 100(3): 43–47.

Watanabe S, Hosomi N, Kitade Y et al (2000) Assessment of the presence and severity of esophagogastric varices by splenic index in patients with liver cirrhosis. Journal of Computer Assisted Tomography 24(5): 788–794.

Woodrow P (2000) Intensive care nursing. London: Routledge.

Further Reading

Fahey S (1999) The experience of women with primary biliary cirrhosis: a literature review. Journal of Advanced Nursing 30(2): 506–512.

This article discusses primary biliary cirrhosis and the experience of women who have it (an ignored minority), including the stigma attached to cirrhosis and adaptation processes. There is an interesting presentation of the symbolic significance of terms associated with liver disease.

McArdle J (2000) The biological and nursing implications of pancreatitis. Nursing Standard 14(48): 46–51.

This is a thorough and critically analytical review of the care of the patient with pancreatitis. Specific nursing issues are considered, especially capillary blood sampling, and protocols are suggested.

McCreaddie M, Neilson M (2001) Hepatitis C: why all the fuss? Nursing Times 97(11): 34–41.

A comprehensive, well presented account of hepatitis C and its implications for nurses and health care.

Robertson G (1999) Individuals' perception of their quality of life following a liver transplant: an exploratory study. Journal of Advanced Nursing 30(2): 497–505.

For those who are interested in examining quality-of-life issues following liver transplantation, this is a very interesting piece of primary research. The researcher uses a reflective, phenomenological approach.

Shovein J, Damzo R, Hyams I (2000) Hepatitis A: how benign is it? American Journal of Nursing 100(3): 43–47.

This article uses a clinical case study as a basis for an approachable but thorough discussion of the nurse's role in caring for a patient with hepatitis A.

Caring for the patient with a nutritional disorder

Sue Lee

Introduction

Metabolism

Meeting nutritional requirements

Recommendations for healthy eating

Factors that influence dietary patterns

Assessment

Obesity

Undernutrition

Undernutrition due to withholding of nutritional support

Nutritional needs of the elderly

Cultural and religious influences on dietary habits

Summary

Introduction

Nutrition is fundamental to growth, good health and well-being, and is a potential cause or contributing factor in illness. Therefore a sound knowledge of the principles of nutrition and the requirements of individuals in health and sickness is vital for nurses to give effective care.

Recent evidence suggests that patients in hospital receive inadequate nutrition (Bond 1997). The incidence of this is unacceptably high (McWhirter and Pennington 1997). Patients at risk of malnutrition are not always recognized as such. Furthermore, needy patients do not receive adequate help or assistance with eating and drinking, leading to a further deterioration in their nutritional status on discharge (Association of Community Health Councils of England and Wales (ACHCEW) 1997).

Nurses should be able to assess a person's nutritional status, relating data from a physical examination to that taken from a dietary history. They must have a knowledge of the requirements of a balanced diet, and the skills to be able to work with clients to devise and implement a plan to meet individual needs.

In 1992, the Government produced the document *The Health of the Nation* (Department of Health 1992a). It set targets for changes in the national average diet, with the purpose of reducing the incidence of coronary heart disease and stroke. This was superseded in 1999 by *Saving Lives: Our Healthier Nation* (DoH 1999). As before, two of the main aims are to achieve a reduction in cancer, heart disease and stroke. The Government recognizes the effect on people of poverty, unemployment, poor education, bad housing and inadequate recreational facilities; it also supports individuals' actions to improve or maintain health by stopping smoking, keeping active and eating sensibly, i.e. following a balanced diet with plenty of fruit and vegetables (DoH 2000).

This chapter identifies the key components of any diet and describes how the body utilizes and metabolizes these nutrients. Means of assessing nutritional status are presented, together with the implications of the findings for nursing care. Recommendations for a balanced diet are identified, as well as a recognition of the needs of those who may be overweight or malnourished. There is a discussion of the ethical and legal difficulties associated with the nutrition of patients who are unable to take food or fluids orally, and who may be unconscious and therefore unable to verbalize their wishes. The cultural and religious influences on diet are considered briefly.

The provision of food and fluids has long been considered part of the nurturing role of nursing, although the evidence does suggest that nurses have neglected this aspect of caring for patients, particularly the elderly. It has been suggested that this may be due to a growing emphasis on the increasingly expanded nurse's role, a lack of knowledge about assessment of nutritional status and a lack of clarity over responsibility and management (Loftus-Hills and Duff 1997). Nurses need to be knowledgeable and skillful, and grasp the full implications of this aspect of care. Liaison with dieticians and other healthcare professionals is vital, but ultimately it is nurses who are uniquely placed to identify needs and deliver appropriate care, whether in hospital or in the community.

Metabolism

Production of energy

Metabolism
See chapter 2.6

Glucose metabolism
See chapter 2.6

Food is essential to provide energy and to supply materials from which cells synthesize chemicals and bodily structures. Energy is required even at rest, when no voluntary physical activity is being undertaken. It is necessary for cellular activity, for the function of the organs of the body, and for growth and maintenance of tissues. The amount of energy needed to maintain these involuntary functions at rest is known as the *basal metabolic rate* (BMR). The BMR varies with age, sex and body size, and is influenced by an individual's hormonal activity (especially the thyroid hormone). It is highest in children and adolescents because of their requirements for growth, and declines with age. Women tend to have a lower BMR than men.

Energy requirements for individuals vary greatly and are related to the BMR. When energy intake equals energy use, bodyweight is maintained.

Food is taken into the gut and broken down by digestive processes into a form in which it can be absorbed into the bloodstream. From the blood it is taken up into tissue cells. Some nutrients will be used by the cells to meet material requirements for the construction of tissue, for growth and repair, or for the production of hormones and enzymes. Much of the food, however, will be broken down to produce the energy the body requires.

Within the cells foods undergo the physical and chemical changes that comprise metabolism. When the cellular activity results in the synthesis of tissue substance, the process is referred to as *anabolism*, or *anabolic metabolism*. The processes that break down the materials into simpler forms and release energy are called *catabolism*, or *catabolic metabolism*.

Energy is stored inside the cells as adenosine triphosphate (ATP). ATP is generated by a mechanism called *phosphorylation* – the addition of a phosphate to adenosine diphosphate (ADP). Briefly, this means that oxygen is consumed in the reaction; lower-energy ADP combines with the energy from the fuel (e.g. fat or glucose) and a phosphate, to form the higher-energy ATP:

$$\text{Fuel} + \text{Oxygen} + \text{ADP} + \text{Phosphate} \rightarrow \text{Carbon dioxide} + \text{ATP} + \text{Water}$$

Glucose metabolism

Carbohydrates are absorbed as glucose, fructose and galactose, and are the body's main energy source. Fructose and most of the galactose are converted to glucose by the liver. Some galactose remains as such, and is one of the components of the myelin sheath surrounding nerve fibres. Some glucose circulates in the blood to maintain a relatively constant blood glucose level.

Once glucose enters the cells it can be metabolized in three main ways:

1. broken down completely to produce ATP
2. converted into glycogen and stored in liver and muscle cells
3. converted into fat and stored in adipose tissue.

The breakdown of glucose within the cells involves two main processes. *Glycolysis* involves the splitting of a glucose molecule into two pyruvic acid molecules and the release of some energy. The pyruvic acid is then broken down in a series of chemical reactions, controlled by enzymes, known as the *Krebs cycle* (or citric acid cycle). The end-result of the metabolism of one molecule of glucose is the production of water, carbon dioxide and energy (Fig. 17.1):

$$C_6H_{12}O_6 + 6O_2 \rightarrow 6H_2O + 6CO_2 + \text{Energy}$$

Some of the energy released is in the form of heat energy; the remainder is stored as ATP. The glucose that is not needed to maintain the blood glucose level or as an immediate energy source is converted to glycogen and stored in the liver or muscles. The muscle cells store it for their own use during contraction. The liver stores glycogen and, as the blood glucose level falls, converts the glycogen back to glucose and releases it into the blood. If the absorbed glucose exceeds what the cells use, and what can be stored as glycogen, it may be converted to fat and stored in the fat depots of the body. Insulin plays an important role in stimulating the deposition of fat.

Fat metabolism

Fat is broken down in the gut into glycerol, fatty acids and monoglycerides. After entering the intestinal mucosa these recombine into new triglycerides, which in turn are coated by phospholipids to become *chylomicrons*. The chylomicrons enter the lymph system and eventually the blood, where they are transported to the cells. Fat may be used by the body as an immediate or future source of energy, or for the

Figure 17.1 Metabolism of food to produce energy.

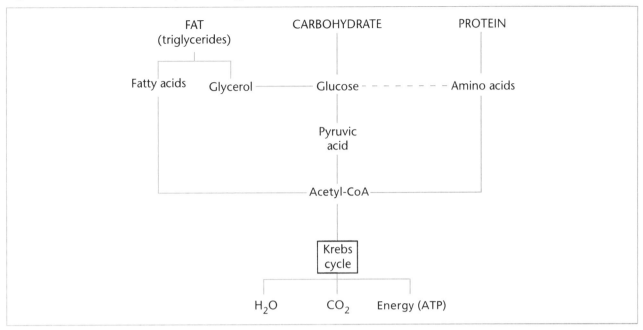

synthesis of fat compounds (e.g. phospholipids, lecithin, steroids and cholesterol). When **fats** are used to provide energy, the triglycerides are first broken down by the liver into glycerol and fatty acids. These may then be stored in adipose tissue as a future energy source.

If required as an immediate source of energy, glycerol is converted to glucose and broken down to pyruvic acid and metabolized via the Krebs cycle (see Fig. 17.1). The fatty acids are split by a series of reactions that occur mainly in the liver. In each reaction two carbon atoms and energy are released. Two carbon atoms combine with coenzyme A to form acetyl-CoA, which then enters the Krebs cycle to produce water, carbon dioxide and energy (ATP). Ketone acids are also produced and move out of the liver to be transported by the blood to cells in need of energy, where they are metabolized via the Krebs cycle. Under normal circumstances the level of ketones in the blood is very low. However, if there is a shortage of glucose in the cells, there may be an increased use of fat as an energy source, resulting in an increase of ketone production. If ketone production exceeds ketone metabolism, *ketosis* will result. This condition may occur in starvation or in diabetes mellitus.

Fat that is not required for immediate use is stored in fat depots in the body. Most of the fat is deposited in the subcutaneous tissue, in the abdomen, especially on the mesentery and omentum, around the kidney and between the muscle fibres.

A certain amount of stored fat is of value. The subcutaneous fatty tissue insulates the body against excessive heat loss and against the cold of the external environment. Fatty tissue also provides a protective cushion for the body against trauma.

Not all the absorbed fat may enter the liver after a meal. Some of it moves directly into the fat depots so that the concentration of fat in the blood is quickly lowered. The fat in the tissues is mobilized when it is needed for energy. There is, therefore, a constant movement of fat in and out of the fatty tissue.

A number of hormones influence fat metabolism. Most of them increase fat mobilization and fat utilization by the cells. These hormones include growth (somatotrophic) hormone, thyroxine, cortisone and adrenaline. Insulin increases fat synthesis and utilization. Oestrogen increases the deposition of fats in the tissues.

Protein metabolism

During digestion, protein is broken down into its constituent amino acids and in this form absorbed into the bloodstream. **Amino acids** are sometimes termed the body's building blocks. They may be built into body tissue (e.g. skin, hair, etc.) or used in the synthesis of functional products, such as enzymes and hormones, or the formation of protein compounds such as plasma proteins.

Protein is not generally used as an energy source, as the essential amino acids are vital for growth and tissue repair. When inadequate carbohydrates or fat is available, for example in starvation, protein may be broken down to provide energy (ATP) (see Fig. 17.1). Thus amino acids are used to:

- build and repair tissue and synthesize functional products
- produce ATP after deamination in liver
- convert into glucose or fat after deamination.

Fats
See chapter 5.1

Amino acids
See chapters 5.1 & 5.2

The liver is the main organ involved in the metabolism of amino acids. In a process called *deamination*, the amino radical is removed from the amino acid, forming ammonia. As ammonia could be toxic to tissue cells, it is combined with carbon dioxide to form urea, which is subsequently excreted via the kidneys. The residual elements of the amino acid are converted into glucose or fat, which may be metabolized to meet energy requirements.

Some amino acids are described as '*essential*', that is they must be provided in the diet because the body cannot synthesize them in adequate amounts. Others, however, may be synthesized in the liver in a process called *transamination*; the amino radical is removed from one amino acid and attached to the molecule of a carbohydrate or fatty acid.

Protein metabolism is influenced by certain hormones. Growth hormone, thyroxine and testosterone stimulate the use of protein in the synthesis of tissue and cell products. The glucocorticoids promote mobilization of amino acids into the blood from cells and their conversion to glucose.

Meeting nutritional requirements

A person requires food for energy and for materials to maintain the structure and functions of the body. These needs will be met by a number of different nutrients. Carbohydrates and fats are used by the body as prime energy sources. Protein may make some contribution to energy production, as will any alcohol consumed. Protein and certain types of fats are essential for growth and maintenance of the body's structure and functions. A number of vitamins and minerals are also essential.

Carbohydrates
See chapter 1.2

Different nutrients have different energy values (Box 17.1). Energy is expressed in joules (the SI unit) or calories. The 'calorie' used in food science is, in fact, a kilocalorie, or 1000 calories. It is equivalent to 4.2 kJ.

Carbohydrates

Sugars, starches and non-starch polysaccharides (NSPs) are known collectively as **carbohydrates**. They all contain carbon, hydrogen and oxygen, in the basic unit of $C_6H_{12}O_6$. A monosaccharide (e.g. glucose) contains one such unit; disaccharides (e.g. sucrose) contain two units, and a carbohydrate with many units is described as a polysaccharide (e.g. starch). Sugars and starches may be broken down by the body to provide energy. NSPs are not used as an energy source, but help to maintain normal

Box 17.1 Energy values of different nutrients	
Carbohydrate provides	17 kJ (3.75 kcal) per g
Fat provides	37 kJ (9 kcal) per g
Protein provides	17 kJ (3.75 kcal) per g
Alcohol provides	29 kJ (7 kcal) per g

bowel function. Dietary fibre is more properly known as *non-starch polysaccharide*, and this is how it is labelled on many nutritional products. However, the term 'dietary fibre' itself has gained currency within the population and government bodies (DoH 1998a).

Starch is found widely in grains, cereals, root vegetables and legumes. It is digested at a slower rate than disaccharides, and therefore releases glucose into the bloodstream at a relatively slow rate. Dietary fibre is present in starchy foods in large quantities. Dietary fibre is a term used to include a number of different substances, each with differing properties. As foods contain varying combinations of dietary fibre substances, it is important to eat a range of high-fibre foods.

Dietary fibre may contribute to good health in a number of ways. An increased consumption of it is directly correlated with an increase in stool weight, which in turn helps to prevent constipation. There is also some evidence that low stool weights are associated with increased risk of bowel disorders such as cancer and gallstones, so that increasing the stool weight may afford some protection (DoH 1991a). Some types of dietary fibre, especially water-soluble components found in oats and beans, may help to lower blood cholesterol levels.

It is advisable to obtain dietary fibre from food rather than from unprocessed wheat bran, which may impair the absorption of some minerals (e.g. iron, calcium, zinc and copper) (DoH 1991a).

Sugars

The food sugars most important in human nutrition are the monosaccharides, glucose and fructose, and the disaccharides, sucrose and lactose. The effect of sugar in the body is determined not only by the type, but also by the source. Sugars may be classified as *intrinsic* or *extrinsic* (Fig. 17.2).

No detrimental effects on dental health or health in general are attributed to lactose in milk and milk products or to intrinsic sugars. Non-milk extrinsic sugars (NMESs), however, play a significant role in the development of dental caries. It is not only the amount of sugar in sweets, drinks and snacks that is relevant, but also the length of time for which sugar is in contact with teeth. Sugar eaten as part of a meal may cause less decay because it is washed away by other food and drink (DoH 1989). It is particularly relevant to note that in people aged 65 years and over, the evidence suggests that the better a person's oral health is, including how many natural teeth they have, the better their diets and subsequent nutritional status. Furthermore, the presence of natural teeth (in people not living in institutions) was significantly related to their intake of protein, intrinsic and milk sugars, fibre, calcium, non-haem iron, niacin and vitamin D. The amount of intake of intrinsic sugars and fibre was also related to the distribution of teeth (DoH 1998a).

Figure 17.2   Classification of sugars.

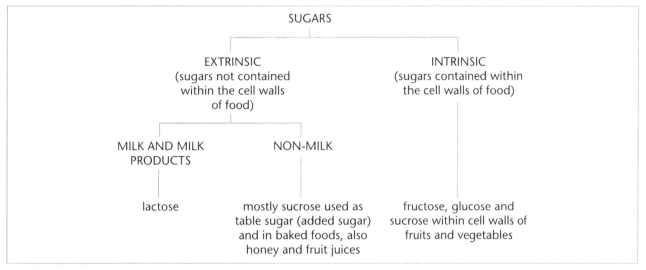

From Department of Health (1991a), with permission.

Fat

Fat, as eaten in foods, is a mixture of triglycerides, each composed of a glycerol molecule and three fatty acid molecules. There are three main types of fatty acid:

- saturated fatty acid (saturates)
- monounsaturated fatty acids (monounsaturates)
- polyunsaturated fatty acids (polyunsaturates).

All fatty foods contain a mixture of these fatty acids, although some are more prevalent in particular foods.

Saturates

These are chemically very stable and are solid at room temperature. They are found mostly in foods of animal origin and in hard margarine. A high intake of saturates may contribute to an increase in blood cholesterol level, one of the main risk factors in the development of coronary heart disease (DoH 1994).

Monounsaturates

These are found to some extent in meat and dairy products; olive oil and rape-seed oil are particularly rich sources. Substitution of saturates by monounsaturates reduces plasma levels of cholesterol but only to about the same extent as substitution by carbohydrates (DoH 1994).

Polyunsaturates

These are chemically less stable. Some polyunsaturated fatty acids are known as *essential fatty acids* because they cannot be synthesized by the body and have to be provided in the diet. Different classes of polyunsaturates appear to have different functions in the body. The n-6 class, principally derived from seed oils and polyunsaturated margarines, reduces plasma cholesterol levels. It also contains essential fatty acids. The n-3 class of fatty acids has an important effect in reducing blood clotting, and therefore reducing a tendency for thrombosis development. These fatty acids are found mainly in oily fish (e.g. mackerel, sardines, herring, pilchard, trout and salmon). The n-3 class also contains essential fatty acids, found primarily in green leafy vegetables.

Cholesterol

Cholesterol is a fat-like structure, essential for cellular functioning. It is also required for synthesis of steroid hormones, bile salts and vitamin D. Most of the body's requirements are synthesized in the liver, although some cholesterol is present in the diet. A high intake of foods rich in saturates increases the synthesis of cholesterol in the liver and slows the breakdown rate, thus raising blood levels. Blood cholesterol levels are influenced more by the total fat content of food than by the amount of cholesterol present in food eaten.

Protein

Protein in the diet is essential, as proteins form part of every cell in the body. Some proteins are required for formation, growth and repair of body tissues, such as hair, skin and muscle. Others are involved in the synthesis of hormones and enzymes. Protein may also be used as an energy source.

Proteins are comprised of amino acids in various combinations. Twenty-two amino acids are used by the body to synthesize the proteins it needs. The liver can interconvert amino acids, that is, it can synthesize some amino acids from others. There are eight amino acids, however, that are described as *essential* because the body cannot synthesize them and they must be provided in the diet.

Proteins that contain all eight essential amino acids have a high biological value. These proteins come mainly from animal sources such as milk, cheese, yoghurts, meat and fish. Proteins from vegetable sources tend to have a lower biological value. However, when proteins from different sources are eaten together, the relative surplus from one source can supplement the relative deficiency in another. The complementary effect is a mixture of proteins of high biological value. This combining of proteins is particularly important in vegetarian and vegan diets.

Vitamins

These micronutrients are required for normal growth and maintenance and are involved in the normal metabolism of other nutrients. Nearly all **vitamins** must be obtained from the diet, as the body cannot synthesize them. They are derived from a variety of sources, and a varied diet is the most important factor in ensuring requirements are met. Some are fat soluble (A, D, E, K); others are water soluble.

Minerals and trace elements

These are incorporated in many body tissues and fluids, and are essential components of many hormones, enzymes and transport molecules.

Vitamins
See chapter 1.2

Recommendations for healthy eating

Dietary reference values

The 1991 Committee on Medical Aspects of Food and Nutrition Policy (COMA) report on *Dietary Reference Values* (DoH 1991b) presents advice on the intake of fat, carbohydrates, protein, salt, vitamins and nutrients. The report introduced a number of new terms, which replaced the previous recommended daily amounts (RDAs). The new terms present an estimate of the average requirements, together with upper and lower limits advocated for good health. These should make it easier to identify a person who is likely to be having insufficient (or possibly excessive) intake.

It is interesting to note that several years after this COMA report food manufacturers still use the term RDA on their products, rather than any of the new terms. This tends to suggest that the terminology explained below is difficult for the general population to understand, and may therefore be inappropriate. However, these terms do occur in the professional literature, hence their inclusion here.

The dietary reference values include the following terms:

- ■ *Estimated average requirement (EAR)* – this is an estimate of the average requirement for food energy of a nutrient. Some people need more and some less than average.

- ■ *Reference nutrient intake (RNI)* – this represents the amount of a nutrient that will be sufficient for about 97% of the population. It is equivalent to the former

RDA. This value will be higher than most people will need, and if individuals are regularly consuming the RNI they are unlikely to be deficient in that nutrient.

- ■ *Lower reference nutrient intake (LRNI)* – this amount of a nutrient will be sufficient for only a few people with the lowest 2–3% of needs. Nearly all the population needs more than the LRNI. If an individual habitually eats less than the LRNI, they are at risk of becoming deficient in that nutrient.

- ■ *Safe intake* – this is the level of a nutrient that is judged to be adequate for almost everyone's needs, but not so large as to cause undesirable effects. The term is used when there is insufficient information to estimate requirements.

- ■ *Dietary reference value (DRV)* – this is a blanket term used to cover all the recommendations. All DRVs refer to the needs of healthy people.

Our healthier nation

In 1999, the Government published its White Paper *Saving Lives: Our Healthier Nation* (DoH 1999). This document suggests that we can improve our own health through physical activity, eating and drinking sensibly, and by not smoking. Interestingly, the DoH recognizes that the advice on how to do this is sometimes confusing and recommends following the chief medical officer's '10 top tips' (see Box 17.2). In nutritional terms, the advice is much less prescriptive than before, focusing on achieving and maintaining health generally, and holistically, by following a balanced diet with plenty of fruit and vegetables.

Box 17.2   *Our healthier nation*: 10 tips for better health

1. Don't smoke. If you can, stop. If you can't, cut down.

2. Follow a balanced diet with plenty of fruit and vegetables.

3. Keep physically active.

4. Manage stress by, for example, talking things through and making time to relax.

5. If you drink alcohol, do so in moderation.

6. Cover up in the sun, and protect children from sunburn.

7. Practise safer sex.

8. Take up cancer screening opportunities.

9. Be safe on the roads: follow the Highway Code.

10. Learn the First Aid ABC: airways, breathing, circulation.

From DoH (1999), with permission.

Table 17.1   Dietary reference values

	Estimated average requirement (kcal/day)		Reference nutrient intake for protein (g/day)		Population average	
					Carbohydrate (as % energy)	Fat (as % energy)
	Male	Female				
0–3 months	545	515	12.5			
4–6 months	690	645	12.7			
7–9 months	825	765	13.7			
10–12 months	920	865	14.9			
1–3 years	1230	1165	14.5			
4–6 years	1715	1545	19.7			
7–10 years	1970	1740	28.3			
			Males	Females		
11–14 years	2220	1845	42.1	41.2		
15–18 years	2755	2110	55.2	45.0		
19–50 years	2550	1940	55.5	45.0	47	33
51–59 years	2550	1900	53.3	46.5	47	33
60–64 years	2380	1900	53.3	46.5	47	33
65–75 years	2330	1900	53.3	46.5	47	33
75+ years	2100	1810	53.3	46.5	47	33
Pregnancy		+200		+6		
Lactation						
1 month		+450		+11		
2 months		+530		+11		
3 months		+570		+11		

From Department of Health (1991b), with permission.

Nutritional requirements and recommendations

In the UK, the estimated nutritional requirements for the population have been described by COMA. The COMA group critically evaluates the evidence and makes recommendations which are then used to inform government policy, such as *Our Healthier Nation* (DoH 1999) and the national service framework for coronary heart disease (DoH 1998b, DoH 2000). The last definitive set of recommendations was formulated in 1991: *Dietary Reference Values for Food Energy and Nutrients for the United Kingdom* (DoH 1991b).

It is important to remember that nutritional requirements are described in technical terms, using the terminology and definitions provided earlier in this chapter. The *estimated average requirements* for calories, protein, carbohydrate and fat in different age groups and sexes are provided in Table 17.1. Nutritional requirements vary from person to person. Each nutrient has a particular function and all are needed in differing amounts. Our individual requirements are related to age, sex, level of physical activity and state of health (British Nutrition Foundation 1998a). However, many people take in more energy than their bodies actually require, resulting in obesity and potential ill-health (DoH 1994). The three main types of nutrient – fat, protein and carbohydrate – all provide energy, as can alcohol – although this should provide no more than 5% of total energy in a person's diet. A poor energy mix in a person's diet may be a factor in some diseases (e.g. coronary heart disease and some cancers) (British Nutrition Foundation 1998a, DoH 1998a).

In 1994 the COMA report on nutritional aspects of cardiovascular disease was published (DoH 1994). This confirmed the Government's targets for reduction of fat intake as appropriate. It also made a number of recommendations relating to dietary intake:

1. *Maintain a desirable weight* – a body mass index (BMI) of 20–25 is associated with an appropriate weight for most people. (See p. 547 for calculation of BMI.)

2. *Carbohydrates should contribute 50% of total daily energy intake*. Non-milk extrinsic sugars (see Fig. 17.2) should form a maximum of 10% of total energy intake. Consumption of complex carbohydrates should be increased (e.g. fruit and vegetables, bread and cereals).

3. *Dietary fibre intake should increase to 18 g/day*. This should follow from the increased consumption of fruit, vegetables and cereals.

4. *Fat should form a maximum of 35% of total daily energy intake*. A maximum 10% of energy intake should come from saturated fats.

5. *Protein intake of 11% of total daily energy intake* should be ample to meet daily requirements. (See Table 17.1 for reference nutrient intake.)

6. *Salt intake should be on average no more than 6 g/day.*

7. *Antioxidant vitamin intake (E, C, β-carotene) should be maintained* as they may afford some protection against coronary heart disease (CHD).

8. *Energy levels should be maintained but daily exercise should increase* (for people of normal weight). Table 17.1 shows the estimated average requirements for total daily energy intake.

The recommendations given in the COMA report (DoH 1994) are designed to reduce risk factors associated with developing cardiovascular disease and stroke. For other potential disease, the risk factors may be reduced; for example, by increasing dietary fibre intake, problems associated with constipation and bowel disease may be decreased.

However, the guidelines are not in a form that is readily accessible to the general public. It is very difficult to know exactly what to eat to enable 35% of the total energy intake to come from fats, or for 50% of the energy requirement to come from carbohydrates. In the past this type of report has been criticized for not enabling people to make the practical changes in their diet that the report advocates.

Food groups

If nurses are to be able to advise clients on a nutritionally appropriate diet, they must be aware of the nutritional value of foods that may be available to the client. For this reason it is useful for nurses to become familiar with the four food groups devised by nutritionalists.

The Nutrition Task Force (NTF) guide emphasizes and clarifies the notion of a 'balanced diet'. However, rather than stating nutritional requirements in terms of DRVs etc., it shows the different food groups and the different proportions a person should eat, including fats and sugary foods (see Box 17.3). This is perceived to be a more user-friendly way of getting the healthy eating message across.

In addition to this, the *Balance of Good Health* document recommends an eight-point plan for achieving a healthy diet (see Box 17.4). These guidelines are useful and relatively easy to understand. However, proportion and types of foods also have to be considered. It is unnecessary to try to achieve a full balance of all nutrients at one meal; instead this should be considered over a full day or even a week (Health Education Authority/Ministry of Agriculture Fisheries and Foods (HEA/MAFF) 1994, British Nutrition Foundation 1998b).

Foods are grouped according to their nutritional content, with foods in the same group having a similar range of nutrients, or similar role in the diet (see Box 17.3). For example, foods in the milk group are a good source of protein, calcium and B group vitamins. For an adult, an

---

Box 17.3 Summary of food groups

Bread, other cereals and potatoes
Recommendations: eat lots.

Milk and dairy foods
Recommendations: eat and drink moderate amounts and choose lower-fat versions whenever you can.

Fruit and vegetables
Recommendations: eat lots (at least five portions a day, excluding potatoes).

Meat, fish and alternatives
Recommendations: eat moderate amounts and choose lower-fat versions whenever you can.

Foods containing fat, foods containing sugar
Recommendations: eat foods containing fat sparingly and look out for the low-fat alternatives.

Foods containing sugar should not be eaten too often, as they can contribute to tooth decay.

From HEA/MAFF (1994).

Box 17.4 Guidelines for a healthy diet

1. Enjoy your food.

2. Eat a variety of different foods.

3. Eat the right amount to be a healthy weight.

4. Eat plenty of foods rich in starch and fibre.

5. Don't eat too many foods that contain a lot of fat.

6. Don't have sugary foods and drinks too often.

7. Look after the vitamins and minerals in your food.

8. If you drink alcohol, drink within sensible limits.

From HEA/MAFF (1994).

---

adequate balanced diet would include a number of portions from each of the five groups.

The size of the portion would depend on the dietary requirements of the individual. Children, adolescents and nursing mothers require more portions (three or four) from the milk group, because of their need for calcium and protein. Within each of the groups there is scope for following or ignoring the general guidance (HEA/MAFF 1994). Within the milk group, for example, a person could eat whole milk or skimmed milk, Cheddar cheese or cottage cheese; the difference in fat content of the alternatives would be substantial. The vitamin content of fruit and vegetables may vary considerably according to the storage and cooking. Nurses should advise on the importance of a balanced diet, including food from all five food groups. Whilst recommendations are to reduce fat intake, fats are essential to health and well-being and are an important source of vitamins. Severe diets, excluding a range of nutrients, may cause health problems of their own.

It should be noted that the dietary reference values (DoH 1991a,b), the HEA/MAFF (1994) guidelines and suggested portions of the five food groups refer to essentially healthy individuals. When illness or disease is present the ability or desire to eat may be absent or limited, and specific dietary regimens may be necessary to promote recovery. Often insufficient attention is paid to the dietary requirements of the ill (Bond 1997), and malnutrition in hospital is not uncommon.

It is therefore vital that nurses thoroughly assess their patients to determine their nutritional status and individual dietary requirements. If, as a result of this initial assessment, there appear to be problems associated with nutrition or metabolism a further assessment by dietician and physician may be required.

Factors that influence dietary patterns

Dietary behaviour is influenced by physiological, psychological, sociocultural and environmental factors, as well as knowledge of food and food requirements. The consumption of food is usually a social activity; eating habits are very complex and are resistant to change as they become an integral part of the individual and family lifestyle.

Physiological factors influencing nutritional needs and eating behaviour include the individual's metabolic rate, growth phase, body excretions, reproductive functions and level of daily physical activity. Increased energy and nutrients are required by the individual during periods of rapid physical growth, pregnancy and lactation, increased metabolic rate (e.g. hyperthyroidism) and increased physical activity. Fewer kilocalories are needed by elderly individuals because of their lower basal metabolic rate and decreased activity, and by those with sedentary lifestyles.

The hypothalamus, the limbic system of the brain and gut hormones regulate food intake by influencing appetite, hunger and satiety. *Hunger* is a physiological phenomenon involving unpleasant sensations of abdominal discomfort and irritability which prompt the individual to search for food. *Appetite* involves the conscious desire to eat. *Satiation* is the pleasant feeling of being fully satisfied after a meal. *Anorexia* is the abnormal loss of the desire to eat, and may be influenced by both physiological and psychological factors.

Emotions are important in determining eating behaviour. Food has different meanings for each individual, and responses to stress or happiness are often expressed as changes in eating habits. Some individuals respond to stress and decreased self-esteem by overeating, whereas others have loss of appetite and decrease their food consumption. It is possible that some people may experience both increases and decreases in consumption depending on the degree of stress perceived. Eating habits are believed to be formed early in life and become fixed responses.

Sociocultural factors influencing eating behaviour include religious and ethnic practices and the use of foods that have special meaning for the individual and family. The media also play an important role in influencing food consumption. Advertisements relating to specific foods have an impact on individuals and families; the portrayal of an 'ideal' body appearance greatly influences dietary intake and patterns of food consumption in girls and young adult females (Gilbert 1999). Sociocultural factors also influence the proportion of meals eaten in restaurants as opposed to the home, and the quality of restaurant chosen. 'Fast food' chains tend to have foods of higher saturated fat and salt than might be consumed in a meal prepared at home. Social class may affect diet, with knowledge about what constitutes a healthy diet being greater in higher social class families.

Environmental factors include the availability, cost and convenience of foods. The individual's income may be inadequate to meet the cost of the essential foodstuffs, or disability may limit a person's ability to prepare food or shop for food. The environment in which food is prepared and eaten also influences eating behaviour. Appetite is usually stimulated when eating takes place in a pleasant and relaxed social milieu.

Knowledge of dietary requirements and food values is an important factor in the individual's or family's eating patterns. In some instances, persons may not understand that in planning a balanced diet expensive food elements can usually be substituted by less expensive items that will meet the essential dietary requirements.

These non-biological influences on the use of food may contribute to the development of nutritional disorders and are important restraining factors when attempting to change eating habits.

Assessment

Health history

Any assessment of a person's nutritional status must obtain details about lifestyle and health status. A number of factors must be considered.

Age and sex Both will influence a person's basal metabolic rate, and therefore their energy requirements, and may influence other dietary needs (e.g. for protein and calcium).

Nationality and religion The types of food eaten may be influenced by family traditions and cultural identity, although people may not adhere strictly to the religious dictates on diet.

Activity and rest The number of calories needed daily will be determined by energy expenditure. Occupation and daily activity should be noted, together with how the person feels following physical activity. Rest and sleep are assessed in relation to the normal pattern.

Elimination Bowel habits are determined, together with information relating to the nature, formation, colour, odour and frequency of stools. The use of laxatives or supplementary fibre is assessed. The volume, frequency and colour of urine is determined, as well as the presence of nocturia or urgency and frequency. Use of diuretics is noted, and urine tested for abnormalities.

Medical history Any existing medical conditions or previous surgery or illnesses are noted, together with the impact (if any) that these have had on the diet consumed and future dietary requirements.

Socioeconomic factors Marital status and family grouping are recorded, as is the usual pattern of taking meals (e.g. in company or alone, eating out or eating at home). Presence or lack of employment may be considered. Other social and economic factors may be relevant (e.g. whether the person has cooking facilities, and whether they are able to store and prepare food independently).

The availability of shopping facilities and the ability to go shopping may be considered, together with economic factors relating to the ability to purchase sufficient food to meet the needs of the person and/or family.

Physical examination

Table 17.2 gives an indication of clues the nurse may pick up to suggest that a nutritional disorder or problem may be present.

- *General body appearance* is observed, including the patient's general stature and posture, distribution of body fat and state of alertness. The skin is inspected for rashes, lesions, petechiae, bruises and change of colour. The oral mucous membranes, tongue, lips, teeth and gums are observed, as well as hair, nails and eyes.

- *Height and weight* are measured and recorded, and changes in bodyweight over given periods are

Table 17.2 Assessment of the patient's nutritional status

	Characteristics of good nutritional status	Characteristics of poor nutritional status
Nutritional intake	■ Usual daily food intake contains basic food groups and all essential nutrients ■ Fluid intake 1500–2000 mL/day ■ Balanced calorie intake for size and activity	■ Some food groups and essential nutrients missing from diet ■ Calorie intake less than or greater than required for body size and activity ■ Fluid intake less than 1200 mL/day ■ Abuse of laxatives and diuretics
Physical examination		
General body appearance	■ Stands erect ■ Alert ■ Abdomen flat	■ Drooped shoulders ■ Inattentive ■ Abdomen protruded
Weight	■ Constant ■ In proportion to height and body size	■ Variable ■ ≥20% under or over suggested weight for height and body type
Body mass index	■ BMI 20–25	■ BMI below 20 or above 25
Skinfold thickness	■ Within 80% of standard value for age and sex	■ ≥20% above or below standard value for age and sex
Circumference measurement	■ Body muscle stores are within 90% of standard value for age and sex	■ Body muscle stores ≤80% of standard value for age and sex
Skin	■ Clean and intact	■ Dry, transparent, scaly with petechiae
Oral mucous membrane	■ Clean, moist and intact	■ Gums swollen and bleeding
Teeth	■ Clean, smooth, regular edges, straight and symmetrical, and intact	■ Dental caries ■ Discoloration ■ Irregular edges ■ Malpositioned and absent teeth
Lips	■ Smooth, intact	■ Red and swollen with fissures
Hair	■ Shiny and clean	■ Dull, listless and brittle
Nails	■ Smooth, shaped and intact	■ Brittle, ridged, irregular edges
Eyes	■ Clean, focused ■ Conjunctiva pink and moist	■ Sunken ■ Conjunctiva pale ■ Discharge

identified. The BMI can be calculated to give an indication of the appropriateness of the weight for height (Box 17.5).

- *Skin-fold thickness* is measured to determine the amount of subcutaneous fat. Callipers are used to measure the skin-fold thickness over the triceps. Results are compared with a table of normal values for age and sex.

- *Mid-arm circumference (MAC)* measurements are taken. The circumference of the mid-arm muscle can be calculated by using this measurement and the triceps skin-fold thickness. This value can then be compared with a table of normal values. These calculations provide information on the body's muscle stores.

- *A functional assessment* may be carried out to determine whether a patient is physically able to hold cutlery and feed him or herself. The patient's ability to chew food (noting whether their own teeth are adequate or dentures are well fitting) and ability to swallow food may also be considered.

Dietary history

As well as assessing a person's health status, it is important to determine the dietary patterns and average food intake of clients before nursing problems can be fully identified and interventions planned.

The nurse may wish to identify:

- all the food and drinks consumed in the past 24 hours, including times of meals and snacks, methods of preparing food and circumstances under which food was consumed

- an estimate of the quantity of foods eaten, using familiar measures (e.g. three egg-sized potatoes, two tablespoons of rice, a large glass of milk)

- details about specific types of food consumed, for example type of milk (whole or skimmed), spread (butter, sunflower margarine, low fat spread), bread (white or wholemeal)

- food preferences or dislikes; food allergies

Box 17.5 Body mass index (BMI)

The BMI is calculated by dividing a person's weight (in kilograms) by the square of their height (in metres):

$$\frac{\text{Weight (kg)}}{\text{Height}^2 \text{ (m)}}$$

BMI <20	underweight
BMI 20–25	normal (desirable) range
BMI 25–30	overweight
BMI >30	obese

From Department of Health (1994), with permission.

- average daily fluid intake; types of drink consumed
- strength or lack of appetite
- history of dieting
- consumption of dietary supplements
- consumption of snacks, type of snack and frequency.

The nurse or dietician may wish to investigate further and the patient may be asked to keep a food record or diary for a few days (e.g. 3 days to 1 week). The dietician may estimate the amount of specific foods consumed daily and convert this into energy and nutrient intake in grams, milligrams or micrograms, using food tables. It is then possible to compare the client's nutritional intake with the dietary reference values, giving an indication of the adequacy of the diet.

As well as establishing what a client eats, the nurse must ascertain what a patient knows about the nutritional and energy values of food regularly consumed.

Diagnostic tests

Depending on the information obtained from the health and dietary histories and physical examination, it may be deemed useful to carry out blood and urine studies. These will reflect changes in the metabolism of carbohydrates, proteins and fats, and may be used to determine the level of vitamins and minerals. Nurses will probably carry out urinalysis routinely, which may reveal the presence of glucose or ketones. However, most tests will be in consultation with a medical practitioner.

Obesity

Obesity may be clinically defined by a person's BMI (see Box 17.5).

The prevalence of obesity in the UK is increasing. In England, in 1994, it was estimated that 43% of men and 29% of women aged 16–64 years were overweight, and of these 13% of men and 16% of women were obese (Colhoun and Prescott-Clarke 1996). This is a 50% increase on 1980 data (Knight 1994). The values for Scotland are similar (Scottish Intercollegiate Guidelines Network 1996), and data for Wales also show an increase (Welsh Office 1996).

Health risks

There may be considerable risks to health from being obese. The incidence of CHD is high in obese men and women, particularly those under 50 years of age (DoH 1994). The distribution of fat about the body appears to be relevant. Men and women with excessive abdominal fat (central obesity) are at greater risk of CHD and diabetes mellitus than when the distribution is focused around the hips and thighs (peripheral obesity) (Effective Health Care 1997). For this reason hip:waist ratio may sometimes be calculated.

Metabolic changes may be related to obesity. The linkage between obesity and type II diabetes is well known (see Ch. 18). Repeated unsuccessful attempts at weight loss may exacerbate these risk factors.

In addition to the metabolic changes and their associated increase in health risk factors there is the psychologically stressful effect of being overweight. There are considerable social pressures to be thin, and those who are sensitive to the pressure to conform to the ideal may suffer from a poor body image and low self-esteem.

Factors related to obesity

Obesity results from an intake of energy that is in excess of the energy expended by the individual. The excess calories are stored, mainly as triglycerides, in the form of adipose tissue. There may be environmental, genetic, behavioural, physiological, psychological and socioeconomic factors influencing the development and/or maintenance of obesity. Of these factors, many are hard to control or influence. Those most readily amenable to change involve:

- the type of diet consumed (energy intake)
- voluntary physical activity (energy expenditure).

BMR is a major factor in determining energy expenditure, but is not amenable to change.

When the level of voluntary physical activity remains the same, it is ultimately the number of calories consumed that will determine the amount of fat stored. It is irrelevant as to which food source the calories come from, but it has been observed that diets high in fat may be more conducive to the development of obesity (DoH 1994). Research has suggested a positive correlation between the proportion of fat in the diet and measures of body fat. In their study Lissner et al (1987) found that in the short term people spontaneously ate more and gained weight if given a high-fat diet, compared with a medium-fat diet. The same subjects spontaneously ate 627 kcal less per day and lost weight when on a low-fat diet, although they consumed 84 g per day more food than on the high-fat diet. Hankey and Lean's (1995) study found that even modest weight loss of 5 kg produced some important health gains.

The cause of obesity for any individual will be a unique combination of factors. Before progress towards weight loss can be made, assessment of the person's health and dietary history is vital.

Assessment

Health history

In addition to the information gathered for a general nutritional assessment (see Table 17.2), the individual should be questioned about their history of weight fluctuations, past attempts at weight control, and any pattern of restricted eating followed by binging. Any history of depression or drug and alcohol abuse or dependency should be noted. A family history of weight problems, hypertension, diabetes mellitus or heart disease should also be identified. The nurse should probe for dissatisfaction regarding bodyweight and shape. It is important to discern the daily pattern of eating, amount of food intake and the exercise pattern.

Physical assessment

Height and weight should be measured and the BMI calculated. Hips and waist may be measured for possible calculation of hip : waist ratio. Blood pressure should be recorded.

Laboratory investigation

Medical assessment should include thyroid function, glucose tolerance, triglyceride, lipoprotein and cholesterol levels. Diagnosis and treatment of medical disorders is essential before actual treatment of obesity.

Identification of patient problems

The exact nature of the problems will vary between individuals, but most are likely to have a mismatch between nutritional intake and body requirements. Self-concept and body image may also be disturbed.

Goals

The goals may be said to have been achieved if the patient is able to:

1. state the components of a nutritionally balanced diet
2. describe the potential effects of excessive weight and body fat on health
3. describe and implement a plan to increase physical activity
4. eat a diet containing essential food groups
5. space intake of food over the day
6. recognize feelings of hunger (as opposed to appetite) and satiety
7. state positive attributes of the body and self
8. resist weight preoccupation
9. state the dangers of severe food restriction.

Nursing intervention

Prevention of overweight and control of obesity are important nursing responsibilities. However, given the many complex and multiple causes of obesity, the effectiveness of interventions will vary. If obesity is life threatening, the treatment of choice may be hospitalization for gastric stapling surgery, calorie restriction and/or appetite-suppressant drug therapy. In this case, the role of the nurse is daily measurement of weight and the monitoring of emotional reactions, food intake, drug effectiveness and side-effects. There is little reported about the long-term maintenance of weight lost after gastric stapling. However, the use of anorectic drugs produces only short-term results.

The majority of people with a weight problem are treated in the community. Nurses have a vital role in assessing clients and supporting them in their attempts to reduce or stabilize their weight. When assessment reveals that an individual's weight problem is related to overeating or lack of activity, the nurse can have an impact through education and support. This will be focused on three major areas: reducing energy intake, maintaining motivation and increasing exercise.

Reducing energy intake

When working with a client on a weight reduction programme there are a number of dietary factors to consider (Effective Health Care 1997):

1. The intake of energy must be reduced from the client's usual.

2. A balanced diet is essential.

3. Foods from each of the five groups should be eaten, but the following advice noted:
   a. *milk and milk products* – use low-fat varieties of products (e.g. semi-skimmed or skimmed milk, cottage cheese, low-fat yoghurts)
   b. *fruit and vegetables* – eat at least five portions daily
   c. *bread and cereals* – eat varieties high in dietary fibre; eat smaller portions
   d. *meat and meat alternatives* – trim all fat off meat, avoid products with high fat content.

4. Fat intake should be reduced (cooking methods may need to be changed).

5. Consumption of non-milk extrinsic sugars (see Fig. 17.2) should be greatly reduced or avoided.

6. Protein levels should be maintained.

7. A regular meal pattern should be established, usually involving three meals a day.

8. A list of foods to be eaten freely and foods to be avoided should be available.

Maintaining motivation

Nurses must consider a client's lifestyle, religious beliefs, financial restrictions and dietary preferences when advising a diet. It is also important to stress the long-term nature of weight reduction and maintenance of a desirable weight. Weight loss need not be dramatic, but changes in dietary habits should be incorporated into a person's lifestyle and be sustainable over a period of time. Motivation is crucial to success. Targets for weight loss should be realistic and encourage the client to persevere with a steady weight loss. Clients should also be made aware that occasional lapses will not lead to excessive weight increases. The guilt feelings that accompany a lapse may cause the client to abandon the diet.

Increasing exercise

Increased exercise will hasten weight loss but, more importantly, will help a client to develop a positive attitude to their body and feel good about themselves. In those who are very obese, exercise should be introduced gradually and should not be strenuous because of the risks to the cardiovascular system. It could include walking instead of using a car or public transport. For those who are only moderately overweight more vigorous exercise may be suggested, but this should be built up gradually and be within the limits of their health. Clients should be aware that vigorous exercise may increase their appetite, but maintaining a reduced energy intake is vital to weight loss.

For some clients who have a history of repeated dieting followed by weight gain, it may be preferable for them actually to stop weight reduction programmes, stabilize eating and increase activity levels.

Evaluation

Prevention of obesity is of primary importance in preventing the usual accompanying risk factors. People with an established weight problem can be helped, but success becomes less likely as the degree of excess weight increases. Frequent evaluation of progress towards goals needs to be carried out by the patient and nurse in order to monitor progress continuously and change the plan as necessary (see Case Study 17.1).

Case Study 17.1   *Obesity*

Mrs S is a 45-year-old woman with a long-standing history of obesity following the birth of her first child. She is 5 feet 6 inches tall and weighs 110 kg. She comes to see the practice nurse for help and advice as she has recently been told she is a 'borderline hypertensive' (blood pressure 165/95 mmHg) by the GP. The GP is reluctant is to start Mrs S on any antihypertensive medication and has advised her to lose some weight. Mrs S is both angry and upset: she states that the GP is judgemental and 'knows nothing about my life'. Previously, she has attended various slimming clubs and lost varying amounts of weight (10–25 kg). However, the weight has always crept back on slowly over time. Mrs S states quite categorically that she will not countenance 'counting calories' and that she doesn't want to do anything like going to a gym or health club as they are too expensive and time consuming and 'they're only for thin people, anyway'.

The practice nurse uses her knowledge, skills and experience to assess Mrs S holistically. She knows that any goals and interventions must be decided upon with Mrs S's full participation and collaboration. She is also aware of the implications for Mrs S of developing hypertension, and the need, therefore, for monitoring and liaison with the GP.

Between them, they decide that Mrs S's goal should be to eat healthily rather than 'go on a diet'. It is important for Mrs S not to become preoccupied with weight loss, so the practice nurse suggests that Mrs S weighs herself only once a week and should aim for a slow (1 kg per week) but steady loss over a long period of time. They discuss Mrs S's normal eating patterns and meal preparation and how these could be altered to make them healthier. Mrs S finds she 'gets the munchies' quite late in the evening when watching TV, so ways of coping with this are addressed (treats are allowed as long as they are in a small amount; try fruit and lower-fat alternatives). They also discuss shopping ideas. The practice nurse also provides some written healthy eating literature with recipes to support the discussion.

Mrs S has a dog and is amenable to taking brisk walks three times a week. The practice nurse encourages her to take her family along, if possible, to make these more sociable and enjoyable.

Finally, Mrs S is encouraged to return to the surgery for weekly, then monthly, weigh-ins and blood pressure recording. The practice nurse also suggests that, as time progresses, she will keep in telephone contact with Mrs S to see how her weight loss and motivation are being maintained.

Undernutrition

Undernutrition occurs when the energy intake is less than the energy expenditure. Body fat is depleted for energy, and protein, mineral and vitamin deficiencies develop. The individual is underweight compared with ideal-weight charts.

Related factors

Undernutrition may result from inadequate food intake or a pathophysiological condition. The cause of inadequate food intake may be:

- famine, unavailability of food

- poverty, which prevents the individual from obtaining sufficient food

- inability to shop for or prepare food, such as may occur in the elderly, disabled or housebound individual

- lack of knowledge of essential nutritional needs

- influence of the mass media in promoting nutritionally unbalanced 'junk foods'

- emotional disturbance (such as eating disorder, extreme fear of fat or desire to be thin)

- pathophysiological conditions. These include those that interfere with ingestion, digestion, absorption and/or metabolism of food; increase the body's requirements for energy; or result in loss of body fluids and their constituents.

Identification of patient problems

The problem will be a nutritional intake of less than the body requirements. The exact cause of this will determine the precise goal and the nature of the nursing interventions.

Goals

The individual will be able to:

1. demonstrate understanding of basic nutritional needs of the body

2. gain weight progressively towards the normal range

3. express awareness of any underlying emotional disturbances

4. comply with the prescribed dietary regimen and, if indicated, with a counselling or psychotherapy programme.

Nursing intervention

Malnutrition from inadequate food intake due to socio-economic factors is a worldwide problem, existing in industrialized countries as well as in developing nations. Alleviation of this problem requires increasing the world's food supply and its distribution, as well as providing economic assistance to those in need. Individuals and families require knowledge of basic nutritional needs as well as assistance in the selection and preparation of foods to ensure an adequate diet within the limits imposed by their sociocultural and economic situations.

For the individual who is underweight because of inadequate intake of food although it is available, nursing interventions include:

- providing information about basic nutritional needs of the body. This may be by discussion and the provision of pamphlets that outline a dietary plan containing the essential food groups (see Box 17.3)

- identifying the causes of inadequate nutrition

- assisting the individual to develop a diet that will promote the development of body tissue.

Being thin may currently be fashionable, and peer pressure tends to reinforce the idea (Crawley and Shergill-Bonner 1995). Simply increasing calorie intake may serve only to increase body fat; the diet should be balanced and contain extra protein as well as carbohydrates and fats. Meals should be regular and between-meal snacks of protein and complex carbohydrates encouraged. Moderate activity serves to build body tissue, but adequate and regular rest is essential to conserve energy and promote weight gain.

When emotional disturbances are the primary factor of malnutrition as, for example, in the patient with anorexia nervosa or bulimia nervosa, intervention is focused on identifying the underlying emotional cause. This is a long-term process that requires counselling and psychotherapy for the patient and usually the family as well. The person needs help to acquire a realistic appraisal of self and body, which may be distorted. Harmful and bizarre behaviours need to be identified and attitudes changed. The patient may have to be admitted to hospital initially.

Evaluation

Weight gain may be seen by the nurse as the ultimate goal of care, but an overemphasis on frequent weighing can cause disillusionment. Developing a knowledge of the nutritional needs of the body and the components of a balanced diet can be seen as progress by the client. Sometimes the resolving of other physical or psychological problems, such as nausea or depression, will result in an improvement in nutritional status in the future (see Case Study 17.2).

Undernutrition in hospitalized patients

Undernutrition in hospital patients has been recognized as a major problem for some time (Butterworth and Blackburn 1975). Hinson (1985) stated that there was convincing evidence that many patients in hospital were malnourished, and Coates (1985) found that patients were not reaching the recommended energy or protein intakes set by the Department of Health and Social Security (1979). However, it seems that the malnutrition continues to be a significant problem (McWhirter and Pennington 1997), yet frequently goes unrecognized and untreated (ACHCEW 1997). Inadequate food intake, especially when linked with illness, reduces a patient's nutritional status, which slows recovery and may be linked to an increase in complications and a reduced quality of life (Bond 1997).

There may be many factors affecting patients' eating habits in hospital, in addition to those directly related to their medical condition. The type of food served, the presentation, quantity and temperature of the meal may stimulate enjoyment of the food, or otherwise. The presence or lack of company, and the position in which the patient eats the meal (leaning sideways out of bed, for example), can affect a person's ability to finish a meal. In many hospitals the distribution of meals and collecting of plates afterwards is carried out by non-nursing staff. Nurses therefore have to be particularly vigilant to observe what patients eat and what they leave on their plates. The

Association of Community Health Councils of England and Wales found that patients who needed help with eating and drinking often did not receive any assistance from the nursing staff; many patients' nutritional status had actually deteriorated on discharge (ACHCEW 1997). To be aware of patients' needs, a nutritional assessment should be made on admission and at regular intervals throughout the hospital stay. Frequent liaison with the dietician is essential, so that action may be taken before patients become malnourished. Measures may be required to improve the nutritional status of many patients, particularly those in intensive care and during the postoperative period.

Case Study 17.2   *Undernourishment in hospital*

Mr B, aged 72 years, was admitted to hospital following a severe stroke. He has a right hemiparesis, including difficulty swallowing and speaking. He also has diet-controlled diabetes (diagnosed last year). Mr B's clothes hang loosely; his daughter says he looks as if he has lost a lot of weight recently; his wife died 6 months ago and he has been depressed ever since.

The staff nurse who admitted Mr B fully understands his nutritional needs and the potential difficulties involved. She knows that it is important to obtain Mr B's body mass index (BMI) so that his progress can be monitored. As Mr B is unable to stand, she ascertains his height by measuring his arm span (Ward and Rollins 1999) and then weighs him using the ward sit-down scales, which are very accurate. A BMI of less than 20 means that Mr B is, in fact, underweight.

Because of Mr B's dysphagia and dysphasia, he is referred to the dietician so that his swallowing reflex can be assessed. Initially, he is commenced on nasogastric feeding but, as his swallowing reflex improves over the next 3 days, the nasogastric feeding is withdrawn and Mr B is given thickened supplements to help him swallow. Daily weighing shows an initial weight loss, however. Mr B also develops two small (2 cm) grade 2 pressure sores: one on his right buttock and the other on his right heel.

The occupational therapist is involved at an early stage and Mr B is provided with specially adapted cutlery and crockery to help him feed himself. At first, a student nurse stays with and helps Mr B cut up his food and eat. It is a time-consuming process: Mr B does not like to feel rushed and it takes him time to chew his food properly. However, the student nurse is very patient and gives Mr B time and support. She also encourages Mr B to choose from the hospital menu. Mr B begins to put weight back on slowly – he has gained 2 kg while in hospital. The pressure sores also show signs of improvement.

Before discharge, the dietician discusses Mr B's dietary requirements with him and his daughter. The daughter is very pleased to discover that her father will not need 'sloppy food' and understands how to use the modified cutlery provided. Future follow-up will include input from the diabetic nurse specialist, the general practitioner, the occupational therapist and the district nurse.

Undernutrition due to withholding of nutritional support

Ethical issues

The withholding of nutritional support from a patient is one of the more controversial dilemmas faced by patients, families, surrogates and healthcare professionals. The provision of food and water holds moral and emotional significance, and the symbolic value of providing nourishment may be far greater than any resulting therapeutic benefit. Advances in medical technology make it possible to offer nutritional support via a nasogastric tube, gastronomy tube or central venous catheter to patients who would otherwise die as a result of their inability to swallow fluids and diet. This poses the dilemma as to when nutritional support should be given, and whether it is ever ethically justifiable to withhold food and fluids.

Legal implications

There are no clear guidelines for doctors or nurses in the UK. The Declaration of Geneva (Internal Code of Medical Ethics) behoves that 'a doctor must always bear in mind the obligation of preserving human life' (British Medical Association 1981). The position in law is unclear, and decisions as to whether nutritional support is given or withheld are generally made by doctors in consultation with the family. The case of Anthony Bland has clarified the situation a little, but left it unclear in other respects.

Anthony Bland was crushed at a football match (the 'Hillsborough Disaster') and suffered brain damage. His brainstem functions were intact, he could breathe unaided, cough, blink and respond to loud noises, but he had no higher brain activity. He remained unconscious and was diagnosed as being in a persistent vegetative state (PVS). He was fed and hydrated via a nasogastric tube. He was not brainstem dead, but there was no possibility of his condition improving. His parents fought to have the artificial nutrition and hydration withdrawn, and the case of Airedale NHS Trust versus Bland was taken to the House of Lords in 1993. The Law Lords upheld both the Court of Appeal and High Court decisions, stating that 'it was not unlawful for doctors to withdraw life-supporting medical treatment, including artificial feeding from a patient in a PVS who had no prospect of any recovery or improvement, when it was known that the discontinuance of treatment would cause the patient's death within a matter of weeks'. The ruling stressed that it was applicable only to the case in question, and that in any future cases an application should be made to the courts. However, shortly afterwards, in the case of Frenchay Health Trust versus S, the courts allowed an emergency declaration that the health authority refrain from providing life-saving treatment for a patient in a PVS, on the basis that it was in the patient's best interests.

The United Kingdom Central Council for Nursing, Midwifery and Health Visiting (UKCC) was asked to give evidence to the Select Committee on Medical Ethics (House of Lords 1993) following the Bland case. The terms of reference stated that the Committee was appointed 'to consider the ethical, legal and clinical implications of a person's right to withhold consent to life prolonging treatment, and the position of persons who are no longer able to give or withhold consent' (House of Lords 1993, p. 140). The UKCC highlighted the dilemma facing many nurses in caring for patients requiring life-supporting measures, and the difficulty in making a distinction between 'killing or letting die', when the action taken in withholding support results in the patient's death. The judgement in the Bland case was made on the basis of the patient's 'best interests', but the UKCC noted that this raises the question of who is to be regarded as the arbiter of the best interests of the patient. The views of relatives may at times be in conflict with those of healthcare professionals. The UKCC recommends that all relevant professionals should discuss the way forward, seeking to take account of those closest to the patient (who may or may not be relatives). If no consensus emerges, then the case may need to be taken to court, but this should not normally be necessary.

Clinical factors

The issue of withdrawal or withholding of nutritional support is related to many more patients than those in a PVS. Patients who have suffered a cerebrovascular accident may have lost their ability to swallow, and patients with cancer of the larynx or oesophagus may be unable to swallow food or fluids. In terminal illness, particularly in the end stages, patients may lose the desire and ability to eat. Patients with acquired immune deficiency syndrome (AIDS) often have severe weight loss in the terminal stages of their illness, and gastrointestinal dysfunction prevents adequate intake of nutrients. Patients who are unconscious for whatever reason will require artificial hydration and nutrition. In every situation where patients are unable to meet their own hydration and nutritional requirements, a decision will need to be taken as to how these requirements will be met.

For each patient there will be a balance between the benefits and burdens of nutritional support. It is important that the patient is consulted; fluids and food should be given, or not given, according to the patient's wishes, provided that he or she is mentally competent to make the decision. Tube feeding causes discomfort and may not be in the best interests of terminally ill elderly patients as it carries the risk of aspiration pneumonia, and diarrhoea is a common side-effect (Payne-James et al 1992).

For terminally ill patients the provision of good nutrition in the end stages is unlikely to prolong life, and the aim is the maintenance of comfort and dignity. There is an ongoing debate as to the merits of continuing to hydrate patients who cannot drink or eat in the last few days of life. Some contend that a reduced fluid intake may result in a potentially painful and distressing state of dehydration, which requires artificial hydration therapies (i.e. administration of intravenous, nasogastric or subcutaneous fluids). Other workers suggest that dehydration may actually benefit patients by relieving distressing symptoms; incontinence may be reduced, and a reduction in pulmonary secretions will lessen coughing and reduce the need for tracheal suction. Sutcliffe and Holmes (1994) found that hospice nurses believed dehydration might relieve symptoms, so that artificial hydration was not necessary. Hospital nurses, however, had a much less positive perception of dehydration (House 1992). Lennard-Jones (2000) makes the relevant and valuable point that thirst, as a symptom, may arise from a dry mouth, and does not necessarily correlate with general dehydration. The more aggressive forms of hydration and nutrition support, such as intravenous feeding, can be distressing to relatives, and they may be afraid of going near the equipment or disturbing it. This may prevent them from getting close to the dying patient. For these patients, it may be that local measures to relieve thirst and a dry mouth, such as sucking ice-chips, may be more appropriate.

Ethical decision-making process

When considering whether artificial nutrition or hydration should be commenced or continued, Fawcett (1993) suggests there are a number of questions that must be addressed:

- Is there a right to terminate medical care?

- What types of care (including nutritional support) can be discontinued?

- From what types of patients can care be discontinued?

- Who should make the decision?

- What are the appropriate criteria for justifying the discontinuation of care?

- What quality of life can the patient expect if care is to be continued?

When it is identified that an individual's nutritional state is inadequate or deteriorating, the nurse should discuss this with the dietician and doctor. If an ethical conflict arises regarding the provision of nutritional support,

all responsible individuals should participate in determining its resolution. Patients and their families may be unaware of the options for nutritional support, and nursing staff should initiate discussion appropriately and facilitate enquiries. If the patient is conscious, every effort should be made to fulfil the patient's wishes, involving them in discussion as appropriate. The intent of a patient's behaviour – when turning their head away, or not opening their mouth, or pulling out tubes – is often difficult to assess, but the team must work alongside the patient and relatives to try to find the most acceptable way forward. If the patient is unconscious the clinical team, together with the relatives, need to make a decision. However, relatives cannot make a decision *on behalf of* a patient (Lennard-Jones 2000). The patient may have made a 'living will', expressing a desire to avoid being dependent on life support systems. These statements, however, rarely refer to nutrition and hydration support. Accurate records summarizing discussions (as fully and clearly as possible) and identified wishes must be kept in the patient's notes.

Intravenous feeding is expensive, and the nursing hours involved in caring for an unresponsive patient for weeks, months or even years are considerable. The cost implications are very significant. The UKCC, in its evidence to the select committee, emphasized its opposition 'to decisions being led on the grounds of cost and economics'. It stresses that 'it must always be the patient's best interests and not the financial position of a purchasing authority or agent that is the determining factor' (House of Lords 1993, p. 141). Fawcett (1993) observes that prolonged nutritional support for patients with AIDS may be financially hard to justify in the light of a very poor prognosis. However, the effect on the patient may be highly significant, giving them strength to finalize any legal and personal matters before they die. In such cases the quality, not the quantity, of life is paramount.

Implications for nurses

The provision of nourishment to patients may be viewed as symbolic of the caring and nurturing nature of nursing. The withholding or termination of nutritional support to patients may provoke strong feelings in the nurse and may be morally offensive. In certain clinical situations, nurses may feel that, by providing food and fluids by technical means, they are prolonging a person's dying rather than supporting life. In other situations, they may feel that the lack of adequate nourishment is contributing to the patient's death.

Ethical decisions about a patient's care should be made by the healthcare team in collaboration with the patient or family. Whilst the decision may be, in the words of the Bland case, 'to withdraw life-supporting *medical* treatment', in practice it is *nursing* care that is being withheld. Nurses must therefore ensure that they are active in continuing to give the patient all the care they require in support of this decision. Moistening the patient's lips and frequent cleansing of the mouth are necessary to prevent and alleviate any feelings of thirst or discomfort. If conscious, oral foods and fluids may be given to the patient who requests them and can tolerate them. Continual psychological support to the patient and relatives is essential.

Nutritional needs of the elderly

There is evidence that a lifelong good diet is an important determinant of good health in older people (DoH 1994). The nutritional requirements of older people vary only a little from those of younger adults, but older people may be more susceptible to malnutrition. There are a number of factors that may influence their desire and ability to eat:

- *Teeth* may be in poor condition or dentures ill-fitting.

- *Appetite* may be reduced.

- *Social circumstances* influence desire to eat: cooking for one and eating alone may seem a waste of effort (pets sometimes eat far better than their owners). Cooking facilities may be limited. Income may be low and ability to purchase a balanced diet limited.

- *Functional ability* may be impaired, and the ability to buy food, cook and eat may be limited in some way.

- *Knowledge* of nutritious foods and requirements of a balanced diet may be poor; individuals may never have needed to cook before their spouse died.

- *Health* – ill-health may impinge on appetite or ability to eat.

The consequences of poor nutrition in elderly people are well documented in terms of susceptibility to infection, increased risk of developing pressure ulcers, delayed wound healing and a variety of deficiency disorders that significantly reduce quality of life (Watson 1994). In a study of readmission to hospital in elderly patients undergoing rehabilitation, the best predictor of readmission was poor nutritional status (Sullivan 1992).

When in hospital, elderly patients may not necessarily eat a good diet. There is evidence of poor nutrition among the general hospital population, and this is particularly true in the elderly. Lipski et al (1993, p. 244), found that 'elderly long-stay hospital patients were grossly undernourished and their dietary intake did not satisfy basal metabolic demands'. Hibbert and Loftus-Hills (1996) stated that elderly people living in continuing care environments are as likely to be as vulnerable to undernutrition as people living at home.

However, it is not only the hospitalized elderly who may be vulnerable. Patients over 80 years of age are particularly at risk of malnourishment (DoH 1992b). Nurses need to be aware of the nutritional needs of their older clients and to be able to advise on ways in which they can maintain a good nutritional status, bearing in mind any limitations of the circumstances or abilities. The dietary requirements are similar to those of any adult. The 1994 COMA recommendations on reducing fat and sugar intake are relevant, but balance is very important. This report stresses that 'adequate energy intake is paramount and advice which may compromise this in people with poor appetites should be avoided' (DoH 1994, p. 150). Although elderly people do sometimes have more difficulty in maintaining a regular bowel habit, increasing their non-starch polysaccharide intake too markedly may reduce their energy intake.

The COMA report *The Nutrition of Elderly People* (DoH 1992b) recommends a diet that moderates plasma cholesterol levels (as the incidences of coronary heart disease and stroke in the elderly are significantly higher than those in the general population). The consumption of fruit, vegetables and fish should be increased, and added salt in the diet reduced. The need to maintain moderate levels of physical exercise, for example walking, is stressed.

For hospitalized patients, nurses have a vital role in assessing nutritional status, liaising with the dietician if appropriate and ensuring that patients receive an appropriate diet. Nurses are responsible for making sure that patients have appropriate food and for recording the amounts of food eaten. If insufficient amounts of food are consumed, dietary supplements may be recommended. However, it seems prudent that supplements should be used by nurses only according to local guidelines or on the specific advice and prescription of a dietician, as recommended in the document *Nutritional Standards and the Older Adult* (Royal College of Nursing 1993). This paper makes a number of other suggestions to help maximize food intake, including paying attention to the mealtime environment in hospitals. With a little consideration to decor, freedom from interruptions and seating arrangements, patients may be tempted to eat a little more of an unexciting meal. Nurses must involve patients whenever possible in menu selection, helping them to choose nutritious and balanced meals, and explaining terms when necessary (lasagne and nut-roast may be unfamiliar to the older patient). In 1997, Loftus-Hills and Duff reported a study investigating the actual implementation of these nutritional standards. They found that the standards could be used effectively as a basis for making 'significant changes' in the way that staff provided nutrition for their elderly patients.

Box 17.6 provides a summary of care for the undernourished patient, and highlights the need for liaison with all members of the multidisciplinary team.

Cultural and religious influences on dietary habits

Food is one of the most obvious aspects of an individual's cultural identity, and is closely related to religious, social and economic circumstances. Within the UK today there

Box 17.6   Critical summary: the undernourished patient

Nurse

1. Record patient's height and weight; calculate BMI (weight in kg/height in metres^2)

2. Weigh patient daily

3. Pressure sore risk calculation; re-assess according to level of identified risk

4. Liaise with multidisciplinary team members

5. Ensure patient has access to food, appropriate cutlery and crockery

6. Monitor and record all food and supplements intake, including snacks

7. Ensure that patient is given time and appropriate assistance to eat; involve relatives (as per patient's wishes)

8. Monitor and record bowel movements, particularly diarrhoea

9. Monitor and record nausea and/or appetite

10. Discuss discharge dietary needs with patient and carers.

Occupational therapist

1. Swallowing assessment within 48 hours (for patients with stroke or motor neurone disease)

2. Assessment and monitoring of consistency of food required

3. Assessment and monitoring of progress of motor coordination and activities of daily living (e.g. muscle strength)

4. Provision of modified cutlery and other aids to assist food intake.

Dietician

1. Calculate and record calorific and metabolic requirements

2. Order dietary supplements and discuss food preferences with patient

3. Liaise with pharmacy redietary supplements and feeds required

4. Calculate actual calorific intake

5. Discuss discharge dietary needs with patient and carers.

Doctor

1. Initiate referrals to multidisciplinary team members

2. Assess and discuss causes for poor nutritional status

3. Prescribe parenteral feeds if necessary

4. Review patient's progress.

Pharmacist

1. Liaise with dietician retype and amount of feeds and dietary supplements required

2. Provide feeds and dietary supplements.

is a wide diversity of ethnic, religious and cultural backgrounds, and a corresponding variety of preferred dietary behaviour. All over the world societies have developed traditional eating patterns, based on locally available foods and influenced by cultural and religious beliefs (Hill 1990).

Healthy aspects of traditional diets

Many of the traditional diets of people from minority ethnic groups now living in the UK would be considered healthy in the light of the 1994 COMA recommendations (DoH 1994). People from Bangladesh, African–Caribbean and Mediterranean countries, for example, have a tradition of eating a large variety of fish and seafood products. The COMA report exhorts us to eat more oily fish. Regular consumption of a great variety of fresh fruits and vegetables is a healthy aspect in the diet of many people from black and minority ethnic groups, again recommended by the COMA report. Many millions of people in the Far East and Asia eat vegetarian diets. These are healthy when nutritionally balanced, and involve complementary foods such as beans or pulses with cereals, and are eaten with adequate fresh fruit and vegetables.

The amount of fat in the average British diet is considered by the Government to be too high. Yet the diets of many people from minority ethnic groups have much lower fat contents and a higher ratio of polyunsaturated to saturated fats. A dietary study of Asian households in Brent and Harrow (London) showed lower intakes of saturated fat and cholesterol, and much higher intakes of polyunsaturated fat, vegetable fibre and β-carotene compared with that of the British population (Coronary Prevention Group 1986). Many people from African and African–Caribbean communities eat soup and stews regularly. These are prepared with cereals, beans and root vegetables, and therefore are high in fibre and low in fat. These cooking methods also help to reduce the loss of some vitamins and minerals.

Possible causes for concern in traditional diets

The diet of many societies evolved over generations is often very healthy. However, the effects of coming to a colder climate, and many traditional foods being unavailable (or expensive), together with the influences of a British diet can have adverse effects on the health of individuals. In some diets, for example in Chinese cuisine and African–Caribbean diets, a lot of salty foods or added salt are used. This may be appropriate in a hot climate to compensate for loss of sodium through perspiration, but can be a contributor to hypertension when sodium loss is minimized. Rickets (caused by vitamin D deficiency) is now relatively uncommon in the white population of the UK, partly due to the fortification of margarine with vitamin D. However, for Asians who use ghee (clarified butter) instead of margarine, and who may be vegetarian, there may be an increased incidence.

The variety of fruit and vegetables may have become severely restricted for many people compared with what they may have been used to. There is often a very good range of traditional fruit and vegetables in shops and markets serving communities where there is a large minority ethnic population, and supermarkets do stock a wide variety. However, because of the need to import the fresh produce, it is generally more expensive. This may lead to vitamin deficiencies.

Although a vegetarian or vegan diet can be nutritionally balanced, there is some risk that there may be deficiencies, particularly of protein, vitamin B_{12}, riboflavin, vitamin D and calcium (Health Education Authority 1991, Miller et al 1991). Deficiencies are more likely in a group that has moved away from its country of origin, as subtle changes may occur, and even if one or two commonly consumed foods are missing this may cause deficiencies. Changes in the source of foods can also have an effect. For example, rice in south-east Asia is a good source of calcium and iron, containing 600% more calcium and 380% more iron than rice quoted in British food tables (Hill 1990, Effective Health Care Bulletin 1997).

There is evidence that people, particularly young people from black and other minority ethnic communities, have an increased consumption of snacks and other processed foods, such as crisps, biscuits and high-fat takeaways. The consumption of refined sugar has also increased, especially of fizzy and sugary drinks, sweets and the consumption of tinned fruit in syrup (Hill 1990, Effective Health Care 1997). This is in marked contrast to the traditional diets in many countries, where fresh fruit would be eaten as snacks rather than commercial products. There is a high incidence of diabetes, coronary heart disease and hypertension in African–Caribbean and Asian communities in the UK. No clear contributory factors have emerged, and their diets do not appear to be, on average, higher in fats than that of Europeans, although there may be a relatively high consumption of refined sugar in some diets. However, it is clear that for many communities in the UK the 'westernization' of their diet may bring increased health risks.

The influence of religion on diet

Food is not only a way of obtaining nutrients. For nearly all people, meals are important, having social and possibly religious significance. Food is central to celebrations and commemorations, but the preparation and presentation of everyday meals are related to social and cultural norms. In many countries cooking is a time-consuming activity and (often) the women in the household may spend a large proportion of their day in food preparation. With changing economic trends and more women in employment, there have been inevitable changes in the pattern of meals consumed and the relative value placed upon them.

For some minority ethnic groups there are special concepts surrounding the nature of food, and for others there are clear religious codes that dictate the preparation and serving of a meal. Some of these may be familiar to nurses. Hindus will not eat beef, and are often vegetarian. Some may eat mutton, poultry, fish and eggs, whereas others follow a vegan diet. Sikhs will tend not to eat beef or pork, but usually eat mutton, poultry, fish, eggs and diary products. Islam provides directives relating to food preparation and eating. Food laws are derived from the Koran, which forbids the consumption of alcohol, pork, carnivorous animals and some birds (see Critical incident, p. 557). All meat consumed by Muslims must be from animals killed by ritual slaughter (Halal), and utensils that have come into contact with pork or pork products cannot be used for cooking (Health Education Authority 1991). Buddhists are vegetarian or vegan, eating no food of animal origin. Jews have strict regulations governing the consumption and preparation of food. They will not eat pig products or shellfish, and only kosher meat from a kosher butcher should be eaten. Milk and meat foods must be kept apart in cooking and eating. All utensils used in the preparation and serving of either food must be washed and kept separately (e.g. crockery, cupboards, ovens, tea-towels). Meat and milk dishes may not be served at the same meal, and a period of 3 hours must elapse after a meat meal before foods containing milk can be consumed.

The importance of balance in traditional diets

The observance of these directives will vary between individuals and communities. There are, however, other concepts that may significantly affect an individual's eating habits, but are unfamiliar in Western diets. These concepts often involve balance. Many people from Bangladesh, India and Pakistan hold to the concept of 'hot' and 'cold' foods. The actual temperature of the food is unimportant. 'Hot' foods are meat, ginger, dates and spices – they have pungent, acidic and salty tastes. 'Cold' foods are milk products, cereals, potatoes, fruits and leafy vegetables. The latter are foods that are sweet, bitter, sour or astringent. Groups of people who use this Unani system believe that sickness is produced by an imbalance of humours. Healing can be achieved by eating foods containing the opposite qualities to those of the humour that is out of balance.

In traditional Chinese medicine, good health similarly depends on maintaining a balance of two opposite elements, 'yin' (cold) and 'yang' (hot). When this balance is altered a person may become ill. To help a person's recovery, an appropriate diet is very important. Some foods have 'heating' (yang) and others 'cooling' (yin) properties. Other foods are neutral. The property of a food is not related to its temperature when eaten, although boiling and stir-frying tends to make foods 'colder' (more yin), and stewing, roasting and deep frying all increase the food's 'heat' (its yang properties). Yang foods include meat, herbs, alcoholic drinks, ginger, pepper, spices, oils and fats. Fish, rice and some vegetables are regarded as neutral (yin yang), and yin food includes some fruits and vegetables (Macauley and Mares 1987).

These concepts may be unfamiliar to Western thinking, where associations with foods do not appear to have any such spiritual or symbolic significance. Yet a knowledge of the Unani (hot–cold) system, and yin and yang concepts is particularly important for people involved in the provision of food to those who are ill. These food beliefs and preferences may strongly affect what people will eat. What may seem a nutritionally appropriate meal to a nurse, may be quite unacceptable to an ill patient. Even in health, it is very important. A pregnant Bangladeshi woman is considered to be in a 'hot condition', and would therefore eat fewer 'hot' foods, such as chicken, meat and eggs, but aim to restore balance in the body by eating more 'cold' foods such as milk, cereals, fruit and vegetables.

Food racism?

There is a relative lack of understanding and provision for the needs of black and other minority ethnic groups within the UK, which has been described as 'food racism' (Hill 1990). Progress is being made and the provision of traditional foods in nurseries, schools, hospitals, day centres and workplace canteens is slowly increasing. In hospitals the provision of adequate food of a type that can be consumed by ill patients is vital. In the community and in hospital, the detection of health problems that may be related to diet is essential, and cultural and religious influences should be considered when a patient is assessed. There has been only a brief consideration here of some of the cultural and religious influences on diet. Nurses, whatever their cultural background, must explore the specific dietary needs of the people with whom they are in contact, and recognize the centrality of food in the maintenance and restoration of health.

Summary

In every contact with clients, in hospital or in the community, nurses have a unique opportunity to assess needs, liaise with other health professionals, plan and implement care to ensure that individuals' nutritional needs are met. To do this nurses must have a knowledge of the metabolic processes whereby food can be transformed and used by the body. Nurses must know how to undertake an assessment of nutritional status and how to use the information

gathered to plan care. They must be familiar with recommendations for a healthy diet and know how these can be related to the diets of clients with whom they are working. There are increasing numbers of obese people in our communities, and nurses should be aware of their needs and how to help individuals maintain a desirable weight. Conversely, there are many who are vulnerable to becoming malnourished and underweight, and nurses have a duty to help this client group. Nurses also have a particular responsibility towards those who are unable to maintain their own nutrition. The provision of nutrients by either enteral or parenteral routes may, however, be surrounded by ethical dilemmas. Nurses should not shy away from these, but must be involved in the resolution of these difficult decisions in each individual case. Nurses should have an awareness of the needs of people whose diet may be influenced by their religious beliefs or their cultural heritage. A detailed knowledge of their eating patterns, beliefs, and possible causes for concern in the diet will help nurses to ensure the individual's needs are met in a positive and supportive manner.

Nutrition is vital to the maintenance of health and well-being, and to the restoration of good health. Nurses must accept that they have a fundamental responsibility to promote good nutrition to achieve an optimal state of health.

Critical incident 'Bring me "hot bread!" '

Mrs K, a 68-year-old Muslim, was admitted to the female orthopaedic ward with a fractured neck of femur at 10 p.m., having been in A&E for 4 hours waiting for a bed. She spoke very little English; her 18-year-old granddaughter acted as an interpreter and informant but was sent home by Sister when Mrs K was settled into the ward.

That night Mrs K slept well but became very agitated at breakfast time when she was given porridge and orange juice on a tray. She spat the porridge out, failed to open the orange juice carton and pushed the tray away, which was then removed. 'Bring me "hot bread!"' she demanded, 'hot bread!'. The nursing staff gave her a bread roll with some butter and jam; this was also refused.

The dietician visited Mrs K later that day as Mrs K had already refused her entire lunch of ham salad, demanding 'hot bread' again. Although the dietician understood the requirements of a Muslim diet, she was unable to ascertain Mrs K's preferences, nor did she understand the request for 'hot bread'.

By this time, Mrs K was very upset and shouting at everyone. She was transferred, still protesting loudly,

(Continued)

Critical Incident (*Continued*)

into a single side-ward. Her family visited early in the evening, just as Mrs K was being served curry and rice (as ordered by the dietician). Mrs K took one bite and refused the rest. She had eaten nothing for 36 hours, and had drunk very little. Urine output via urinary catheter was poor. Vital signs were at the lower end of the normal range.

Mrs K's granddaughter spoke to the nurse in charge and explained that her grandmother did not like very spicy food. She was appalled and very annoyed that her grandmother had been offered a ham salad. She also explained that 'hot bread' meant 'toast'. A letter of complaint was received by the hospital 2 days later: it alleged neglect, lack of knowledge and racism.

Reflection

■ What are the issues here and who for?

■ How and when could these needs and problems have been identified?

■ What nursing actions could have prevented these problems arising?

■ What potential physiological complications could ensue here?

See Appendix 2 for guidelines on reflection.

References

Association of Community Health Councils of England and Wales (1997) Hungry in hospital. London: ACHCEW.

Bond S (1997) Eating matters: a resource for improving dietary care in hospitals. Newcastle upon Tyne: Centre for Health Services Research.

British Medical Association (1981) Handbook of medical ethics. London: BMA.

British Nutrition Foundation (1998a) Nutritional requirements. Online. Available: www.nutrition.org.uk/Facts/energynut/requirements

British Nutrition Foundation (1998b) Achieving a balanced diet: putting the advice into practice.Online. Available: www.nutrition.org.uk/Facts/nutandhealth/balanceddiet

Butterworth CE, Blackburn GL (1975) Hospital malnutrition. Nutrition Today 10: 11.

Coates V (1985) Are they being served? London: Royal College of Nursing.

Colhoun H, Prescott-Clarke P, eds (1996) Health survey for England 1994 (a survey carried out on behalf of the Department of Health). London: HMSO.

Coronary Prevention Group (1986) Coronary heart disease and Asians in Britain. London: Confederation of Indian Organisations.

Crawley H, Shergill-Bonner R (1995) The nutrient and food intakes of 16–17-year-old female dieters in the UK. Journal of Human Nutrition and Dietetics. 8: 25–34.

Department of Health (1989) Dietary sugars and human disease. Committee on Medical Aspects of Food Policy. Report on Health and Social Subjects 37. London: HMSO.

Department of Health (1991a) Dietary reference values – a guide. London: HMSO.

Department of Health (1991b) Dietary reference values for food energy and nutrients for the United Kingdom. Committee on Medical Aspects of Food and Nutrition Policy. Report on Health and Social Subjects 41. London: HMSO.

Department of Health (1992a) The health of the nation: a strategy for health in England. London: HMSO.

Department of Health (1992b) The nutrition of elderly people. Committee on Medical Aspects of Food and Nutrition Policy. Report on Health and Social Subjects 43. London: HMSO.

Department of Health (1994) Nutritional aspects of cardiovascular disease. Committee on Medical Aspects of Food and Nutrition Policy. Report on Health and Social Subjects 46. London: HMSO.

Department of Health (1998a) Committee on Medical Aspects of Food and Nutrition Policy (COMA) 1998 annual report. London: HMSO.

Department of Health (1998b) Health service circular HSC 1998/074: national service frameworks. Leeds: NHS Executive. Online. Available: www.open.gov.uk/doh/coinh

Department of Health (1999) Saving lives: our healthier nation. London: HMSO. Online. Available: www.doh.uk/ohn.ppopver

Department of Health (2000) National service frameworks. Coronary heart disease: modern standards and service models. London: HMSO.

Department of Health and Social Security (1979) Recommended daily amounts of food energy and nutrients for groups of people in the United Kingdom. London: HMSO.

Effective Health Care (1997) The prevention and treatment of obesity. vol. 3, no. 2. York: NHS Centre for Reviews and Dissemination, University of York.

Fawcett H (1993) Interpreting a moral right: ethical dilemmas in nutritional support for terminally ill patients. Professional Nurse 8(6): 380.

Gilbert H (1999) Weight watching. Nursing Standard 14(6): 12.

Hankey C, Lean M (1995) The benefits of weight reduction and the maintenance of weight loss. Edinburgh: Royal College of Physicians of Edinburgh Working Group on Obesity.

Health Education Authority (1991) Nutrition in minority ethnic groups. Briefing paper. London: HEA.

Health Education Authority/MAFF (1994) The balance of good health. London: HEA.

Hibbert A, Loftus-Hills A (1996) Eating well: quality matters for older people. Nursing Standard 10: 49.

Hill SE (1990) More than rice and peas. London: The Food Commission.

Hinson LR (1985) Nutritional assessment and management of the hospitalized patient. Critical Care Nurse 5(2): 53.

House N (1992) The hydration question: hydration or dehydration of terminally ill patients. Professional Nurse 8(1): 44.

House of Lords (1993) Minutes of evidence taken before the select committee on medical ethics: Tuesday 15 June 1993. United Kingdom Central Council for Nursing, Midwifery and Health Visiting. London: HMSO.

Knight I (1994) The heights and weights of adults in Great Britain. London: HMSO.

Lennard-Jones J (2000) Legal and ethical aspects of feeding. NT Plus 96(17): 7.

Lipski PS, Torrance A, Kelly PJ, Kames OFW (1993) A study of nutritional deficits in longstay geriatric patients. Age and Ageing 22: 244–255.

Lissner L et al (1987) Dietary fat and the regulation of energy intake in human subjects. American Journal of Clinical Nutrition 46: 886–892.

Loftus-Hills A, Duff L (1997) Implementation of nutrition standards for older adults. Nursing Standard 11(44): 33–37. Online. Available: www.nursing-standard.co.uk/vol11-44/research

Macauley D, Mares P (1987) Nutrition education in a multiracial society. London: National Extension College Training in Health and Race.

McWhirter JP, Pennington CR (1997) Incidence and recognition of malnutrition in hospital. British Medical Journal. 309: 345–348.

Miller PR et al (1991) Vitamin B_{12} status in a macrobiotic community. American Journal of Clinical Nutrition 53: 524.

Payne-James J et al (1992) Artificial nutritional support in hospitals in the United Kingdom: second national survey. Clinical Nutrition 11: 187.

Royal College of Nursing (1993) Nutritional Standards and the Older Adult. RCN Dynamic Quality Improvement Programme. London: RCN.

Scottish Intercollegiate Guidelines Network (1996) Obesity in Scotland. Integrating prevention with weight management. Edinburgh: Scottish Intercollegiate Guidelines Network.

Sullivan D (1992) Risk factors for early hospital readmission in a select population of geriatric rehabilitation patients: the significance of nutritional status. Journal of the American Geriatrics Society 40: 792.

Sutcliffe J, Holmes S (1994) Dehydration: burden or benefit to the dying patient. Journal of Advanced Nursing 19: 71.

Ward J, Rollins H (1999) Screening for malnutrition. Nursing Standard 14(8): 49–53.

Watson R (1994) Nutritional standards and the older adult. Journal of Advanced Nursing 20: 205.

Welsh Office (1996) Health Statistics Wales, 1995. Cardiff: Welsh Office.

Further Reading

Bond S (1997) Eating matters: a resource for improving dietary care in hospitals. Newcastle upon Tyne: Centre for Health Services Research.

This is clear and well written. It provides practical suggestions and standards to improve nursing and multidisciplinary team management of nutritional needs of patients in the hospital setting. It is an extremely influential piece of work which is widely quoted.

Ellis J, Cooper A, Davies D et al (2000) Making a difference to practice: clinical benchmarking part 2. Nursing Standard 14(33): 32–35.

This is the second of two articles that explore the use of clinical benchmarking in nursing practice. Nutrition benchmarking factors and benchmark statements of best practice are identified. The article is relevant to nurses who are thinking of benchmarking as a way of addressing continuous quality improvement, and ensuring the effectiveness of nursing practice.

Effective Health Care (1997) The prevention and treatment of obesity. vol. 3, no. 2. York: NHS Centre for Reviews and Dissemination. University of York.

This bulletin was produced in 1997, and some new research evidence should be available by now. However, it is a comprehensive and useful review of the research literature which assesses the effectiveness of interventions for obesity.

Johnson B, Hackett AF, Bibby A, Cross J (1999) An investigation of the face validity of a food intake questionnaire: lessons for dietary advice. Journal of Human Nutrition and Dietetics 12(4): 307–316.

A primary research study carried out by dieticians in the north-west of England. The authors aimed to find out the extent to which current expert (dieticians') opinions matched the Food Intake Questionnaire (FIQ), which is frequently used to assess a person's intake. The results showed that, even amongst professionals, there is some confusion in terms of 'translating' DRVs into recommending which foods to eat.

Lennard-Jones J (2000) Ethical and legal aspects of fluid and nutrients in clinical practice. Nursing Times Clinical Monograph no. 37. London: NT Books.

This monograph is excellent value at £4.95; it summarizes the legal and ethical positions succinctly and in jargon-free language. The author links the underpinning pathophysiology with the professional concerns.

Loftus-Hills A, Duff L (1997) Implementation of nutrition standards for older adults. Nursing Standard 11(44): 33–37.Online. Available: www.nursing-standard.co.uk/vol11-44/research

A widely available and easily accessible primary research study which assesses the implementation of the Royal College of Nursing's nutrition standards for the older person. The management of the change process is evaluated. The implications for nursing practice are identified and this may well be useful for others seeking to improve practice in their own clinical areas.

18

Caring for the patient with a disorder of the endocrine system

Mike Walsh

Introduction

Disorders of the endocrine system

The person with diabetes

The person with a disorder of the thyroid gland

The person with a disorder of the parathyroid glands

The person with a disorder of the pituitary gland (hypophysis)

The person with a disorder of the adrenal cortices

The person with a disorder of the adrenal medullae

Summary

Introduction

A gland is an organ that extracts substances from the blood and produces one or more new chemical substances, referred to as secretions. Glands may be classified as exocrine or endocrine. The secretion of an *exocrine gland* is carried along a duct into a body cavity or to the external surface of the body. Examples of such glands are the salivary, gastric, mammary and sweat glands. *Endocrine glands* do not have ducts; their secretions, which are called *hormones*, pass directly into the blood and act on remote tissues.

The glands usually cited as composing the **endocrine system** are shown in Figure 18.1. Unlike other body systems in which the component organs are located close together and are connected, the glands are situated in various parts of the body.

Coordination and integration of the development and functions of the body that maintain homeostasis are dependent upon the nervous system and the endocrine system. The endocrine system is concerned mainly with growth, maturation, metabolic process and reproduction. The action of each hormone is specific. One hormone may modify the activity of all body cells (e.g. thyroxine); others affect the activity of only one particular organ (e.g. adrenocorticotrophin). The site of action of any hormone is referred to as the *target organ* or *tissue*.

Target cells contain *receptors* for which specific hormones have an affinity. Some hormones are necessary for survival (e.g. adrenocorticoid hormone); others are not essential to life (e.g. gonadal secretions).

Mechanism of hormone action

Hormones are transported in the blood either freely in solution or in combination with a carrier protein. The water-soluble hormones bind with the receptors on the surface of the target cells. The steroids and thyroid hormones require a carrier for transportation to the target cells and bind with intracellular receptors.

Hormones that bind with surface receptors on the target cells act by altering a membrane-bound enzyme which stimulates the production of a 'second' messenger in the cell; the second messenger then activates enzymes within the cell to produce the specific cellular functions. The second messenger is believed in most instances to be cyclic adenosine monophosphate (cAMP).

Steroid hormones cross the membrane of cells containing their specific receptors and bind with the intracellular receptors. The receptor is altered by the hormone, allowing it to enter the cell nucleus and combine with the chromatin of certain genes. The messenger ribonucleic acid (RNA) is formed and migrates to the cell cytoplasm where it influences the synthesis of specific peptides and proteins. These peptides and proteins carry out the metabolic functions of the cells that were in the past attributed to the steroid hormones.

Endocrine system
See chapter 2.6

Hormone action
See chapter 2.6

Figure 18.1 Endocrine glands in the body.

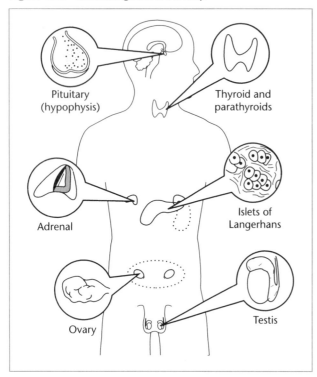

Figure 18.1 Endocrine glands in the body.

Pituitary
See chapter 2.6

Pituitary hormones
See chapter 2.6

Regulation of secretion

The production of endocrine secretions is generally controlled according to the need for their action; that is, production and release into the bloodstream are stimulated when their action is needed and are inhibited when the effect is achieved. Secretions by the pituitary gland are regulated by either hormonal or nervous signals originating in the hypothalamus. The control mechanism may be influenced by the blood concentration of the target organ, or by physicochemical processes. For example, regulation of secretion by the thyroid, adrenal cortices and the gonads is maintained by hormones that are produced by the anterior pituitary gland and liberated in response to the blood concentration of the hormones of those glands. A hormone that stimulates the secretion of another hormone is referred to as a *trophic hormone*.

Dysfunction

Disorders of an endocrine gland may incur an excess or deficiency of its hormone(s). Signs and symptoms of the disorder are predominantly manifestations of dysfunction in the target organ or tissues. Enlargement or outgrowths of a gland may also impose on neighbouring structures, interfering with their function(s).

Pituitary gland (hypophysis)

The **pituitary** gland is a very small gland located at the base of the brain in the sella turcica, a depression in the sphenoid bone. It is attached to the hypothalamus by a stalk, the *infundibulum*, which contains nerve fibres and blood vessels. The gland has two distinct parts: the anterior lobe (or anterior pituitary) and the posterior or neural lobe (posterior pituitary).

The cells of the anterior pituitary are truly glandular in that they extract substances from the blood and secrete new chemicals (hormones). The posterior pituitary consists mainly of many terminal nerve fibres which originate with nerve cells (neurones) in the hypothalamus. The hormones released by the posterior pituitary are secreted by the neurones of the hypothalamus and are released at the nerve endings in the posterior pituitary.

Anterior pituitary lobe (adenohypophysis)

The anterior pituitary secretes the following **hormones**:

- *thyroid-stimulating hormone* (TSH)
- *growth hormone* (GH)
- *prolactin* (PRL), which affects lactation
- *adrenocorticotrophic hormone* (ACTH), which stimulates the adrenal cortex and related peptides – β-lipotrophin (β-LPH), α-melanocyte-stimulating hormone (MSH), which increases pigmentation of the skin and mucous membranes, and β-endorphin (a substance with morphine-like actions)
- *follicle-stimulating hormone* (FSH), which stimulates the development of mature Graafian follicles in women and stimulates spermatogenesis in men
- *luteinizing hormone* (LH), which stimulates the development and maintenance of the corpus luteum in women; in men, where it is called *interstitial cell-stimulating hormone* (ICSH), it affects secretion of testosterone.

The hormones TSH, ACTH, FSH and LH stimulate other glands; GH, PRL and MSH act directly on tissues of the body.

Regulation by hypothalamic hormones

Hypothalamic hormones control, by stimulation or inhibition, the release of hormones from the pituitary gland. The hypothalamic hormones comprise:

- growth hormone-releasing hormone (or factor) (GHRF)
- growth hormone release-inhibiting hormone (somatostatin; GHRIH)
- thyrotrophin-releasing hormone (or factor) (TRH)
- corticotrophin-releasing hormone (CRF)
- gonadotrophin-releasing hormone (GnRH)
- prolactin release-inhibiting hormone (PIH).

Functions of the anterior pituitary hormones

Figure 18.2 summarizes the metabolic functions of anterior pituitary hormones.

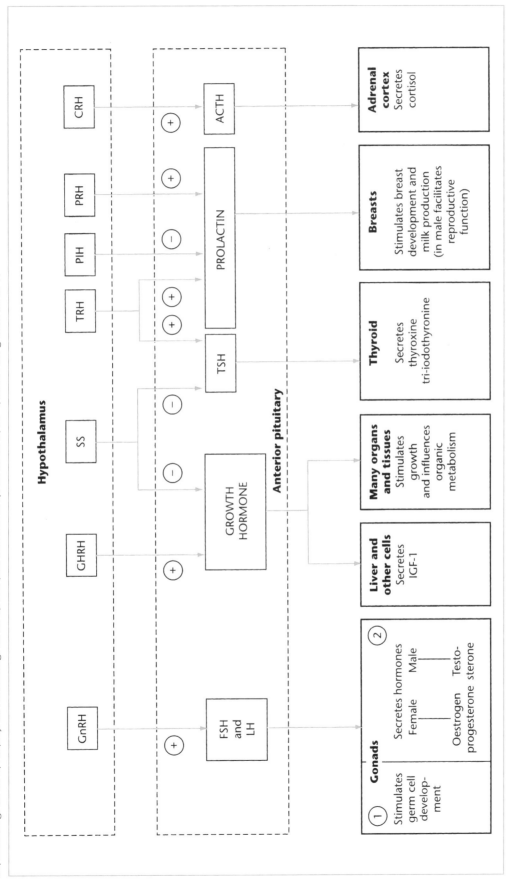

Figure 18.2 Summary of the hypothalamic–anterior pituitary system. GnRH, gonadotrophin-releasing hormone; GHRH, growth hormone-releasing hormone; SS, somatostatin; TRH, thyrotrophin-releasing hormone; PIH, prolactin release-inhibiting hormone; PRH, prolactin-releasing hormone; CRH, corticotrophin-releasing hormone; FSH, follicle-stimulating hormone; LH, luteinizing hormone; TSH, thyroid-stimulating hormone; ACTH, adrenocorticotrophic hormone; IGF-1, insulin-like growth factor 1.

Modified from Vander et al (1990). Reprinted by permission of the McGraw-Hill Companies, Inc.©

Growth hormone

Growth hormone is concerned with the growth of the body and plays an important role in determining a person's size. The most striking effect of the hormone is evidenced in the skeleton. Bones increase in length and thickness until late adolescence, the muscles enlarge and there is a corresponding growth of the viscera. Growth is also dependent upon the secretion of normal amounts of other hormones. The thyroid hormones are necessary to maintain an adequate metabolic rate, and insulin must be available to promote glucose metabolism for the provision of energy. Growth hormone is diabetogenic; it increases the breakdown of glycogen in the liver, promotes the release of glucose into the blood and also produces an anti-insulin effect in muscles. This promotes the synthesis and conservation of protein, conservation of glucose and utilization of fat.

The secretion of GH is controlled by the hypothalamus, which produces two regulating hormones: one stimulates the release of GH and the other, somatostatin, inhibits the release of GH by the anterior pituitary. The secretion of GH is influenced by the state of nutrition; hypoglycaemia, fasting, exercise, stress and trauma increase its production. Hyperglycaemia and high concentrations of cortisol decrease the secretion.

Thyroid
See chapter 2.6

Thyroid-stimulating hormone

Thyroid-stimulating hormone promotes the growth and secretory activity of the thyroid gland, the function of which is the production of hormones that regulate the metabolic rate of all tissues. The production of TSH is regulated by a negative-feedback mechanism. A decrease in the blood concentration of thyroid hormones increases the secretory output of thyrotrophin; conversely, when the thyroid hormones reach a normal or above normal level, there is a reciprocal decrease in the release of thyrotrophin.

Adrenocorticotrophic hormone

Adrenocorticotrophic hormone has as its target organ the adrenal cortices, influencing their secretory output of several cortical secretions. ACTH secretion is regulated by an ACTH-releasing factor produced in the hypothalamus in response to a decreased blood level of cortisone, or to nerve impulses initiated by biological stress (e.g. trauma, pain).

Follicle-stimulating hormone

Follicle-stimulating hormone causes the development of the ovarian follicle and the secretion of oestrogen. The secretion of FSH is inversely related to the blood level of oestrogen.

Luteinizing hormone

Luteinizing hormone promotes ovulation and is necessary for the formation of the corpus luteum in the ruptured follicle. When the corpus luteum develops and secretes progesterone, the production of LH is suppressed. In the male, this hormone may be called the interstitial cell-stimulating hormone (ICSH) because it stimulates the production of the male hormone testosterone by the interstitial cells of the testes.

Prolactin

Prolactin stimulates the corpus luteum to secrete progesterone and initiates and stimulates the secretion of the mammary glands which have undergone preparatory changes in response to the oestrogen and progesterone blood levels. It is similar to LH.

Posterior pituitary lobe

Functions of the posterior pituitary hormones

Two hormones, antidiuretic hormone (ADH) and oxytocin, are released by the posterior pituitary gland.

Antidiuretic hormone

Release of ADH by the posterior pituitary lobe is regulated by osmoreceptors in the hypothalamus. When the osmotic pressure of the blood is increased, for example because of dehydration, the neurones sensitive to changes in the osmotic pressure of the blood transmit impulses to the posterior pituitary to release ADH into the circulating blood. This reduces urine output as a result of increasing water reabsorption in the kidneys. ADH has this effect by increasing the permeability of the distal and collecting tubules. This hormone therefore plays an important role in maintaining normal fluid balance.

Oxytocin

Oxytocin excites contractions of the pregnant uterus, especially during the latter part of gestation. This hormone also plays an important role in lactation; suckling initiates afferent nerve impulses which, on reaching the hypothalamus, bring about the liberation of oxytocin from the posterior pituitary gland. The hormone is carried by the blood to the mammary glands, stimulating the release and flow of milk.

Thyroid gland

The **thyroid** is situated in the neck and consists of two lateral lobes, one on each side of the trachea immediately below the larynx. These lobes are connected by a band of tissue, the thyroid isthmus, lying across the anterior surface of the trachea (Fig. 18.3). The lobes contain numerous vesicles or follicles, and the walls of the follicles are composed of a layer of secreting cells. The follicles contain a clear, colloidal protein–iodine compound called *thyroglobulin*. The gland has an abundant blood supply; paired superior and inferior thyroid arteries arise from the external carotid and subclavian arteries.

Figure 18.3 (a) Front and (b) back views showing the position of the thyroid.

Hyoid bone

Thyroid cartilage

Cricoid cartilage
Lobe of thyroid
Isthmus

Trachea

First rib

Sternum

(a) Front

Pharyngeal wall from the back

Lobe of thyroid

Parathyroid

Trachea, anterior to oesophagus

Oesophagus

(b) Back

Three hormones are produced and released into the blood:

- tri-iodothyronine (T$_3$)

- thyroxine (T$_4$)

- calcitonin (thyrocalcitonin; TCT).

Tri-iodothyronine and thyroxine are produced by the follicular cells, and calcitonin is secreted by the parafollicular (c) cells. Thyroxine (T$_4$) occurs in greater amounts than T$_3$.

The thyroid hormones (T$_3$ and T$_4$) increase the metabolic rate in most of the cells by stimulating oxidative processes. There is a notable increase in cellular activity, oxygen consumption and heat production. The hormones are essential for normal physical growth, maturation and mental development. The production and release of the thyroid hormones are controlled by TSH secreted by the anterior pituitary. A negative-feedback relationship exists between TSH and the thyroid hormones. When the blood concentration of the thyroid hormones decreases, the hypothalamus produces a releasing factor (TRH) which alerts the anterior pituitary to release TSH.

Calcitonin is secreted in response to an above-normal increase in the blood level of calcium or an excess of glucagon in the blood. It lowers the serum calcium and phosphate levels by promoting their excretion in urine and movement into the bones.

Parathyroid glands

The parathyroid glands are small oval bodies attached to the posterior surface of the lateral lobes of the thyroid.

The number may vary but is usually four. The principal secretion of the parathyroid glands is **parathyroid hormone** (PTH), which regulates the concentration of calcium and inorganic phosphorus in the blood through its action on the intestine, bone tissue and kidneys. It promotes absorption of calcium in the intestine, and the demineralization of bone and movement of the calcium into the extracellular fluid. In the kidneys, the hormone increases the excretion of phosphorus by decreasing its reabsorption from the glomerular filtrate and, conversely, the reabsorption of calcium is increased, decreasing its excretion in urine.

A normal concentration of calcium is essential for the normal structure of bones and teeth, coagulation of blood, maintenance of normal cardiac rhythmicity, normal neuromuscular excitability and cellular membrane permeability. The greater part of the absorbed calcium is deposited in bones.

The rate of secretion of the PTH is controlled by the concentration of calcium in the blood. When the calcium level rises above normal, the glands are inhibited and less hormone is produced. A fall in the blood calcium level stimulates the glands, resulting in an increased output of PTH.

Adrenal glands

The two adrenal, or suprarenal, glands are situated immediately above the kidneys. Each is enclosed within a capsule and consists of two distinct parts: the cortex and the medulla. The adrenal glands have an abundant blood supply through branches of the aorta and the inferior phrenic and renal arteries.

Parathyroid hormone
See chapter 2.6

Adrenal glands
See chapter 2.6

Adrenal cortex

The **cortex** forms the outer part as well as the greater portion of the gland and produces hormones essential to life. These are steroids and collectively are called the *adrenocorticoids*, corticosteroids or corticoids. Those secreted in physiologically significant amounts fall into three classes: mineralocorticoids, glucocorticoids and sex hormones. The steroids in each of these classes have some predominant characteristics or actions, but may overlap into another class.

Mineralocorticoids

Mineralocorticoids are essential to life. The most significant is *aldosterone*, which influences electrolyte concentrations and fluid volume.

The secretion of aldosterone is regulated in the interest of maintaining a normal sodium concentration and normal fluid volume. Factors that influence the amount of aldosterone released are the blood sodium and potassium levels and the blood volume. A decrease in the sodium concentration stimulates an increased output of aldosterone, and vice versa. Aldosterone acts by stimulating the renal tubules to reabsorb sodium and excrete potassium; consequently the effect of changes in serum potassium levels is the reverse of that of sodium. Decreases in renal arterial blood pressure such as occur in shock, physical trauma and haemorrhage increase renin secretion by the kidneys. The production of angiotensin II that results from the release of renin stimulates the adrenal cortex to secrete aldosterone.

Adrenal cortex
See chapter 2.6

Adrenal medulla
See chapter 2.6

Pancreas
See chapter 2.6

Glucocorticoids

Several glucocorticoids have been recognized, but *cortisol* (hydrocortisone) is considered to be the most important, because it is more potent and is produced in much greater amounts than the other cortical hormones. Cortisol influences the metabolism of glucose, protein and fat, and is involved in the body's responses to physical and mental stress. Its actions are complex and not clearly understood; for example, it enables a person to deal more effectively with stress, but how this is achieved is not known. Cortisol increases the blood sugar level and the liver glycogen stores are increased. Tissue protein is broken down and the amino acids are converted to glycogen or glucose in the liver (gluconeogenesis). Fat is also mobilized, some of which is also converted to glucose.

Glucocorticoids are secreted in response to circulating ACTH. In turn, the production and release of ACTH by the anterior pituitary depends upon the release of corticotrophin-releasing hormone (CRH) which is secreted by the hypothalamus. The production of CRH is influenced by a negative-feedback mechanism; that is, a low concentration of adrenocorticoid secretions in the blood initiates the hypothalamic responses. With an increase in the blood level of glucocorticoids, the output of ACTH is depressed. Physical and psychological stress and hypoglycaemia also stimulate the release of CRH through impulses delivered from the cerebral cortex or midbrain to the hypothalamus.

A concentration of cortisol in excess of the normal is of clinical significance because it suppresses local inflammatory responses to irritating substances (anti-inflammatory effect), delays healing through depressed fibroplasia and reduces tissue sensitivity reactions to antigens (antiallergic reaction). Other effects also associated with an excess of cortisol include a decreased production of antibodies and an increased secretion of gastric hydrochloric acid and pepsinogen which predisposes to the development of ulcers.

Adrenal sex hormones

The adrenal cortices of both sexes secrete both male and female hormones: *androgens, oestrogen* and *progesterone*. Oestrogen and progesterone are produced in lesser amounts than the androgens but, normally, the quantity of any of these hormones is considered to be physiologically insignificant compared with the amounts produced by the gonads.

Adrenal medulla

The **medulla** forms the central portion of each adrenal gland and is composed of specialized neurones which secrete two hormones, *adrenaline* and *noradrenaline*. Because of their chemical composition, they are frequently referred to as *catecholamines*. During any stress or threat to the organism, the hormones are released and serve with the autonomic nervous system to produce defensive reactions throughout the body. Their production is controlled by nerve impulses transmitted to the medullae by sympathetic nerve fibres, and their effects are similar to those produced by sympathetic innervation.

Adrenaline causes constriction of the peripheral and renal blood vessels and dilatation of the coronary and skeletal muscle blood vessels. The rate and force of contraction of the heart and skeletal muscle is increased. The smooth muscle of the bronchioles, gastrointestinal tract and urinary bladder relaxes. The dilator muscle fibres of the irises contract, resulting in dilatation of the pupils. The blood sugar level is raised by increased glycogenolysis (conversion of glycogen to glucose) in both the liver and skeletal muscles. The metabolic rate is accelerated and there is an increased alertness and awareness due to stimulation of the brain. Adrenaline also promotes the release of ACTH, which in turn increases the secretion of glucocorticoids.

Noradrenaline causes a more generalized vasoconstriction and does not produce dilatation of any vessels. Because of this action, it is more effective in raising the blood pressure; both systolic and diastolic blood pressures rise.

Pancreas (islets of langerhans)

The **pancreas** is both an exocrine and an endocrine gland. Its exocrine secretions are carried by a system of ducts to the duodenum and contain enzymes that play an important role in digestion. The islets of Langerhans form the endocrine component of the pancreas and consist of irregularly scattered groups of cells that are totally independent of the pancreatic system of ducts. The islets are highly vascularized and consist of four types of cell:

1. *α cells*, which secrete the hormone **glucagon**

2. *β cells*, which produce **insulin**

3. *δ cells*, which may secrete small amounts of gastrin and **somatostatin** (growth hormone release-inhibiting hormone) (GHRIH)

4. *F cells*, which secrete pancreatic polypeptide.

Insulin and glucagon are proteins and are rendered inactive in the gastrointestinal tract by the proteolytic enzymes; when prescribed, they must be administered parenterally.

Secretions and functions

Insulin

This hormone plays a dominant role in carbohydrate, fat and protein metabolism, especially in the liver and muscular and adipose tissues. Knowledge of the ways in which insulin promotes specific metabolic cellular activities is incomplete, but it has been established that it binds to receptors in cell membranes and stimulates the following actions:

1. the transfer of glucose into most cells and its metabolism by those cells

2. the formation of glycogen by the liver and muscle cells

3. the synthesis of fatty acids and storage of fat in adipose tissue

4. the uptake and incorporation of amino acids into cell proteins

5. an increased uptake of potassium by cells.

These activities result in a lower concentration of glucose in the blood.

The concentration of blood glucose is the major controlling factor in the secretion of insulin. An increase raises the production of insulin and, conversely, a decrease below the normal blood level of glucose suppresses its secretion. Thus, a positive-feedback mechanism is established which controls the output of insulin in order to maintain the blood sugar level within a normal range. The synthesis of insulin is also stimulated by an excess of growth hormone and glucocorticoids, but somatostatin is an inhibitor of both insulin and glucagon secretion. The amount of insulin circulating in the blood increases when carbohydrate foods are ingested; this is attributed to the effect of the gastrointestinal hormones on the β cells. Glucose given intravenously does not produce the same effect as when it is taken orally.

Other factors that result in an increased insulin level include vagal nerve stimulation and oral hypoglycaemic agents.

Glucagon

This hormone may also be referred to as the hyperglycaemic factor, because its primary effect is stimulation of glycogenolysis (the conversion of glycogen to glucose) and the release of glucose into the blood by the liver to increase the blood glucose concentration. Its secretion by the α cells is stimulated by a low blood sugar level. An oral intake of proteins initiates an increased secretion of glucagon, greater than that seen in response to the intravenous administration of amino acids. This suggests a gastrointestinal hormone that stimulates the secretion of glucagon. Sympathetic nervous stimulation of the pancreas also increases the glucagon output.

Somatostatin (growth hormone release-inhibiting hormone; GHRIH)

This hormone is found in cells of the hypothalamus, where it passes down the portal vessels to the anterior pituitary, gastrointestinal tract and islets of Langerhans. It inhibits the secretion of insulin, glucagon, pancreatic polypeptide, GH and various gastrointestinal hormones. It interferes with carbohydrate absorption and possibly with the absorption of protein and fat.

Pancreatic polypeptide

This hormone is known to decrease glycogen concentration in the liver and to slow the absorption of food. Release of the hormone is stimulated by protein ingestion, fasting, exercise and hypoglycaemia.

Blood sugar level

The normal blood sugar (glucose) level 3–4 hours after a meal varies from approximately 6.5 to 7.5 mmol/L. Fluctuations occur as a result of energy expenditure and the ingestion of foods. The types of food taken also influence the degree of change; obviously, a meal high in carbohydrate produces a greater concentration of glucose for a period of time than a meal with a low carbohydrate content. An increase in the blood sugar level above the normal is known as *hyperglycaemia*. A level below normal is referred to as *hypoglycaemia*. Blood sugar level is therefore determined principally by the hormones secreted in the islets of Langerhans, although some other endocrine secretions also have an effect, such as the glucocorticoids.

Disorders of the endocrine system

General

Signs and symptoms of endocrine dysfunction may be non-specific, resulting from changes in the widespread

Glucagon
See chapter 2.6

Insulin
See chapter 2.6

Somatostatin
See chapter 2.6

target tissues and are common to many disorders. They include the following.

Alterations in growth *Delayed growth* can occur from endocrine and metabolic disorders as well as genetic factors. Delayed growth from endocrine disorders usually occurs during a specific period of development. *Excessive growth* may result from endocrine disorders in which an excess of adrenal, ovarian or testicular, or pituitary hormones is produced. Excessive pituitary secretion of growth hormone causes gigantism.

Obesity Obesity can be associated with hormonal disorders and may be a causative factor (as in diabetes) as well as a result of a disorder.

Appetite changes These include anorexia and polyphagia. Excessive eating (polyphagia) is most often seen with uncontrolled diabetes, hyperthyroidism and occasionally with a hypothalamic disorder.

Polyuria and polydipsia Excessive urinary output and abnormal thirst are frequently the result of uncontrolled diabetes mellitus.

Weakness and exhaustion Excessive weight loss, muscle wasting, weakness and exhaustion may be seen in patients with uncontrolled disorders of the pancreas, thyroid or adrenal glands.

Skin pigmentation Changes in skin pigmentation may develop in patients with disorders of the pituitary, parathyroid and adrenal glands.

Hirsutism Changes in the distribution and texture of body hair occur with several endocrine disorders. Facial hair in the female may occur with adrenal or ovarian disorders.

Sexual disturbances Impotence, menstrual disorders and infertility may be associated with endocrine disturbances. Impotence may occur in men who have had diabetes mellitus for several years. The onset of puberty and delay in the development of secondary sex characteristics may occur with deficiency of growth hormone and gonadal dysfunction.

Bone and joint disorders These may accompany changes in the secretion of growth hormone, thyroid hormones and adrenocorticoids.

Renal colic and stones These may be associated with excess secretion of parathyroid hormone leading to hypercalcaemia.

Hypertension This occurs as a result of hyperactivity of the adrenal cortex.

Personality changes Behavioural changes, including lethargy, confusion, nervousness, restlessness, convulsions and coma, may result from acute metabolic disorders associated with uncontrolled diabetes mellitus as well as with disorders of secretions of the pituitary gland, adrenal gland and thyroid.

Diabetes mellitus
See chapter 2.6

The person with diabetes

Diabetes mellitus

Diabetes mellitus is a heterogeneous group of disorders of carbohydrate, fat and protein metabolism characterized by chronic hyperglycaemia, degenerative vascular changes and neuropathy. It tends to accelerate degenerative changes throughout the body by widespread vascular changes in the large blood vessels and the microvessels.

Characteristics and epidemiology

Diabetes is diagnosed when the patient has the symptoms of diabetes (such as polyuria, unexplained weight loss and excess thirst) and a casual plasma glucose level ⩾11.1 mmol/L. Casual refers to the fact that the blood sample has been taken at any time of the day regardless of the last meal. A fasting plasma glucose ⩾7.0 mmol/L (no food in the previous 8 hours) in the presence of the classical symptoms is also diagnostic of diabetes (Watkins 1998).

There are two principal types of diabetes which have different aetiologies. *Type 1* or *insulin-dependent diabetes mellitus* (IDDM) is caused by the destruction of β cells in the islets of Langerhans. The destruction is an autoimmune response associated with environmental and genetic factors. This process starts early in life and it may be several years before symptoms begin to appear. The onset can then be very rapid.

Type 2 or *non-insulin-dependent diabetes mellitus* (NIDDM) covers a multitude of different disorders. The basic problem is that either the islets of Langerhans gradually diminish their insulin output or there is increased peripheral resistance to the action of insulin. The onset tends to be slow. Obesity and lack of exercise are the commonest causes of insulin resistance and hence of type 2 diabetes (Springhouse Corporation 2000). The most common age of onset is 50–70 years. There is a strong genetic influence, and as a result certain families and ethnic groups are much more likely to have type 2 diabetes. For example in the UK, Pakistanis and Bangladeshis are more than five times as likely as the general population to have diabetes, while Indians are three times more likely (Erens et al 2001).

There are approximately one million people in the UK with diabetes. The ratio of type 1 : type 2 is 3 : 7, but of patients with type 2 (NIDDM) approximately 50% remain undiagnosed (Haslett et al 1999). The complications of diabetes are a greater public health problem than any infectious disease, particularly as many of the patients who develop complications do so before their diabetes is even diagnosed.

In addition to primary diabetes (types 1 and 2) there is also secondary diabetes. This is due to a range of conditions such as pancreatic disease or hormonal disorders such as Cushing's syndrome (see p. 604), or it occurs as a side-effect of medication such as steroid therapy.

Whatever the cause, the result is a deficiency of insulin or inadequate insulin function. This leads to an inadequate transfer of glucose into the cells; the utilization of glucose for energy and cellular products and its conversion to glycogen or fat and storage as such are depressed. Glucose accumulates in the blood, causing hyperglycaemia.

Fat may be mobilized from adipose tissue and broken down to provide a source of energy. The mobilized fat is withdrawn from the blood by the liver and broken down to glycerol and fatty acids. The fatty acids are oxidized by the hepatic cells to ketone bodies, which are then circulated and may be metabolized by cells to produce energy, carbon dioxide and water. Only a limited amount of ketone acids can be utilized by the cells. If ketogenesis proceeds rapidly, exceeding the rate at which they can be metabolized, the ketone acids accumulate in the blood, causing ketosis or ketone acidosis.

Tissue protein may also be broken down to amino acids which are used in gluconeogenesis, contributing to the hyperglycaemia. Both the uptake of amino acids by the cells and body protein synthesis are decreased.

The patient excretes an excessive volume of urine (*polyuria*) as a result of the increased concentration of glucose in the glomerular filtrate. The glucose increases the osmotic pressure of the filtrate, preventing the reabsorption of water. As a result of the excessive water loss, the patient experiences a persisting thirst (*polydipsia*), and dehydration and electrolyte imbalance may develop. The blood glucose concentration exceeds the capacity of the renal tubules to reabsorb it from the glomerular filtrate, and glucose is excreted in the urine (*glycosuria*). The maximum capacity of the renal tubules to reabsorb glucose represents what is referred to as the glucose renal threshold. The normal value is 10–12 mmol/L.

Weakness and fatigue are common complaints because the glucose cannot be utilized to produce energy. There is a loss of weight which is attributed to the mobilization of fat from adipose tissue and the breakdown of protein. Some patients also experience an increased appetite (*polyphagia*).

Female patients may develop pruritus of the vulva, usually due to infection by fungi (candida) that thrive on the glucose deposit from the urine. The vulva becomes swollen and inflamed. Balanitis is a similar problem affecting the glans penis in men.

Table 18.1 lists the clinical characteristics of persons with the two major types of diabetes mellitus.

Chronic complications of diabetes

The blood vessels of practically all diabetics undergo degenerative changes to some extent. These changes may be both microvascular and macrovascular. Hyperinsulinaemia and/or increased insulin resistance is considered to be fundamental to vascular complications in diabetes (Winters and Jernigan 2000). Microalbuminuria is a significant marker for many vascular problems being a precipitating factor in insulin resistance, along with raised low-density lipoprotein (LDL) cholesterol levels and hypothyroidism (see p. 588). These three factors are important indicators or markers for microvascular and macrovascular complications according to Winters and Jernigan (2000).

Microvascular degenerative changes

Microvascular degenerative changes are specific to diabetes; the basement membrane in the capillaries and arterioles thickens. The retinae, kidneys and skin are the areas most affected by microvascular changes. The long-term quality of diabetic control plays a major part in determining the rapidity of onset of such complications.

Diabetic retinopathy occurs in the form of minute aneurysms in the retinal vessels. These dilatations are prone to rupture and cause a haemorrhage into the eye. The resultant visual loss varies with the location and proliferation of the lesions. Poor diabetic control, increased diastolic blood pressure, impaired renal function, deterioration in motor nerve conduction and raised triglyceride levels increase the risk for diabetic retinopathy. It is estimated that comprehensive screening and treatment for diabetic retinopathy could prevent 260 new cases of blindness per year in the UK (York CRD 1999).

Renal function may be slowly impaired by changes in the glomerular capillaries (intercapillary glomerulosclerosis, or Kimmelstiel–Wilson syndrome) and by sclerotic changes in the larger renal vessels. There may be no clear symptoms

Table 18.1 Classification of diabetes mellitus

	IDDM (type 1)	NIDDM (type 2)
Synonyms	Juvenile onset	Maturity onset
Age of onset	Usually before 30 years	Usually after 40 years
Type of onset	Frequently sudden	Usually gradual
Presentation	Polydipsia, polyuria	Often asymptomatic
Bodyweight	Thin	Usually (80%) obese
Ketoacidosis	Ketosis-prone	Ketosis-resistant
Control of diabetes	Difficult; brittle	Generally easy
Control by diet alone	Not possible	Frequently possible
Control by oral agents	Not possible	Frequently possible
Long-term complications	Frequent	Frequent

reported by the patient until renal disease is far advanced and the kidneys are close to failure. Approximately 25% of patients with type 2 diabetes have microalbuminuria and a further 15% have proteinuria (Melville et al 2000). Diabetic renal disease is also associated with hypertension, which exacerbates further renal damage, setting up a vicious circle. This explains the recommendation by the York CRD (2000) that diabetic patients with above normal levels of albumin in their urine should be commenced on angiotensin-converting enzyme (ACE) inhibitors, whatever their actual blood pressure reading.

Macrovascular degenerative changes

Macrovascular degeneration involves the development of *atherosclerosis* (deposits of the fatty substance cholesterol) in the arteries, narrowing their lumen. Atherosclerosis of the coronary arteries frequently leads to angina pectoris and myocardial infarction, especially in older persons.

Defective circulation due to vascular changes in the lower limbs may lead to abnormal coldness of the extremities, numbness, discoloration, muscular cramps, weakness, burning pain or a small ulcer that does not heal. Proteinuria indicates a high risk of such large vessel disease (Watkins 1998). Something as trivial as a wrinkled sock or a poorly trimmed toe nail, a superficial injury or a pressure sore on the heel may precipitate an infected lesion and ultimately gangrene, leading to the amputation of a foot or leg. A combination of poor peripheral blood supply and/or nerve damage (diabetic neuropathy; see below) leads to some 15% of people with diabetes developing foot ulcers. Infected diabetic foot ulcer is the second most common reason for amputation after trauma (York CRD 1999). It is estimated that some 40–50% of lower-limb amputations in diabetic patients are, however, avoidable (Umeh et al 1999). Screening for the two main predictors of gangrene and amputation – peripheral vascular disease and peripheral neuropathy – should therefore form part of the long-term management of all diabetic patients.

Diabetic neuropathy

Neuropathy may be defined as a non-inflammatory, non-specific pathological or functional disorder of the peripheral nervous system. This complication affects all parts of the nervous system except the brain. Peripheral neuropathy is usually bilateral and worsens at night. The patient may experience muscular cramps, tingling and burning sensation as well as pain.

Deep tendon reflexes are absent and the patient's vibratory and positional senses may be impaired. Foot problems are most common due to accidental injury as the person gradually loses sensation in the lower limbs. Injuries are compounded by poor circulation, which delays healing (see above). A Diabetic Foot Screen tool is available for screening peripheral sensation and involves the use of a calibrated nylon filament mounted on a handle that buckles at 10 g of pressure when applied perpendicular to the skin. This monofilament is applied systematically to

---

> **Box 18.1** Risk markers for diabetic vascular complications
>
> - Sedentary lifestyle
> - Obesity
> - Increased blood viscosity
> - Raised blood glucose and haemoglobin A levels
> - Hypothyroidism
> - Tobacco use
> - Hyperlipidaemia
> - Raised blood pressure
> - Microalbuminuria and proteinuria
> - Vision changes
> - Skin lesions on feet and diabetic neuropathies.

---

each foot at the required pressure while the patient has their eyes closed. The foot is 'at risk' if the patient cannot consistently and accurately report the touch of the monofilament as it is applied (Umeh et al 1999). Autonomic neuropathy is not common but leads to diarrhoea, vomiting and postural hypotentsion. Impotence and retrograde ejaculation may occur in the male.

Box 18.1 shows the main risk markers for vascular complications in diabetic patients. The prevention of complications depends upon identifying which of these are present and working with the patient to reduce or eliminate them (Winters and Jernigan 2000).

Prevention of diabetes mellitus

Primary prevention

Diabetes mellitus is not a single entity but a group of heterogeneous disorders caused by a combination of genetic, environmental and viral factors. With the knowledge now available, primary preventive measures are limited but measures can be taken to prevent and/or correct obesity and stop smoking. This is especially important for those with a family history of diabetes. Haslett et al (1999) point out that the only cost-effective way to deal with diabetes is to prevent it. This observation is of major importance for nurses, especially as the majority of non-insulin-dependent diabetics are either obese at the time their disease is manifested or have a history of obesity. Health promotion aimed at reducing obesity and increasing fitness could therefore be of immense benefit to the whole population.

Secondary prevention

Once diabetes has been diagnosed in a patient, health education aimed at preventing or at least delaying the development of complications is worthwhile. Such secondary prevention can greatly improve the quality of life of the patient and bring about enormous savings in cost to the National Health Service. Once again, nurses are in the forefront of such work, especially practice nurses who have developed considerable expertise in the field of diabetic care.

Management and education of the diabetic patient and family

Although inroads are being made in the prevention of diabetes, to date no cure exists. Individuals must therefore live with this chronic disorder and the potential complications. The diabetic patient may be dependent on health professionals for restoration of health when the disease is first diagnosed and during episodes of acute illness. As the individual acquires knowledge and skill to make alterations in lifestyle to regulate the hyperglycaemia, greater independence may be achieved. Individuals with diabetes mellitus must alter their lifestyles and health behaviours to regulate their blood glucose levels if they are to minimize the impact of the disease

Management of diabetes mellitus

The principal aim of management is to establish and maintain metabolic control in order that treatment may:

■ save life

■ alleviate symptoms

■ prevent long-term complications.

This also involves reducing risk factors such as obesity, smoking and hypertension

The main therapeutic interventions aimed at achieving these goals consist of diet, insulin, other medication aimed at reducing blood glucose levels, and lifestyle modification such as weight reduction, smoking cessation and exercise. Ideally this should all be carried out within a framework of patient self-care, allowing individuals to take the maximum responsibility for managing their condition.

Blood glucose levels are controlled by balancing the person's energy intake with energy utilization or output. *Dietary measures*, *medication* and *physical activity* are adjusted to achieve the best possible glycaemic control for the individual.

Diet

The patient's *goals* are:

1. to restore and maintain blood glucose and lipid levels to normal

2. to prevent wide fluctuations in blood glucose levels throughout the day

3. to attain and maintain a desirable bodyweight

4. to prevent or delay the development of cardiovascular, renal and neurological complications.

Diet is a major factor in the control of diabetes and is the first line of management in type 2 diabetes. The prescribed 'diabetic diet' has been replaced by an individualized diet regimen with the patient assuming responsibility for planning, implementing and adjusting the diet to needs and lifestyle. The diet should be quite similar to that advocated for the non-diabetic and must provide sufficient variety to make it appetizing and palatable.

The *dietary plan* indicates the number of calories required each day and the proportions of these calories to be allocated to carbohydrate, protein and fat. The number of calories is determined by the person's ideal and present weight, age, sex, activity and previous dietary intake. Initially, if the non-insulin-dependent patient is overweight, the number of calories must be lower than the value indicated as needed for their ideal weight. The objective is to bring about a gradual and steady loss of weight until the normal weight is achieved. Appropriate increases in the food plan are usually made as the weight approaches normal. The insulin-dependent diabetic has impaired protein and fat synthesis as well as inefficient use of glucose and so an overall increase in calorie intake is required until better control achieves weight gain.

Generally, the proportion of prescribed calories allocated to each food type is approximately 50–55% carbohydrate, 10–15% protein and 30–35% fat (Haslett et al 1999). Some authorities argue that all sugar should be eliminated from the diet (Watkins 1998), although others permit concentrated forms of simple sugars, such as sugar, sweets, jam, ice cream, pastries, cake and sweetened beverages in strictly limited quantities. These sugars should only be taken as part of a meal to prevent rapid increases in blood sugar levels that might otherwise occur. Unrefined carbohydrates with fibre, such as wholegrain breads and cereals, fruit and vegetables, should be substituted for the refined carbohydrates. It is believed that foods with a high soluble fibre content improve glucose tolerance, lower insulin secretion, reduce glycaemia and glucosuria, and reduce LDL levels. Foods high in soluble fibre include oat, rice and corn brans, legumes and lentils. Carbohydrate intake is distributed over the day to avoid abnormal fluctuations in blood glucose concentrations. In the selection of fat, the substitution of unsaturated for saturated fats is recommended because of the diabetic's predisposition to the development of atherosclerosis and vascular lesions. As public awareness of the benefits of soluble fibre and low-fat diets increases, recipes and products using soluble fibre and less fat are becoming more readily accessible to consumers.

Food exchange information provides help for patients and their families to select a varied diet. Food intake is usually best divided into at least three main meals. If an oral hypoglycaemic drug or insulin is used, the carbohydrate intake is usually divided across meals and snacks distributed throughout the day and evening.

Diabetes management
See chapter 2.6

Careful education and the availability of good eating guides or exchange lists permit the diet to be varied and take into account the availability of foods as well as the person's preferences. Cookery books, extensive information about food values, and general dietary guidelines are available from Diabetes UK. This material can be useful in supplementing the basic but individualized food plan that will be given to each person on diagnosis by the local dietetic team.

It must be impressed upon the person that all of the daily food allowance should be eaten, especially if insulin or a hypoglycaemic drug is being taken. If the insulin-taking patient is unable to take his or her usual diet, the carbohydrate requirement is made up in some way (e.g. orange juice, milk). Meals should be taken regularly: the delay or missing of a meal may upset the blood glucose level and promote the breakdown of fat. Foods of no significant nutrient value, or 'extra' foods that the person may have as desired, include clear broths and consommé, clear tea and coffee, and artificially sweetened carbonated beverage. Non-caloric sweeteners such as aspartame and saccharin may be used safely by diabetics. These sweeteners are found in many low-calorie beverages and prepared foods.

Sorbitol (a sugar alcohol) has been used as a sweetening agent, as has fructose (crystalline fruit sugar). Both are virtually all absorbed and metabolized, but the rate of absorption from the gut is slow and so sorbitol and fructose have less effect on blood sugar levels than glucose. Both are often used in the manufacture of 'diabetic' jams, boiled sweets, biscuits and chocolate. Because they do not offer any energy savings, they should not be used for slimming purposes or by diabetics whose main therapeutic aim is to reduce weight. They also have the disadvantage of possibly lulling the patient into a false sense of security with regard to diet. The use of artificial non-nutritive sweeteners and the bulk nutritive sugar substitutes are not necessary in the management of diabetes, but many people find their use improves the quality of their life and helps make dietary restrictions more acceptable.

The diabetic person's diet is very much an individual affair. After the initial dietary plan, the patient is followed closely to determine whether it is satisfactory; the blood glucose levels are checked several times a day, weight is recorded daily, and general reactions (physical and psychological) are noted. Adjustments in the total calorie intake and distribution of food throughout the day are often necessary. Adherence to a diet can be very difficult and it is not uncommon for patients to fail to keep to the recommended diet. Common problems experienced by patients include the need for continual self-discipline, the influence of other people especially when eating out, time constraints and dealing with their own emotions and self-image. To increase compliance with dietary regimens, patients therefore need assistance with self-management

Insulin action
See chapter 2.6

techniques and require psychosocial support during the adjustment period. Above all a non-judgemental, non-confrontational approach is needed to build a rapport with the patient. Even though dietary adherence may be poor in the short term, it is still possible to build up a therapeutic relationship with the patient that will improve adherence in the long term.

The individual's perception of adherence and good diabetic control may be different to that of the health professional. This is illustrated in a study by Richmond (1993) of a sample of young patients with IDDM. She chose a sample of 70 patients aged 16–30 years and sent them a questionnaire, achieving a response rate of 74%. One of her striking findings was that 27% of respondents rated their control as good yet also admitted that they maintained their blood glucose at high levels, which is a contradiction in terms. This demonstrates that the patient's perception of good control is very different to the medical perception, as running a high blood glucose level is poor control. This is a key point in diabetes care (and many other areas of health education) as the patient's view may be very different from that of the nurse or doctor. In Richmond's study, 46% of subjects stated that they experienced regular hypoglycaemic attacks (see p. 580), and 34% had work disruption as a result (e.g. being sent home after an attack). Hypoglycaemia disrupted the social life of 36% of subjects. The close relationship between diet, diabetic control and everyday life is vividly shown by these findings and you must be fully aware of them before attempting health education work with any diabetic patient.

The key dietary points important for individuals with diabetes mellitus to note are listed in Box 18.2.

Medication

The *goal* of drug therapy is that the patient will maintain therapeutic glucose levels by increasing endogenous insulin production and utilization; or by maintaining serum insulin levels through the administration of exogenous insulin.

Insulin

Insulin is prescribed for all insulin-dependent diabetics. Non-insulin-dependent diabetics may require insulin during periods of stress (e.g. infection, surgery, pregnancy or emotional crisis). Insulin is prescribed for the individual whose plasma glucose level cannot be controlled at acceptable levels despite weight control and adherence to dietary regulation, and for the treatment of ketoacidosis and non-ketotic hyperglycaemia. The main actions of insulin are summarized in Box 18.3.

Insulin may be prepared from the pancreas of pigs (rarely from beef) or, most commonly, synthetically by genetic engineering. Because it is a protein, insulin is destroyed in the gastrointestinal tract by proteinases; therefore, it must be given parenterally. Several types are available and may be classified as rapid acting with a

Box 18.2 Key points regarding diet for the person with diabetes mellitus

■ The diet provides approximately 55–60% of calories as carbohydrate, 12–20% as protein and less than 30% as fat

■ Total calorie intake will be adjusted as necessary for the individual to achieve and maintain a desirable weight

■ Calorie intake is adequate to provide for optimal growth and development (childhood, pregnancy and lactation)

■ Carbohydrate intake is evenly distributed throughout the day and consistent from day to day

■ The diet should consist of normal foods, with a preference for foods that contain unrefined carbohydrates and are high in soluble fibre

■ Food intake is adjusted to accommodate changes in lifestyle (e.g. illness, physical activity, emotional stress, eating out and travel)

■ Meal plans are individualized and consider social, cultural and ethnic values of the patient and family.

Box 18.3 Main actions of insulin (adapted from Walton and Brand 1994)

1. Stimulates glucose uptake by cells, thereby making it available for energy production.

2. Increases the storage of glucose as glycogen in liver and muscle.

3. Inhibits release of glucose from glycogen stores.

4. Stimulates conversion of glucose into glycerol, which then combines with fatty acids to form triglycerides which are stored in adipose (fatty) tissue.

5. Increases uptake of amino acids by cells and hence facilitates protein synthesis.

---

shorter duration of action, as intermediate acting with a longer duration of action, or as long acting with a prolonged duration of action. The *rapid-acting* preparations include unmodified, clear solutions such as soluble insulin. The *intermediate-acting* insulins include isophane insulins and insulin zinc suspensions. *Long-acting* insulins, which have an extended effect on lowering blood glucose, are mostly prolonged-action insulin zinc suspensions. Table 18.2 gives the onset and duration of action of each

type of insulin. These values are approximate, because individual differences in responses occur.

In addition, biphasic insulins are available which are a mixture of rapid-acting and long-acting insulins. The use of two different insulins has the advantage of combining an immediate effect with a more long-lasting sustained effect. Commonly used bipahsic insulins include Humalog Mix 25 (25% insulin lispro, 75% insulin lispro protamine), Human Mixtard (soluble and isophane insulin) and Humulin (soluble insulin and isophane insulin). Human Mixtard and Humulin are differentiated by the different recombinant technologies used in the production of the isophane insulin. Each is available in different proportions of the two types of insulin it contains.

It is important for the nurse caring for or counselling diabetics to be familiar with the action characteristics of the various types of insulin so that appropriate instruction can be given and the patients assisted in monitoring their medication.

Administration of insulin Insulin is measured in units. Each patient's regimen is determined individually in relation to a particular schedule and diet plan in an attempt to achieve a normal physiological level of glucose throughout a 24-hour period. The regimen is organized so that insulin action coincides with major meals and also provides action overnight. Diet and activity may have to be readjusted with the insulin routine to facilitate physiological control. Blood glucose levels are normally lowest during the night and begin to rise in the early morning hours. Most insulin regimens consist of combinations of rapid-acting and intermediate-acting insulin. Patients may use a multi-injection regimen with an intermediate-acting insulin given at bedtime and a rapid-acting insulin administered immediately before meals. Most patients can be taught to adjust or supplement their insulin regimen in response to changes in their blood glucose levels, changes in activity, eating patterns, stress or illness.

Insulin is given by subcutaneous injection below the subcutaneous fat to prevent lipodystrophy. The arms, thighs and abdomen are the areas used (Fig. 18.4). Injections should be at least 2.5 cm apart until the full site is completely used. The site is then rotated. Too frequent use of one site causes fibrosing and scarring, which delay absorption as well as make the injection more difficult. Disposable syringes with non-detachable needles of fine gauge are used with a capacity of either 0.5 mL (50 units insulin) or 1 mL (100 units). The site should be clean, but there is no need to swab it with an alcohol wipe as this has no effect on the normal bacterial population living on the skin and may lead to hardening of the skin. The injection should be given at 90° to the skin.

The use of an injection 'pen' makes the process of injecting more convenient and discreet (Watkins 1998). The device, similar to an ordinary cartridge pen, is loaded with a prefilled cartridge of insulin. The 'nib' of the pen is

Table 18.2 Examples of commonly used insulins

Category	Preparation	Source[a]	Onset	Peak	Duration
Rapid acting	Human Actrapid	Human	0.5	2–4	8
	Humulin S	Human	0.5	2–4	8
	Velosulin	Pork	0.5	2–4	8
	Pork Actrapid	Pork	0.5	2–4	8
Intermediate acting	Lispro	Human	0.5	2–4	8
	Humulin I	Human	1–2	4–8	16–35
	Hypurin Porcine Isophane	Pork	1–2	4–8	16–35
	Insulatard	Pork	1–2	4–8	16–35
	Human Insulatard	Human	1–2	4–8	16–35
Long acting	Human Monotard	Human	2.5	6–16	24
	Humulin Zn	Human	3	6–16	24
	Lentard MC	Pork and beef	3	8–18	24
	Human Ultratard	Human	4	8–30	36

The "Action (hours)[b]" header spans the Onset, Peak, and Duration columns.

[a]All pork and beef insulins are highly purified.
[b]Times of action vary in different patients and according to the source of insulin. Human insulin may have a more rapid onset than pork or beef insulin.

Figure 18.4 Sites for insulin injection.

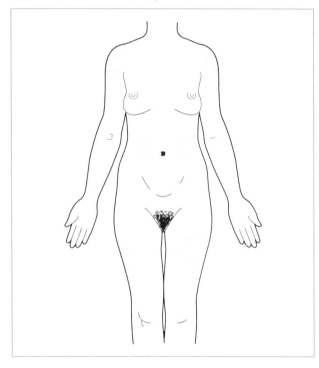

a disposable needle. The dose of insulin required is selected on the dial on the body of the pen, or clicks are counted, and the insulin is injected at the usual site. Individual regimens are planned with the patient according to needs and abilities. An alternative is subcutaneous administration via a small electrically driven pump attached to a belt. The patient 'tops up' the insulin level with a subcutaneous injection just before meal times. It is a very expensive technique and the pumps are prone to break down, leading to ketoacidosis. There are additional problems of increased infection risks. Problems such as these mean the technique is available at only a small number of specialist centres.

All insulin other than the soluble clear insulin must be thoroughly mixed before use to ensure uniform suspension and concentration throughout. This is done by rotating the bottle and inverting it slowly from end to end; vigorous shaking is avoided to prevent the formation of froth.

Some patients require a combination of extended-acting insulin with soluble insulin. If soluble and extended-acting insulin are to be mixed in the same syringe before injection, the following procedure should be adopted:

1. Inject air into cloudy insulin (lente, isophane).

2. Inject air into clear insulin (soluble).

3. Draw up correct dose of clear insulin and remove all bubbles of air.

4. Draw up correct dose of cloudy insulin.

If too much extended-acting (cloudy) insulin is drawn up into the syringe, do *not* inject it back into the vial, as the syringe contains a mixture of insulins, but dispose of the contents of the syringe and start again.

If soluble insulin and insulin zinc suspension (lente, ultralente) are mixed in the syringe, they must be given immediately. This is because excess zinc in the lente and ultralente preparations can delay the effect of the soluble insulin after mixing.

Soluble insulin and isophane (NPH) insulin can be mixed in the syringe and then stored in a refrigerator for up to 5 days, but it is normal practice to use them the same day. Before injecting the insulin it is important that the syringe is rotated between the hands for 10–15 seconds to ensure that the insulin is well mixed.

Each bottle of insulin bears an expiry date beyond which the content should not be used. Insulin should be kept in a cool place, preferably a refrigerator; freezing is avoided. Extremes of temperature and exposure to sunlight are likely to cause deterioration.

Complications of insulin therapy Various local and general reactions to insulin may occur. The *local reactions* are minor in nature and include local sensitivity, lipodystrophy and fibrosis. Frequently, when insulin therapy is first started, sensitivity may be manifested at the site of injection because the insulin is a foreign protein and antigenic. The area becomes red, swollen and itchy, but the response is generally temporary and disappears as the patient becomes desensitized by the repeated doses of insulin.

The local action of insulin on the adipose tissue cells may incur a swelling of the fatty tissue followed by atrophy, which leaves a hollow space in the area. These atrophic areas are not serious but present an undesirable cosmetic effect. Management may consist of switching the patient to a more purified pork insulin. Frequent and repeated injections into one area of tissue may result in hypertrophy of tissue and eventual fibrosing. Fibrous tissue has poor vascularization which decreases the rate of absorption of insulin. This complication may be prevented by systematic rotation of the injection sites and avoiding the use of any one spot more often than once every 4 weeks.

Oral hypoglycaemic drugs

Several groups of drugs are used in conjunction with dietary control in the treatment of type 2 diabetes. Avoidance of accidental hypoglycaemia is a high priority whichever drug is used. The term 'non-insulin-dependent diabetes' is misleading as up to 50% of patients with type 2 diabetes ultimately require insulin therapy (Barnett 2001). The main drugs used are described briefly below.

Sulphonylureas They stimulate the β cells in the islets of Langerhans to secrete more insulin and as a result can be very effective in reducing blood glucose levels in the early part of the disease. Commonly used examples are gliclazide, glipizide and glibenclamide, although the latter readily causes hypoglycaemia if taken in excess.

Biguanides The biguanides act by reducing the production of glucose in the liver and increasing glucose uptake in muscle. The person has to be manufacturing at least some insulin for these drugs to work. The only member of this group licensed in the UK is metformin, which has the disadvantage of causing gastric side-effects (nausea, vomiting, etc.).

α-Glucosidase inhibitors Intestinal enzymes known as α-glucosidases are important in breaking down carbohydrate molecules into short sugar chains. Competitive inhibition of these enzymes has a mild effect in reducing blood glucose levels. The only UK-licensed drug in this group is acarbose, which has the problem of causing severe flatulence.

Meglitinides The first drug in this group to be used in the UK is repaglinide, which is a derivative of glibenclamide. It is taken just before a meal, has a short duration of action and can be used with metformin (British National Formulary 2000).

Thiazolidinediones (glitazones) These recently introduced drugs increase the sensitivity of the body to insulin, thereby having an insulin-sparing effect. The two licensed UK products are rosiglitazone and pioglitazone, and they should be used in conjunction with either a sulfonylurea or metformin.

Barnet (2001) reports that a new group of products should be licensed for UK use very soon, known as the non-sulfonylurea insulin secretagogues, the first of which is likely to be *nateglinide*. The drug should be taken immediately before each meal and in the presence of food; it appears markedly to enhance insulin secretion, thereby reducing sharp rises in glucose level immediately after a meal.

Activity

The *goals* of activity and exercise for the person with diabetes mellitus are to:

1. establish a daily activity and exercise pattern to promote metabolic control

2. reduce the risk for cardiovascular and peripheral vascular complications

3. assist in weight control.

Physical activity promotes health and its importance is shown by the fact that 25% of diabetes is attributable to lack of exercise (Lehmann 1998). Apart from reducing obesity, activity promotes the uptake of glucose to muscle for a period several times longer than the period of exercise and hence reduces blood glucose levels (Pullen 2000). It also stimulates and improves the circulation, helps to maintain muscle tone, and promotes a sense of well-being. Some diabetics have sufficient exercise in their occupation, but those in sedentary jobs or who are retired should have a planned programme which is introduced gradually. As the prescription for diet and a hypoglycaemic agent is based on the patient's physical activity, the regimen should be approximately the same each day to minimize fluctuations in the blood glucose concentration. When variations in daily energy expenditure are necessary, adjustments in the diet may be needed. Extra carbohydrate in the form of fruit, milk or bread may be added if activity is increased, or even more concentrated carbohydrate forms may be required if activity is strenuous or prolonged. When the usual amount of activity is decreased for some reason (other than illness or infection), some decrease in the calorific and carbohydrate intake is usually indicated.

Active exercise at regular intervals is encouraged during hospitalization if at least a moderate degree of glycaemic control has been achieved. With an anticipated increase of activity on discharge from the hospital, the insulin dosage may be decreased and the food plan amended accordingly. For the older diabetic a daily routine of walking and light home chores (house and garden) is recommended.

The aim is to maintain a balance between energy expenditure and the prescribed treatment (diet with or without insulin or oral hypoglycaemic). More than the usual amount of exercise lowers the blood glucose level; less than the usual amount will raise it. Patients must be cautioned that exercise may aggravate the glycaemic state, causing hyperglycaemia and hyperketonaemia, when the person's glycaemic control is poor (if the blood glucose level is greater than 11 mmol/L).

The diabetic participating in strenuous activity, particularly if on insulin therapy, is likely to face several problems. The impaired physiology of diabetics may mean that they tire very quickly. If the person is insulin dependent, injected insulin is not inhibited by adrenaline and noradrenaline as happens with the normal person, lowering insulin levels, during exercise. Abnormally high levels of insulin therefore inhibit three normal mechanisms of energy release: growth hormone and cortisol release, the conversion of fatty acid glycerol to glucose and glucagon production (Pullen 2000). Hypoglycaemia may ensue as the uptake of glucose by muscles is unimpaired but the ability to mobilize glucose is poor. Careful, controlled experimentation under medical supervision with diet and insulin and frequent blood glucose monitoring are essential if the diabetic person is to achieve optimum performance in sporting events. However, the remarkable Olympic achievements of the oarsman Steve Redgrave are a testimony to what can be achieved.

Patient and family education

The overall *goals* of diabetic education are to:

1. impart the knowledge and skills necessary to maintain optimal glycaemic control

2. develop and foster the attitudes, beliefs and behaviours that are conducive to metabolic control

3. promote a quality of life whereby the individual's disease and lifestyle are harmoniously balanced.

The person with diabetes mellitus has a chronic lifelong disease. To achieve a state of health and an acceptable level of functioning, the person must learn to coordinate the treatment regimen of diet, activity and medication into a daily routine of work or school and recreation to achieve and maintain normal physiological blood glucose levels. The diabetic is ultimately responsible for the self-management of health care. To do this,

adequate knowledge and skill to be able to make informed decisions about health problems are required.

Nursing intervention

The nurse, with the doctor, dietician and pharmacist, is responsible for assessing learning needs, helping the patient to set realistic goals, providing knowledge, teaching necessary skills, identifying relevant learning resources and evaluating the outcomes of teaching. Diabetic education programmes benefit from a team approach.

All nurses should possess a sound working knowledge of diabetes as, whatever area of care you practice in, a significant proportion of your patients will be diabetic. Some nurses have, however, built up considerable levels of expertise in the specialist field of diabetic care and manage patients in primary care with a high degree of autonomy.

Assessment of learning needs

Assessment of what the patient already knows, learning capability and lifestyle factors that will influence learning and cooperation with the therapeutic plan is important before a learning plan can be developed. For a previously diagnosed diabetic, information is required about the usual diabetic routine at home, work or school, how usual activities have changed, community resources used, and what further information and skills are needed.

Assessment should include the patient's perceptions (which may be very different from the nurse's), their interpersonal relations, the social systems they live within (family, work, etc.), and finally the health state and usual capabilities of the person. This is a holistic approach to health that, while maintaining the importance of key physiological parameters such as blood glucose levels, brings in a host of other psychosocial factors that influence the health of persons with diabetes and their ability to cooperate with treatment. The patient's own goals for diabetes management can be made visible in this way. Coping strategies therefore need to be explored carefully with the patient as part of the assessment process. How the person lives with diabetes should be a major concern of the nurse.

Educating a patient does not, however, guarantee that there will be any observable change in behaviour. McIntyre and McDowell (1994) described an illuminating case study involving a 55-year-old Asian Muslim woman, Mrs R, who had had diabetes for 17 years. She was considered to be at risk of developing foot problems, so a teaching programme was instituted concerning foot care. The authors concluded that after 9 weeks her knowledge of diabetic foot care had increased significantly; however, her practice of it remained minimal. Similar findings were made for other aspects of self-care resulting in consistently high blood glucose levels and continued smoking. McIntyre and McDowell considered that Mrs R had not accepted that diabetic care was within her own control and consequently did not take responsibility for her own self-care. They speculated whether her Muslim religion encouraged a fatalistic view of life and health care, perhaps explaining her lack of self-care. This case study underlines two important points:

- Diabetes care and health education in general must encompass the whole individual and their psychosocial framework.

- Outcomes must be demonstrated that show changes in behaviour and health status before any health education programme can be claimed a success. Simply increasing patient knowledge is not sufficient on its own.

The patient's responses to diagnosis and treatment influence readiness to learn. Initial responses to the diagnosis may include fear, withdrawal or anger. Assessment of learning needs continues as patients work through their immediate reactions to reach a phase in which they may talk about their feelings and are prepared to listen and accept the reassurance that their disease can be controlled and that the necessary treatment and care can soon become a routine part of their life without seriously altering it.

Development of a teaching plan

Once learning needs have been identified, the nurse, with the patient and family, sets priorities. These may be dictated by the fact that the patient will be discharged in a few days and will be responsible for preparing meals and/or administering insulin. The knowledge and skill necessary for safe functioning assumes priority and must be adjusted according to the readiness of the patient to learn. Information available from Diabetes UK may provide further support after discharge home.

In planning the instruction, it is necessary to know the patient's background so that care can be adapted as much as possible to normal living patterns. The amount of information given at one time depends on the patient's ability and willingness to receive it. Generally, brief periods of discussion are more effective than the presentation of a large amount of information at one time. Group instruction may be used in the hospital or clinic for some topics, but it must be remembered that each diabetic's treatment and lifestyle are unique. A large part of the discussion must be on an individual basis. Patient negotiation and learning contracts are useful strategies to assist individuals with the development of self-management skills.

Teaching is begun as soon as possible to avoid giving too much at one time, leading to confusion and discouragement, and to allow time for the patient to practise self-care, read and ask questions.

Explanations are made in simple lay terms, and demonstrations are broken into steps, made slowly, repeated as often as necessary, and sufficient opportunity is provided for the patient to practise. Follow-up discussion of signs and symptoms experienced during episodes of

---

Box 18.4 Areas to be covered in an education programme for the patient with diabetes

- An explanation of diabetes – types and effects on everyday living

- Diet – meal plans, foods to avoid, a plan to achieve correct bodyweight

- Insulin therapy or oral hypoglycaemic agents, if appropriate – demonstrate correct technique for insulin injection, explain storage, time and dosage of insulin, or explain name, dosage and timing of oral hypoglycaemic drug

- Activity – balance of insulin and exercise

- Assessment of glycaemic control – explain and demonstrate technique for blood glucose monitoring, explain significance of variation in blood glucose levels

- Metabolic emergencies – discuss causes of hypoglycaemia and hyperglycaemia, and strategies to prevent or cope with problems

- Diabetic identification card

- Special personal care

- Regular health supervision – discuss long-term complications, signs to look out for and how to prevent them

- Sources of information and assistance.

---

hypoglycaemia and hyperglycaemia, and responses to interventions, helps the patient to develop the problem-solving skills needed for self-management. Illustrations, videos and written material should be used for clarification and reinforcement of teaching. The Diabetes UK website is a source of excellent teaching material.

An educational programme should cover the areas listed in Box 18.4.

Implementation of the teaching plan

How the learning plan is implemented depends upon the immediate patient situation and the agreed goals and plan. Rarely does one nurse have the opportunity to work with a patient and family throughout the learning process. Teaching carried out in hospital, whether with the newly diagnosed diabetic or with an established diabetic patient and family, requires evaluation and supplementation in the community as the person has the opportunity to apply knowledge and skill and learning needs continue to evolve.

The following is presented as an example from which the nurse can select the content relevant to an individual patient in a given situation.

What is diabetes mellitus? A simple basic explanation is made of the nature of diabetes, relating it to the symptoms experienced by the patient. To illustrate, the patient may be told that sugar and starches (such as bread and cereal) are converted by digestion to a simple form of sugar called glucose, which is the body's chief source of energy. In order for the cells to extract glucose from the blood and use it, the chemical insulin is necessary. There are two types of diabetes. In type 1 diabetes, there is not sufficient insulin being produced to use the amount of sugar and starches being taken, so glucose accumulates in the blood in excess of the normal. The kidneys remove some of the excess, which is why the diabetic voids a lot of urine that contains sugar. The loss of large amounts of urine results in thirst. Weakness, fatigue and hunger occur because the sugar is not being 'burned' to produce energy. The body, in an effort to provide energy, may break down body tissue, causing a loss of weight. Daily insulin injections and dietary measures are necessary to control this disorder.

With type 2 diabetes enough insulin to handle the amount of sugar may be produced but the cells cannot effectively utilize the glucose. This type of diabetes can usually be controlled by diet and activity to achieve a desirable bodyweight. Some patients may require an oral hypoglycaemic agent.

Diet The prescribed diet must be clearly and carefully interpreted to the patient and family. The initial instruction is usually given by a dietician, but considerable clarification and reinforcement by both ward and community nurses is necessary. The dietician explains the prescribed diet and reviews the foods allowed each day and how these may be distributed into meals and snacks. It is helpful for the patient to plan meals for several days. The purchase and preparation of food and how it may be worked in with the family meals are discussed.

The patient and health professional discuss and agree on a target or ideal bodyweight for the person. A plan to achieve and/or maintain the desirable weight is mutually developed and should include plans for regular weight checks.

Adjustment of diet and medications in relation to increased stress and changes in lifestyle is important. Diabetic patients can be taught to adjust their diet and medication in relation to change in demand for glucose and insulin. Blood glucose monitoring by patients has made it possible for them to achieve good glycaemic control during illness and to be more flexible in their eating patterns, activity and travel.

Eating out and delayed meals may also necessitate changes in food intake. Whenever possible, diabetics should maintain their usual eating pattern, including the time of meals and the content of each meal. They quickly learn to select appropriate meals from menus or from the selection offered by friends and relatives. When eating out, the diabetic should be prepared for delays and the possibility of hypoglycaemia by carrying sugar lumps or other sources of quickly absorbable carbohydrate. When aware that meals will be delayed, the patient is instructed to have a small snack before leaving home. Insulin-dependent diabetics with good understanding of their disease and its management may be provided with guidelines from their doctor on the use of compensatory insulin supplements before large meals. Patients using insulin pumps and blood glucose monitoring quickly learn to take an extra bolus of insulin with an unusually large meal.

The patient is encouraged to read and obtain for personal use books and pamphlets that contain considerable detail on diabetic dietary plans.

Drug therapy If the patient is on *insulin* therapy, advice is required on equipment and where it may be obtained. An explanation is made of what insulin is, types available, the name and nature of the insulin prescribed, and how it is identified. Unit dosage is explained and measurement by units is demonstrated. The injection technique (see p. 574) is described and demonstrated to the patient who is the encouraged to practise under supervision until competent. Storage and maintenance of an adequate supply of insulin are discussed. Automatic injectors are available which may be of assistance to patients who find injection of the needle difficult. The injector has a mechanically controlled spring which, when released, pushes the needle quickly through the skin. The need to plan and break down all this information into small logical teaching units or blocks is again emphasized. If discouragement and frustration are evident, further instruction is delayed and another approach considered.

If an *oral hypoglycaemic agent* is prescribed, the importance of taking the drug in the exact dosage at the times ordered is stressed. Written directions are given, and the patient is advised that if headache, nausea, vomiting or other disturbances are experienced, the general practitioner should be contacted. The patient is reminded not to experiment with the dosage of the drug and that adherence to the prescribed diet is most important even though medication is also being received.

Illness will affect drug medication. Diabetics are instructed on how to manage their disease during illness. If nausea and vomiting are present, the diet plan may be converted to liquids. A balanced diet may still be obtained. Vegetables and fruit may be ingested in the form of juices or soups. If oral intake is not possible, parenteral fluids are administered. The insulin-dependent diabetic and patients on oral hypoglycaemics should continue to take their medication during an illness. Larger doses of insulin with more frequent supplementary doses may be required. Insulin dosage should be adjusted according to prescribed guidelines in relation to blood glucose determinations. Insulin may be switched to soluble, short-acting insulin for the duration of illness.

Travel may also necessitate changes in drug therapy. The insulin-dependent diabetic needs to take precautions to avoid hypoglycaemia while travelling. If travelling by car, snacks or juices are kept available. On planes and trains, while meals may be obtained if delays occur, it is still important to carry some food in the hand-baggage in case there are problems. Additionally, luggage in the baggage hold of an aircraft can experience very low temperatures which may damage insulin. Travelling through several time zones should not pose any difficulties, provided a plan is developed ahead of time. The insulin-dependent diabetic must remember to carry insulin and syringes and be prepared to inject insulin wherever required. It is important for the patient to take a sufficient quantity of insulin and supplies for insulin administration and blood glucose monitoring or urine testing for the duration of any stay, as products may vary or be difficult to obtain in different countries. Insulin should be refrigerated whenever possible but will be quite safe if kept in a small insulated container to prevent exposure to high temperatures and bright light.

Activity Regular activity is beneficial and an integral component of the person's diabetic control. The nurse and patient should review usual activity patterns and develop plans for the person to receive consistent exercise. The person who participated in extended exercise activities before diagnosis is helped to develop a modified routine until glycaemic control is achieved and the skill of balancing diet and insulin in relation to activity has been learnt.

Precautions to avoid exercise-induced hyperglycaemia and hyperketonaemia include:

■ regulation of food and insulin intakes in conjunction with exercise

■ regular monitoring of blood glucose levels

■ a readily available source of carbohydrate

■ a decrease in insulin dosage before extended exercise

■ use of an injection site that is not active during exercise (e.g. the abdomen)

■ regular monitoring of blood glucose levels

■ avoiding exercise when glycaemic control is poor.

Skin integrity Diabetes increases the individual's risk for infection and skin breakdown. The person is taught to keep the skin clean, warm and free of irritation and pressure as far as possible. Precautions are taken to prevent cracks and breaks in the skin. Scratches, cuts and abrasions are cleaned and protected with a dressing. The use of strong antiseptic (such as iodine) and adhesive is avoided. Prolonged exposure to sunlight and the use of local heat applications (hot water bottle) are discouraged.

The adult diabetic's feet require regular special attention because of the increased susceptibility to circulatory disorders and loss of sensation. The patient is directed to bathe the feet daily with warm (not hot) water, using a mild soap and a small amount of bath oil, and to dry them thoroughly, especially the areas between the toes,

using gentle pressure rather than vigorous rubbing. Talcum powder may be used sparingly if the feet tend to be moist and perspire; if they are dry and scaly, a light application of lanolin or prescribed lotion is rubbed into the skin. The toenails are cut straight across with scissors. Calluses and corns should be treated by a state-registered chiropodist who is advised of the person's diabetes. The patient is cautioned against attempting to remove them by cutting or applying commercial preparations. Stockings or socks should fit well to avoid any constriction or wrinkles that might cause irritation or pressure, and are changed daily. To prevent possible interference with the circulation, garters are not worn. Shoes should be well fitting so there is no irritation or pressure on any part of the foot, and new shoes are worn only for brief periods until 'broken in'. Walking barefoot and the application of heating appliances are discouraged. The feet should be examined daily for breaks in the skin, discoloration, dryness and drainage. Numbness, persisting coldness, discoloration, a burning feeling, pain or any unusual condition of the lower limbs should be reported to the doctor.

Assessment of glycaemic control Urine testing has been the traditional method of monitoring diabetic control but more recently monitoring of capillary blood glucose has taken over as the method of choice.

Urine glucose monitoring is not adequate to enable good control of glycaemia. It does not identify hypoglycaemia and may not reveal hyperglycaemia; the latter is detected only when the blood glucose levels exceed the renal threshold, which is variable and may change in older diabetics and those with renal complications. Testing the urine for ketones is, however, useful when the blood glucose test result is raised, during periods of illness or stress, in pregnancy, or when oral hypoglycaemic therapy is being commenced.

Recent evidence (York CRD 2000) suggests that people with type 2 diabetes should have their urine screened twice yearly for proteinuria and, if this is negative, for microalbuminuria. A positive finding indicates damaged kidneys associated with microvascular pathology and raised blood pressure, which should be treated with ACE inhibitors whether the blood pressure is within a normal range (140/90 mmHg) or not (Melville et al 2000).

Blood glucose monitoring is easily perfected by most patients once they have adjusted to the invasive aspect of pricking their finger to obtain a drop of blood. Self-monitoring of blood glucose levels facilitates understanding of diabetes and gives the patient an active role in the management of the disorder. Satisfaction is generally high; infections and other complications due to self-monitoring are negligible.

Most monitors are intended to be used only with capillary blood and therefore should not be used with either venous or arterial blood as they will give false readings due to the differing partial pressure of oxygen that the sample will contain. Results can also be affected by abnormal haematocrit readings, and equipment will have a stated range within which the machine should be used. This is particularly important in areas such as intensive care and maternity (Batki 1999).

Monitoring of blood glucose levels may be done continually to build up the blood glucose profile of a 'typical day' to assess glycaemic control. This allows adjustment of diet, exercise and medication to achieve better control of blood glucose levels. It may also be done as a spot check for hypoglycaemia or during episodes of illness or when other problems occur. Self-monitoring of blood glucose is carried out using a reagent strip and a machine that gives a digital display of the result. It is important to follow the manufacturer's instructions precisely, particularly with regard to calibration, accuracy and timing. It is a common mistake to use the test strips after the recommended expiry date or to fail to store the strips in the airtight container.

The hand is washed in warm water to improve circulation and remove any contamination from the skin which, if transmitted to the blood drop, can affect the reading. A single-prong lancet pricks the skin either manually or as part of an automated device. A drop of blood large enough to cover the reagent pad is placed on a reagent strip, which is inserted into the machine and left for the period of time recommended by the manufacturer. The machine provides a digital readout of the result.

The person should be given information and teaching on the various types of equipment and their use. Pamphlets, audiovisual presentations and individualized instruction are usually available from the supplier. The newly diagnosed diabetic patient may not grasp the significance of the results initially; however, involvement in the decision making process about disease management will help to promote responsibility for self-care. The person should begin to keep a record of the results of the blood glucose tests while in hospital. The nurse and doctor discuss these with the patient each day, comparing results with the previous day and exploring factors that influenced any changes. This process is continued after discharge.

A very important method of assessing diabetic control is to measure glycated haemoglobin ($HbA1_c$) concentrations. Measurement of this fraction of haemoglobin gives a good indication of overall blood glucose levels over the previous 6–8 weeks and offers a validation check on the results the patient produces in their own diary. The results are expressed either as the percentage of $HbA1_c$ alone (normal value 4–6%) or as the percentage of total glycated haemoglobin (HbA1) including all other subfractions (a + b + c), which gives a normal range of 5–7% (Watkins 1998).

Knowledge of metabolic emergencies (hypoglycaemia and hyperglycaemia) The diabetic who is receiving insulin or an oral hypoglycaemic agent should know that under certain circumstances the blood glucose level may fall below normal, resulting in what is called an insulin or *hypoglycaemic* reaction. The patient and family should be familiar with the symptoms, which usually begin to appear when the blood glucose level falls below 3.3 mmol/L. A hypoglycaemic reaction in a person receiving rapid-acting insulin usually occurs approximately 2–6 hours after the injection. In a person receiving intermediate-acting insulin, the reaction happens more commonly in the afternoon or evening. Hypoglycaemic reactions to slow-acting insulin generally occur during the night or the following morning. It is possible for persons receiving oral hypoglycaemic drugs to develop hypoglycaemia.

Symptoms vary from one person to another, but each individual usually has similar symptoms with each reaction. The early signs and symptoms include sweating, tremor, apprehension, hunger, weakness, rapid pulse and palpitations. More advanced symptoms are faintness or dizziness, blurring of vision or diplopia, headache, slow reactions, uncoordinated movements, twitching, disorientation and confusion. The possible causes of hypoglycaemia are the delay or omission of a meal following administration of insulin or oral medication, excessive energy expenditure with prolonged and/or strenuous exercise, an overdose of insulin, anorexia, vomiting or diarrhoea, increased utilization of glucose and weight loss without readjustment of insulin dosage.

The person is instructed that on experiencing early symptoms carbohydrate should be taken immediately. With more pronounced symptoms, a quick-acting form of carbohydrate will be required, for example two or three cubes of sugar, tea or coffee with two or three teaspoonsful of sugar, two or three small sweets, orange juice or grape juice (120 mL) or two teaspoonsfuls of honey or syrup may be used. If the symptoms do not disappear in 10 minutes, the administration is repeated. The patient on insulin is advised always to carry lump sugar, boiled sweets or glucose tablets.

The family should know that, if the diabetic cannot swallow or retain sugar, glucagon should be administered or a 999 call made. Friends and associates as well as the family should know that the person takes insulin and may experience a reaction. Hypoglycaemic attacks should be reported to the doctor as the insulin dosage or diet may require adjustment.

The patient should also be able to recognize early symptoms of uncontrolled diabetes, which cause *hyperglycaemia*. If not corrected in the early stage, hyperglycaemia may lead to the serious complications of diabetic ketoacidosis or hyperosmolar non-ketotic coma. Hyperglycaemia and dehydration with or without ketosis develop more slowly than hypoglycaemia, usually over several days. The disturbance is usually manifested by loss of appetite, nausea, vomiting, thirst, weakness, drowsiness and general malaise. Glucose will be present in the urine and blood glucose levels are greatly increased. They are frequently associated with infection or stress, or may be due to prolonged dietary indiscretion or omission of insulin or oral hypoglycaemic agent. The patient is advised that the general practitioner should be contacted as soon as symptoms are experienced. Until medical attention is obtained the patient should remain in bed, keep warm, and try to drink clear fluids *without sugar*, to avoid dehydration and electrolyte imbalance, even if this causes vomiting. If possible, someone should remain with the patient.

Health management The newly diagnosed diabetic will be required to make more frequent visits to the general practitioner or diabetic clinic. These will become fewer as the disease and treatment are stabilized. The nurse in either situation checks how the patient is managing and gives the patient the opportunity to ask questions. Some aspects of care may require repetition and reinforcement. Before leaving the hospital, the importance of keeping appointments is stressed. In the case of older persons, assistance may be necessary in making arrangements for transport to the clinic.

It is advisable for the diabetic to have an annual *eye examination* because of the risk of diabetic retinopathy, which is the most common cause of blindness in advanced industrial countries. Up to 40% of people with diabetes have some retinopathy when type 2 diabetes is first diagnosed (York CRD 1999).

Every diabetic should carry a *diabetic identification card* at all times so that their condition can be made known quickly in the event of a reaction, illness or accident. Cards that carry appropriate information are available from the hospital, doctors, the diabetic clinic and Diabetes UK or its local branches. The patient should be informed about available *sources of help and information*. These include the national and local diabetic associations, which patients are encouraged to join. This entitles them to the regular periodical and additional literature published by Diabetes UK.

Evaluation of patient and family teaching

Studies of diabetic education use a variety of outcome measures to evaluate the effectiveness of education programmes and individual teaching. *Knowledge* of the disease and its management can be evaluated using tested tools. However, this knowledge has to be translated into positive behaviour. Auditing the frequency of hospital admissions, A&E attendances or clinic visits related to diabetes control and complications also gives a useful indication of how well the person is managing their diabetes.

Glycaemic control can be evaluated using blood glucose levels. These are useful for daily monitoring by the patient as well as by health professionals. The determination of glycosylated haemoglobin levels (see above) gives an accurate picture of long-term glucose control over the preceding 2 months. It is possible that the patient may

have deliberately recorded false values, showing much lower levels, in their diary. Such a situation needs great tact and good communication skills if it is to be resolved satisfactorily.

Attention must be given to the *patient's attitudes to diabetes* and what it means to them. Patient education should help diabetics achieve the highest standards of glycaemic control, but this should be accompanied by satisfactory emotional adjustment and social fulfilment. Diabetes educators need to address the affective or attitudinal aspects of coping with this lifelong condition.

The nurse in any clinical setting should always use the best source available to evaluate the effectiveness of *teaching the patient and family*. Only the patient and those close to him or her can determine whether the knowledge and skills taught meet their needs and whether the teaching contributed to their psychological and social adjustment to diabetes.

Two clinical situations are described in Case Studies 18.1 and 18.2.

Case Study 18.1

Grace Cook is a relatively inactive 60-year-old woman who enjoys baking and gardening. She is 10 kg overweight. She has been having a problem with a cut on her right middle finger that 'just won't heal'. She has also been experiencing blurring of her vision, has less energy than usual and, when questioned, thinks that she has been urinating more frequently. Her fasting blood glucose level was 13 mmol/L and negative for ketones when tested by her practice nurse.

Mrs Cook's doctor refers her to a dietician for dietary assessment and a diet for type 2 diabetes. The dietician finds that Mrs Cook is drinking a lot of fruit juices. She skips breakfast but eats a very large evening meal with her husband and continues to eat snacks throughout the evening while watching television.

Discussion

Mrs Cook is typical of many persons with type 2 diabetes. Her symptoms developed slowly, she has the major risk factor of obesity and she is within the age group of 40–65 years, when over 50% of non-insulin-dependent diabetics are diagnosed. Symptoms of hyperglycaemia experienced by Mrs Cook included decreased energy, urinary frequency, blurred vision and impaired healing. Her fasting blood glucose level was raised.

The patient's overall goals were to return to a normal bodyweight for her age and height, and to have blood glucose levels within normal limits.

Goals

Mrs Cook will:

1. decrease her bodyweight by 10 kg over the next 6–8 months

2. establish a regular pattern of exercise

3. alter her eating habits to decrease calorie intake, increase dietary carbohydrate and fibre, and eat three meals a day

4. have a blood glucose level of <9 mmol/L.

Intervention and evaluation

The dietician prescribed a weight-reducing diet which included three meals a day. She helped Mrs Cook to select foods that were high in complex carbohydrate and fibre. She told her to drink water or diet fizzy drinks rather than fruit juices for thirst. Mrs Cook was able to lose 1 kg in the first month of her diet and her fasting blood glucose level dropped to 10 mmol/L.

Exercise recommendations for type 2 diabetics include low-intensity exercise over 40–60 minutes on at least 5 days each week. Mrs Cook began taking a walk after breakfast. She did this for 30 minutes almost every day and was able to lose a further 0.5 kg in the second month. Her fasting blood glucose dropped to 8.7 mmol/L.

Case Study 18.2

Tom Tolly is a recently married 22-year-old construction worker. He has experienced a weight loss of 9 kg in the past 2 weeks, has been very thirsty and has been urinating large amounts. He has been getting up at night to urinate and to drink fluids. He states that his vision is blurred and that he is tired and lacks energy. His appetite has been very poor for the past few days and he has experienced nausea and stomach pain.

Tom went to his general practitioner whose practice nurse carried out a random capillary blood glucose measurement, which was over 30 mmol/L. His urine tested positive for glucose and ketones. Tom was sent to hospital for blood glucose tests. The results were: blood glucose 36 mmol/L, positive ketones; pH 7.0; and bicarbonate level 17 mmol/L.

Tom was admitted to hospital with a medical diagnosis of severe diabetic ketoacidosis. The medical goals of care are to rehydrate him and to treat his diabetes with insulin.

The priorities for nursing care relate to the patient's hyperglycaemic state. Although diabetic ketoacidosis can be resolved in 24 hours, it may be life threatening. Nursing actions included immediate and continuous assessment of Tom's metabolic state and the identification of associated health problems, as well as collaborative activities related to the implementation and evaluation of medically directed care. The long-term goal for Tom and his wife is to control and achieve self-regulation of his diabetes.

Tom's hyperglycaemia is related to diabetic ketoacidosis and is due to inadequate production of insulin associated with his undiagnosed type 1 diabetes mellitus. He demonstrates the characteristic clinical picture of a person with diabetic ketoacidosis. His symptoms, which developed over a 2-week period, include thirst, polyuria, blurring of vision, weakness, loss of appetite, nausea and gastrointestinal discomfort. The results of diagnostic tests show that Tom has glycosuria, as evidenced by the presence of glucose and ketones in his urine, and that he is hyperglycaemic; his blood glucose level is raised and ketones are present. His bicarbonate level is decreased (normal range 24–32 mmol/L) and his pH is below normal (normal 7.35–7.45). As the nurse, you expect to observe changes in respirations. *Kussmaul breathing* (rapid, deep respirations) is usually present in diabetic ketoacidosis when the pH is below 7.2. When the bicarbonate level decreases, hyperventilation occurs in order to drive off excess carbon dioxide in an attempt to maintain the pH at a physiological level. When the pH is less than 7.0, the compensatory mechanisms change and slower respirations result. Tom is in a very vulnerable state with a pH of 7.0.

The nurse must also be alert for the development of drowsiness and confusion as Tom's metabolic state is no longer compensated and increases in the partial pressure of carbon dioxide (P_{CO_2}) will have a depressing effect on his central nervous system.

The actual and potential *patient problems* on admission to hospital are listed in Table 18.3.

The *goals* for Tom on admission in hospital are that:

1. he will achieve fluid, electrolyte, acid–base and metabolic balance

2. he and his wife will develop a basic understanding of his diabetes and resulting ketoacidosis.

Table 18.3 presents the care plan developed for a patient with ketoacidosis.

Evaluation

On admission to hospital Tom was acutely ill and required skilled care from knowledgeable, experienced nurses. The nurses worked in collaboration with the doctors to manage the acute medical problems. Many of the patient problems discussed in Table 18.3 fall primarily into the realm of

Table 18.3   Care plan for a patient with ketoacidosis

Goals	Nursing intervention	Rationale
Patient problem 1: Fluid volume deficit due to polyuria and glycosuria		
1. Fluid intake and urine output will be in physiological balance 2. Mucous membranes will be moist 3. Blood glucose levels will decrease towards normal	Administer 0.9% saline at 650 mL/h for the first 2 h as ordered. Adjust rate as indicated	The severe dehydration is life threatening. Isotonic fluids are administered rapidly to restore the intravascular volume and increase cardiac output
	Accurately record fluid intake and output hourly	
	Assess for signs of fluid overload: dyspnoea, pulmonary crackles and wheezes, increased central venous pressure	
	Assess blood pressure, pulse and respirations hourly	Hypotension and tachycardia occur in response to hypovolaemia and decreased tissue perfusion
	Record patient's temperature 2–3 hourly	Dehydration produces a rise in body temperature
	Provide mouth care regularly	
Patient problem 2: Metabolic imbalance: ketoacidosis related to decreased production of insulin		
1. Serum glucose level will be 5.6–7.8 mmol/L 2. Serum acetone level will be 51.6–344.0 mmol/L 3. Urine will be negative for glucose and ketones	Administer regular insulin by continuous i.v. infusion (8 units/h) and adjust rate as ordered	Low-dose infusions of insulin are effective in decreasing the catabolic process and promoting glucose uptake by the cells. The rate of flow (dosage) is determined by blood glucose levels and decreased ketosis
	Monitor blood glucose and acetone levels, urine glucose and ketones and urinary output hourly	
	Assess hourly for signs of hypoglycaemia	Sudden reduction in blood glucose levels can cause tachycardia and symptoms of hypoglycaemia
Patient problem 3: Ineffective breathing pattern related to hyperventilation in response to metabolic acidosis		
1. Respirations will be 20–24/min and regular 2. Blood gases, pH and bicarbonate levels will return to normal range	Assess respiratory rate, depth and rhythm hourly	Hyperventilation occurs with acidosis. Respirations decrease with pH less than 7.0
	Change position 2-hourly and assess response to position change	
	Administer oxygen by nasal cannulae as ordered	To increase tissue perfusion
	Evaluate blood gas level	
Patient problem 4: Sensory/perceptual deficits due to ketoacidosis, central nervous system depression, and blurring of vision		
1. pH will be within normal limits 2. Serum glucose levels will be within normal limits 3. Patient will respond appropriately to the environment and to verbal commands	Assess level of consciousness and pupillary responses, reflexes and behavioural responses 2-hourly and record	Cognitive and perceptual changes are multifactorial in origin and can develop in response to aggressive rehydration and treatment of acidosis
	Call by name	
	Explain all procedures and activities and describe what is happening	
	Explain that vision will clear when diabetes is controlled	Awareness that blurring of vision is transient helps to decrease fear
	Keep cot sides in place on bed	

(Continued)

Table 18.3   (*Continued*)

Goals	Nursing intervention	Rationale
Patient problem 5: Alteration in nutrition: intake less than body requirement due to inability to utilize glucose as a result of insulin deficit, loss of appetite, nausea and gastrointestinal discomfort		
1. Abdominal distension and discomfort will be absent	Assess for abdominal distension and signs of increased abdominal discomfort	Gastric mobility is impaired with ketoacidosis
2. Gastrointestinal sounds will be present on auscultation	Pass nasogastric tube	To decompress gastrointestinal tract and reduce discomfort
3. Patient will take oral fluids with no discomfort	Document amount and colour of aspirated gastric content	
	Following removal of nasogastric tube, administer small amounts of clear fluid and assess for distension and discomfort	
	Answer questions regarding diabetic diet and explain that the dietician will see the patient before discharge	
Patient problem 6: Impaired physical mobility related to weakness, fatigue and restrictions of treatment		
1. Peripheral pulses will remain palpable	Assess peripheral skin colour and peripheral pulses 2-hourly	Patient is at risk for developing vascular thrombi due to decreased intravascular volume with dehydration and acidosis, increased blood viscosity, decreased tissue perfusion, decreased cardiac output and increased adhesiveness of platelets
2. Peripheral skin will be normal and warm to touch	Provide antiembolic stockings if prescribed	
3. Patient will move to bedside chair within 24 h	Perform passive leg exercises 2-hourly while awake until fully mobile	
4. Rehydration will be evident by urine output of >1.5 L/day and normal vital signs	Mobilize patient as soon as possible	
Patient problem 7: Lack of knowledge about diabetes mellitus, ketoacidosis and their management		
1. Patient and family will be able to describe the causes of ketoacidosis and signs of hyperglycaemia	Assess level of understanding of diabetes and ketoacidosis	If the patient and family are knowledgeable about the signs and symptoms of hyperglycaemia and appropriate interventions, future episodes of ketoacidosis are largely preventable
2. Patient and family will verbalize plans to begin learning about diabetes and its management	Provide explanations of all procedures and activities	
	Answer questions from patient and family	
	Develop an initial learning plan with the patient and family as soon as they are able to participate	

nursing. The patient usually makes a good recovery with prompt care and is normally awake, self-caring and mobile within 48 hours of admission.

Teaching plan

A teaching plan is developed with Tom and his wife. Teaching will be carried out in short intervals throughout the day to accommodate his limited physical tolerance and shortened attention span. Teaching sessions with the dietician, pharmacist and nurse are arranged for late afternoons when Mrs Tolly will be present. Because of the overwhelming quantity of new knowledge and skills faced by Tom and his wife, care is taken to limit teaching to that which they need to know to function safely on discharge. The following expectations are agreed to.

Goals

The reader is referred to the list on page 577. Additional goals which might be incorporated in a teaching package include the ability for Mr and Mrs Tolly to:

1. experience a gradual increase in weight for Tom from his present 65.5 kg to his ideal bodyweight of 72 kg

2. understand how insulin works

3. describe the role of exercise in diabetes management

4. discuss with health professionals the adjustments to insulin dose as a result of changes in blood glucose levels

5. verbalize awareness of complications of diabetes

6. describe the relationship between diabetes control and the development of complications

7. talk about the meaning of the diabetes to themselves, their new relationship and their future lifestyles

8. confirm that their major concerns have been addressed

9. describe an agreed plan for continuing education and medical supervision on discharge.

Tom's major expressed difficulties are: (1) how he can continue his current job, which often does not have regular coffee and lunch breaks and is very physically demanding; and (2) acceptance of the fact that he has diabetes when he is a young, healthy man, recently married and enjoys sports and drinking alcohol with friends.

The nurse should discuss Tom's concerns with him and arrange for the dietician to talk with him about possible solutions to the irregular meals and snacks he will experience at work. It will be possible for him to learn to adjust his insulin administration when he knows that meals will be delayed. He can also carry snacks with him to take when meals are delayed. Although his present insulin dosage is being regulated according to his restricted activity in hospital, this will be increased and regulated according to the demands of his usual work activity. He should be referred to the occupational health department in his place of work. He should be told that he will still be able to participate in active sports. It is important that Tom has regular, consistent exercise. When exercise is extended or excessive, he will have to take glucose supplements such as fruit and sweets and adjust his insulin. He is assured that he will have the opportunity to learn these skills once metabolic control is re-established and after he has learnt the basics of diet, insulin and exercise management. The doctor will help him with regulation of the insulin and a referral will be made for the diabetic nurse specialist to work with Tom and his wife when he returns home.

Another area to explore with Tom concerns sex, as he may have experienced difficulty in maintaining an erection due to his diabetes. It should be explained that the severely high blood glucose levels he experienced with the uncontrolled diabetes may cause impotence and that this will resolve when metabolic control is re-established. The diabetes will not affect his sexual desire but when the diabetes is uncontrolled he may be unable to achieve or maintain an erection. As this problem may impede progress, alter self-concept and affect his new role as a husband, the nurse should encourage him to discuss this with his wife. The initial and later changes in sexual function associated with diabetes can represent the most difficult adjustments faced by persons with diabetes. The reality of impotence, concerns about infertility and the stress these place on the relationship are major concerns for any patient and family. The nurse may give Tom a pamphlet on sexual health and diabetes, and plan to reassess his concerns and discuss them further before his discharge.

Acute metabolic emergencies

Diabetic ketoacidosis

Diabetic ketoacidosis is a serious metabolic complication that develops when there is too little insulin and an excess of glucose.

The cause of insulin deficiency may be inadequate production of insulin in the undiagnosed diabetic, inadequate administration of insulin or an increased need for insulin resulting from emotional or physical stresses such as infection. Excess glucose may result from increased hepatic production of glucose, decreased utilization of glucose by peripheral tissue and increased ingestion of glucose in the diet.

The production of **ketone bodies** involves processes occurring in adipose tissue, liver and muscle. The glucose in the blood cannot be utilized by the cells, and fat is broken down to provide energy. Fat is mobilized and broken down rapidly, producing ketone bodies (acetoacetic acid, β-hydroxybutyric acid and acetone) in excess of the ability of tissue cells to metabolize them. Alterations in liver metabolism lead to further ketone production. This process is accelerated when glucagon levels rise. An associated decrease in the ability of muscle tissue to utilize these organic acids further contributes to ketoacidosis. The acids and acetone accumulate in the blood. At first the normal pH is maintained by the buffer systems, but eventually the alkali reserve becomes depleted and the pH of the body fluids falls, resulting in acidosis. At the same time, the increased concentration of glucose causes an increased output of urine (osmotic diuresis), and dehydration develops. The increased osmotic pressures of the extracellular fluid result in the movement of fluid out of the cells accompanied by electrolytes. Serious sodium, potassium and phosphate deficiencies develop.

Ketones
See chapter 2.6

Symptoms

Ketoacidosis has an insidious onset over several days, being preceded by symptoms characteristic of uncontrolled diabetes (polyuria, thirst, glycosuria, weakness). The symptoms related to the accumulation of ketones and reduced alkalinity of body fluids include anorexia, nausea, vomiting, deep and rapid respirations, drowsiness, weakness which progresses to prostration, and abdominal pain or muscular cramps. The skin and mouth are dry, and the eyeballs are soft because of dehydration. The patient may appear flushed in the early stages but later becomes pale owing to hypotension. The pulse is rapid and may be weak because of severe dehydration and the reduced intravascular volume. Unless the condition is recognized and treated promptly, the blood pressure falls, the patient becomes comatose, and brain damage will occur unless the situation is reversed quickly. Even though the patient may be fully conscious and walking when presenting in the health centre or medical admissions unit, he or she is seriously ill with the risk of a rapid deterioration in their condition leading to coma, brain damage and possible death.

The patient's urine shows a high concentration of glucose, while blood glucose levels are well above normal. Ketones will be found in the urine related to increased levels of ketones in the blood. Reduced serum bicarbonate levels ($<12\,$mmol/L) indicate severe acidosis associated with the raised ketone levels in plasma. The patient's reserves of sodium, potassium and chloride are greatly reduced as a result of the loss of fluid and dehydration. The leucocyte count is generally raised as part of the stress response. There may be no correlation between the blood glucose levels and the severity of the ketoacidosis; only moderately increased blood glucose levels may be associated with a life-threatening ketoacidosis.

Treatment and nursing intervention

The treatment and nursing intervention for the patient with diabetic ketoacidosis requires emergency care that is directed toward stimulating the utilization of glucose by the cells and decreasing the production of ketone bodies by the administration of insulin, and correction of dehydration and the electrolyte imbalance. Any causative disorder is also treated.

An indwelling catheter may be inserted if the patient is comatose, to enable monitoring of urinary output. If the patient is stuporous or comatose, a nasogastric tube is passed to avoid risk of aspiration of vomitus. The patient receives an intravenous infusion of soluble (rapid acting) insulin. Continuous cardiac monitoring is necessary to detect cardiac arrhythmias due to abnormal blood potassium levels. Intravenous fluids are given to correct electrolyte deficits as well as dehydration. The initial solution used is usually normal saline, 1 litre in 30 min, followed 0.5 litre in 30 min and then 0.5 litre in 1 hour. As potassium moves out of the cells in this situation, first the serum concentration may be misleadingly normal or even raised. With the administration of the intravenous infusions and insulin, plasma potassium moves into the cells and hypokalaemia develops, which may necessitate the administration of potassium chloride supplements to the intravenous infusion. Repeated blood electrolyte, glucose and ketone determinations are necessary. When the blood

glucose level approaches normal, the frequency of administration and the dosage of insulin are decreased, and an intravenous glucose solution (5% in water or saline) may be ordered. If the patient's blood pressure is low and shock is present, plasma or plasma expanders may be given. Unless the cause of the ketoacidosis was evident at the onset, efforts are made to determine why it occurred.

A clinical situation of diabetic ketoacidosis is described in Case Study 18.2.

Hyperglycaemic, hyperosmolar, non-ketotic diabetic coma

This serious metabolic complication is characterized by severe hyperglycaemia with no significant ketosis or acidosis. Serum osmolarity is increased; insulin is deficient but not absent; and severe dehydration and hypovolaemia exist.

Hyperglycaemic, hyperosmolar non-ketotic **coma** is most likely to occur in elderly people and carries a mortality rate of 40% or more (Haslett et al 1999). The patient may not even have been diagnosed as a diabetic when they present in a collapsed condition, usually to A&E or a medical emergency admissions unit. The onset of hyperglycaemic, hyperosmolar non-ketotic coma is insidious, occurring over several days. The patient demonstrates weakness, polyuria and polydipsia. As intracellular dehydration progresses and fluid shifts to the extracellular spaces, symptoms of neurological involvement, lethargy, confusion, convulsions and eventually coma develop.

Treatment

Treatment is directed toward reversing the hyperosmolar state with fluid replacement and correcting underlying causes. The prognosis for patients with this condition is generally poor but is improved with prompt treatment. Treatment differs in three ways from that of ketoacidosis:

1. Hypotonic saline solutions (0.45%) are given intravenously instead of the isotonic solutions (0.9%) used to treat ketoacidosis. Central venous pressure monitoring serves as a guide to the rate of infusion.

2. Insulin is administered intravenously, but lower doses are required than for ketoacidosis.

3. Thromboembolic problems are common; therefore heparin should be given.

Nursing intervention

Nursing intervention is similar to that outlined in Table 18.3 for the patient with diabetic ketoacidosis. Careful monitoring and recording of the large volumes of hypotonic parenteral solutions that are administered is important. The patient is assessed for signs of fluid overload, which include dyspnoea, pulmonary crackles and wheezes, and increased central venous pressure. The low doses of insulin prescribed are administered using an infusion controller to regulate the dosage carefully.

Coma
See chapter 2.6

Observations should be made for signs of hypoglycaemia as a precaution.

Care of the patient with altered levels of consciousness is discussed in Appendix 1. Nursing intervention includes measures to maintain a patent airway, personal safety and pressure area care.

The patient and family's level of understanding of diabetes, the causes of metabolic complications, general disease management and actions to take when complications occur are assessed. An individualized teaching plan is developed, implemented and evaluated; referrals are made to the community nurse where appropriate. Attempts are made to determine the factors precipitating the episode and to institute measures to prevent future episodes of hyperosmolar, non-ketonic coma.

Hypoglycaemia

Hypoglycaemia implies an abnormally low blood glucose concentration. The onset of symptoms varies with individuals and consequently different people develop symptoms at different blood glucose. Both type 1 and type 2 diabetics can have hypoglycaemic episodes; the most frequent cause of the problem is inadequate patient education. The patient may take their normal medication but miss or delay a meal or eat a meal that is inadequate in carbohydrate content. Unexpected exercise or excess alcohol intake can also provoke an episode. Errors in self-medication or deliberate self-harm caused by manipulation of the dietary or hypoglycaemic medication regimen may also lead to hypoglycaemia. Nocturnal hypoglycaemia may occur if the patient has a poorly designed insulin regimen.

A hypoglycaemic reaction in a patient receiving rapid-acting (soluble) insulin usually occurs approximately 2–6 hours after the injection. In the patient receiving an intermediate-acting insulin given in the morning, it happens more commonly in the afternoon or evening. Hypoglycaemic reaction to a slow-acting insulin generally occurs during the night or early in the morning of the following day. It is also possible for the patient receiving an oral hypoglycaemic agent to develop hypoglycaemia. It develops insidiously and may occasionally go unrecognized.

The signs and symptoms manifested by an abnormally low blood glucose level are a reflection of its effect on the central nervous system. The brain is very dependent on a constant, adequate supply of glucose. Any deprivation, even for a relatively brief period, may seriously impair cerebral activity and result in permanent damage. Similarly, repeated occurrences of hypoglycaemia, even of short duration, especially in children, may incur some permanent cerebral impairment. The manifestations of hypoglycaemia vary from one patient to another but tend to be the same with each reaction for the same person, which makes it more easily recognizable by the individual. The earlier signs and symptoms include sweating, tremor, apprehension, hunger, weakness, tachycardia and palpitation. Symptoms usually do not appear until the blood glucose level is 2.8–3.3 mmol/L. More advanced symptoms are faintness or dizziness, blurring of vision or diplopia, headache, slow reactions, uncoordinated movement which occasionally leads to mistaking the patient's condition for alcohol intoxication, muscular twitching that may progress to convulsions especially in children, disorientation and confusion, stupor and eventual loss of consciousness. The urine is usually negative for glucose although, occasionally, a trace may be found if the bladder has not been emptied for a few hours. All diabetics, their immediate family and close associates should be familiar with the early signs and symptoms of hypoglycaemia and should know what to do.

If the patient can still swallow, some form of rapidly absorbable concentrated sugar should be given; 10–20 g of carbohydrate are usually sufficient to restore the blood glucose level. Two teaspoons of sugar or 200 mL of milk contain 10 g of glucose. Hypostop Gel ampoules can also be used, or spoonfuls of jam or honey. After eating, the person should measure the blood glucose level 15–20 minutes later. If there is no improvement, the administration is repeated. If the patient is unconscious or uncooperative, 30–50 mL of 50% glucose are given intravenously. Glucagon (1 unit) subcutaneously may be ordered to promote hepatic breakdown of glycogen (glycogenolysis) and subsequent increase in blood glucose. It also stimulates the secretion of insulin. Family members may be taught to administer the glucagon. A venous or capillary blood specimen is collected as soon as possible and is repeated at frequent intervals for blood glucose determinations until the patient is stabilized.

Following a reaction, the patient is encouraged to rest for several hours in order to decrease the utilization of blood glucose. Carbohydrate administration may be repeated and some form of protein (cheese or milk) should be given to the patient to provide additional glucose that is produced gradually as a result of protein metabolism. The nurse should check with the doctor before giving the next scheduled dose of insulin. If the patient is at home, instructions should be given not to take more insulin or hypoglycaemic agents at that time. Adjustments are usually made in the carbohydrate content of the diet and in the insulin dosage.

Most diabetic patients and their families are taught which symptoms signal hypoglycaemia or hyperglycaemia. Evidence suggests that people miss hypoglycaemia or hyperglycaemia symptoms and erroneously believe that their blood glucose levels are within normal range, or feel they are hypoglycaemic or hyperglycaemic when they are not. Self-monitoring of blood glucose, while readily available and used by many diabetic patients, is not necessarily used appropriately to confirm subjective symptoms. The individual's ability to distinguish good predictors of blood glucose levels can be improved through systematic

Hypoglycaemia
See chapter 2.5

training. The person may be helped to review documented daily blood glucose levels and associated symptoms and to identify which cues are predictive of the actual blood glucose levels. This problem-solving approach requires that the patient and a family member or close associate be knowledgeable of the symptoms, the measurement of blood glucose levels, the associated risk factors and the treatment of hypoglycaemia. The patient and family member will learn from the experience if encouraged to examine the reaction in retrospect. A discussion of the possible cause and the early symptoms may be helpful in preventing further reactions and in having the patient recognize hypoglycaemia at the onset.

The *Somogyi effect* occurs in insulin-dependent diabetics who are treated too aggressively in an attempt to normalize blood glucose levels. The hypoglycaemia resulting from administration releases counter-regulatory hormones, producing a rebound hyperglycaemia. The insulin produces a decrease in blood glucose concentration, which triggers the sympathetic nervous system to release ACTH. The liver releases glycogen and the blood glucose level rises. Further administration of insulin causes a repeat of the cycle. Sudden falls in blood glucose levels followed by rebound hyperglycaemia are characteristic of the Somogyi effect. Treatment consists of gradually decreasing the insulin dosage. The phenomenon is less common in patients whose diabetes is controlled by insulin infusion pumps.

Thyroid disorders
See chapter 2.6

Hypothyroidism
See chapter 2.6

The person with a disorder of the thyroid gland

Disease of the thyroid may cause a hyposecretion or hypersecretion of the thyroid hormones and a change in the size of the gland. A deficiency in the secretion is called *hypothyroidism*; an excessive secretion is referred to as *hyperthyroidism*. The normally functioning gland is referred to as *euthyroid*.

Assessment

Assessment of the person with a disorder of the thyroid gland begins with a comprehensive health history. The health problems experienced by the individual usually develop gradually and are vague and general in nature. Knowledge of the clinical characteristics of altered thyroid function assists the nurse to organize data collection, to formulate specific questions for the health history and to identify patterns of responses demonstrated by the patient. Table 18.4 lists the common health problems experienced by persons with thyroid disorders and the clinical characteristics of hypothyroidism and hyperthyroidism.

Health history

The patient is asked about changes in physical appearance, activity tolerance and energy level, skin moisture, muscle tone, bodyweight, diet, menstrual cycle and thought processes. Specific questions related to usual and current daily routine and activity patterns and how the individual organizes the day may provide clues to subtle changes and how the person is compensating. With questioning, the person may recognize that they have become more forgetful and have compensated for the changes by instituting reminders for themselves to keep appointments and fulfil commitments. They may also recognize insidious changes in physical activity and usual exercise patterns. Other specific information includes any difficulty in swallowing, episodes of palpitations, prescription and non-prescription medications taken and any family history of thyroid disease. It is important to identify the onset and duration of the symptoms.

Physical examination

Physical examination begins with observation of the person's *general appearance*. Changes that may indicate decreased thyroid function are paleness, facial puffiness and a non-expressive appearance. The person with increased thyroid function may appear anxious and agitated and their eyeballs may protrude. The *skin* and *hair* are inspected for dryness, brittleness and texture. The density and pattern of hair distribution are noted. *Vital signs* are measured because changes in respiratory rate and depth, blood pressure and cardiac rate and rhythm may be present.

Hypothyroidism

Hypothyroidism is a common disorder characterized by a hypometabolic state. It is more common in females and can occur at any age but the incidence is higher in the elderly.

Causes and contributing factors

The deficiency of thyroid hormones may be primary, due to a disorder in the thyroid itself, or may be secondary as a result of a pituitary or hypothalamic disturbance. If the dysfunction is congenital or develops in infancy or early childhood, it gives rise to cretinism which is characterized by a failure to achieve normal physical growth and mental development. In the adult it produces myxoedema.

Primary hypothyroidism accounts for about 95% of the cases of hypothyroidism in adults. It is due to destruction of thyroid tissue by disease, surgery or radioactive iodine treatment of hyperthyroidism. Autoimmune thyroid disease (Hashimoto's thyroiditis) is the most common cause of hypothyroidism.

A less common cause is iodine deficiency, which produces an enlargement of the thyroid gland known as a goitre. The enlargement of the thyroid in iodine deficiency occurs because of stimulation by an increased release of thyroid-stimulating hormone (TSH) by the anterior pituitary in response to the low thyroxine concentration of the blood. The follicles increase in number and size and the thyroid becomes more vascular.

Table 18.4   Assessment of the person with altered thyroid function

	Clinical characteristics	
	Hypothyroidism	Hyperthyroidism
Nutrition and metabolism	Pulse rate decreased Blood pressure low Respirations decreased Appetite poor Weight gain Serum cholesterol raised	Pulse rapid and bounding Palpitations Increased blood pressure Respiratory rate increased Appetite increased Weight loss Serum cholesterol decreased
Activity tolerance	Weakness and fatigue Slow movements Dyspnoea Decreased muscle tone and reflexes	Weakness and fatigue Weakness of eyelid muscles Shortness of breath on exertion Tremor of hands Increased muscle tone and reflexes
Skin integrity	Skin dry, thick and pale Eyelids oedematous Lips and tongue enlarged Hair coarse and sparse Interstitial oedema	Increased sweating Skin warm and moist Eyelids retracted Hair loss
Thought processes and emotional responses	Slow mental processes Increased sleep and lethargy Speech hoarse, slow and monotonous Depression Mental disturbance	Anxiety, apprehension Restlessness Irritability Emotional instability Insomnia
Bowel elimination	Decreased gastrointestinal motility Constipation	Increased gastrointestinal motility Diarrhoea
Thermoregulation	Sensitivity to cold Decreased body temperature	Sensitivity to heat Increased body temperature
Sexuality patterns	Metrorrhagia Amenorrhoea Low sex drive Infertility	Oligomenorrhoea or amenorrhoea Low sex drive Impotence

A deficiency in the natural supply of iodine in the water and soil occurs in inland areas distant from the sea. The addition of iodine to the salt used in food has largely eliminated this once endemic cause of hypothyroidism in the UK.

Clinical characteristics

A decreased production of tri-iodothyronine (T_3) and thyroxine (T_4) influences most metabolic processes of the body, resulting in many and varied manifestations.

The symptoms and the rate at which they develop correspond to the degree of thyroid inactivity. An abnormal decrease in thyroid hormone causes a general reduction in cellular metabolism, producing mental and physical sluggishness. The person gradually exhibits apathy and slowness in responses. An abnormal deposition of a mucopolysaccharide, which tends to hold water, occurs in the subcutaneous tissues, giving the person an oedematous appearance. The skin becomes dry and thick, the face

(particularly the eyelids) appears puffy and the lips and tongue enlarge. The person experiences weakness, fatigue and an increased sensitivity to cold, and appetite is poor although there may be a gain in weight. The temperature, pulse and blood pressure may be abnormally low. Mental processes are slow and the patient sleeps a great deal. Impaired function of the reproductive system is manifested by menstrual disorders, such as metrorrhagia and amenorrhoea, and loss of sexual drive. Hoarseness and slow, monotonous speech may be noted (Elliot 2000). Because of complacency and dull mental processes, the condition may appear to be of much less concern to the patient than to the family or friends witnessing the changes. Allowed to progress, the disorder may lead to cardiac insufficiency, depression or the patient may pass into a comatose state.

Older persons with hypothyroidism are more predisposed to develop coma, particularly in response to cold weather when body temperature may fall to hypothermic levels and respiratory insufficiency may develop.

With a goitre, the enlarged gland may cause disfigurement which creates embarrassment for the person. More serious symptoms are pressure on the larynx and trachea, manifested by a chronic cough and respiratory difficulty, interference with swallowing, and compression of nerves in the area.

Treatment

Hypothyroidism is treated with thyroid hormone replacement therapy, usually thyroxine in uncomplicated cases. In cases where there are complications, such as ischaemic heart disease, tri-iodothyronine (T_3) may be given. T_3 acts very rapidly, but the effect is sustained for a shorter period than that of thyroxine (T_4), which is not fully effective before 7–10 days. The dosage is usually small to start with and is increased gradually to guard against too sudden and excessive a demand on the heart by rapid acceleration of metabolism. The pulse is checked and recorded frequently until the maintenance dose is established. Symptomatic relief for the patient will usually be reported within 2–4 weeks of beginning replacement therapy, but it takes up to 6–8 weeks for steady-state levels of thyroid hormones to be achieved (Elliot 2000). Patient and family should therefore be advised that there will be only a gradual improvement in symptoms. Adverse effects are almost entirely related to under-replacement, with the symptoms of hypothyroidism remaining, or to over-replacement, producing symptoms of hyperthyroidism. Allergic reactions are rare.

The maintenance dose is individualized on the basis of the person's responses and on levels of TSH and T_4 and T_3. Elderly persons usually require smaller doses. Drug replacement is lifelong.

Nursing intervention

It may be necessary for the nurse to explain the condition to the patient and family and emphasize that replacement therapy must be continued indefinitely. The patient may neglect to take the medication if feeling better. During the myxoedematous state, it is important that the family appreciate that the patient's lethargy and dullness are a part of the disease. The nurse, the patient and the family must be tolerant of this slowness, and encouragement and time should be given to complete responses and activities. Early indications of improvement and response to the drug therapy may be pointed out as reassurance that the physical condition is reversible, although depression does not always resolve.

Much of the nursing care is symptomatic. For example, extra warmth is provided because of the patient's lower heat production and consequent decreased tolerance to cold. Without extra clothing and bedding, the person may be uncomfortable in an environmental temperature that is comfortable to others. A minimum of soap is used on the patient's skin, and oily lotions or creams are applied to relieve the dryness. The diet should be low in calories to decrease and/or maintain bodyweight; low in fat and cholesterol because of the accompanying increase in serum cholesterol concentration; and high in fibre with increased fluid intake to promote bowel function. Laxatives or enemas may be necessary to maintain adequate bowel elimination. The hypothyroid patient is seen at the outpatient clinic or by the general practitioner at regular intervals; adjustment of the drug dosage is necessary from time to time.

The patient with hypothyroidism must learn self-management in relation to the drug therapy and symptom control. Teaching is individualized and planned according to the identified needs of the individual. This takes into account the severity of symptoms, the impact the disorder is having on the person's life and daily functioning, and the ability of the family to adjust to the changes in the patient before control is achieved and during episodes when readjustment of the treatment plan is necessary.

Despite treatment, survey evidence from O'Malley et al (2000) suggests that 75% of patients remained overweight whereas 80% reported still feeling depressed even though their thyroid hormones had been returned to normal levels. The areas of weight and mood therefore remain problematical even though other symptoms will probably be largely relieved by hormone therapy. A clinical situation of hypothyroidism is described in Case Study 18.3.

Case Study 18.3

Jane Green is a 34-year-old wife, mother and office manager. She and her husband Robert, an engineer, usually share household tasks and childcare activities and like to participate in outings which include their 4-year-old and 8-month-old sons.

Jane makes an appointment to see you as practice nurse. She tells you that she is having difficulty balancing her job and her family life since returning to full-time work after the birth of her last child. She is constantly tired and falls asleep each evening while reading bedtime stories to the children. She feels pressured by the demands of her job and is concerned that she is becoming forgetful and disorganized.

You question Jane about any physical and emotional changes she has experienced since the birth of the baby and discover that Jane has not been able to lose the extra weight she had gained; her menstrual periods are still not regular; her hair and skin have become very dry; she feels cold and wears an extra sweater, socks or other clothing to keep warm; she is frequently constipated; and she feels she is pushing herself to get through the day. She states that her husband complains about her disinterest and feels that she is not fulfilling her share of household tasks. Following discussion with the GP you take blood, and arrange for Jane to see her GP.

On Jane's next visit to the surgery, her GP, on reviewing the health history and the results of laboratory tests, concludes that Jane has primary hypothyroidism. Jane is to begin thyroid replacement treatment with thyroxine 0.025 mg daily. The dose is to be adjusted in 3–4 weeks according to her serum TSH level and response to drug therapy.

You meet with Jane and mutually set the following learning objectives. Jane will be able to:

- understand the reasons for the physical and behavioural changes she has been experiencing

- take her prescribed hormone replacement regularly, safely and knowledgeably

- recognize the clinical signs and symptoms of hypothyroidism

- discuss actions to take to alleviate the health problems she is experiencing related to changes in activity tolerance, temperature regulation, nutrition, constipation, skin integrity, sexual pattern and thought processes.

Jane's lethargy, decreased attention span and distress at her diagnosis are impeding her ability to comprehend instructions at this time. It was agreed that you will review her medication plan and answer immediate concerns.

Thyroid hormone replacement

The medication is taken daily on an empty stomach. Jane decides that she will take her tablet as soon as she wakes up each morning. You tell her not to exceed the prescribed dose and explain the importance of continuing with drug therapy. You review the signs of under-replacement, which are the same symptoms that Jane is presently experiencing. The half-life of thyroxine is 6–7 days, so Jane should not expect immediate relief from her symptoms. You explain to Jane that her blood pressure and pulse rate will be monitored on each visit. She is currently hypotensive and her pulse is slow at 60 per minute. As her hormone levels rise, her pulse and blood pressure should return to her usual levels. As Jane is not taking any other prescription or non-prescription medications she does not need to be cautioned about the fact that thyroxine potentiates the effects of anticoagulants, insulin and oral hypoglycaemic agents.

It is agreed that at a later visit you will discuss the symptoms of over-replacement and any concerns Jane has after starting her hormone replacement.

Evaluation

Jane returns to the surgery in 3 weeks with her husband. At this time her symptoms are beginning to abate. She is still extremely tired and sensitive to cold but is taking more interest in family and work activities. You discuss the function of the thyroid gland and its hormones, and help Jane and her husband to understand the cause of her symptoms. You emphasize that, although she will require hormone replacement for life, her symptoms can be controlled and she should return to her previous level of functioning. She requires regular medical supervision to monitor her control and to make periodic adjustments in hormone replacement.

Jane's husband is encouraged to learn about her responses to decreased thyroid hormone levels and the symptoms of hyperthyroidism so that he can help Jane to recognize changes and seek further medical evaluation. An appointment is made for Jane to meet the dietician to discuss her dietary needs. She is taking her medication regularly. The increase in the dose prescribed by her GP is explained to her. Her blood pressure is 115/80 mmHg and her pulse rate is 72 per minute. Arrangements are made to review Jane's learning needs on her next visit.

Hyperthyroidism

Hyperthyroidism implies an excessive secretion of the thyroid hormones and may be called *thyrotoxicosis, toxic goitre, exophthalmic goitre* or *Graves' disease*. The terms exophthalmic goitre or Graves' disease are reserved for hyperthyroidism that is accompanied by exophthalmos (see p. 592) and extreme nervousness.

Hyperthyroidism
See chapter 2.6

Causes

The exact cause of hyperactivity of the thyroid in most patients is not clear. In many cases it is thought to be due to autoimmunity. Thyroid-stimulating immunoglobulins (TSIs) are found in almost all people with Graves' disease. There may also be a genetic factor in Graves' disease (Springhouse Corporation 1998). Excessive secretion of TSH by the pituitary gland may also cause enlargement of the thyroid gland and thyroiditis. Over-replacement of thyroid hormones is the most common iatrogenic cause of hyperthyroidism. Hyperthyroidism affects females more often than males, and is rare in childhood.

Clinical characteristics

Some enlargement of the gland may be evident owing to a diffuse hyperplasia of the gland or the development of one or more adenomas. It may be readily seen to move upward with the larynx in swallowing.

The increased blood level of thyroid hormones accelerates the metabolic rate. The patient's appetite increases and, unless the food intake keeps pace with the rapid metabolic rate, there is a loss of weight. Lowered heat tolerance and excessive sweating are manifested. The hyperthyroid patient is uncomfortably warm in an environmental temperature acceptable to others.

Nervousness, apprehension, emotional instability and restlessness are evident, and the hands are *warm* and moist in contrast to the *cold*, moist extremities associated with anxiety. Despite eating more, the patient may complain of weakness and fatigue. The pulse is rapid and exhibits a sharp rise on exertion. The increased pulse rate is due to the increased metabolic demands and the effect of thyroxine on the sympathetic nervous system. Shortness of breath on exertion and palpitation are experienced as a result of the increased metabolic rate. The diastolic blood pressure is usually lower than normal because of widespread vasodilatation. A fine, rapid tremor develops in the hands and is accentuated when they are outstretched. Diarrhoea, resulting from increased gastrointestinal activity, may be troublesome. Menstrual disorders, such as oligomenorrhoea (scant flow) or amenorrhoea, are common.

Eye changes may appear in hyperthyroidism. *Exophthalmos* may be evident when the upper eyelids are retracted, showing the upper sclerae, and the eyes appear to be protruding. This is due to the accumulation of mucopolysaccharides and fluid in the retro-orbital tissues, which forces the eyeball outwards. The lids fail to follow the movement of the eyes when the person looks down (lid lag).

Treatment

Hyperthyroidism may be treated by antithyroid drugs, radioactive iodine (^{131}I) or surgery.

Drug therapy

The drugs most commonly used suppress the formation of the thyroid hormones. They may be used alone or as an interim treatment before surgery; they include carbimazole and propylthiouracil, although much larger doses of the latter drug are required. The drug is generally taken over a prolonged period of 1–2 years if the patient remains free of side-effects. These antithyroid drugs are potentially toxic. Side-effects that may develop are dermatitis, agranulocytosis and fever. The patient is advised to report promptly a sore throat, swollen tender 'neck glands', fever or a rash. The patient must be taught the importance of taking the drugs regularly and at the hours suggested in order to obtain the desired effect and prevent a remission. Some compensatory enlargement of the gland may occur and the patient is reassured that this is not serious.

The patient is followed closely; weekly visits to the general practitioner or clinic are usually required for 4–6 weeks and the interval is gradually lengthened. A blood specimen is taken for determination of serum levels of T_4, T_3 and TSH, and a leucocyte count is made on each visit. The reports may indicate a need for an adjustment in the dosage of the antithyroid drug.

Short-term drug therapy may be given to reduce the cardiac effects of excess T_3 and T_4 levels and other symptoms; for example, a β-adrenergic blocking agent may be prescribed to decrease the heart rate.

Radiation treatment

Iodine-131 therapy of hyperthyroidism is widely used. Treatment by radioiodine is very simple. It is given orally and is trapped in the thyroid, where its radiation destroys tissue, reducing the functioning mass. Improvement is usually evident in 3 weeks and the metabolic rate is expected to reach a normal level in 2–3 months. Antithyroid drugs are usually prescribed during this period. Radioiodine is never given during pregnancy. The therapeutic dose is not considered large enough to constitute a radiation hazard to those in the person's environment.

The patient is observed closely for signs of aggravation of the disease and thyroiditis, manifested by tenderness and soreness in the area of the gland. Rarely, a thyroid crisis may develop (see p. 596). After receiving the ^{131}I, regular visits to the clinic or the doctor are necessary. The patient is examined for remission of the disease and for hypothyroidism, which can frequently occur as a side-effect. The serum T_3, T_4 and TSH levels are determined. If hypothyroidism is indicated, a replacement preparation (e.g. a thyroxine preparation) is prescribed.

Surgical therapy

A partial thyroidectomy may be done if radioactive iodine is contraindicated, for example if the patient is young, if antithyroid drug therapy has failed, if there is the possibility of carcinoma, if sensitivity precludes its prolonged administration, or if the gland is very large, causing disfigurement or pressure on the respiratory tract or oesophagus. In hyperthyroidism, approximately three-quarters of the gland is removed; in the case of cancer of the thyroid, a complete thyroidectomy is done, which necessitates continuous replacement drug therapy during the remainder of the patient's life. The patient must be euthyroid before surgery can be undertaken.

Nursing assessment

An accurate record of the person's temperature, pulse and respirations is made at least every 4 hours, and the responses and degree of restlessness and agitation are noted frequently. This is necessary so that an early indication of increasing thyrotoxicosis and cardiac insufficiency may be recognized and receive prompt attention. The patient is told that the vital signs will be checked at regular intervals, to avoid undue apprehension associated with such frequent checking. The patient is weighed daily or every second day to determine whether calorie intake is keeping pace with metabolic rate.

Patient problems

The patient with hyperthyroidism is expending energy in excess of the body's ability to produce energy. Metabolic processes are increased, requiring more calories to prevent excessive weight loss. Environmental stimuli increase energy demands further. Health problems that are experienced by the person with hyperthyroidism are listed in Table 18.4 (p. 589).

Goals

The patient and family will be able to:

1. understand the reasons for the physical and behavioural changes

2. recognize the clinical signs and symptoms of hyperthyroidism

3. describe the prescribed medication and/or treatment plan

4. describe the expected and possible adverse responses to therapy

5. discuss actions to take to alleviate the health problems experienced in relation to changes in thought processes and emotional responses, nutrition, activity tolerance, thermoregulation, skin and eye integrity, sexual pattern and body image

6. describe plans for ongoing therapy and health supervision.

Nursing intervention

Altered thought processes and emotional responses

The *goal* is that the patient will appear less anxious:

■ *Environment* – Because of the patient's nervousness and hyperexcitability, quietness is very important. An established routine may prevent unnecessary disturbance, which only aggravates the condition. If the patient is being cared for at home, the family is made fully aware of these needs. They are advised that irritability, restlessness and emotional lability are characteristic of the illness and are helped to develop coping strategies to avoid upsetting the individual. In the hospital careful consideration should be given to placement on the ward. Exposure to very ill, talkative or otherwise disturbing patients should be avoided.

■ *Information* – You should explain all procedures and medical treatment to the patient and family and answer questions regarding care, and work in a calm, quiet, competent manner.

■ *Identification of additional stresses* – You should work with the patient and family to identify additional stresses that may have resulted from the patient's illness or may have existed previously. Referrals to community resources are made if relevant.

■ *Visitors* – Visitors and family members require information on the need for limiting visitors and suggestions as to how they can best contribute to the patient's well-being and avoid aggravating the condition.

Altered nutrition

The *goal* is that the patient will maintain or increase bodyweight:

■ *Diet* – The patient requires a high-protein, high-carbohydrate, high-calorie diet (4000–5000 kcal) to prevent tissue breakdown caused by the high metabolic demand and to satisfy the patient's increased appetite. A snack between meals and at bedtime is provided. Tea and coffee are usually restricted to eliminate caffeine stimulation. Decaffeinated coffee may be used as a substitute.

■ *Fluids* – The patient's excessive heat production and resultant perspiration increases fluid loss, necessitating extra fluids. Also, there is an increased production of metabolic wastes, requiring dilution for elimination by the kidneys. A minimum fluid intake of 3000–4000 mL daily is recommended, unless contraindicated by cardiac or renal dysfunction. An explanation of the importance of this amount of fluid is made to the patient to gain cooperation, and a variety of fluids is provided.

Hyperactivity and fatigue

The *goal* is that the patient will decrease energy expenditure:

■ *Rest and activity* – Activity is restricted because it increases the metabolic rate, but the patient's nervous excitability makes it difficult to rest. Efforts are made to engage the patient's interest in activities which expend little energy. The occupational therapy department may be very helpful in this goal. The patient is helped to plan activities and daily routines to obtain sufficient rest. Activities requiring fine motor movements are kept to a minimum. When necessary, assistance is provided by the family or nurse.

Altered thermoregulation

The *goal* is that the patient will state that he or she feels comfortably cool.

As the patient is producing more than the normal amount of body heat, comfort will be achieved only in an environment of lower temperature than normal. Lightweight clothing is used and the room is kept well ventilated and cool.

Altered skin and eye integrity

The *goals* are that the patient will maintain skin integrity and avoid injury to the eyes:

■ *Skin care* – A daily bath is necessary because of the profuse perspiration. If the patient is extremely restless, has lost weight and has decreased mobility, special attention is given to the pressure areas.

■ *Eye care* – If the patient has exophthalmos, the eyes should be protected from irritation by sunglasses. Methylcellulose (a conjunctival lubricant) drops (0.5–1%) may be recommended to prevent drying of the conjunctiva and cornea. The patient's vision is tested frequently, especially if the exophthalmos is progressive; compression of the optic nerve and artery may occur, with ensuing visual impairment.

Altered sexual patterns and self-image

The *goal* is that the patient will express concerns regarding alterations in body image and changes in sexual patterns.

The patient and partner are helped to understand that the changes in menstrual cycle, low sex drive and/or impotence are a result of the hyperthyroidism and that they will abate or disappear once thyroid hormonal balance is achieved.

Repeated explanations of the causes of the physical changes and assurance should be given. There is a prolonged phase of gradual improvement of the eyes once the hormone imbalance has been corrected. It should be said, however, that the eyes may not return to the normal state. Good grooming and attractive dress promote self-confidence and the feeling of wellness.

Lack of knowledge about the disease process, therapeutic plan and self-management

The *goal* is that the patient will achieve self-management of the therapeutic regimen and self-care.

The patient and family are given information about hyperthyroidism, causes, manifestations and treatment. Learning needs are assessed and they are assisted in developing a plan for home care of the patient. The dietician may be consulted about diet and meal planning.

Evaluation

The physical and behavioural changes that the person is experiencing should begin to diminish with treatment. With drug therapy, clinical improvement should be apparent after several weeks. The dose of the medication will then be decreased by the doctor according to symptomatic changes and decreases in the T_4 level. The person should begin to regain weight. As weight approaches the person's desirable level, and energy expenditure is consistent and within usual parameters, the diet is adjusted and calorie intake decreased.

The patient and family should demonstrate understanding of the hyperthyroidism, the treatment plan and medication regimen. They should be able to describe and implement measures to alleviate symptoms by: (1) the provision of a quiet, cool environment; (2) the avoidance of undue stress; (3) provision for sufficient rest and sleep and decreased physical activity; (4) adequate calorie and fluid intake; (5) maintenance of dry clean skin; and (6) protection of the eyes. The person should verbalize a decrease in anxiety and begin to take responsibility for self-care.

The person having thyroid surgery

In caring for the patient who has had a thyroidectomy, pertinent factors to be kept in mind are:

- the location of the gland in relation to the trachea and larynx
- its proximity to the recurrent laryngeal nerve, which controls the vocal cords
- its abundant blood supply
- that the parathyroid glands, which influence neuromuscular irritability through their control of the blood calcium level, lie on the posterior surface of the thyroid. The nurse must be constantly alert for manifestations of disturbances due to these factors.

Preoperative preparation

The hyperthyroid patient who is to have surgery is given an antithyroid drug for several weeks before operation to reduce the metabolic rate and return the gland to as near the euthyroid state as possible. During this period, whether at home or in the hospital, the care cited in the preceding section is applicable. The antithyroid drugs produce some compensatory enlargement of the gland and an increased blood supply. When the metabolic rate has been reduced to a satisfactory level, the drug is discontinued. Then, in a few days, a course of potassium iodide is commenced and continued for approximately 10 days. This reduces the size and vascularity of the gland, facilitating surgery and lessening the problem of bleeding. As potassium iodide has a disagreeable taste and may also irritate the mucous membrane, it is well diluted in fruit juice or milk.

Preparation includes electrocardiography to obtain further information about the patient's cardiac status, and blood typing and cross-matching for transfusion. The female patient may have some concern regarding the cosmetic effect of the operation. She is assured that consideration is given to this and that the scar becomes barely perceptible in a few months. During the interval, it may be concealed by a scarf or necklace. Remembering that the hyperthyroid patient may be hyperexcitable and apprehensive, judicious explanations are made of what may be expected after the operation. Demonstration and practice in supporting the head with the hands while turning in bed is carried out to decrease stress on the neck.

Preparation to receive the patient after operation

Special equipment to be assembled and ready for use when preparing to receive a patient following a thyroidectomy includes:

1. sandbags or small firm pillows to immobilize the head

2. suction equipment and catheters for clearing mucus from the throat

3. sterile clip removers or stitch cutters in case of a haematoma at the site of surgery obstructing the trachea by compression

4. a humidifier to relieve tracheal and laryngeal irritation and facilitate the removal of mucus

5. intravenous infusion equipment

6. a sterile emergency intubation and tracheostomy tray in the event of respiratory obstruction

7. equipment for obtaining a blood specimen quickly for blood calcium determination

8. ampoules of calcium chloride or calcium gluconate, with the necessary equipment for intravenous administration in the event of the complication of tetany (hypocalcaemia) due to inadvertent parathyroid damage.

Postoperative care

Patients are usually very apprehensive, and serious complications may *develop rapidly*. They should therefore be placed on the ward in a position where they are readily visible at all times.

Assessment

Vital signs are recorded every 15 minutes; the frequency is gradually reduced if the patient remains stable. The body temperature is recorded every 4 hours. The degree of restlessness and apprehension is noted and, if not relieved by the prescribed sedation, is brought to the surgeon's attention. Particular attention is paid to the patient's respirations; any complaint or sign of respiratory distress and cyanosis is reported promptly, because it may indicate laryngeal paralysis or compression of the trachea by accumulating blood. Some hoarseness is common and is due to irritation of the larynx by the operation and the endotracheal tube used in maintaining the airway during surgery. The doctor is advised if the hoarseness and weakness of the voice persist beyond 3 or 4 days. Potential patient problems are listed in Box 18.5.

Goals

Following thyroid surgery, the patient will be able to:

1. maintain a patent airway

2. state that pain is absent

3. show vital signs within normal limits

4. assume self-care activities

5. achieve and maintain desirable bodyweight

6. demonstrate ability to perform neck exercises safely

7. describe a plan for follow-up care.

Box 18.5 Potential patient problems following thyroid surgery

- Obstructed airway, because of:
  — oedema, decreased head and neck mobility and tracheal–bronchial secretions from the anaesthetic, which all contribute to difficulty in expectorating secretions
  — haematoma formation behind the wound site pressing on the trachea

- Pain related to surgical intervention

- Impaired mobility of head, neck and shoulders related to surgical intervention, pain and discomfort

- Inadequate nutrition because of difficulty in swallowing

- Complications as a result of the surgical intervention (e.g. haemorrhage, respiratory distress, loss of voice or tetany)

- Inadequate knowledge about follow-up care

Nursing intervention

Potential obstruction of the airway

The *goal* is that the patient will maintain a patent airway:

- The patient is assisted to a sitting position with support given to the head and neck in order to help the patient to cough and expectorate. Suction of the oropharynx is carried out if the accumulation of secretions is severe. Deep breathing and coughing should be encouraged several times each hour. Pulse oximetry may be used to monitor oxygen saturation.

- You should observe the wound and ensure free drainage from the wound drains is maintained to prevent the formation of a haematoma.

Pain

The *goal* is that the patient will state that pain is absent. Opioid analgesia and an antiemetic may be required to keep the patient comfortable and less apprehensive during the first 48 hours. Analgesia should be administered regularly and consistently to control pain. Respirations are assessed for evidence of a decrease in rate or depth.

Wound healing

The *goal* is that the wound will heal and the patient will maintain the range of movement of the neck.

After recovery from the anaesthetic, the patient is placed on his or her back and the head of the bed is moderately elevated to facilitate breathing. The head and neck are supported by a pillow and are positioned in good alignment, preventing flexion and hyperextension. When the patient's position is changed, the nurse lifts and supports the head, preserving good alignment. The patient is taught to lift and support the head by placing the hands at the back of the head when wishing to move.

The patient often returns from the operating theatre with surgical drains inserted. These should be checked at intervals to ensure that they are functioning. While a large accumulation of blood behind the wound site can cause respiratory obstruction, smaller haematomas may increase vulnerability to infection and delayed wound healing.

If the vital signs are stabilized and normal, the patient is assisted out of bed on the first postoperative day. After removal of the drains, sutures or skin clips and firm healing of the incision, head exercises, which include flexion (forward and lateral), hyperextension and turning, are gradually introduced with the surgeon's approval. To prevent contraction of the scar, the patient may be taught to massage the neck gently twice daily, using lanolin, cold cream or an oily lotion.

Inadequate nutrition

The *goal* is that the patient will maintain adequate food intake.

Some difficulty in swallowing is usually experienced for a day or two, but fluids by mouth are encouraged as soon as tolerated. Intravenous fluids are given until an adequate amount can be taken orally. The patient progresses through a soft diet to a full diet in 2–3 days.

Potential complications

The *goal* is that complications will be promptly identified and corrected.

The nurse must be aware that haemorrhage, respiratory difficulty, loss of voice and tetany are serious complications that may occur following thyroid surgery. The first three may develop with startling rapidity and are usually seen within 48 hours of operation.

Haemorrhage may be manifested by a rapid pulse, fall in blood pressure and evident bleeding. The bleeding may be discovered only by frequent checking of the dressing and by sliding the hands under the shoulders and behind the neck. Blood may collect quickly within the tissues and cause pressure on the trachea. The patient may complain of a choking sensation and shortness of breath; cyanosis and dyspnoea develop and, unless the pressure is relieved quickly, asphyxia may occur. The surgeon is notified immediately at the earliest sign of change. The dressing is loosened to promote freer, outward drainage. Instruments for removing the sutures or skin clips should already be at the bedside and the emergency tracheostomy tray is made ready, because the surgeon may consider an immediate tracheostomy necessary. On reporting the situation, the nurse may be instructed to remove the skin clips to allow the escape of blood. A thick sterile dressing is then applied until the surgeon arrives. The patient will probably be returned to the operating theatre to bring the bleeding under control.

Occasionally, *injury to one or both recurrent laryngeal nerves* may occur during thyroid surgery. These nerves control laryngeal muscles, the opening of the glottis and voice production. Injury to one nerve produces hoarseness and weakness of the voice but no serious respiratory disturbance. Bilateral nerve injury causes paralysis of muscles on both sides of the larynx, resulting in closure of the glottis and respiratory obstruction. The patient is unable to speak and stridor occurs (i.e. respirations become shrill and crowing), cyanosis develops and loss of consciousness ensues unless respirations are quickly re-established. Prompt endotracheal intubation or emergency tracheostomy is done, and oxygen is administered via either tube. The injury and paralysis are rarely permanent; function is usually gradually restored, and the tracheostomy tube is removed.

During surgery, interference with the blood supply to the parathyroid glands or injury or removal of parathyroid tissue may occur which depresses secretion by the glands. Decreased parathyroid hormone concentration leads to *hypocalcaemia*, resulting in increased neuromuscular irritability and the condition known as *tetany*. Early signs of this complication include complaints of numbness and tingling in the hands or feet, muscle twitching and spasms, and gastrointestinal cramps. A change may be evident in the voice; it may become high pitched and shrill, because of spasm of the vocal cords. A blood specimen is obtained for serum calcium determination with the appearance of early symptoms. Calcium gluconate 10% may be slowly administered intravenously by the doctor; then, an oral preparation is given until normal parathyroid function resumes. The patient is encouraged to take milk and calcium-containing foods.

Thyrotoxicosis or thyroid crisis rarely complicates the postoperative period following a thyroidectomy. This emergency situation is attributed to: (1) the release of a large amount of thyroid hormone into the circulation to produce a hypermetabolic state, and (2) adrenergic hyperactivity which may potentiate the hypersecretion of thyroid hormone. The patient's symptoms develop abruptly and include irritability, tremor, tachycardia, vomiting, visual disturbance, vascular collapse, hypotension, pyrexia, coma and death. Rapid notification of medical staff, electrocardiography (ECG), temperature and vital sign monitoring are essential as this is a rare but life-threatening crisis (Springhouse Corporation 1998).

Inadequate knowledge concerning follow-up care

The *goal* is that the patient will verbalize understanding of a plan for post-hospital care and follow-up.

The patient's hospitalization is usually brief if no complications develop. Information regarding the amount of activity that may be resumed is discussed with the patient. Extra rest will still be necessary, and the patient is advised to continue neck exercises until there is freedom of movement without any feeling of pulling.

Follow-up is usually at the outpatient clinic for about a year, checking for any residual laryngeal damage, hypoparathyroidism, recurring hyperthyroidism or developing hypothyroidism. If no problems develop during that year, an annual check-up is then recommended. Information is provided on the administration and effects of prescribed thyroid hormone replacement. Following a total thyroidectomy, hormone replacement will be lifelong.

Evaluation

The patient should show absence of complications; the serum calcium level will be within the normal range. There will be no muscle twitching, hoarseness or breathing difficulties. The patient and family will describe plans for follow-up care and demonstrate understanding of the prescribed neck exercises, medication schedule and other self-care activities.

The person with a disorder of the parathyroid glands

Primary hyperparathyroidism has a prevalence of about 1 in 800 and is found predominantly in people aged over 50 years, in women more often than men, and is usually caused by a single parathyroid adenoma (Haslett et al 1999). Serum calcium levels increase in response to the excess parathyroid hormone (PTH) secretion. Secondary hyperparathyroidism occurs when the gland secretes excessive amounts of PTH to try to compensate for hypocalcaemia caused by any abnormality that inhibits the effect of PTH, such as chronic renal failure, thiazide diuretic use or vitamin D deficiency. Hypoparathyroidism occurs due to a rare autoimmune genetic disorder or more frequently due to damage to the glands during thyroid surgery.

Assessment of parathyroid function

The *health history* begins with the collection of information related to the health problems experienced by the individual. Table 18.5 lists health problems common to individuals with increased and decreased parathyroid function. The nurse asks specific questions to determine the presence, duration and severity of the associated signs and symptoms; vitamin D and calcium intake; the use of drugs such as thiazide diuretics; and any history of renal calculi.

Hypoparathyroidism

Clinical characteristics

The deficiency of parathyroid homone (PTH) causes hypocalcaemia. Symptoms of increased neuromuscular excitability and tetany are usually the first manifestations

*Hypoparathyroidism
See chapter 2.6*

Table 18.5   Assessment of the person with altered parathyroid function

	Clinical characteristics	
	Hypoparathyroidism	Hyperparathyroidism
Activity tolerance	Muscular cramps and spasms Numbness and tingling of extremities Tetany	Muscle weakness and fatigue Decreased muscle tone Bone tenderness and pain on weight-bearing Pathological fractures
Thought process and emotional response	Irritability, agitation Depression Psychosis Slow mental processes Anxiety	Lethargy Drowsiness Impaired memory Disorientation
Nutrition	Nausea and vomiting Abdominal cramping	Loss of appetite Nausea and vomiting Abdominal discomfort Weight loss
Elimination	Constipation or diarrhoea	Constipation Increased urinary output
Skin integrity	Skin coarse, scaly and dry Alopecia Loss of eyebrows Nails brittle with horizontal ridges	
Breathing pattern	Laryngeal spasm Wheezing	

(muscle cramps, carpopedal spasms, laryngeal spasm affecting the voice, dysphagia, convulsions). Wheezy respirations may be heard due to bronchospasm. Less calcium than normal is excreted in the urine because of the low blood calcium level, and the bones tend to become more dense. Renal excretion of phosphorus is reduced and the serum phosphate level is raised, which predisposes the patient to acidosis. If the hormone deficiency is prolonged, calcium deposition may develop in the lens and conjunctiva of the eyes, the brain, lungs or gastric mucosa. The hair becomes thin and grey, areas of alopecia and loss of eyebrows are common. The skin becomes coarse and scaly and the nails are brittle and have horizontal ridges. Mental changes include depression, fatigue, psychosis and intellectual impairment.

Treatment

The hypocalcaemia is corrected initially by the intravenous administration of 20 mL calcium gluconate 10%. The patient is then given regular oral doses of a calcium salt, such as gluconate or lactate, along with a preparation of vitamin D to promote the absorption of the calcium. The patient is followed closely; frequent determinations of blood phosphorus and calcium levels are made in order to adjust vitamin D dosage. Overdosage may cause renal damage. Phosphorus-containing foods may have to be limited to avoid complications: these are principally dairy products. An alternative may be the prescription of aluminium hydroxide gel which binds the phosphorus in the intestine, preventing its absorption. The patient is encouraged to take extra fluids to promote renal excretion of phosphorus.

Hyperparathyroidism
See chapter 2.6

Hyperparathyroidism

Clinical characteristics

The high PTH concentration in the blood causes decalcification of the bones, and hypercalcaemia occurs. The blood level of inorganic phosphorus falls as its renal excretion increases, and the concentration of calcium in the glomerular filtrate is higher than normal, predisposing to the formation of renal calculi. Neuromuscular excitability is depressed and loss of muscle tone is evident. Demineralization of the bones may be so marked that fibrous cystic areas develop which frequently lead to deformities and pathological fractures. In some instances bone tumours consisting of an overgrowth of osteoclasts develop. When bone changes occur, the disorder may be referred to as *von Recklinghausen's disease* or *osteitis fibrosa cystica*, and the patient may experience tenderness and pain in the bones, especially with weight-bearing. Muscular weakness, loss of appetite, nausea, vomiting and constipation may develop. The urinary volume is usually increased because of the excessive amounts of calcium and phosphorus to be excreted. Renal function may become impaired; the tubular epithelium may be

damaged by the excessive excretion of calcium or the formation of renal calculi. Frequently, the disease is recognized only when some deformity develops or a pathological fracture occurs.

Treatment

If the patient is very ill as a result of increased serum calcium levels (malignant hypercalcaemia), rehydration with up to 6 litres of normal saline is needed. Biphosphonates (e.g. i.v. pamidronate) are given to reduce serum calcium levels, together with further i.v. saline and furosemide (frusemide) to achieve a forced diuresis aimed at further reduction of serum calcium concentration. Fluid intake and output are monitored carefully. Foods containing calcium are restricted in the diet.

Hyperparathyroidism is treated by surgical excision of all four glands. Normal residual parathyroid tissue may be allografted into a muscle to preserve as much of the patient's parathyroid function as possible. After operation the patient is observed closely for the early signs of possible hypocalcaemia (tetany). Frequent serum calcium and phosphorus determinations are made. A diet high in calcium and phosphorus may be necessary to restore normal bone structure.

The person with a disorder of the pituitary gland (hypophysis)

Assessment

The signs and symptoms of pituitary dysfunction are varied and reflect not only the increase or decrease in the production of one or more of the pituitary hormones, but also the resultant changes in the target tissues. Pituitary hormones, their functions and associated disorders are listed in Table 18.6.

Health history

The health history should include questions related to the following:

- *Growth and development* – Questions relate to changes in growth pattern and perceived changes in appearance or clothing size. The development of secondary sex characteristics and abnormalities of secondary sex characteristics may be explored. A great deal of sensitivity is required as these are all very personal areas. For the female, questions are asked about changes in the menstrual cycle. For the male, questions relate to sexual dysfunctions, in particular difficulties in attaining and maintaining an erection and any changes in body hair growth and distribution.

- *Appetite and bodyweight* – Recent changes in appetite and the pattern of weight gain or loss are determined. It is important to ask questions about the volume of fluid intake, and whether thirst is relieved. Alteration

Table 18.6   Pituitary gland hormones

Hormone	Functions	Disorders
Anterior pituitary		
Growth hormone (GH)	Growth; aids in determining size; accelerates metabolism; diabetogenic	Panhypopituitarism Gigantism – increase in GH level in childhood Acromegaly – increase in GH level in adulthood Short stature – decrease of GH level in childhood
Thyroid-stimulating hormone (TSH)	Promotes secretory activity of thyroid	Hyperthyroidism secondary to increase of TSH Hypothyroidism secondary to decrease of TSH
Adrenocorticotrophic hormone (ACTH)	Stimulates secretion of adrenal cortices	Cushing's syndrome and excess TSH Addison's disease secondary to pituitary disorder
Gonadotrophins: a. Follicle-stimulating hormone (FSH)	In women: development of ovarian follicle and secretion of oestrogen In men: promotes production of spermatozoa	Tumours Amenorrhoea Infertility
b. Luteinizing hormone (LH)	In women: induces ovulation, stimulates secretion of progesterone In men: stimulates production of androgens	
c. Prolactin	Initiates and sustains lactation	Galactorrhoea Infertility
Melanocyte-stimulating hormone (MSH)	Pigmentation of skin cells	Increase in pigmented areas
Posterior pituitary		
Antidiuretic hormone (ADH)	Increases permeability of distal and collecting tubules of kidneys (i.e. increases reabsorption of water)	Tumour
Oxytocin	Contracts pregnant uterus; stimulates release and flow of milk	

in heat tolerance may also be present with metabolic changes.

- *Elimination patterns* – Changes in the volume, frequency and pattern of urinary elimination are determined. The person is asked specifically about getting up at night to void. Changes in bowel habits, constipation and/or diarrhoea are identified.

- *Skin and hair* – Alteration in skin colour, texture, dryness, bruising and ability to heal may be caused by pituitary dysfunction. The patient can validate the nurse's observations as he or she is in the best position to recognize changes.

- *Activity tolerance* – Questions are asked about feelings of tiredness or exhaustion related to usual daily activities and on exertion. Knowledge of the person's usual pattern of daily activity provides a basis for comparison.

- *Cognitive/perceptual function* – Changes in memory, ability to concentrate, decreased attention span and visual losses may result from pituitary disorders or altered function of the target tissues. How the person

usually responds to stressful physical and emotional events is elicited in detail and recent changes in these responses are also recorded.

Physical examination

The following areas are assessed:

- *General appearance* – The patient's general appearance, body build and fat distribution provide valuable information about pituitary abnormalities and overall growth and development of the individual.

- *Bodyweight and vital signs* – The patient's weight, height and vital signs are recorded.

- *Skin, hair and nails* – The skin is observed and palpated for pigmentation, dryness, oiliness, elasticity, hydration, temperature and breaks in the integrity and any resulting discharge. The pattern of distribution and amount of body hair are observed and the texture and dryness noted. Nails are observed for thickness and changes in growth.

- *Genitalia and breasts* – The genitalia of the male and female are observed for size and shape, and the breasts are examined to assess development and maturation.

- *Neurological examination* – Changes in sensation, pain, discomfort and muscle tone are noted. The patient's speech is carefully listened to for huskiness, slurring, hoarseness, volume and pitch, and rationality.

Diagnostic measurements

Apart from taking bloods to measure hormone levels, medical staff may carry out other tests such as those involving the osmolality of urine and serum which are influenced by ADH levels. A key investigation is the adrenocorticotrophic hormone (ACTH) stimulation test, which is used if there is suspicion of a pituitary tumour. It will also help to diagnose primary or secondary adrenal insufficiency. The patient receives an intramuscular injection of 250 µg tetracosactrin and blood samples are taken immediately and 30 minutes later to assess plasma cortisol levels. In normal people the response should be a plasma cortisol level greater than 550 nmol/L 30 minutes after the injection. Such a result indicates normal adrenal function (Haslett et al 1999).

Radiological studies

These include magnetic resonance imaging (MRI) and computed tomography (CT). Larger tumours may be identified with CT, but MRI is needed for smaller microadenomas.

Acromegaly
See chapter 2.6

Patient problems

Problems associated with disorders of the pituitary vary greatly, depending on which lobe is involved, the nature of the disease (hyperplasia, neoplasm or destruction of tissue) and the particular type of cell of the anterior pituitary that is involved. Dysfunction may be manifested in one or more of the gland's target organs, reflecting either an excessive or deficient output of one or more pituitary hormones. Secondary neurological disturbances may also occur as a result of pressure on neighbouring brain tissue by a pituitary neoplasm. For example, early manifestations may include altered perceptual/visual function. The visual disturbances frequently occur because of the proximity of the visual tract. Conversely, primary pathological lesions in the brain, especially in the hypothalamic region, may cause secondary involvement of the pituitary.

The more commonly recognized disease entities associated with the anterior pituitary include:

- gigantism, the result of an excessive secretion of growth hormone (GH) in childhood

- acromegaly, due to an excessive secretion of GH commencing in adulthood

- dwarfism, resulting from a deficiency of GH in childhood

- Cushing's disease, the result of a hypersecretion of ACTH

- Simmonds' disease (panhypopituitarism), which occurs when there is a deficiency of all the anterior pituitary hormones.

Hyperthyroidism (Graves' disease) may also be secondary to an excessive production of TSH or an abnormal form of the hormone, and is discussed in the section on disorders of the thyroid.

The most common disorder associated with the posterior pituitary is *diabetes insipidus*, which is a result of a deficiency of ADH.

Hypersecretion of growth hormone: acromegaly

An overproduction of GH before closure of the epiphyses and skeletal maturity causes a rapid overgrowth of the bones, producing the condition known as *gigantism*. **Acromegaly** results from an excess of growth hormone after puberty, usually due to a GH-secreting pituitary adenoma. It is a rare condition affecting four people per million of the population. The person has usually had the disease for several years before diagnosis, typically around the age of 40 years (Carr 2001).

Clinical characteristics

A person with gigantism may attain a height of 2.1–2.4 metres. Most cases are attributed to an adenoma. When the person passes adolescence, acromegaly is superimposed on the gigantism.

If the adenoma develops after the epiphyses have closed, longitudinal growth cannot occur, but marked thickening of the bones occurs and acromegaly develops. Enlargement of the head, jaws, hands and feet becomes apparent. Increased growth of cartilage produces an increase in the size of the nose, ears, costal cartilages and larynx. Hypertrophy of the larynx may be accompanied by a deepening of the voice, and the change in the costal cartilages results in an increase in the thoracic circumference. The skin, subcutaneous tissues and lips thicken, the chin lengthens and the lower teeth separate because of the overgrowth of the mandible. Viscera enlarge and may become overactive, leading to disturbances.

As well as the evident skeletal changes and alteration in appearance, the patient experiences lethargy, weakness, increased metabolic rate and excessive sweating due to hypertrophy of the thyroid. Common complaints are joint pains, stiffness in the limbs, and tingling or numbness in the hands. Impaired carbohydrate metabolism and hyperglycaemia develop owing to the diabetogenic effect of GH. Pressure from the causative expanding neoplasm may cause headache, insomnia, and loss of visual acuity and fields. Increased gonadal function may be associated with the early stage of acromegaly but, later, loss of libido and amenorrhoea are common. Osteoporosis (rarefaction of bones due to loss of calcium) may develop, especially in the vertebrae, and kyphosis (forward curvature of the spine) may be seen in the advanced stage. Hypertension is a common complication. The course of the disease varies considerably from one patient to another; it may develop slowly over many years in some, but in others it may prove fatal in 3–4 years. Destruction of pituitary tissue by progressive growth and spread of the tumour may cause a general hypopituitarism.

Diagnostic investigation involves radiography of the skull in which the sella turcica is checked for widening.

Treatment

Acromegaly may be treated surgically by a hypophysectomy or transphenoidal microsurgery to remove the hyperfunctioning tissue. A nasal, trans-sphenoidal approach is used by the surgeon. Radiotherapy is a second line of treatment. Internal radiation may be achieved by the implantation of radioactive yttrium (^{90}Y) seeds in the pituitary; a proton beam may be used for external irradiation. Patients may require long-term injections of somatostatin (hypothalamic release-inhibiting hormone) anologues, which lower GH levels. Octreotide or lanreotide are licensed for use but they have significant adverse gastrointestinal side-effects. During treatment, GH-producing pituitary tumours can still expand and the patient should be monitored carefully for reports of visual disturbance which would indicate such a problem is developing (British National Formulary 2000). Substitution hormonal preparations are prescribed if a hypophysectomy is done or if the patient manifests insulin, thyroid, adrenal or gonadal insufficiency in the advanced stage of the disease. Treatment arrests further changes but the changes in bony structures are irreversible.

Nursing intervention

Health problems experienced by the person with acromegaly vary with the stage and type of therapy, the impact of the disorder and treatment on the individual's lifestyle. Common problems include the following:

- *anxiety* related to the operation and treatment

- *altered self-esteem* related to changes in physical appearance

- *sexual dysfunction* related to possible amenorrhoea, decreased libido or impotence

- *altered nutrition* related to increased physical growth and metabolic rate

- *perceptual deficits* related to visual impairment

- *knowledge deficit* related to surgery or radiation therapy and possible long-term hormone replacement therapy

- *social and career disruption* caused by frequent visits to hospital and time off work due to symptoms such as joint pains.

Long-term support and counselling are needed. The reasons for the physiological changes are explained and the patient is taught about both short- and long-term therapy. The nurse helps the patient and family to develop a self-care plan that includes a diet that is well balanced but high in calories and plans for long-term hormone replacement therapy.

Panhypopituitarism (Simmonds' disease)

This disease denotes a deficiency of all the anterior pituitary hormones. The condition may be the result of a primary lesion, such as a tumour or cyst, within the anterior lobe itself, or it may be secondary to a space-occupying lesion in neighbouring structures or to interference with the blood supply to the gland. The latter may occur with thrombosis of the hypophyseal vessels associated with postpartum shock. This remains the most likely cause of Simmonds' disease (Rees and Williams 1995). A tumour will compress and destroy the secreting cells as it enlarges. Surgical excision or irradiation of the gland for the purpose of suppressing the secretion of certain hormones in the treatment of carcinoma of the breast or acromegaly may incur hyposecretion of all the adenohypophyseal hormones.

Clinical characteristics

The multiple hormone deficiency results in a lack of stimulation to the thyroid, adrenal cortices and gonads. Secondary atrophy and hyposecretion of their hormones ensue. If the condition occurs in childhood, failure of the secretion of GH along with the other hormones produces dwarfism. Growth and development are arrested, the skin becomes wrinkled and the child develops an appearance characteristic of a 'wizened old person'.

In the adult, there is also a general wasting of all body tissues and the person exhibits emaciation and severe weight loss. The skin is dry and wrinkled and may assume a yellowish cast. The body hair becomes sparse. Decreased thyroid activity causes a reduction in the metabolic rate, leading to a subnormal temperature and extreme weakness. Arrested function of the gonads results in failure of ovulation and amenorrhoea in the female, and an absence of spermatogenesis and impotence in the male. Concomitant hypoglycaemia and hypotension are seen and may lead to shock and coma. The low blood sugar level is attributed to the decreased GH and adrenocorticoid secretions. If the panhypopituitarism is due to an expanding neoplasm, the posterior pituitary and the infundibulum may become involved, manifested by polyuria and extreme thirst, which is characteristic of a deficiency of antidiuretic hormone (ADH). An expanding lesion may impose itself on the optic tract, impairing vision. The hypothalamus may also be affected, and varied neurological disturbances become evident; for example, the patient may experience severe anorexia.

Treatment

Treatment includes the administration of substitution hormones of the target glands. The patient receives corticosteroids and thyroid hormone in dosages adjusted to individual needs. Thyroid hormone is prescribed only when the patient is receiving corticosteroids. Gonadal hormones may be prescribed, depending on the patient's age. Testosterone (male hormone) may be administered to both sexes for its anabolic effect. Oestrogen may be used in the female to preserve female secondary sex characteristics.

If the cause is a tumour, it is removed by transsphenoidal microsurgery and/or treated by irradiation.

Nursing intervention

The nurse assists the patient and family in setting realistic long-term goals to promote adjustment to the chronic endocrine dysfunction. Patient and family concerns are identified and explored in depth, because the disorder has profound effects on both the individual and family, particularly if it is after a postpartum haemorrhage.

The nurse plays an important role in encouraging patients at home to take a high-calorie, high-vitamin diet. As anorexia is a common problem, resourcefulness is necessary to ensure adequate nourishment. Various methods and approaches must be tried. It is usually helpful to provide small servings of high-calorie foods at frequent intervals. Varying the foods, adding concentrates to fluids, determining the patient's preferences, having favourite 'dishes' prepared at home, eating with others and a change of environment are just a few suggestions that may prove beneficial.

The lethargy and apathy generally associated with Simmonds' disease predisposes to the patient's immobility. Prompting the patient to change position and exercise is necessary to stimulate circulation and prevent complications.

Diabetes insipidus
See chapter 2.6

ADH hyposecretion: diabetes insipidus

Causative factors

The causative factor in this disorder may be a deficiency of antidiuretic hormone (ADH; vasopressin) or failure of the renal tubules to respond to ADH. A deficiency of ADH is most commonly due to hypoactivity or destruction of a part of the hypothalamic–posterior pituitary system resulting from primary or metastatic neoplasms or infection, such as encephalitis, meningitis or brain injury. In some instances, no apparent cause can be identified.

Clinical characteristics

Diabetes insipidus is characterized by a very large urinary output (polyuria) and extreme thirst (polydipsia). The daily output may range from 5 to 20 litres and the patient may experience anorexia, headache, muscular pains, loss of weight and strength, and electrolyte imbalance. The urine has an abnormally low specific gravity and does not contain any abnormal constituents. If fluid is withheld or does not keep pace with the output, an excessive loss of urine continues, leading to severe dehydration and shock. The persisting symptoms of polyuria and polydipsia day and night interfere with rest and normal activities.

Diagnosis

Investigation of the disorder usually involves water deprivation tests. A period of 8 hours without any fluids to drink will produce a significant rise in urine concentration in the normal person, but not in a person with diabetes insipidus.

Investigative procedures may also include neurological examination, radiography of the skull, visual field tests and CT.

Treatment

The patient is treated by replacement therapy with hypotonic parenteral fluids and unlimited oral fluids; a preparation of posterior pituitary extract or vasopressin is prescribed. The preparation used is normally desmopressin, an analogue of vasopressin. It is given as either an intranasal spray (10–40 µg daily in one or two doses) or by injection.

The patient is usually hospitalized during diagnostic investigation and regulation of medication.

Nursing intervention

Nursing care focuses on the two major health problems demonstrated by individuals with diabetes insipidus: (1) dehydration due to polyuria; and (2) a lack of knowledge concerning hormone replacement therapy.

Dehydration

The nurse is responsible for the ongoing assessment of the person's fluid balance and for teaching the patient and family to recognize signs of dehydration and hypovolaemia. Vital signs, mental status, intake and output, urine specific gravity and skin integrity are assessed and recorded regularly. Daily weights are determined.

Provision of adequate fluid intake is achieved by the intravenous administration of hypotonic fluids, which serve to reduce the existing hypertonic state, and unlimited oral fluids. When the thirst mechanism is intact, the person will seek fluids, which should be readily available. If the person lacks the desire to drink, the nurse must be creative to ensure that the oral intake is maintained and/or supplemented with parenteral fluids.

Patient and family teaching

Lifelong dependence upon medication is not an easy fact for the patient to accept. The nurse can help the patient to plan for necessary readjustments, while giving reassurance that a normal pattern of life can be resumed.

The patient and a family member are taught the details of how to administer the drug. The instructions are also given in writing. Further explanation of the disorder may be required for appreciation of the importance of regular administration of the drug, and it should be advised that vasopressin is ineffective when taken orally because of inactivation by digestive enzymes. The patient is advised to record the weight every 2 or 3 days, and to note the urinary volume. Water retention indicated by weight increase and scanty urine may necessitate a decrease in vasopressin dosage.

ADH hypersecretion: syndrome of inappropriate antidiuretic hormone (SIADH)

Causes

Inappropriate production of antidiuretic hormone (ADH) may be caused by malignant tumours, respiratory and central nervous system infections, head trauma or positive-pressure ventilation. The exact mechanisms producing the excessive ADH secretion are not fully understood.

Clinical characteristics

The clinical characteristics of SIADH are those of water intoxication. The blood volume increases, haemodilution results, and serum sodium level and osmolality are decreased. Oedema is absent as a result of the hypo-natraemia. The person's urine is concentrated and the volume is diminished. Weight gain, nausea and vomiting, a decreased level of consciousness and seizures may be present.

Treatment

Treatment depends on the severity and duration of the water intoxication. In an emergency situation, intra-venous hypertonic saline solutions are administered along with diuretic drugs such as furosemide (frusemide). In less acute situations, the restriction of fluids to 500 mL daily may be sufficient. Demeclocycline may be pre-scribed because it inhibits the renal response to ADH. The underlying cause of the increased ADH secretion must be treated.

Nursing intervention

Nursing care is directed toward: (1) management of the fluid volume excess; (2) assessment and control of the altered thought processes that occur as water moves into the cerebral cells; and (3) patient teaching for the person with chronic SIADH.

Fluid volume excess

Assessment of the person's fluid balance includes moni-toring vital signs, serum electrolytes, urine osmolality, fluid intake and output, bodyweight and mental status. Oral fluids are restricted to 500 mL a day. Intravenous infusions are monitored closely and administered slowly to prevent further fluid overload and aggravation of the neurological manifestations.

Mental status

The patient's level of consciousness is assessed regularly. If it declines or if seizures are likely, safety precautions are implemented. The side-rails should be up on the bed and the patient should be visible at all times.

Patient and family teaching

The patient and family are helped to understand the disease and to recognize signs and symptoms of water toxicity. Information is provided about Medic Alert iden-tification. The patient is instructed to monitor body-weight and changes in the amount of urine output.

Pituitary ablation

The anterior and posterior pituitary gland may be removed or destroyed because of hyperfunction or a neoplasm of the gland. Hypophysectomy is also employed in the treat-ment of cancer of the breast and prostate, and is often supported by the sex hormones oestrogens and androgens respectively. Removal of the source of gonadotrophic hor-mones reduces support for the primary neoplasm and its metastasis. Withdrawal of the hormones does not cure the disease, but usually produces a remission for a period of several months.

Pituitary ablation may be carried out by radiation ther-apy, surgical excision or destruction by cryosurgery (freezing). Irradiation may be from an external source or radioactive yttrium-90 may be implanted. Access to the gland is usually by a nasal–trans-sphenoidal approach, but a transfrontal approach may be used if the tumour is large and has spread.

Hypophysectomy results in the withdrawal of ACTH, TSH and probably ADH, as well as the gonadotrophins. In some instances, the neural stalk, which transmits the nerve fibres from the hypothalamus to the posterior pituitary gland, may be preserved at operation, thus pre-venting diabetes insipidus. The patient requires cortisone, thyroxine and possibly ADH replacement for the remain-der of his or her life. Gonadal function ceases and the patient becomes infertile. If the operation was done because of disease of the pituitary gland, the male patient may be given testosterone to prevent impotence.

Preoperative preparation

The patient and family are likely to be very apprehensive. The nurse should therefore encourage them to talk about their fears and ask questions, and provide necessary emo-tional support. The permanent results of the operation will have been explained by the doctor, but the nurse, knowing what the patient has been told, should be pre-pared to answer questions and explain the hormonal replacement.

The patient is advised that nasal packing will be inserted if a trans-sphenoidal approach is used. The patient is taught deep-breathing techniques, encouraged to practise mouth breathing before operation and is cautioned against nose-blowing, sneezing and coughing after surgery. A cor-ticosteroid preparation is usually given the day before operation and again before going to the operating theatre.

Postoperative care

The care following a hypophysectomy is similar to that of any patient who has had intracranial surgery. Close observation is made for early signs of acute adrenal insufficiency (see below) or fluid imbalance. An adrenocorticoid steroid is given intravenously until the patient can tolerate it orally. The dose is gradually decreased until the maintenance dose is established. Vasopressin may be necessary to control the fluid loss; the dosage is adjusted to the urinary volume. Thyroid extract may be started orally on the second or third postoperative day.

The intravenous infusion is usually discontinued the morning after operation. Oral fluids may be started the evening of surgery or the next morning. If a transsphenoidal approach was used, the incision will be above the front teeth. The patient is instructed not to brush the teeth until the incision is healed and the sutures are removed. Mouthwashes are used to maintain dental and oral hygiene. The patient is taught to carry out meticulous oral hygiene regularly until healing has taken place in about 4–6 weeks. The period of hospitalization is relatively short; instruction about the taking of the necessary hormones (cortisone, vasopressin and thyroxine) is carried out throughout the postoperative period and, if necessary, a referral is made for follow-up instruction and supervision by a community nurse.

The person with a disorder of the adrenal cortices

As with other endocrine glands, dysfunction of the adrenal cortices may involve hyposecretion or hypersecretion of their hormones. Adrenocortical hypofunction produces Addison's disease. Hyperfunction may cause Cushing's syndrome or primary aldosteronism.

Assessment of adrenocortical function

Assessment of the person with altered adrenocortical function includes the identification of health problems common to persons with increased or decreased production of the adrenocortical hormones (Table 18.7).

Common characteristics identified during the *health history* include progressive fatigue and weakness, and changes in appetite and weight. The patient and family are questioned regarding changes in emotional responses including irritability, lability or depression. Questions are posed to identify changes in sexuality patterns in both males and females.

Table 18.7　Assessment of the person with altered adrenocortical function

	Clinical characteristics	
	Adrenocortical insufficiency (Addison's disease)	Adrenocortical hyperfunction (Cushing's disease)
Nutrition and metabolism	Hypoglycaemia Anorexia, nausea Abdominal pain Weight loss	Hyperglycaemia Abdominal discomfort Weight gain
Fluid and electrolyte balance	Dehydration Increased serum potassium level Decreased serum sodium level Hypotension	Oedema Decreased serum potassium level Increased serum sodium level Hypertension
Skin and hair	Skin dusky, bronze Increased pigmentation	Purple striae Bruising Thinning of skin and hair Hirsutism
Activity tolerance	Weakness Constant fatigue	Weakness, fatigue Muscle atrophy
Potential for infection		Delayed wound healing Suppression of usual signs of infection
Sexuality patterns	Decreased pubic and axillary hair in females	Secondary male sex characteristics in females Amenorrhoea Development of breasts in males
Individual coping	Depression Irritability Restlessness	Depression Apathy Mood changes

The *physical examination* focuses on observation of the skin and secondary sex characteristics.

The *skin* is inspected for signs of oedema or dehydration; increased bruising and pigmentation may be present on the palms and exposed body surfaces, joints, genitalia and oral mucosa. The abdomen is observed for the presence of purple striae. The development of a 'moon face' and the existence of fat deposits, particularly a 'Buffalo hump' (cervicodorsal fat), are characteristic signs that may be observed.

Changes and deviations in the structure of the breasts and in the distribution and amount of body hair, particularly scant pubic and axillary hair and excessive facial hair in the female, are noted.

Body height and weight are measured and alterations in normal growth and development assessed.

Adrenocortical insufficiency (Addison's disease)

Causes

Primary failure of the adrenal cortices to produce corticosteroids is rare; it is most often the result of atrophy of the glands but may also be caused by congenital adrenal hyperplasia, tubercular infection, adrenal haemorrhage or a neoplasm. Atrophy of the glands is attributed to an autoimmune reaction and affects females twice as often as males. Secondary hypofunction of the adrenal cortices occurs with hypopituitarism and the concomitant deficiency of ACTH, and with excessive administration of steroids. Adrenal insufficiency may also occur in patients with acquired immune deficiency syndrome (AIDS) as a result of fungal or cytomegalovirus infections.

Clinical characteristics

In Addison's disease there is a deficiency of cortisol which interferes with the maintenance of a normal blood sugar level; the body cannot compensate by gluconeogenesis, liver glycogen is depleted and hypoglycaemia develops, especially between meals. There is a general depression of metabolic activity and energy production. The ability to cope with even mild stress is greatly diminished and minor infections, slight injuries, exposure to extremes of temperature or emotional problems that are relatively insignificant to the normal person may prove very serious to these individuals.

The patient complains of weakness and constant fatigue, which becomes progressively more severe and incapacitating. Listlessness, irritability and impaired mental ability may be manifested. Anorexia, nausea, abdominal pain and constipation alternating with diarrhoea are common complaints. Increased sensitivity to cold develops. The patient loses weight. The skin takes on a dusky, bronze hue and brown pigmented areas appear, especially in sites normally exposed to light, pressure or friction. Patchy areas of pigmentation may also be observed in the oral mucosa and conjunctivae.

The adrenocortical insufficiency causes an outpouring of the hormone ACTH, which is similar in chemical structure to the melanocyte-stimulating hormone (MSH) and, in high concentration, may produce similar effects. As a result, pigmented areas of the skin are common in the patient with Addison's disease.

The aldosterone deficiency leads to decreased reabsorption of sodium by the renal tubules with a consequent excessive loss of water as well as sodium in the urine. Severe dehydration may develop, leading to a depletion of the intravascular volume and ensuing reduced cardiac output, hypotension and shock. Hypotension is invariable and it would be unlikely that someone with a systolic blood pressure above 110 mmHg would have the disease. The patient is often diagnosed only after presenting in a collapsed and critically ill condition known as an *Addisonian crisis* (see below).

Treatment and nursing intervention

Addison's disease is treated by maintenance doses of corticosteroid preparations. The glucocorticoids are replaced by the oral administration of a cortisol preparation (hydrocortisone) two or three times daily. The deficiency of mineralocorticoid (aldosterone) associated with primary adrenocortical insufficiency is met by giving fludrocortisone (synthetic aldosterone) orally once daily. The patient with secondary adrenocortical insufficiency does not require the aldosterone replacement.

Addison's disease
See chapter 2.6

The nurse caring for a patient receiving corticoid preparations must be familiar with the potential adverse effects of these drugs. If the patient receives corticoids in doses even slightly in excess of the amounts normally secreted, certain changes are likely to occur, especially with prolonged administration. Constant observation is necessary for early signs of side-effects. Restlessness, insomnia, euphoria and swings in mood may be manifested. The patient's susceptibility to infection may be markedly increased by the drug's suppression of lymphocyte and antibody production and local inflammatory responses. Muscle wasting and weakness may occur as a result of an excessive protein breakdown and increased loss of potassium in the urine. Sodium and water retention may be evidenced by oedema. Increased fat deposition on the trunk and face may develop, changing the patient's general appearance. Increased fullness and rounding of the face produces the characteristic change referred to as the 'moon face'. Females may develop secondary male characteristics accompanied by growth of hair on the face, and growth of the breasts in males is occasionally seen. Prolonged administration of corticoids in excess of normal secretion may produce hyperglycaemia and glycosuria. The patient also becomes predisposed to the development of gastrointestinal lesions, such as peptic ulcers.

The patient with Addison's disease is encouraged to take a high-carbohydrate, high-protein diet. The danger of hypoglycaemia which may occur with glucocorticoid deficiency may be offset by the patient taking nourishment between meals and at bedtime. In primary adrenal insufficiency the patient may require additional sodium chloride. A directive as to the amount of salt to be included in the diet should be received from the doctor; the average amount served with meals may be sufficient. The patient with secondary adrenocortical insufficiency will not require additional salt.

Acute corticoid insufficiency, which is also referred to as *Addisonian crisis*, may develop when corticoid replacement is inadequate or omitted, or it may be what brings the patient for medical attention before the disease is diagnosed. Frequently a crisis is precipitated by some physical or psychological stress such as infection, exposure to extremes of temperature, gastrointestinal upset (e.g. vomiting and diarrhoea), fever, profuse perspiration, strenuous activity, anxiety or grief. Acute insufficiency is serious and, unless treated promptly, can rapidly lead to death. Early symptoms are nausea, vomiting, diarrhoea, abdominal pain, fever and extreme weakness. Severe hypoglycaemia and dehydration develop rapidly; the blood pressure falls, and shock and coma may follow. Blood glucose, sodium and cortisol levels are low and the potassium and urea concentrations are markedly increased.

Addisonian crisis is treated by continuous intravenous infusion of normal saline to which hydrocortisone (cortisol) is added for at least the first 24 hours. Intravenous dextrose is required if hypoglycaemia is present. Hydrocortisone is also given orally as replacement medication. The large doses of hydrocortisone that the patient receives usually exert a sufficient sodium-retaining effect, eliminating the need for supplementary administration of a mineralocorticoid preparation such as fludrocortisone in the short term.

Frequent recordings of the blood pressure, temperature, pulse respirations and level of response are made. The patient is kept at absolute rest to avoid expenditure of energy and is turned, bathed and fed by the nurse. He or she is kept flat and any change of position is made slowly because of the hypotension. Frequent high-carbohydrate feedings are given as soon as they can be tolerated. When the patient's blood pressure and other vital signs have returned to normal and are sustained, and the condition that precipitated the crisis has been controlled, the corticoid dosage is gradually reduced to maintenance level.

Patient and family teaching

The overall goals are to learn self-regulation of the disease and to maintain a satisfactory level of functioning.

Goals

The patient and family will be able to:

1. state the purpose of lifelong steroid replacement therapy

2. describe a plan for taking medications daily and state the names, dosage, frequency, actions and side-effects of each prescribed medication

3. describe the effects of stress on the disease and plans to minimize stress

4. discuss plans to minimize exposure to infection

5. describe symptoms that indicate Addisonian crisis and actions to take if symptoms develop.

Nursing intervention

As primary adrenal insufficiency requires lifelong replacement therapy, an important nursing function is teaching the patient and family about the disease and necessary care. A simple explanation is given of the nature of the condition with reassurance that, although hormone replacement will be necessary for life, if the prescribed therapeutic regimen is followed, a relatively normal life can be expected.

Activity tolerance

The importance of regular and adequate hours of rest, stopping activities short of fatigue and avoiding exposure to cold are stressed, indicating the effect of exposure and overexertion on cellular activity and the blood sugar level.

Medication therapy

No medications, including laxatives, except those ordered by the doctor should be taken. Detailed teaching is carried out regarding the taking of prescribed corticoid preparations, including the importance of talking the exact amounts at the correct times. The patient is warned of the dangers of being without medication. Increased doses of medication may be recommended during periods of stress.

Nutrition

The high-carbohydrate, high-protein diet with the amount of sodium recommended by the doctor is discussed in detail, explaining the need for nourishment between meals and at bedtime to maintain a normal blood sugar level.

Prevention of infection

The patient and family are advised of the need to avoid contact with those with an infection as much as possible, and suggestions are made as to how this may be achieved.

Individual coping

Patients should understand that a stressful situation or illness demands more corticoids. To prevent a serious crisis or acute corticoid insufficiency, prompt medical attention is necessary with any disorder such as a respiratory infection, vomiting, diarrhoea, fainting or sudden weakness. The role of worry and emotional situations in precipitating a crisis is emphasized.

Safety measures

The patient with Addison's disease should always carry a steroid card or wear a Medic Alert bracelet or pendant that clearly indicates the presence of corticoid insufficiency and what should be done in the event of injury or sudden collapse.

In teaching, the nurse does not attempt to provide all the necessary information at one time. The instruction is planned to cover several sessions; salient points are clarified and reinforced by repetition, and opportunities are provided for the patient and family members to ask questions and to participate actively in the learning process.

Evaluation

The patient and family should be able to administer the prescribed corticosteroid replacement therapy safely and to recognize side-effects of over- or under-replacement. The patient should be able to describe plans to receive adequate rest, to decrease exposure to infection, to minimize the effects of added physical and emotional stress and for ongoing health care and supervision. The patient should maintain a desirable bodyweight and quickly identify fluctuations in weight pattern.

Adrenocortical hyperfunction (Cushing's syndrome)

Causes

This is a rare disorder which is more common in females and results from an excessive secretion of adrenal corticoids. It may be due to primary hyperfunction of one or both of the adrenal cortices or may be secondary to a pathological hypersecretion of ACTH by the anterior pituitary gland. Primary hyperactivity of the adrenal cortex is usually caused by a neoplasm, most frequently an adenoma, but may also occur as a result of unexplained hyperplasia. The most common cause, however, is iatrogenic: the excessive administration of ACTH.

Clinical characteristics

These will vary in individuals according to age and the amount of corticoid being produced in excess of the normal. The increased output of cortisol causes excessive protein catabolism, gluconeogenesis, an abnormal distribution of fat and atrophy of lymphoid tissue. The person manifests a decreased glucose tolerance, hyperglycaemia, and muscle wasting and weakness. The appearance changes because of the increased deposition of fat on the trunk, thin wasted limbs, and a round, bloated-looking face ('moon' face). Purple striae may appear, notably on the abdomen, buttocks and thighs, and are due to increased fragility of the blood vessels and atrophy of the skin. Ecchymoses are common. The production of lymphocytes is suppressed, increasing the patient's susceptibility to infection. Osteoporosis may occur, usually

in the vertebrae, because of calcium mobilization; the patient frequently complains of backache.

The excessive secretion of mineralocorticoids results in electrolyte, fluid and acid–base imbalances. Hypernatraemia, water retention and hypokalaemia develop. The increased reabsorption by the renal tubules of sodium ions in exchange for hydrogen ions depletes the acid ions, producing alkalosis. The low blood level of potassium may cause extreme weakness and cardiac dysfunction. Hypertension due to the sodium and water retention is common.

As a consequence of the increased production of androgens, women develop secondary male characteristics. There is a marked growth of hair on the face, the voice deepens, breasts atrophy, amenorrhoea occurs and the clitoris may enlarge.

If the disease is secondary to a hypersecretion of ACTH, the disturbances are associated principally with an excessive production of the glucocorticoids only.

Treatment and nursing intervention

The treatment of Cushing's syndrome is urgent as the disease carries a 5-year mortality rate of 50% (Haslett et al 1999). This depends upon whether the hypersecretion of corticoids is due to primary dysfunction of the adrenal cortices or is the result of a hypersecretion of ACTH. In the case of an adrenocortical neoplasm, the affected gland is removed. If the disease is pituitary dependent, a bilateral adrenalectomy is usually done, whereas a pituitary adenoma can be removed surgically via the transsphenoidal route. The patient is prepared medically with drug therapy before operation to reduce cortisol levels, and then receives hormonal replacement therapy after surgery as outlined for Addison's disease. If the condition is secondary to a pituitary tumour, the tumour is usually treated by irradiation or surgical removal.

Nursing care of the patient with Cushing's syndrome is mainly symptomatic (Table 18.7). Precautions are necessary to prevent accidental falls, which may occur because of weakness. The fluid intake and output are recorded to determine the amount of water retention, and sodium intake is restricted. The blood pressure and pulse are taken at regular intervals so that early changes may be detected. Changes in mood and behaviour are common and should be recorded. Exposure to persons with infection is avoided because of the patient's lowered resistance.

Hyperaldosteronism

An excessive production of aldosterone occurs rarely and is usually caused by an adenoma or hyperplasia of the particular adrenocortical cells that secrete the hormone. The most striking features of the disease are the excessive renal loss of potassium, retention of sodium and hypertension. The person experiences severe generalized muscular weakness due to the hypokalaemia. Depletion

*Cushing's syndrome
See chapter 2.6*

of the body potassium reduces the kidneys' ability to concentrate the urine, and polyuria occurs. Despite an increased retention of salt, there is no corresponding retention of water or oedema. This is attributed to an increased glomerular filtration rate and the polyuria. As a result of the hypernatraemia and polyuria, the person usually experiences severe thirst. An increase in arterial blood pressure is characteristic. In addition to hypernatraemia and hypokalaemia, laboratory investigation reveals raised urinary and plasma aldosterone levels and normal renin concentration. Treatment consists of surgical removal of the adenoma or affected gland preceded by administration of potassium salts.

Secondary hyperaldosteronism due to an excessive secretion of renin by the kidneys may occur. It may be treated with spironolactone, an aldosterone antagonist, or renal surgery.

The person with a disorder of the adrenal medullae

Assessment of adrenal medullary function

The *health history* focuses on identification of the person's usual responses to stress and documentation of episodes of excessive stress reactions (flight or fight reaction).

Physical examination involves the documentation of fluctuations in and excessively high blood pressure readings.

Phaeochromocytoma
See chapter 2.6

Excess of adrenaline and noradrenaline (phaeochromocytoma)

Disease of the adrenal medullae is rare and most commonly occurs in the form of a neoplasm known as a **phaeochromocytoma**, which produces an excessive amount of adrenaline and noradrenaline. The tumour is usually unilateral and benign, and causes hypertension, hyperglycaemia and hypermetabolism. The increased liberation of large amounts of the hormones is usually paroxysmal at first, lasting from a few minutes to hours, but is likely eventually to become persistent. The patient frequently complains of a pounding headache, nausea, vomiting, palpitation, air hunger, nervousness, tremor and weakness. Sweating, pallor, dilatation of the pupils, tachycardia and a sharp rise in the blood pressure are also manifested. The increased glucogenolysis and subsequent raised blood sugar level may result in glucosuria.

Tests used to establish the diagnosis of phaeochromocytoma include the estimation of the blood and urinary content of the hormones or their major metabolite, vanillylmandelic acid (VMA). CT is carried out to localize the tumour.

The patient with phaeochromocytoma is treated by surgical removal of the tumour of the affected gland. Sympathetic blocking agents are administered before operation to decrease blood pressure and reduce other symptoms.

Nursing in adrenal surgery

Surgery of the adrenal glands may be performed on patients with hypersecretions of hormones due to hyperplasia or tumours of one or both glands. The procedure may involve the removal of both adrenal glands (bilateral or total adrenalectomy), the removal of one gland (unilateral adrenalectomy) or resection of part of a gland (subtotal adrenalectomy). Bilateral adrenalectomy is occasionally undertaken in patients with cancer of the breast and occasionally in those with cancer of the prostate. Malignant disease of these organs is dependent to some extent on sex hormones, and because the adrenal cortices produce both oestrogens and androgens removal of the cortices eliminates a source of the supporting hormones. In the case of cancer of the breast, adrenalectomy is preceded by oophorectomy (removal of the ovaries). Occasionally the patient with cancer of the prostate undergoes orchidectomy (removal of the testicles) before adrenalectomy is considered.

Preoperative preparation

Preparation of the patient for adrenal surgery includes the general preparation cited in Chapter 10. Blood studies are done to determine electrolyte concentrations, and corrections are made as indicated. Because of an excessive potassium excretion, a solution of potassium chloride may be ordered to restore the normal level of potassium in the blood. The blood sugar level and glucose tolerance are investigated. The patient is given a high-protein diet because of the protein depletion due to excessive glucocorticoid secretion. The fluid intake and output are measured, and the balance is noted. The blood pressure is recorded at least once daily to serve as a postoperative comparative baseline. The patient with hyperfunction of the adrenal cortices frequently has experienced hypertension for some time. Phenoxybenzamine hydrochloride (an alpha-blocker) may be prescribed before surgery for 6 weeks to reduce vasomotor tone and restore normal plasma volume.

If both adrenal glands are to be removed, the patient and the family must understand that constant hormone replacement will be necessary for the remainder of the patient's life.

After operation, the patient's respirations tend to be shallow because the incision is close to the diaphragm. Careful teaching about postoperative breathing and coughing exercises are therefore essential.

The surgeon's approach to the adrenal gland is usually through a high flank incision or occasionally through the abdomen. When a bilateral adrenalectomy is carried out, two incisions are made, unless the transabdominal approach is used.

Hydrocortisone may be administered before and during as well as after the operation to prevent adrenal insufficiency in the immediate postoperative period. An intravenous solution is run slowly and continuously.

This is in preparation for prompt administration of corticosteroids or a vasopressor, as indicated.

Postoperative care

Assessment and management of medication and fluid therapy

During the first few postoperative days, and until the maintenance dosages of hydrocortisone and fludrocortisone are established in the case of adrenalectomy, special attention is paid to the patient's blood pressure, **fluid balance** and blood chemistry. Constant nursing care is necessary until the vital signs and the corticoid, sodium and potassium concentrations are stabilized. The blood pressure, respirations and pulse are recorded every 15 minutes for several hours and the interval is gradually lengthened if they remain satisfactory. Any rapid or significant fall in blood pressure, dyspnoea or tachycardia is reported promptly. The fluid intake and output are accurately measured, and any imbalance is brought to the doctor's attention. Frequent checks are made of the blood sodium, potassium and glucose levels, which influence the amount of corticoids given. Vomiting, increased weakness, dehydration, hypotension and an increased temperature may indicate acute corticoid insufficiency.

Intravenous corticoids are given continuously for a day or two with the dosage and rate of flow adjusted to the patient's clinical condition and electrolyte and fluid balances. Oral doses of hydrocortisone and fludrocortisone are started as soon as tolerated by the patient. The dosage of both corticoid preparations is gradually tapered off until maintenance amounts are established. When the intravenous corticoids are withdrawn, an intravenous infusion of glucose in water or normal saline is continued slowly even though the patient may be tolerating fluids by mouth. The purpose of this is to keep the route available for quick administration of corticoids or a vasopressor (e.g. metaraminol or noradrenaline (norepinephrine) acid tartrate) if needed. The patient's condition tends to be labile and may change quickly. The nurse must be constantly alert for signs of corticoid insufficiency or indications of excessive corticoid administration.

When surgery is performed to remove a phaeochromocytoma, monitoring of the blood pressure is necessary every ½–1 hour for at least 36–48 hours; severe fluctuations may occur. A marked rise may occur during or immediately after operation because of excessive liberation of catecholamines from the tumour during removal. An adrenergic blocking agent such as phentolamine is kept available for quick intravenous administration to neutralize the medullary hormones.

More often the problem following surgery is severe hypotension and concomitant shock. The blood pressure is maintained by giving a vasopressor such as noradrenaline (norepinephrine) acid tartrate or metaraminol in an intravenous solution. The rate of flow must be carefully controlled and adjusted according to frequent blood pressure recordings and the doctor's directives. The patient is kept flat and any change in position achieved slowly.

When unilateral adrenalectomy or a subtotal resection of one or both glands is done, the patient may receive some hydrocortisone following operation. Less will be required than in total adrenalectomy, and it is gradually withdrawn.

After adrenal surgery the patient usually stays in bed until the blood pressure remains at a satisfactory level. Before commencing ambulation, the head of the bed is elevated and the blood pressure checked. The patient should not be left unattended during mobilization and frequent blood pressure checks should be carried out. If a significant decrease in blood pressure occurs, the patient is returned to bed and kept flat.

Patient teaching

In preparation for discharge, the patient who has had a bilateral adrenalectomy receives the same instruction as the patient with Addison's disease. If one gland has been removed or a subtotal resection done, the patient is cautioned to avoid overfatigue, exposure to extremes of temperature (especially cold), infections and emotional disturbances as much as possible. It is possible that stress may precipitate an acute adrenal insufficiency or crisis because the remaining adrenal tissue cannot meet the increased hormonal demand. If the patient experiences weakness, fainting, fever, or nausea and vomiting, the general practitioner should be contacted immediately; a corticoid supplement will be required.

After any adrenal operation the patient should resume activity very gradually and is followed closely as an outpatient. Usually several months are required to adjust the hormonal replacement satisfactorily. The patient who has had hypertension due to phaeochromocytoma may not regain a stable blood pressure level for 3–4 months.

Fluid balance
See chapter 2.6

Summary

The endocrine system contributes to the homeostatic control of many body functions. Disorders of the endocrine system and its interrelated components are of three major types:

1. Increased production of one or more hormone(s).

2. Decreased production of one or more hormone(s).

3. Failure of the target organ or tissue to respond to the hormone.

Clinical characteristics of endocrine disorders are varied, subtle and slowly progressive. The patient and family are the best source of assessment information as they are usually aware that something is wrong before a pattern of characteristic signs and symptoms can be recognized. The health problems common to most persons with endocrine disorders include: altered nutrition and metabolism, changes in activity tolerance, altered thought processes and emotional responses, altered sexuality patterns, altered fluid balance, impaired skin integrity and impaired thermoregulation.

The person with a hormone imbalance is at risk for the development of life-threatening as well as chronic complications. The nurse provides intensive care during acute episodes and assists the patient and family to recognize the early warnings of endocrine imbalances and actions to take to prevent complications.

The discussions in this chapter focus on the more common endocrine disorders of type 1 and type 2 diabetes mellitus, and hypothyroidism and hyperthyroidism. Individuals with disorders of the pituitary gland, parathyroid and adrenal glands experience similar and equally devastating problems. Many persons with endocrine disorders require lifelong hormone replacement therapy as a result of decreased production of hormones with disease and/or therapeutic destruction of the involved gland. All are faced with the need to make major adjustments in their lives. The patient ultimately becomes responsible for self-management of the endocrine disorder.

The growing body of nursing knowledge available to resolve patient health problems is useless if it is not transmitted to patients and their families to enable them to assume control of their own care. Throughout this chapter the importance of patient and family teaching is stressed. Emphasis is placed on the provision of information about the survival skills or the basic knowledge and skill the person requires to function safely. Nurses are also responsible for evaluating the effectiveness of health teaching and for determining whether the patient and family understand the need for continuing therapy.

Advanced teaching and counselling skills are needed to help people change their habits and lifestyles. Although all nurses do not have the opportunity to follow individuals for an extended period of time to enable them to provide this level of teaching, they can ensure that all persons with long-term endocrine disorders are aware of the many resources available in the community.

References

Barnett A (2001) New therapies for the management of type 2 diabetes. Nursing Times 97(6): 34–36.

Batki A (1999) Selecting blood glucose monitoring systems. Professional Nurse 14(10): 715–723.

British National Formulary (2000) British National Formulary. London: British Medical Association/Royal Pharmaceutical Society of Great Britain.

Carr S (2001) Acromegaly management in the community. Nursing Times 97(2): 32–33.

Elliot B (2000) Diagnosing and treating hypothyroidism. Nurse Practitioner 25(2): 92–105.

Erens R, Primatesta P, Prior G (2001) Health survey for England; the health of minority ethnic groups. London: DoH.

Haslett C, Chilvers E, Hunter J, Boon N (1999) Davidson's principles and practice of medicine, 18th edn. Edinburgh: Churchill Livingstone.

Lehman R (1998) The effects of exercise on cardiovascular risk factors in type 2 diabetes mellitus. Practical Diabetes International 15(5): 151–156.

McIntyre M, McDowell J (1994) Educating a patient with diabetes about foot care. British Journal of Nursing 3(2): 75–78.

Melville A, Richardson R, Lister-Sharp D (2000) Complications of type 2 diabetes: renal disease and the promotion of patient self management. Nursing Times 96(17): 37–38.

O'Malley B, Hickey J, Nevens E (2000) Thyroid dysfunction: weight problems and the psyche, the patients perspective. Journal of Human Nutrition and Dietetics 13(4): 243–248.

Pullen M (2000) Exercise for the person with diabetes. Professional Nurse 16(2): 888–891.

Rees P, Williams D (1995) Principles of clinical medicine. London: Edward Arnold.

Richmond J (1993) An investigation into the effects of hypoglycaemia in young people aged 16–30 years. Journal of Advanced Nursing 18: 1681–1687.

Rodgers J (2000) Pharmacological interventions in type 2 diabetes: the role of the nurse. British Journal of Nursing 9(13): 866–870.

Springhouse Corporation (1998) Handbook of medical–surgical nursing. Springhouse, PA: Springhouse Publishing Corporation.

Springhouse Corporation (2000) Handbook of pathophysiology. Springhouse, PA: Springhouse Publishing Corporation.

Umeh L, Wallhagen M, Nicoloff N (1999) Identifying patients at high risk for amputation. Nurse Practitioner 24(6): 5670.

Vander AJ, Sherman JH, Luciano DS (1990) Human physiology: the mechanism of body function, 5th edn. New York: McGraw-Hill.

Walton J, Brand S (1994) Diabetes mellitus: implications for nursing care. British Journal of Nursing 3(9): 442–445.

Watkins P (1998) ABC of diabetes, 4th edn. London: BMJ.

Winters S, Jernigan V (2000) Vascular disease risk markers in diabetes: monitoring and evaluation. Nurse Practitioner 25(6): 40–65.

York CRD (1999) Complications of diabetes: screening for retinopathy, management of foot ulcers. York: York NHS Centre for Review and Dissemination.

York CRD (2000) Complications of diabetes: renal disease and the promotion of self-management. York: York NHS Centre for Review and Dissemination.

Caring for the patient with a disorder of the renal system

Mike Walsh

Introduction

The renal system and urinary tract

Assessment of renal function

Clinical characteristics of renal dysfunction

The person with impaired renal function

The person with a disorder of the urinary system

Tumour of the bladder

Summary

Introduction

Understanding the renal and urinary systems is complex and challenging. Renal and urinary tract anatomy and physiology are intricate, yet delivery of expert, comprehensive care to the person with a disorder in either system involves understanding the full impact of that disorder on the individual's quality of life. The purpose of this chapter is to give an overview of the normal kidney and urinary tract and how disorders affect the rest of the body. This will assist the nurse to understand the impact of disease and how to deliver care to the person within a holistic framework.

The renal system and urinary tract

Structure of the kidneys

The kidneys are paired organs that lie retroperitoneally against the dorsal abdominal wall. Each kidney is enclosed in a fibrous capsule and is embedded in fatty tissue. It consists of approximately 1 000 000 *nephrons, collecting tubules,* and a *pelvis*. The kidney is anatomically divided into an outer portion called the *cortex* and an inner section lying between the cortex and the pelvis called the *medulla* (Fig. 19.1). The blood vessels, nerves and ureter enter or leave the kidney at the *hilum*, the indentation on the medial surface.

Nephron

The nephron is the functional unit of the kidney. It consists of a narrow, convoluted tubule and a tuft of capillaries referred to as a *glomerulus*. The upper end of the

Figure 19.1   Cross-section of the kidney.

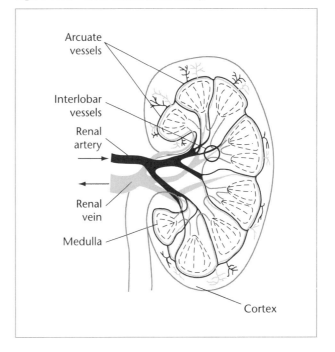

- Arcuate vessels
- Interlobar vessels
- Renal artery
- Renal vein
- Medulla
- Cortex

Renal function
See chapter 5.4

Structure
See chapter 5.4

tubule is dilated and invaginated to envelop the glomerulus and is called *Bowman's capsule*.

The tubule is divided into three segments: the *proximal convoluted tubule*, the hairpin-like *loop of Henle* and the *distal convoluted tubule* (Fig. 19.2). A major function of the tubules is to convey water and solutes in either direction

Figure 19.2   A renal unit, or nephron, of the cortex of the kidney.

Renal function
See chapter 5.4

Filtration
See chapter 5.4

across the tubular cells between the interstitial fluid and the tubular content. The thickness and structure of the walls differ from one segment to another; this arrangement accounts for different substances being reabsorbed and secreted in different sections of the tubule.

The proximal convoluted tubule is the longest portion of the nephron and has thin walls consisting of a single layer of cells. The loop of Henle varies in length and lies mainly in the medulla. Its terminal portion approximates the glomerulus of the nephron, of which it is a part, and its afferent arteriole. The distal convoluted tubule is shorter than the other portions of the tubule. The cells in most of the tubule are sensitive to the concentration of antidiuretic hormone (ADH) and adrenocortical steroids, which influence reabsorption of substances by the distal tubule.

Collecting tubules

The distal tubules coalesce to form straight collecting tubules, which unite to form progressively larger collecting tubules. Groups of the larger tubules come together to form a pyramid-like structure in the medulla. The apex of each pyramid is known as the *papilla* and contains the terminations of collecting tubules through which the urine passes into a cup-like pouch (calyx) of the renal pelvis. The ureter drains the kidney via the renal pelvis.

Blood supply

The renal artery to each kidney arises from the abdominal aorta. When the artery enters the kidney, it progressively subdivides to become afferent arterioles. Each *afferent arteriole* enters a nephron to form a glomerulus. The glomerular capillaries unite to form the *efferent arteriole*,

which terminates in a second capillary network in which the tubule is invested. The blood pressure in this second set of capillaries is much lower than that in the glomerulus. The blood is then collected into venules and eventually into a renal vein which carries it to the inferior vena cava.

A large volume of blood is circulated continuously through the kidneys. It is estimated that the renal blood flow averages about 1000–1200 mL per minute in an adult. Receiving an adequate blood supply under the appropriate driving pressure is critical to maintaining kidney function.

A group of special cells is located just before the afferent arteriole becomes the glomerulus. These are known as *juxtaglomerular cells*. They are responsible for the production of the chemical *renin*.

Renal function

Normal functioning of the body cells is greatly dependent upon a relative constancy of the internal environment. The kidneys play a major role in maintaining this constancy by regulating the water and electrolyte content and the acid–base balance of the body; they *conserve* appropriate amounts of essential substances vital to normal cellular function (e.g. glucose) and *excrete* excesses, the waste products of metabolism, toxic substances and drugs in the urine.

The kidneys also have an important *endocrine role*: the production of renin and erythropoietin, and their release into the blood when needed. In addition, the kidney is the major organ responsible for the production of the most active vitamin D metabolite (calcitriol). Its major effect is to stimulate calcium absorption from the gut, thereby assisting in the maintenance of healthy bone. The processes involved in these functions performed by the kidneys are filtration, selective reabsorption, the transport of substances from the interstitial fluid to the tubule and endocrine secretion (Box 19.1).

Filtration

The permeability of the glomerular capillaries is greater than that of capillaries elsewhere in the body. The same principles that govern the movement of fluid out of the arteriolar ends of the capillaries throughout the body are applicable to the filtration process in the glomeruli. The hydrostatic pressure of the blood in the glomerular capillaries is approximately 60 mmHg, which is considerably higher than that in the other capillaries of the body. This hydrostatic pressure is opposed by the osmotic pressure of the blood proteins (approximately 28 mmHg) plus the hydrostatic pressure in Bowman's capsule (about 18 mmHg). The net filtration force is 14 mmHg: hydrostatic blood pressure (60) − colloidal osmotic pressure (28) − capsular hydrostatic pressure (18) = 14 mmHg.

The average volume of filtrate in both kidneys is estimated to be about 180 litres each day. The glomerular filtration rate (GFR) is directly proportional to the filtration

Box 19.1   Renal functions

Overall function

Homeostasis – the maintenance of a suitable environment for optimum cellular function

Principal function

To regulate the volume and composition of the extracellular fluid

The kidney maintains homeostasis by performing the following roles:

1. *Production*:
    vitamin D metabolite (calcitriol)
    erythropoietin
    renin.

2. *Regulation*:
    volume of water in extracellular fluid
    concentration of electrolytes in extracellular fluid
    osmolality of extracellular fluid
    concentration of hydrogen ions in the extracellular fluid.

3. *Excretion*:
    endogenous – end-products of protein catabolism
    exogenous – medications.

force; the normal rate is approximately 125 mL per minute. Factors that may alter the GFR include:

- change in glomerular capillary hydrostatic pressure, which may be incurred by an increase or decrease in systemic blood pressure or by constriction or dilatation of the afferent and efferent arterioles

- increase or decrease in renal artery blood volume

- increase or decrease in the hydrostatic pressure within Bowman's capsule due to compression by ureteral obstruction or disease within the kidney, causing swelling confined within the renal capsule

- decrease or increase in the oncotic pressure (concentration of plasma proteins)

- increased glomerular permeability due to disease, such as nephrotic syndrome

- decrease in glomeruli due to pathological destruction.

Many solutes escape from the blood in the glomerular filtrate, but small amounts of only a few of them appear in urine. The formed elements and plasma proteins of the blood do not normally pass out of the glomeruli; the composition of the filtrate is the same as that of plasma minus the plasma proteins.

Tubular reabsorption

Reabsorption and secretion are complex renal activities. The composition and volume of the filtrate that enters the Bowman's capsule differ markedly from those of urine.

Of the 180 litres of filtrate produced in 24 hours, only about 1.5 litres are excreted as urine. Most of the water and many of the solid constituents of the filtrate are needed by the body to maintain homeostasis and normal cell metabolism. Other substances, such as urea, creatinine, uric acid, sulfates and phosphates, are waste products of metabolism and are excreted in the urine. The tubule cells selectively reabsorb according to the body's needs. Certain substances, such as glucose and amino acids, are completely reabsorbed when their plasma concentrations are within normal range but appear in the urine when the normal is exceeded. About 99% of the water in the filtrate is reclaimed. Reabsorption of the inorganic salts (e.g. sodium, chloride, calcium, potassium, bicarbonate) is variable, depending mainly on their plasma levels.

The *proximal convoluted tubule* is responsible for the greatest amount of reabsorption. All of the glucose and amino acids and a large proportion of the water and other essential substances are reabsorbed here. Only about 35% of the total volume of filtrate enters the loop of Henle.

The *loop of Henle* seems to be concerned principally with the transport of sodium chloride ions and water. The ascending limb is impermeable to water. It actively transports sodium and chloride ions out into the interstitial fluid, and the tubular fluid becomes hypotonic. The descending limb of the loop of Henle is permeable to water; water moves out to the interstitial fluid which has become hypertonic. At the same time sodium and chloride ions diffuse into the descending limb.

The maintenance of the volume and concentration of body fluids within a narrow range is largely controlled by the ability of the kidney tubules to concentrate or dilute the urine. When body fluids are diluted by an excess of water or diminished solute intake (especially sodium), the urine becomes dilute and the volume is increased. Conversely, if the concentration of body fluids is raised to above the normal level by an excessive intake of solutes or an extrarenal loss of water, water reabsorption from the filtrate is increased, concentrating the urine and decreasing the output volume.

The dilution and concentration of urine depend principally on two factors: (1) the osmotic pressure of the peritubular fluid, which in turn is mainly dependent on the normal functioning of the loop of Henle and the distal convoluted tubules, and (2) the concentration of ADH in the blood.

The fluid entering the distal tubule is hypotonic, but the volume and osmolality are modified selectively as the fluid proceeds through the distal and collecting tubules.

Reabsorption of water from the hypotonic filtrate in the distal convoluted and collecting tubules is regulated by ADH. This hormone is produced by the hypothalamus in the brain, and is stored and released into the blood by the posterior pituitary gland (see p. 564).

The reabsorption of sodium by active cellular transport in the distal and collecting tubules is influenced by the

Reabsorption
See chapter 5.4

adrenocortical hormone *aldosterone*. A high concentration of aldosterone stimulates the distal tubular cells to reabsorb increasing amounts of sodium. Aldosterone also affects the amount of potassium reclaimed and excreted. Increased concentrations of the hormone promote excretion of potassium, and a deficient amount of aldosterone produces excessive retention of potassium.

Tubular secretion and excretion

Tubular cells are capable of actively transporting some substances from the blood into the filtrate – a reverse process to that of reabsorption. The potassium concentration of plasma is regulated by this process. Practically all of the potassium that escapes from the plasma into the filtrate is reabsorbed in the proximal tubule. Any excess in the blood is then actively secreted by the distal tubules and is excreted in exchange for sodium ions.

Cells of the distal tubules play an important role in maintaining a normal *acid–base balance* in the blood and extracellular fluid. In association with the respiratory system, the kidneys regulate the body's systemic arterial pH within a narrow range of 7.35–7.45.

The first lines of defence against alteration in body pH are the extracellular and intracellular buffers. The major extracellular buffer is bicarbonate and the buffering capacity of the HCO_3–CO_2 system is greatly extended by the regulation of carbon dioxide gas tension by the respiratory system.

The kidney's role in acid–base homeostasis is to stabilize the balance between H^+ and HCO_3^- in the blood. This is accomplished by four processes:

1. secretion of hydrogen ions
2. reabsorption of sodium and bicarbonate ions
3. acidification of phosphate salts
4. synthesis and secretion of ammonia.

All these mechanisms serve to restore the hydrogen ion concentration so that the pH of the blood is maintained within normal limits.

Endocrine renal secretions

The kidney produces two endocrine secretions: renin and erythropoietin.

Renin reacts with an inactive precursor fraction of the plasma globulin (angiotensinogen), producing a substance called angiotensin I which is converted to angiotensin II by another enzyme in the lungs. As angiotensin II circulates it causes vasoconstriction of the systemic arterioles and stimulates the secretion of aldosterone and, to a lesser extent, glucocorticoids.

The principal mechanism responsible for the release of renin is a drop in blood pressure and circulating blood volume, although falling sodium and chloride levels in the distal tubule can have the same effect.

A second hormone produced by the kidneys is the *renal erythropoietic factor* (REF; erythrogenin). It is produced and secreted into the blood mainly in response to hypoxia and functions in the maintenance of normal erythrocyte production by the bone marrow. REF reacts with a plasma globulin to produce *erythropoietin*, which stimulates the bone marrow to produce and release blood cells.

Characteristics and composition of urine

When the filtrate flows into the main collecting tubules and renal pelvis, it becomes **urine**. The average volume excreted in 24 hours is approximately 1.5 litres, but varies with fluid losses through other channels (e.g. sweat) and fluid intake. The reaction of urine is usually acid, with a pH of about 6.0, but may range from 4.5 to 8.5 with a varied dietary intake. The acidity increases with high protein ingestion and tissue catabolism, whereas a vegetable diet produces an alkaline urine.

The specific gravity, which gives a rough estimate of the concentration of solids, ranges from 1.003 to 1.040. The composition of urine varies with dietary intake and metabolic wastes produced. Normally, about 90–95% of urine is water. The chief solutes are urea, creatinine, uric acid and the chlorides, phosphates and sulfates of sodium, potassium, calcium, magnesium and ammonia.

Ureters, bladder and urethra

Ureters

Each of the two **ureters** is a tube, made up mainly of muscle tissue, 25–30 cm in length, extending from a kidney to the bladder. They are situated behind the parietal peritoneum and enter the posterior wall of the lower half of the bladder obliquely. The slanted entrance forms a flap in the bladder wall which serves as a valve to prevent a reflux of urine as the bladder fills or contracts.

The function of these tubes is simply to convey urine from the kidneys to the bladder. Contraction of the ureteral muscular tissue produces peristaltic waves which move the urine along the tube and into the bladder in spurts.

Bladder

The urinary bladder serves as a temporary reservoir for the urine, which it expels at intervals from the body. It is a collapsible muscular sac that lies behind the symphysis pubis. Three layers of plain muscle tissue form the bladder walls. The fibres are arranged in longitudinal, circular and spiral layers. Collectively, these layers are referred to as the *detrusor muscle*. The ureteral orifices in the posterior wall and the urethral opening outline a triangular area called the *trigone*. When the bladder is empty, the mucous membrane lining falls into folds (rugae) except in the area of the trigone (Fig. 19.3).

Urethra

The **urethra** is a slender tube that conveys urine from the bladder to the exterior. It has a thin layer of smooth muscle tissue and is lined with a mucous membrane which is continuous with that of the bladder. The opening from

Urine production
See chapter 5.4

Ureters
See chapter 5.4

Urethra
See chapter 5.4

Figure 19.3   The bladder, ureters, urethra and prostate in (a) females and (b) males.

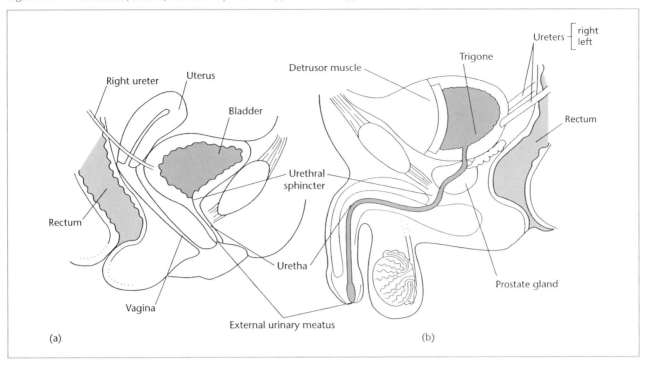

the bladder is controlled by two sphincters: an internal one which is under autonomic (involuntary) nervous system control, and an external one which is voluntarily controlled by the cerebral cortex. The external urethral orifice is known as the *urinary meatus*.

In the female, the urethra is about 4 cm long and lies anterior to the vagina. The male urethra is approximately 20 cm in length and, on leaving the bladder, passes through the prostate gland. As well as conveying the urine, the male urethra receives the semen from the ejaculatory ducts of the reproductive system, transmitting it through the meatus (see Fig. 19.3).

Micturition

This is a term used for the elimination of urine from the bladder. The process involves both autonomic (involuntary) and voluntary nervous impulses. When 300–400 mL of urine collect in the bladder, receptors that are sensitive to stretching initiate impulses that are transmitted by afferent nerve fibres into the lower part of the spinal cord. A reflex response via parasympathetic nerves to the bladder results in contractions of the detrusor muscle and relaxation of the internal sphincter.

The initial impulses from the stretch receptors are also relayed via a spinocortical tract to the cerebral cortex, producing an awareness of the need to void. When a person is prepared to empty the bladder, voluntary impulses are initiated that descend the cord and are carried out to the external sphincter, causing it to relax. With both sphincters relaxed, the detrusor muscle contracts and urine flows from the bladder through the urethra. Voluntary micturition may also be accompanied by relaxation of the

perineal muscles and contraction of abdominal muscles. Infants and very young children empty their bladder whenever the micturition reflex is initiated, as they have not yet developed voluntary control over the external sphincter. Obviously, any interruption of the spinocortical impulse pathway interferes with control of the external sphincter, resulting in involuntary voiding or retention.

Assessment of renal function

The investigation of renal dysfunction may include examination of urine specimens (which may be voided or obtained by bladder or urethral catheterization), blood chemistry determinations, renal function tests, radiography and ultrasonographic procedures.

Urine output

Perhaps one of the most crucial nursing functions in the care of the person with renal dysfunction is the accurate measurement of urine output and fluid balance.

Urine colour

It is important that the nurse be aware of the colour of the urine being eliminated. Changes from the normal amber, clear urine can be an indication of many things, such as urinary tract infection (cloudy urine), bleeding into the urinary tract (blood-stained urine) or dehydration (darker, more concentrated urine).

Routine urinalysis

Routine **urinalysis** is usually a nursing responsibility; it is relatively fast, simple and accurate because of the wide

Micturition
See chapter 5.4

Urinalysis
See chapter 5.4

availability of reagent strip tests that allow the nurse to test for protein, glucose, ketones, acetone, blood and bilirubin, as well as to measure pH.

Urine for bacteriological examination

This is achieved by culturing the urine; the organism is identified by means of a microscope. Sensitivity to antibiotics is determined by placing impregnated discs of specific agents upon the culture plate and observing the colonization pattern. Areas where colonies of microorganisms fail to grow indicate sensitivity to the specific antibiotic.

Urine specimens for bacteriological examination should be fresh, or refrigerated after collection. The first morning specimen is the most concentrated and therefore most likely to reveal abnormalities. A clean-catch mid-stream specimen (MSU) is the most effective method of obtaining urine for bacteriological examination. The patient should be given clear instructions on how to prepare himself or herself and which part of the urine stream should be collected. The individual should start passing urine and, once the urine is being voided, a sterile container should be used to collect it. The last part of the stream should be avoided. In the catheterized patient the specimen should be obtained using a syringe and needle from the rubber portal on the collecting tube, not from the reservoir or collecting bag.

Glomerular filtration rate
See chapter 5.4

24-hour urine collection

A 24-hour urine specimen means collection of all the urine that a person produces in a 24-hour period. Collection is begun first thing in the morning, with the urine of the first void being discarded. For the next 24 hours all the urine must be saved and collected in a container, including the first void of the next day. Serious errors in the results may occur if strict attention is not paid to timing the 24-hour period or if the patient voids urine that is not collected. The urine can be examined to determine the amounts of specific substances that the person's kidney is capable of excreting, based on calculations that include height, weight and total volume excreted during the 24-hour period. By making a quantitative determination of the 24-hour creatinine clearance, a statement can be made about the glomerular filtration capacity of the kidney. The container should be refrigerated during the period of collection. Some 24-hour collections may be needed for specific tests, and a stabilizer or preservative may be added to the receptacle before collection.

Blood chemistry determinations

Impaired glomerular filtration and loss of the tubular ability to reabsorb and excrete discriminately lead to alterations in plasma composition. Blood specimens may be requested to determine the concentration of a number of substances. The nurse is often the first healthcare provider to be informed of results, and should therefore have an understanding of normal serum concentrations so that abnormal levels can be promptly passed on to medical staff. The following normal values are of particular importance for patients with renal disorder:

- urea nitrogen – normal: 2.5–6.6 mmol/L
- creatinine – normal: 55–120 μmol/L
- urate – normal: 0.42–0.48 mmol/L.

Haematological tests

The haemoglobin concentration and haematocrit are determined, as anaemia is a common problem. If infection is suspected a leucocyte count is done, and a platelet count and prothrombin time may be needed in advanced chronic renal failure.

Renal function tests

Renal function tests may be classified according to the kidney function being evaluated. In renal function, the removal or clearance of substances from the blood is achieved by glomerular filtration and tubular cell activity. If a substance passes freely through the glomeruli, and is neither reabsorbed or secreted by the tubules, the quantity appearing in the urine is the same as that filtered by the glomeruli. The 24-hour urine collection test referred to earlier is used for renal function tests, usually to estimate creatinine clearance. By measuring the amount excreted in the urine in a specified period of time, information is obtained about the efficiency of glomerular filtration.

The nurse needs to understand what is involved in these tests for two reasons: first, to ensure the patient is properly prepared and cared for before and after any procedure; second, to reduce anxiety and fear by answering questions and giving explanations to the patient.

Glomerular filtration rate

To determine the **glomerular filtration rate** (GFR), creatinine or ^{51}Cr-labelled ethylenediamine tetra-acetic acid (EDTA) clearance tests are used most frequently.

Creatinine clearance test

In the creatinine clearance test, the patient maintains normal but not excessive activity, because endogenous creatinine is produced in muscular activity. No special diet is necessary but excessive intake of tea, coffee and meat is avoided for a 24-hour period before the test. A 24-hour specimen of urine and a venous blood specimen are collected for determination of creatinine concentration. The rate of urinary excretion per minute is calculated. The normal amount of creatinine excreted in 24 hours varies with age: in an adult the normal range is about 1.2–1.7 g, and in a child it is approximately 0.36 g. Calculations are made to determine the volume of plasma cleared of creatinine per minute, which is the GFR.

^{51}Cr-labelled EDTA clearance test

EDTA labelled with ^{51}Cr, a radioactive isotope, is given intravenously into one arm. Blood tests from the other arm are taken hourly for 3 hours and, from the rate of clearance from the plasma, the GFR is calculated.

Tubular function

To maintain homeostasis, normal kidneys are able to vary the concentration of solid wastes and the volume of urine according to the volume of body fluids. When there is an excessive loss of body fluid by other channels or a restricted intake, more water is reabsorbed by the renal tubules; the solid wastes are excreted in a smaller volume of urine and the specific gravity is high. Conversely, with a large fluid intake, less water is reabsorbed by the tubules, the volume of urine is greater and the specific gravity and osmolality are lower than usual. This ability to vary the volume and concentration of the urine appropriately is impaired when there is tubular damage.

The standard test involves collecting an early morning sample for estimation of osmolality (normal value 550 mosmol/kg or above; younger people usually have values of 750 mosmol/kg or above). Below-normal values indicate the need for concentration tests to estimate specific gravity. Protocols vary between hospitals, so you are advised to consult your own pathology laboratory directions.

Renal scanning

The use of radioisotope scanning techniques may demonstrate areas of renal dysfunction and is becoming increasingly widespread as an investigative procedure.

Ultrasonography

There is no preparation for ultrasonography, and no X-rays or injections are needed, although if the person is not anuric a full bladder may be requested as it provides a good 'landmark' for the radiographer. The examination is used to look at the size and structure of the kidneys and other organs. Renal lesions seen in polycystic kidney disease and hydronephrosis can be distinguished. Ultrasonography is also widely used in determining the position of a kidney for renal biopsy.

Intravenous pyelography (IVP) or intravenous urography (IVU)

This procedure involves the intravenous administration of a radio-opaque contrast medium. This fluid concentrates in urine and, as it is excreted through the kidney (pyelography) and the ureters and bladder (urography), radiographs are taken. Patient preparation varies, but fluids are usually restricted 4 hours before the procedure; sometimes a laxative is administered the night before the examination. This avoids bowel content or gas obscuring the outline of the urinary tract. It is important to ascertain whether the individual has a history of allergies, particularly to iodine preparations, as severe reactions to the contrast medium can occur.

Ultrasonographic investigations are replacing IVP and IVU in many centres.

Cystoscopy and retrograde pyelography

Cystoscopy involves the passage of a cystocope through the urethra into the bladder. The instrument is equipped with a light which permits direct visualization of the internal surface of the bladder. A long, fine catheter may also be introduced into each renal pelvis through the cystoscope (ureteric catherization), and a urine specimen collected from each kidney. Ureteric catheterization may be used to obtain specimens from one or both kidneys for microscopic examination and culture, or in renal function tests when the function of each kidney is to be determined.

A radio-opaque iodide preparation may then be introduced into the catheters, and radiographs which outline the renal pelvis and ureters are taken. This procedure is referred to as *retrograde pyelography*. The examination is used to exclude or delineate a ureteral obstruction when excretion of contrast by the kidney during an IVP is poor.

Preparation of the patient for a cystoscopy includes an explanation of the procedure. The patient's signature indicating consent for the examination is required. The procedure may be performed under local, epidural or general anaesthetic; food and fluid therefore are restricted for 6–8 hours preceding the examination and intravenous fluid is administered to ensure hydration and hence urinary flow.

If a general anaesthetic is contraindicated, the procedure may be performed under sedation. Increasingly, it is possible to perform cystoscopy with a flexible cystoscope under sedation without discomfort.

Upon completion of the examination, the person rests in bed for a few hours. Additional fluids are encouraged. It is important that the nurse examine the urinary output for haematuria, and any severe pain or persisting bright blood in the urine is reported to the doctor. Should the individual report inability to pass urine it may be necessary for an indwelling catheter to be inserted. Severe haematuria may necessitate catherization and irrigation of the bladder with fluid to control bleeding and flush debris and blood clots.

Computed tomography

Computed tomography (CT) is used in the detection of renal tumours and cysts. The patient is given an oral contrast medium before the scan to opacify the bowel; food is not allowed for 4 hours before the procedure.

Renal angiography

Renal blood vessels may be outlined on an X-ray film following the administration of a radio-opaque substance into the vascular system. The procedure is performed under local anaesthesia by a radiologist; it is used to explore the blood supply to the kidneys. The main indication for renal angiography is for a diagnosis of renal artery stenosis or to differentiate renal masses (e.g. tumours or cysts). As the person may be sensitive to the radio-opaque iodide preparation, the same precautions as cited for intravenous urography should be followed. Preparation of the patient is similar to that for intravenous urography.

After the procedure, the site of catheter introduction into the femoral artery has a firm dressing applied and frequent inspections are made for bleeding. The person may be on bedrest for several hours after the procedure to reduce the risk of bleeding. The site is also observed for local swelling, redness and tenderness. The temperature of the lower limbs is noted and the popliteal and pedal pulses are checked so that any indication of impaired circulation may be reported promptly.

Magnetic resonance imaging

This technique is also being developed to permit investigation of the kidneys and has been shown to have an important role in the detection of abnormalities of renal tissue.

Percutaneous renal biopsy

A biopsy is a valuable test in diagnosis and assessment of the effects of treatment but carries with it the risk of haemorrhage. It is frequently used to determine the underlying pathology of renal dysfunction so that appropriate treatments may be selected. Renal biopsy is also performed in selected cases in renal transplant patients in order to diagnose rejection. It is contraindicated if the person has hypertension, a bleeding tendency, only one kidney, or suspected perirenal abscess. Before a person is booked for renal biopsy, coagulation, bleeding and prothrombin times are determined. If these are satisfactory, the person's blood is grouped and cross-matched, and compatible blood is kept available in the event of haemorrhage. An explanation is given to the person of what to expect and that he or she will be put in the prone position over a firm pillow (kidney elevator) for a brief period.

The exact location of the kidney is identified by radiography, which may include intravenous urography or ultrasonography, and the position is indicated on the skin surface. The skin is cleansed and local anaesthesia is infiltrated. The person is instructed to hold the breath during insertion of the needle and the actual taking of the specimen. Following removal of the biopsy needle, pressure is applied to the site for a few minutes.

The blood pressure and pulse are recorded every 15 minutes for 1 hour, then every 30 minutes for a period of 1–2 hours, and then every 4 hours for 24 hours. The risk of heavy bleeding after the procedure is very real, so the nurse must observe the person carefully for signs of shock, and assess the urine for prolonged haematuria.

Micturition disorders
See chapter 5.4

Any undue pain, haematuria or change in vital signs should be reported immediately. The person is kept on bedrest in the dorsal recumbent position for 18–24 hours or until the urine is cleared of blood.

Clinical characteristics of renal dysfunction

In impaired kidney function, the constancy of the internal environment (homeostasis), which is essential for the normal functioning of all body cells, is disrupted. The normal volume, composition and reaction of the body fluids may be altered by the inability of the kidneys to conserve essential substances and excrete excesses, metabolic wastes and toxic substances; disturbances in the functioning of other organs readily develop. Consequently, the signs and symptoms of renal insufficiency are varied, and many are not directly referable to the urinary system. Whether the disease is acute or chronic, and whether it affects the glomeruli or the tubules, will also affect the manifestations.

As the nurse assesses the patient the physical signs listed in Box 19.2 must be borne in mind as evidence of significant renal dysfunction. The nurse should be alert to the possible psychological sequelae of these clinical signs as such effects may be a cause of great distress requiring urgent nursing intervention, for example a change in the colour of a person's urine.

Abnormal urinary volume

Oliguria or anuria may develop, especially in acute and advanced renal failure:

- *Oliguria* means that less than 500 mL of urine is formed in 24 hours.

Box 19.2   Physical signs of renal dysfunction

- Abnormal urinary volume
- Abnormal constituents in the urine (e.g. protein, blood, casts, pus, organisms)
- Abnormal urine colour
- Uraemia
- Fluid, electrolyte and pH imbalances
- Changes in vital signs
- Gastrointestinal disturbances
- Headache and pain
- Visual disturbances
- Neurological manifestations
- Skin changes
- Haematological changes.

- *Anuria* implies a urinary output of less than 250 mL in 24 hours and is sometimes referred to as a renal shutdown.

The diminished urine formation may be associated with decreased glomerular filtration due to renal disease (e.g. glomerulonephritis), hypotension as in shock and dehydration, decreased renal blood flow or an obstruction within the tubules.

Polyuria, a volume of urine in excess of the normal (over 2000 mL in 24 hours), may also indicate renal disturbance in which the ability of the tubules to reabsorb water and concentrate the solid wastes is limited. It is seen most often in patients with chronic kidney disease, or may be secondary to diabetes insipidus as a result of a deficiency in the secretion of vasopressin (antidiuretic hormone). Polyuria may not be a manifestation of renal disease but may indicate a disorder elsewhere. Frequently, polyuria is the symptom that may cause an individual to go to a doctor where, on investigation, diabetes mellitus is diagnosed.

Nocturia (voiding during the night) usually accompanies polyuria and the person becomes desperate for undisturbed sleep. Inability of the kidneys to reabsorb the normal amount of water and to concentrate the wastes may be referred to as *hyposthenuria*. As well as the excessive volume, a low specific gravity of the urine persists because the impaired tubules cannot concentrate or vary the amount of solids.

Abnormal constituents in the urine

Abnormal constituents revealed in urinalysis vary with the underlying renal disease. They include protein (usually albumin), blood, casts, pus and organisms.

The large molecular structure of serum albumin inhibits its filtration through normal glomeruli. *Albuminuria* usually indicates inflammation and almost always indicates damage to the glomeruli. If significant amounts of protein are lost in urine, this leads to the development of nephrotic syndrome. Protein loss leads to a range of symptoms of which oedema, increased risk of blood clotting, raised cholesterol levels and increased infection risk are the most common (Haslett et al 1999).

Haematuria denotes blood in the urine and may be macroscopic or recognized only by microscopic examination after a positive dipstick test. Fickenscher (1999) comments that false-positive dipstick test results may occur in the presence of contaminants such as bleach or peroxidase released by bacteria or if a woman is menstruating at the time the test is carried out. Haematuria indicates a systemic problem (such as a clotting disorder or excess dosage of warfarin) or some pathological process within the kidneys or the urinary collecting system. A clear history from the patient may give important clues about the possible cause of such a finding. For example, the most common cause of macroscopic haematuria in men aged over 60 years is benign prostatic hyperplasia (BPH). A history of difficulty in passing urine coupled with haematuria in a man of that age suggests BPH as a probable cause. Conversely, in a young woman haematuria is most likely to be due to a bacterial infection of the urinary tract (Fickenscher 1999).

Urinary casts are microscopic cylindrical structures formed in the distal and collecting tubes by the agglutination of cells and cellular debris in a protein matrix. They are moulded or cast in the shape of the tubule. Depending on their composition, casts are usually classified as red blood cell, epithelial, hyaline, granular or fatty. They point to the presence of some inflammatory or degenerative process within the tubules. Obviously, *pus* and *bacteria* in the urine indicate infection in the kidneys or urinary tract.

The presence of protein, blood and casts together in the urine is strongly suggestive of disease of the renal parenchyma, especially in the presence of peripheral oedema and/or hypertension.

Abnormal urine colour

Abnormal discoloration of urine may be associated with infection within the urinary tract, but more often occurs with a disorder extrinsic to the kidneys and urinary tract. Examples of disorders in which the urine is discoloured are: obstructive jaundice, where the urine appears a dark colour due to the presence of bilirubin; haemoglobinuria, which may develop following a blood transfusion reaction in which there is a breakdown of erythrocytes and the release of haemoglobin; and melanoma, a skin neoplasm characterized by excessive pigmentation.

It should be remembered that urine can sometimes be discoloured by the contrast media used in intravenous X-ray examination, or by the eating of foods such as beetroot.

Uraemia

Metabolic wastes accumulate in the blood when renal function is impaired. Urea, creatinine and uric acid levels are usually raised. In acute failure and anuria, the levels rise rapidly. In chronic kidney disease, even though there may be polyuria, the blood urea progressively rises as the kidneys are failing to excrete the waste products of metabolism.

Fluid, electrolyte and pH imbalances

Generalized *oedema* may be one of the early symptoms of renal insufficiency and usually becomes apparent first around the eyes. It may be due to decreased glomerular filtration and the retention of water and sodium, or to an abnormal permeability of the glomeruli to plasma proteins, especially serum albumin. The loss of plasma protein causes a decrease in the colloidal osmotic pressure of the blood, and an excess of water remains in the interstitial spaces. The urine is high in albumin, and the plasma protein concentration is abnormally low.

In some instances of chronic renal failure due to impaired tubular function, the excessive volume of urine excreted (polyuria) may lead to *dehydration* unless there is a corresponding increase in the water intake. Fluid balance is an important sign which must be monitored carefully in any acutely ill patient, whatever the cause. Daily fluid loss of up to 800 mL can occur in evaporation from the skin and in exhaled air, together with a further 100 mL in faeces. Urine output alone therefore does not convey an accurate picture of the patient's true fluid balance (Sheppard 2000).

Deficiencies or excesses of electrolytes may occur, depending on the nature of the renal disturbance and the degree of tissue damage. Failure of impaired tubules to secrete potassium ions is a serious development in renal insufficiency. Abnormal concentrations of sodium and calcium as well as hyperkalaemia may develop, and may seriously affect cardiac function and threaten the patient's life.

Failure of the kidneys' capacity to excrete hydrogen ions by the formation and excretion of acid sodium phosphate and ammonia results in their accumulation in the blood, causing *acidosis*.

Vital signs

An increase in **blood pressure** occurs in most patients with renal insufficiency associated with parenchymal disease of the kidneys. It is attributed to an increase in the blood volume as a result of the retention of sodium and water, or to a decrease in the renal blood flow and consequent secretion of renin by the juxtaglomerular cells. The renin results in the formation of angiotensin I and II, which cause vasoconstriction of the arterioles and increased aldosterone release.

Blood pressure
See chapter 4.2

Central venous pressure (CVP) monitoring is an invasive technique for monitoring fluid load and how well the heart is coping with the work it has to do. The CVP is obtained by measuring blood pressure in the venous circulation and it is used in critical care areas (see p. 269). Jugular venous pressure (JVP) may be measured without any specialist equipment and gives an estimate of fluid overload or dehydration. It is therefore a useful guide, in the same way as the CVP reading. A raised JVP indicates fluid overload, whilst dehydration is associated with a lowered JVP. The technique is described by Walsh et al (1999), and advanced practice nurses such as nurse practitioners are learning this medical skill to assist in patient assessment.

The *pulse* may become weak because of heart failure, which may result from hypertension, excessive fluid load or electrolyte imbalance.

The patient may experience *dyspnoea* due to pulmonary oedema. *Kussmaul's breathing* (deep rapid respirations), characteristic of acidosis, may be manifested. In advanced renal failure, the breath has an ammoniacal or 'uraemic' odour.

Pyrexia is associated with infection in the kidneys or secondary infection, such as pneumonia, that may develop readily if pulmonary oedema is present.

Gastrointestinal disturbances

The patient experiences anorexia and, in the later stages of renal dysfunction, nausea and vomiting. Diarrhoea may also be troublesome in the acute stage. Hiccups may develop in advanced failure, and the oral mucosa may become sore and ulcerated.

Headache and pain

Headache is an early complaint as a result of the hypertension and cerebral oedema. Pain and tenderness in the back between the lower ribs and iliac crest occur in acute kidney disease because of the stretching of the renal capsule.

Visual disturbances

The patient may complain of 'spots before the eyes' or blurred vision, which are attributed to oedema of the optic papillae (papilloedema).

Neurological manifestations

Signs of both irritation and depression of the nervous system appear in renal failure. The patient becomes irritable, lethargic and drowsy. Family members may be distressed at perceived personality changes in the person. Short-term memory may also be affected, hence clear explanations and repetition will be necessary. It is important to assess the level of consciousness as the person may become disoriented and progress to a comatose state. Muscular twitching may be noticeable and, in advanced kidney disease, may be an indication of ensuing convulsions.

Skin changes

Dehydration alone leads to turgid, dry skin, a dry tongue and oral membranes (Sheppard 2000). However, in progressive renal insufficiency, the skin may take on a yellowish-brown appearance. Dryness and scaliness, known as *xerosis*, are common with chronic disease and polyuria. The patient may complain of pruritus, and excoriated lesions may appear from scratching. Pruritus is often persistent and there is no treatment that appears to have a lasting effect. Consequently, pruritus can be a debilitating and depressing experience.

In advanced failure, urea frost may be manifested, although this will be seen only in those persons for whom dialysis intervention is not possible. As the individual becomes progressively uraemic, deposits of small white crystals of urea are excreted by the sweat glands. The frost is usually first seen around the mouth.

Haematological changes

Most patients with prolonged renal disease show a reduction in the production of red blood cells, a shortened red cell survival time with a resultant anaemia. Normal kidneys, as well as the liver, contribute erythropoietin which stimulates erythropoiesis. In renal dysfunction, this activity may be decreased.

With uraemia, the patient develops a bleeding tendency; the platelets are defective and the bleeding time increases. Petechiae, purpura or bleeding from mucous membranes, particularly the gums, may be present. The person with renal dysfunction is most likely to notice an increased propensity to bruising.

The person with impaired renal function

Renal dysfunction may be due to a primary disease within the kidneys or may be secondary to a disorder elsewhere in the body. When kidney function is impaired, dysfunction of extrarenal systems ultimately develops. Similarly, primary dysfunction in other systems may readily affect renal function.

Renal failure

When the kidneys are unable to excrete metabolic wastes and perform their role in fluid, electrolyte and acid–base balance, renal failure exists. Homeostasis of the internal environment is no longer maintained. The retention of the waste and excess products normally excreted in the urine may be referred to as *uraemia*. The latter is not a disease but rather a syndrome or complex of symptoms reflecting failure of the kidneys to carry out their role in regulation of the fluid volume, acid–base and electrolyte balances, and excretion of metabolic wastes. Renal production of renin, erythropoietin and vitamin D_3 is also disturbed. With failure of fluid volume regulation, the patient becomes either oedematous or dehydrated and the acid–base imbalance leads to metabolic acidosis. Electrolyte imbalances occur and an accumulation of nitrogenous wastes produces increased blood levels of non-protein nitrogenous substances such as urea, creatinine and uric acid. The disturbance in the secretion of hormones leads to alterations in blood pressure, erythrocyte production and calcium absorption by bone tissue. As renal efficiency diminishes, symptoms develop reflecting impairment of function in other body systems. Renal failure may be acute or chronic.

The population of patients in renal failure is ageing, in line with the general population. Bevan (2000) estimates that 60% of patients in Europe receiving kidney transplants are over 65 years old. The nursing care of the person with renal failure, whether acute or chronic, is complex. The working relationship between patient and nurse must begin with an assessment and baseline physical examination to establish appropriate, individualized healthcare needs.

Health assessment

In assessing the patient, the nurse needs to explore the physical, psychological and social effects of the illness on the person's normal functioning. Not only should the patient's self-caring or adaptive abilities and family resources be examined, but it is also important to discover the patient's own perceptions and understanding of the illness and health status.

Physical assessment

The physical assessment of the patient with acute or chronic renal failure will focus upon collecting information on the effects of renal impairment on extracellular fluid volume and the body systems. The nurse should begin by making careful observation of the person's overall appearance, noting the skin's colour, turgor, intactness and texture. General activity and comfort level should be assessed by noting posture, movement, gait, strength and restlessness. Mental status is assessed by noting the level of consciousness, orientation, anxiety and any signs of agitation.

As fluid volume assessment is critical in acute and chronic renal failure, the nurse looks for distinctive changes that might suggest circulatory overload or dehydration. Records of fluid intake, urine output and daily weights might show trends that indicate gains or losses. The nurse then assesses the pulse and blood pressure for hypertension. Circulatory overload may manifest as breathing difficulties, such as dyspnoea and orthopnoea. Pulmonary congestion and oedema can result from renal disease. The nurse should observe the individual for breathlessness, alteration in respiratory effort, restlessness, sounds accompanying breathing, and engorgement of jugular veins.

The skin at the base of the spine should be inspected for oedema, particularly in the patient who is critically ill and is in a dependent position in bed: extracellular fluid expansion may manifest itself in oedema at the base of the spine rather than at the periphery. It is crucial for the nurse working with the hospitalized renal patient to perform a fluid volume assessment on at least a daily basis.

The increasing number of older people who reach end-stage renal failure means that, when assessing patients, changes that occur naturally with ageing must be taken into account, such as loss of skin turgor. Older people have a raised thirst threshold; therefore they have a reduced thirst response when dehydration develops. Although the GFR declines with age, so does muscle and body mass, and as a result lower levels of creatinine excretion are not the problem they might be in a younger person. Sodium excretion slows down with age, whereas potassium is more readily lost – factors that are important in considering the effects of diuretics (Bevan 2000).

Acute renal failure
See chapter 5.4

Acute renal failure (ARF)

Acute renal failure is a sudden, severe interruption of kidney function that, in most instances, is a complication of another disorder and is reversible. A biochemical definition of ARF is an increase in plasma creatinine concentration to above 200 μmol/L (Haslett et al 1999). As ARF is often associated with serious other pathology, mortality rates are high although, if the patient survives, renal function frequently returns to normal.

Causes

The primary or initiating causes of ARF are many but the basic mechanisms causing the failure, in most instances, are tubular necrosis due to inadequate tissue perfusion and hypoxia, or acute inflammation of glomeruli. Causes may be classified as prerenal, intrarenal or postrenal.

Prerenal

Prerenal refers to extrarenal disorders that cause inadequate renal perfusion as a result of a decrease in vascular volume or cardiac output or obstruction of a renal artery. The renal insufficiency is secondary to a condition that reduces the blood supply to the kidneys. The condition may be haemorrhage, dehydration, shock (due to major trauma, cardiac failure or burns) or renal artery occlusion by thrombosis. The frequent association of ARF with major trauma leads to many situations where the patient suffers major tissue destruction and hence is in a hypercatabolic state. As Garrett (1995) points out, the patient's energy requirement may be much greater than the normal supply, leading to breakdown of fats and proteins to make good the shortfall in energy supply. This process is known as *catabolism* and, when it exists alongside ARF, it poses major problems.

Intrarenal

Intrarenal refers to disorders in which there is actual renal tissue irritation and destruction which impairs renal function; examples are acute inflammation of the glomeruli (glomerulonephritis), acute tubular necrosis, and acute inflammation of the kidney tissue and renal pelvis (pyelonephritis). The primary renal tissue damage may be induced by a chemical or biological product or an infectious agent.

Renal failure may be the result of glomerulonephritis which is secondary to an extrarenal *Streptococcus haemolyticus* infection. The antigen complexes formed in response to the infection are trapped in the glomeruli and initiate the inflammatory process.

Nephrotoxic agents that are possible causes of a renal shutdown may be endogenous or exogenous in origin. Epithelial cells are destroyed; the tubular lumens are obliterated by swelling and oedema of the tissues as well as by casts formed from the sloughed cells. Examples of endogenous nephrotoxins are haemoglobin, released in haemolysis of erythrocytes following incompatible blood transfusion, and myoglobin, released from muscle cells in crushing injuries. The molecules of haemoglobin pass through the glomeruli and become concentrated in the tubules, obstructing the flow of filtrate. Similarly, the tubular necrosis that follows a crushing injury is attributed to the.myoglobin accumulating in the tubules and causing an obstruction, as well as to shock. The individual who has been 'pinned down under a weight' for a period of time or who has been subjected to limb ischaemia may appear to be in a satisfactory condition when released, but should be put to bed under close observation. Severe shock, acute renal failure and gross oedema of the injured part may develop hours later.

Exogenous nephrotoxins may be poisonous chemicals or drugs. Poisons, which may be taken accidentally or with suicidal intent, include carbon tetrachloride, ethylene glycol (a constituent of antifreeze), bichloride of mercury, chloroform and lead. Common pharmaceuticals that may prove toxic and damaging to the tubules include sulfonamide preparations (e.g. sulfadiazine), analgesics such as aspirin, non-steroidal anti-inflammatory agents, a cephalosporin and furosemide (frusemide) combination, and aminoglycoside antibiotics (e.g. kanamycin, gentamicin, tobramycin). Interstitial nephritis may be produced by methicillin and some analgesics. Obstructive disorders may result from cytotoxic drugs.

Postrenal

Postrenal causes of acute renal failure are conditions that result in an obstruction to the outflow of urine. Calculi, a neoplasm or prostatic hypertrophy may obstruct collecting tubules, the pelvis, a ureter or the bladder; the accumulation of fluid within the kidney compresses blood vessels and nephrons, seriously reducing kidney function.

Clinical characteristics

Patients with acute renal failure fall into two distinct categories:

1. Those who are oliguric, passing less than 500 mL of urine per day.

2. Those who are never oliguric but who continue to pass 1000–1500 mL of dilute urine per day.

The effects of a decreased urinary output are retention of an excess of certain biochemical substances in the blood and a decrease in the pH of body fluids, indicating increasing acidosis. Additionally blood urea and serum creatinine, potassium and sodium chloride concentrations are raised.

The first sign of acute renal failure may be oliguria, which may progress rapidly to anuria. The oliguric phase may last for 7–10 days and the urine contains blood and protein. An output of less than 30 mL per hour is an indication for concern and should be reported immediately. If oliguria and anuria persist for a few days, manifestations of water retention and disturbances of blood chemistry are likely to develop. Sodium and water retention cause oedema and, unless the fluid intake is controlled, overhydration may lead to cardiac failure and pulmonary oedema.

The increase in serum potassium concentration becomes a serious threat to cardiac muscle. In addition to the fact that potassium is not being eliminated by the kidneys, haemolysis and the breakdown of tissue cells by the primary condition (trauma, burns, sepsis, etc.)

increase the concentration of potassium ions in the blood. Metabolic acidosis, which also develops in acute renal failure, promotes the movement of potassium out of the cells. Cardiac arrhythmias are common, and cardiac arrest may occur.

The rate of the accumulation of nitrogenous wastes (urea and creatinine) in the blood varies with the cause of the renal insufficiency. If there is rapid catabolism, as in infection, fever and pathological destruction of tissue, the blood concentration of nitrogenous wastes may rise more quickly. The onset of the uraemic state is usually marked by mental changes, nausea and vomiting, and probably hiccups. The patient may complain of pruritus.

Metabolic acidosis develops because the hydrogen ions produced in metabolism are not being eliminated by the renal tubules. Respirations are increased in rate and depth, and an acidotic odour of the breath becomes noticeable.

Leucocytosis may be present and anaemia is likely to develop fairly quickly. If the renal failure persists, the patient may develop a bleeding tendency. Ulcerated areas in the mouth are common and may bleed. Vomit and stools may contain blood, and petechiae and ecchymoses may appear. As the condition worsens, disseminated intravascular coagulation (DIC) may develop (see p. 421).

The patient becomes drowsy and may progress to a comatose state. Muscle twitching and convulsions may also develop.

The outcome in acute renal failure is unpredictable. Many patients do recover; tubular healing and repair occur within 2–6 weeks and there is no serious functional impairment. Those who do not recover do not necessarily die from renal failure alone; frequently, the cause of death is the severity of the underlying cause or the combination of several associated disorders and complications. The patient with renal insufficiency is very susceptible to infection, especially pulmonary. Fluid in the alveoli (pulmonary oedema) and the retention of secretions due to inability to cough because of weakness predispose to pneumonia. Early recognition of renal insufficiency and prompt treatment are important. The nurse may play an important role in early recognition by being familiar with the possible causes of renal failure and by being alert to any significant decrease in a patient's urinary output.

Diuretic phase

If the renal failure is reversible, the patient experiences a period of diuresis following the oliguric period; large volumes of urine are excreted. The tubules are unable to concentrate urine and serum creatinine and blood urea levels remain raised. A diuretic phase may not be observed if the patient has been treated by dialysis.

Recovery phase

Improvement in renal function continues over 3–12 months. As function returns, the urine becomes more concentrated but some residual impairment often remains.

Complications

Complications that commonly develop in renal failure include hyperkalaemia, cardiac insufficiency, convulsions and coma.

Hyperkalaemia

Normal serum potassium levels of 3.5–5.0 mmol/L can be maintained until the 24-hour urine output falls below 500 mL with a decreased GFR. There are few visible signs of hyperkalaemia that the nurse may observe until the serum concentration reaches 7–8 mmol/L. At this increased level, severe electrocardiographic changes may rapidly occur. Cardiac function becomes impaired, and failure or sudden cardiac arrest may occur.

The nurse should be aware of the possible clinical symptoms of potassium intoxication which include:

- generalized muscular weakness
- shallow respirations
- complaints of a tingling sensation or numbness in the limbs and around the mouth
- a slow irregular pulse
- a fall in blood pressure.

Electrocardiographic (ECG) changes are an important indication of potassium intoxication. The critical aberrations include tall, tented T waves, ST segment depression, prolonged P–R interval and broadening of the QRS complex, with eventual ventricular fibrillation and cardiac standstill.

As the outcome of hyperkalaemia can be life threatening, its management focuses on prevention, early detection and treatment of emergencies.

As well as ensuring that no potassium is ingested in fluid or food, preventive measures may include the oral or rectal administration of a cation-exchange resin, such as calcium resonium. The resin preparation combines with the potassium in the gastrointestinal secretions, preventing its absorption. Care must be taken to give a stool softener with it, as constipation and occasionally bowel obstruction are complications. Potassium loss via the gastrointestinal tract is effective only if a regular and effective bowel habit is established.

If hyperkalaemia develops, an intravenous infusion of 50 mL glucose (50%) with a dose of human soluble insulin may be given if hyperglycaemia occurs. Alternatively a 10–20% glucose solution may be given 4–6 hourly. This is to promote the deposition of the glucose as glycogen, a process that utilizes potassium. A solution of 1.26% sodium bicarbonate (500 mL 6–8 hourly) may be given to correct acidosis, and 10–20 mL calcium gluconate (10%) given intravenously to reduce the risk of cardiac arrest (Haslett et al 1999). An antiarrhythmic drug may also be prescribed. The only permanent and effective way for potassium to be removed from the body is by dialysis.

Cardiac insufficiency

Heart failure may occur as a result of the retention of sodium and water (see Ch. 12). If hypertension is associated with the renal failure, it may also be a factor in heart failure. Urgent fluid removal by ultrafiltration is required to ensure the safety of the patient.

Convulsions

Convulsions may occur and are usually preceded by muscular twitching, persisting severe headache, severe hypertension, increasing oedema and rising blood urea level. Benzodiazepines (e.g. diazepam) may be prescribed to control the seizures.

Coma

Increasing drowsiness may indicate increasing uraemia and may progress to disorientation and coma. The delirious patient requires constant attendance, and a sedative such as diazepam may be prescribed. If the patient becomes comatose, the care appropriate for any unconscious patient is applicable. At this stage an urgent decision needs to be made either to refer the patient for dialysis or to institute palliative care.

Management

Medical management of acute renal failure is aimed at regulating fluid and electrolyte balance, controlling nitrogen imbalance, maintenance of nutrition and treatment of the underlying cause. Dialysis is initiated before the uraemic state develops to re-establish a normal homeostatic environment for tissue repair and restoration of renal function. Haemodialysis is considered necessary to deal with the hypercatabolic state encountered in severe renal failure (see p. 622). (See discussion of haemodialysis and peritoneal dialysis on page 629.)

Daily dialysis is usually required but the frequency will vary according to the rate of catabolism and the fluid imbalance. Excess fluid may be removed by haemofiltration using continuous, slow ultrafiltration. The use of ultrafiltration filters permits continuous fluid removal from the patient's intravascular content without the side-effects of sudden fluid loss, and without altering serum osmolality as occurs with diffusion dialysis. *Ultrafiltration* can be monitored by the nursing staff in an intensive care unit and has the advantage of allowing intravenous fluids and medications to be given to treat the cause of the patient's acute renal failure while controlling the fluid balance.

Fluid intake is restricted to 500 mL plus the previous day's output. The dietary protein should not be severely limited to decrease the production of nitrogenous wastes but maintained to provide adequate resources for tissue repair, and the patient should be dialysed as often as necessary to keep nitrogenous wastes at an acceptable level. In other word, dialysis is performed as often as needed to 'make room' for a healthy protein intake. This will often mean daily dialysis. The calorie intake is maintained by the administration of glucose. The electrolyte balance is closely monitored, sodium and potassium are restricted and dialysis is used to lower the potassium level.

Patient problems

The nursing management of persons with acute renal failure is challenging and complex. Virtually every body system will be affected and the nurse must be able to assess how the disease process is affecting the patient as a whole. Table 19.1 lists actual and potential health problems and outcome criteria for care relevant to most persons with acute renal failure.

Nursing intervention

Assessment

The patient with acute renal failure is seriously ill and requires constant nursing care and *close observation* for changes, which may occur suddenly.

Fluid intake and output

Accurate measurements are essential. The daily fluid intake is limited to 500 mL plus an amount equal to the urinary output of the preceding 24 hours. The 500 mL replaces the obligatory loss through the skin and lungs. The fluid that may be given will depend on the laboratory findings. An explanation of the fluid restriction is essential if the patient is to understand the reasons for such severe limits on fluid intake.

Vital signs and blood tests

The *pulse*, *respirations* and *blood pressure* are checked frequently. Cardiac function may be impaired by the retention of potassium and fluid or by hypertension, which may accompany renal parenchymal disease. Blood tests are carried out at least every 4 hours to detect changes in the serum potassium level (hyperkalaemia). Continuous ECG monitoring may be established if the plasma potassium level remains raised.

Any oedema is noted, and the patient's weight recorded daily as a gain usually indicates fluid retention. Breathing is observed for signs of developing pulmonary oedema, which may result from overhydration and cardiac failure. A noticeable increase in the volume and depth of respirations may point to acidosis.

The blood pressure is recorded at frequent regular intervals to provide information on the patient's progress. A progressive rise in excess of normal levels is reported to the doctor; it may point to increasing fluid volume. The temperature is taken every 4 hours, even if normal, as a sudden increase may occur and indicate complicating infection.

Frequent laboratory determinations of blood urea and serum creatinine levels and electrolytes are followed closely. The sodium and potassium levels are especially important in decisions relating to the types of solutions to be

Table 19.1   Actual and potential health problems of persons with acute renal failure

Patient problem	Goals	Outcome criteria
1. Excess circulating fluid volume due to inability of kidneys to excrete water	The patient will achieve a state of fluid balance with intake and output within normal limits	The patient's weight will be stable and within 2 kg of usual weight Fluid intake and output are balanced and within normal volumes
2. Alteration in electrolyte levels, particularly life-threatening hyperkalaemia, due to inability of kidneys to maintain normal serum electrolyte levels	Electrolyte levels will be within normal limits	Serum electrolyte concentrations, pH and osmolality will be within normal range
3. Loss of lean body mass due to malnourishment	No loss of lean body mass will occur	The patient experiences no true weight loss Serum creatinine and blood urea nitrogen levels are within an acceptable range for the patient
4. Potential impairment of oral mucosa and skin integrity due to oedema and increased excretion of waste through the skin	Patient's skin and oral mucosa will be clean and intact	The oral mucosa will have a normal healthy appearance
5. Potential for infection and bleeding due to effects of uraemia on patient's resistance to infection and clotting mechanism	Infection and bleeding will not occur	Temperature < 37°C; respiration < 20/min No evidence of petechiae, haematuria or melaena
6. Anxiety due to lack of knowledge and loss of control over events	Patient will be able to talk about anxieties and ask questions	The patient states that he or she is less anxious and shows some understanding of the disease process and its implications
7. Potential for injury due to confusion	No injury will occur	The patient does not injure self despite altered cognition or level of consciousness
8. Dehydration due to excessive fluid loss associated with diuresis or diuretic therapy	The patient will not become dehydrated	The patient will be in fluid balance Signs of dehydration (e.g. dry mouth, loss of skin elasticity) will be absent
9. Lack of knowledge about plans for future management	Patient will be aware of long-term implications of the illness for future life	The patient and family understand how to manage convalescence The patient is aware of support services within the community and how to use them to promote recovery

administered, and the patient's fluid balance and weight are used to determine the daily volume of fluid to be given.

Responses to drugs

Patient responses to medications are carefully assessed. Administering a drug to a patient in renal failure requires knowledge of the metabolic and excretory course of the drug, that is, what happens to it within the body. Drugs with which renal cells normally react or which are excreted by the kidneys are not given or, if used, are administered in a lower dosage than usually prescribed, and levels are monitored. Drugs containing potassium or sodium are not given.

Neurological signs

Muscular twitching, increasing drowsiness and disorientation are recorded, as they may be manifestations of uraemia, cerebral oedema and approaching convulsions and coma.

Nutrition

A minimum of 100–200 g of potassium-free carbohydrate is given daily to reduce the amount of tissue protein and fat broken down for energy. The patient may lose 250–300 g of protein per day from muscle breakdown (catabolism), yet even when dialysed patients can cope with only 70–100 g of protein daily. Intakes in excess of these amounts will therefore only exacerbate uraemic symptoms (Haslett et al 1999). Often patients initially do not tolerate large amounts of food and so are fed nasogastrically or intravenously until they have a desire to eat.

Essential amino acids as well as hypertonic glucose may be provided by the administration of total parenteral nutrition (TPN). Adequate protein is necessary for the synthesis of body tissues, enzymes and antibody production. The delivery of these nutrients requires the administration of a considerable volume of fluid, so parenteral administration of nutrients is used if the patient is treated by ultrafiltration to remove the excess fluid and prevent overloading the heart.

Activity

Activity is not restricted but most patients are initially very ill and therefore need help with all activities. Early involvement of the physiotherapist and occupational therapist is important, so a coordinated exercise regimen, including active and passive exercises and use of appropriate devices and aids, is used to support and assist activities and so enhance independence. The family should be consulted to determine the usual level of pre-illness function. Preparations for rehabilitation and discharge should be initiated early, involving other appropriate healthcare professionals and referral to community services so that recovery is supported both in hospital and at home.

Skin and oral mucosa

Mouth
See chapter 5.1

In renal failure, the **mouth** requires special care. The tongue becomes coated, salivary excretion is reduced, and the mucosa and lips are dry and frequently encrusted. Ulcerative lesions may develop, and the patient may be distressed by the disagreeable taste frequently associated with uraemia. Mouth lesions predispose to respiratory infection, local mouth infections and parotitis.

Frequent cleansing of the mouth is necessary. Petroleum jelly or cold cream is applied to the lips. The limited fluid intake and dry mouth are frequently a source of great distress to the patient. Resourcefulness on the part of the nurse may reduce the discomfort. Rinsing the mouth with ice-cold mouthwash or water is more acceptable than using lukewarm solutions. Occasional rinsing of the mouth with ice-cold fruit juice or ginger ale provides a change.

The patient is bathed daily to remove the increased wastes that may be excreted in sweat and to provide comfort. Regular assessment of pressure risk should be carried out, with inspection of at risk areas at frequent intervals. Meticulous pressure area care is essential.

Anxiety

Acute renal failure that is secondary to some serious disorder heightens the patient's fear and anxiety. Giving information to the patient and creating time in which the patient can ask questions or just talk about feelings are essential aspects of care. Relatives are kept informed of the patient's progress and encouraged to visit. They require support in understanding changes observed in the patient's behaviour and level of awareness.

Potential for injury

Cot sides may be kept in position because the uraemic patient may become drowsy and disoriented. Uraemia frequently leads to convulsions and coma, but regular dialysis will prevent this.

Fluid volume deficit (diuretic phase)

Improvement in renal function is manifested by a steady increase in the volume of urine. The latter may rise rapidly to as much as 6000–8000 mL in 24 hours. The diuresis is accompanied by marked losses of potassium, sodium and water because the tubules have not yet regained their ability to regulate the volume and composition of urine. Frequent serum electrolyte determinations continue, and necessary replacements are made either orally or intravenously. The fluid intake is increased to cover the volume lost. The nitrogenous waste concentration (urea) decreases more slowly.

The patient is offered a soft diet and then a light diet. The nurse continues to record the intake and output.

Patient education

Preparation for discharge requires a multidisciplinary approach in order for the anticipated needs of the individual, family and significant others to be met. The patient and family should be actively involved in discharge preparation to promote a sense of personal control and to ensure cooperation with ongoing management. The nurse may be a key member of the team, ensuring coordination and reinforcing information so that it is fully understood. Early involvement of the dietician is important so that that dietary restrictions can be discussed against a background of the individual's food preferences, usual eating patterns and food preparation practices at home.

Education should include information concerning recognition of the signs and symptoms of volume overload and hyperkalaemia, and monitoring of dialysis access sites for bleeding and infection. Written and verbal information and contact addresses and telephone numbers should be provided. Community services such as district nursing should be discussed and organized. Again, written and verbal communication with the community services will assist in ensuring continued and appropriate support. Discharge planning should also include outpatient follow-up plans so that the person clearly understands when the doctor will need to review progress and plan further care.

The prolonged convalescence frequently causes socioeconomic problems for the person and family. The nurse may be able to assist by a referral to a medical social worker. It is important to understand the uncertainty of this period because many patients may be discharged before renal function is fully recovered. Consequently, the nurse who is working with the individual, planning the discharge, must be sensitive to the need for continued emotional support of the patient within the community.

Chronic renal failure (CRF)

Chronic renal insufficiency is due to progressive disease of both kidneys. Irreversible damage to nephrons occurs which eventually leads to the retention of many waste and toxic products of metabolism, fluid and electrolyte imbalances, metabolic acidosis, anaemia, hypertension and decalcification of bone tissue (renal osteodystrophy).

Causes

The most frequent causes of CRF are given below with approximate percentages (Haslett et al 1999):

- *Glomerulonephritis* (19%) – This involves a variety of immunologically induced diseases that cause inflammation, fibrosis and destruction of glomeruli, with tubular degeneration.

- *Diabetes mellitus* (17%) – Diabetic nephropathy involves extensive glomerular and arteriolar impairment. The glomeruli lose their structure and no longer act as filters.

- *Interstitial disease* (14%) – Includes chronic pyelonephritis and reflux nephropathy.

- *Polycystic kidney disease* (7%) – Progressive enlargement of the cysts compresses functional renal parenchyma, increasing renal insufficiency in this inherited disease.

- *Vascular disease* (6%) – Renal artery stenosis.

- *Hypertension* (4%) – This involves a nephrosclerosis secondary to hypertension.

- *Other causes* (15%).

- *Cause uncertain* (18%).

It should be noted that the incidence of *diabetes* varies substantially in different ethnic groups. Diabetes is five times more common amongst Asians living in the UK than amongst caucasian UK citizens. It is not surprising, therefore, that end-stage renal failure is six times more common and death from renal failure three times more common amongst Asians than amongst caucasians in the UK (Whyte 2000).

Clinical characteristics

Regardless of the cause of the chronic renal failure, the disease progresses through three stages:

1. *Diminished renal reserve*, characterized by an asymptomatic decrease in renal function.

2. *Renal insufficiency*, demonstrating slightly raised serum creatinine and blood urea levels, and a GFR of about 25% of normal.

3. *End-stage renal failure or uraemia*, which occurs when the GFR is less than 10% of normal, and functional disturbances are apparent.

The patient may pass through the early stage of chronic kidney impairment without the renal disease being recognized. It may first be discovered in a routine physical examination, revealed by an increase in blood pressure and by albuminuria. The rate of destruction of functional tissue varies among individuals and with the primary causative factor. Some persons live a normal active life for many years because the functioning nephrons compensate for those destroyed. Others, whose disease progresses rapidly, may enter the advanced uraemic phase in a matter of a few months. In compensation, the GFR per nephron is increased, as are the reabsorption and secretory functions of the tubules. However, a deficit still exists which progressively increases.

Gradually, with increasing nephron destruction, the patient enters the phase in which renal compensation can no longer maintain homeostasis. The normal total GFR for an adult is 80–120 mL/min; when this rate has dropped to 20 mL/min or less, symptoms become apparent. Filtration is impaired and there is a loss of tubular ability to vary the composition and volume of urine according to the need to conserve or eliminate urinary solutes and water.

The signs and symptoms vary considerably in individuals in the early stages of uncompensated insufficiency, but tend to become similar in the more advanced stage when all the body systems become affected (Box 19.3). An increase in blood pressure, lassitude, headache and loss of weight may be the earliest manifestations. Urinalysis reveals albumin due to increased permeability of glomeruli. The loss of plasma protein as the disease progresses may be severe enough to produce the nephrotic syndrome (see p. 642). As more and more nephrons are destroyed, decreased filtration results in the retention of metabolic wastes. The blood urea and serum creatinine levels rise and a formal medical diagnosis will be made depending upon the GFR.

With a progressive decrease in GFR and the development of hypertension, the patient experiences increasing fatigue and lassitude, more severe headaches and loss of weight. Nausea, especially in the mornings, and anorexia become troublesome. Fat and glucose metabolism are impaired, as well as protein metabolism. Serum triglyceride levels increase and a moderate hyperglycaemia occurs as a result of increased sensitivity to insulin.

Initially, in chronic renal failure the 24-hour urinary volume is increased and the patient experiences nocturia as a result of tubular inability to concentrate the glomerular filtrate. The concentration of solutes in the

Chronic renal failure
See chapter 5.4

Box 19.3   Physiological alterations related to chronic renal failure

Fluid and electrolyte alterations

- Volume overload or depletion
- Hyperkalaemia or hypokalaemia
- Metabolic acidosis
- Hypercalcaemia and hypocalcaemia
- Raised serum phosphorus concentration.

Cardiovascular and pulmonary alterations

- Arterial hypertension
- Heart failure
- Pericarditis
- Pulmonary oedema.

Neurological alterations

- Fatigue, lassitude
- Headache, irritability
- Impaired cognition
- Seizures
- Peripheral neuropathy.

Gastrointestinal alterations

- Anorexia, nausea and vomiting
- Weight loss
- Peptic ulcer
- Gastrointestinal bleeding.

Haematological alterations

- Anaemia
- Bleeding tendency
- Increased potential for infection.

Musculoskeletal alterations

- Muscular twitching and weakness
- Renal osteodystrophy
- Calcium deposition in muscle tissue.

Skin alterations

- Pruritus associated with xerosis
- Thinning, loss of elasticity
- Increased potential for bruising
- Increased potential for skin breakdown and infection
- Calcium deposition in the skin.

Metabolic and endocrine alterations

- Hyperlipidaemia
- Sex hormone disturbances
- Secondary hyperparathyroidism
- Hyperglycaemia.

urine is invariable, producing a fixed specific gravity. If the fluid intake does not cover the increased fluid loss, the patient develops a negative fluid balance and the retention of solid wastes is increased.

Tubular destruction causes electrolyte imbalances. There is usually an excessive loss of sodium, which may produce hyponatraemia unless there is adequate replacement. Potassium retention is not usually a problem until the terminal oliguric phase. In moderately severe failure, metabolic acidosis develops and hypocalcaemia may also be a problem, contributing to muscular twitching and general weakness.

Eventually, the urinary output is reduced, hypertension becomes severe, and the nitrogenous waste and potassium blood concentrations rise sharply. The patient is pale, and the haematocrit and haemoglobin determinations indicate anaemia, which accounts in part for the fatigue and reduced activity. In chronic renal failure a bleeding tendency is also manifested; the thrombocyte count is low and the prothrombin time is abnormal. Petechiae, ecchymoses and bleeding of mucous membranes may be observed.

The central nervous system is affected by the retained wastes: the person is irritable; memory, reasoning and judgement are impaired and the attention span is shortened. In the advanced uraemic stage, the patient manifests confusion, disorientation, drowsiness and stupor. Restlessness and twitching may be observed and frequently precede convulsive seizures. Retention of phosphate and decreased synthesis of the active metabolite of vitamin D by the kidney alter bone metabolism, producing renal osteodystrophy (osteomalacia, osteitis fibrosa, soft tissue calcification and osteosclerosis).

Pruritus may be a severe problem for the person with renal failure; it is attributed to the precipitation of retained phosphates into the skin.

Alterations in ovulatory and menstrual patterns occur in women experiencing renal failure. Although pregnancy has been reported, few women can successfully continue a pregnancy to term because of the overwhelming physiological changes in the body. Both women and men often experience changes in sexual desire and expression. This is for a variety of reasons but fatigue, lowered self-esteem and changed perceptions of attractiveness to their partners appear to play a great part.

Late symptoms are anuria, generalized oedema, persistent headache of increasing severity, nausea and vomiting, hiccups, diarrhoea, muscular twitching, convulsions, ulceration of the mouth, fetid breath, rapid deep respirations indicating acidosis, drowsiness, disorientation and coma. As a result of the severe hypertension and water retention, a cerebrovascular accident or cardiac failure and pulmonary oedema may supervene.

Management

It is necessary to create a positive relationship so that the nurse and patient can work together to meet patient-centred goals effectively. The more involved the patient is, the more successful therapy is likely to be.

The primary cause of renal failure is treated to retard progression of the disease (e.g. hypertension, pyelonephritis). The therapeutic plan includes measures to correct the body biochemistry and modify symptoms.

Conservative treatment

Conservative treatment is reserved for patients who can be maintained without dialysis or kidney transplantation. The dietary and fluid intake are adjusted to maintain water and electrolyte balance and to reduce the retention of nitrogenous waste. Dietary protein may be decreased to around 60 g per day and limited to proteins high in essential amino acids (eggs, meat, fish and poultry) and to proteins from vegetables and grains. Carbohydrate intake is increased to provide adequate calories and to prevent the catabolism of body protein. Polyunsaturated fats are recommended and cooking with fats is avoided. A normal sodium intake is maintained if the patient has no signs of oedema or hypertension, but is restricted if these symptoms develop. Dietary potassium is usually restricted and potassium-exchange resins are prescribed if hyperkalaemia persists. Serum phosphate levels are controlled by the use of phosphate binders such as *aluminium hydroxide gel* and restricting the intake of high-phosphate foods such as cheese and milk. Multivitamin tablets are prescribed daily to prevent deficiencies of water-soluble vitamins which may develop when the diet is low in protein and potassium. Serum calcium concentration is monitored closely and, if generalized bone pain, muscle weakness or radiological evidence of bone changes are present, vitamin D in the form of 1α-hydroxycholecalciferol is given and calcium supplements may be prescribed if the phosphate level has been lowered. Balancing the sometimes contradictory requirements outlined above in a diet that prevents malnutrition, and which the patient can adhere to, is often very difficult.

The patient is monitored closely for symptoms of complications, and treatment is initiated promptly to control hypertension, fluid and electrolyte imbalances, metabolic acidosis, anaemia and altered bone metabolism.

Dialysis

When conservative treatment will no longer adequately control the blood concentration of wastes and the fluid and electrolyte balance within limits compatible with life, regular *dialysis* may be employed to maintain the patient, and a kidney transplant is considered.

The person undergoing dialysis

When the person with renal failure is being cared for on a conservative therapeutic regimen, he or she will be monitored closely for manifestations that suggest that dialysis needs to be initiated. When the serum creatinine level reaches 800–1200 μmol/L, dialysis will probably need to be instituted. However, blood concentrations alone do not indicate clinical need for dialysis. The signs and symptoms that the nurse must be aware of and that should be reported are progressive hypertension, fluid retention, anorexia, nausea, vomiting, twitching and/or pruritus. These symptoms are often experienced to a degree of debilitation that indicates that dialysis needs to be initiated.

Dialysis is a therapeutic procedure used in acute and chronic renal failure to lower the blood level of metabolic waste products (urea, creatinine, uric acid) and toxic substances, and to correct abnormal electrolyte and fluid balances. Two methods currently in use are *continuous ambulatory peritoneal dialysis* (CAPD) and *haemodialysis*. The latter dialysis takes place outside of the body using a dialysis machine to which an artificial kidney is attached. Although the procedures in the two types of dialysis differ, the purposes and principles are basically the same. In haemodialysis a semipermeable membrane separates the patient's circulating blood from a specially prepared solution known as the *dialysate*. In CAPD, the peritoneum is the membrane that separates the dialysate from the person's interstitial fluid, the dialysate being introduced into the peritoneal cavity. By using the principles of osmosis and diffusion, the dialysis procedure can partially replace some of the excretory and regulatory functions of the nephrons of the kidney. It is important to understand that the endocrine function of the normal kidney cannot be replaced by either haemodialysis or peritoneal dialysis.

Continuous ambulatory peritoneal dialysis (CAPD)

This technique may be used for most people with symptomatic renal failure and a healthy peritoneal surface area. The dialysate is introduced into the peritoneal cavity, which is lined by a membrane, the peritoneum. This acts as a dialysis membrane. Osmosis removes fluids whilst other metabolites are also gradually removed. CAPD is effective in removing small and middle-sized molecules, sodium, potassium and water, and in controlling hypertension and anaemia. The dialysate is replaced four times a day. Scheduling of exchanges is flexible and the equipment is portable to permit travel, work and schooling. This method is used particularly in children and the elderly, and patients may be maintained for up to 10 years with CAPD. A recent innovation involves automated peritoneal dialysis, which consists of a machine able to perform the exchanges during the night while the patient

Figure 19.4 Continuous ambulatory peritoneal dialysis. (a) Fluid flows from bag into peritoneal cavity through permanent access tube. (b) Patient wears bag around waist or leg and resumes normal activity. (c) Bag is lowered and fluid drains out. Bag is then discarded and the procedure is repeated with fresh fluid.

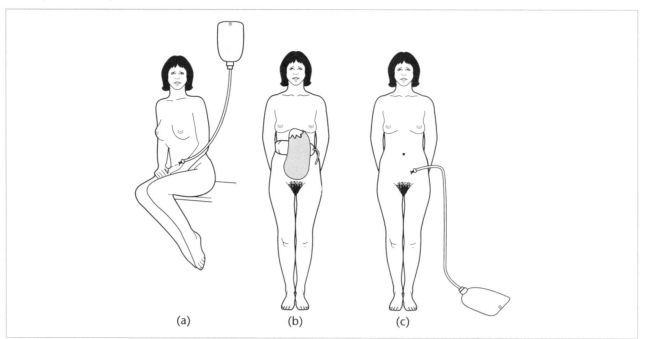

(a)   (b)   (c)

is asleep. As a result the patient does not have to dialyse during the day.

CAPD involves the following steps:

1. Connection of the catheter to tubing from a plastic bag containing the dialysate solution

2. Instillation of the dialysate

3. Folding of the plastic bag into a waist, leg or pocket pouch worn under the clothing

4. Drainage of the peritoneal cavity by gravity into the plastic bag about 6 hours later

5. Disposal of the filled bag

6. Connection and instillation of a fresh bag of dialysate (Fig. 19.4).

Bags containing 2 litres of dialysate are exchanged four times a day, 7 days a week. The exchange schedule may be adjusted allowing 6 hours between two exchanges, 4 hours between the next exchange and an 8-hour interval at night to permit uninterrupted sleep.

Peritoneal catheters

A permanent peritoneal catheter is required for CAPD. A catheter with several openings in the tip, such as the Tenckhoff catheter is inserted into the peritoneal cavity. Tissue cells (fibroblasts) grow into the two Dacron cuffs on the subcutaneous section of the catheter in 2–3 weeks, stabilizing the catheter position and decreasing the incidence of infection and escape of fluid. The procedure is usually carried out in the operating theatre under either a local or a general anaesthetic.

Dialysis cycles

Each exchange of dialysate is divided into three stages:

1. instillation time

2. dwell time

3. drainage time.

The solution is warmed to body temperature and infuses fairly rapidly into the peritoneal cavity by the force of gravity.

The *instillation time* for the 2 litres of solution usually used for an adult requires approximately 10 minutes. *Dwell time* is the period of time the dialysate remains in the peritoneal cavity. For CAPD this varies from 4 to 8 hours, and exchanges are carried out continuously, 7 days a week. Smaller molecules such as blood urea nitrogen equalize in 2–3 hours; larger molecules take longer to equalize. The osmolarity of the solution influences the dwell time required to remove water. Dextrose concentrations above 1.5% increase the osmolarity of the dialysate above that of the plasma and promote water removal. Higher concentrations of dextrose (4.25%) remove larger volumes of water in less time than solutions of 1.5% dextrose. *Drainage time* is the period in which the solution drains from the cavity. It takes up to 20 minutes.

Complications of peritoneal dialysis

Peritonitis This is the major complication of peritoneal dialysis. Symptoms include abdominal pain and tenderness, cloudy effluent, fever, and occasionally vomiting and paralytic ileus. The peritoneal effluent is cultured for identification of organisms and white blood cell count.

Antibiotic therapy is required and if this is not successful the catheter may require resiting.

Catheter complications Leakage around the catheter, obstruction of the catheter, retention of fluid and infection of the exit site are the most common complications associated with the catheter. Maintenance of regular bowel elimination helps to prevent problems with the flow of solution into the peritoneal cavity.

Dehydration This may result from use of large volumes of 4.25% dextrose dialysate. The patient will be hypotensive, manifesting pallor, weakness, fainting and a rapid, weak pulse, and will experience muscle cramps and may also be hyperglycaemic.

Pain This may be due to the tip of the catheter pressing on viscera or overheating of the dialysate.

Nursing care of the person undergoing long-term peritoneal dialysis

Because of its relative simplicity, nurses often make the assumption that the person undergoing long-term peritoneal dialysis should adjust quickly and easily. However, it is wrong to imply that peritoneal dialysis is 'easy', as it involves skill, problem-solving ability and fine motor coordination. Learning the technique takes time and the patient needs a gradual, well supported, approach. By careful assessment the nurse can begin to work with the patient to promote self-care as independently and safely as possible. The nurse can assist patients to develop new methods of self-care which are unique to their particular needs and situation. At all times the nurse must be aware of the patient's perspective of the illness.

Before dialysis is started, an explanation of the procedure and its purpose is given to the patient and family. Assessment of their continued education needs is crucial, because the effects of uraemia, by interfering with cerebral function, may prevent the patient from understanding what is being taught.

While the patient is learning CAPD, frequent assessment is very important and should include recording of blood pressure, pulse, respirations, temperature and weight in order to establish a baseline for physical signs. Signs of oedema, respiratory distress and dehydration should also be noted. The area around the exit of the catheter is observed for redness, drainage and infection. It is important to assess how the patient is feeling and how the forthcoming dialysis is viewed. When outflow is completed, the volume of fluid drained should be measured and recorded in order to ensure all dialysate is drained. Long-term complications reported by Bevan (2000) in older patients include hernia formation, constipation and the potential for malnutrition due to excess protein loss in the dialysate draining from the peritoneum

Haemodialysis

Haemodialysis can remove water and catabolic wastes at a faster rate than CAPD. Because of this efficiency, it may not always be used for patients who are haemodynamically unstable, as can be the case in certain cardiac diseases. It is a complex procedure that requires expensive and sophisticated equipment.

In haemodialysis an extracorporeal dialysing system is used to remove toxic wastes. During haemodialysis the person's uraemic blood is purified by drawing it from an artery, passing it through a sterile extracorporeal circulation, through a dialyser in which dialysis takes place, and returning it to the venous system in its purified state. It is within the dialyser that the actual exchange of material across the dialysis membrane takes place. Figure 19.5 illustrates the relationship of the patient to the equipment. During routine haemodialysis, clearance of body toxins and filtration of water occur simultaneously.

In haemodialysis, both solute and solvent transfer across the membrane under the force generated by hydrostatic pressure, in addition to that created by osmotic pressure.

The dialysate is an aqueous solution that contains varying concentrations of the body's normal extracellular and intracellular cations and anions. The cations commonly found in dialysate are sodium, potassium, calcium and magnesium. The anions found in dialysate may be acetate, bicarbonate and glucose.

The concentrations within the dialysate solution promote the removal of toxic substances, such as excess urea, creatinine and uric acid, from the body, as well as excess potassium, sodium, phosphate and water. Because of the semipermeable nature of the dialysis membrane, it readily allows the passage of small molecules such as urea, potassium and sodium, while retaining such large entities as proteins, glucose and red blood cells. The small molecules that can pass through the pores of the membrane will always travel from the area of greater to lesser concentration so that there is equal composition and concentration on both sides of the membrane. Because of the hydrostatic pressure across the membrane, excess water can be removed as the water flows toward the dialysate solution, which is of greater osmolality.

Vascular access

Maintenance haemodialysis requires direct access to the circulating blood by the extracorporeal dialysing system. The requirement for vascular access in persons with renal failure can be either permanent or temporary. Patients using long-term haemodialysis will need a permanent access because the duration of the treatment will be months or many years. Access is usually via an arteriovenous fistula. Each access requires specialized nursing care, the focus of which should include assessing the access for patency, pain, signs of infection, tissue trauma or oedema, and bleeding. The nurse will also work with the patient to ensure that he or she can monitor the vascular access thoroughly and independently. The need for long-term vascular access is often problematic in older

Figure 19.5   (a) Diagrammatic representation of haemodialysis. (b) Relationship of the patient to the equipment.

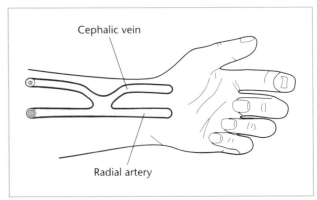

patients because of the adverse effects of ageing on their blood vessels.

Arteriovenous (AV) fistula This is surgically constructed by a side-to-side or end-to-end anastomosis between an artery and a vein in the forearm. The anastomosis may be between the cephalic vein and the radial artery, or between the cephalic vein and brachial artery (Fig. 19.6). This redirects arterial blood through the vein, thereby causing enlargement of the vein in response to the increased rate of blood flow and the higher pressure of arterial blood now passing through it. This engorgement of the arterialized vein requires 6–12 weeks to 'mature' before it is able to withstand the changing pressures against its vessel wall and the repeated insertion of dialysis needles.

Haemodialysis with an AV fistula involves the insertion of two needles into the vein. One needle is inserted at least 2 cm above the anastomosis and is connected to the arterial line of the dialyser. The second needle is inserted 3–4 cm above the outflow needle and is connected to the tube that returns the blood from the dialyser. Blood flows out from the distal needle through the dialyser and back via the proximal needle (Fig. 19.7). The limb in which an AV fistula is developed should not normally be used for taking blood pressure or blood samples, as either may jeopardize the patency of the fistula.

Figure 19.6   An arteriovenous fistula.

The AV fistula is the preferred access for long-term haemodialysis because it has several distinct advantages. It is completely subcutaneous, thus lessening the possibility of infection and reducing the risk of haemorrhage and thrombosis during everyday activity. Temporary vascular access can be gained via alternative methods in some clinical situations. For example, the normal access may have failed and the patient may need urgent dialysis before a permanent access can be re-established. In these cases, the patient may undergo haemodialysis with a *subclavian catheter* or preferably a *femoral catheter*. In either case, access is gained to the circulation by percutaneous insertion of a cannula.

Figure 19.7 The position of needles when an arteriovenous fistula is established for haemodialysis.

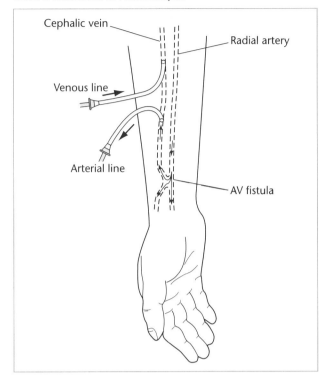

Cephalic vein

Radial artery

Venous line

Arterial line

AV fistula

Box 19.4   Guidelines for nursing care of the patient with a permanent or temporary vascular access for haemodialysis

1. Elevate affected arm or leg on pillow to minimize tissue swelling.

2. Check dressing for any bleeding; document and report to the doctor.

3. Check warmth, colour and mobility of fingers or toes for circulation.

4. Oedema is expected after operation but excessive oedema should be reported to the doctor.

5. Access insertion is a painful procedure, so analgesia should be given as required during the postoperative period.

6. Teach the patient to monitor own access for bleeding and swelling, and to report pain.

7. No blood specimens, intravenous infusions, blood pressure monitoring, etc. to be performed on access arm.

8. Psychological support should be given to the patient at all times.

Box 19.4 outlines issues for the immediate postoperative care of the patient with a newly created AV fistula or temporary access.

Nursing intervention in haemodialysis

Nurses responsible for the care of patients receiving dialysis require specialized preparation. Dialysis is a complex therapeutic procedure used to correct a life-threatening body dysfunction. Staff on general medical and surgical units and in the community should also have an appreciation of the implications for and the concerns of the renal patient and family. Personnel working in dialysis units usually assume responsibility for the specialized needs of dialysis patients being cared for in other areas of the hospital.

Emotional and socioeconomic concerns When the person's chronic renal failure necessitates haemodialysis, it is natural that the patient and family will be concerned. The need for dialysis is likely to have many implications; knowing that the disease has progressed to this stage and that life has become dependent upon the procedure is extremely threatening. Severe anxiety may be manifested due to concern for the future and life expectancy. Acceptance may be very difficult for some patients and they may show resentment and anger at first, followed by a period of depression. A regular schedule of dialysis two or three times weekly imposes modifications on the patient's and family's life pattern. Treatment may mean changing occupation or giving up employment or, at best, working only part-time unless home dialysis can be provided. The adjustments that have to be made may cause both social and economic changes for family members. The patient may be the main source of income or the mother, or combine both roles. Special diet requirements and transport to and from the dialysis unit or the need to accommodate dialysis equipment in the home may incur worrisome additional expense. A referral to a social worker may be helpful.

It is important for the nurse to be a willing listener and encourage the patient and family to reveal their concerns and problems; these vary from person to person and from family to family. An understanding of their situation and recognition of their reactions are essential to providing the appropriate support and care, and in assisting them to accept necessary modifications in lifestyle. A positive attitude on the part of the healthcare team promotes realistic patient and family acceptance and adaptation. Many people obtain support and pleasure through socialization and the establishment of close relationships with other dialysis patients.

Gradually, as the uraemic toxicity is reduced, the person experiences physical and emotional improvement and, by degrees, becomes more active and interested in living and may lead a relatively normal productive life.

Predialysis responsibilities The patient and family should receive a simple explanation of the purpose of dialysis and what to expect during the procedure. Many units have prepared brochures and audiovisual programmes to provide information and reinforce verbal explanations and instruction. If the patient is to be dialysed at home, an extensive home-training programme is planned. Prior to the initial treatment, if the patient's condition permits, he or she should visit the dialysis unit, meet the dialysis staff and may have the opportunity to chat with a patient on a regular dialysis programme. Such preparation is helpful in reducing the person's fear.

For dialysis, the patient is positioned comfortably in a bed or a reclining chair with the limb with the AV fistula exposed and supported. Temperature, pulse, respirations, lying and standing blood pressure and weight are recorded before the dialysis is commenced to provide a baseline. Blood specimens are obtained when the needles are introduced (or cannulae are opened) for laboratory determination of the haematocrit, electrolyte (K^+, Na^+), blood urea and creatinine levels, and clotting time. Anxiety is often greatly reduced if the patient and a relative are actively involved, even for the first dialysis. This might mean helping to set up the machine or preparation of the patient's dialysis access. A working knowledge of the equipment often greatly reduces fear.

The vascular access site is examined for signs of a haematoma or infection. Observations are made of the person's colour and the condition of the skin (dryness, turgor, abrasions) and for oedema. Weight is compared with that recorded following the last dialysis to check fluid accumulation. Weight changes, as well as blood chemistry and physical findings, determine the desired fluid loss and the appropriate dialyser, dialysate and flow rate.

Responsibilities during dialysis During dialysis the patient is monitored continuously for indications of the effectiveness of treatment and signs of complications. Each unit or home programme will have a schedule for observing and recording vital signs, equipment used, rate of flow, composition and temperature of dialysate, heparinization and blood-clotting times, as well as ongoing monitoring of the functioning of the equipment. The person is observed closely for signs of dehydration or overhydration. Changes in blood pressure and respirations are recorded and the flow rate through the dialyser is regulated accordingly. If there is a rapid, excessive loss of water into the dialysate, the ensuing reduction in the intravascular volume causes a sharp fall in the blood pressure. Overhydration may be indicated by respiratory distress, moist sounds and an increase in the blood pressure.

Headache, vomiting and twitching may develop if the patient becomes dehydrated and should be brought to the doctor's attention. The first dialysis should be short (i.e. 2–3 hours) to allow a gentle clearance of nitrogenous waste. This prevents the complication of cerebral oedema associated with disequilibrium syndrome, which may be present as disorientation or a convulsion.

The length of time the patient is kept on the dialyser varies with the patient's condition and type of machine used. The average range is 4–6 hours. The frequency also varies with patients. In acute renal failure, daily dialysis may be necessary until renal function is re-established. Persons with chronic renal insufficiency are dialysed two

or three times weekly and may lead a relatively normal, productive life for the remainder of the week. The dialysis programme may be long term, extending over years, or may be a temporary measure for the individual who is awaiting a kidney transplant.

Postdialysis care Upon completion of the dialysis the arterial line is clamped and as much blood as possible in the dialysing circuit lines is returned to the patient. Dressings are applied to the needle sites and the area observed until there is no evidence of bleeding; it may be necessary to apply some pressure for a brief period. The patient's weight, blood pressure (lying and standing), pulse and temperature are recorded for comparison with the original baseline observations.

Patient education When a regular dialysis programme is recommended, the person and a relative receive detailed instruction concerning diet and fluid intake, care of the fistula site or cannulae, activity, and recognition of disturbances that should prompt immediate notification of the doctor or dialysis unit. The brochure given out by the dialysis unit that explains dialysis also discusses these factors.

The diet prescribed varies from person to person and with doctors. The food intake must be balanced with the renal capacity to eliminate protein waste and prevent excesses of electrolytes (K^+, Na^+) and water. The protein content may be 60–80 g per day, allowing 0.75–1 g per kg bodyweight if dialysis facilities are limited; otherwise a normal diet is encouraged and dialysis hours are adjusted to control nitrogenous waste.

Nursing the person with chronic renal failure

Patient problems

Patients are particularly vulnerable to reactive depression, feelings of powerlessness and loss of control, social isolation and a whole host of physiological complications. This is illustrated by the work of McCann and Boore (2000). They found fatigue and lack of vitality associated with sleep problems, poor physical health, anxiety and depression were closely interrelated in a study of 39 adult patients undergoing haemodialysis. Box 19.5 lists actual and potential health problems common to most patients with chronic renal failure. The needs of patients and their families will also vary as the disease progresses.

Nursing intervention

Altered fluid and electrolyte balance

Assessment of fluid and electrolyte balance is continuous. The patient and family should be taught to identify signs and symptoms of fluid excess or dehydration and to adjust fluid intake accordingly. The patient is also taught to recognize the signs of hyperkalaemia and other electrolyte imbalances and to adjust diet as necessary.

Fluid balance
See chapter 2.6

In the early stages of chronic renal failure, tubular reabsorption of water is decreased so the intake must be increased to approximately 2000 mL per day to avoid dehydration. When oliguria is present the fluid intake is limited to 400–500 mL plus the measurable loss (e.g. urine and vomit). Fluid restriction may be minimal for the person on CAPD because fluid is removed continuously; however, fluid restrictions may be introduced if the individual on CAPD exhibits signs of fluid volume expansion that could jeopardize cardiovascular integrity.

Nutrition

The prescribed diet varies with the severity of disease and the type of maintenance treatment used. In the early stages, protein restrictions may be based on the glomerular filtration rate (GFR), but when the GFR decreases to 4–5 mL/min, protein restrictions are no longer effective in reducing the retention of nitrogenous wastes and dialysis is required. Protein is lost during CAPD and the loss is greater if peritonitis develops. Less protein is lost during haemodialysis, but some free amino acids escape with this treatment. The protein intake must be adjusted to compensate for the loss and prevent catabolism of body protein. Calorie intake must be sufficient to permit activity without breakdown of tissue protein.

Electrolyte balance is maintained by adjusting the dietary intake according to serum electrolyte levels. As impaired tubular reabsorption results in an excessive loss of sodium, salt is not restricted in the diet unless there is oedema or hypertension. Dietary sodium is restricted following a transplant as corticosteroid therapy leads to sodium and water retention. Foods high in potassium are restricted for most renal patients because potassium is not effectively removed by impaired kidneys. The serum phosphate level is usually controlled by the use of phosphate binders, such as an aluminium hydroxide antacid, and avoidance of foods high in phosphorus.

Nutritional management in chronic renal failure is complex. As diet is such an important part of disease management, the individual and family require considerable teaching and prolonged support from the nurse as well as the dietician. It is essential that a person's previous meal patterns and food preferences be incorporated into any management plan.

Dietary management becomes more complex for the person with chronic renal failure who experiences sudden stress such as infection, surgery or trauma. Food and fluid intake must be closely monitored and adjusted to body needs.

Preventing infection and bleeding

Immunosuppressive drugs or uraemia affect white cell activity, making the person prone to infection. Preventive measures and prompt treatment of infection are essential. Uraemic blood also has altered clotting ability and the patient therefore needs to be monitored for signs of bleeding from the dialysis access, mucous membranes or surgical sites.

Activity intolerance

The individual with chronic renal failure experiences considerable fatigue and lethargy; anaemia may contribute to the decreased energy. The anaemia may be due to decreased erythropoietin production, depression of the bone marrow associated with uraemia, or to blood loss due to increased tendency to bleed and through dialysis. It develops gradually and may not be symptomatic at first.

The nurse working with haemodialysis patients should therefore take precautions to minimize blood loss during dialysis. Promising research results suggest that the monitored administration of a manufactured form of erythropoietin, *recombinant human erythropoietin*, may be instrumental in increasing haemoglobin concentrations. This will improve the person's energy level and quality of life dramatically.

Enquiry should be made concerning joint and muscle pain and any changes in range of motion or mobility. Signs of hypocalcaemia, tetany, carpopedal spasm, seizures, numbness and tingling of extremities, or confusion should be noted and reported to medical staff.

Skin and oral mucosa

Assessment of the skin of the patient with chronic renal failure may show pallor, a yellow–grey colour, dryness, bruising and decreased sweating. The patient complains of itching. The hair is dry, becomes brittle and the nails are rigid and dry. The mouth should be inspected regularly for signs of inflammation and bleeding.

The patient is taught to care for skin, mouth, hair and nails; this includes following the dietary regimen to control serum calcium and phosphorus levels and avoiding tissue trauma.

Clouding of consciousness

Changes in the patient's level of awareness usually develop gradually as uraemia increases. Rapid progression of the disease produces severe disturbances in behaviour and cognition. Dialysis should be started before the progression of these neurological complications.

Early symptoms may include headache, lethargy, dizziness, euphoria, depression, apathy, sleeplessness or drowsiness. Recent and remote memory and attention span are decreased and decision making is impaired. In the late stages of renal failure, confusion, slurred speech, stupor, coma and convulsions may develop.

The patient is assessed for orientation to time, place and person. Changes in behaviour as perceived by the patient and family are noted and relatives are helped to understand that the patient cannot always control behaviour.

Cognitive abilities should be evaluated before patient teaching is started. Explanations of procedures should be simple, broken down into steps and repeated frequently. It is possible that the patient's home environment may need modification to promote safety.

Coping patterns

Adaptation to chronic renal failure is a complex process and varies with each patient, the degree of loss of renal function, the type of treatment selected and support available.

Assessment of the patient's coping includes learning about pre-illness personality and the degree of independence in daily life. The patient will have to cope with many losses such as loss of job and financial security; position in the family; stamina; and sense of well-being. The patient will experience a loss of freedom due to dependence on a machine coupled with loss of self-esteem, and will have to cope with a reduced life expectancy. Further changes in family roles and relationships are increased by decreased sexual function. The previously independent person has the most difficulty in adjusting initially, but measures to prevent feelings of helplessness and dependence can be effective.

Information about how the patient coped with stress in the past helps in assessing present coping responses and in developing new coping strategies. Some coping mechanisms used every day are dangerous when employed by the person with chronic renal failure. For example, a period of denial or non-adherence to the management plan is often seen in persons with chronic illness as they strive to deal with the staggering life changes necessary. The nurse should accept this as the patient works through the denial period, and should work with the person in exploring thoughts and feelings about the impact of chronic illness on lifestyle.

Changes in cognitive ability and behaviour affect the patient's perceptions of the illness, ability to comprehend what is happening, to understand and adhere with treatment and make informed, rational judgements about care.

Chronic fatigue and lethargy together with increased dependency on others further impair the patient's ability to cope. The presence of family and other support groups enhances positive coping; consequently family members are very important in supporting the patient. The family requires knowledge of the disease, understanding of the patient's responses and understanding of the treatment plan so that they can be informed participants in care and support.

The patient starting dialysis must acknowledge dependence on machines to sustain life. Transplantation usually results in an initial state of euphoria, which is followed by reactions to living with a foreign body, before eventual acceptance of the graft occurs. These patients live with a lifelong need for medication and constant fear of graft rejection. Even with a successful transplantation the patient needs help adjusting to the changes imposed by this lifelong process.

Lack of knowledge

As the patient and family must assume the responsibility for following the prescribed regimen, formal and informal instruction is planned. Patient education is started at the time of diagnosis and the teaching is adjusted as the patient's needs change with progression of the disease and revision of the treatment plan. The decision about home or hospital dialysis influences the degree of responsibility the patient and family assume for self-care and the resources needed to help them.

When a patient with chronic renal failure is admitted to hospital it is important that the nursing staff assess the patient's understanding of care and support the individual's achievements by encouraging active patient participation in care. Taking away the patient's control on each hospital admission retards progress already made and contributes to feelings of dependency.

Goals for education should be established for each patient and teaching should draw upon a range of different methods such as pamphlets, detailed instructions for technical tasks, videos, group sessions and practical demonstrations. Content includes the function of the kidneys, types of treatment (dialysis or transplant), self-care measures and lifestyle adaptations.

Necessary alterations to lifestyle Helping the person adjust his or her lifestyle is an individual process. The teaching programme includes consideration of the following:

- *Work*. The person's treatment plan, chronic fatigue and lethargy may limit the ability to retain gainful employment. Liaison with the individual's employer and occupational health service, if available, or employment counselling may assist the person to continue working.

- *Sexuality*. Counselling of the patient and partner helps them to understand the reasons for changes in sexual desire and expression. Many persons do not ask about the effects of renal disease on this aspect of their lifestyle. The nurse therefore needs to be sensitive to the couple's need to discuss this issue. Contraceptive information is necessary because pregnancy is possible, although there is a high likelihood of spontaneous abortion in the second trimester. Many couples affected by renal disease are able to have a satisfying sexual relationship by exploring alternative ways of expressing affection. The nurse should encourage the couple to participate in decision making and care, and assist them in establishing and maintaining open communication, thereby fostering the solidarity of the emotional and sexual relationships.

- *Holidays*. The person and family are helped to plan holidays and are informed of resources available. These include portable machines that may be borrowed, a directory of renal units in other cities nationally and internationally, and trips and camping facilities available through the local or national Kidney Foundation.

- *Exercise*. The patient is helped to plan an activity schedule that includes moderate exercise and is taught that regular exercise improves circulation and appetite and promotes rest and a sense of well-being.

- *Social activities*. Alterations in social activities, such as eating and drinking, that are required by the treatment regimen need to be discussed fully. Encouragement from staff and family is needed for the person to initiate and increase social interaction.

Kidney transplantation

The development of donor selection by tissue typing and the steady progress that has been made in managing the rejection process have resulted in an increase in the number of kidney transplants.

An advantage of a kidney transplant for the person who has severe renal failure is the discontinuance of the demanding dialysis schedule; considerable time is saved, and the individual's employment is uninterrupted and more productive. Dietary restrictions are lifted and constraint of activity is slight. The patient must be aware of the possible adverse effects as well as the benefits of transplantation before deciding on this mode of treatment. Some experience few complications and their quality of life is greatly improved. Others experience side-effects from the drugs used to control the rejection process and graft rejection. Transplantation requires major surgery and a lifelong dependency on immunosuppressive drugs. Rejection of the transplant necessitates return to dialysis and consideration for retransplantation.

Transplant recipients

The patient and family should be informed of the available types of treatment for chronic renal failure and the risks and benefits of each, as well as the implications for their well-being and quality of life. Given such understanding, the person makes the final decision whether to have the transplant or not.

The criteria for the selection of transplant candidates have become more liberal in the past few years. However, demand far exceeds supply and as of March 2000 there were 5704 people awaiting kidney transplant in the UK (Whyte 2000). A set of evidence-based rules has therefore been introduced to decide priorities when kidneys become available for transplant. Certain patient groups are prioritised immediately, such as children and people with high levels of sensitization to human leucocyte antigens (HLA, see below). A points-scoring system is also used with factors such as length of time on waiting list, similarity in age with donor organ, ease of matching, distance between donor and recipient centre and the success rate of the recipient centre (UK Transplant Support Service Authority 2000).

Immunological factors

The greatest hazard associated with any organ or tissue transplant from another person is the incompatibility of the recipient's tissue with that of the donor, and the ensuing rejection process. Secondary to this are the effects of the immunosuppressive drugs used to depress the rejection process; the most formidable is the recipient's increased susceptibility to infection.

The rejection process is an antigen–antibody reaction or immune response; the recipient's immune system recognizes the graft as a foreign substance, and specific antibodies and sensitized lymphocytes attack the foreign tissue.

The antigenicity and compatibility of the donor and recipient in tissue and organ transplants are determined by heredity. The antigens of concern, being determined by genes, are specific for each individual and are located on the surfaces of nucleated cells and red blood cells. Erythrocyte antigens compose the ABO antigen system used in blood typing and matching in blood transfusions, and may be present in vascular endothelium of the graft. Blood groups must be identical in the UK for organ transplant.

The donor–recipient relationship is an important factor in influencing acceptance or rejection of a graft. The closer the relationship, the greater the possibility of compatibility. Because cellular proteins and antigens are specific for each individual, donor tissue is rejected by the recipient's body unless it is taken from an identical twin. In this case, the transplant is compatible because the antigens of both the host and donor are identical, having been determined by the same genetic blueprint of a single fertilized ovum. Such a graft (with identical cellular proteins and antigens) is referred to as an *isograft*. A graft between two genetically dissimilar persons is known as an *allograft* or *homograft*.

Organ transplant
See chapter 6.2

The antigens located on the nucleated cells belong to the system designated HLA (human leucocyte antigen). These antigens, present on cell membranes of most tissues, are easily detected on leucocytes, which are readily accessible for tissue typing and clinical tests for histocompatibility of potential donor tissue. Histocompatibility may be understood as the ability of cells to be accepted and to function in a new situation. Normally, the HLA antigens would be recognized as foreign by the T lymphocytes of the recipient's immune system. This would lead to the production of killer T-cells and subsequently antibody-secreting B lymphocytes.

Tissue typing is the typing of antigens of the recipient and each potential donor. Antigens are identified by mixing lymphocytes with a series of standard sera that contain HLA antibodies. The reaction of the donor's and patient's cells to each serum is observed; lysis of the cells indicates that the antigen is specific to the known antibody. The patient's HLA typing is then compared with that of the donor. The closer the match, the less the T-cell response and the better the chance of a successful outcome. It is estimated that this technique improves the success rate by at least 10% or, put another way, permits some 200 extra transplants each year in the UK alone (Dyer 2000).

The importance of HLA tissue typing becomes apparent when the high incidence of renal failure amongst the Asian population of the UK is recalled (see p. 627). Because of the presence of certain very low frequency HLA antigens in the Asian population, tissue typing is difficult. The situation is exacerbated by the low frequency of donors amongst the Asian population owing to the mistaken belief that their religion forbids it. The opposite is true as Hinduism, Islam and Sikhism all approve of the practice (Whyte 2000). As Dyer (2000) has pointed out, this means that if transplant centres are to carry out transplants on Asian patients they have to accept an HLA mismatch and possibly lower success rates.

ABO blood typing identifies the red blood cell antigens present in the recipient and donor. Antigens are identified when agglutination occurs on exposure of red blood cells to serum containing identified antibodies.

Donor

In early transplants the kidney was always obtained from a live blood relative. Now, cadavers serve as the principal donor source. The cadaver is frequently an accident victim or someone who has had a sudden death and who is known to have been in good health.

If a living donor is used, he or she is usually related to the patient. The donation is more likely to be successful if the relative is close (e.g. sibling, parent) than if the donor is a genetically non-related person (e.g. cousin, uncle by marriage).

The demand for kidneys is much greater than the supply, and locally available kidneys may not be immunologically compatible. An established central service or register is maintained; persons with end-stage renal failure are registered with their tissue and blood types. When a locally available kidney is not compatible, one that matches may become available in another part of the country and is obtained through the UK transplant centre based in Bristol. Because of the demand for kidney transplants, various educational programmes have been organized to alert the public to the need for donors.

Legal and ethical considerations include the need for donation consent and the determination of death. Organ donation cards making a gift of any organ for the purpose of transplantation in the event of death can be completed and carried at all times. These cards are available from surgeries, most healthcare settings and public buildings, and are sometimes displayed in shops and public houses. Nurses can play a significant role in encouraging the general public to participate in this programme, particularly by working with Asian communities where the problem is most acute (see above). The next of kin may also provide written authorization for the donation of organs if death is imminent. Laws in most countries define brain death, and policies are established to ensure independence of the doctors treating the donor patient from the transplant team. Most regions now have a transplant coordinator who is responsible for coordination of organ transfer. This person will often meet the potential donor, next of kin and ward staff, and is responsible for feedback of information to them after the transplant. The coordinator also has a very important role in the education, not only of the medical and nursing staff, but also of the general public to encourage greater referral of potential donors.

When death occurs, the kidneys are removed with their arteries, veins and ureters. The blood vessels are flushed out with an 'extracellular' electrolyte solution such as Ringer's lactate.

The organs are kept cool during transport and storage, until implantation. Transplantation should be done within 72 hours of obtaining the kidney from the donor. Storage for up to 2–3 days requires pump oxygenator perfusion. When a cadaver kidney is used in transplant, the source remains anonymous to the recipient and the family.

Transplant procedure

The donor kidney is placed in the recipient's iliac fossa, usually on the side opposite to that from which it was taken: that is, a left donor kidney is placed in the recipient's right iliac fossa (Fig. 19.8).

The patient's own kidneys are removed if there is recurrent infection or uncontrolled hypertension. Polycystic kidneys may need to be removed to provide room for the graft. Usually this will have been performed while the patient awaits transplantation.

When a person is selected as a candidate for a renal transplant, a full and detailed discussion with the surgeon is necessary. The patient and family are informed of

Figure 19.8   Location of a transplanted kidney.

Normal kidney location

Location of transplanted kidney

what is entailed in the operation: that the kidney graft may be rejected, necessitating the resumption of a maintenance dialysis programme; that continuous drug therapy and close supervision will be needed; and that precautions against infections will be necessary. The patient is encouraged to be as fit as possible whilst awaiting a transplant. This may involve taking calorie supplements to improve nutritional status.

If the patient's anaemia is severe, blood transfusions may be given. Controversy exists as to whether blood should be given; transfusions are believed to increase graft survival but may also cause presensitization.

The patient's family's level of anxiety is assessed. The patient receiving a cadaver graft will have little notice before the actual operation. Preparations must be made quickly but opportunity is provided for the person to review the decision and to ask questions and share feelings. A consent form will be completed.

Deep breathing and coughing are taught and practised and the patient is informed about what to expect after the operation. If the person is known to have respiratory problems, baseline blood gases will be measured before surgery. Immunosuppressive drug therapy is commenced before operation and maintained afterwards. The most common regimen consists of azathioprine, prednisolone and ciclosporin (Hasselder 1999). A central venous pressure line will be established under anaesthetic so that the intravascular fluid volume can be monitored during and after operation. A retention (Foley) catheter is introduced into the bladder in the theatre under strict aseptic conditions for accurate monitoring of urine output.

Nursing intervention

The nursing care of the patient who has received a kidney transplant includes measures to maintain fluid balance, kidney function, prevention of infection and assessment for possible graft rejection and other complications. The

immediate care is the same as that for any patient recovering from anaesthesia.

Assessment

Vital signs, urinary output, fluid intake and electrolyte concentrations are monitored, and frequent observations are made for bleeding from the wound and early signs of infection and rejection. A renal scan is performed the day after operation to provide a baseline for graft function.

Maintenance of fluid balance and kidney function

The retention catheter is connected to a sterile closed-drainage system; the urinary output is recorded hourly. Frequent urinalyses and cultures are made and 24-hour urine specimens may be obtained for measurement of creatinine clearance.

The transplanted kidney usually begins to excrete urine soon after the operation. The volume may increase rapidly, resulting in profuse diuresis. The patient may experience bladder spasm and pain with the large urine volume, because the bladder has not been used to receiving urine for some time before surgery. If the transplant fails to excrete sufficient urine for several days, haemodialysis or peritoneal dialysis may be used until kidney function improves. Fluid and electrolyte restrictions are required until adequate urine volume has been achieved. Once kidney function appears to be stabilized, the hourly measurement can be discontinued. The catheter is removed, normally at about 4–5 days. The person is encouraged to void frequently to avoid overdistension of the bladder and pressure on the ureteral implantation area. If the patient's own kidneys have been retained, consideration must be given to their usual output when assessing the function of the graft kidney. The patient's weight is recorded daily and changes noted.

Prevention of infection

The person is receiving immunosuppressive medications and is at greater risk of infection. The application of good asepsis is stressed; thorough handwashing is important before each contact with the patient. Infection risk remains high in the long term and problems such as pneumonia, food poisoning, chickenpox, urinary tract infections and late infection with cytomegalovirus (CMV) some 6 months after transplant are cause for particular concern. Late CMV infection is an opportunistic infection that can lead to loss of the transplanted organ (Hasselder 1999).

Because the patient's immune system is suppressed, normal inflammatory responses to infection may not occur. The patient's skin and oral mucosa are examined frequently for redness, swelling, drainage, warmth and tenderness. The temperature is taken every 4 hours and the patient is asked to report any pain or discomfort. The white blood cell count is monitored frequently and, if severely depressed, protective measures may be instituted and immunosuppressive therapy decreased for a brief period.

Fluid balance
See chapter 2.6

The patient is required to carry out regular frequent periods of deep breathing and coughing, and ambulation is encouraged. Early removal of central venous lines and the urethral catheter eliminates potential sources of infection and facilitates ambulation. Mouth care should be carried out regularly, particularly after meals.

Rejection

Early manifestations of the rejection process may occur on the second or third day. There may be swelling and increasing tenderness over the kidney, fever, general malaise, headache, an increase in the leucocyte count, anorexia, decreased urinary output, hypertension, oedema and raised levels of serum creatinine, sodium and potassium, and of blood urea concentration.

The intensity of the rejection process and the rapidity with which it develops correspond to the degree of difference between the recipient's and donor's cellular antigens; the greater the difference, the more severe and rapid is the rejection:

Hyperacute rejection occurs within minutes or hours of the **transplant**, due to preformed antibodies attacking the homograft. This severe type of reaction may be attributed to presensitization to donor antigens as a result of previous transfusions or several pregnancies.

Acute or early rejection may develop up to months after the transplantation. Oliguria and increasing blood urea and creatinine levels are manifested. Rejection can usually be reversed by increased dosage of immunosuppressive drugs.

Late rejection develops insidiously after 3 or 4 months, or it may occur several years after the homograft was received. This type of rejection is characterized by arterial impairment due to intimal hyperplasia. It is attributed to chronic reaction between circulating antibodies and the antigens of the vascular endothelial cells. This process cannot be reversed with medication.

Prevention of rejection

The dosage of azathioprine and prednisolone is adjusted according to the leucocyte count and the patient's reactions to these drugs. It is necessary for the nurse to be familiar with their side-effects. Azathioprine may depress the bone marrow production of leucocytes and produce leucopenia. Ciclosporin A is severely nephrotoxic and so blood levels are monitored closely. It may also produce hepatic impairment and lymphomas.

Immunosuppression can lead to the development of glucose intolerance in 20% of patients and even diabetes in some; consequently blood glucose levels should be monitored closely. (Hasselder 1999)

When rejection is suspected, the patient is given higher doses of prednisolone, which may be given intravenously as well as orally. Plasma exchange may be carried out to remove antibodies and immune complexes and thus reduce the rejection response. This will depend on the patient's original disease. If the reaction is severe and there is marked fluid retention and an increase in serum potassium and creatinine and blood urea levels, dialysis may have to be resumed. Fluid intake and dietary restrictions may also be necessary.

If the rejection process is irreversible, the immunosuppressive drugs are discontinued and the graft may be removed. The patient may well become discouraged and the nurse should be prepared to offer support and reassure the patient that a second graft may be considered.

Other medications

Most medications are eliminated through the kidneys, so as few drugs as possible are given following renal transplantation. Small doses of an analgesic may be prescribed, if necessary, for the relief of pain and discomfort when nursing measures do not provide adequate palliation.

Patient education for health management

The patient may become apprehensive about leaving the hospital and becoming independent. The need to follow a prescribed pattern of living indefinitely and be constantly alert for early signs of rejection and complications may provoke considerable anxiety. Consequently a good teaching programme for both patient and family is essential. The patient should fully understand the drug regimen that will be required after discharge. Careful self-monitoring of weight and fluid output is essential, and the patient should be advised about simple measures to reduce the risk of infections (e.g. regular handwashing).

The early signs of rejection are reviewed with the patient and family. By this time the patient is usually quite familiar with them and realizes that prompt action is necessary. The patient and family are cautioned to report immediately a cold, sore throat, fever, dysuria, frequency or other disturbance that may indicate infection. The patient is also urged to contact the unit promptly if there is a sudden gain in weight (e.g. 1 kg in 1 day), swelling of the ankles or puffiness of the face, pain, tenderness and/or swelling in the area of the graft, decrease in urinary output, headache, unaccounted for fatigue, or increased temperature.

After discharge, the patient is followed closely by visits to the outpatient department at least once a week, because constant surveillance plays an important role in progress and the development of acceptance of the situation with less fear. If progress is satisfactory, and understanding and efficient management of care are demonstrated, the intervals between visits are gradually lengthened. The patient and family may appreciate information regarding self-help organizations such as the British Kidney Patient Association.

Complications

The 1-year transplant survival rate is 87%, and 64% survive for 5 years. Complications include all those associated with steroid therapy and the risk of rejection. In addition, Hasselder (1999) cites evidence that there is an

Transplant
See chapter 6.2

Immunosuppression
See chapter 6.2

increase in the risk of developing cancer associated with immunosuppression, particularly of the skin.

Other disorders of renal function

Glomerulonephritis

This disease is usually characterized by a diffuse, non-infectious inflammation of the glomeruli of both kidneys. As the blood supply that supports the tubules normally passes through glomerular capillaries before reaching them, fibrous scarring and obliteration of some glomeruli lead to secondary degenerative changes in the associated tubules, blood vessels and interstitial tissues.

Causes

The glomerular injury is usually caused by immunological processes. Three major immunological mechanisms are recognized:

1. Antigen–antibody complexes formed extrarenally are trapped in glomeruli and initiate the inflammatory process; this is a common reaction responsible for glomerulonephritis.

2. Antibodies are formed against an antigen in or produced by the glomerular basement membrane, initiating glomerular inflammation.

3. Activation of the alternative complement pathway.

A common cause of glomerulonephritis is the β-haemolytic streptococcus, although a wide range of other infectious organisms have been implicated as possible causes. The patient's history usually reveals that the renal disturbance follows an infection, such as a sore throat or respiratory infection of some form, by a latent period of 2–4 weeks. In some instances, the infection may have been so mild that little or no attention was given to it at the time.

Clinical characteristics

The onset of glomerulonephritis is generally abrupt but in some instances may be insidious. The affected glomeruli are partially or completely obstructed, resulting in reduced filtration. Some glomeruli rupture, permitting the escape of blood into the tubules. The permeability of the glomeruli that remain patent is increased. The scant output of urine is cloudy and contains albumin, blood cells and casts.

Oedema develops and is usually seen first in the periorbital areas and ankles. The patient complains of pain and tenderness in the back, headache and weakness. Visual disturbances may also be manifested. The blood pressure is raised, and decreased filtration results in a gradual accumulation of nitrogenous wastes in the blood; the blood urea and serum creatinine levels may be increased.

Neurological signs and symptoms corresponding to the degree of hypertension may be present (see Ch. 20).

Unless the renal insufficiency is reversed, uraemia, pulmonary oedema and cardiac failure may ensue.

Management

The treatment of patients with acute glomerulonephritis consists mainly of rest, fluid and diet regulation, and chemotherapy to eliminate possible residual streptococcal infection. The daily fluid intake is restricted to 400–500 mL in excess of the urinary output of the previous 24 hours. The blood chemistry is followed closely and the sodium, potassium and chloride intake regulated according to the findings. The patient receives a high carbohydrate diet to reduce the breakdown of tissue protein. Protein may be provided in the form of essential amino acid or keto analogues to achieve nitrogen balance. Similarly, salt restriction in the diet is regulated according to the degree of oedema and hypertension.

If the low output of urine is prolonged and the blood potassium and nitrogenous waste levels are progressively increasing, diuretic therapy is initiated or peritoneal dialysis or haemodialysis may be instituted.

Plasma exchange may be carried out to remove antibodies and immune complexes because the disorder is usually caused by immunological processes. Precautions are necessary to protect the patient from exposure to infection. A superimposed infection could aggravate the disease or cause pneumonia that could prove fatal.

The frequent association of glomerulonephritis with respiratory infections emphasizes their potential danger and the importance of prevention and prompt, adequate treatment of such infections. Too often they are ignored, considered as unavoidably seasonal and treated very lightly. Women who have a history of acute glomerulonephritis are advised to consult a doctor before planning a pregnancy, as they are more likely to develop toxaemia and eclampsia.

The majority of patients with acute glomerulonephritis associated with infection (e.g. streptococcal) recover with no residual kidney disease. These patients generally show an increase in the volume of urine and a decrease in the blood pressure and serum urea levels within 1 week. The albuminuria and microscopic haematuria may persist for much longer. A few patients progress through a subacute phase to chronic glomerulonephritis. Others may be asymptomatic for a period of months or years and then experience an insidious development of the chronic disease which may progress to chronic renal failure.

Pyelonephritis

This is an inflammation of the pelvis and parenchymal tissue of the kidney due to infection. The predominant causative organism is *Escherichia coli*. Other causative agents are the *Proteus* species, *Klebsiella*, staphylococci or streptococci. The infective organisms have usually invaded the lower urinary tract and ascended to the kidney via the

Glomerulonephritis
See chapter 5.4

ureters. In rare instances the pathogen, such as the staphylococci or streptococci, may be bloodborne.

Significant predisposing factors are defective urinary drainage and reflux of urine from the bladder into the ureters. Obstructions to the flow of urine from the kidney may be the result of a renal calculus, neoplasm, stricture of a ureter due to pressure, scarring or congenital anomaly. Stasis of urine in the lower urinary tract due to bladder or urethral dysfunction may increase the intravesical pressure sufficiently to produce a reflux into the ureters.

Pyelonephritis is more common in females than males. The incidence is relatively high in female infants and children, due perhaps to faecal soiling and *E. coli* contamination of the urethral meatus. Its frequent occurrence in pregnant women is attributed to stasis of urine incurred by pressure from the enlarging uterus and atonia of the ureters due to the effect of progesterone. It may also occur following urethral catheterization; infection introduced into the bladder may ascend through the ureters to the kidney. Pyelonephritis in males in the later years of life is generally associated with defective urinary drainage as a result of an enlarged prostate.

Clinical characteristics

The onset is usually sudden. In children it may be accompanied by a convulsion. Manifestations include chills, fever, headache, nausea and vomiting, pain and tenderness in the loins, leucocytosis, and frequent and painful micturition (dysuria). The urine is cloudy and contains bacteria, pus, blood and epithelial cells.

Treatment

The patient is encouraged to take liberal amounts of fluid unless there is complete obstruction of urinary drainage. An accurate record of the fluid intake and output is necessary. A culture will be made of the urine and the causative organism antibiotic sensitivity determined. Antibiotic therapy is prescribed.

Unless there is complete eradication of the infection, pyelonephritis may become chronic with insidious destruction of nephrons, leading to chronic renal failure and uraemia. After the initial episode of acute pyelonephritis, the patient generally undergoes a thorough investigation for a predisposing obstructive lesion. Antimicrobial therapy and a high fluid intake are needed beyond the disappearance of acute signs and symptoms in order to ensure complete eradication of the infective organism. Specimens of urine are examined and cultured at regular intervals after the antimicrobial drug is discontinued.

Tuberculosis of the kidney

Tubercular infection in the kidney is usually secondary to tuberculosis elsewhere in the body; most often the primary site is a lung or lymph node. It is, however, very rare in the UK. The tubercle bacilli are carried by the blood to the kidneys. Scattered characteristic granulomatous lesions (tubercles) develop, eroding renal tissue and leaving cavitations. The infection may spread to involve the bladder and multiple strictures may develop in the urinary tract.

The patient receives a prolonged, intensive course of antituberculous drugs and should be observed for possible reactions to the drugs, which may take the form of dermatitis, fever, dizziness and impaired hearing. A nutritious full diet is encouraged without restrictions if there is adequate renal function to prevent oedema, hypertension and the accumulation of wastes in the blood. Frequent urine smears and cultures are made to determine the progress of the patient's disease. Treatment is continued for a period of 12–18 months even if the cultures become negative for tubercle bacilli.

The nephrotic syndrome (nephrosis)

The characteristic symptoms of the nephrotic syndrome are proteinuria (more than 3.5 g protein in 24 hours), hypoproteinaemia and oedema. It may develop in a patient with primary renal disease, or may be associated with other conditions in which kidney involvement is secondary. Systemic disorders (e.g. diabetes mellitus, systemic lupus erythematosus and amyloidosis), circulatory disturbances and infections are some of the causes.

The proteinuria, which is chiefly albumin, is the result of some change in the glomeruli that causes an increase in their permeability to the plasma proteins. Obviously, the loss of the proteins reduces the colloidal osmotic pressure of the blood, contributing to increased movement of fluid into the interstitial spaces as well as to its decreased reabsorption into the capillaries. The resulting decrease in intravascular volume leads to retention of sodium and water by the kidneys.

The urine is reduced in volume and usually contains casts as well as large amounts of albumin. In contrast to other forms of impaired renal function, the blood pressure and nitrogenous waste levels of patients usually remain within a normal range in the absence of advanced damage to glomeruli.

The severity of the nephrotic syndrome is variable. In some, the oedema may cause only slight puffiness in the periorbital areas and ankles, yet in others it may be so extreme that ascites (accumulation of fluid in the peritoneal cavity) and pleural effusion develop. The oedematous areas are generally soft and readily pit on pressure. The patient is usually pale, may be breathless, complains of fatigue and may experience anorexia, which further complicates the problem of hypoproteinaemia. Susceptibility to infection increases and the incidence of venous thrombosis is greater as anticoagulant substances are lost in the urine. The onset may be insidious or abrupt.

Treatment

When the nephrotic syndrome is secondary, the treatment is directed towards the likely prime cause and inducing diuresis, reducing oedema, producing and maintaining a normal serum albumin level. Diuretics will help reduce oedema and the patient's diet should contain a full quota of protein.

The patient is particularly susceptible to infection because of the lowered resistance of oedematous tissues and reduced plasma γ-globulin which is essential in the formation of antibodies. Precautions are necessary to avoid exposure to infection.

The patient is not usually hospitalized once a satisfactory therapeutic regimen has been established, nor confined to bed; activity is encouraged. Treatment is generally required over a long period, and frequent medical check-ups are necessary.

Nephrolithiasis (renal calculi)

Stones or small concretions may develop in the collecting tubules, calyces or the pelvis of a kidney. They are formed by the precipitation of various substances in the urine; if retained, the initial precipitation forms a nucleus or matrix which promotes further precipitation and calculus enlargement. The substances commonly involved in calculus formation are calcium, oxalate, phosphate, uric acid, cystine, xanthine and ammonia, but most often the stones are of mixed composition (e.g. mixed phosphates and oxalates). They vary in size from tiny particles to large smooth or irregular masses. The irregular stone that forms in the pelvis and has projections into the calyces is referred to as a *staghorn calculus*. The usual composition of the latter type of calculus is phosphate.

Causes

The constituents of renal calculi are present in normal urine; any condition that increases their concentration, reduces their solubility or promotes retention of the urinary salts favours their precipitation, calculus formation and possible obstruction to urinary flow. Conditions favourable to their formation include hypercalcaemia, as occurs with hyperparathyroidism, excessive vitamin D, an excessive ingestion of milk or an alkali, and prolonged immobilization. Other causes include dehydration, a highly acid urine and infection by *Proteus* (Gram-negative bacteria usually associated with faeces). *Proteus* infection makes the urine alkaline; this results in the precipitation of phosphates, forming what may be referred to as a *struvite calculus*.

Symptoms

The manifestations of renal calculus depend upon the size of the stone and whether it remains stationary. It may remain latent over a long period, producing no symptoms. Small gravel-like stones may be passed without any disturbance.

The majority cause some pain, haematuria, infection and, if large, kidney damage and renal insufficiency. Renal calculi may obstruct renal drainage by impaction of the tubules, by completely filling calyces and the pelvis, or by lodging in a ureter. The urine accumulates in the pelvis and tubules, dilating them and creating a back pressure; this condition is known as *hydronephrosis*. Compression of the blood vessels and nephrons by the mass of fluid leads to their destruction and obliteration, and to renal insufficiency.

The patient may complain of pain in the back, which may be caused by irritation of tissues by movement of the stone or by the back pressure and accumulation of fluid if the stone is obstructing renal or ureteral outflow. A small stone may enter the ureter and initiate *ureteric colic*. The patient complains of excruciating pain radiating from the back to the front along the groin into the genitalia; this may be associated with pallor, sweating, restlessness and vomiting.

Haematuria results from injury to the membranous lining of the pelvis or ureter. Infection is frequently associated with a calculus and, if present, chills, fever, leucocytosis and pyuria are likely to be manifested.

Complete obstruction of the kidney outflow is eventually reflected in renal insufficiency and a palpable mass in the renal area as a result of the hydronephrosis. The total volume of urine is less than normal, and blood investigations indicate reduced elimination of waste products.

Investigation of the patient for nephrolithiasis includes: midstream specimen of urine for culture and sensitivity, ultrasonography, abdominal radiography, intravenous urography or pyelography, and sometimes cystoscopy with retrograde pyelography. Serum calcium and uric acid levels are determined and renal function tests may be done. Investigation includes 24-hour urine studies for calcium, phosphorus, uric acid, creatinine and sodium oxalate.

Calculi
See chapter 5.4

Treatment and nursing intervention

If the urogram indicates that the calculus is small and may be passed by the patient, activity and large amounts of fluids are encouraged. All urine is strained through several layers of gauze or a filter paper and is observed. All sediment or solid particles passed are saved and submitted for identification of their composition.

During an attack of ureteric colic, the patient usually receives an analgesic, such as pethidine, to relieve the pain, and an antiemetic. When the pain subsides, fluids should be encouraged once nausea is no longer a problem.

Modern techniques have made direct surgical removal of stones rare events. Percutaneous stone removal involves the introduction of a needle and other instrumentation under radiographic control, through the loin and into the kidney. Laser or ultrasound probes can be used to disintegrate the stone, permitting its piecemeal removal. This technique can be employed with access being gained via the urethra and bladder (retrograde removal). An alternative approach is known as *extracorporeal shockwave lithotripsy* (ESWL). Ultrasound shockwaves are focused on the stone to shatter it, the fragments then being passed naturally.

Calculi are prone to recur in patients with a history of previous episodes. In an effort to prevent the formation of new stones or the enlargement of existing stones a high fluid intake of at least 3000 mL daily is essential to maintain a dilute urine. A portion of this should be taken at bedtime and during the night to prevent the concentration of urine that normally occurs at night. High levels of uric acid are associated with calcium oxalate stones in some patients, and the administration of potassium citrate may help. This makes the urine alkaline and increases the solubility of uric acid, reducing the risk of uric acid crystals acting as the nuclei of new stones.

If the patient should become ill, prolonged immobility should be avoided as the effects of immobility on calcium metabolism increase the probability of stone formation.

Neoplasms in the kidneys

Neoplasms in the adult kidney are of lower incidence than those in many other areas of the body. When they occur, they are usually malignant and are seen more often in males than in females. Tumours may arise in parenchyma or the collecting system of the kidney. The most common form of parenchymal tumours in adults is adenocarcinoma. It readily invades the blood vessels, causing early metastases to bones, lungs or liver, which may be the lesion that brings the person to the doctor. Tumours that arise in the renal pelvis and ureter are the same histologically as bladder cancer; 85% are transitional cell in origin, the remainder being squamous cell or adenocarcinoma-type cancers. Tumours of the renal pelvis and ureter are ten times less common than those developing in the bladder.

Clinical characteristics

In the adult, the first symptom is usually haematuria. As the neoplasm enlarges, the kidney becomes a palpable mass and the patient experiences pain, abdominal discomfort from pressure, anorexia and loss of weight. Ureteric colic may occur as a result of a blood clot entering the ureter. Polycythaemia develops in some patients because of an overproduction of erythropoietin by the affected kidney. Others may have marked anaemia.

A cystoscopy with ureteric catheterization is done to determine whether the source of the bleeding is unilateral or bilateral. Radiological studies are undertaken, using intravenous or retrograde pyelography to determine filling defects and the location of the neoplasm. Renal angiography may also be done to assess the extent of blood vessel involvement. Renal ultrasonography may be performed to assess the nature of the lesion and allow visualization of the lesion to facilitate aspiration.

Treatment

Nephrectomy is the usual treatment for parenchymal tumours; treatment may also involve local lymph node dissection. Embolization of the kidney may be used to prevent or relieve symptoms of metastatic disease when nephrectomy is not performed. Radiotherapy may be used but its effectiveness with these tumours is debatable, except for prophylaxis of metastatic symptoms. Chemotherapy, immunotherapy, hormone manipulation and the use of interferon are currently being investigated to determine their value in treating these cancers.

Polycystic disease of the kidneys

This disorder is characterized by the widespread distribution of cysts of varying sizes throughout both kidneys. The disease is congenital and familial, and affects both sexes. It is predominant in infants and adults over 40 years of age. In infants and young children, other abnormalities may be present. The disease is often found in more than one member of the family and in successive generations. Because of the distinct difference in the age of the groups in which the disease is manifested, it is suggested that there are two different genetic types. When it occurs in infants and young children, it is considered to be autosomal recessive, but the polycystic disease that becomes manifest in adults is autosomal dominant.

The person with a disorder of the urinary system

Clinical characteristics

Clinical characteristics of impaired bladder function and urinary elimination include abnormal constituents in the urine and altered patterns of urinary elimination (functional, reflex, stress, total and urge incontinence, and urinary retention). Alterations in voiding may be related to infection in the urinary tract, emotional stress, a neurological disorder, bladder calculi, obstructive disease of the bladder or urethra and, rarely, chemicals excreted in the urine.

Abnormal constituents in urine

Blood, pus, microorganisms and mucus may be present in the urine as a result of inflammation, tissue necrosis or a malignancy in the lower urinary tract. The urine may be cloudy or blood coloured and have an ammoniacal odour.

Alteration in patterns of urinary elimination

Symptomatic changes in voiding include:

- frequency
- urgency
- dysuria
- residual urine
- alterations in urinary stream
- retention
- incontinence.

Frequency, urgency and dysuria

Irritation of the bladder or urethral mucosa may give rise to an abnormally frequent desire to void, urgency and painful micturition. Frequency due to a urological disturbance is generally accompanied by an *urgency*, which implies that there is an intense desire to void immediately. The normally voluntary control to retain the urine cannot be maintained, and some urine may escape before the person can reach the toilet or use a bedpan. *Dysuria* refers to the abnormal discomfort, pain, burning or smarting sensation that may accompany voiding. *Strangury* is a term used occasionally when the dysuria is unusually severe and there is increasing frequency of decreasing amounts of urine.

Residual urine

Micturition may not completely empty the bladder, leaving a residue of urine. This problem is diagnosed, and the amount determined, by catheterizing the patient immediately after voiding. Residual urine is usually the result of an obstruction to the bladder outlet and causes a stagnation that predisposes to bladder and kidney infection and calculus formation.

Alterations in the urinary stream

The person may have difficulty in initiating the urinary flow. This symptom of hesitancy is usually due to some obstruction in the bladder–urethral orifice or the urethra. Pressure within the bladder must be increased beyond the normal to force the urine past the obstructing lesion. Because of resistance to the urinary outflow, the muscle tires before the bladder is empty; after a few moments, it contracts again and voiding is resumed.

Retention of urine

The inability of a person to void is a relatively common problem. The distension of the bladder and stasis of urine predispose to the development of ureteric back pressure, reflux of urine into the ureters, and infection of the bladder and kidneys. The reaction of the bladder to progressive obstruction of the outflow is hypertrophy of the detrusor muscle. Diverticulae may develop; these are saccular protusions of the mucosa between the muscle fibres. The sacs fill with urine, which becomes stagnant and readily infected. Calculi may also form within the diverticula.

Retention of urine is suspected if the person has had a normal fluid intake and has not voided within a period of 8–10 hours or if there is distension of the lower part of the abdomen. A distended bladder may also be present with frequent voiding of small amounts (30–50 mL), which is termed *retention with overflow*. The person may experience a constant desire to void but efforts to do so are ineffective.

Urinary incontinence

Estimates of the prevalence of urinary **incontinence** give a wide range of values. This is due to the difficulty in defining exactly what is meant by the term and reliance upon self-reporting with little external validation. Notwithstanding this difficulty, Dorey (2000) cites evidence showing a range of estimates of between 3.6% for men aged over 45 years up to 28% in men aged 90 years or more. The figures seem to be higher in women, and Brittain et al (2001) present data from various studies showing a range from 9% in women aged 20–59 years to 47% in a sample of women aged 30 years or more, the average being around 25–30%. It is difficult to extrapolate from these studies to the whole population with any precision, but we can estimate that several million people are affected by problems of urinary continence in the UK.

Incontinence probably goes untreated or unassessed because of embarrassment associated with social interaction and can exert severe stress both on the individual, partner and carers. Urinary incontinence presents a real challenge to nurses to assist in improving the quality of life of a significant proportion of the population.

The classification of types of urinary incontinence can be confusing. It is better, therefore, to focus on the causes, which may be grouped under three headings (Cheater 1995):

- physiological causes
- extrinsic factors affecting bladder function
- intrinsic factors affecting bladder function.

Incontinence
See chapter 5.4

Physiological causes

Instability of the detrusor muscle leading to spontaneous contraction or contraction in response to a stimulus such as coughing leads to micturition occurring with little or no warning. Urgency, frequency and substantial volumes of residual urine (i.e. urine left in the bladder after micturition) occur commonly.

Genuine *stress incontinence* is the other main physiological cause. It occurs when pressure in the bladder exceeds that in the urethra and is usually associated with a sudden rise in intra-abdominal pressure (e.g. sneezing or laughing). It is more common in females.

Other causes include damage to the spinal cord (neurogenic bladder) and obstruction of urinary outflow which leads to large volumes of residual urine and overflow.

Extrinsic causes

Limited mobility and dexterity, difficulty of access to toilet facilities, low expectations of carers and confusion can all contribute to incontinence.

Intrinsic causes

Faecal impaction can lead to compression of the bladder, exacerbating continence problems. A urinary tract infection or an endocrine disorder such as diabetes which causes polyuria can cause incontinence.

Urinary incontinence is a major health problem. It brings with it many hardships; not only is there the cost, but also the effort involved in maintaining hygiene and containing the problem, together with the emotional hardships in relation to the isolating and demeaning aspects of the problem.

It is generally acknowledged that most people with urinary incontinence can benefit from treatment, yet many receive only palliative remedies of protective pads and urinary appliances while the basic problem remains unidentified and untreated.

Nursing assessment

Urinary elimination is a personal and private activity; social norms and personal habits influence how individuals respond when problems develop with urinary emission. Patients may be uncomfortable and embarrassed discussing their problems and delay seeking assistance until some event finally triggers action. The main triggering events found by Brittain et al (2001) amongst a sample of 112 patients were:

- raised awareness of the issue and a service that could help as a result of publicity

- deterioration of their symptoms

- personal factors such as emotional difficulties, embarrassing events, anxiety over hygiene and awareness of age

- worries about their health

- the impact of incontinence on their social life.

The key findings here are that publicity campaigns which raise awareness of the problem can lead to many people seeking help. In assessing the patient, the nurse has to be sensitive to the personal significance of the problem to the patient and the impact it has on significant others in their life. Assessment should therefore include the individual's level of anxiety, feelings of discomfort or embarrassment; the nurse should acknowledge awareness of these feelings and reassure the patient that everything possible will be done to ease any embarrassment and provide privacy. It is also important to establish the terms and expressions used by the patient to describe the act of voiding and to ensure that the terminology used by the nurse is understood.

Patient history and subjective data

The person should be asked about their perception of the problem and how it effects their life. Tactfully, they should be asked to describe the symptoms they experience and to estimate how often and how much leakage occurs. Bowel habit should be discussed together with any previous surgical or medical history. Particularly relevant are any *family or personal history* of urinary system disorders or infections, diseases affecting the urinary system such as diabetes mellitus or hypertension, and the past use of drugs (either prescribed or bought over the counter). Women should be asked about their obstetric

history because of the effects of pregnancy on the pelvic floor muscles. Functional factors such as whether a male patient is able to stand to void, ease of access to toilet facilities, and manual dexterity with buttons and zips should be explored (Dorey 2000).

Specific information about the person's usual and present *pattern of urinary elimination* is obtained. Information includes frequency of voiding, volume of urine excreted at each voiding and in a 24-hour period, and usual times of voiding. Any changes in the usual pattern of elimination such as nocturia or frequency are identified. The person is asked about the colour, odour and clarity of urine and whether there is any discomfort or pain associated with voiding. It is important to determine for how long the incontinence has been present.

Factors influencing urinary elimination

- *Past experiences and attitudes*. Urinary habits vary with each individual. The nurse should discuss the person's usual habits and attitudes to urinary elimination. The person may associate urinary incontinence with loss of control of body function, and see the problem as regression towards infancy; sensitivity on the nurse's part is therefore of paramount importance.

- *Diet and fluid intake*. The volume of fluid intake has a direct effect on the urinary output. The person who suffers from incontinence may well restrict fluid intake in order to try to reduce the problem. Unfortunately, this may lead to dehydration and an increased risk of urinary tract infection (UTI). For patients with renal disorders it is important to identify usual eating habits and the relative amounts of protein and sodium in the daily diet.

- *Lifestyle factors* that influence elimination include accessibility of toilet facilities, privacy and any unusual stresses associated with voiding.

- *Activity, mobility and dexterity*. Physical activity is necessary to maintain muscle tone and normal amounts of calcium in the bones. Bedrest and immobility predispose to the formation of calculi. Impaired mobility and dexterity may interfere with the individual's ability to get to the toilet quickly enough to use it effectively.

- *Level of awareness and orientation*. Confusion, disorientation and difficulty following directions may interfere with the individual's ability to respond appropriately to the urge to void as well as to meet fluid and nutritional needs.

- *Medications*. The name, dosage, frequency and duration of use of any medications being taken are recorded. Diuretics have a direct effect on urine production, whereas sedatives may alter cognition.

Physical assessment

General appearance

The patient is observed for general state of health, lethargy, fatigue and degree of alertness.

Urinary meatus and perineum

The urethral orifice is observed for signs of drainage, oedema, redness or ulceration, and underclothing is examined for urine or other stains.

Bladder

The bladder is not normally palpable but may be felt if it is overdistended. With the person supine, gently palpate the area just above the symphysis pubis; the distended bladder feels smooth and firm. Palpation of a distended bladder causes increased discomfort for the patient.

Assessment of functional status

The person's mobility, manual dexterity and communication skills are determined.

Box 19.6 lists the basic skills required by an individual to achieve control of micturition. The nurse and patient collectively identify which of these basic skills the patient possesses, where difficulties are encountered in the course of daily activities, and what measures and techniques the patient uses to compensate for these deficits and their effectiveness.

Analysis of medical and nursing assessments may demonstrate the need for further evaluation by members of the multidisciplinary team such as continence nurse adviser, occupational therapist or speech therapist. Early referral to the continence nurse adviser may assist in the appropriate management of the incontinence, the supply of appliances or aids, and liaison with community services in anticipation of discharge to ensure continuity of care. The occupational therapist will evaluate the home environment and toilet facilities in relation to the patient's mobility, dexterity and awareness. Difficulties manipulating clothing are also identified. The speech therapist will assess communication skills and recommend means by which the patient can communicate needs. The role of nursing staff and relatives in contributing to the patient's incontinence is also assessed, especially in the institutionalized, the elderly and the disabled. An expectation of incontinence will probably result in incontinence: it becomes a self-fulfilling prophecy. Assistance to allow a schedule of regular voiding may be lacking, resulting in incontinence. Staff and family attitudes and relationships with the patient can be changed by helping them define expectations, set goals and develop strategies for dealing with the individual problem.

Clinical diagnostic measurements

Urine tests

A random or midstream urine (MSU) specimen may be sent to the laboratory for routine and microscopic analysis. Cook (1995) has pointed out that cleansing of the external urinary meatus before collecting a MSU sample is no longer considered necessary.

Residual urine determination

To identify overflow incontinence associated with urinary retention, an in-and-out catherization is performed immediately after voiding. The amount of urine that remained in the bladder after the person voided is measured and recorded.

Urodynamic investigations

These studies provide information on bladder sensation and detrusor muscle and urethral sphincter function. The tests consist of:

1. urine flow studies
2. pressure studies of both bladder and urethra (filling and voiding cystometrography, urethoral pressure profile)
3. video studies.

Urine flow studies measure the rate and volume of urine passed and usually include determination of the amount of residual urine in the bladder following voiding. *Cystometrography* is a method of recording the bladder's responses to increasing distension. Synchronous video pressure flow cystourethrography is a newer, more sophisticated and expensive method of evaluating bladder and urethral function; it provides information on the appearance of the bladder during the micturition cycle. Patients can find these studies very embarrassing owing to the intimate nature of the procedure and lack of privacy leading to severe anxiety (Shaw et al 2000).

> **BOX 19.6**   Basic skills required to achieve urinary continence
>
> - The ability to initiate micturition voluntarily at an appropriate time
>
> - The ability to delay, temporarily, the onset of micturition
>
> - Perception of the urge to urinate well in advance of reflex voiding
>
> - Awareness of socially acceptable places and/or circumstances to urinate
>
> - The ability to communicate needs and interpret oral directions and written signs to get necessary assistance or locate the toilet
>
> - The physical mobility and manual dexterity to reach the toilet, to assume and maintain body posture during micturition, adjust clothing, deal with doors, locks, flushing systems, seats and washing facilities.

Incontinence voiding record or diary

Documentation of the person's ability to void and episodes of incontinence may be obtained in the form of a patient diary or record kept by the individual, carers or nurse. The data are collected for several days to 2 weeks to enable analysis of the frequency of the incontinence and its relationship to fluid intake and physical and social activities and events. This record is useful in helping to develop a management programme appropriate to the needs of the individual.

Management

Interventions to reduce or manage urinary incontinence include:

- drug therapy
- pelvic floor exercises
- behavioural interventions
- protective pads and appliances
- surgery.

There are also a number of general measures that should be used in conjunction with these interventions to alleviate any contributing factors. These are listed in Box 19.7.

Medication

Many drugs are available that influence the activity of the detrusor muscle and urethral sphincter but their use is limited because of the other generalized effects of these drugs and the unpleasant side-effects produced.

Pelvic floor exercises
See chapter 5.4

Box 19.7   General measures directed to the alleviation of contributing factors to urinary incontinence

1. Weight reduction if the person is overweight.
2. Maintaining a fluid intake of at least 2000 mL per day.
3. Decreasing fluid intake if it has been excessive.
4. Review of medication for possible contributing factors and adjustment of these medications if necessary.
5. Adjustment of any diuretic therapy so that the action of the drugs occurs during the day.
6. Decrease in alcohol intake.
7. Institution of measures to suppress a chronic cough.
8. Treatment of any underlying urinary tract infections.
9. Increase in daily physical activity.
10. Prevention or treatment of constipation.

Anticholinergic agents decrease smooth muscle activity of a hypertonic bladder and may be used to treat urge incontinence related to neurogenic impairment and detrusor muscle instability.

The association of stress incontinence with a chronic cough is such that treatment of the respiratory problem with drug therapy may relieve the incontinence (Torrance and Jordan 1995).

Pelvic floor exercises

Kegel exercises increase the tone of muscles involved in micturition. They may be taught to control stress incontinence in women. The person sits with the feet on the floor and knees apart and is instructed to tighten the perineal muscles, as if stopping the flow of urine, and to hold the muscle contraction and then relax. This exercise is repeated several times every 2–4 hours throughout the day. During voiding, the patient is instructed to stop and start the urinary stream by contracting the perineal muscles. A feedback device may be used for patients who lack sensory input as it provides them with pressure readings, demonstrating the effectiveness of the muscle contractions.

Behavioural interventions

A *bladder training programme* is developed whenever possible with the active participation of the patient and family. Kennedy (1992) presents a strong case for the effectiveness of bladder training in her review of the research literature. A detailed chart or diary of urine frequency and volume, fluid intake, the times of fluid intake and voiding, and the circumstances surrounding incidents of incontinence is kept for several days. From this information, the nurse and patient can develop a voiding schedule and a plan that considers the person's needs and daily activities. Voiding normally occurs on arising in the morning, before or after meals, and before retiring in the evening. The voiding schedule may begin by having the person void every 1 or 2 hours, with the intervals increased gradually as control is acquired. The person's level of awareness and perception of the urge to void influence the degree of personal control that can be expected. When a patient is confused and disoriented, it is necessary for others to prompt the patient to follow the schedule and to provide assistance in tasks such as getting to the toilet and manipulating clothing.

Fluid intake of at least 2000 mL daily is maintained throughout the programme to avoid the risks of dehydration and urinary tract infection. Physical activity is increased.

Toilet facilities, a commode chair, bedpan or urinal should be within reach of the person, and privacy provided. An assessment of the home environment is done and recommendations made if necessary for modifications to the home or the purchase or loan of a commode chair or bedpan. A night light should be provided. Voiding should always take place in the usual sitting posture for females and standing posture for males, with the nurse or a relative providing the necessary assistance.

For those with flaccid, hypotonic bladders, *Credé's manoeuvre* is taught. The hands are placed flat over the abdomen below the umbilicus. Manual pressure is exerted over the bladder to initiate flow of urine. Suprapubic tapping or stroking of the thighs may also be used to stimulate reflex voiding when incontinence is the result of neurogenic dysfunction (reflex incontinence).

Suggestions are provided for adapting clothing for the person with impaired manual dexterity or the individual who has minimal time between the sensation or urge to void and the act of voiding (urge incontinence). The person may need instruction and practice with the manipulation of zippers, buttons or other aspects of clothing.

Positive reinforcement or contingency management is a behavioural approach using positive verbal and social reinforcement to establish continent behaviours. *Prompted voiding* and socialization are behavioural techniques that have been used effectively with female nursing home residents to decrease episodes of incontinence (Creason et al 1989). The technique used involved asking residents whether they needed to void and, if so, assisting them with toileting. The schedule for prompting must be established for each individual in relation to their voiding pattern and activities.

Biofeedback, used alone or in combination with bladder training and positive reinforcement, has been shown to be effective in the treatment of stress and urge incontinence. This procedure provides the person with information about bladder and abdominal pressures which is useful in learning to inhibit bladder contractions voluntarily. This method is most effective when used with cognitively aware individuals.

Protective pads and appliances

Various aids are used in the management of incontinence. Self-control of continence cannot be achieved for every patient. Some may continuously require protective measures. Others may require protective measures during assessment and treatment or during periods of illness. Many protective devices and aids are available.

Protective pants and pads Underpads may be used on bedlinen or furniture, or pads are available to be worn by the person. Various types of waterproof pants and pads are also available. Each type is designed to meet a specific need and the absorbency of the various pads varies. The marsupial pants (Kanga pants) are designed with a waterproof pouch to hold the pad in place. Most products are available in a variety of sizes and styles, and some are disposable while others are washable. Use and selection of pants and pads must be individualized and requires the individual's interest and cooperation. Protection of clothing allows the patient to dress normally and participate in social functions. The use of pads or plastic or rubber pants for adults may be demeaning and serve to promote feelings of dependence and withdrawal if their use is not discussed and agreed with the person. Sanitary towels are not designed to contain urine and are inappropriate, ineffective and an expensive means of containing incontinence.

The need for careful assessment of different types of aid, rather than a blanket use of one or two types only, is shown by the work of Gibbs and Wong (1994). Their research indicated that a wide range exists in the comfort and dryness achieved by different aids, depending largely on the sex of the patient and the heaviness of voiding. They concluded that males were less well served than females by the pants and pads approach to continence management.

External urinary drainage devices A condom with an attached drainage bag is useful for men. It may be worn only at night or during the day under clothing; care must be taken to select an appropriately sized condom. The penis is checked frequently for oedema, redness or excoriation. A female external urine collecting device is available. It has an adhesive plate similar to a stoma wafer with an integral pouch which can be attached to a collecting bag. Wear times achieved by this device vary and mobility can be restricted. In order to achieve adherence, the skin around the external genitalia is shaved and a skin-protective gel is applied.

Catheter Catheterization as a means of controlling incontinence is not considered until other alternatives have been tried. An indwelling catheter may be used in some instances to permit increased independence for the patient. For long-term use the catheter should be made of silicone or coated with silicone-elastomer or hydrogel as this produces less tissue inflammation. The smallest size possible should always be used.

A study by Getliffe (1995) of 34 long-term catheterized patients found little embarrassment about having an indwelling catheter. Her research indicated that, for this group of patients, long-term catheterization was acceptable because of the benefits it brought.

Although the development of urinary tract infections in long-term catheterized patients has a certain inevitability about it, no increase in mortality or morbidity rates associated with UTI in such patients has been shown (Getliffe 1995).

Intermittent catheterization is an alternative to an indwelling catheter; the person or carer is taught to perform the procedure. The risk of infection is reduced with intermittent catheterization as opposed to an indwelling catheter. It is performed on a regular schedule which is determined in a similar manner to the bladder training schedule.

Electrical devices Electrical stimulators are receiving moderate attention as a means of increasing the tone of pelvic muscles. They create continuous contraction of the pelvic muscles which is relieved by releasing the electrical stimulation to facilitate voiding when desired.

Occlusive devices These are not satisfactory for long-term use. Penile clamps and an inflatable pad which applies pressure against the perineum to close the penile urethra are available for men.

Occlusive devices for females are vaginal tampons and an inflatable vaginal balloon which elevate the bladder neck and apply pressure on the urethra through the vagina and may be useful for minor stress incontinence or during periods of physical activity.

Surgery

Surgical intervention for incontinence is directed to the correction of anatomical defects that contribute to the incontinence (e.g. correction of obstructions in the urinary tract, repair of a cystocele, or uterine prolapse, or prostatic hypertrophy). Urethrovesical resuspension may be performed in women with severe stress incontinence. This procedure increases the support for the bladder and restores the closure of the bladder outlet. Sometimes urinary diversion is performed for uncontrollable incontinence. This is occasionally necessary following radiotherapy for bladder cancer, where the bladder becomes atrophied with a small capacity, or for congenital malformations of the bladder (e.g. ectopic vesicae), or in spina bifida.

Artificial urethral sphincters can be implanted in men and women. Various types of devices are available but they generally consist of a cuff filled with fluid and a mechanism for diversion of the fluid when voiding is desired.

Nursing intervention

Effective management of urinary incontinence usually involves the collaborative efforts of a multidisciplinary team and the active participation of the individual and carers. The nurse is an important member of this team and is often in the best position to initiate and coordinate activities (Case Study 19.1).

Case Study 19.1

Betty Jarvis is a 76-year-old woman who was admitted to hospital for a total knee replacement. After the operation the nursing staff noted that she was requesting the bedpan frequently and was often incontinent by the time they got to her.

Mrs Jarvis had a 10-year history of problems with urgency, frequency and incontinence of urine. She had had bladder surgery 8 years ago but this was effective only for the first year. When her symptoms returned she consulted her doctor who told her there was nothing further to be done and she would have to learn to live with it.

Assessment

Bladder A postvoiding residual volume was requested to determine how well Mrs Jarvis was emptying her bladder. A toileting routine was instituted for the next 48 hours to assess the amount and frequency of voiding. Mrs Jarvis voided 50–75 mL every 2 hours and the frequency increased in direct relation to her intake. In the initial postoperative phase she had an intravenous infusion at 100 mL per hour and was voiding every half hour; once the infusion was stopped this decreased to every 2 hours.

Bowel Mrs Jarvis stated that her bowels had not moved since before the operation 5 days previously. An abdominal assessment and rectal examination were done. Her abdomen was distended, with bowel sounds present, and was firm on palpation. The rectum was full of very hard, constipated stool.

Once the assessment was complete it was determined that Mrs Jarvis was voiding small amounts frequently with a normal postvoiding residual volume and was considered to have detrusor instability. The instability was being further exacerbated by her faecal impaction.

Intervention

Mrs Jarvis was put on a bowel programme to resolve the constipation. She was also started on an anticholinergic medication to reduce the irritability of her bladder, thus allowing an increase in voided volumes and the time between voiding. A postvoiding residual volume was determined 5 and 10 days after the start of the anticholinergic treatment to ensure that she was not in retention.

Evaluation

Mrs Jarvis was discharged home 3 weeks after operation and was delighted to have regained her continence after so many years.

Assessment

Assessment is the key to identification of the problem and to determining accurately the type of incontinence and the contributing factors. The nurse plays a vital role in the assessment process in identifying individuals at risk for or with incontinence and in promoting recognition that a problem exists. The nurse is able to document the person's patterns of urinary elimination over a period of time and identify factors associated with the incontinent episodes. The nurse assumes responsibility for ongoing patient assessment and thus reassesses the need for indwelling catheters and ensures that they are removed as early as possible once the reason for their insertion is resolved.

Development of the patient plan of care

The nurse should collaborate with the person and family to develop an effective plan to manage the person's urinary incontinence. Patient and family input is necessary to establish realistic goals and to develop a plan to meet the needs, activities and lifestyle of the patient and family members.

Self-concept

Urinary incontinence has a negative impact on the individual's self-esteem and self-concept. Studies of the prevalence of incontinence recognize that many cases are hidden. They are not identified because the person is reluctant to disclose the information. One of the more constructive interventions the nurse can perform is to get the person and family to talk about the problem and to recognize that incontinence is not a normal consequence of ageing or childbirth and that something can be done to help them. Plans for managing the incontinence should consider the impact of the problem on the person's social activities and include strategies for increased socialization.

Patient and family teaching

Patients and families generally lack information about the nature of urinary incontinence and its management. Patients and families need help to develop self-care skills related to the numerous products and appliances used to control the incontinence. Roe (1990) found that patients lacked basic knowledge of their indwelling catheters and that teaching by nurses about catheter care was not comprehensive or consistent. She recommended the use of information booklets to enable learning to take place over time. Not all patients want to learn or are capable of learning about their incontinence and its management. Assessment of learning needs should be ongoing to identify when and whether the patient is ready for further information.

Urinary retention

Urinary retention means the person is unable to empty his or her bladder fully. It is characterized by a distended bladder and a sensation of bladder fullness. The person may be unable to void when fluid intake has been adequate, may experience difficulty with starting a stream of urine, or bladder emptying may be incomplete. The person may void frequent small amounts of urine and may experience dribbling. It may be described as a type of incontinence (urinary incontinence with overflow).

Retention may be related to obstructive disease of the bladder or urethra (usually due to enlargement of the prostate gland with ageing in men; see below), surgical intervention or neurogenic disease (Box 19.8).

Benign prostatic hypertrophy

Obstructive disease of the bladder is caused by benign prostatic hypertrophy (BPH), a common condition in later life which affects a high proportion of men. As the

---

> **Box 19.8** Causes and characteristics of urinary retention
>
> *Causes*
>
> - Obstructive disease of the bladder or urethra
> - Surgical intervention
> - Neurological disease
> - Embarrassment or fear
> - Constipation.
>
> *Clinical characteristics*
>
> - Frequent voiding of small amounts (overflow)
> - Absence of voiding in 8–10 hours with adequate fluid intake
> - Bladder distension
> - Urgency and persistent desire to void
> - Restlessness
> - Pain and discomfort in the region of the bladder and/or kidney.

---

prostate gland enlarges it interferes with normal urinary outflow from the bladder. The condition is insidious in onset with the person becoming aware of increasing difficulty in passing urine; dribbling and frequency may develop. In time, chronic retention may occur where the person has a large residual volume of urine in the bladder which then becomes prone to infection. Alternatively acute retention may intervene; in this situation the patient will have a distended lower abdomen and be in acute pain and distress as he is unable to pass any urine.

It is important, therefore, in assessing any man aged over 50 years, to enquire carefully about any changes in micturition, remembering the possible embarrassment this may cause the patient. It is interesting to note that a national survey by the British Market Research Bureau (Nursing Standard 1991) found that, although the symptoms of BPH were widespread, knowledge of what the condition involved and its treatment were poor. Only 28% of persons with symptoms had consulted a general practitioner, and only 2% stated that they had consulted a nurse about the problem. This is an area where the nurse has a vital role in the early detection of symptoms and referral for medical treatment in addition to having a strong health education role.

The surgical treatment of BPH involves *transurethral resection of the prostate* (TURP), whereby a cutting diathermy instrument is introduced via a cystoscope and under direct vision the hypertrophied prostate is tunnelled through to enlarge the opening from the bladder and allow normal urinary drainage. Postoperative care is concerned with ensuring that drainage from the catheter is

Retention
See chapter 5.4

kept free and not blocked by any clots that may form and lead to clot retention. Bladder irrigation using a two-way catheter is therefore required and care must be given to ensuring that the patient regains normal bladder control when the catheter is removed (p. 793).

Assessment

The time of last voiding, the volume of fluid intake and the volume of urinary output are determined. Fluid loss by channels other than urinary is also considered. The patient's lower abdomen is examined for distension of the bladder. The patient may complain of low abdominal pain or the distress of feeling the need to void but being unable to initiate voiding.

Nursing intervention

The *goal* is that the patient will establish and maintain a flow of urine from the bladder (see Case Study 19.2).

Case Study 19.2

Frances Lee is an 80-year-old woman who was admitted to hospital in a diabetic crisis in an effort to stabilize her blood sugar level. She was incontinent of large amounts of urine over the first 24 hours and the nursing staff requested an indwelling catheter. They were concerned that prolonged incontinence would put her at risk for skin breakdown and increase the number of linen changes that would be required.

Mrs Lee complained of an ongoing problem with incontinence that had started several years before but had worsened in the past few months.

Catheterization
See chapter 5.4

Assessment

Bladder Inserting an indwelling catheter at this point would simply postpone the problem of determining the cause of her incontinence and the appropriate treatment. Instead, a postvoiding residual was done to determine the extent to which Mrs Lee was able to empty her bladder completely.

Mrs Lee voided 100 mL and was catheterized for a residual volume of 1000 mL. She did not even seem to be aware that she had to void or that her bladder was so overdistended.

Bowel An abdominal assessment and rectal examination determined that she was having difficulty emptying her bowels and was in fact constipated.

Mrs Lee was in urinary retention secondary to three factors: diabetic neuropathy which reduced her sensation of filling; faecal impaction which was partially obstructing her urethra; and immobility which made it very difficult for her to get to the bathroom so she often lost the urge to void or ignored it.

Intervention

Mrs Lee was started on a programme of intermittent catheterization four times a day until her residual volumes reduced to 350 mL, when catheterization was reduced to three times a day. As her bladder tone returned, she began voiding again and her residuals were reduced to twice daily.

The faecal impaction was initially treated with a series of enemas and, once resolved, Mrs Lee continued on a regular bowel programme.

Evaluation

Mrs Lee's condition stabilized over the next few days and she was then transferred to a rehabilitation setting to improve her mobility and evaluate her ability to look after herself. Her urinary retention resolved slowly and she was still on daily residuals when discharged. These were done by the district nurse for further 2 weeks before they were low enough to be discontinued.

Promotion of spontaneous voiding

Nursing measures used to induce voiding include increasing the fluid intake (unless contraindicated), providing privacy, pouring warm water over the perineum, letting the patient hear running water and, unless contraindicated, assisting the patient to assume the normal position for voiding. Women are encouraged to use a commode at the bedside; men may stand beside the bed. A warm bath may prove effective with some patients.

Urinary retention in a postoperative patient may result from incisional pain and discomfort or be associated with embarrassment at the lack of privacy. Analgesics are administered before offering the patient a bedpan or urinal or assisting them to a sitting position, commode chair or to the bathroom. Privacy should be maintained at all times.

Urethral catheterization

Emptying of the bladder by the insertion of a catheter into the urethra and bladder may be done on an intermittent or continuous basis. Urinary **catheterization** may be performed for reasons other than urinary retention; it may be necessary to assess urinary output accurately in a critically ill patient, to promote healing following surgery in the perineal region, or to measure the volume of residual urine remaining in the bladder following micturition. Before inserting a catheter, the need for it should be thoroughly assessed and documented. Because of the increased risk of infection, as well as the patient's discomfort and loss of dignity, the catheter should be removed as soon as possible.

The procedure and the purpose for it are explained to the patient and privacy is provided throughout the procedure. Precautions are taken to avoid the introduction of organisms and trauma of the mucosa; sterile gloves are worn, and strict aseptic technique is observed throughout the procedure. Sterile anaesthetizing gel should be introduced into the urethra at least 2 minutes before the catheter. This lubricates the passage of the catheter and reduces sensation. This practice has traditionally been reserved for male patients because of the much longer male urethra, but, as Mackenzie (1994) has pointed out, there is no reason why women should not also have the benefit of local anaesthesia during catheterization.

The catheter is handled with great care in order to minimize trauma. If the retention has been acute and severe, not more than 1000 mL of urine are removed initially. The sudden, complete emptying of an overdistended bladder may result in an atonic bladder wall. The sudden release of pressure on the blood vessels in the bladder region causes a sudden inflow of blood, and sometimes capillary bleeding may occur. Rarely, the patient may experience faintness. The catheter is removed or may be clamped after 1000–1500 mL has been drained, and then reopened to allow further drainage at a later time.

Management of an indwelling urethral catheter

A closed drainage system is used to maintain a continuous urinary flow and decrease the potential for the entry of organisms into the system. The catheter is attached to tubing and a collecting bag with a drainage valve, or to a leg bag that contains a valve to prevent backflow of urine into the bladder. The leg bag or regular drainage bag is kept below the level of the bladder and attached to a hanger or hook on the side of the patient's bed or chair. A leg bag is used for the patient who is mobile because it is less cumbersome and can be worn under clothing. The drainage system should not be disconnected unnecessarily for fear of introducing infection to what should be a closed, sterile system.

The drainage system is assessed frequently for patency; kinks in the tubing and tension on the catheter and tubing are avoided. In women, the catheter is taped to the inner thigh; in men the catheter is taped laterally to the upper thigh or abdomen to prevent pressure on the penile–scrotal angle. The latter is an important preventive measure as erosion of tissue at the penile–scrotal angle may develop if tension is applied to the catheter, and the resulting fistula can be corrected only by plastic surgery.

Indwelling urethral catheters are changed at varying intervals and may be left in place for 4–6 weeks depending on the type of material used in the catheter; information is usually available on the catheter package. Collecting tubing and drainage bags are changed every 2–7 days. Urethral catheters are inconvenient for the patient, but should not interfere with the performance of usual daily activities. Showers are generally permitted.

Measures to prevent the development of urinary tract infections from catheter use are discussed on page 654.

Patient teaching

Individuals requiring retention catheters during periods of hospitalization require information about the purpose of the catheter and general principles of care and the importance of preventing infections. They are taught to keep the

drainage bag below the level of the bladder, to prevent tension on the catheter and to maintain a closed system.

The person requiring intermittent or continuous catheterization at home requires detailed instruction about the supply and care of equipment, and the performance of the procedure if necessary. The inevitability of infection in long-term catheterized patients has already been discussed. It appears that a biofilm consisting of microorganisms and their extracellular products forms and adheres to the catheter and drainage bag. The biofilm protects live bacteria from antimicrobial agents, making eradication impossible (Mulhall et al 1993).

Referrals are made to the community nurse or continence adviser to assist the person and family in managing the catheter. At home, the drainage tubing and bag required for night use may be cleaned with soap and water and stored dry during the day before reconnection at night. With intermittent self-catheterization it is also possible to wash through the catheter and store it in a clean dry place until required again. Good clean technique is necessary whatever system is adopted.

Management of the person after removal of the catheter

An indwelling catheter is removed as soon as possible to lessen the trauma to urethral sphincters and the loss of muscle tone that ensues. After the catheter is removed, the person is encouraged to pass urine hourly for a few hours and the time and amount of each voiding are recorded, as well as the fluid intake. The patient is assessed for any discomfort, dribbling of urine due to dilatation of the sphincter by the catheter, sensation of urgency or stress incontinence. If the person is unable to void in 6–8 hours and has had an adequate fluid intake, intermittent catheterization may be necessary. If only small amounts of urine are voided, catheterization may be done to measure the amount of residual urine. A bladder training programme may be instituted if difficulties persist after a few days.

Suprapubic catheterization

The insertion of a catheter into the bladder through the suprapubic area is a surgical procedure and requires local or general anaesthesia. Nursing care of the patient with a suprapubic catheter and closed drainage system is similar to that of the patient with an indwelling urethral catheter. The suprapubic catheter is sutured in place and then taped to the abdomen to prevent tension on the catheter. The exit site is cared for as a surgical incision. Stomahesive can be used to protect the skin around the insertion site or a transparent, sealed dressing (e.g. Opsite) is used.

Lower urinary tract infection

Lower urinary tract infection (UTI) refers to an acute or chronic infection and inflammation of the bladder (*cystitis*) and the urethra (*urethritis*). It is a common health

Catheter care
See chapter 5.4

Lower urinary tract
See chapter 5.4

problem affecting at least 20% of women during their lifetime, with about 3% experiencing recurrent infections. The incidence is less in men but increases after 65 years of age, probably as a result of obstructive disorders and the loss of bactericidal activity of prostatic secretions.

Causes

Lower UTI is most often due to infection caused by the ascent of organisms by way of the urethra, but may also be associated with the administration of certain drugs (e.g. cyclophosphamide) and radiation therapy of the lower abdomen. Predisposing factors are the use of indwelling catheters, trauma of the tissues, stagnation of the urine, and distortion or compression of the bladder by an enlarged neighbouring organ. The latter condition is a factor in cystitis that not infrequently develops in the pregnant woman, especially in the last trimester; the enlarging uterus compresses the bladder. The higher incidence in females is attributed to the shorter urethra of a relatively wide calibre. Sexual intercourse and the type of contraception, particularly diaphragm use, are precipitating factors. Poor bladder emptying is a precipitating factor in older women. Organisms from rectal and vaginal discharge can enter readily. In the male, it is usually secondary to prostatic hyperplasia or infection or to congenital malformation (e.g. hypospadias).

Clinical characteristics

Frequency, urgency, dysuria and abnormal urine constituents are the primary characteristics of a UTI. The inflammation is generally confined to the mucosa and submucosa, which are hyperaemic and oedematous. Scattered haemorrhagic areas are present, and small ulcerative lesions may develop as a result of sloughing of the lining tissue of the bladder. The urine contains blood cells, pus, bacteria and mucus. If the UTI becomes chronic, the inflammation may extend into the detrusor muscle. Fibrosis of the tissues occurs with persisting inflammation, which reduces the bladder capacity and increases the problem of frequency.

Treatment

In some instances, a UTI is of brief duration, being resolved spontaneously. There is always the danger that the infection may ascend via the ureters and cause pyelonephritis. In uncomplicated cases involving women, a short, 3-day course of trimethoprim or amoxycillin is usually adequate. A urine specimen obtained before any antimicrobial drug is given may be cultured to determine the infective organism and its drug sensitivity. Potassium citrate may help by reducing the acidity of the urine. Warm baths may reduce bladder spasm and provide relief. The person is encouraged to drink liberal amounts of fluids, which should include citrus fruit juices.

If the condition persists, the UTI is suspected of being secondary. The patient is then investigated for a primary condition which might be pyelonephritis, a bladder calculus, urethral stricture or, in the case of the male, an enlarged prostate.

As UTI is frequently the result of an ascending infection and occurs readily in females, good personal hygiene and efficient cleansing of the perineum, especially after defaecation, are extremely important and require emphasis in health teaching. Adequate cleansing is often very difficult for the ill person who is weak or handicapped and confined to bed. It becomes the nurse's responsibility to see that the patient is cleansed thoroughly.

Prevention of urinary tract infections

The nurse has responsibilities for health promotion and patient teaching to decrease the development or recurrence of UTI in individuals at risk and to prevent and/or decrease episodes of catheter- or therapy-induced UTI.

Patient teaching

Handwashing and personal hygiene

As most UTIs result from bacteria that originate in the gastrointestinal tract, frequent handwashing, especially after defaecation, is an important preventive measure. Women should be taught to wipe the perineal area from the front to the back and then dispose of the tissue. This avoids contamination from the rectal area and should be practised after each bowel movement.

Sexual intercourse

This is a contributing factor in the development of UTI in women. For women who experience repeated UTI associated with sexual intercourse, both partners should wash their genitals before intercourse and the female should empty her bladder just before and again after intercourse. She should be taught to drink lots of fluids to keep the urine dilute. The use of condoms should be discussed.

Treatment of altered patterns of urinary elimination

Elimination disorders that result in retention and stasis of urine predispose the individual to UTI. If complete emptying of the bladder is not possible, a programme of intermittent catheterization may be indicated. It is important to identify and treat persons with urinary incontinence and retention.

Catheter-induced urinary tract infections

Use of urinary catheters

Catheters are a major cause of UTI. They allow entry of microorganisms to the bladder, they offer a surface for the organisms to grow, they are a foreign body and therefore interfere with the body's immune responses, and they may cause chemically induced inflammation of the urethral and bladder mucosa. Catheters also stretch the urethral orifice and injure the tissues. Obstruction of a catheter produces increased intravesicular pressure, promoting the spread of organisms across the mucosa and up into the ureters.

Because of the risk associated with urinary catheters the following precautions should be taken:

■ The need for catheterization, either intermittent or indwelling, should be assessed and documented before the procedure. A catheter should be used only if essential.

■ Indwelling urinary catheters should be removed as soon as possible.

■ External urinary devices, such as condom catheters for men, should be used in place of urinary catheters whenever feasible.

■ Intermittent self-catheterization may be used in preference to indwelling catheters, especially where spinal cord injury is causing bladder dysfunction.

In hospitals or other institutions, strict aseptic technique is required when inserting any catheter. Patients can be taught intermittent self-catheterization, to be performed at home using clean, non-sterile technique.

Care and management of urinary catheters

■ When an indwelling catheter is in place, a closed system should be maintained to decrease infection.

■ Urine specimens should be obtained from the designated port of a closed catheter system using a syringe with a small-bore needle. The system should not be opened to obtain a specimen.

■ Wash hands and wear gloves before handling the catheter system and teach patients to wash their hands before touching the catheter and attached drainage receptacles.

■ When emptying the drainage bag ensure that the tap does not come into contact with other surfaces, thereby reducing the risk of infection.

■ The site of the catheter insertion at the urethral opening provides a port for the entry of organisms. Many topical antiseptic agents and cleansing procedures have been tested to decrease contamination of the urinary meatus. There is no evidence to warrant the adoption of any of these protocols in clinical practice.

■ The addition of bactericidal agents to urine drainage bags has been frequently tested. Most well designed studies have failed to show any benefits from this practice.

■ Bladder instillations are claimed to maintain the patency of catheters by dissolving and flushing away encrustations. Roe (1993) points out that in many cases there is no sound underlying rationale for their use, and conclusive evidence as to their efficacy is lacking.

In view of the above guidelines, it is worth noting that Mulhall et al (1993) in a study of nurses' techniques of catheter care found that closed drainage systems were disconnected on 11% of occasions and incorrect techniques for bag emptying were observed on 6.7% of occasions. Of the 334 patients in this study, 88 developed bacteriuria. Mulhall et al were, however, pleased to report that in many areas nursing technique had greatly improved when compared to the worrying findings of Crow et al (1986) (e.g. cross-infection precautions).

Bladder injury

Accidental injury of the urinary bladder, causing perforation and ensuing extravasation of the urine (escape of urine from the bladder), is not uncommon. It may occur when the pelvis is fractured or as a result of direct blows to the lower abdomen. If the bladder is full and distended at the time of accident, it is more vulnerable.

If the laceration occurs in the upper portion, the rupture is intraperitoneal. Urine escapes into the peritoneal cavity and produces peritonitis. The patient becomes shocked and experiences abdominal pain and tenderness, with a rigid distended abdomen and usually a paralytic ileus.

Rupture of the lower part of the bladder is usually extraperitoneal; urine escapes into the surrounding tissues, and infection, cellulitis and necrosis of tissue may ensue. Occasionally an abdominal or perineal fistula develops.

When there is a history of an injury or blow to the lower abdomen followed by pain and tenderness, injury to the bladder is suspected. A urine specimen is obtained promptly, either by having the patient void or passing a catheter, to determine whether there is haematuria. If blood is present in the urine, cystography may be done to confirm the diagnosis and locate the laceration.

Treatment

The injury is a serious threat to life and requires prompt treatment. The shock and haemorrhage are treated with a blood transfusion and intravenous infusions. An indwelling catheter is inserted into the bladder, and the patient is prepared for abdominal surgery. The site of injury is repaired and a temporary cystostomy (incision of the bladder and introduction of a suprapubic catheter) is carried out to establish urinary drainage and prevent the possibility of pressure on the repair suture line. If the rupture was intraperitoneal, the extravasated fluid is aspirated before closure.

After surgery the patient is observed closely for signs of infection. Antibiotics may be administered immediately. An accurate record of the fluid intake and all drainage is very important. (See section on nursing care of the patient having had a cystostomy, p. 657. For the care of the patient with peritonitis and paralytic ileus, see Ch. 15.)

Tumour of the bladder

Tumours in the bladder may develop at any age but occur more frequently after the age of 50 years and are twice as common in males as females. The majority arise from the epithelial lining (transitional cell) as papillomas and may be benign or malignant. Those that are benign and recur tend to become malignant eventually. Others appear as ulcers which are usually malignant and are more invasive of deeper tissue layers.

Risk factors

Prolonged occupational exposure to aniline dyes is recognized as a predisposing factor. It is recommended that the period of working with these chemicals should be limited to 3 years and that during this period such persons should have urinary examinations for malignant cells. Workers are also advised of the importance of prompt reporting of any blood in the urine or slight bladder irritation. Smoking has also been cited as a predisposing cause of bladder cancer.

Clinical characteristics

The first symptom is usually intermittent painless haematuria, or cystitis may be the initial factor that brings the person to a general practitioner. The lesion may encroach on the urethral orifice, giving rise to hesitancy and a decreased force and calibre of the urinary stream. Suprapubic pain and a palpable mass generally indicate that the condition is in an advanced stage. The person may experience pain in the flank region if the growth obstructs a ureteral orifice which causes hydronephrosis. The lesion ulcerates, which accounts for the haematuria, and readily becomes infected. If the infection is severe and anaemia has developed, the patient manifests weakness and loss of weight.

Diagnostic tests

Diagnostic procedures include the following:

- cystoscopy and biopsy
- urine specimen for cytology and midstream specimen for culture and sensitivity
- intravenous urography to identify obstruction or defects of the urinary system
- computed tomography to identify invasion of other organs by tumour.

Treatment

The treatment used depends upon whether the neoplasm is benign or malignant and, in the case of malignancy, upon the stage and the depth of the tissue involved. Surgery, radiation, chemotherapy, or a combination of these, may be used. Small papillomatous growths may be treated by transurethral resection followed by electrocoagulation of the base tissue. An indwelling catheter may or may not be inserted in the bladder on completion of the operation. The urinary drainage is observed frequently for possible bleeding. Bladder spasm and irritability may cause considerable discomfort which may be reduced by a warm bath. The patient is encouraged to take a minimum of 2000 mL of fluids daily.

As papillomas, benign as well as malignant, tend to recur, these patients are followed closely for 5–6 years. They are advised to report any bleeding or bladder irritability promptly. A cystoscopic examination is usually done every 3 months during the first year after the resection, every 6 months during the second year, and then annually for 3 or 4 years.

If the neoplasm is malignant, a partial resection of the bladder or total cystectomy (removal of the bladder) may be done.

Partial cystectomy

A partial cystectomy is used only if the cancer is in the upper part of the bladder, well above the urethral orifices. At operation, a tube or catheter is placed in the bladder and brought out through the incision, and an indwelling catheter is also introduced through the urethra. Removal of a part of the bladder obviously reduces its capacity. Adequate drainage in the postoperative period is necessary to prevent distension and possible disruption of the suture line. The tube in the incision may be connected to gentle intermittent suction. The length of time it remains in the bladder will depend on the rate of healing.

The urethral catheter usually remains in place for approximately 2–4 weeks. On its removal, frequency becomes a problem for the patient because of the reduced bladder capacity. This may lead to discouragement and depression; consequently, understanding support from the nurse is essential. Any attempt to reduce the frequency by cutting down fluid intake must be guarded against. The importance of a minimum fluid intake of 2000 mL to prevent dehydration, and the spacing of the fluids so that the intervals between voiding may be increased during certain periods (e.g. at night), should be discussed with the patient. The traumatized bladder gradually becomes less irritable and increases its capacity.

Cystectomy

A total cystectomy with ureteric transplantation for permanent urinary diversion is used when the tumour is situated in the lower part of the bladder or is quite extensive. Permanent urinary diversion may be achieved by continent ileal urinary pouch or the formation of an ileal conduit (Fig 19.9).

Continent ileal urinary pouch

Several surgical procedures (e.g. Koch, Camay, Mitroffonoff, Indiana) are being done to create a continent ileal or internal reservoir from an isolated segment of ileum which is then connected to the abdominal wall. A nipple-like valve is created to allow insertion of a catheter to drain urine.

Figure 19.9 Methods of permanent urinary diversion. (a) Pyeloileostomy. (b) Classical.

The internal pouch replaces the external urine collecting bags worn by persons without the built-in reservoir.

Ileal conduit (ureteroileostomy)

This involves removal of a segment of the ileum with its mesentery and blood supply. The open ends of the ileum left by the resection are anastomosed to re-establish intestinal continuity. One end of the resected ileal section is closed. The open end is brought through the abdominal wall to the skin surface and secured. The detached ends of the ureters are implanted in the ileal segment near its closed end. Approximately 1000 such procedures are performed each year in the UK (Black 1994).

Radiation

Internal or external radiation may be used in treating cancer of the bladder. It may be used alone, as an adjunct to surgery, or with chemotherapy. External radiotherapy may be used to treat the tumour as an adjunct to surgery, or prophylactically to reduce pressure symptoms or tumour mass. During treatment the individual is likely to experience gastrointestinal disturbance (nausea, vomiting and diarrhoea) and cystitis. This should be discussed with the person before commencing therapy. Information booklets may be useful in reinforcing verbal information. Long-term side-effects of radiotherapy include chronic urinary disturbance, telangiectasia of the bladder mucosa with chronic haematuria, and usually loss of erectile function in men and decreased orgasmic sensation in women.

Intracavity radiation may be achieved by the enclosure of a radioisotope (e.g. ^{60}Co, ^{198}Au) in a catheter balloon which is placed within the bladder. The catheter is connected to a drainage receptacle, and all urine is saved and sent to the radioisotope department. In some instances, radon seeds or radiotantalum (^{182}Ta) needles may be implanted around the lesion. Safety precautions are necessary in the handling of these radioactive materials. Internal radiation causes cystitis, and the patient usually experiences considerable bladder spasm and discomfort. Fluids are given freely and analgesics may be necessary. The application of heat over the bladder region may provide some relief.

In advanced carcinoma of the bladder, and when metastases are suspected, chemotherapy may be used as well as surgery and irradiation. Local or intravesical chemotherapy can be used for the control of some bladder cancers. This can be performed on an inpatient or outpatient basis. The management of this procedure is often performed by nurses, and safety precautions in relation to the handling of cytotoxic drugs should be observed (see Ch. 11).

Bladder surgery

Operative procedures used in the treatment of **bladder** disease may be transurethral or by open surgery. Transurethral operative procedures may be performed to obtain a biopsy, remove a neoplasm or calculus, or resect the prostate gland. The resectoscope, which is used to resect tissue, is similar to a cystoscope but has insulated walls and is equipped with a wire loop which is activated by a high-frequency current to cut tissue and control haemorrhage by electrocoagulation (diathermy). The procedure is referred to as a *transurethral resection of the prostate* (TURP). A lithotrite, which is a special crushing instrument, is used to remove a stone, and the procedure is called *litholapaxy*.

Open surgery on the bladder may be undertaken for repair of a perforation or laceration, the removal of a neoplasm, calculus or the prostate gland, or a segmental resection or removal of the bladder. The open operative procedures include *cystotomy* (an incision into the bladder and closure without a drainage tube), *cystostomy* (an incision into the bladder and the insertion of a drainage tube which is brought out on to the abdominal surface), *segmental resection* (the removal of a section of the bladder) and *total cystectomy* (the removal of the bladder, involving urethral transplantation and urinary diversion). A suprapubic approach is most commonly used in open bladder surgery, with the bladder being opened below the peritoneum.

Nursing care of the patient having bladder surgery

Preoperative preparation

Unless the bladder is injured or there is acute retention that cannot be relieved by urethral catheterization, the patient who is to have bladder surgery usually undergoes investigation and preparation. Kidney function is assessed and certain blood chemistry levels are determined (e.g. urea, creatinine, potassium, sodium, chloride, calcium). The urine is examined microscopically and, if infection is present, a urinary antiseptic or an antibiotic is prescribed. The patient is encouraged to take 2500–3000 mL of fluid daily unless a large amount of fluid is contraindicated by cardiac or renal insufficiency. The fluid intake and output are recorded and the balance noted. The patient's nutritional status frequently requires attention. Many of

Bladder
See chapter 5.4

these patients are elderly and the existing condition may have contributed to their lack of interest in food, resulting in deficiencies. In encouraging the patient to take nourishment, its importance in recovery is explained. Dietary adjustments and supplements may be necessary to meet nutritional needs.

During the preparatory period, an indwelling catheter may be used to provide adequate drainage and reduce the residual urine. The patient is usually encouraged to remain ambulatory.

Psychological support in the preoperative phase is equally as important as physical care. Opportunities should be provided for the discussion of feelings and concerns, and for the patient to ask questions. The patient and family are advised as to what may be expected after the operation. If the patient is to have a partial cystectomy, this explanation will include a discussion of the frequency of voiding that will be experienced when the tubes are removed because of the reduced capacity of the bladder. Reassurance is given that this gradually becomes less troublesome.

The immediate preparation for open bladder surgery is similar to that for any patient having abdominal surgery (see Ch. 10).

Postoperative nursing intervention

Preparation to receive the patient after operation includes the assembling of sterile tubing and drainage receptacles ready for prompt connection to an indwelling urethral catheter and a cystostomy tube. A tray of sterile equipment and solution for irrigating the catheters in the event of obstruction by clots should be readily available. Goals for the patient following a cystotomy, cystostomy or segmental bladder resection are listed in Table 19.2.

Maintenance of urinary elimination

The patient returns from the operating theatre with an indwelling urethral catheter which is secured to the upper thigh to prevent traction. It is connected to sterile tubing leading to a closed sterile drainage receptacle. The length of the tube should allow for turning and moving the patient without tension being exerted on the catheter.

If there is a cystostomy as well, a tube is anchored in the bladder by a suture at the time of operation. The cystostomy tube is attached to a sterile tube and receptacle.

Both drainage systems are checked frequently (at least hourly for the first 36–48 hours) for patency. The characteristics (colour, consistency, and content or sediment) of the drainage are noted at the same time. The urine will be blood-stained for the first 2–3 hours, gradually becoming lighter. The drainage is best examined in the plastic connecting tubes before it becomes mixed with what is already in the receptacles.

The cystostomy tube, urethral catheter or tubing may become obstructed by a blood clot. The drainage system is checked for patency. If blockage of the tubing is indicated, it may be 'milked' or changed. If the obstruction is within

Table 19.2 Identification of problems relevant to the patient who has just had a cystotomy, cystostomy or segmental bladder resection

Patient problem	Goals
1. Altered pattern of urinary elimination related to bladder incision, urethral catheter and cystostomy tube	Patient will achieve fluid balance
2. Ineffective airway clearance related to anaesthesia and decreased mobility	Patient will show normal respiratory function
3. Impairment of skin integrity related to surgery and possible leakage of urine	Wound will heal without complications
4. Pain related to surgical intervention and bladder spasms	Patient will be free of pain
5. Alteration in nutritional and fluid balance related to surgery and discomfort	Patient will maintain nutritional status
6. Altered bowel elimination related to surgery and discomfort	Patient will have normal bowel actions
7. Lack of knowledge concerning fluid intake, catheter care and health supervision	Patient will show understanding of condition and requirements after discharge

the catheter tube in the bladder, an order may be given to irrigate with sterile normal saline. Some 50–75 mL of the fluid are introduced; if the initial fluid does not return, no more fluid is instilled and the surgeon is consulted. Adequate postoperative drainage is very important to prevent bladder distension and pressure on the suture line.

Bladder irrigation systems are available that may be used to prevent clots blocking the catheter. Specially made-up sterile bags of sterile irrigation fluid may be run into the bladder under gravity and then allowed to drain. It is important to ensure that fluid instilled is drained off before any further fluid is run into the bladder, for reasons discussed above. This procedure is particularly important after TURP.

The drainage from each system is measured and recorded every 4 hours. Care of the tubing and drainage bag varies with local policy. It may be replaced daily with a fresh sterile set or changed every second day or twice weekly.

The cystostomy tube usually remains in place from 4 to 7 days, depending on the patient's healing. The urethral catheter is generally left for a few days longer or until the incisional opening in the bladder heals. When the cystostomy tube is removed, some urine will escape on to the dressing for a few days until the fistula heals over.

After removal of the urethral catheter, a close check is made of the patient's frequency of voiding and the volume of the daily output for several days. The ambulant patient should be encouraged to record the necessary information. When a urethral catheter that has been in place for several days is removed, dribbling is a frequent problem because the bladder–urethral sphincters have been continuously dilated for a period of time. Frequent perineal exercises, which consist of contracting the abdominal, gluteal and perineal muscles while continuing to breathe normally, may help the sphincters recover their tone and control. Occasionally, a patient may not be able to void and catheterization may be performed if voiding has not occurred within 8 hours.

A permanent cystostomy is sometimes done as a palliative measure for a patient who has an inoperable obstruction of the urethra (e.g. advanced carcinoma of the urethra, bladder neck or prostate). A urethral catheter is not inserted in this patient; bladder drainage is entirely dependent upon the cystostomy tube.

Assessment

As well as frequent checking of the drainage system(s), the patient's blood pressure, pulse, colour and level of consciousness are noted and recorded at frequent intervals, which are gradually lengthened if the vital signs are satisfactory. Haemorrhage and shock are possible complications following either transurethral resection or open bladder surgery. Bleeding may be evident in the drainage, but the dressing, surrounding skin areas and groins are also examined.

The daily fluid intake and output are recorded for a longer period than with most surgical patients. The ratio of the intake to the output is examined by the nurse so that he or she is alert to possible renal insufficiency or retention of urine. The characteristics of the urine are noted for a period of 10–14 days. The appearance of sediment, blood, shreds of mucus-like material, cloudiness or the presence of an unusual odour is reported. Sloughing and ensuing bleeding may occur 8–10 days after the removal of a lesion.

Maintenance of airway clearance

The reader is referred to Chapter 10 for a discussion of the importance of avoiding respiratory and cardiovascular complications in the postoperative period.

Impairment of skin integrity

Compared with other abdominal surgery, the dressing is changed earlier and more frequently for patients who have had open bladder surgery. There is almost certain to be some leakage of urine through the incision and around the tube. The skin is cleansed of urine frequently and is kept as dry as possible to prevent excoriation and infection. The application of a skin protection preparation may aid in preventing excoriation. If excoriation occurs, the use of stoma or hydrocolloid dressing wafers may help in preventing further skin breakdown and encourage healing. Early referral to the stoma care nurse or wound care specialist nurse (if available) may help obviate problems.

The lower back, buttocks, groin, inner thighs and perineum are examined each time the dressing is changed. If any areas are moist with urine drainage, they are washed and dried thoroughly to prevent excoriation. The bedding is changed as often as is necessary to ensure dryness and comfort.

Control of pain

Bladder trauma and irritation cause bladder spasms which are very painful, and the patient may also experience the desire to void frequently, even though the bladder is emptied by tube drainage. In the case of the sensation of frequency, it may be necessary to explain to the patient that the bladder is empty and that trying to void only increases bladder spasms and pain. An analgesic such as pethidine is usually necessary at regular intervals during the first 48 hours. If the pain and discomfort are not relieved, the surgeon is consulted. Either the catheter or cystostomy tube may require adjusting to relieve the pressure of its tip on the bladder wall.

Maintenance of fluid balance and nutrition

A daily fluid intake of at least 2500–3000 mL (unless contraindicated by other coexisting disease) is necessary to ensure adequate irrigation of the bladder as well as to maintain satisfactory hydration. Most of it usually has to be administered by intravenous infusion during the first day or two. A soft diet is given and is progressively increased to a regular diet as tolerated.

Maintenance of bowel elimination

The patient may be given a mild laxative after 2 days, or an enema may be given. **Constipation** and straining at stool should be avoided as they tend to increase the patient's pain.

Patient education

Most patients who have had a cystotomy or cystostomy remain in the hospital until the wound is healed and normal micturition is re-established. The nurse should discuss the resumption of their previous activities with them and explain any restrictions indicated by the doctor. They are advised to continue taking a minimum of 2000–2500 mL of fluid daily. Some may require reassurance that no special care of the wound is necessary and that they may resume baths.

If the cystostomy is permanent or a urethral catheter is to remain in place, the patient and a family member are given detailed instruction about the necessary care. This instruction is given over several days and should be completed soon enough for the patient to demonstrate satisfactory self-care before going home. This gives confidence and provides the opportunity to clarify certain points. Verbal and written instructions will include an

Fluid balance
See chapter 2.6

Constipation
See chapter 5.1

explanation of the necessary equipment, its use and maintenance, how it may be acquired, and any precautions to be observed in its use. An inconspicuous plastic leg bag that can be strapped to the thigh may be required by the patient if an indwelling catheter is to be used. The lower end of the bag has a valve that permits emptying of the bag into the toilet at necessary intervals. The importance of thorough washing of the hands with soap and running water before connecting or disconnecting the equipment is stressed to reduce the possibility of ascending infection. The patient and a relative are also taught how to anchor the tube that is in the patient to the abdomen or thigh to prevent traction on it.

The patient is reminded of the need to continue taking at least 2000–2500 mL of fluid daily to provide adequate bladder irrigation. Odour is likely to be less of a problem with more dilute urine, and there is less danger of infection with constant washing out of the bladder.

A referral may be made to the district nurse for assistance and supervision when the patient goes home. This is likely to be needed when the patient is elderly and finds it difficult to cope with the necessary care. The patient and family are advised how often the catheter needs to be changed and should be referred to the community continence adviser where possible.

Evaluation

On discharge from hospital, the patient should be able to perform usual daily activities with minimal discomfort and only temporary changes in activity tolerance. The patient and family should be aware of expectations for self-care and community resources available. They should be able to describe plans for follow-up health supervision.

Urinary diversion

Complete removal of the bladder necessitates establishing a new urinary outlet; this may be achieved by ileal conduit (ureteroileostomy) or an internal continent ileal pouch.

After operation, the patient who undergoes a cystectomy and ureteral transplant is seriously ill. The amount of surgery usually involved predisposes the patient to shock. Frequently, considerable surrounding tissue is resected with the bladder (e.g. lymphatics, prostate gland), and if the ileal conduit procedure or internal ileal pouch is used an intestinal resection and anastomosis are done. The patient will have a large vertical or transverse incision through which the bladder is removed, the ureters are freed for transplant, and the intestine is resected. The stoma through which the urine will drain is made separately in the right abdominal wall and an internal pouch may be created. Care of the patient requires consideration of the needs incurred by the cystectomy, the intestinal surgery, the ureteric transplantation and urinary diversion, as well as the individual patient's psychological and physiological responses to such radical surgery.

Preoperative preparation

The operative procedure and the permanent change in urinary drainage that will ensue should be explained to the patient and family by the surgeon and stoma therapist. This is likely to produce considerable anxiety and despair and will prompt many questions. The nurse needs to show acceptance of these understandable concerns and provide opportunities for the patient and family members to express their feelings and ask questions and, when they are ready, the necessary adjustments and care associated with urinary diversion are outlined in simple terms. They are told that a relatively normal, active life is possible. This may be reinforced by having a person who has had a permanent urinary diversion and has made a successful adjustment talk with them. If such a person is not available, someone with an ileostomy may prove helpful. The nurse who is willing to take time to talk freely with the patient, discussing future plans, and is patient in repeating answers and reinforcing what has probably already been said can provide immeasurable support. A rapport can be developed that contributes to acceptance of the situation and the development of positive attitudes on the part of the patient and family.

The sexual implications of the surgery should be discussed with the individual and partner, together with the treatment options available should difficulties arise after operation. Whenever sexual issues are discussed, sensitivity and tact are of the utmost importance because of the personal nature of this subject and the potential threat to self-image and self-esteem. Many men and women who undergo surgery of this type fear rejection and abandonment by their partners or, if single, believe they will never have a physical relationship again. The following changes can result from radical bladder surgery: in men, sexual desire and genital sensation is often normal, orgasm intensity may be reduced, ejaculation dry, and erectile dysfunction may be present; women may experience dyspareunia and reduced vaginal secretion but orgasm normally remains the same. Treatment options for men include intercavernosal self-injection technique, penile prosthesis, or use of vacuum devices. Women who experience painful intercourse may wish to try different positions for lovemaking, extended foreplay, or the use of lubricants (e.g. water-soluble gel). Vaginal dilators may be useful to dilate the vagina. Some women respond to replacement hormone therapy.

As part of the physical preparation for surgery, kidney function is assessed and the blood levels of nitrogenous wastes, potassium, sodium and chloride are determined. The patient usually receives a blood transfusion during and probably after the operation, so typing and crossmatching are necessary. At least 2500 mL of fluid daily are given unless contraindicated by cardiac insufficiency or urinary obstruction.

If the intestine is to be entered, the patient may receive a low-residue diet for 3 or 4 days, then clear fluids only for

2 days before operation to reduce the faecal content. The reasons for these restrictions are explained in order to gain the patient's cooperation and acceptance. Laxatives and enemas are also used for cleansing purposes, and a course of an antimicrobial drug that is poorly absorbed from the gastrointestinal tract is given orally to destroy intestinal organisms (e.g. neomycin). A nasogastric tube is passed at operation to provide drainage of secretions and prevent intestinal distension after the surgery. The remainder of the preparation is similar to that for any major abdominal surgery (see Ch. 10).

The operation is a lengthy procedure; relatives should be informed about when they may call to enquire about the person's condition and/or visit.

Management of the patient with a urinary diversion

A large part of the required care is essentially the same as that for any patient having an intestinal resection (see Ch. 15). Table 19.3 lists goals relevant to the patient with a urinary diversion.

Maintenance of urinary elimination

On completion of the operation a disposable clean plastic ileostomy bag is secured to the skin around the stoma. This allows for vizualization of the stoma and drainage. Ileostomy bags have a valve system to prevent reflux over the stoma and leakage (Black 1994). They can be connected to larger-volume bags, which reduces the frequency of emptying. A cessation of drainage may indicate occlusion of the stoma by mucus or by swelling and oedema of the tissues, and the surgeon is notified immediately. A sterile catheter may be inserted periodically to determine whether there is residual urine.

Maintenance of integrity of stoma and peristomal skin

The appliance should be removed gently to prevent trauma to the peristomal skin. A tissue or wipe can be used to cover the stoma to collect urine. The skin is gently washed with mild soap and water, and dried. Barrier creams, adhesive preparations and skin sealants may be used on intact skin. A new appliance is applied carefully, ensuring correct fit around the stoma. Transient erythema is usual on appliance removal but this should rapidly resolve. Any persistent redness, broken skin, complaints of discomfort or allergic reactions should be investigated and rapidly treated. The stoma should be monitored for signs of oedema, bleeding, excoriation, ulceration, unusual drainage or discoloration. (See Care of the individual with faecal diversion, Ch. 15.)

Odour control may be a problem for some individuals. Advice should be given concerning the avoidance of foods that produce strong odours in urine. Introduction of a few drops of vinegar or commercial deodorizer into the appliance via the outlet spout may reduce stale urine odours.

Abdominal pain, distension or rigidity, nausea, vomiting or fever is reported promptly. Any of these symptoms

Table 19.3 Identification of problems relevant to the patient with a urinary diversion

Patient problem	Goals
1. Altered pattern of urinary elimination related to formation of a ureteroileal conduit	The patient will maintain urinary elimination
2. Potential impairment of skin integrity (stoma and peristomal skin) due to surgical intervention and irritation	The integrity of stoma and peristomal skin will be preserved Infection will not occur
3. Alteration in mobility related to surgical intervention and pain	The patient will be pain-free Normal mobility will be regained
4. Alteration in nutrition and fluid balance related to surgery on intestine, bladder and ureters	The patient will maintain nutritional status and fluid balance
5. Disturbance in body image related to the urinary diversion and creation of the abdominal stoma	The patient will demonstrate a healthy body image
6. Disturbance in sexual functioning related to damage to nerves, surgical excision of tissue, and trauma to reproductive system	The patient will demonstrate understanding of potential alterations in sexual functioning
7. Lack of knowledge about self-care of the urinary diversion and follow-up care	The patient will show knowledge, skills and resources to manage healthcare regimen

may indicate peritonitis, resulting from the escape of intestinal content from the site of the intestinal anastomosis or from a leakage of urine from the ileal conduit or ureters into the peritoneal cavity.

Maintenance of mobility and physical function

As the ileal conduit opens on to the right side of the abdomen, more complete drainage occurs when the patient is on the right side or back with the trunk elevated. With each change of position, the bag and tubing are checked for any kinks or compression.

Early ambulation is encouraged to foster adequate drainage and prevent complications.

Good pain relief is essential and the nurse carries the main responsibility for ensuring the patient is pain-free in the postoperative period.

Maintenance of nutritional status and fluid balance

The nasogastric tube remains in place for 3–4 days and the patient is given intravenous fluids. The patient is observed for any signs of distension. Once bowel sounds indicate the re-establishment of peristalsis, and there is no distension, the nasogastric tube is removed. The intake of clear fluids is gradually increased and the diet progresses through soft foods to a light solid diet. Gas-forming foods are avoided for 4–6 weeks and then added gradually as tolerated.

Promotion of a healthy body image

The person with a urinary diversion must deal with the altered body structure of an abdominal stoma that is initially red, swollen and tender, the loss of control of urine, and the perceived effects on social interactions and sexual activity. Acceptance of body image changes takes place slowly. It is important that the nurse encourages the patient to talk through concerns and discuss them with both partner and family.

Initially patients are often uncomfortable looking at the stoma. The nurse can support them in looking and talking about it as care procedures are being performed. The person will need support to touch the stoma and gradually to assume self-care activities. Some patients benefit from talking with others who have learned to manage their urinary diversions and sharing experiences related to care and the resumption of social activities. Information regarding self-help groups should be offered. Before discharge, patient concerns related to sexual function should be assessed and addressed. If the actual or perceived concerns are beyond the scope of the nurse, plans may be made for further assistance from specialists or resources in the community or hospital.

Patient and family education

The patient and a family member are taught the care of the stoma, skin and appliance following the same plan as that outlined for the ileostomy patient in Chapter 15. Emphasis is placed on the precautionary measures necessary to prevent infection. Once the oedema subsides and the stoma shrinks, the stoma is measured for a permanent appliance (approximately 7 days). The patient is taught to measure the stoma in order to adjust the size of the appliance as healing continues to take place.

If a continent internal pouch has been constructed, the individual is taught to insert a catheter through the valve to drain the urine. The nurse helps the person to develop a schedule and to adapt it to usual daily activities as control is established. During this period the importance of continuing a daily intake of 2500–3000 mL to keep the ureters and ileal conduit patent should be emphasized. The patient and family are cautioned that the doctor is to be consulted immediately if there is a decrease in urinary drainage, abnormal constituents such as blood in urine, fever, pain in the back or abdomen, severe skin excoriation or general malaise. Mucus from an ileal conduit or internal pouch is normally present in the urine. This should be explained to avoid distress or concern. The patient is followed closely after hospital discharge. A referral may be made to the district nurse and community

stoma care nurse, and the patient is seen at regular intervals at the clinic or by the general practitioner. These visits may be frequent at first, and the intervals are gradually increased to 3–6 months if the patient's progress is satisfactory.

Urinary diversion: summary

Factors to be considered in caring for a patient who undergoes permanent urinary diversion, regardless of the method used, include the following:

- The individual's psychological reaction to a change in body image and normal pattern of function requires thoughtful understanding on the part of the nurse, with sincere efforts to reduce the patient's despair and promote acceptance and adaptation.

- Preoperative cleansing and 'sterilization' of the bowel are necessary if the operative procedure involves resection of or entry into the intestine.

- Maintenance of continuous, adequate urinary drainage from the ureters after operation is essential to prevent renal complications.

- Drainage of urine through an opening on to the skin necessitates special skin care to prevent excoriation and maceration.

- A daily fluid intake of 2500–3000 mL of fluid is important to provide good internal irrigation of the renal pelvis and ureters.

- A planned programme of teaching the care of the stoma, skin and appliance or drainage of the pouch is given to the patient and a relative. It should take place over a period of time that will allow them to acquire a satisfactory understanding and competence by the time the patient leaves the hospital. The instruction includes an explanation of the need for ample fluids and prompt reporting of decreased urinary drainage and significant symptoms.

- Information about the person's previous employment is obtained, and consideration is given as to whether it is possible for previous employment to be resumed or whether a referral to a social worker would be of assistance in finding other employment.

- The person requires close follow-up. Frequent home visits by a district nurse, especially during the first few weeks after leaving the hospital, can provide assistance and considerable support to the patient and family. Regular visits to a clinic or the general practitioner are necessary.

Summary

This chapter provides an overview of the structure and function of the kidneys, the formation and composition of urine, and the mechanisms of urinary elimination.

The nursing management of persons with acute and chronic disorders of renal function are discussed.

Urinary incontinence is a prevalent health problem, especially in elderly women. Comprehensive assessment of the person with urinary incontinence is essential to define accurately the type of incontinence and the contributing factors. The nurse plays an important role in the assessment process and in promoting effective patient management. Participation of the patient and family in the care process enables the development of a relevant and realistic management programme and facilitates acceptance of the plan of care. Urinary catheters are identified as the major cause of nosocomial infection. The nurse has a responsibility to prevent urinary tract infections from being acquired as a result of catheter use. Permanent urinary diversions cause a disturbance in self-image and necessitate skilled patient and family teaching by the nurse.

Throughout this chapter, emphasis is placed on the impact of renal disorders and altered urinary function on the quality of life of the person and the resulting effects on the family. The nurse plays a vital role in identifying the impact of the disorder on the patient and family, in teaching them self-management skills and in helping them to develop appropriate coping patterns.

References

Bevan M (2000) The older person with renal failure. Nursing Standard 14(32): 48–52.

Black P (1994) Stoma care: a practical approach. Nursing Standard 8: 34.

Brittain K, Perry S, Williams K (2001) Triggers that prompt with urinary symptoms to seek help. British Journal of Nursing 10(2): 74–86.

Cheater F (1995) Promoting urinary continence. Nursing Standard 9(39): 33–37.

Cook R (1995) Urinanalysis. Nursing Standard 9(28): 32–35.

Creason NS, Grybowski JA, Burgener S et al (1989) Promoted voiding therapy for urinary incontinence in aged female nursing home residents. Journal of Advanced Nursing 14(2): 120–126.

Crow RA, Chapman RC, Roe BH, Wilson JA (1986) A study of patients with indwelling urinary catheters and related nursing practice. Guildford: University of Surrey Nursing Practice Research Unit.

Dorey G (2000) Male patients with lower urinary tract symptoms. 2: Treatment. British Journal of Nursing 9(9): 553–558.

Dyer P (2000) Kidney transplantation for Asian people; does biology discriminate? Nursing Times 96(23): 39–40.

Fickenscher L (1999) Evaluation adult hematuria. Nurse Practitioner 24(9): 58–64.

Garrett B (1995) The nutritional management of acute renal failure. Journal of Clinical Nursing 4: 377–382.

Getliffe K (1995) Long-term catheter use in the community. Nursing Standard 9(31): 25–27.

Gibbs H, Wong G (1994) How to choose: nurse's judgements of the effectiveness of a range of currently marketed continence aids. British Journal of Nursing 3: 77–86.

Haslett C, Chilvers E, Hunter J, Boon N (1999) Davidson's principles and practice of medicine, 18th edn. Edinburgh: Churchill Livingstone.

Hasselder A (1999) Renal transplant; long term effects of immunosuppression. Professional Nurse 14(11): 771–776.

Kennedy A (1992) Bladder re-education for the promotion of continence. In: Rose B, ed. Clinical nursing practice. London: Prentice Hall.

McCann K, Boore J (2000) Fatigue in persons with renal failure who require maintenance haemodyalisis. Journal of Advanced Nursing 32(5): 1132–1142.

Mackenzie J (1994) Questioning the assumption that urinary catheterization is a pain-free event for women. Journal of Clinical Nursing 3: 64.

Mulhall A, King S, Lee K, Wiggington E (1993) Maintenance of closed urinary drainage systems: are practitioners more aware of the dangers? Journal of Clinical Nursing 2: 135–140.

Nursing Standard (1991) Clinical news. Nursing Standard 5(10): 15.

Roe BH (1990) Study of the effects of education on patients' knowledge and acceptance of their indwelling urethral catheters. Journal of Advanced Nursing 15(2): 223–231.

Roe B (1993) Catheter associated UTI: a review. Journal of Clinical Nursing 2: 197–203.

Shaw C, Williams K, Assassa P, Jackson C (2000) Patient satisfaction with urodynamics; a qualitative study. Journal of Advanced Nursing 32(6): 1356–1363.

Sheppard A (2000) Monitoring fluid balance in acutely ill patients. Nursing Times 96(21): 39–40.

Torrance C, Jordan S (1995) Bionursing: assessment of stress incontinence. Nursing Standard 10(4): 29–31.

UK Transplant Support Service Authority (2000) The new national kidney allocation scheme; first monitoring report summary. UKSSTA User's Bulletin 35: 5.

Walsh M, Crumbie A, Reveley S (1999) Nurse practitioners; clinical skills and professional issues. Oxford: Butterworth Heinemann.

Whyte A (2000) Organ recital. Nursing Times 96(23): 28–29.

Winder A (1990) Intermittent self-catheterization. Nursing Times 86(43): 63–64.

20

Caring for the patient with a disorder of the nervous system

Douglas Allan

Introduction

The nervous system

Assessment of neurological function

The person with a neurological disorder

The person with a cerebrovascular disorder

The person with trauma of the nervous system

The person with a neoplasm of the nervous system

The person with a degenerative disorder

The person with a paroxysmal disorder

The person with an infection of the nervous system

The person with a peripheral nerve disorder

Summary

Introduction

Neuroscience nursing is concerned with caring for those with a disorder of or trauma to the nervous system. As a result many clients will display neurological impairments and the nurse will encounter these in differing situations, ranging from the seriously head-injured patient requiring emergency surgery and intensive care to control raised intracranial pressure (ICP) to the client with a chronic neurological disorder being cared for and supported in the community.

The nervous system

The **nervous system** is an integrated, multipurpose system made up of many parts. It contains the higher human functions such as memory and reasoning, controls and coordinates all parts of the body, and provides a complex communication system between the body's internal and external environments.

Classification

The nervous system can be divided into discrete parts for the purpose of description, as outlined in Figure 20.1. However, in reality, the activities of each division are interrelated to harmonize the many complex functions of the whole system.

Structurally, the nervous system is composed of two parts: the **central nervous system** (CNS) and the *peripheral nervous system*. The CNS consists of the brain and the spinal cord, whereas the peripheral system consists of the spinal and cranial nerves. The two functional divisions of the nervous system are the somatic or voluntary nervous system and the autonomic or involuntary nervous system. The *somatic system* is concerned primarily with the transmission of impulses to and from the non-visceral parts of the body such as the skeletal muscles, bones, joints, ligaments, skin, eyes and ears. Its activities are usually conscious and willed responses. The **autonomic system** is concerned with regulation of the activities of visceral muscles and glands.

Nervous system
See chapter 2.1–2.5

Central nervous system
See chapter 2.2

Autonomic nervous system
See chapter 2.5

Neurone
See chapter 2.1

Nerve impulses
See chapter 2.1

Action potential
See chapter 2.1

Figure 20.1   Organization of the nervous system.

Figure 20.2   Structure of a typical neurone.

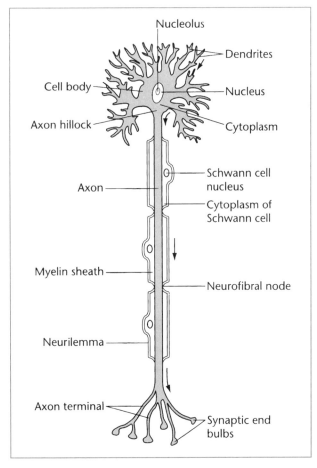

Neurone

The **neurone**, or nerve cell, is the structural and functional unit of the nervous system (Fig. 20.2). The cell body contains a nucleus and other structures and masses concerned with cell maintenance and activity. The cytoplasmic processes include a single axon and one or more dendrites.

The *axon* is a tubular process that conducts nerve impulses away from the cell body, out to the dendrites of other neurones or to muscles and glands. Near its end, the axon divides into numerous fine branches, each of which has a specialized ending called the *presynaptic terminal*. *Dendrites* are short, thin projections that receive stimuli and carry impulses generated by the stimuli toward the nerve cell body. Most stimuli affecting nerve cells are chemical messengers (neurotransmitters) that are secreted from one neurone to an adjacent neurone. The profuse branches of dendrites increase the surface area over which impulses may be picked up.

Neurones are classified according to their function into three types:

- motor (efferent or effector) neurones
- sensory (afferent or receptor) neurones
- connecting (internuncial) neurones.

The axons of *motor* neurones transmit impulses from the CNS to stimulate muscle or glandular tissue. Axons of *sensory* neurones transmit impulses to areas of the brain or spinal cord from the periphery. *Connecting* neurones, which occur only in the grey matter of the brain and spinal cord, convey incoming stimuli to neurones of various integrating centres of the CNS. The connecting neurones form the association areas in the cerebral cortex. They have an important role in the CNS because they 'decide' the responses to the sensory impulses and promote the initiation of the appropriate motor neurone response.

Neurones are designed to initiate, receive and react to stimuli, transmit impulses, process and store information. Neuronal activity results in a wide variety of responses ranging from a simple reflex to complex behaviour requiring central coordination.

Unlike most body cells, neurones lose their ability to undergo mitosis early in life. They lose their viability if denied a supply of oxygen or glucose for more than a few minutes. When neurones are destroyed in the peripheral system, neuronal processes may be replaced under favourable conditions. However, in the CNS neurones are not replaced. These unique properties of nerve tissue have important implications for the nursing care of patients with neurological dysfunction.

Nerve impulses

The functions of the nerve cells are to receive, initiate and conduct 'messages' known as **nerve impulses**. An impulse is a combination of physical and chemical processes which are initiated at the point of stimulation. It occurs as the result of a mechanical, chemical or electrical change at some point in the immediate environment of the neurone. This change temporarily alters the permeability of the cell membrane at that point and is referred to as the *stimulus*. The series of events that result

Figure 20.3 Action potential in neurones.

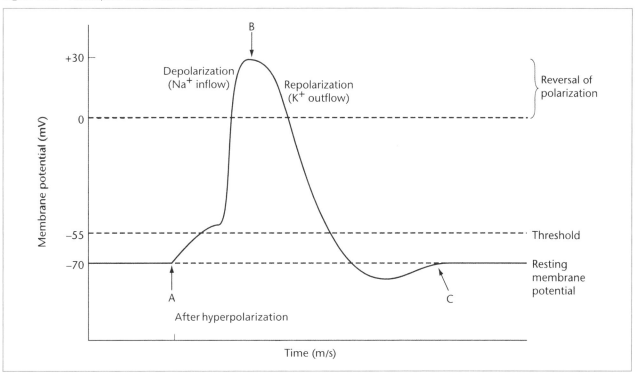

from the change in the membrane permeability produces an electrical current (Fig. 20.3).

When a normal neurone is in a resting state, the outer surface of its membrane is positively charged and the inner surface is negatively charged. As a result, it is described as being *polarized*. This electrical polarity is attributed to the selective action of the cell membrane by which a higher concentration of sodium ions is maintained outside the cell. The positive sodium ions, which are normally attracted to the negative ions within the cell, are not allowed to cross the membrane; if they do so, they are ejected by the cell membrane. The negative electrical charge within the cell is mainly due to the non-diffusable protein anions and retained chlorine ions and measures -70 mV (point A, Fig. 20.3). This is known as the *resting membrane potential*. When a stimulus occurs, i.e. one that is sufficient to achieve a threshold of -55 mV, the membrane becomes permeable to sodium. The influx of cations depolarizes the membrane; a reversal of the electrical potential develops as the outer surface of the membrane becomes negatively charged and the inner surface becomes positively charged at 30 mV. This change alters the electrical relationship of the excited area to the adjacent portions; the shift of ions acts as a stimulus and a wave of depolarization passes along the length of the neuronal process (point B, Fig. 20.3). In a fraction of a second, following depolarization, the membrane recovers its normal permeability by the outward flow of potassium and the resting electrical polarity is restored, i.e. *repolarization* (point C, Fig. 20.3).

The velocity of impulse transmission is determined by the diameter of the neuronal process (nerve fibre) and the presence or absence of a myelin sheath, a white lipid and protein insulating cover. Nerve fibres enclosed in a myelin sheath are referred to as *myelinated*. Larger myelinated fibres conduct more quickly than smaller unmyelinated ones. Neural impulses move at a maximum of 100 metres per second in large fibres.

Synapses

A synapse is the junction between the axon of one neurone and the dendrite of another (Fig. 20.4). A release of chemicals at the synapse provides for the transmission of impulses from neurone to neurone. The termination of a nerve fibre in a muscle cell is called a *neuromuscular junction*. This is basically similar to the synapse between two neurones. The synapse of each axon terminal of a motor neurone on a voluntary muscle cell is referred to as a *motor endplate*.

Chemicals released from the terminal portion of the axon may have an excitatory or an inhibitory effect on the transmission of impulses across a synapse and are called *neurotransmitters*. There is evidence that about 30 different neurotransmitter substances exist (Table 20.1).

Reflexes

A **reflex** is an involuntary, stereotypic response mediated by the nervous system. It serves as a defence mechanism and may involve the contraction of muscle tissue or the

Reflex
See chapter 21

Figure 20.4   A synapse.

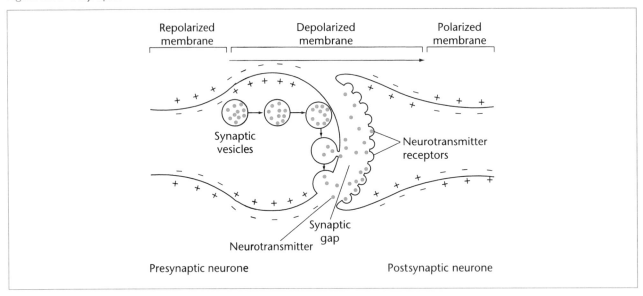

Table 20.1   Neurotransmitters

	Action
Acetylcholine	Usually excitatory but can have an inhibitory effect on some of the parasympathetic nervous system
Serotonin	Inhibitor of pain pathway in the spinal cord. Has role in control of mood and sleep
Noradrenaline	Usually excitatory although sometimes inhibitory. Located in the brainstem
Dopamine	Found in the midbrain and usually inhibitory
γ-Aminobutyric acid (GABA)	The most common inhibitory neurotransmitter found in the brain
Glutamate	Excitatory effect found in the brain
Glycine	Inhibitory effect found in the spinal cord
Encephalin	Excitatory to systems that inhibit pain
Endorphin	Excitatory to systems that inhibit pain
Substance P	Excitatory effect found in sensory nerves, spinal cord pathways and parts of the brain associated with pain transmission

secretion of a gland. Although reflexes occur without voluntary or willed initiation, the person usually becomes conscious of the reflex activity because the impulses reach the cerebral cortex and are interpreted as sensation. The pathway over which nerve impulses pass is called a *reflex arc* (Fig. 20.5). The arc is comprised of receptors, an afferent pathway (sensory nerve fibres), CNS connections, motor neurones, efferent pathway (motor nerve fibres) and effector organ (muscle fibres or glandular cells). The simplest reflex arc consists of two neurones: a sensory and a motor neurone. The patellar reflex ('knee jerk') which is elicited by tapping the tendon of the quadriceps femoris muscle is an example of this type of reflex.

A *receptor* consists of bare nerve endings or specialized structures sensitive to specific stimuli. An *effector* is muscular or glandular tissue. When a receptor is stimulated by a change in its environment (e.g. pressure, temperature, chemical, stretching), it evokes an impulse in the nerve fibres. The impulse is carried through the cell body of the sensory neurone and along its axon into the CNS. Here, it may pass through one, several or many connecting neurones before it excites a motor neurone whose axon (efferent or motor fibre) carries the impulse out of the CNS to the effector tissue or organ. The terminal portion of the efferent fibre releases a chemical at its junction with the effector, initiating its response. For example, this response is contraction in the case of muscle, and is secretion if it is a gland that is innervated.

Figure 20.5   Component structures of a reflex arc.

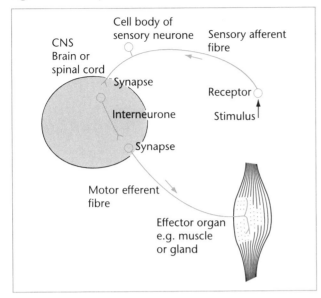

Reflex responses are either protective or postural. Protective reflexes are produced in response to irritating or painful stimuli. Examples include the closing of the eyelid when the cornea is touched lightly (blink reflex) and the rapid withdrawal of a hand from a hot stove (withdrawal reflex).

Postural reflexes maintain an appropriate degree of muscle tone which is essential in supporting the body against gravity and maintaining an upright position. The body can stay upright because muscles exert a continual pull on bones in the opposite direction to gravitational forces. Reflex mechanisms that regulate the muscle contraction necessary to oppose gravity are the stretch reflex and impulses originating in the inner ear (see p. 748).

There are four groups of clinically important reflexes:

1. *Superficial (or skin and mucous membrane) reflexes* – these include the sneeze reflex, the gag reflex, the abdominal reflex and the plantar reflex.

2. *Deep (or myotatic) reflexes* in which receptors are located in deeper tissue such as tendons. An example is the biceps reflex, which produces flexion at the elbow when the biceps tendon is struck.

3. *Visceral (or organic) reflexes* – examples are pupillary reflexes, such as constriction in response to pressure over the eyeballs, and the oculocardiac reflex, which slows the heart rate and blood pressure in response to pressure over the carotid sinus in the neck.

4. *Pathological (or abnormal) reflexes* – these are usually elicited only when neurological disease is present. Primitive defence responses, normally suppressed by cerebral inhibitory influences, are frequently present in these reflexes.

Neuroglia

Neuroglial cells provide structural support for the neurones. They lack axons and comprise about 40% of the total volume of the brain and spinal cord. There are several different types of neuroglial cells; some form the myelin sheath around the axons of peripheral neurones (Schwann cells) and others are involved in the production of cerebrospinal fluid (CSF).

As strong intracellular substances such as collagen and elastin are lacking in neuroglial cells, fresh brain and spinal cord tissue appears soft and jelly-like. In contrast to neurones, neuroglial cells retain their mitotic abilities throughout the lifespan of the individual. From a clinical viewpoint, neuroglial cells are important because they are the most common source of primary tumours in the nervous system.

The central nervous system

Meninges

The brain is protected by the skull and three layers of connective tissue membranes known as the meninges. There are three **meninges** called, from the outer layer inward:

1. the dura mater

2. the arachnoid mater

3. the pia mater.

Meninges
See chapter 2.2

The dura mater

This is a thick, inelastic, collagenous double membrane. One layer is attached to the skull and the other is adjacent to the arachnoid. Two potential spaces associated with the dura are the *extradural space* between the cranium and the periosteal layer of the dura, and the *subdural space* between the dura and the arachnoid. This latter is said to contain a thin film of fluid.

The tentorium cerebelli separates the superior surface of the cerebellum from the occipital lobes, defining the *supratentorial* and *infratentorial cranial compartments*. The opening in the tentorium through which the brainstem passes is known as the *tentorial notch* or *tentorial incisura*. The notch is of clinical significance when intracranial pressure increases.

The arachnoid

The arachnoid ('spider-web-like') is a thin, avascular, delicate membrane. It conforms to the general shape of the brain. A *subarachnoid space*, filled with CSF, is located between the arachnoid and pia mater.

The pia mater

The pia mater is a thin, vascular, elastic membrane that adheres closely to the brain and spinal cord, following every sulcus and gyrus. The choroid plexuses arise from the vascular structure of the pia mater.

Brain

The human **brain** is the organ concerned with thought, memory and consciousness. It is also concerned with a range of sensory experiences, with motor activity, with the regulation of visceral, endocrine and somatic functions, and with the use of symbols and signs that underlie communication. For descriptive purposes the brain may be subdivided into the cerebrum, basal ganglia, thalami, hypothalamus, midbrain, pons, medulla oblongata (known collectively as the brainstem) and cerebellum.

Cerebrum

The **cerebrum** accounts for 80% of the total weight of the brain. It is divided into two hemispheres by the *longitudinal fissure*. The two hemispheres are joined at their bases by bands of neuronal fibres collectively forming the *corpus callosum*. It is believed that the corpus callosum transfers information from one hemisphere to the other (see Fig. 20.6).

In selected higher functions, one cerebral hemisphere appears to be the 'leading' one and is referred to as the *dominant hemisphere*. Cerebral dominance tends to be most complete in relation to the complex aspects of language. Handedness also is related to cerebral dominance, although its relationship is less clearcut than previously believed. In true right-handed persons it is nearly always the left hemisphere that is dominant and governs language, but the converse of this is not necessarily true. Each hemisphere, independently, contains the ability to learn but the right hemisphere has a superior role in intuitive and creative responses and in spatial perception.

The brain contains areas of grey and white matter. The *grey matter* is a collection of neuronal bodies and unmyelinated processes. *White matter* consists primarily of myelinated fibres coming off cell bodies. Grey matter, which forms the surface of the cerebrum, is called the *cerebral cortex*. The cortex is believed to contain about 100 billion neurones. It is 2–5 mm thick and is arranged in a series of convolutions or coil-like elevations called *gyri*. Shallow crevices between the gyri are called *sulci*. The folding into gyri and sulci has the effect of increasing the surface area of the brain. Sulci that are particularly deep are called *fissures*.

The cerebral cortex of each hemisphere is made up of primary sensory areas, primary motor areas and association areas. Primary sensory areas are receptive areas for incoming impulses. Primary motor areas are concerned with dispatching outgoing impulses to prompt action responses in peripheral structures.

The motor area that initiates all voluntary movements of the body occupies the strip of the frontal lobe immediately anterior to the central fissure. In general, the motor area in one hemisphere controls the movements on the opposite side of the body. The size of the cortical area representing the body parts is proportional to the complexity and functional importance of the part.

The sensory impulses that enter the cerebral cortex are transmitted to specific areas of the cortex, depending on their origin. Impulses concerned with the somataesthetic senses such as touch, pressure, temperature, pain, and the sense of body position and its parts are transmitted to the parietal lobe immediately posterior to the central fissure.

The primary receptive area for vision is located in the posterior part of the occipital lobe. The primary auditory receptive areas or centres for hearing are located in the superior parts of the temporal lobes.

Brain
See chapter 2.2

Cereburm
See chapter 2.2

Figure 20.6   Frontal view of the brain.

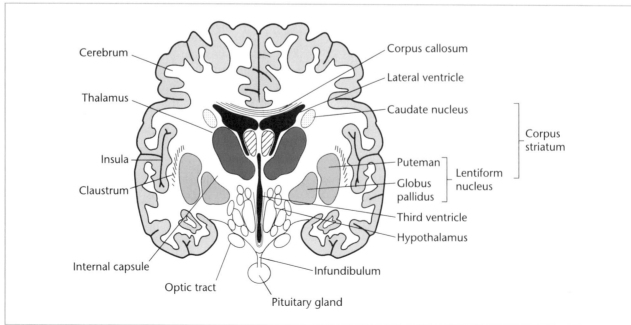

Cerebrum — Corpus callosum — Lateral ventricle — Thalamus — Caudate nucleus — Corpus striatum — Insula — Puteman — Lentiform nucleus — Claustrum — Globus pallidus — Third ventricle — Hypothalamus — Internal capsule — Infundibulum — Optic tract — Pituitary gland

The frontal lobes contain the motor area. Other areas in the frontal lobes are the premotor cortex, the prefrontal areas and Broca's area. The premotor cortex is also known as the motor association or secondary motor area. The prefrontal areas of the frontal lobe are concerned with memory and ability to concentrate, and ability to think in abstract terms. They are also concerned with personality, emotional reactions, initiative and sense of responsibility for socially acceptable standards. *Broca's area* is categorized as an association area because it aids in the formulation of words.

Beneath the grey cerebral cortex, the cerebrum is composed mainly of white matter. Myelinated neuronal processes are arranged in functionally related bundles called tracts. These are classified as commissural, association and projection tracts:

- *Commissural tracts* transmit impulses between the two hemispheres.

- *Association tracts* carry impulses from one area of the cortex to another in the same hemisphere.

- *Projection tracts* are ascending and descending pathways from one level of the central nervous system to another. One of the most important of these is the *internal capsule*, a massive bundle of efferent and afferent nerve fibres connecting the various subdivisions of the brain and spinal cord.

Basal ganglia (nuclei)

Basal ganglia are groups of nerve cell bodies deeply embedded within the white matter of each cerebral hemisphere. The functions of the basal ganglia are complex and not clearly understood. The system operates, along with the motor cortex and cerebellum, as a total unit, and individual functions cannot be ascribed solely to the various parts of the system. One of the general functions of the basal ganglia is inhibition of muscle tone throughout the body.

Thalami

The **thalami** are a pair of egg-shaped masses of grey matter at the base of each hemisphere. Each mass is referred to as a thalamus and forms part of the lateral walls of the third ventricle. The thalami form the main relay centre for sensory impulses and cerebellar and basal ganglia projections to the cerebral cortex.

Hypothalamus

This is an important grey mass that lies beneath the thalamus. It forms the floor and part of the wall of the third ventricle. It contains nuclei of the autonomic nervous system for the control of most of the body's involuntary functions as well as many aspects of emotional behaviour. There are neuronal links between the **hypothalamus** and the posterior pituitary gland (see p. 562). The hypothalamus is also concerned with gastrointestinal and feeding regulation. Hunger centres and a satiety centre have been identified in this grey mass. In addition, it activates feeding reflexes such as licking the lips and swallowing. It is also known to affect responses such as pleasure and fear.

Brainstem

The **brainstem** is composed of the midbrain, pons varolii and medulla oblongata. The *midbrain* forms the upper portion and is the location of the nuclei of origin of cranial nerves III and IV. The *pons varolii* is located between the midbrain and medulla. It consists of numerous tracts that link various parts of the brain and serve as conduction pathways.

The *medulla oblongata* lies between the pons and the spinal cord. It is composed of ascending and descending conduction pathways. Autonomic centres that regulate such vital functions as breathing, cardiac rate and vasomotor tone as well as centres for vomiting, gagging, coughing and sneezing reflex behaviours are located in the medulla.

Reticular activating system

This is a diffuse system of motor and sensory fibres and nerve cells that forms the central core of the brainstem. It has widespread afferent connections, receiving sensory impulses from all over the body. The cerebral cortex can stimulate this system. It is known to be associated with initiation and maintenance of wakefulness and alertness.

Cerebellum

This lies beneath the posterior portion of the cerebrum, posterior to the pons and medulla. It is separated from the cerebrum by a fold of meningeal membrane (dura mater) called the tentorium cerebelli. Direct input is received from the spinal cord and brainstem and conveyed to the deep cerebellar nuclei and cerebral cortex.

The **cerebellum** is integrated into many connective pathways throughout the brain for the provision of muscle coordination in the body. All sensations are relayed through the cerebellum, thus providing information about muscle activity. The functions of the cerebellum are essentially to control fine movements and balance, to control coordination of movement and maintain feedback loops to correct movement, and to coordinate the action of muscle groups. Dysfunction of the cerebellum can result in gait disturbance, equilibrium ataxia (overstability or understability) and tremors.

Blood supply to the brain

The ever-active brain receives about one-fifth of the blood pumped by the heart and consumes about 20% of the oxygen utilized by the body. The brain requires a continuous **flow of blood** because it can store only minute quantities of glucose and oxygen, and derives its energy almost exclusively from the metabolism of glucose delivered by the blood. Its blood requirement is the same whether one is mentally active or sleeping.

Basal ganglia
See chapter 2.2

Thalami
See chapter 2.2

Hypothalamus
See chapter 2.2

Brainstem
See chapter 2.2

Reticular activating system
See chapter 2.2

Cerebellum
See chapter 2.2

Cerebral circulation
See chapter 2.2

Brain cells are extremely sensitive to hypoxia, particularly those of the cerebral cortex. Interruption of blood supply to the brain produces loss of consciousness in seconds. Irreversible brain damage occurs if the blood supply is interrupted for 2–4 minutes. Brainstem neurones are less sensitive to hypoxia than cortical cells; individuals experiencing prolonged hypoxia may survive because the vital centres in the medulla are more resistant and recover, but irreversible cortical damage persists, resulting in damage. The arterial blood supply to the brain is derived from two internal carotid arteries and two vertebral arteries. The vertebral arteries unite to form the basilar artery. The internal carotid arteries supply blood, via the anterior and middle cerebral arteries, to most of the hemispheres excluding the occipital lobes, the basal ganglia, and the upper two-thirds of the diencephalon.

Although the vertebral basilar arterial tree and the internal carotid arterial tree are essentially independent, some anastomotic connections between the two systems exist. Small posterior communicating arteries connect the two systems to form an arterial crown known as the cerebral arterial circle of Willis. The anterior communicating artery that connects the two anterior cerebral arteries completes the circle. It allows blood to reach all parts of the brain even after one or more of the four supplying vessels is obstructed. Most venous blood drains into the internal jugular veins at the base of the skull.

Blood–brain barrier

This is a unique relationship between the capillary walls in the brain and the glial cells. It is believed that the **blood–brain barrier** limits the entry of substances that may be harmful into the extracellular space of the brain around the neurones. This barrier phenomenon effectively keeps microorganisms out of the brain. However, it is equally effective in keeping most antibiotics out, thus complicating therapy for intracranial infections.

Ventricles and cerebrospinal fluid

The ventricular system is a series of cavities within the brain (Fig. 20.7). Each cerebral hemisphere contains a lateral ventricle, which communicates with the third ventricle by means of an intraventricular foramen. The third ventricle is a slit-like space between the thalami and is continuous with the fourth ventricle through a narrow channel called the cerebral aqueduct. The medial opening

Blood–brain barrier
See chapter 2.1

Cerebrospinal fluid
See chapter 2.2

Figure 20.7 Path of flow of cerebrospinal fluid.

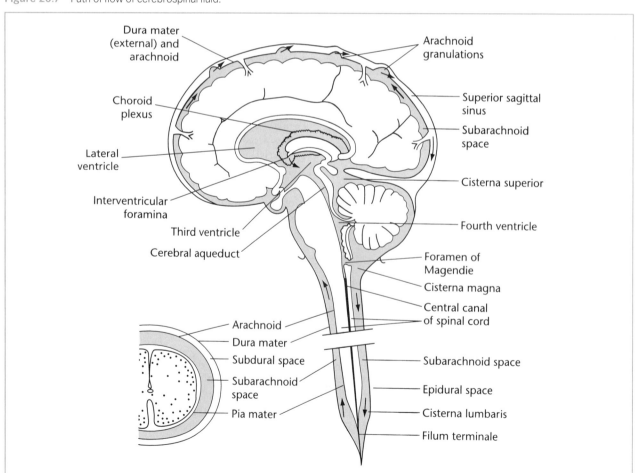

Based on an illustration by R.J. Demarest in Noback CR (1967) The human nervous system. New York: McGraw-Hill.

of the fourth ventricle allows CSF to circulate around the spinal cord. Two lateral openings channel fluid around the brain. This distribution of CSF provides a protective cushion for the brain and cord.

The ventricular system is filled with CSF. Each ventricle contains a *choroid plexus,* which is a rich network of blood vessels covered by a layer of ependymal cells that secrete CSF continuously. The CSF is a clear, colourless, water-like fluid with a specific gravity of 1.007. It contains occasional lymphocytes and traces of the minerals and organic materials found in blood. The glucose concentration is normally 2.8–4.5 mmol/L and protein concentration is 0.1–0.4 g/L at the lumbar level. The total volume of CSF in the adult ranges from 125 to 150 mL. Normal pressure is 40–180 mmH$_2$O.

The CSF circulates through the ventricular system and around the brain and cord in the subarachnoid space. It is steadily reabsorbed into the arachnoid villi, which are projections from the subarachnoid space into the venous sinuses of the brain. Any interruption within the CSF circuit results in an excessive accumulation of fluid within the ventricles. The condition is referred to as *hydrocephalus.* The brain tissue becomes compressed between the skull and the expanding volume of fluid resulting in increased intracranial pressure.

Spinal cord

The **spinal cord** is a long, cylindrical structure of grey and white matter within the vertebral column. It is continuous with the medulla oblongata, originating at the foramen magnum of the skull and extending to the first or second lumbar vertebrae. It tapers off into a fine, non-neural cord called the *cauda equina,* which continues inferiorly (caudally) to its attachments in the coccyx. A small canal (central canal) extends the full length of the cord; it contains CSF, and the upper end opens into the fourth ventricle. The cord is surrounded by the three meninges, which are continuous with those encapsulating the brain. The meninges extend to the level of the fifth lumbar vertebra.

The grey matter (cell bodies) in the spinal cord is concentrated in its interior, roughly in the form of an H. White matter, composed of nerve tracts and fibres, surrounds the H-shaped grey matter (Fig. 20.8). Afferent impulses are received by neurones in the posterior columns or horns of grey matter. Efferent impulses are discharged by neurones in the anterior columns or horns of the grey matter. The grey matter also contains neurones that may transmit impulses from one lateral half of the cord to the other, from posterior to anterior and to other levels of the CNS.

Nerve fibres emerge from the spinal cord in uninterrupted series of posterior (sensory or afferent) and anterior (motor or efferent) rootlets which unite to form 31 pairs of posterior and anterior roots. In the area of an intervertebral foramen, a posterior and an anterior root meet to form a *spinal nerve* (Fig. 20.9) which supplies innervation to a segment of the body. The cord has two enlargements: cervical and lumbar. The cervical enlargement (plexus) is associated with nerve roots that innervate the upper limbs, and the lumbar enlargement (plexus) innervates the lower limbs.

The spinal cord has three major functions:

1. It carries impulses via sensory nerves through ascending tracts up to the brain.

2. It carries impulses from the brain via motor nerves through descending tracts to nerves supplying effector organs (muscle and glands).

3. It functions as a centre for reflex actions.

Nerves and tracts

Nerves are bundles of neuronal processes that extend beyond the CNS, whereas tracts are bundles of processes within the CNS. Nerves consisting only of afferent fibres, which transmit impulses from the periphery to the CNS, are called sensory nerves. Motor nerves are composed entirely of efferent fibres, which transmit impulses from the CNS out into the periphery. Many nerves (e.g. all

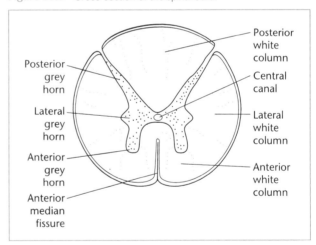

Figure 20.8 Cross-section of the spinal cord.

*Spinal cord
See chapter 2.2*

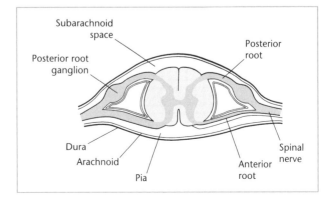

Figure 20.9 The spinal nerve: its posterior root ganglion, posterior root and anterior root.

spinal nerves) contain both efferent and afferent fibres and are known as *mixed nerves*.

Structurally, three types of nerve fibres or processes occur:

1. Myelinated or medullated fibres are enclosed in a lipoprotein sheath (myelin) and an outer membranous sheath called the neurilemma (sheath of Schwann).

2. Non-myelinated (non-medullated) fibres have no myelin sheath but do have a neurilemma. Most non-myelinated fibres belong to the autonomic nervous system, which is concerned with visceral activity.

3. A third type has a myelin sheath but lacks the neurilemma. All fibres within the CNS, as well as the optic and auditory nerves, are of this type. Neuronal processes lacking the neurilemma cannot regenerate following injury.

Nerve tracts transmit impulses that are usually similar in origin, termination and function. The origin and destination may be determined from the name of the tract. For example, the corticospinal tract carries impulses originating in the cerebral cortex to the spinal cord; the spinothalamic tract transmits sensory impulses from the spinal cord to the thalamus.

The peripheral nervous system

The peripheral nervous system is composed of nerves and ganglia. The nerves may be divided into two main groups, *cranial* and *spinal* nerves, according to whether they emerge from the CNS at the cranial or spinal level.

Cranial nerves

There are 12 pairs of **cranial nerves** that are considered to be part of the peripheral nervous system. They emerge from the undersurface of the brain and are named according to their function or distribution. The origin and functions of cranial nerves are described in Table 20.2.

Spinal nerves

Thirty-one pairs of nerves arise from the spinal cord. They are numbered and named according to the order in which

Cranial nerves
See chapter 2.2

Spinal nerves
See chapter 2.2

Table 20.2   Name and functions of the cranial nerves (12 pairs)

Number	Name	Function
I	Olfactory	Olfactory sense (sense of smell)
II	Optic	Vision
III	Oculomotor	Movements of the eyeball and upper eyelid; size of the pupil of iris; control of ciliary muscle to regulate degree of refraction by the lens
IV	Trochlear	Movement of eyeball by superior oblique muscles
V	Trigeminal Largest cranial nerve has three sensory divisions: ophthalmic, maxillary, mandibular	Motor function: mastication Sensory function: sensations (pain, touch, temperature) of the face, nose, teeth and mouth
VI	Abducens	Movement of the eyeball by lateral rectus muscle
VII	Facial	Motor function: contraction of facial and scalp muscles (facial expression); secretion of saliva by submaxillary and sublingual glands Sensory function: taste (from anterior two-thirds of tongue)

VIII	Vestibulocochlear
	Has two divisions:
	   Vestibular
	   Cochlear
		Sensory function:
		   vestibular branch: equilibrium (position, balance)
		   cochlear division: sense of hearing

IX	Glossopharyngeal	Motor function: swallowing reflex, control of blood pressure through connection with carotid baroreceptors; salivary secretion by parotid glands Sensory functions: taste and oral and pharyngeal sensations
X	Vagus Has very wide distribution	Motor function: muscles of pharynx, larynx, thoracic and abdominal viscera (e.g. regulates gastrointestinal motility of peristalsis; influences cardiac rate); secretion by gastric, intestinal and pancreatic glands Sensory function: sensations in pharynx, larynx, and thoracic and abdominal viscera
XI	Accessory	Movement of shoulder and head by trapezius and sternocleidomastoid muscles
XII	Hypoglossal	Movements of the tongue

they arise and the vertebral level at which they emerge. There are 8 cervical, 12 thoracic, 5 lumbar, 5 sacral pairs and 1 coccygeal pair.

All spinal nerves are mixed (sensory and motor) and each has two origins which are referred to as anterior and posterior roots (see Fig. 20.9). The anterior roots carry two types of motor fibres:

1. The *general somatic efferent fibres* which have axons originating from lower motor neurones (anterior horn cells in the spinal cord) and which innervate voluntary striated muscles.

2. The *general visceral efferent fibres* (autonomic nerves) which innervate visceral and cardiac muscle, and regulate glandular secretions.

The posterior roots convey sensory input via two types of sensory fibre:

1. The *general somatic afferent fibres* which carry impulses for pain, temperature, touch and proprioception from the body wall, tendons and joints into the CNS.

2. The *general visceral afferent fibres* which carry sensory impulses from the viscera into the CNS.

After emerging from the vertebral canal, each spinal nerve divides into two major branches: the anterior and posterior rami. The branches of the anterior rami tend to form intricate networks of interlacing nerve branches before proceeding to the structures they innervate. These networks are referred to as *plexuses*. Spinal nerves lose their individuality after passing through a plexus and they emerge as peripheral nerves. Four major plexuses are formed by the anterior rami of spinal nerves: the cervical, brachial, lumbar and sacral plexuses. The *cervical plexus* gives rise to peripheral nerve branches that innervate muscles of the neck and shoulders. It also gives rise to the phrenic nerve which supplies the diaphragm. Important peripheral nerves that arise from the *brachial plexus* are the musculocutaneous, median, radial and ulnar nerves, all of which supply the upper limbs. The *lumbar plexus* generates the femoral, saphenous and obturator nerves which innervate the lower abdominal wall, external genitalia and parts of the thigh and leg. The nerves leaving the *sacral plexus* supply the buttocks, perineum and lower extremities. The most important nerve derived from this plexus is the sciatic, the longest and largest nerve in the body.

Ganglia

A ganglion is a group of nerve cell bodies located outside the CNS. The **ganglia** that form the posterior or sensory roots of the spinal nerves lie just outside the spinal cord within the vertebral column. These are the spinal or posterior root ganglia. Other ganglia are associated with the autonomic nervous system and mostly lie adjacent to the vertebral column.

Autonomic nervous system

The **autonomic nervous system** controls the visceral functions of the body. This system helps to control such phenomena as arterial blood pressure, gastrointestinal motility and secretion, urinary bladder emptying, sweating and body temperature. It carries only efferent impulses and the responses are involuntary.

The autonomic system is largely activated by centres located in the spinal cord, brainstem and hypothalamus. In addition, parts of the cerebral cortex can transmit impulses to the lower centres and in this way influence the autonomic system. Often, the autonomic system operates by means of visceral reflexes. That is, sensory signals enter the centres in the CNS and these in turn transmit appropriate reflex responses back to the organs via the autonomic system to control their activities.

The autonomic nervous system is divided into the *parasympathetic* and *sympathetic* systems. Most viscera have a nerve supply from each division; impulses delivered from one system excite visceral activity, and those originating with the other division inhibit activity (Table 20.3).

Parasympathetic nervous system

The **parasympathetic** fibres leave the CNS through several cranial nerves (75% are in the vagus nerve) and through the pelvic nerves. The responses to parasympathetic stimulation are localized and specific for parts of the body.

Generally, parasympathetic innervation promotes a normal state; it is concerned with the restoration and conservation of body energy and elimination of body wastes (Table 20.3).

Sympathetic nervous system

The **sympathetic** nerves originate in the thoracic and lumbar regions of the spinal cord. The sympathetic nerves leave the spinal cord via the anterior roots and form the white communicating rami of the thoracic and lumbar nerves. Through these, nerves reach the trunk ganglia of the sympathetic chain.

The sympathetic system produces generalized physiological responses rather than specific, localized ones. It responds to stress, strong emotions, severe pain, cold, or any threat. The purpose of the responses induced is to mobilize the body's resources for defensive action ('fight or flight') (Table 20.3).

Stimulation of the sympathetic nervous system results in stimulation of the adrenal medullae. Increase in secretion of adrenaline and noradrenaline results and this augments the body defence responses mediated by the sympathetic nervous system.

Chemical mediators

In both the sympathetic and parasympathetic nervous systems the transmission of impulses from the preganglionic

Ganglia
See chapter 2.1

Autonomic nervous system
See chapter 2.5

Parasympathetic nerves
See chapter 2.5

Sympathetic nerves
See chapter 2.5

Table 20.3   Autonomic effects on various organs of the body

Organ	Effect of sympathetic stimulation	Effect of parasympathetic stimulation
Eye:		
Pupil	Dilated	Constricted
Ciliary muscle	Slight relaxation	Contracted
Glands:		
Nasal	Vasoconstriction and slight secretion	Stimulation of thin, copious secretion (containing many enzyme-secreting glands)
Lacrimal		
Parotid		
Submaxillary		
Gastric		
Pancreatic		
Sweat glands	Copious sweating (cholinergic)	None
Apocrine glands	Thick, odoriferous secretion	None
Heart:		
Muscle	Increased rate	Slowed rate
	Increased force of contraction	Decreased force of atrial contraction
Coronary arteries	Dilated (β_2): constricted (α)	Dilated
Lungs:		
Bronchi	Dilated	Constricted
Blood vessels	Mildly constricted	Dilated
Gut:		
Lumen	Decreased peristalsis and tone	Increased peristalsis and tone
Sphincter	Increased tone	Relaxed
Liver	Glucose released	Slight glycogen synthesis
Gallbladder and bile ducts	Relaxed	Constricted
Kidney	Decreased output	None
Bladder:		
Detrusor muscle	Relaxed	Excited
Trigone	Excited	Relaxed
Penis	Ejaculation	Erection
Systemic blood vessels:		
Abdominal	Constricted	None
Muscle	Constricted (adrenergic α)	None
	Dilated (adrenergic β)	
	Dilated (cholinergic)	
Skin	Constricted	None
Blood:		
Coagulation	Increased	None
Glucose	Increased	None
Basal metabolism	Increased up to 100%	None
Adrenal cortical secretion	Increased	None
Mental activity	Increased	None
Piloerector muscles	Excited	None
Skeletal muscle	Increased glycogenolysis	None
	Increased strength	

Neurotransmitters
See chapter 2.5

fibres to the ganglia is dependent upon the release of acetylcholine by the preganglionic axon terminals. Acetylcholine is rapidly deactivated by cholinesterase. The postganglionic fibres of the parasympathetic system also release acetylcholine at their junction with the effector organs to facilitate the transmission of their impulses. The **neurotransmitter** that is released by the postganglionic nerve terminals in the sympathetic system is noradrenaline, which is deactivated by enzymes (e.g. monoamine oxidase) or taken up again by the nerve terminals.

Motor and sensory systems

Contraction of skeletal muscles normally results only from impulses discharged by motor neurones within the CNS and transmitted along peripheral nerve fibres to the muscle. As the motor centres lie within the cerebral cortex, contractions are usually produced voluntarily. Involuntary contractions occur in the form of reflex responses.

The process whereby a nerve impulse is converted into a muscle action current is referred to as *neuromuscular transmission*. Each nerve fibre terminates at a specialized region of the muscle fibre, called *myoneural* or *neuromuscular function* or *motor endplate*. The endplate is a localized specialization of the sarcolemma. Essentially, the release of acetylcholine at the endplate and its rapid destruction by the enzyme cholinesterase is at the basis of electrical and chemical reactions and the release of mechanical and heat energy in the contraction of muscle fibres.

Voluntary movement

Normal voluntary movements are the result of controlled contraction and relaxation of groups of muscles. All willed movements depend upon excitation of neurones within the cerebral cortex (upper motor neurones) as well as at a lower level (lower motor neurones). Those at a lower level may be the motor components of cranial nerve nuclei in the brainstem or they may be in the spinal cord. Two major neuronal pathways in the CNS are involved in voluntary muscle activity: the *pyramidal tract* and the *extrapyramidal system*.

Pyramidal tract (corticospinal tract)

The **pyramidal** tract arises in the sensorimotor cortex of the cerebrum and is one of the major pathways whereby motor signals are transmitted from all the motor areas of the cortex to the anterior motor neurones of the spinal cord.

Voluntary movement begins with the stimulation of a discrete area of neurones in the motor area of the cerebral cortex. If the movement applies only to muscles on one side of the body, then only the motor area of the cerebral hemisphere on the opposite side will be involved. The motor fibres pass downward through the brainstem, and in the lower medulla approximately 90% decussate (cross over) to form the pyramids of the medulla. These fibres descend in the lateral corticospinal tract of the cord and terminate in posterior horns of cord grey matter. Fibres that did not decussate earlier continue on the same side (ipsilaterally) in the anterior corticospinal tracts and cross over further down the cord.

At various levels in the cord, the fibres synapse with neurones in the anterior horns of grey matter. The axons of these neurones form the motor fibres of the peripheral nerves whereby the impulses are delivered to muscle fibres. Some fibres in the tract may synapse in the brainstem with nuclei of cranial nerves. The impulses are then carried out to a muscle by motor fibres of a peripheral cranial nerve.

The neurones of the cerebral cortical motor area are referred to as the *upper motor neurones*. Those with which the axons of upper motor neurones synapse are called *lower motor neurones*. The cell bodies of lower motor neurones reside within the CNS and their axons carry the impulses to skeletal muscles in the periphery.

Extrapyramidal system (extrapyramidal tracts)

This system includes all the tracts exclusive of the pyramidal tract which transmits motor signals from the brain to the spinal cord. Unlike the pyramidal tract, which is a direct link from the cerebral cortex to the spinal cord, the **extrapyramidal system** conveys its influences to the cord via multineuronal and multisynaptic linkages involving the cortex, basal ganglia, thalami, cerebellum, brainstem and related structures. Extrapyramidal impulses are initiated in several areas of the brain below conscious level and all are transmitted by reticulospinal tracts to lower motor neurones. The lower motor neurones provide the final common pathway for all the afferent impulses (both pyramidal and extrapyramidal) to skeletal muscles. Inhibition, facilitation and coordination essential for smooth, precise muscle activity is normally provided by the extrapyramidal system.

An imbalance in the interactions within the complex circuitry of the extrapyramidal system occurs with malfunction of various nuclear complexes. The motor disorders resulting from the improper functioning of the extrapyramidal system and associated nuclei include various abnormal movements such as paralysis agitans, athetosis and chorea.

Voluntary muscle activity involves the pyramidal and extrapyramidal tracts in concert. The pyramidal tract transmits the impulses that are consciously initiated to produce a given movement. The other essential components of the movement such as reciprocal relaxation of certain muscles, correlation, stabilization and adjustment in posture are automatically contributed by the extrapyramidal system.

The complex interrelationship of the nervous system means that when considering disorders this cannot be done in isolation. A patient with a head injury may survive the initial trauma but may die from infection or sustain epilepsy as a complication. For the purpose of explanation, the disorders that can affect the nervous system are described as follows:

- trauma including traumatic brain injury (head injury) and spinal cord injury

- cerebrovascular disorders including stroke and cerebral aneurysm

- neoplasms

- epilepsy, both as a disorder and as a symptom of other disorders

Motor system
See chapter 2.3

Pyramidal
See chapter 2.3

Extrapyramidal
See chapter 2.2

- meningitis
- degenerative disorders including acquired immune deficiency syndrome (AIDS), dementia, multiple sclerosis, Parkinson's disease and motor neurone disease.

This is not an exhaustive list of disorders but is representative of those that patients are most likely to present with.

Assessment of neurological function

Accurate assessment such as monitoring level of consciousness will inform effective nursing interventions and medical management. More complex diagnostic investigations such as angiography necessitate neuroradiological intervention using specialist technology. Other procedures require cooperation between different groups of healthcare providers, for instance medical staff will institute continuous intracranial pressure (ICP) monitoring and nursing staff monitor the data.

Assessment of cognitive status

The neurological examination is the part of the physical examination that evaluates the function of the cerebrum and the cranial nerves as well as the motor and sensory status, reflex status and the status of the autonomic nervous system.

Cranial nerves
See chapter 2.2

Cerebral function

Evaluation of cerebral function includes information obtained from observing the patient, evoking responses and questioning family and friends. It relates to the appropriateness of the individual's appearance, behaviour, level of consciousness, mood, attitude and flow of speech. Cognitive functions such as orientation, speech comprehension, general intelligence, attention and concentration, memory retention and immediate recall, vocabulary, judgement and abstract reasoning are also evaluated. Deterioration in one or more of these functions commonly occurs with cerebral dysfunction.

Disease involving the CNS may affect the patient in many ways. The patient's family may report a change in appearance, particularly facial expression, posture and personal grooming. Disordered emotional reactions may be evident in the patient's fluctuating attitudes. There may be inappropriate laughing, crying, irritability or unprovoked expressions of anger. Sharp mood swings may occur; the patient who is withdrawn and depressed or anxious may suddenly become excited or euphoric. Impaired reasoning, unjustified fears, distortion in perception and loss of memory may occur. The attention span may be abnormally short and there may be inability to do very simple calculations or to identify normally familiar objects or sounds. Confusion or disorientation as to time, place or person may occur with a cerebral lesion.

The patient's response to stimuli may vary from a coherent verbal response to no response of any sort, even to painful stimuli.

Speech dysfunctions which occur with cerebral lesions vary with the location, size and nature of the lesion. Aphasia, dysphasia, agnosia and apraxia are examples of speech disorders that may occur.

Aphasia refers to the loss of ability to understand words or to use them to communicate. Difficulty in using words to communicate due to lack of coordination and ability to put words in order occurs more commonly and is referred to as *dysphasia*. Aphasia may be classified as *motor* (*expressive, Broca's*) or *sensory* (*receptive*). Motor aphasia implies that the person understands spoken and written words and knows what he or she wants to say but cannot speak the words. Motor aphasias include any loss of communication by writing, speaking or making signs. Sensory aphasia implies that the comprehension of written and spoken words is affected. A patient may suffer auditory aphasia (word deafness) which is the inability to make sense of sound because of an inability to comprehend symbolic communication associated with sound. Some may experience visual aphasia ('word blindness') which means loss of ability to understand the symbolic content of written words or figures and, even though they can see them, they cannot read them. In many instances of aphasia, elements of both expressive and receptive communication are lost.

Certain areas of the cerebral cortex are essential to the recognition of objects by sight, sound, feeling, smell and taste. Cerebral dysfunction may result in the inability to recognize objects through any of the senses and is referred to as *agnosia*. Agnosia may be visual, auditory or tactile. A cerebral lesion may also result in *apraxia*, which is the inability to carry out purposeful, useful or skilled acts in the absence of paralysis, or use objects correctly. *Dyslexia* means inability to comprehend written words.

Cranial nerves

Cranial nerves are referred to by specific name or number (see Table 20.2). Most arise from the brainstem, and much information can be obtained by testing cranial nerve function. Evaluation of cranial nerve function involves the following test procedures.

Olfactory (I) nerve

The patient is asked to close the eyes and identify a series of odorous substances such as coffee, peppermint or oil of cloves. Each nostril is tested separately. Inability to identify the substances (in the absence of a cold or allergy) may suggest a lesion in the frontal lobe such as a tumour of the olfactory groove.

Optic (II) nerve

This is tested using ophthalmoscopic examination and evaluation of visual acuity and visual fields. Visual acuity may be grossly evaluated by asking the person to read from a printed page or distant sign both with and without corrective lenses if such are used. See assessment in Chapter 21.

Ophthalmoscopic examination may reveal papilloedema, which is oedema of the area where the optic nerve and blood vessels enter and leave the eyeball, and is a classical sign of increased intracranial pressure.

Oculomotor (III), trochlear (IV) and abducens (VI) nerves

These nerves are usually tested together because they are all involved in the muscles that rotate the eyeball, constrict the pupils and elevate the eyelids. On examination, pupils should be round and equal in size and shape. Each pupil is tested, in a darkened room, for the direct light reflex. A light is directed into each pupil and the response observed. The normal pupil constricts briskly in response to light stimulus. The consensual light reflex is also tested. This is a slightly weaker constriction of one pupil when the other is stimulated by light.

Accommodation is tested by asking the person to look at a distant spot and then follow the examiner's finger to within 15 cm of the person's nose. Visualization of a distant object causes pupillary dilatation, whereas viewing a near object produces constriction and convergence. Abnormal pupillary responses suggest neurological dysfunction.

The range of ocular movements is evaluated by asking the person to follow the examiner's finger as it moves up, down, medially and laterally. Inability to move the eyeball in a particular direction may result in *diplopia* (double vision). Normal eyes move conjugately (track together). Disconjugate movement implies failure of function of one or more of the eye muscles. Abnormal eye movements can result from injury to the nerves themselves or their nuclei in the midbrain and pons. During examination of ocular movements, observations for *nystagmus* are made. This is an involuntary rhythmic movement of one or both eyes in a lateral or vertical direction. It may occur in normal persons with severe myopia or fatigue or it may occur with neurological disease. *Ptosis* (drooping) of the eyelid may occur with paralysis of the levator palpebrae muscle due to damage of cranial nerve III.

Trigeminal (V) nerve

The trigeminal nerve has sensory and motor components. The sensory function is assessed by testing both sides of the face and mouth for touch, temperature and pain sensations while the person's eyes are closed. The motor function is evaluated by having the person make chewing and biting movements. The ophthalmic branch of the trigeminal nerve controls the corneal reflex. If this reflex is intact, the person blinks briskly when the cornea of each eye is lightly touched with a wisp of cotton wool. The corneal reflex is one of the last to disappear when the patient's condition is deteriorating.

Facial (VII) nerve

The facial nerve has a sensory and motor component. The sensory component is tested by seeing whether the person can recognize the taste of sweet and salty substances when applied to the anterior part of the tongue. The motor divisions are tested by asking the person to use the facial muscles in such expressions as smiling, frowning, closing the eyes tightly and puckering the lips.

Vestibulocochlear (VIII) nerve

This nerve has two divisions: the cochlear nerve and the vestibular nerve. The cochlear nerve is tested for hearing acuity by whispering in one ear, using a ticking watch and a tuning fork. Loss of hearing or reports by the patient of constant or abnormal recurring sounds described as roaring, ringing, buzzing or swishing should be recorded and reported to the doctor. The vestibular nerve, concerned with equilibrium reflexes, is tested by rotating the patient and performing the caloric test. Dizziness and loss of position balance (equilibrium) may occur with disturbance in the semicircular canals of the internal ear, of the vestibular part of the auditory nerve, or pathway within the brain.

Glossopharyngeal (IX) and vagus (X) nerves

These nerves are usually examined simultaneously because of their overlapping innervation of the pharynx. In response to touching of the pharynx with a tongue depressor, a brisk gag reaction should be elicited. Ability to swallow water is assessed and the posterior third of the tongue may be tested for taste. Absence of the gag or swallowing reflex occurs in neurological damage and renders the person vulnerable to aspiration. To assess the vagus nerve, the ability to speak and to cough is evaluated. Ineffectual cough and a weak, hoarse voice suggest possible vagal involvement.

Motor control
See chapter 2.2

Accessory (XI) nerve

This nerve is tested by inspecting the sternocleidomastoid muscle and the upper portion of the trapezius muscle for symmetry, atrophy and strength. The person is asked to elevate the shoulders with and without resistance from the examiner's hand, and to rotate the head to each side against the pull of the chin to the midline by the examiner's hand.

Hypoglossal (XII) nerve

This nerve is assessed by observing various movements of the tongue and examining it for symmetry, atrophy and tremor when protruded.

Motor function

This is evaluated by examining muscle symmetry, size, shape, tone and movement. Muscle function, balance accuracy and muscle strength are assessed. Inspection and comparison of muscles on both sides of the body, palpation and measuring the circumferences of areas with a tape measure provides information about size and shape and can reveal abnormalities such as atrophy or hypertrophy. Muscle tone is assessed by palpating muscles at rest and noting the resistance to passive movement. Excessive resistance (*spasticity*), a constant state of resistance (*rigidity*) and decreased muscle tone (*flaccidity or hypotonia*) are examples of abnormal muscle tone.

Movements are examined for 'fine' and 'gross' abnormalities. Fine muscle abnormalities are *fasciculations* which are involuntary ripples, or twitches, that occur when the person is relaxed. They suggest lower motor neurone disease. Gross abnormal movements may indicate extrapyramidal disease and include athetoid, choreiform and dystonic movements, spasms, myoclonus, tics and tremors.

Athetoid movements These are involuntary, repetitive, slow and writhing. They may be unilateral or bilateral and follow a definite pattern in the individual patient, ceasing only during sleep. Athetosis is commonly seen in persons with cerebral palsy.

Choreiform movements These are involuntary, rapid, rhythmic and jerky. They begin abruptly, are variable in pattern and distribution, and may occur during sleep. The limbs, face and tongue are most often involved, and difficulty in speaking, chewing and swallowing may be present. The forcefulness of the movements may lead to injury unless protection is provided.

Spasms or cramps These are sudden, violent, involuntary contractions of a muscle or muscle groups which result in pain, interference with function and voluntary movement. Muscles of the limbs and neck are most frequently affected. The cause may be a lesion within the CNS, such as degenerative changes in the extrapyramidal system, a deficient blood supply to the muscle(s), overstretching and injury of the muscle fibres or a blood calcium or sodium deficiency.

Dystonic movements These involve spasms in portions of the limbs as well as the trunk. The result is usually slow, grotesque, twisting movements and abnormal posture.

Myoclonus This is shock-like contractions of a portion of a muscle, an entire muscle or group of muscles restricted to one area of the body or appearing synchronously or asynchronously in several areas (seen most commonly in epilepsy).

Tics Tics are frequently of psychogenic origin. They are stereotyped, repetitious, purposeless movements that vary from individual to individual. Twitching of a cheek is an example of a tic.

Tremors These are involuntary shaky movements, particularly of the limbs, which may have a physical or psychological aetiology. A fine, rapid tremor, particularly of the hands, may be associated with anxiety, fatigue or toxic conditions such as thyrotoxicosis, uraemia and alcoholism. *Intention tremor* occurs when a voluntary movement is initiated and progressively intensifies, especially with precision movements. *A resting tremor* is one that diminishes with voluntary movement and disappears during sleep.

Muscles are further evaluated by putting all the joints through a full range of passive movement. Pain, contractures and muscle resistance are abnormal findings.

Muscle strength may be assessed by flexion and extension and other movements, first without resistance and then with the examiner offering resistance. In addition, the person may be asked to hold the arms straight in front with the palms up and the eyes closed for 20–30 seconds. If one arm moves downward or one hand begins to pronate, a *drift* is said to be present, suggesting muscle weakness in that arm. Drift can be tested in the lower limbs by asking the person to raise both legs off the bed while in a supine position.

Coordination, balance and accuracy of muscle function is mediated largely by the cerebellum. These attributes may be assessed by point-to-point tests (e.g. with the eyes open, then repeated with the eyes closed, the person repeatedly touches the examiner's finger and then his or her own nose). Coordination and balance may also be assessed by observing the person's gait while the eyes are open and again when closed. Locomotion depends upon a normal degree of tone, close integration and coordination of the involved muscles of the lower limbs and trunk. These factors are primarily dependent upon normal innervation.

Various abnormal gaits may be observed in the presence of neurological dysfunction:

- The *ataxic gait* is an unsteady, uncoordinated walk. With the feet placed far apart to provide a wide base for support, each foot is lifted abnormally high and slapped down with each step. The steps are unsure, unevenly spaced and may deviate to one side. Ataxic gait is associated with a loss of proprioceptive sense and a lack of coordination of muscle action. It tends to be more pronounced in the dark, as visual influences diminish.

- The *stepping gait* (foot-drop gait) is characterized by foot drop due to paralysis of the anterior tibial muscles, usually secondary to lower motor neurone disease. The person looks as though he or she is walking upstairs, because the advancing leg is lifted abnormally high to avoid dragging the foot and stumbling.

- *Cerebellar ataxia* is staggering, unsteady and wide based. Turns are made with difficulty. The person is unable to stand steadily with the feet together, whether the eyes are open or closed. It is associated with damage in the cerebellum or related tracts.

- *Parkinson's gait* is characteristic of patients with the basal ganglia defects of Parkinson's disease. With this gait, the trunk is stooped forward, the knees are slightly flexed, steps are short and often shuffling and the speed of walking progressively accelerates.

Paralysis or loss of motor function is a common occurrence in neurological disease or injury. Paralysis may be partial and exhibited by weakness (paresis) or complete and may be classified according to the extent of the involvement:

- Monoplegia refers to paralysis of one limb.

- Hemiplegia means paralysis of one side of the body. There is loss of muscle power in the limbs and the muscles of the face on the same side. If the side of the face opposite to that of the paralysed limbs is affected, the term alternate hemiplegia may be used.

- Paraplegia denotes paralysis of the legs or the lower half of the body.

- Quadriplegia or tetraplegia refers to paralysis of the trunk and all four extremities.

Isolated paralysis indicates the loss of the contractile ability of one muscle of a group. It is frequently associated with peripheral nerve damage and is usually accompanied by loss of sensation in the area supplied by the injured nerve.

Paralysis may also be classified as that due to an upper or lower motor neurone lesion. Damage to the motor areas of the cerebral cortex or their projection pathways (corticospinal or pyramidal tracts) produces paralysis due to an upper motor neurone lesion or what may also be termed spastic paralysis. As the lower motor neurones and reflex arc are intact, the affected muscles are still capable of reflex movements and exhibit hypertonicity (spasticity) as well as exaggerated reflexes. There is increased activity of postural (stretch) and protective reflexes. Paralysis resulting from injury of the motor neurones in the nuclei of cranial nerves or in the anterior horns or columns of grey matter in the spinal cord or damage to their axons in the periphery may be referred to as that due to a lower motor neurone lesion or as flaccid paralysis. Flaccidity occurs because the reflex arc is interrupted: there is a lack of reflex innervation and responses.

Serious abnormal postures that may develop with some cerebral and brainstem disorders are decerebrate rigidity and decorticate rigidity (Fig. 20.10). Normally, primitive reflex spinal mechanisms that initiate involuntary muscular responses are kept inactive by cerebral control. These primitive involuntary responses may be referred to as spinal automatisms. When control from the higher centres is abolished, sustained rigid posturing develops.

Sensory function

This includes assessment of the visual, auditory, olfactory, gustatory, touch, proprioceptive, pain and temperature senses. Most of these have been discussed in conjunction with assessment of the cranial nerves. The body areas usually tested for touch, pain and temperature are the face, hands, arms, trunk, thighs, feet, perineal and perianal regions. The patient is asked to close the eyes and

Figure 20.10   (a) Decorticate rigidity (spastic flexion). (b) Decerebrate rigidity (spastic extension).

each side of the body is compared with the other. Sensitivity to touch (a wisp of cotton wool), superficial pain (a pin prick), deep pressure pain, heat and cold, vibration and position is tested. In addition, the patient is asked to differentiate among various textures.

Sensory tests are often difficult to evaluate and a great deal depends upon the cooperation of the patient. Neurological lesions more often result in a diminution of sensation than in total anaesthesia. A sensory disturbance may be localized in one particular area of the body because of the different sensory pathways being associated with different parts. Hyposensitivity or hypersensitivity in the area may provide information about the location of a lesion.

Reflex status

Evaluation of **reflexes** provides valuable information about the nature, location and progression of neurological disorders in both the conscious and unconscious patient. Exaggeration or diminished responses of normal reflexes and the presence of pathological reflexes are frequently among the earliest indications of neurological disturbance. Reflexes most commonly tested are the deep tendon or muscle stretch reflexes, superficial reflexes and pathological reflexes. The part of the body tested should be relaxed and the stimulus applied with the same intensity to each side of the body. Rapidity and strength of the muscle contractions are noted.

The *deep reflexes* are tested by tapping briskly on a tendon over a bony prominence, evoking an instantaneous stretching of certain muscles and their resulting contraction. The maxillary, biceps, brachioradialis, triceps, patellar and Achilles reflexes are the most common tested. *Superficial reflexes* are elicited by light, rapid stroking of a particular area of the skin or mucous membrane with an object. The corneal and pupillary reflexes, the pharyngeal or gag reflex, abdominal and plantar

Reflexes
See chapter 2.1

reflexes are the common superficial reflexes tested. Diminished superficial reflex responses occur on the opposite side of the body when lesions are present above the decussation of the corticospinal tract. Loss of these reflexes occurs on the same side as the lesion when the lesion is below the corticospinal tract decussation.

The *Babinski reflex* is a useful pathological reflex suggestive of neurological disease, particularly of the pyramidal tract. In response to light stroking of the lateral aspect of the sole of the foot, an extension or dorsiflexion of the big toe and fanning of the other toes occurs.

Consciousness

Consciousness is defined as the complete awareness of self and environment, with appropriate responsiveness to stimuli. It is a dynamic experience involving a series of different elements whose relationship changes incessantly. The precise limits are hard to define as consciousness is inferred from a person's appearance and behaviour.

Two physiological components affect conscious behaviour. These are *content* and *arousal*. Mental activities involve the contents of sensation, perception, attention, memory and volition. Analysis and synthesis of information, along with emotional implications, also occur. The content aspects generally refer to those mental functions carried out in the cerebral cortex. The arousal aspects are reflected in the person's appearance of wakefulness. Cognitive functions are not possible without some degree of arousal. Arousal can exist without the emotional and thinking components of content.

The system of consciousness is driven by an arousal mechanism. Full consciousness depends upon the interaction between the cerebral cortex and the reticular activating system. Neurones in the reticular activating system receive collateral nerve fibres from all sensory pathways that enter the brain via the upper spinal cord or cranial nerves. It has been demonstrated that if the sensory pathways are blocked impulses travel by the collaterals to the reticular activating system, then to the thalamus and on to innervate the cortex. This activation of the cortex produces a state of alertness. Further, it has been postulated that impulses are conducted via a feedback loop back to the reticular activating system, which in turn stimulates the cortex. This continuous circuitry of arousal maintains the state of readiness of the cortex to receive and interpret incoming sensory impulses. A further function of the reticular activating system is to screen and modulate incoming messages so that the cortex is able to process significant information.

Consciousness
See chapter 2.2

Sleep
See chapter 2.2

Sleep

Normal **sleep** is a periodic depression of the physiological function of the parts of the brain concerned with consciousness from which a person can be aroused to awareness. Sleep occurs in two ways: first, as a result of decreased activity in the reticular activating system, which produces *slow-wave* or *normal sleep*. This is a restful type of sleep during which the respiratory and pulse rates and blood pressure fall, the pupils constrict and react more slowly to light, the eyes deviate upwards and tendon reflexes are abolished.

The second way by which sleep occurs results from the abnormal channelling of brain signals and is referred to as *paradoxical* or *desynchronized sleep*. Short episodes of paradoxical sleep usually occur about every 90 minutes throughout a night. Heart and respiratory rates and blood pressure alter, cerebral blood flow increases, clonic jerks may occur and rapid eye movements (REM) take place. Most dreams occur during paradoxical sleep.

During normal sleep, activity of the reticular activating system is decreased, whereas in paradoxical sleep some cerebral areas are active while others are suppressed.

During sleep a person may be easily aroused to wakefulness or consciousness by cerebral arousal through stimuli such as pain or unaccustomed noise. The return to wakefulness shows that the reticular activating system is still functioning and capable of screening and discrimination.

Continuous intracranial pressure monitoring

Direct measurement of intracranial pressure (ICP) is possible with the placement of a pressure-sensitive probe within the intracranial cavity.

The pressure-sensitive probe measures the physical pressure at the selected location and this is converted, with the aid of a transducer, into an electrical signal. The result is a reading displayed as numerical data on a monitor or as a pressure waveform.

ICP monitoring is most commonly used following head injury, especially in patients with evidence of raised ICP but who do not have a focal lesion. ICP monitoring is more fully described on p. 697.

Diagnostic tests

Neurodiagnostic procedures supplement and add precision to clinical data. As with any procedure, the patient needs both physical and psychological preparation to promote confidence in unfamiliar personnel and procedures. A routine test to the nurse can be a bewildering and frightening experience for the patient.

Neurodiagnostic tests can be classified as invasive or non-invasive, although this can be slightly misleading; for example, computed tomography is considered non-invasive but some patients may be given an intravenous contrast to enhance the image. Psychological care and patient teaching are very important, as ever. The aim is to reduce any stress that the patient may experience. Patient teaching is the key to achieving this, and the information for each test should include the following:

- use of the test's proper name avoiding the use of abbreviations

- an explanation as to why the test has been ordered

- who will perform the test and when and where it will be performed

- the length of time that the test normally takes

- the preparation procedure for the test, particularly that which is required of the patient

- an explanation of what will happen during the test

- information on whether, if appropriate, the patient will experience any discomfort or pain

- the aftercare routine and why this is necessary.

Some of this information may duplicate information given by medical staff to the patient during the process of obtaining consent. An additional factor to consider is that, with some neurological disorders, the patient's ability to understand explanations may be impaired. This needs to be assessed and taken into consideration when explanations are provided.

Additional precautions are required before tests are performed. It is necessary to ascertain whether the patient has an allergy to iodine if contrast is to be used and, if female, whether there is any possibility of pregnancy. This information should be documented and reported to medical staff where appropriate.

Non-invasive neurodiagnostic procedures

Non-invasive procedures pose minimal risks to the patient but may still provoke a high level of anxiety. This level of anxiety can be decreased following the advice given in the introduction above. This can be done using various media including charts, diagrams, pamphlets and audiovisual materials. Once the material is reviewed, patients should be encouraged to ask questions in order to clarify any misconceptions. A signed consent is not usually required before the test, but if a contrast medium is injected intravenously during the procedure a signed consent will be required.

Neuroradiography

Conventional radiographs of the skull and spine are frequently the first investigation in neurological disease. A wide spectrum of abnormalities may be demonstrated, including fractures, bone destruction, calcification and congenital lesions. In fact, they may give specific clues to the nature of the underlying problem.

Computed tomography

In *computed tomography (CT)* the scanner circles the patient's head taking multiple radiographs which a computer translates into cross-sectional brain images. These images are based on tissue density and can detect a range of intracranial lesions including contusions; atrophy; hydrocephaly; inflammation; space-occupying lesions such as tumours, haematomas, oedema and abscesses; and haemorrhages. An intravenous contrast may be administered to enhance the image of certain lesions.

An intravenous iodinated water-soluble contrast medium may be used if a plain scan reveals an abnormality or if specific lesions are thought to exist. These would include arteriovenous malformation, acoustic neuroma or intracerebral abscess. The intravenous contrast will show areas with increased vascularity or with impairment of the blood–brain barrier. Intrathecal water-soluble contrast medium combined with CT will outline the basal cisterns, the spinal cord and the lumbosacral nerve roots. Three-dimensional reconstructed images are now possible with sophisticated computer programs and can be rotated on a monitor screen. This is known as dynamic CT.

Magnetic resonance imaging (MRI)

During scanning, the patients should not have any metal objects on them as this will interfere with the procedure. MRI has several advantages over CT, notably in investigating the posterior cranial fossa and the spinal cord. It also more clearly demonstrates certain brain lesions, such as the demyelinating plaques of multiple sclerosis. Obtaining images can be a slow process in comparison with CT – taking up to 1 hour to complete. The test requires patients to be enclosed in a long cylindrical tube, often giving a sensation of claustrophobia.

Carotid Doppler ultrasonography

This non-invasive diagnostic study is used to assess the blood flow through the carotid arteries and the extent of sclerotic vascular change that may be partially or completely obstructing the normal flow of blood to the brain. The study may be done on persons who are considered at risk of stroke because of attendant signs and symptoms (e.g. transient ischaemic attacks).

The study involves the placing of a probe over the carotid area. The probe gives off ultrasound waves and receives them back as they rebound from erythrocytes flowing through the carotid arteries.

Single-photon emission computed tomography (SPECT)

This is a form of radionucleoide imaging using compounds labelled with γ-emitting tracers. A rotating γ-camera is used and multidetector systems have now been introduced. A two-dimensional image is produced depicting the radioactivity emitted. The most popular tracer used rapidly diffuses across the blood–brain barrier and thus presents a picture of cerebral blood flow. SPECT can be used for detection of early ischaemia, blood flow changes in dementia and evaluation of patients with intractable epilepsy.

Another form of radionucleoide imaging is positron emission tomography (PET). In this, the radioactive emissions (positrons) of the tracer are picked up by sensitive detectors around the head as it distributes in the brain. PET provides safe, rapid scanning of blood flow in the brain, as well as biochemical mapping. It can be used to study diseases related to chemical changes in the brain and to localize the area of action in the brain.

Electroencephalography (EEG)

The EEG is a recording of the brain's electrical activity. Several small electrodes are placed superficially on the scalp in standard positions. The electrodes are attached to an amplifier and recorder. The electrical activity of neuronal dendrites of the superficial layers of the brain are responsible for the low-voltage electrical waves. If the patient has been prescribed an anticonvulsant drug it is usually withheld for 24 hours or more before the test. The patient needs assurance that an electric shock will not occur during the test and that the machine cannot 'read the mind'. The technician cleans the scalp and applies the electrodes with collodion. In some instances needle electrodes are inserted into the scalp, which necessitates cleansing the scalp before the needles are inserted. The patient lies or sits in a quiet, dimly lit room. In order to evoke or accentuate certain abnormal wave patterns the patient may be asked to hyperventilate, or the technician may flash bright lights before the eyes. Some abnormalities become evident only during sleep; therefore, a sedative may be prescribed and recordings made before, during and after sleep.

The EEG may take up to an hour to complete. After the test the patient may need assistance in using acetone to remove the collodion from the hair and scalp. The EEG is particularly useful in evaluating seizure disorders and it may help to localize tumours.

An ambulatory EEG may be performed over a 24-hour period, using a portable recorder attached to the patient's waist. This is used to diagnose petit mal, temporal lobe epilepsy or seizures of unknown origin.

EEG telemetry is frequently used as with this method the patient can be observed with a video camera, while at the same time the EEG tracing can be seen and recorded. This method gives essential information on seizure type and patients' behaviour.

Electromyography (EMG)

This is a record of the electrical currents produced by skeletal muscles. Small needle electrodes are inserted into a muscle and the electrical currents are recorded with the muscle at rest and during activity. The test is useful to monitor changes in peripheral nerve dysfunction, to determine types of primary muscle disease and to identify defective transmission at the myoneural junction. The patient usually experiences some discomfort when the needle electrodes are inserted, and if many muscles are tested some discomfort may persist.

Neuropsychological tests

These tests are done when deficits in adaptive abilities are suspected. Motor, perceptual, language, visual–spatial, cognitive and other abilities can be assessed to determine the extent of impairment in brain functions. The tests measure deficits in coping skills by evaluating these skills directly rather than indirectly. They require several hours to complete and may result in recommendations concerning educational and vocational placement.

Lumbar puncture
See chapter 2.2

Invasive neurodiagnostic procedures

Invasive procedures carry a greater risk for the patient, thus preparation, both physically and in terms of information giving, is crucial. Signed consent is required for all these procedures.

Lumbar puncture (LP)

This involves the insertion of a spinal needle into the lumbar subarachnoid space of the spinal canal. The needle is passed through the intervertebral space between the third and fourth or fourth and fifth vertebrae. Indications include the measurement of lumbar CSF pressure, to obtain specimens of CSF for analysis or to inject drugs such as anaesthetics or antibiotics. Only drugs specifically manufactured for intrathecal injection are used. The patient lies in the lateral recumbent position, with the back on the edge of the bed, and flexes the knees to the chest so that they touch the chin, in order to widen the interspineous spaces. The nurse should be prepared to support the patient behind the neck and knees. The skin is prepared, local anaesthetic injected and a spinal needle is inserted using an aseptic technique. The needle is advanced until the tip is in the subarachnoid space and CSF is obtained (Fig. 20.11). If required, a manometer is attached and the lumbar pressure measured (normal pressure 40–180 mmH$_2$O). Specimens of CSF are collected in the appropriate container as required. When collection is complete, the needle is removed and a small sterile dressing applied once it has been ascertained that there is no leakage of CSF.

Figure 20.11 Lumbar puncture.

Third lumbar vertebra
Dura mater
Subarachnoid space
Cauda equina

The advantage of this procedure is that it permits direct observation of CSF and withdrawal of fluid for examination, thus aiding diagnosis. It is contraindicated in the patient with raised ICP. Removal of CSF may cause herniation of the brain leading to damage affecting the brainstem as medial brain structures are forced through the tentorial notch in response to the increased pressure gradient. After the procedure the patient may experience a transient difficulty with voiding urine; temperature increase due to meningeal irritation; pain, oedema or haematoma at the site of the puncture, and headache may also occur.

There are some specific nursing interventions to implement. The patient is required to remain on bedrest for 6–24 hours after the procedure. Remobilization will occur as the patient feels able. Increased frequency of neurological observations for the first 12 hours are required to detect any deterioration. Complications such as difficulty with voiding, raised temperature and headache are dealt with as they arise. Mild analgesia, cold compress and bedrest will relieve the headache.

Cisternal puncture

This is done if an LP is contraindicated or if there is a block in the spinal subarachnoid space. A short needle is inserted into the cisterna magna (a small sac of CSF between the cerebellum and medulla) just beneath the occiptal bone. Because this puncture is close to the brain and the patient's cooperation is necessary, anxiety-reducing and supportive measures are essential. The nape of the neck is shaved, the patient is positioned on the side and the head is flexed forward and held firmly by the nurse, or the patient may be sat upright, resting the arms on pillows on a bed-table. Observation is necessary for signs of respiration difficulty, which may suggest that the needle has made contact with the medulla. Usually the patient resumes normal activity soon after the procedure.

Cerebral angiography

This is performed by injecting radio-opaque material into the carotid and vertebral arteries. While this can be done by a direct puncture of the vessel, the method of choice is by a catheter, manipulated into the origin of the vessel via the femoral artery. Under local anaesthesia, sterile technique and with the patient sedated, a suitably shaped catheter is passed retrogradely up to the aorta over a guidewire. Selective catheterization of the carotid and vertebral arteries can be undertaken as indicated. During the injection, radiographs are obtained in rapid sequence. After removal of the needle, a sterile gauze pad is applied over the injection site and firm pressure is applied for 5–10 minutes to prevent haemorrhage and haematoma formation.

Following angiography the patient remains on bedrest for at least 8 hours. Neurological observations are carried out frequently and the pressure dressing is checked for bleeding. A cold compress or ice-bag may be applied to the injection site to control oedema and discomfort and to reduce the possibility of bleeding. If a limb was used for the puncture site (e.g. femoral artery), the distal part is checked for colour, temperature and presence of a pulse. Vasospasm, thrombosis or formation of a haematoma can occur, obstructing the blood supply to the distal portion.

Rarely, cerebral angiography may precipitate a stroke, seizure, allergic reaction to the contrast substance, or other serious complications. Any signs of deterioration in the patient's condition must be reported to the doctor immediately.

Myelography

This is an X-ray examination of the spinal cord and vertebral canal following injection of a radio-opaque contrast substance into the spinal subarachnoid space. It is used to detect and localize lesions that may be compressing the spinal cord or nerves. Water-soluble, non-ionic contrast medium is injected into the CSF surrounding the spinal cord and emerging nerve roots. The most common access site is the lumbar region (as for lumbar puncture), but when pathology is suspected in the cervical region a lateral puncture of the dura may be made, between the spinous processes of C1 and C2.

As with all procedures, an explanation is given so that the patient will know what to expect and can cooperate more fully. A history of any allergy is recorded and brought to the doctor's attention. Food and fluid are withheld for up to 6 hours before the procedure and sedation may be prescribed 1 hour beforehand. The lumbosacral area of the back is shaved if necessary.

After the procedure, the patient rests supine in bed, with the head and trunk at 45°. This position minimizes the volume of contrast that enters the CSF surrounding the brain. Serious complications of myelography are fortunately rare, particularly with the use of the new non-ionic contrast media. However, the neurological status of the patient should be kept under review after the procedure; persistent headache, pain and/or the development of neck stiffness should be reported.

The person with a neurological disorder

The highly complex nature of the nervous system is revealed through its numerous and diverse disorders. The dysfunctions that result depend primarily on the area(s) of the nervous system affected, the extent of the lesion and, to a lesser degree, the nature of the pathological process. For this reason, it is difficult for healthcare professionals to predict outcomes and thereby develop outcome criteria. The focus of nursing activity includes disease stabilization, health promotion and prevention. The family is an integral part of patient care and members are encouraged to participate in all aspects of care, including decision making, to the degree that they are able.

Pathology of the CNS often compromises intellectual and reasoning process, hence the added importance of family involvement and the need for nurses to be aware of concepts such as maintenance of dignity and need for advocacy. There are recurrent legal and ethical issues inherent in the care of patients with neurological dysfunction. Issues such as brain death, persistent vegetative state and surrogate decision making are only some examples where nurses face ethical dilemmas.

The following sections will consider the common disorders most often encountered in nursing practice.

The person with a cerebrovascular disorder

Cerebrovascular disorders are among the most common of all neurological disorders. The greater number may be classified as ischaemic or haemorrhagic. Either may cause a cerebrovascular infarction, which is commonly known as a stroke or may also be referred to as a cerebrovascular accident (CVA).

Stroke (cerebrovascular accident)

Incidence

Stroke
See chapter 2.2

Strokes are a leading cause of death and disability. They have their highest incidence in those over 60 years of age.

A stroke or CVA involves an interruption of the blood supply to a part of the brain and the development of neurological deficits. If the ischaemia persists, necrosis of the deprived area follows, the infarcted area eventually liquefies and is absorbed, and the neurological deficits remain. The cause of the stroke may be atherosclerosis, cerebral thrombosis or embolism, or intracranial haemorrhage. The artery that ruptures is usually vulnerable due to degenerative vascular changes (atherosclerosis) or the presence of an aneurysm. A haemorrhagic stroke may be precipitated by increased blood pressure and is usually associated with some physical or emotional stress.

According to the rate of development and permanence of the neurological effects, a stroke may be categorized as a transient ischaemic attack, stroke in evolution or completed stroke. Gradual development of stroke symptoms over a period of several hours or days is usually associated with a cerebral thrombosis or slow leak in a cerebral artery. This type of stroke is referred to as a stroke in evolution. A stroke is classified as a completed stroke when the neurological deficits remain longer than 3 or 4 days.

Cerebral atherosclerosis

This is a chronic degenerative process of the cerebral arteries in which the intimal layer gradually develops atheromas (fibrous fatty plaques). These narrow the vascular lumen, damage the underlying layer of tissue media and tend to undergo calcification, ulceration with overlying thrombosis and intraplaque haemorrhage, which worsen the luminal narrowing or cause total occlusion. These degenerative changes result in interference with cerebral perfusion. Although the brain represents only about 2% of the body's weight, it consumes 20% of its oxygen. As the brain cannot store energy nor temporarily exist by anaerobic metabolism, deprivation of oxygenated blood for even a very few minutes leads to neuronal death.

Atherosclerosis affects the larger vessels at the base of the brain first, particularly at the points of vessel branching, and tends to develop silently. The incidence increases with increasing age. Its presence is manifested when it is well advanced by the following signs and symptoms:

1. the development of ischaemia of vital organs (e.g. deterioration of mental faculties)

2. episodes of local neurological dysfunction, which are referred to as transient ischaemic attacks

3. predisposition to thrombosis, which may give rise to emboli

4. weakening of an arterial wall resulting in an aneurysm.

Occasionally, on routine physical examination, a noise or bruit may be heard through a stethoscope placed over the carotid artery when there is turbulent blood flow due to irregularities in the vessel wall.

Because the cause of atherosclerosis continues to elude scientists, interventions are directed to reducing the risk factors. This diagnosis can promote much anxiety and uncertainty in the patient and family, who will consequently require information about risk factors, such as smoking, cholesterol (low-density lipoprotein; LDL) and obesity, and a discussion about possible changes in lifestyle that will decrease the level of risk. Risk factors that are the target of educational interventions include:

- diets high in cholesterol and saturated fat
- hypercholesterolaemia
- hypertension
- cigarette smoking
- diabetes.

Controversy continues with regard to the control of atherosclerosis by modification of diet and blood lipid values. In addition, some defend and others deny a role for control of blood sugar levels in the progression of atherosclerosis, but the desirability of controlling hypertension and cigarette smoking is unquestioned. An anticoagulant (e.g. aspirin, warfarin) may be prescribed.

Surgical therapy for atherosclerosis causing cerebral ischaemia involves a carotid endarterectomy or cerebral artery bypass (see p. 687).

Cerebral thrombosis and embolism

This is the most common cause of stroke and is usually due to atherosclerosis of the carotid, vertebral or larger cerebral arteries. The narrowing of the lumen of the vessel by atherosclerotic plaques leads to thrombus formation, occlusion of the artery, and ischaemia of the respective brain area. Inadequate delivery of blood to the brain and subsequent thrombosis may be secondary to cardiac insufficiency, shock or to reduced intravascular volume as occurs in haemorrhage and severe dehydration.

Embolic material, which may be a thrombus or atherosclerotic plaque that becomes free in the bloodstream, lodges in a cerebral artery, occluding the vessel and resulting in a cerebral infarction (stroke). The middle cerebral artery is the most frequent location. The occlusion occurs suddenly; there is no warning or time for the development of collateral circulation. Anticoagulant therapy may be prescribed to prevent a second stroke.

Transient ischaemic attacks

A large proportion of patients with an atherothrombic stroke have a history of transient ischaemic attacks. These episodes of local neurological dysfunction may last for a few seconds to several hours; most last for 5–10 minutes. There may be only a few attacks or as many as several hundred before an actual stroke. These transient attacks are due to focal ischaemia incurred by temporary occlusion of an artery by vasospasm, microemboli or insufficient blood supply. They are usually associated with atherosclerosis.

Transient attacks are warning signs of impending complete stroke. Manifestations include transient paresis or hemiplegia, visual deficits (decreased vision in one eye), difficulty in or loss of speech, difficulty in comprehension, dizziness, unsteadiness and sudden falls.

Lack of knowledge in the patient experiencing transient ischaemic attacks is a major concern. It is a nursing responsibility to assess the patient's understanding of the episodes and to urge prompt medical attention. Timely and appropriate therapy can reduce the number of these attacks and may reduce the risk of a disastrous stroke in the near future.

The therapeutic regimen may involve a low-fat diet, control of hypertension, no smoking and an anticoagulant drug such as warfarin or aspirin. Selected patients are treated surgically by a carotid endarterectomy or cerebral artery bypass.

Endarterectomy

Endarterectomy of the internal carotid artery involves the removal of the atheroma from the intima. A venous graft or Dacron prosthesis may be necessary to reinforce the vascular area from which the plaques are removed.

Not all patients with atherosclerosis or experiencing transient ischaemic attacks are candidates for surgery; those who are very elderly and have extensive vascular disease, or who have serious heart or renal problems, are a high risk.

Nursing intervention

Preoperative preparation of the patient for an endarterectomy follows that for neurosurgery outlined later (see p. 713). A specific directive may be received concerning skin preparation.

Postoperative nursing care follows that for the neurosurgical patient. Additional interventions include:

- *frequent monitoring of blood pressure* – an increase may place stress on the operative site and cause severe haemorrhage. Hypotension predisposes to thrombus formation within the artery at the surgical site

- *frequent observation of the operative site* for evidence of bleeding or oedema in the area.

The neck circumference is observed frequently for swelling due to internal bleeding. Respiratory distress is reported promptly: swelling due to oedema or clot formation may compress the trachea and interfere with respirations. Assessment of neurological function may follow that outlined in Table 20.4.

The patient is kept at rest and quiet with a minimum of stimuli during the first 24 hours; all exertion is avoided. After this period, the patient is gradually mobilized if vital signs are satisfactory and stable.

An anticoagulant is prescribed and is usually continued for about 6 months after operation. Regular checking of prothrombin time is necessary. On discharge from the hospital, the patient is advised to report any blood in the urine or stool, bleeding of gums or discoloured bruised areas (ecchymoses). Former activities are resumed very gradually.

Cerebral artery bypass

Cerebral artery bypass surgery may be performed on patients who have lesions in the smaller arteries inside the skull that cannot be corrected by endarterectomy. Using microsurgical techniques and a craniotomy just above the ear, a large scalp artery (e.g. superficial temporal) is anastomosed to a blocked artery in order to supply blood beyond the stenosis.

Nursing intervention

Nursing care after operation is similar to that outlined for endarterectomy.

The major complications following bypass surgery include interruption of blood flow through the graft, stroke and subdural haematoma due to bleeding at the surgical site. The patient is positioned off the operative side with the head of the bed elevated 30°. Anticoagulant therapy may be continued for several months after surgery. Long-term benefits and indications for cerebral bypass have not been firmly established but there is some evidence of decreased stroke rate and improvement in the quality of life of patients who have had a bypass.

Table 20.4 Organization of a functionally oriented nursing neurological evaluation

Functional category	Examples of specific function which may be tested
Consciousness	
Arousing (reticular activating system)	Arousability, response to verbal and tactile stimuli
Mentation	
Thinking (general cortical function plus specific regional functions)	Educational level Content of conversation Orientation Fund of information Insight, judgement, planning
Feeling (affective)	Mood and affect Perception and reaction to ability, disability
Language	Content and quantity of speech Ability to name objects Ability to repeat phrases Ability to read, write, copy
Remembering	Attention span Recent and remote memory
Motor function	
Seeing (cranial nerves, II, III, IV, VI)	Acuity Visual fields Extraocular movement Pupil size, shape, reactivity Presence or absence of diplopia, nystagmus
Eating (cranial nerves, V, IX, X, XII)	Chewing Swallowing Gag (if swallowing impaired)
Expressing (facially) (cranial nerve VII)	Symmetry of smile, frown
Speaking (cranial nerves VII, IX, X, XII)	Clarity, presence or absence of nasality
Moving (motor and cerebellar systems)	Muscle tone, mass, strength Presence or absence of involuntary movements Coordination: heel-to-toe walk, observing during dressing Posture, gait, position
Sensory function	
Smelling (cranial nerve I)	Ability to detect odours
Blinking (cranial nerve V)	Corneal reflex
Hearing (cranial nerve VII)	Acuity, presence or absence of unusual sounds
Feeling (sensory pathways)	Pain – pinprick Touch, stereognosis Temperature – warm, cold

Cerebral aneurysm

An aneurysm is a saccular dilatation of an arterial wall, thought to be caused most often by the congenital absence of muscular and elastic tissue in the wall of that area of the vessel. It may also develop as a result of degenerative vascular changes. The most common cerebral aneurysm is referred to as a *berry aneurysm* because it is a rounded out-pouching on a stem. The majority occur at the base of the brain in the circle of Willis at points of bifurcation. The lesion does not always produce symptoms and may be single, or there may be several (Fig. 20.12).

Aneurysms are the cause of death in over 50% of all fatal cerebrovascular lesions in persons under the age of 45 years. Although the weakness in the arterial wall is congenital, actual distension of the vessel occurs much later in life. The distension may produce localizing symptoms by pressure on adjacent structures (e.g. paralysis due to pressure on cranial nerves). Rupture of the artery

Figure 20.12   Circle of Willis and sites of saccular aneurysms.

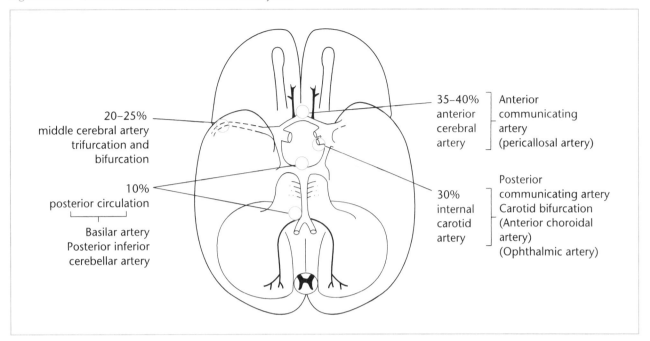

20–25%
middle cerebral artery
trifurcation and
bifurcation

10%
posterior circulation

Basilar artery
Posterior inferior
cerebellar artery

35–40%
anterior
cerebral
artery

Anterior
communicating
artery
(pericallosal artery)

30%
internal
carotid
artery

Posterior
communicating artery
Carotid bifurcation
(Anterior choroidal
artery)
(Ophthalmic artery)

is the most serious consequence. It may be preceded by a series of small leaks over several weeks manifested by headache and stiffness of the neck, but more often the rupture occurs without any warning. The most vulnerable persons are those aged 35–60 years and those with hypertension or polycystic disease of the kidneys. Rupture may be precipitated by physical or emotional exertion and the bleeding may occur into the subarachnoid space, cerebral substance or both those areas.

Assessment

Clinical characteristics

Rupture of a cerebral aneurysm forces blood under arterial pressure into the brain tissue and subarachnoid space giving rise to an explosive headache, nausea, vomiting and, in some, rapid loss of consciousness. Symptoms of meningeal irritation will also be present, which include pain and neck rigidity, positive Kernig's sign (inability to extend the knees without pain while in supine position with hips flexed), positive Brudzinski's sign (person in supine position bends the knees to avoid pain when the neck is flexed), photophobia, blurred vision, irritability, restlessness and possible temperature increase. The presence and severity of symptoms are determined by the location and extent of the bleeding.

Investigation

If a patient is suspected of having had a subarachnoid haemorrhage, the investigative approach will differ depending upon the presence of coma or focal signs. If the patient is obeying commands with no focal signs and access to a CT scanner is not possible, lumbar puncture will

be performed. If the CSF is clear, no further investigation will occur. Uniformly blood-stained CSF or xanthochromia (straw-coloured supernatant due to the breakdown products of haemoglobin) is indicative that a subarachnoid haemorrhage has occurred. The patient would now be referred for an urgent neurosurgical opinion. The patient showing signs of coma or focal neurological signs will not have a lumbar puncture performed because of the risk of herniation due to raised ICP. Instead CT is indicated along with an urgent neurosurgical referral. Cerebral angiography is carried out at the earliest opportunity, although in some instances this may have to be delayed because of the patient's condition. CT will confirm the diagnosis of subarachnoid haemorrhage, identify other associated lesions (e.g. hydrocephalus) and help in the identification of the site of the aneurysm rupture. These investigations will assist in determining the grade of the haemorrhage as this is important in relation to outcome. A number of grading systems exist; an example of one incorporating the Glasgow Coma Score is included in Table 20.5.

Prognosis

Predicting prognosis following subarachnoid haemorrhage depends on a number of factors. The natural history of ruptured aneurysm shows that, of 100 people with aneurysmal subarachnoid haemorrhage treated conservatively, 15 will die before reaching hospital. Of the remaining 85, further 15 will die within the next 24 hours. This pattern repeats itself until, at the end of 2 years, only 25 patients are still alive from the original 100. This is described as a high initial mortality rate that gradually declines with time. Neurosurgical intervention can impact on these figures. Of patients surviving the initial

Table 20.5   Grading of subarachnoid haemorrhage

Grade	Glasgow Coma Score	
I	15[a]	Neurologically intact (except for cranial nerve palsy)
II	15	Neurologically intact (except for cranial nerve palsy) with neck stiffness, headache or both
III	13–14	(a) Without focal neurological deficit (b) With focal neurological deficit
IV	8–12	With or without focal neurological deficit
V	3–7	Unresponsive coma with or without abnormal posturing

[a]Glasgow Coma Scale scoring is calculated as follows:

Eye opening	Spontaneous	4 points
	To speech	3 points
	To pain	2 points
	None	1 point
Motor response	Obeys commands	6 points
	Localizes	5 points
	Flexion	4 points
	Abnormal flexion	3 points
	Extension	2 points
	None	1 point
Verbal response	Oriented	5 points
	Confused	4 points
	Inappropriate words	3 points
	Incomprehensible sounds	2 points
	None	1 point

bleed and admitted within 3 days to a neurosurgical unit, a third die within the following 3 months. Almost half make a good recovery and regain former employment, although, in a proportion, minor personality change and intellectual deficit persist. Factors that provide a prognostic guide include age of the patient, loss of consciousness, clinical condition on admission, and the presence of pre-existing hypertension or arterial disease.

The intracranial complications of subarachnoid haemorrhage are as follows:

■ *Rebleeding* – the patient may experience rebleeding, which is a major problem. The risk of death following rebleeding is twice that of the initial bleed.

■ *Cerebral ischaemia/infarction* – this most frequently occurs between the day 4 and day 10 after the bleed. It is a serious complication in that 50% of the patients who develop it die. The aetiology is complex and not fully understood, although it is known that vasospasm (arterial constriction) is a major factor. The clinical effects of cerebral ischaemia/infarction may be widespread and devastating, including the development of incontinence, confusion, dysphasia and hemiplegia depending upon the area of the brain affected.

■ *Hydrocephalus* – drainage of CSF may be impaired by the presence of blood clots.

■ *Intracranial haematoma* – the development of a haematoma as the result of the initial bleed may be exaggerated by the presence of brain swelling.

■ *Epilepsy* – can occur at any stage and adopt either a generalized or partial format.

Medical management

If surgery is indicated, the patient will be assessed carefully for risk factors. If conservative treatment is considered appropriate this will include bedrest until asymptomatic, analgesia for headache, and control of other symptoms (e.g. nausea) as they arise.

The purpose of the operation is to avoid rebleeding. Clipping the neck of the aneurysm is the only certain method of preventing a rebleed. This can be done in a number of ways. Direct clipping using a metal, self-closing spring-clip following careful dissection of arachnoid tissue around the neck is the commonest. Wrapping the fundus of the aneurysm with muslin gauze is an alternative option if clipping proves difficult. Sometimes a solidifying acrylic agent is applied over the muslin to strengthen it. A third technique is trapping: distal and proximal vessels leading to the aneurysmal sac are clipped. A newer technique has been developed involving the induction of a thrombosis.

The timing of surgery has been much debated over the years. Traditionally, it was noted that the longer the delay, the better the results from surgery; however, a long delay also increases the patient's chance of dying from rebleeding. Therefore, surgery was planned to take place between 6 and 14 days after the initial bleed. Operating within 48 hours has the advantage of avoiding the risk from rebleeding but increases the operative mortality rate. However, it is now suggested that grade I patients should be operated on sooner rather than later as the risk of dying from rebleeding is greater than the small additional risk of early operation.

Antifibrinolytic agents may be used before operation. These include transexamic acid and ε-aminocaproic acid. The aim is to prevent rebleeding by delaying clot dissolution around the fundus of the aneurysm.

Nursing care

Assessment

Vital signs and neurological status are assessed at frequent intervals (15 or 30 minutes) during the acute stage. A decrease in the level of consciousness, disorientation and other neurological changes are recorded and reported promptly to the doctor. The blood pressure is followed very closely because a rise may increase the bleeding or precipitate rebleeding.

Patient problems

The problems of the patient treated *conservatively* include:

- Potential for continued intracranial bleeding or for recurrence of bleeding.

- Loss of self-care abilities.

- Headache.

- Anxiety and ineffective coping. Fear of the circumstances and concern for the outcome.

- Potential for injury secondary to altered level of awareness, disorientation and immobility.

- Alteration in food and fluid intake due to nausea, vomiting and restricted fluid intake.

- Alteration in urinary and bowel elimination secondary to reduced level of awareness, decreased intake and enforced immobility.

- Potential for complications – rebleeding, hydrocephalus and vasospasm.

- Potential for residual mental and/or physical impairment resulting in need for rehabilitation.

Goals

Patient goals are to avoid the complications associated with the above problems and to achieve maximum independence and self-care.

Nursing intervention

If the patient's level of consciousness is decreased, the measures already discussed are implemented as part of nursing care.

Observe for bleeding or a rebleed

The patient is kept on complete bedrest with one pillow under the head or the head of the bed elevated about 30° to promote venous drainage and prevent increased intracranial pressure, although in some instances enforced bedrest heightens the patient's anxiety. The blood pressure is monitored frequently; it is important that it remains within the extreme low range of normal. Certain restrictions may be placed on visitors; these should be limited and cautioned against being too lively.

Because self-care requires exertion, which increases the blood pressure predisposing to rebleeding, assistance is provided with activities such as bathing. However, to maintain dignity, patients who are able can perform some of these tasks for themselves (e.g. eating meals). In change of position, the patient is cautioned against physical effort.

If the patient is unable to rest, a mild sedative may be prescribed but used only with caution because it may mask neurological changes. The essential immobility predisposes to venous stasis and thrombophlebitis; the application of antiembolic stockings to the lower limbs may be recommended.

Vomiting and coughing are controlled because they increase the intracranial pressure. If the patient is nauseous and vomiting, oral fluids and food are withheld and an antiemetic prescribed. Deep breathing is encouraged at regular intervals to promote pulmonary ventilation.

Alteration in comfort

The severe headache that the patient experiences causes restlessness, nausea and vomiting. Nursing measures include keeping the patient at rest and as quiet as possible. Cold applications to the head may help and a mild analgesic (e.g. codeine) is usually prescribed.

Anxiety and ineffective coping

The patient will probably be very fearful and concerned for the future. It is important, therefore, to allow and encourage the patient to talk about these fears and answer questions openly. If the patient is alert, it will be helpful to explain the serial assessments, procedures, enforced immobility and restrictions. A calm, reassuring approach can be therapeutic.

The family's perception of the illness, their expectations and coping patterns are assessed. Their role in keeping the patient quiet and at rest is explained to them. They are kept informed as to the patient's progress, and opportunities are provided for the expression of feelings and for questions. Tests and procedures are explained to them.

Fluids
See chapter 2.6

Potential for injury

Impairment of awareness may occur resulting in disorientation. If so, cot sides are kept up and frequent close observation made for confusion and restlessness; a mild sedative may be necessary. It may be necessary to have someone remain constantly with the patient to avoid personal injury.

When the comatose patient regains consciousness, frequent orientation to place and circumstances is necessary as well as reassurance as to care and progress.

Potential pressure sores

The regular assessment of pressure areas and an appropriate regimen of prevention is necessary.

Fluid and food intake

When tolerated, the patient receives a soft diet initially. The **fluid** intake may be limited to a specific volume per 24 hours to promote a reduction in cerebral oedema and in intracranial pressure. This varies from unit to unit. Some units have a policy of a 3-litre minimum intake in 24 hours. An accurate record of the fluid intake and output is maintained.

Urinary and bowel elimination

Voiding urine in the supine position may be problematic. Rather than exert the patient by attempting to use a bedpan, it is easier for the patient to get out of bed and go to the toilet – provided they are able to do so safely.

A mild laxative or stool softener may be prescribed after 3–4 days to prevent **constipation** and straining at stool. Enemas are contraindicated.

Potential complications

The complications previously outlined will manifest themselves as changes in level of consciousness and vital signs, together with the symptoms of paresis, paralysis or speech impairment. If the spasm persists, infarction of the brain tissue occurs, causing serious neurological deficits.

Treatment of secondary hydrocephalus may involve a cranial burrhole and the placing of a tube in a ventricle (ventriculostomy) for external drainage of the CSF. If the hydrocephalus persists, a permanent ventriculoatrial or ventriculoperitoneal shunt may be done to drain the CSF.

Residual impairment

The patient may recover and be left with brain damage that results in reduced physical and/or mental capacity. This clearly has long-term social and psychological implications for the patient and family which must be addressed realistically and with the support of a wide range of agencies.

The patient treated by surgery

The care outlined in the sections on preoperative and postoperative care should be referred to (see p. 713).

Effects of a CVA on the patient

Whether the CVA was due to atherosclerosis, thrombosis, embolism or a ruptured cerebral artery, it may produce a wide range of severe effects, leading to the following range of problems:

- alteration in level of consciousness
- headache and vomiting
- neuromuscular deficits
- incontinence
- eye changes
- impairment of speech
- mental impairment
- unfavourable vital signs.

Alteration in level of consciousness

The patient may experience only a decrease in responsiveness to stimuli, confusion or clouding of consciousness, whereas other patients may suddenly or gradually become unconscious. The coma may last a few hours to days; the gravity of prognosis tends to increase if the coma extends beyond 36 hours.

Headache and vomiting

If remaining conscious, the patient may complain of severe headache as a result of increased intracranial pressure. **Vomiting** frequently occurs with the initial onset and may be recurring in the conscious patient.

Neuromuscular deficits

The immediate onset may be accompanied by convulsive movements which may be local or general. The effects of the impairment of neuromuscular control by stroke vary from only a muscular weakness to complete paralysis. Hemiplegia (paralysis of one side of the body) is one of the most common effects of a stroke and indicates interruption of motor pathways. The axons of motor neurones which initiate willed movements in each hemisphere converge into the internal capsule. The motor fibres from each hemisphere cross over in the medulla; as a result, paralysis of one side of the body indicates that the cerebral lesion is on the other side; that is, a stroke in the right side of the brain causes paralysis of the left arm and leg. For a few days, there is a marked loss of tone in the affected muscles and an absence of normal reflexes. Even if the patient is in coma, a greater loss of tone in the affected limbs is recognizable (when flexed the limb falls more quickly in a limp, lifeless manner). Later this flaccidity is replaced by spasticity.

One side of the face may be paralysed, which causes the alternating abnormal distension and retraction with each respiration. The mouth is also drawn to one side.

When conscious, the patient may experience difficulty in swallowing (dysphagia), indicating some paralysis of the swallowing muscles.

Incontinence

Urinary and bowel **incontinence** are common in the early stage. The bladder is atonic and the patient does not experience the desire to void. Later, tone returns and the bladder may become spastic and the patient experiences frequency and urgency. Unless the cerebral damage is extensive, involving both hemispheres, bladder control may be re-established with training. The patient may be insensitive to the defaecation reflex, resulting in incontinence.

Eye changes

The pupils may be unequal in size; the larger of the two is on the side of the lesion. The eyes as well as the head tend to turn to the side of the lesion in the early stage; later the deviations may be reversed. Hemianopia (loss of vision in half of the visual field) occurs and may be temporary. In the unconscious patient, the corneal and pupillary reflexes may be absent and the fundus may reveal papilloedema due to increased intracranial pressure or hypertension.

Impairment of speech

There may be complete or partial loss of the ability to communicate. The speech centre is in the dominant cerebral hemisphere; if the stroke occurs on that side, aphasia is likely to occur. The left hemisphere is dominant in the

Constipation
See chapter 5.1

Vomiting
See chapter 5.1

Incontinence
See chapter 5.4

majority of persons. The patient may not only be unable to communicate verbally but may manifest some impairment of comprehension of either or both written or verbal communication.

The aphasia may take various forms (Box 20.1). In motor or expressive aphasia, the person understands and knows what he or she wants to say but cannot utter the words. In receptive aphasia the person does not comprehend either written or spoken words. If there is total loss of speech and communication it is referred to as global aphasia and indicates a serious, massive lesion.

Mental impairment

A stroke may impair the patient's memory, comprehension, and the ability to reason and make judgements. There may be inability to recognize previously familiar objects or sensory impressions (agnosia) and to use objects correctly (apraxia).

Emotional lability is common: the patient may cry or laugh inappropriately.

Vital signs

The respirations are usually slow and stertorous or may be Cheyne–Stokes. The pulse is usually slow, full and bounding in the initial phase. The temperature may be normal during the first few hours and then become raised. Hyperpyrexia is an unfavourable sign.

Diagnostic procedures

When a stroke occurs, procedures may be carried out to identify the underlying cause because the therapy for an ischaemic stroke differs from that for a haemorrhagic stroke. Diagnostic procedures also may reveal the extent and location of involvement. They may include the following:

- CT – a collection of blood, cerebral oedema or an infarcted area will show up because of a change in density. The scan will also demonstrate the displacement of tissue.

- EEG – to determine the amount of brainwave activity and differentiate a thrombotic or haemorrhagic stroke. High-voltage slow waves are characteristic of a haemorrhagic stroke; if the cause is thrombosis, the tracing usually shows low-voltage slow waves.

- Rarely, a lumbar puncture is done, and in the case of a stroke and infarction there is an increase in the leucocyte count in the CSF; the presence of blood in the CSF indicates haemorrhage.

Ongoing assessment

An initial assessment of the vital signs and neurological status establishes a base for ongoing evaluations and prompt recognition of changes. During the acute phase, vital signs, level of consciousness, and motor and sensory functions are monitored at frequent intervals.

After the acute stage the patient's motor functions and level of awareness are assessed daily. Some improvement may occur day to day as the cerebral oedema and pressure are reduced and collateral circulation is established. The regaining of function tends to follow a pattern in which the facial and swallowing muscles recover first, then those of the lower limbs. Usually, speech and arm function return more slowly and less completely. Observations are made frequently for early signs of complications such as contractures and pressure sores.

Patient problems

- **Coma**

- Alteration in **respiratory process**:
  — ineffective breathing pattern
  — ineffective airway clearance
  — impaired gas exchange

- Potential increased intracranial pressure secondary to cerebral oedema and haemorrhage

- Headache and **vomiting** due to increased intracranial pressure

- Alteration in elimination processes:
  — possible urinary retention with overflow
  — incontinence
  — potential **constipation**, faecal impaction and bowel incontinence

- Alteration in fluid and food intake: deficit due to coma, vomiting and/or dysphagia. The taking of food may also be influenced by difficulty with mastication as well as swallowing

- Potential for injury secondary to neurological deficits, confusion or fits

- Potential **pressure sores** related to immobility and incontinence

- Self-care deficits due to coma, paralysis, impaired cognition and awareness

Glasgow coma Scale
See chapter 2.2

Dyspnoea
See chapter 5.3

Vomiting
See chapter 5.1

Constipation
See chapter 5.1

Pressure sores
See chapter 6.1

Box 20.1 Common types of aphasia

- *Auditory aphasia* – inability to comprehend the spoken word. May be referred to as *word deafness*.

- *Expressive aphasia* – individual understands spoken and written words and knows what he or she wants to say but cannot speak the words. Also referred to as *motor* or *Broca's aphasia*.

- *Global aphasia* – complete aphasia involving both sensory and motor functions that provide all forms of communication.

- *Receptive aphasia* – inability to comprehend spoken, written or tactile symbols. Also referred to as *sensory aphasia*.

- Impaired verbal communication – aphasia

- Impairment of mobility – occurs in varying degrees, ranging from weakness to complete paralysis

- Cognitive dysfunction – impaired awareness, confusion, loss of memory, reasoning and judgement

- Emotional lability – inappropriate responses, for example inappropriate outbursts of anger, crying and laughing. If awareness is not impaired, the patient usually manifests the characteristics of the grieving process (denial, anger, depression, gradual acceptance and resolution)

- Lack of knowledge about rehabilitation and home management.

Goals

In the acute phase the goals are that the patient will not develop complications related to the problems stated above, while in the convalescent and rehabilitative phase additional goals involve the recovery of maximum independence and adaptation to reduced function.

Nursing intervention

A great deal of patience is needed to support both family and patient in striving to meet these goals.

The degree of recovery after a stroke is determined by the size of the haemorrhage and infarction, and is influenced by the patient's age, available rehabilitation programmes, and the individual's personality and behavioural responses. Improvement can occur but deficits that are present after 6 months are usually permanent. Early, sustained and intensive therapy for the highly motivated patient with strong professional and family support frequently results in independence and a very satisfying recovery and quality of life.

Treatment and nursing care of a patient with a thrombotic stroke will differ somewhat with that of a haemorrhagic stroke and, of course, it varies with the degree of cerebral damage and ensuing neurological deficits. In the case of a thrombotic stroke, in evolution, an anticoagulant such as heparin may be administered and efforts are directed to maintaining a normal level of blood pressure. The patient is kept on bedrest with minimal disturbance and environmental stimuli to reduce the potential for haemorrhage. Surgical removal of the thrombus may be undertaken. When the stroke is due to a cerebral haemorrhage, therapy and nursing involve efforts directed towards relief of the increased intracranial pressure, life support measures, relief of hypertension to prevent further bleeding and the prevention of complications.

The care required by the stroke patient during the acute phase following the initial onset differs from that required during the convalescent and rehabilitative phase. The care will also vary with the severity of the CVA and extent of brain damage. During the acute phase, intervention is directed principally towards maintaining life and preventing increased neurological deficits and complications.

Much of the nursing care surrounding problems such as diminished level of consciousness, altered respiratory processes, headache, elimination, personal hygiene and pressure care has already been discussed. Care must be taken with nutrition.

When consciousness is regained, the gag reflex is tested before giving any fluids orally. If the patient can swallow, a soft diet is given and increased progressively to a full balanced diet as tolerated. The hemiplegic patient may have to be fed at first if the dominant arm is affected but, with the necessary assistance, is encouraged to feed unaided as soon as possible to establish independence.

If one side of the face is paralysed, food is placed in the opposite side of the mouth. Mouth care is then given following each meal to remove retained food particles from the affected side to prevent aspiration and the development of ulcers.

Protection from injury is necessary because of the motor deficits and possible seizures. Contractures and deformities may develop as flexor muscles take over and loss of range of joint movement occurs. Limbs are supported in a natural position. Passive movements of all joints are carried out at regular intervals, for example when changing the patient's position.

Sensory function may also be impaired; as well as a reduced sensitivity to pressure, pain and temperature, there may be loss of the ability to know the location of parts of the body in space (impaired spatial perception). Cot sides are kept up; the patient may be disoriented and also, if turning in bed, may not have the normal reflexive muscular responses that would maintain balance and prevent the patient falling from the bed. When allowed up, precautions are taken to prevent falls and accidents (sufficient assistance, hand-rails, walking frames or sticks).

As soon as the condition has stabilized, opportunity is provided for the patient to regain as much independence as possible as active assistance is gradually withdrawn while giving support and encouragement. The call light or buzzer, water, toilet articles and other needed items are placed within the patient's reach. The nurse should encourage the patient to be aware of and to use the affected side if possible.

Heparin or warfarin may be prescribed. The INR (international normalized ratio) blood estimation will be necessary at frequent intervals, initially on alternate days until the correct level of anticoagulation is achieved (normal, 1; controlled, 2.5–3). Care should be taken to ensure that the patient is not taking other drugs that could prolong the clotting time (e.g. aspirin or one of the non-steroidal anti-inflammatory drugs). If the blood pressure is raised, an antihypertensive or diuretic drug may be prescribed. The blood pressure is monitored at frequent, regular intervals; a low normal blood pressure is desirable.

If there is a confirmed diagnosis of cerebral thrombosis or embolism, an anticoagulant such as heparin may be prescribed.

Family assessment

Once a family assessment has been carried out and problems or concerns are identified, the family will require some assistance in developing both short- and long-term plans. Questions may arise about community resources, self-help groups, rehabilitative facilities, home adaptations, social security payments and possibly employment prospects, to name but a few of the areas of long-term concern for the patient and family.

Rehabilitative phase following stroke

Rehabilitation really commences with the initial onset and acute phase: certain aspects of the care received in the early stage of the illness play an important role in the patient's rehabilitation. As soon as the patient is well enough, an assessment is made of residual disabilities and remaining capacities. A multidisciplinary team then becomes involved in plans to assist the patient to develop maximum potential and independence, and to assist the family with the necessary adjustments. Both patient and family should participate in setting achievable goals. Attainment of the goals usually requires months of perseverance and patience. The patient and family naturally experience periods of frustration, depression and pessimism. Activities are taken in steps so that achievement is experienced. Complete restoration to previous functional ability may not be possible but much can be done to restore the patient to a degree of independence that makes life more tolerable.

Impaired communication

The aphasia associated with a stroke is usually expressive in type, although variants do occur. The sudden loss of the ability to communicate creates fear and frustration in the patient; feelings of isolation, insecurity and loneliness develop. The nurse endeavours to allay some of the anxiety by anticipating the patient's needs as much as possible, acknowledging the difficulty and concern and indicating time and willingness to work through the problem. The patient is likely to benefit psychologically from knowing that someone understands and will help. Many aphasic patients recover the ability to communicate to some degree. It is not possible to predict this at the onset; speech is usually recovered very gradually and slowly and requires the assistance of those around the patient. The nurse avoids conveying what may be false optimism at first but reassures the patient and family that special assistance will be given to minimize speech and other neurological deficits. In the early stage, gestures to indicate needs and wishes may be encouraged but should not be accepted indefinitely as established use of them inhibit efforts to speak.

If the services of a speech therapist are available, a retraining programme is planned. In many situations, the nurse will be mainly responsible for helping the patient recover the ability to communicate. It is necessary, as soon as possible, to determine whether the patient can express ideas verbally or by the written word, and whether the spoken and written word is understood. Comprehension may be limited to short simple phrases or single words. Rarely, intellectual impairment occurs (e.g. receptive aphasia) that precludes speech rehabilitation. It is important to talk normally and with ease to the patient; auditory stimulation and socialization can play important roles and are considered as valuable as structured remedial drills.

Loss of speech is no indication that intelligence, comprehension and hearing are impaired. The patient should be included in conversation at all times. Short simple sentences, kept at a functional level relating to present and immediate needs and environment, are used if there is evidence of difficulty in comprehension. When encouraging the patient to try, emphasis is placed on nouns and simple responses such as 'yes' and 'no' at first; then progression through verbs and adjectives to short sentences is made. The necessary retraining in many instances is much the same as the process used with the young child learning to communicate. The use of several sensory avenues is usually more effective than the use of just one at a time. Hearing words in direct association with the objects and the printed words that represent them contributes to recovery.

During speech therapy, the patient should be rested and relaxed and in a quiet undistracting setting. The periods of instruction are kept brief as the patient may tire easily and have a short attention span. Emphasis on exact pronunciation is unnecessary and may lead only to frustration and discouragement.

Early in the illness, the family members and others are helped in understanding the patient's communication problems and their role in the recovery of speech. The importance of conversing normally with the patient, expecting a response, making every effort to understand and giving plenty of time to respond should be emphasized to the family, who should be fully involved in speech therapy. At least one member should be given the opportunity to observe a teaching session carried out in the hospital or rehabilitation unit. The need for patience and the need for providing opportunities for the patient to practise and use what speech he or she has are stressed. The family is advised that progress may be slow and is cautioned against making excessive demands on the patient. Progress should be acknowledged because it encourages and prompts motivation for continued effort.

Impaired mobility

The muscles of affected limbs are flaccid for a few days after CVA, then become spastic. The paralysed arm becomes adducted and flexion occurs at the elbow, wrist, fingers and thumb joints. The lower limb assumes a position of external rotation at the hip, flexion of the thigh and leg, and plantar flexion of the foot. With **immobility**, muscles atrophy and the collagen fibres of the connective tissue of the tendons, ligaments and joint capsules tend to

Immobility
See chapter 3.1

shorten and become dense and firm. The process may be hastened by circulatory stasis, oedema and trauma. As a result, if the affected limbs are permitted to remain immobile in the positions they automatically assume, contractures and reduced range of joint motion may become permanent. Deformities are created which actually increase the person's disability and make rehabilitation difficult. Liaison with the physiotherapist is essential when caring for the stroke patient.

Maintenance of joint motion, support to prevent the pull of gravity on joints and subsequent subluxation, and positioning to prevent contractures and maintain good alignment are essential from the onset of the stroke.

When lying on the unaffected side, the patient's unaffected shoulder is brought slightly forward and the arm should lie straight, in line with the trunk. The unaffected leg should be straight. A pillow is placed under the affected arm, which is straightened at the elbow; the hand is straightened, with the fingers spread over the upper part of the pillow. The affected leg is flexed at the knee and hip, with a pillow underneath for support. A pillow is placed along the back of the patient for support.

When the patient is lying on the affected side, a reverse, similar position is adopted, except that the unaffected arm is flexed at the elbow, with the hand towards the edge of the bed. The affected leg is flexed slightly at the knee. Pillows are this time placed under the unaffected, not the affected, limbs for support and to prevent friction and pressure. A pillow at the back should support the patient.

Marked spasticity of the affected hand may necessitate the application of a padded splint, especially at night, to prevent flexure contractures of the wrist and fingers. A support may be provided to prevent foot drop.

The limbs are passively moved through a full range of movements two or three times daily. While the patient is dependent and confined to bed, the position is changed and passive movements are carried out every 2 hours.

The stroke patient is usually assisted out of bed for progressively increasing periods as soon as the condition has stabilized. Balance should be assessed and improved (if possible) before walking is commenced. Being up reduces the possibility of complications and may help to promote a more positive attitude on the part of the patient towards the future. When the patient is up, support of the affected arm in a sling may sometimes be necessary to prevent subluxation of the shoulder joint. A pillow may be used to support the arm when sitting in a chair.

Most hemiplegic patients fortunately experience extensor spasm of the affected knee and hip muscles with weight-bearing, which stabilizes the leg as the unaffected leg is carried through a forward step. Some patients do experience spasm of flexor rather than extensor muscle in the affected leg and as a result, when the patient attempts to walk, the knee and hip flex and do not support him or her. This necessitates the application of a leg brace for stabilization. When assisting the patient who is walking, the nurse or family member provides support from the affected side. An aid, such as a walking frame, may be required to help regain independence. When plantar flexion and toe-dragging interfere with walking, a drop-foot splint may be used. A few hemiplegic patients suffer ataxia and loss of balance which may prevent walking and confine the patient to a wheelchair.

As soon as possible the retraining for self-care is begun. Retraining carried out by the occupational therapist and the nurse includes the simple useful functions on which every person is dependent in normal living. Examples are dressing and undressing, opening doors, using the telephone, writing and the handling of various articles (e.g. cutlery). The hemiplegic patient is taught how to change position in bed (turn, sit up, transfer to a chair, stand up). The bed is lowered and made stationary when transfer techniques are carried out. A schedule of exercises is established to strengthen the trunk and unaffected limb muscles. The programme includes the affected limbs; if the muscles are weak, active assistive and active exercises are used. If the muscles are unresponsive, passive movements are carried out to prevent contractures and ankylosis.

Sensory deficits

The patient is assessed for possible impairment of sensory functions such as pain, pressure and temperature. There may also be loss of the ability to know the location of parts of the body in space (proprioception deficit) making the judging of distances and movements more difficult. The patient's vision may also be impaired by the loss of function in the corresponding halves of the visual fields (homonymous hemianopia) in both eyes. The inability to recognize objects by touch, sight or hearing may be manifested. The necessary precautions are established to prevent accidents such as falls and burns, and become an important part of the rehabilitation programme.

Patient teaching

The patient may be required to continue taking an anticoagulant; therefore it is important to teach both patient and family its purpose and the importance of prompt reporting of signs of bleeding. A balanced diet with less fat content may be recommended and a dietary plan reviewed with the patient and family that will meet caloric needs according to weight and energy expenditure. The patient is strongly advised against smoking. It is recommended that younger female patients should not take contraceptive pills.

Predischarge planning

The total care and rehabilitation programme should be fully discussed with a member of the family. The importance of encouraging and permitting the patient to do things unaided is emphasized. Family and friends find it difficult to stand back while the patient struggles and perseveres with activities. Before discharge, the patient may be encouraged to spend 1 or 2 days at home (e.g. at the weekend) and a home assessment may be carried out by appropriate personnel.

After discharge from hospital, both patient and family still require considerable support and assistance; referrals should be made to appropriate support and community services. Modifications of the home may be necessary to facilitate the development of independence and prevent accidents. Handrails in the bathroom, placement of articles for ready accessibility, and making the bed stationary are a few examples of adjustments that may be made.

The assistance of social services may be necessary to help solve the problems imposed by the illness and residual disabilities. The family should be taught to recognize signs of resentment at loss of independence by the patient. By listening to their points of view, by explaining the patient's condition and unusual patterns of behaviour, and by helping the family to organize themselves so that all share in the increased responsibility, complete rejection of the patient may be prevented.

Social contact

The patient is encouraged to develop interests and worthwhile hobbies and gradually to assume responsibility for domestic tasks as far as possible. The performance of some useful tasks promotes the patient's morale and greater harmony within the family.

Friends are encouraged to visit and the patient should be included in the social activities of the family. Domestic arrangements may, however, be less than ideal. The patient may live alone in a large house with no close family or live in a small flat in considerable poverty. Elderly patients may have several concurrent medical problems as well as social problems to contend with. Whatever the difficulties, nurses should not be judgemental about families who refuse to have an elderly relative to live with them after a CVA; this will serve no useful purpose for the patient, and antagonism between family and hospital staff is in nobody's interests. The patient may now have to face leaving a home they have lived in for many decades, losing their independence in the process, although this is to be avoided if at all possible – hence the importance of community care.

The person with trauma of the nervous system

Head injuries

Accidents on the roads, in industry and sports, and violence on the streets and in the home are the major causes of head injury, which ranks high on the list of causes of morbidity, mortality and permanent disabilities, particularly in young adults. Frequently, head injury is only one of the major problems seen in the traumatized patient and priorities of care are established on the basis of the assessment of the patient as a whole person.

The classification of head injury is underpinned by the pathological processes that have occurred as a result of injury (e.g. a skull fracture). However, all these processes are influenced in one way or another by the level of intracranial pressure (ICP) and cerebral perfusion pressure (CPP).

Intracranial pressure

This is defined as the measurable pressure exerted by the **CSF** within the ventricles of the brain. It is a phenomenon that constantly changes with transient rises during sneezing and coughing. Raised ICP or intracranial hypertension is when the pressure is increased as the result of trauma or disease and remains so for a period of time. It can be a very serious – sometimes fatal – complication of traumatic brain injury as a result of haemorrhage, brain swelling and/or oedema. These complications can also occur in disorders such as neoplasm where a tumour can act as a space-occupying lesion.

The normal ICP is 0–15 mmHg. This is dependent on normal functioning of the brain, CSF and cerebral blood volume within the rigid bony skull. An increase in the volume of any one of these (brain, blood or CSF) causes an increase in the ICP and a comparable decrease in the volume of one or both of the other contents. The response may be:

CSF
See chapter 2.2

1. Displacement of CSF.

2. A compromise in cerebral blood supply which causes cerebral ischaemia. The latter leads to hypoxia, hypercapnia and acidosis at cellular level, resulting in interruption of cell metabolism.

3. Displacement of brain tissue (herniation).

As ICP begins to rise, compensatory mechanisms come into play. These include the removal of CSF from the intracranial cavity into the distensible spinal sac; reduction of cerebral blood flow by constriction of the cerebral blood vessels (autoregulation); and shifting of brain tissue to produce internal herniation. The volume–pressure curve (Fig. 20.13) demonstrates this phenomenon. The flattened part of the curve represents the compensatory mechanisms, while the steepened part of the curve represents their exhaustion in a process known as decompression. The timescale over which this occurs will vary. In a patient with a severe head injury it may only be minutes, whereas for the patient with a slow growing tumour it may be years.

Cerebral perfusion pressure is the pressure required to maintain perfusion of the sensitive nervous tissue. This is necessary to maintain adequate oxygenation of the brain and the provision of essential glucose. Normal CPP is in the range 70–100 mmHg, and reductions below this level in the neurologically impaired patient can have a deleterious effect on brain functioning.

If pressure is distributed unequally between two compartments, tissue will move from the area of higher pressure to the lower one. This is known as herniation or coning, and occurs in several stages (Fig. 20.14). Initially there is a shift of tissue across the brain from the side where the space-occupying lesion is located. This results in the displacement of structures found in the midline. These include the lateral ventricles and the falx cerebri; thus this is termed a subfalcine herniation. This is referred to as a right to left or left to right midline shift, as appropriate. Once the pressure in the supratentorial compartment has equalized, it is greater than that in the posterior fossa below, thus downward herniation follows. This is termed tentorial herniation and may occur on one or both sides. One consequence of this is that pressure is now applied

Figure 20.13 Intracranial volume–pressure curve.

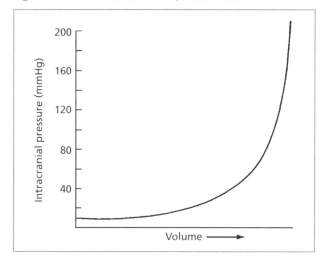

Figure 20.14 Herniation of brain tissue.

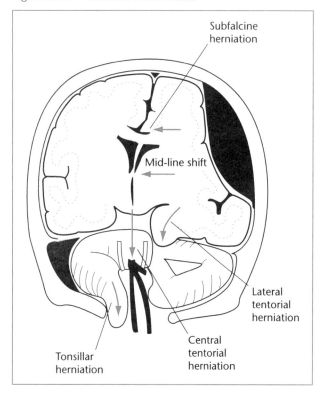

directly to the third cranial nerve (oculomotor nerve). This controls constriction of the pupil; thus, when the nerve is compressed it no longer functions and the pupil becomes fixed and possibly dilated. Pressure is now beginning to build on the brainstem where the vital centres are located. Changes seen at this late stage would include a widening pulse pressure, a slowing of the heart rate, and a reduction in the respiratory rate and possibly apnoea.

Another type of herniation may occur, known as *tonsillar herniation*. A space-occupying lesion in the posterior fossa compressing the cerebellum may force the cerebellar tonsils to herniate downwards with a similar effect on the brainstem.

Causes of increased ICP are swelling of the brain, increased CSF volume and increased blood volume. Swelling of the brain may be due to haemorrhage following trauma, a tumour (increased mass of tissue cells), abscess, inflammatory exudate or cerebral oedema. An increase in the cranial volume of CSF is usually associated with a disturbance in the absorption or outflow of the fluid; it accumulates in the ventricles, compressing brain tissue and blood vessels. An increase in the intracranial blood volume may be due to compression of the venous sinuses or jugular veins, vasodilatation of the cerebral vessels or be associated with trauma.

Classification of head injury

Head injuries may be classified as open or closed, coup or contrecoup, and primary or secondary:

1. *Closed head injury* refers to injury in which there is no break in the tissues (scalp and skull) that separate the intracranial cavity from the external environment (e.g. subdural haematoma).

2. *Open head injury* means that a break exists in the tissues that separate the intracranial contents from the external environment (e.g. perforating skull fracture).

3. *Coup and contrecoup injuries* result from direct trauma to the head in which the sequence of intracranial events resembles an acceleration–deceleration phenomenon:
   a. *Coup* refers to bruising of the brain tissue that directly underlies the site of impact and that rebounds against that portion of the cranium.
   b. *Contrecoup* is brain injury on the side opposite the site of impact. It is due to the wave of pressure created by the impact, compressing the brain substance against the bony ridges and opposite wall of the cranium. For example, a fall on to the back of the head may cause injury to the frontal and temporal cerebral lobes. Injury to the nerve fibres and blood vessels in the brainstem results from the stress of shearing forces.

The mechanisms of head injury are described in Fig. 20.15.

Primary head injuries

Fracture of the skull

A skull fracture is particularly significant if there is communication between the intracranial contents and the outside (open head injury), or there is depression of a piece of skull, compressing the brain below. If the fracture involves the base of the skull, CSF leakage occurs and there is potential communication between the oropharynx and the meninges, leading to the risk of infection entering the meninges, known as *meningitis*.

No specific treatment is used for a simple linear or comminuted skull fracture, but the patient is kept at rest and under close observation because of potential bleeding and haematoma. Meningeal blood vessels may have been torn and incur extradural, subdural or subarachnoid haemorrhage. Concussion or contusion of the brain is a frequent result.

Early surgical exploration is indicated when a depressed fracture occurs. Skull fragments are elevated and splinters and debris removed. Severe fragmentation and depression may necessitate removal of that area of the skull. Later, a cranioplasty may be done: a plate of inert material (e.g. titanium) is inserted to protect the brain and improve the patient's appearance.

Brain injury

Injury to the brain may result from a blow to the head and may or may not be associated with a fracture of the skull. A head injury may cause concussion, cerebral contusion or laceration, haemorrhage and/or compression.

A brain injury may be mild and reversible or may be severe and irreversible, leaving residual neurological deficits if the patient survives. Oedema of the brain and intracranial haemorrhage increase intracranial pressure which, if severe, may compress the brainstem and its vital centres (supratentorial herniation). Initially, *every head injury is considered serious.* It must be emphasized that, regardless of outward appearance, the person requires close observation for evidence of developing secondary brain damage that could result in permanent disability or death.

Concussion

Concussion is characterized by a brief period of unconsciousness due to jarring of the brain and its sudden forceful contact with the rigid skull. The period of unconsciousness is usually at most only a few minutes, depending on the severity of the injury. When the patient regains consciousness, he or she may be confused, dazed and restless, and be unable to recall events that preceded the accident. Headache is a common complaint. If there is no haemorrhage or brain tissue damage, no abnormal neurological findings are present: normal reflexes and muscle tone return.

Nursing intervention

This includes observation for evidence of neurological deterioration if the patient is admitted and, if discharged, ensuring that a reliable person is available. The responsible person is instructed to remain with the patient. If the patient becomes increasingly drowsy or difficult to rouse, or if he or she experiences headache, vomiting, visual

Figure 20.15   Mechanisms of head injury.

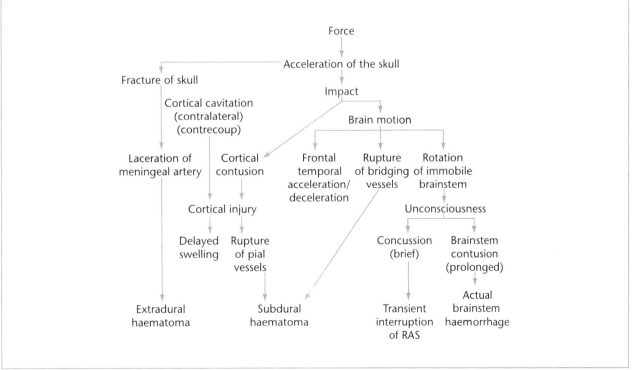

disturbances, seizures or a reduction in limb strength, the patient should be brought back to hospital by ambulance immediately. It is advisable to provide instructions in writing for the responsible person because anxiety may affect the ability to recall what has been said. Recovery following an uncomplicated concussion occurs within a short period of time, although some side-effects may persist for weeks.

Cerebral contusion and laceration

Cerebral contusion and laceration refers to bruising and tearing of superficial brain tissue. The multiple areas of tissue damage may give rise to a wide variety of patient responses. It must be emphasized that a patient with a head injury may have significant trauma and still be alert initially. Lesions of the brainstem are usually the most serious. Level of consciousness may be altered for several hours or weeks. A variety of other neurological abnormalities is usually present on both sides of the body. If neurological signs are present on one side of the body, it is probable that a secondary event such as the development of a haematoma has occurred. The tissue injury is usually accompanied by brain swelling and oedema. Recovery may be a lengthy process; permanent tissue damage and scarring may result in permanent disability if the patient survives.

Secondary events following head injury

Intracranial haemorrhage

Haemorrhage within the cranium and the formation of a haematoma following a head injury frequently leads to a rapid deterioration in the patient's condition. The bleeding may be extradural, subdural, subarachnoid or intracerebral. The clinical characteristics presented are due to increased intracranial pressure and compression of areas of the brain.

Extradural haematoma

An extradural haematoma is an accumulation of blood between the dura and skull (Fig. 20.16) and is a serious complication. As the meningeal artery is frequently torn, extradural bleeding is at arterial pressure. The brain is compressed and displaced, and the ICP rises rapidly. The patient may be comatose for a brief period, regain consciousness, then gradually develop serious neurological symptoms (disturbed vision, dilated pupil and loss of reflex to light in the eye on the affected side, severe headache, confusion, decreased motor and sensory function, seizure, vomiting) and loss of consciousness. Prompt treatment is essential. If an extradural haemorrhage is not recognized and promptly treated, the rapidly increasing ICP may cause tentorial herniation, pressure on vital centres and death within a few hours.

Subdural haemorrhage

Subdural haemorrhage is another possible complication of head injury. Blood accumulates in the subdural space (Fig. 20.16), gradually forming a haematoma which compresses the brain and increases intracranial pressure.

The bleeding may occur following a seemingly minor head injury. As the bleeding is usually at venous pressure, the development of symptoms may be delayed and vague but progressively worsen and, eventually, increasing ICP and brain compression lead to coma.

All head injuries should therefore be treated initially as serious and a potential threat to life.

Subdural haemorrhage may be subacute or chronic in patients of advanced age or with cortical atrophy. In these patients, evidence of increased ICP usually appears very gradually and intermittently.

Subarachnoid haemorrhage

Subarachnoid haemorrhage is bleeding of cerebral vessels into the space between the arachnoid and pia mater. The clinical characteristics are similar to those presented by the patient with a subdural haemorrhage and depend on the area of the brain involved. This is rarely seen in trauma and is much more likely to be due to a cerebral aneurysm.

Intracerebral haemorrhage

Intracerebral haemorrhage is bleeding resulting from a torn or diseased vessel within the cerebrum. It may occur as a result of contrecoup injury, a penetrating wound such as a gun-shot or stabbing, or a CVA (stroke). The symptoms depend on the particular vessel and cerebral area (Fig. 20.16).

Medical management

The head-injured patient with raised ICP can present in a number of different ways. They may be fully alert and oriented presenting with a history of injury accompanied by very mild and transient symptoms, or they may arrive with full paramedical support deeply unconscious. Neurological deficits can usually be found, for example alteration of conscious level, occurrence of a seizure or onset of confusion. Depending on the severity of injury, the initial assessment will be aided if the following information can be ascertained (Lindsay and Bone 1997):

- *Period of loss of consciousness* – relates to the severity of brain damage (i.e. the longer the patient is unconscious, the more severe the damage).

- *Period of post-traumatic amnesia (PTA)* – the period of permanent amnesia that occurs after head injury; it is an indicator of the severity of brain damage (i.e. the longer the period of PTA, the worse the brain damage).

- *Cause and circumstances of the injury* – this may indicate whether other extracranial injuries exist.

- *Presence of headache or vomiting* – these would indicate the possibility of intracranial haemorrhage.

Table 20.6 (p. 702) lists the signs and symptoms of raised ICP.

A head-injured patient should initially be assessed and managed according to clear principles and standards as embodied in the Advanced Trauma Life Support (ATLS)

Subarachnoid
haemorrhage
See chapter 2.2

Figure 20.16 Cranial haematomas. (a) Extradural haematoma. (b) Subdural haematoma. (c) Intracerebral haemorrhage.

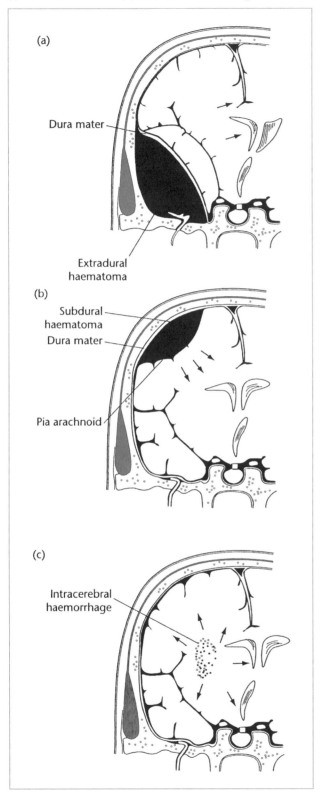

assessment of conscious level, pupil response, limb weakness and eye movements.

Investigations include skull radiography (to demonstrate fractures), computed tomography (CT) and magnetic resonance imaging (MRI) (may demonstrate cerebral contusions or lacerations and/or an intracranial haematoma) (Hickey 1997).

Intracranial pressure monitoring

A typical system comprises a fibreoptic transducer-tipped catheter, which can be placed in the lateral ventricle, subdural space or extradural space. Less emphasis is now placed on the data obtained from ICP monitoring. It is suggested that the maintenance of CPP is more important (CPP = mean BP − ICP) than just treating raised ICP. This is because it has been shown that patients with a high ICP, low blood pressure and low CPP make a poorer recovery. Measures to reduce ICP must not be used indiscriminately and several guidelines have been issued on this. It is suggested that ICP and CPP monitoring are most relevant for the patient with a flexion response (or worse) to painful stimuli, but this policy will vary depending on a number of factors. The aim is to maintain CPP at more than 70 mmHg.

A number of approaches may be adopted in the management of the patient, and these can be regarded as a menu from which some or all are selected to treat a particular individual depending upon the circumstances. They include the use of hyperosmolar agents, controlled hyperventilation, fluid management, sedatives and surgical intervention.

Hyperosmolar agents

These act by establishing an osmotic gradient between the plasma and brain tissue, thus removing water from the oedematous brain tissue to the blood. An intravenous infusion of 100 mL of 20% mannitol over 15 min is a typical adult dose. This will 'buy' time to allow the patient to be prepared for transfer to a specialist unit or for operation. However, if repeated boluses are administered the effect of the drug is neutralized, leading to a rebound increase in ICP (Davies and Lucatorto 1994).

Controlled hyperventilation

To achieve this, the patient needs to be paralysed, intubated and mechanically ventilated. Vasoconstriction is achieved as the result of reducing the arterial partial pressure of carbon dioxide ($Paco_2$), which in turn reduces cerebral blood volume and ICP. It is suggested by Lindsay and Bone (1997) that the resultant reduction in cerebral blood flow may itself cause brain damage. Maintaining the blood pressure and CPP appears to be as important, if not more so, than lowering ICP. It is necessary to measure the amount of oxygen extracted from the brain using a jugular bulb catheter to determine whether or not the brain can withstand further vasoconstriction.

system and, for children, the Advanced Paediatric Life Support (PALS) system (Scottish Intercollegiate Guidelines Network 2000). Clinical assessment will include seeking evidence of injury including basal skull fracture signs,

Table 20.6 Signs and symptoms of raised intracranial pressure

Sign/symptom	Reasons
Early	
Deterioration in conscious level	The most highly specialized cells of the brain are the most sensitive to the oxygen deprivation that occurs with raised ICP. The response to this is that the patient becomes more drowsy
Pupillary dysfunction	Compression of the third cranial nerve (oculomotor) as a result of herniation causes pupillary dilatation, usually on the same side as the space-occupying lesion causing the rise in ICP
Motor weakness	A weakness (hemiparesis) on one side can occur, usually on the opposite side to the space-occupying lesion
Headache	This is initially mild and is thought to occur because the pain-sensitive structures at the base of the brain are distorted. It is usually described as being worse in the morning and improves as the day proceeds. This is because it is known that ICP rises during REM sleep
Papilloedema	Caused by raised ICP when the optic nerve becomes swollen and congested. May be present as an early sign in the patient with a slowly progressing rise in ICP
Later	
Continuing deterioration in the level of consciousness	As ICP continues to rise the patient becomes drowsier and eventually comatose
Vomiting	Thought to be caused by direct pressure on the vomiting centre and is unusual in adults. The mechanism is not fully understood. When it does occur, it tends to be projectile and is not accompanied by nausea
Hemiplegia, decerebration, decortication	This is a later stage to the process described in motor weakness above. Hemiplegia is paralysis of the limbs on one side of the body
Alterations in vital signs	With pressure on the brainstem increasing, changes in blood pressure and pulse become evident. In an attempt to ensure that the brain remains adequately perfused in the face of a rising ICP, blood pressure rises also and eventually the pulse pressure (i.e. the difference between the systolic and diastolic pressures) begins to widen. This is referred to *Cushing's response*. For similar reasons, the pulse becomes full and bounding, and becomes slower
Respiratory irregularities	The brain's attempt to boost the supply of oxygen in response to a rising ICP results in a rise in the respiratory rate quickly followed by a reduction until eventually apnoea supervenes
Papilloedema	May be late finding in some patients when the ICP is markedly increased
Impaired brainstem reflexes	In the latest stages, sustained pressure on the brainstem as a result of herniation results in dysfunction of brainstem reflexes. The testing of these reflexes forms the basis of brainstem death testing

Fluid management

This approach to treatment has been the subject of much debate over time. Some advocate restricting fluid in order to induce slight dehydration. By controlling intake, the extracellular fluid, including that of the brain, is decreased thus reducing ICP. The intake may be set at 1–2.5 litres per 24 hours. However, some now advocate achieving normovolaemia or increasing fluids. Doing this increases cerebral blood flow and thus improves oxygen delivery to the brain.

Sedatives

Traditionally patients with a head injury were never sedated for fear of masking important signs relating to conscious level. However, there are now special circumstances under which sedation might be used. If ICP fails to respond to standard measures then sedation may help under carefully controlled conditions (Lindsay and Bone 1997). Drugs that may be used include propofol and etomidate, although each has associated ill effects that must be countered. Propofol causes vasodilatation that may need to be counteracted to prevent blood pressure from falling and a reduction in cerebral perfusion. Etomidate inhibits steroid synthesis, and so steroid cover is required.

Surgical intervention

Surgery may be performed to remove a focal mass lesion such as an expanding haematoma, and this may be combined with decompression. Withdrawal of small aliquots of CSF via a ventricular catheter results in a reduction of ICP but this provides only temporary relief. To be effective, drainage would require to be continuous, but this is often impractical.

Nursing assessment: altered consciousness

The priority in nursing assessment following head injury is assessment of conscious level.

Interruption of impulses from the reticular activating system, or failure of the cerebral cortical neurones to respond to incoming impulses, produces a loss of consciousness. Other than destruction of the cortical or cortical activating cells (reticular formation) by trauma, the basic factors contributing to unconsciousness are considered to be oxygen and glucose deprivation. Neurones require a constant supply of both of these substances for cellular activity. A deficiency of oxygen for even a few seconds decreases neuronal metabolism to a point at which unconsciousness ensues. Fig. 20.17 describes the effects of alterations in level of consciousness from a state of normal awareness to coma or unconsciousness.

Causes

The patient's level of consciousness may be depressed due to the effects of abnormal metabolic processes or disease, including trauma, involving the brain or brainstem:

1. Processes that may interfere with the *metabolism* of the brainstem and cerebral cortex:
   a. hypoglycaemia or diabetic ketoacidosis, which produces a deficiency of glucose that is essential for cerebral neuronal functioning
   b. respiratory failure, which produces cerebral hypoxia
   c. renal and hepatic failure, which cause an accumulation of metabolic wastes
   d. electrolyte imbalance
   e. infections and autoimmune disorders
   f. drug overdose.

Patients' manifestations resulting from altered metabolism show symmetrical changes in motor function.

2. *Space-occupying lesions* affecting the brain may alter the level of consciousness, and include cerebral haemorrhage from vascular diseases and trauma, tumours, abscess and haematoma from skull injuries. Manifestations are usually unequal on each side and may include hemiplegia and small reactive pupils which later become fixed.

3. *Brainstem lesions* that may cause unconsciousness include cerebral haemorrhage and brainstem infarction, tumours and abscesses, as well as trauma that produces direct pressure on the reticular formation tissue in the brainstem. Symptoms include loss of reflexes and pupillary reactions. Patients with trauma or metabolic disturbance will show signs of generalized brain dysfunction rather than focal signs;

Figure 20.17   Signs of altered consciousness.

NORMAL CONSCIOUSNESS

1 Eyes open, oculomotor activity is normal
Spontaneous interaction with environment; oriented normal speech

Normal voluntary motor and reflex function

2 Eyes open to speech
Talks but is disoriented about time and/or place and person
May still obey commands slowly with repeated requests

3 Opens eyes to painful stimulus
Conversation is not initiated or sustained; words are inappropriate
Tries to remove painful stimulus or flexes to pain

4 Eyes generally closed
Moans and groans but no recognizable words
Flexes or extends to painful stimuli

COMA

5 No response

Glasgow Coma Scale
See chapter 2.2

it is important to assess overall brain function and vital signs frequently.

Assessment of level of consciousness

Decrease in responsiveness to stimuli indicates progressive deterioration in brain function. The chance of complete recovery decreases with increase in the duration of impaired consciousness; decrease in responsiveness to stimuli must be reported immediately in order that measures can be implemented to reduce the risk of irreversible neurological dysfunction or death.

A standardized approach to the measurement of conscious level is essential for improved patient care. Use of a standardized system eliminates confusing language in the description of conscious level and permits efficient transfer of information from one observer to another. An approach that takes this into account is the **Glasgow Coma Scale** (GCS).

Glasgow coma scale

The GCS provides for evaluation of eye opening and the best verbal and motor responses. Within each of these three parameters, there is a variety of responses which are arranged in scales of increasing dysfunction, as outlined in Figure 20.18. Each aspect is assessed independently of the others.

Figure 20.18   Glasgow Coma Scale record sheet.

					Date
Name					
Record No.					Time
C O M A S C A L E	Eyes open	Spontaneously			Eyes closed by swelling =C
		To speech			
		To pain			
		None			
	Best verbal response	Orientated			Endotracheal tube or tracheostomy =T
		Confused			
		Inappropriate words			
		Incomprehensible sounds			
		None			
	Best motor response	Obey commands			Usually record the best arm response
		Localize pain			
		Flexion to pain			
		Extension to pain			
		None			

Eye opening

- *Spontaneous opening* (4). The nurse approaches the patient's bedside and notes whether the eyes are open or closed. Spontaneous opening of the eyes indicates that the arousal mechanism in the reticular activating system of the brainstem is functioning.

- *Opening to speech* (3). If the patient's eyes are closed, the observer speaks, addressing the patient by name. If there is no response to a normal speaking voice, the volume should be increased.

- *Opening to pain* (2). Physical stimulation, in the form of pressure on the fingernail bed using a pencil or pen, is applied. It is important that observers use the same method of applying physical stimulation to ensure consistent, accurate findings.

- *No eye opening* (1). If no response is demonstrated in either eye to increased pain stimuli, there is depression of the arousal system.

The patient may be sufficiently alert to respond by opening his or her eyes, but is restricted by swelling of the eyelids. If the eyelids are swollen shut, the observer records this as a 'C'.

Best verbal response

The patient's ability to speak and to understand the language spoken are determined. If the patient is intubated or has a tracheostomy, verbal response cannot be observed and 'T' is recorded. Speech is first used to stimulate a verbal response by asking the patient simple, direct questions. If there is no response, a painful stimulus is applied. The recommended method for this is illustrated in Figure 20.19. The patient's responses are rated as follows:

- *Oriented* (5). The patient is able to respond as to who he or she is, where he or she is, and can give the year, month and day.

- *Confused* (4). The patient is not fully oriented to time, place and person.

- *Inappropriate* (3). The patient utters words in a disorganized way, swears or does not engage in meaningful conversation.

- *Incomprehensible* (2). Responses are limited to moaning, groaning or mumbling sounds with no recognizable words.

- *No response* (1). No sounds are made in response to noxious stimuli.

Figure 20.19   Fingernail-bed stimulus.

Best motor response

The best possible motor response in either arm is observed and recorded. The patient is asked to raise the arms and hold them outstretched for 10 seconds. The ratings in order of decreasing levels of function include the following:

- *Obeys commands* (6). The patient understands verbal, written instructions or gestures and performs the requested movement.

- *Localization to pain* (5). There is no response to command. When a painful stimulus is applied, such as pressure on the fingernail bed, the patient moves a limb in an attempt to locate and remove the stimulus.

- *Flexion to pain* (4). The arms bends at the elbow in response to fingernail bed pressure. Leg flexion is not a reliable gauge because, with brain death, a spinal reflex may be present causing the legs to flex in response to localized pain.

- *Abnormal flexion* (3). The arm flexes at the elbow and sometimes pronates, making a fist.

- *Extension to pain* (2). The elbow straightens and the arm abducts (usually with internal rotation) in response to localized pain applied to the fingernail bed.

- *No response* (1). No detectable movement or change in the tone of the limbs is observed in response to repeated and varied stimuli.

Abnormal flexion, extension and no response are all abnormal.

Other neurological parameters

Assessment of pupil responses and limb movements provides information and assists in localizing lesions; for example, if the pupil starts to dilate, pressure on the third cranial nerve is present, and neighbouring parasympathetic fibres that control pupillary constriction are affected. This may indicate coning or herniation of brain tissue through the tentorial hiatus.

Pupils

Each pupil is examined for size and reaction. Normally, the pupils are round in shape, equal in size, and constrict in response to direct light. The *size* of each pupil is measured by comparing it with the pupil scale, as illustrated in Figure 20.20. Pupil *reaction* is measured in response to light; the beam of a pentorch is brought in from the patient's side and directed on one eye at a time.

The surroundings should be dimly lit and the light beam of adequate intensity to obtain accurate results.

Limb movement

Verbal commands are used to elicit movement in each limb. When the patient does not respond to commands, painful stimuli are applied to the nailbed of a finger or great toe. Responses in order of decreasing function are recorded as:

- *Normal power* – the limb movements are appropriate to the normal muscle strength for the patient.

- *Mild weakness* – one limb shows normal strength but its opposite is weaker.

- *Severe weakness* – the difference between two limbs is very much marked.

- *Spastic flexion* – there is slow, stiff movement of the arm with the flexed forearm and hand held against the body.

- *Extension* – the elbow or knee are straightened in response to painful stimulation.

- *No response* – painful stimulation produces no movement and the limb remains limp.

It is important to compare each side and to record differences between right and left limbs and changes in the responses of an individual limb.

Vital signs

Changes in the pulse rate and rhythm and in blood pressure provide information about possible increased ICP, internal bleeding or shock. A decrease in the respiratory rate indicates pressure in the respiratory centre in the brainstem as a result of raised ICP.

It should be remembered that any changes in the patient's cerebral condition will manifest first as changes in level of consciousness, hence the importance of frequent and accurate observation, using the Glasgow Coma Scale.

The symptoms are summarized in Box 20.2. It should be remembered that a decreased level of consciousness is the first warning of an expanding brain lesion.

Emergency care

Priorities require to be established as follows:

1. Assessment of respiratory status and correction of deficits (airway and breathing).

2. Assessment of conscious level and other neurological parameters including the risk of neck injury.

3. Assessment of other injuries.

Figure 20.20   Record sheet for other neurological parameters.

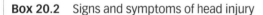

Pupil scale (mm)			

Pupil scale (mm): 1, 2, 3, 4, 5, 6, 7, 8

Blood pressure and pulse: 240 230 220 210 200 190 180 170 160 150 140 130 120 110 100 90 80 70 60 50 40

Respiration: 30 26 22 18 14 10 6

Temperature °C: 40 39 38 37 36 35 34 33 32 31 30

PUPILS	Right	Size
		Reaction
	Left	Size
		Reaction

Limb movements	Arms	Normal power
		Mild weakness
		Severe weakness
		Extension
		No response
	Legs	Normal power
		Mild weakness
		Severe weakness
		Extension
		No response

+ reacts
− no reaction
c.eye closed

Record right (R) and left (L) separately if there is a difference between the two sides

---

Box 20.2   Signs and symptoms of head injury

- Loss of consciousness, which may develop at the time of injury and last for a varying length of time

- Recurrence of unconsciousness following a lucid interval

- Drowsiness and stupor progressing to coma

- Severe headache or dizziness

- Disturbed vision

- Dilatation and failure to react to light of one or both pupils

- Motor and sensory deficits, seizures, nuchal rigidity, speech impairment, disorientation, changes in vital signs indicative of increasing intracranial pressure (see p. 707)

- The escape of CSF from the ear or nose

Glasgow Coma Scale
See chapter 2.2

Patient problems

The following is a list of some of the main problems encountered in the early stages of recovery from brain injury:

- Respiratory dysfunction secondary to:
  — loss of patency of airway
  — injury to or compression of the respiratory centre in the brainstem.

- Alteration in **level of consciousness**.

- Alteration in comfort when conscious – mild to severe headache.

- Motor and sensory deficits due to brain compression and damage.

- Alteration in level of awareness of self and environment.

- Potential for injury related to reduced level of consciousness, confusion, motor and sensory deficits or seizures.

- Impairment of skin integrity secondary to scalp wound or immobility (pressure sores).

- Alteration in fluid and food intake secondary to comatose state, fluid intake restrictions per 24 hours, or anxiety.

- Alteration in elimination patterns:
  a. **urinary** (incontinence, retention)
  b. bowel (**constipation** and potential impaction).

- Self-care deficits affecting personal hygiene secondary to unconsciousness, enforced immobility or motor deficits.

- Anxiety related to confusion and loss of memory of previous events.

- Lack of knowledge about diagnostic and therapeutic procedures, condition, hospitalization and post-hospital care.

Goals

The fundamental goal is that the patient will regain consciousness with no long-term deficits. This involves a series of short-term goals, such as a normal breathing pattern and patent airway, avoiding further injury and the complications of having a decreased level of consciousness leading to confusion and immobility. Goals relating to normal body function such as fluid intake and output should also be set.

Nursing intervention

The special considerations previously described for nursing the patient with an altered conscious level, raised ICP, and preoperative and postoperative care are applicable to the head-injured patient.

The head-injured patient is at risk of infection if an open scalp wound is present; the wound is cleansed, debrided if necessary, and sutured. A reinforcing dose of tetanus toxoid may be prescribed as a prophylactic measure, or human tetanus immunoglobulin may be given.

Loss of the corneal reflexes, periorbital oedema and ecchymoses are common problems with a head injury. If the corneal reflex is absent, the eyelid may be taped shut with non-allergic tape to protect the cornea from drying and abrasions. The tape is removed every 2 hours and the eye irrigated with normal saline and artificial tears instilled before retaping. If the eyelids are swollen, it may be necessary for a second nurse to hold the lids open while pupillary reflexes are assessed. If the lids cannot be opened, the doctor is notified; it is important that pupillary changes be detected in sufficient time to institute treatment.

Hyperthermia may develop following head injury due to a disturbance of the temperature control centre in the hypothalamus leading to temperatures of 40°C or more. Vigorous interventions are required to reduce such extremely high temperatures.

Nursing interventions following head injury will be determined by the extent and circumstances of the patient's injury. Interventions can be considered as those required in the acute or emergency phase immediately after the injury, in the ongoing phase immediately following the acute one, and finally discharge/rehabilitation requirements. The timespan over which this continuum extends can be as little as a few days to several months. Within the continuum there are four significant care events that may be required. These include:

1. caring for the patient with raised ICP

2. caring for the unconscious patient

3. caring for the patient requiring neurosurgical interventions and/or intensive care

4. meeting the needs of the head-injured patient, including those required to achieve an optimal outcome.

Caring for the patient with raised ICP following head injury

Head-injured patients with raised ICP may appear to have sustained no injury initially but can become drowsy or confused, or develop speech problems or limb deficits. The immediate nursing aim is to prevent further damaging rises in ICP. The care plan (see Table 20.7) outlines the principal interventions and their rationale. The presence of other injuries can alter the management of the patient depending upon the initial survey in the acute phase.

For the patient with increased ICP, treatment may be medical, surgical or a combination of both. Surgical intervention usually deals with the specific cause and may involve ventricular drainage. Medical treatment includes the intravenous administration of osmotic diuretics (e.g. mannitol) and the corticosteroid dexamethasone to try to reduce cerebral oedema.

Assessment

The effects of rising ICP on the patient will vary with the speed at which pressure is rising and hence the nature of the lesion itself. The pressure may increase very rapidly, as with an extradural haemorrhage, or it may increase very gradually, as with a slow-growing tumour.

Early symptoms include headache that progressively becomes more severe, drowsiness, slowing of responses and vomiting, which may not be preceded by nausea. It is important that the nurse obtain information from the family about the patient's normal behaviour as a baseline against which to compare current functioning. With further development there is decreasing consciousness, an increase in the systolic blood pressure with a widening pulse pressure, change in respiratory pattern, eye changes (pupillary dilatation, loss of reflex to light stimulus), papilloedema and bradycardia (see Table 20.6). The patient's vital signs and neurological status are assessed to provide a baseline against which any signs of deterioration may be detected. Assessment of the patient's neurological status also includes observations for involuntary movements (twitching, tremors or convulsion), restlessness, rigidity and posturing (decerebrate or decorticate rigidity) (see Fig. 20.10).

Urinary problems
See chapter 5.4

Constipation
See chapter 5.1

Table 20.7   Care plan for patient with raised intracranial pressure

Area of care	Nursing interventions	Rationale
Neurological status	Assess baseline neurological observations including conscious level and reassess as determined by patient's status. Assess vital signs particularly temperature. If raised, institute measures to reduce to normal	Changes in neurological status, no matter how subtle, can herald rising ICP and thus risk of brain damage if not detected. A raised temperature will create greater demand for oxygenation, thus raising ICP
Respiratory status	Assess rate, depth and pattern of respirations. Check breath sounds. Monitor arterial blood gases. Suction as required for maximum of 15 s. Preoxygenate for up to 1 min before suctioning with 100% oxygen. Manage assisted ventilation (if required). Provide tracheostomy care (if required)	Patients with raised ICP require adequate oxygenation to ensure that brain is properly perfused. Attention to factors that may impede this will ensure that ICP is not raised further and the outcome from injury will be better
Avoiding increased ICP due to poor positioning or activities	Nurse patient in a 30° head-up tilt. Prone position and extreme hip flexion are contraindicated. Maintain head in a neutral position with sandbags if required. Ensure patient's head does not fall to one side or that tracheostomy tapes are not too tight around the neck. If patient conscious, ask to exhale when turning in bed. Instruct patient not to press down with hands on the bed when moving. Plan nursing activities to avoid clustering of these. Reposition patient regularly and provide skin care	Elevating head of bed and achieving neutral head position ensures adequate venous drainage from head, thus avoiding raises in ICP. Exhaling on turning avoids Valsalva's manoeuvre which raises ICP. Pushing down produces isometric contraction which will result in raised ICP due to intiation of Valsalva's manoeuvre. Clustering of nursing activities have been shown to raise ICP
Elimination	Monitor volume and specific gravity of urine. Monitor stools. No enemas or suppositories	Indicates diuresis and dilution. Diabetes insipidus indicated by a falling specific gravity and increased output may occur following injury and require treatment. Avoiding constipation prevents initiation of Valsalva's manoeuvre, which can occur when straining at stool or as the result of an enema
Ventricular drainage	Manage ventricular drainage system. Note correct position of drainage bag. Maintain strict asepsis. Maintain closed system	Correct position of bag will result in optimal drainage of CSF. If bag too low, too much CSF will drain resulting in brain herniation; too high means that drainage will not take place thus increasing ICP
ICP monitoring	Manage system. Record data. Maintain asepsis	Recording and reporting data will result in appropriate interventions to avoid further rises in ICP
Seizures management	Maintain seizure precautions	Avoids further rises in ICP. Avoids patient injury

It is important to assess the patient's level of understanding of the current situation and communication skills, and how the family is reacting to the situation.

The physical assessment should include a careful check on the patient's skin to assess for signs of dehydration and pressure area breakdown.

Patient problems

The following is a list of potential problems frequently encountered by patients suffering raised ICP.

- Alteration in respiratory function related to:
  — ineffective clearance of airway
  — injury or compression of the respiratory centre
  — obstruction of the airway by the tongue or aspirate, if unconscious
- Potential for injury due to disorientation and impaired awareness, restlessness, seizures
- Severe headache
- Potential hyperthermia
- Alteration in cardiac function secondary to compression and ischaemia of vital centres in the medulla
- Potential for skin breakdown due to immobility and possible restlessness and hyperthermia
- Potential fluid imbalance due to osmotic diuretic, inadequate intake and vomiting
- Nutritional deficit due to inadequate intake and increased metabolic rate with hyperthermia and injury
- Alteration in elimination – bowel and urinary
- Self-care deficit in personal hygiene due to reduced level of consciousness and motor and sensory changes.

Goals

The goals for the patient revolve around being free from any of the complications outlined in the above list of problems, having the maximum possible insight into the situation and a satisfactory standard of personal hygiene and comfort.

Nursing intervention

Ineffective respiration

If the patient with raised ICP has impaired respiration, then less oxygen is available to perfuse the brain. It is therefore important to ensure optimal respiratory status. The patient may require full artificial ventilatory support. Assessment will include the rate, depth and pattern of respiration. A respiratory rate below 14 or above 24 breaths per minute would give cause for concern. Irregularities in the rate and/or rhythm are indicative of a rising ICP. Assessment might also include pulse oximetry and monitoring of arterial blood gases.

Based on the assessment, appropriate interventions are identified from a menu of activities. These include:

- *Positioning* – normally semiprone with a 30° head-up tilt unless contraindicated. The head-up tilt also assists with minimizing rises in ICP by encouraging venous drainage.

- *Use of respiratory aids* – a Guedal airway is inserted if required. If artificial ventilation is indicated, endotracheal intubation will be required.

- *Suctioning* – oropharyngeal and tracheal suctioning is applied only as required to remove secretions. Excessive suctioning raises ICP. Suctioning is limited to 10–15 seconds per pass and the patient is allowed to recover between suctioning. Pre-oxygenation with 100% oxygen prior to suctioning may be considered to prevent a buildup of carbon dioxide.

- *Oxygen administration* – this is administered as prescribed via the appropriate route.

- *Artificial ventilation* – full ventilatory support involves additional specialized nursing care.

Potential for injury

Increased intracranial pressure

Planning and implementation of care must take into consideration the prevention of further increase in the intracranial pressure as well as the reduction of the existing increased intracranial pressure.

Positions and activities that raise the ICP are avoided. The head of the bed is usually elevated about 30°; the patient with potential or actual increased ICP is never placed in a head-low position but is positioned to prevent any impediment of cerebral venous return. The head is aligned with the spine; flexion and twisting of the head, anything tight around the neck that might compress the jugular veins, and extreme hip flexion are avoided. When moving or changing position, the conscious patient is instructed not to push with the feet or to push or pull with the arms, and to breathe out through the mouth. The latter prevents the Valsalva manoeuvre, which quickly raises the ICP. Clustering of nursing activities should be avoided to minimize rises in ICP.

The corticosteroid dexamethasone may be used to help reduce ICP. The patient receiving dexamethasone is observed for possible side-effects and complications, because corticosteroids suppress the immune response making the patient more susceptible to infection and may also cause gastrointestinal bleeding. An antacid or antisecretory agent such as the H_2-receptor antagonist cimetidine is prescribed to prevent peptic ulceration.

Disorientation and impaired cognitive function

The patient's orientation, judgement, level of consciousness and mobility may change quickly. Protection from injury is necessary. Cot sides are kept in position unless someone stays at the bedside with the patient. Following an intracranial disorder and increased ICP, patients are frequently subject to spells of dizziness or lapses of orientation, or may be slow in regaining their postural reflexes.

Restlessness

This may be due to cerebral hypoxia or increasing rise in the ICP, but restlessness may also be associated with retention of urine, pain, an uncomfortable position, the regaining of consciousness, or fear and concern about the situation. The cot sides are padded for protection. Efforts are made to determine the cause if the patient is restless and to eliminate it if possible. If there are neurological symptoms and changes in vital signs that indicate a further increase in the ICP, they are reported promptly so that further treatment may be undertaken. If the restlessness occurs with the regaining of consciousness, the patient is reoriented to the situation; if the cause of the restlessness is thought to be the patient's anxiety, explanations and reassurance are necessary.

Nursing measures such as position change and staying with the patient and encouraging expression of concerns may promote comfort and reduce restlessness. The environment should be quiet and the lighting subdued. In extreme restlessness a mild sedative may be prescribed to prevent exhaustion.

It should be remembered that the patient with reduced consciousness may be able to hear and comprehend although not able to respond. It is important that those caring for the patient continue to communicate with the patient and guard against inappropriate conversation. Verbal communication provides cerebral stimulation and information; it can be comforting and reassuring to the patient. Non-verbal communication by touch and presence is also reassuring to both patient and family. Family members are advised of the possibility of the patient hearing and are encouraged to communicate with the patient even though unresponsive.

Headache

The patient usually experiences headache with the onset of increased ICP which progressively becomes more severe as the pressure rises. A mild non-narcotic analgesic such as paracetamol may be prescribed. The patient may find that cold applications provide some relief. As the ICP increases and the patient loses consciousness, pain perception diminishes. A quiet room, subdued lighting and a minimum of environmental stimuli are important, and sudden movements should be avoided.

Alteration in body temperature

Compression of the temperature-regulating centre as a result of increased ICP may result in a marked increase in the temperature and, at the same time, the normal physiological heat-dissipating mechanisms are suppressed (dilatation of superficial blood vessels and perspiration). The metabolic rate is increased in proportion to the fever: with a temperature of 40.5°C, there is an increase in metabolism of approximately 50%. Oxygen demands are increased and carbon dioxide production increases.

The room is kept at 18–20°C and a light cotton sheet used to cover the patient. If the temperature is raised, the sheet is arranged to cover only the lower half of the body. An antipyretic such as aspirin, administered by rectal suppository, may be prescribed. The patient should not be cooled too quickly; shivering must be prevented because it increases metabolism, oxygen consumption and the production of carbon dioxide and other metabolites that increase ICP.

Alteration in cardiac function

The compression and ischaemia caused by increased ICP may seriously affect the cardiac and vasomotor centres. Close monitoring of the pulse for irregularity and changes in the rate and volume is necessary. A decrease in cardiac output reduces cerebral perfusion to a greater degree, resulting in ischaemia, increased P_{CO_2} and vasodilatation, and an ensuing increase in ICP. Continuous cardiac monitoring may be established and an antiarrhythmic drug prescribed if necessary. The excessive loss of body fluid as a result of osmotic diuretic therapy may cause a reduction in intravascular volume and a corresponding reduction in cardiac output. Cardiac failure is more likely to occur if the patient has a pre-existing cardiac problem.

Potential for skin breakdown

Maintenance of **skin** integrity requires special attention because of the patient's immobility and possible restlessness and hyperthermia. The patient's position is changed from side to back (only if conscious) to side every 2 hours unless contraindicated by the location of the patient's intracranial lesion or surgery. For example, if a relatively large space-occupying lesion has been

Fever
See chapter 6.1

Skin assessment
See chapter 6.1

Fluid balance
See chapter 2.6

Constipation
See chapter 5.1

removed, the patient is not permitted to lie on the operative side to prevent a shifting of the brain into the remaining space.

Pressure area care is discussed fully in Ch. 25.

Potential fluid imbalance

The fluid intake is usually restricted to a stated volume distributed over 24 hours to maintain slight dehydration which reduces the extracellular volume and ICP. Intravenous fluids are infused slowly and must be monitored closely; rapid infusion could cause a serious, rapid rise in the ICP.

An osmotic diuretic may be prescribed to dehydrate the brain; the drugs administered for this purpose are principally hyperosmolar solutions which are given intravenously (e.g. mannitol). They promote the transfer of fluid from the brain tissue into the vascular compartment by osmosis and increase the urinary output.

Fluid intake is usually calculated every 8–12 hours according to the output; 400–500 mL are added to the output volume to cover insensible loss. Intravenous infusion is usually necessary owing to an inability to take sufficient fluid orally because of nausea, vomiting or coma.

Nutritional deficit

The headache, nausea, vomiting or loss of consciousness results in the patient's inability to take adequate food, which is reflected in changes in strength and muscle mass. Nasogastric feeding may be given every 4 hours to provide necessary fluid and calories. If the patient is febrile, the increased metabolic rate requires more calories; if the caloric requirement is not met, the patient becomes seriously debilitated.

Alteration in elimination

Bowel elimination

The patient is discouraged from straining to defaecate because the effort involved raises ICP. A mild bulk laxative or stool softener may be given, or a bisacodyl (Dulcolax) suppository may be used as faecal impaction must be avoided.

Urinary elimination

If the patient is unresponsive, incontinence is a problem, making a retention catheter necessary so that an accurate assessment can be made of the output, as well as to maintain skin integrity. The output is noted every 1–2 hours to evaluate the effectiveness of the osmotic diuretic.

The fluid intake and output are monitored for oliguria and water retention or an excessive volume of urine with a low specific gravity. The excessive output may develop as a result of a disturbance in the secretion of antidiuretic hormone (ADH) by the posterior pituitary lobe. An increase in ADH causes decreased urine formation, whereas a deficiency of ADH causes large volumes of urine to be excreted, necessitating the administration of vasopressin (Pitressin).

The catheter is removed as soon as possible because of the risk of urinary tract infection. For this reason, the use of a condom-type catheter is preferable.

Self-care deficit in personal hygiene

The nurse provides the personal care that the patient would normally carry out unaided, such as bathing, cleaning of teeth and mouth, combing of the hair and feeding. Nursing care should be carried out with undisturbed intervals between to permit adequate rest. If the eye reflexes are absent, the eyes may be irrigated with sterile normal saline and hypromellose drops (artificial tears) instilled three or four times daily to keep the surface of the eye clean and moist. If one or both eyes remain open, a protective shield is applied.

If permitted, the limbs are moved slowly and gently through their range of motion to preserve joint movements.

Ventricular drainage in increased intracranial pressure

A ventricular puncture may be done via a burr-hole in the skull and a tube inserted into a ventricle to establish drainage of CSF to lower the ICP. Externally, the tube is attached to a sterile closed system. The level at which the tubing and bag are placed is prescribed by the doctor. The bed is usually kept flat unless otherwise indicated by the doctor. The rate of drainage is monitored very closely; too rapid drainage is to be avoided and blockage of the tube is to be reported promptly. Strict asepsis must be observed in handling the tubes and the dressing at the burr-hole. The patient may be given an antibiotic as a prophylactic measure. If the patient complains of severe headache or a neurological disturbance (e.g. disturbed vision) develops that was not experienced before the ventricular puncture, the doctor is notified.

The person with altered level of consciousness

Patient problems

Problems relevant to the patient with an altered level of consciousness are:

- alteration in sensation – visual, auditory, kinaesthesic, gustatory, tactile and olfactory
- alteration in thought processes
- ineffective airway clearance
- impaired physical mobility
- potential for injury
- potential impairment of skin integrity
- nutrition at intake less than body requirements
- incontinence of urine
- incontinence of faeces
- inability to maintain self-care – feeding, bathing/hygiene, dressing, grooming and toileting.

Goals

These principal problems lead to a set of patient goals which involve the patient avoiding harmful complications, maximizing independence and adapting to altered functioning in the above areas.

Nursing Intervention

Identification of changes in neurological function

Monitoring of the patient's level of consciousness, pupillary responses, limb movements and vital signs is carried out continuously. If the patient's condition is changing, data are recorded every 15 minutes. When the patient's neurological status stabilizes, recordings are gradually made less often. Early signs of increasing ICP should be reported promptly to ensure immediate action to prevent cerebral coning. The first sign of increasing ICP is a decrease in the level of consciousness, as measured on the Glasgow Coma Scale – hence the importance of these observations.

Maintenance of body functions and prevention of complications

Maintenance of a patent airway

The first priority in caring for an unconscious patient is the establishment of a patent airway. As the patient's level of consciousness decreases, the ability to maintain a clear airway is limited. The cause may be obstruction of the airway by the tongue when the jaw and tongue relax, vomit, blood or other inhaled foreign material such as dentures. Ineffective ventilation may occur due to depression of the respiratory centre, accumulation of secretions and foreign material, as a result of depression of the cough reflex, and immobility and weakness of respiratory muscles.

The unconscious patient is placed in a lateral or semi-prone position (unless contraindicated by a chest or spinal injury), with the neck aligned with the spine. If the patient is unconscious as a result of a head injury, a spinal injury should be assumed to be present until proven otherwise. See page 718 for movement of spinally injury patients. Either position facilitates the drainage of mucus and vomit, and prevents obstruction of the airway by the relaxed tongue and jaw. If mucus collects in the oropharyngeal cavity, frequent suctioning with a flexible catheter is necessary. The catheter is moistened with water before insertion and is handled gently during insertion and on withdrawal to avoid trauma to the delicate tracheal mucous membranes.

If the patient has lost the gag reflex, an artificial airway will be needed. An oropharyngeal airway or an endotracheal tube may be inserted to maintain the airway and facilitate the removal of secretions by suctioning.

Oxygen may be administered by nasal cannulae or mask, or mechanical ventilation may be instituted. If the patient is able to follow instructions, deep breathing is practised hourly. Hard, sustained coughing is contraindicated because it causes an increase in ICP. If coughing is necessary to remove secretions and the patient is able to do so, staged coughing is taught. This involves the patient taking a deep breath while relaxing the abdominal muscles, holding the breath, and then exhaling in short, staged intervals involving four or five expirations. Postural drainage and chest percussion and vibration are carried out several times a day by the physiotherapist to promote drainage of respiratory secretions.

The patient's position should be changed every 2 hours to prevent pressure sore formation and facilitate the removal of secretions from the lungs. Observations are made following each change of position to determine the effect on respirations. Chest expansion is observed and the rate and rhythm of respirations are noted, as well as the patient's colour and general status.

Care of the eyes

Loss of the corneal reflex and depression of lacrimal secretion may result in prolonged exposure, drying and injury to the cornea which may lead to ulceration. The eyes should be examined regularly for signs of inflammation or injury. Contact lenses are removed. Ophthalmic solutions may be prescribed to irrigate the eyes three or four times a day. The eyes may be covered with dressings to protect them.

Catheterization
See chapter 5.4

Care of the mouth

Dentures should be removed only if they pose a danger. The mouth is cleansed several times a day and teeth are cleaned by brushing when possible. The lips are moistened with a water-soluble ointment or cream. The mouth should be inspected daily for signs of crusting or ulceration of the mucosa.

Positioning

When the patient is placed in the lateral or semiprone position, attention is given to good body alignment and to the prevention of contractures, foot and wrist drop, muscle strain, joint injury, and interference with circulation and chest expansion. The head should be positioned so that the neck is aligned with the spine. The arm that is uppermost is flexed at the elbow and rested on a pillow to prevent drag on the shoulder and wrist drop. The arm that is down is drawn slightly forward, flexed at the elbow, and lies on the bed parallel with the neck and head. The lower limb that is uppermost is flexed at the hip and knee, and supported on a firm pillow; the other lower limb is slightly flexed. The feet are positioned at a 90° angle to the leg and care is taken that *no* pressure is applied by firm objects placed against the feet.

Joint movement

The extremities are passively moved through their normal range of motion at least twice daily to preserve joint function and prevent circulatory stasis. Active exercises are initiated as soon as the patient is able to follow instructions.

Protection from injury

The cot sides of the bed are always maintained in the up position when the patient is unconscious unless someone is in constant attendance on the patient. It may be necessary to pad the sides of the bed if the patient is restless and thrashing about. Alternatively, the patient may be nursed on a mattress on the floor. A very agitated patient may climb over cot sides and suffer serious injury from the ensuing fall. Placing mittens on the hands may be necessary if the patient is restless, scratches, or pulls on the nasogastric or intravenous tube or the urethral catheter. The mittens are removed at least twice daily; the hands are bathed, the nails are kept clean and short, and the fingers put through their normal range of motion by passive exercise.

The nurse should not attempt to force resisting extremities (such as in spastic flexion or extension) to assume a different position. Forcing a rigid extremity into a different position could result in a fracture of that limb. The use of depressant drugs to control agitation is contraindicated as they may further depress the arousal system.

When the patient is ambulatory but has some impairment of awareness, a safe environment should be provided. Scatter rugs and objects are removed from the patient's path to prevent falling. Sharp objects are removed from the immediate environment.

Fluids and nutrition

The patient is assessed for a gag reflex; as soon as it is present, and the patient is conscious, oral feeds are initiated. When the patient is unconscious or the gag reflex is absent, the patient's nutrition may be sustained by intravenous infusion or feeds given via a nasogastric feeding tube. The liquid feed given by tube contains the essential food elements and the amount is individually calculated to provide adequate caloric intake for the patient's size and metabolic activity. The dietician should be consulted for advice. Frequency of feeding varies from slow continuous to every 4 hours. If there is any regurgitation (fluid welling up around the tube into the mouth), the volume given at one time is decreased and the frequency of the feeds is increased. If the patient's condition permits, it is helpful to elevate the head of the bed slightly during the feeding and for a brief period afterwards. The tube is rinsed with 30–45 mL of water after each feeding.

The presence of the tube in a nostril tends to irritate the mucous membrane and stimulate mucus secretion. The area is cleansed twice daily with applicators that have been moistened with normal saline, and is then also lubricated lightly. The tube should be secured loosely enough so that it does not press continuously on any one area of the nostril.

Elimination

The unconscious patient has urinary incontinence. An indwelling **catheter** is inserted initially only if it is necessary to facilitate accurate monitoring of output or if retention of urine occurs. The catheter is removed as soon as possible to prevent complications and promote the return of normal bladder functioning. Condom drainage is established with the male patient as soon as his condition is stable. While the catheter is in place it is taped to the thigh to prevent undue traction. The complete set of tubes and drainage receptacle constitutes a closed sterile system.

If a catheter is not used, frequent attention is necessary to protect the skin. Incontinence pads are used to absorb the urine and are changed promptly after voiding. The skin is washed after each voiding and dried thoroughly. A barrier cream may be applied to the skin. The bed linen is changed as necessary.

The patient may be incontinent of faeces, particularly if receiving tube feedings. Prompt cleansing and changing of soiled pads and bedding are necessary.

Skin care

The unconscious patient is predisposed to the rapid development of pressure ulcers (see p. 929 for preventive measures).

Care should be taken to maintain daily personal hygiene. This includes hair and face washing and shaving. Families should be encouraged to help in these activities if they feel comfortable about it. It is important for families to be included as part of the caring team.

Maintenance or restoration of sensation, perception and awareness

Fluctuations in consciousness affect the patient's ability to receive a stimulus, interpret its meaning and respond with appropriate behaviour. The arousal mechanism may be affected so that repeated stimulation may be required to elicit a response. Sensory stimulation is an important aspect of the care of every patient experiencing alterations in the level of consciousness. The type of stimulation, how it is structured and presented, and its complexity must be planned for each individual according to the level of consciousness, the cause of the decreased consciousness, and the relevance and meaning of the stimulus to this particular individual.

Types of stimuli include auditory, olfactory, visual, tactile, kinaesthetic, vestibular and oral. The nurse should always speak to the patient by name and explain what is being done, and the patient should be informed before procedures such as feeding and turning occur. Touch is used as much as possible. Environmental noise is decreased and night orientation is practised to provide rest. Multisensory stimuli sessions may be carried out three or four times a day. Each method of stimulation is introduced one at a time in a form that is meaningful to the patient.

Caring for the patient requiring neurosurgical interventions and/or intensive care

Following neurosurgery the overall goals of care for patients are:

- continuous assessment of the patient's neurological status

- instituting measures to avoid secondary brain damage

- administration of appropriate therapies.

The main complications of neurosurgery are outlined in Table 20.8.

Skin assessment
See chapter 6.1

Preoperative nursing care

Assessment

If the preoperative period extends over several days, the patient is observed for possible neurological changes from day to day which may indicate a worsening of the condition. The vital signs are followed closely; pupils are checked regularly for size, equality and reaction to light, and the patient's alertness, orientation, sensory perception, motor ability and strength of limbs are noted.

Vital signs and neurological observations are recorded to provide a baseline for measuring progress in the postoperative period.

Patient problems

The patient faces all the usual problems associated with surgery, plus the following problems which are unique to

Table 20.8 Complications of neurosurgery

Complication	Cause	Interventions
Altered conscious level	Increased ICP due to cerebral haemorrhage/oedema	Frequent assessment of neurological status
Limb weaknesses	Increased ICP due to cerebral haemorrhage/oedema	Frequent assessment of limb movements
Speech problems	Increased ICP due to cerebral haemorrhage/oedema	Frequent assessment of verbal responses
Respiratory problems	Increased ICP due to cerebral haemorrhage/oedema	Frequent assessment of respiratory status
Loss of swallowing reflex	Increased ICP due to cerebral haemorrhage/oedema	Frequent assessment of swallowing reflex
Onset of seizures	Cerebral irritation	Observation of seizures. Interventions to ensure patient safety
Loss of corneal reflex	Increased ICP due to cerebral haemorrhage/oedema	Frequent assessment of corneal reflex
Periorbital oedema	Direct result of surgery	Observe for swollen/bruised periorbital tissues

intracranial surgery:

- anxiety related to the intracranial surgery and the outcome
- potential for intracranial infection due to surgery
- fluid deficit due to the administration of an osmotic diuretic because of increased ICP
- potential increased ICP
- potential for respiratory depression and thrombophlebitis
- embarrassment and concern related to shaving of the head.

Goals

Patient goals involve avoiding the potential problems outlined above and being able to talk freely about fears and anxieties, including appearance after head shaving.

Nursing intervention

Anxiety

Any impending surgery is perceived as a threat to the person and generates anxiety, but that involving the brain is even more threatening. The alert patient and the family are usually very fearful of a fatal outcome or permanent changes, disability, and a loss of intellect and competence. Expression of doubts and concerns is encouraged; time and opportunities for questions and answers are provided. The patient is not left alone for long periods; contact with others interrupts concentration on the operation and provides the opportunity to express fears. Visits are limited to family members and friends who can control their anxiety and show a quiet, reassuring presence with the patient.

It is necessary to explain to the patient and family the need for the operation, the nature of the procedure, the risks and possible outcome. The nurse should be able to answer questions, clarify misconceptions and refer, if appropriate, any special problems to others. The sort of information the family requires is that patient may have temporary oedema and discoloration of the face and eyes, and possible neurological deficits such as facial paralysis and aphasia after the operation. The fact that these signs are common after surgery will help to reduce the anxiety they generate. Particular sensitivity must be shown over the issue of head shaving. Shaving of the head is usually left until the patient is anaesthetized. The patient should be advised that a wig of choice will be supplied free once the head dressings and sutures have been removed. It is advisable to ask the appliance officer to visit the patient before operation so that a wig may be chosen and ordered in readiness.

Fluid balance
See chapter 2.6

Potential for infection

Because of surgical interruption of the integrity of the scalp and cranium, the head must be cleansed and prepared to minimize the possibility of infection. Unless it is an emergency, the hair is washed the day before the operation.

Fluid deficit

There is usually concern if a preoperative patient manifests dehydration, and efforts are made to re-establish normal hydration. A fluid deficit in the patient who is to have intracranial surgery may be an important therapeutic measure. A restricted fluid intake may be necessary to control ICP, or an osmotic diuretic such as mannitol to reduce increased ICP may be given.

No attempt is made to increase the fluid intake without a specific directive. The patient may have water up to 4 or 5 hours before the operation unless otherwise indicated.

Common intracranial surgical procedures

Intracranial surgery necessitates an opening in the skull. The size and location of the opening depend upon the nature and site of the lesion and the amount of exposure needed for the operation. If the lesion is in the cerebrum, it is referred to as being *supratentorial* and the incision is well above the hairline. If it is in the cerebellar or brainstem regions, it is designated as *infratentorial* and the incision is usually in the occipital region.

The surgical procedures include the following:

- *Burr-hole.* This is a small circular opening into the cranium made with a bone drill. The purpose may be to obtain tissue for a biopsy, aspirate CSF from a ventricle, or relieve pressure caused by swelling and oedema of the brain or a tumour.
- *Craniotomy.* In this procedure a scalp incision and two or more burr-holes are made over the area to be explored. The bone between the burr-holes is incised, allowing elevation of a bone flap to provide access to the brain. The opening is curved so that the scalp and bone flap can be folded back to expose the affected brain area.
- *Craniectomy.* This involves excision of a portion of the skull and may vary from a small burr-hole to a sizeable area of several square centimetres. The craniectomy may be done to remove shattered bone or to relieve pressure by expanding cranial contents.
- *Cranioplasty.* This is a replacement of a section of the cranium with a synthetic material such as titanium to re-establish the contour and integrity of the skull. In some instances, the bone flap that was initially separated from the skull is replaced; this is referred to as an *osteoplastic craniotomy*.

Postoperative nursing care

As all patients suffer some increase in ICP following brain surgery, the nursing care described for increased ICP as well as the care of the unconscious patient are applicable in the postoperative phase.

Assessment

Vital signs and neurological status are determined when the patient is returned from the operating theatre as a baseline against which progress can be assessed. If the patient is conscious, alertness, orientation, speech and ability to move limbs are checked. The required frequency of these observations may be indicated by the neurosurgeon but usually begins with 15–30-minute intervals which are gradually lengthened to 1 hour, then to 4 hours if the evaluations indicate stability. Care should be taken to assess for pain, headache or other discomfort, as well as for signs of fear and anxiety.

Assessment of the patient's status includes observations for involuntary movements: twitching, tremor, seizure, restlessness, rigidity and posturing (decerebrate rigidity or decorticate rigidity).

The head dressing is examined for security, for moistness suggesting leakage of CSF, and for evidence of bleeding. There may be a drain attached to a gentle negative-pressure system; if so, the amount and type of drainage should be noted as a baseline.

Patient problems

After intracranial surgery, much of the care cited for the patient with increased ICP and for the unconscious patient is applicable, together with care applicable to any patient after operation. Consideration is also given to the following problems:

- The potential for further increased ICP due to the reaction to the trauma imposed by the operation.

- Potential for injury (risk of injury due to malpositioning or disorientation).

- Potential for infection due to open wound and lowered resistance.

- Hyperthermia secondary to the disturbance of the temperature-regulating centre.

- Knowledge deficit – the patient and family require assistance in making necessary adjustments and planning home management.

Goals

The principal patient goal is a safe recovery from surgery, avoiding the potential problems outlined above and the other general problems related to any postoperative patient or person with reduced consciousness.

Nursing intervention

Potential for increased intracranial pressure

All patients experience some increase in ICP following brain surgery because of the oedema and swelling that result from the trauma and inflammation incurred by surgery. Frequent vital signs and neurological evaluations are necessary to recognize significant changes indicating increased ICP.

The head of the bed may be elevated about 30° to promote cerebral venous return unless contraindicated by shock or a specific directive from the surgeon. A small pillow may be necessary under the head to maintain good neck alignment, which promotes cerebral venous return. Following infratentorial surgery (cerebellum or brainstem) the bed is generally kept flat for 2–3 days to prevent pressure on the brainstem and its vital centres.

The fluid intake is usually restricted to a stated volume, distributed over 24 hours to maintain slight dehydration which reduces extracellular fluid and ICP. Intravenous fluids are infused slowly and monitored closely; rapid infusion could cause a rapid rise in ICP. An osmotic diuretic may be prescribed to dehydrate the brain.

Potential for injury

After intracranial surgery, the patient is at risk of injury from malpositioning. The required position depends on the patient's level of consciousness and the location and nature of the operation.

While unconscious, the patient is positioned to promote cerebral venous return as well as to prevent obstruction of the airway and aspiration of secretions. The limbs are positioned and supported in the normal way for an unconscious patient. The head of the bed may be elevated 25–30° and the head aligned with the spine. The patient with potential or actual increase in ICP is never placed in a head-low or prone position. Flexion or twisting of the head and extreme hip flexion are avoided because this may increase ICP.

If a relatively large space-occupying lesion has been removed, the patient is not permitted to lie on the operative side in order to prevent a shifting of the brain into the remaining space. Following infratentorial surgery, the patient lies on either side using a small pillow under the head to maintain alignment. Keeping the patient off the back for 2–3 days prevents pressure on the incision, as well as possible forward flexion on the incision. A specific directive as to positioning may be given by the surgeon.

The position is changed at regular intervals (e.g. every 2 hours) from side to side to back to side unless contraindicated. When repositioned, the patient is turned slowly with adequate support for the head, so that the head and trunk are turned as if they were one unit. Sudden movement and jarring are avoided at all times.

Trauma to the brainstem may depress the gag and swallowing reflexes, predisposing to aspiration. When oral fluids are permitted, only a very small amount is given at first to test the swallowing reflex.

Potential for infection

Following intracranial surgery the risk of **infection** arises from the open wound, from the patient's lowered resistance as a result of the illness and its related stresses, and from the possible administration of a steroid preparation (e.g. dexamethasone). As infectious processes increase

infection
See chapter 6.1

the rate of metabolism, waste products such as carbon dioxide and lactic acid are produced in greater amounts. Waste products in increased amounts cause cerebral vasodilatation, which increases intracranial blood volume and pressure. Strict asepsis is essential when the head dressing is changed. The wound is inspected for redness, swelling, offensive odour and drainage; signs of infection are reported promptly and a swab of the wound drainage is taken for culture purposes. Immediate treatment to prevent meningitis, encephalitis or brain abscess is essential; an antibiotic is prescribed.

Hyperthermia

The patient may develop an increased temperature. To counteract this tendency, the room temperature is kept at 18–20°C and only a cotton sheet and bedspread are used as covers. An antipyretic (e.g. acetylsalicylic acid) is presribed and administered by rectum.

Decreased intellectual function

In some instances, there may be some residual neurological deficit following an intracranial surgical procedure. A rehabilitation programme is planned and instituted as soon as possible with the goal of restoring the patient to independent useful living within his or her potential. This may involve the physiotherapist, speech therapist, occupational therapist and social worker as well as the doctor and nurse. The patient may have to relearn the performance of ordinary daily activities, and progress from the simple to the more complex much as a child learns. It is frequently a slow process and both the patient and family are likely to have periods of depression and discouragement. The nurse assists them in making their plans for home management and the necessary activities and exercises. A referral is made to appropriate support services so that support and guidance are continued.

Rehabilitation: meeting the needs of the head-injured patient

Rehabilitation forms a crucial part of the recovery process. The aim is to maintain and promote function, improve or prevent further deterioration, and also to prevent further complications from occurring. The challenge in this process is to overcome the neurological deficits that can impede progress during the rehabilitation process. These include motor and sensory impairment, communication disability, psychological disability, social disability, and educational or vocational disability.

Grant and Grinspun (1994) highlight the need for a safe and predictable environment for rehabilitation. Realistic goals are set and the rehabilitative process may take months or years to achieve. Not all patients will respond to rehabilitation, or their condition is so severe that rehabilitation is impossible. The patient's needs are assessed by the multidisciplinary team along with the family, with a view to identifying and providing the optimal care and support to achieve an optimal outcome. Often, the patient's role within the family changes. He or she may previously have been the provider within a family, and now have to revert to being dependent on others. For some, a return to work is impossible as their ability to undertake their normal work may be impaired. Some employers provide assisted support to enable such employees to return to different work or reduced hours. Employment difficulties can have long-term financial implications for the family. An alteration to the patient's personality may affect relationships within a family, resulting in much stress and disagreement. Some families will report that the person has completely changed and is now different from the person they knew before. A family support programme to assist families of head-injured survivors is described by Acorn (1995).

Often, repeated explanations of the patient's change in behaviour toward the family are required, as family members find this change distressing. The reaction of the family can range from apparent calm acceptance to rudeness and verbal aggression towards nursing staff. As the time for discharge approaches, many patients and their families are particularly anxious. Much of this anxiety can be allayed if adequate preparation and reassurance are provided, along with an effective plan for discharge. The residual problems that may persist vary widely, ranging from headache to major behavioural changes with or without neurological deficits. The degree of residual difficulty will determine what action is required in the discharge plan. Other influences may include whether the patient requires further surgery or other therapies, necessitating attendance at a hospital or rehabilitation centre. Brief predischarge visits home may be considered and will help to identify potential problems.

It is not usually until the patient is at home that the family fully appreciates the difficulties that may be encountered. Some of the home routine may need to be adjusted and, while this may be easy in the early stages, it becomes more difficult to accept in the long term. Other members of the family often view the disruption to their personal lives negatively and eventually much of the early support gradually disappears. If the patient is still at a stage in which support is required, this withdrawal can be catastrophic. Very often the patient's partner is left to shoulder the burden alone, and in this situation a support group such as Headway may help. This organization seeks to provide help and assistance to the patient and family. Regular meetings and other special outings are arranged, along with helpful literature. Relatives can be provided with a forum for discussion of the problems that they face, and many appreciate sharing their problems with others who are similarly placed. Some families have to acknowledge a sense of failure should the patient have to be admitted for institutional care in either the short or long term. They may feel that they have let the patient down and do not like to admit that they are unable to cope.

Spine and spinal cord injury

Spinal cord injury is a major cause of serious disability, particularly in males aged between 15 and 30 years. Motor vehicle accidents continue to be a major cause of spinal injuries, and frequently alcohol and drugs are involved. Other causes are falls, diving accidents and sports injuries, particularly horse riding and rugby.

Types of injury

A spinal injury may or may not involve injury to the spinal cord. Fracture of one or more vertebrae may occur with no displacement of fragments, resulting in the cord escaping injury. However, rupture of the ligaments holding the vertebrae in alignment may allow displacement of the vertebral column, leading to serious cord injury, even if no fracture occurs. Injury may be the result of:

- sudden forceful angulation of the spine (hyperextension, hyperflexion or hyperextension–hyperflexion) with or without rotational forces

- excessive force applied along the axis of the spine causing burst fractures and vertical compression (e.g. landing on the feet or buttocks from a height)

- a direct blow to the area of the spine.

Effects of spinal injuries

Injuries to the vertebrae may result in spinal cord contusion, laceration and compression. Bleeding into the tissues and oedema occur, causing swelling and compression of nerve tracts. The damage may be slight and completely reversible or it may leave a minor degree of residual impairment. Oedema and bleeding in the cervical cord area is very serious; compression may interrupt innervation of the diaphragm incurring respiratory failure. A laceration that transects the cord or causes severe compression may result in complete, irreversible interruption of ascending or descending tracts. Destruction of the cord resulting in interruption of its tracts is not always due to transection. Injury may incur haemorrhage, circulatory stasis, extravasation of fluid and blood cells, ischaemia and necrosis of the tissue. Interruption of ascending tracts causes loss of sensation below the site of injury. This means that pain, pressure and temperature sensation may be dulled or lost and the patient may be unable to appreciate the position of affected limbs due to interference with proprioception impulse pathways. Interruption of descending tracts results in **paralysis** of the parts deriving their innervation from the cord below the level of the lesion. Flaccid paralysis and an absence of reflexes occur first and are usually followed by spastic paralysis and exaggerated tendon reflexes. Bladder, bowel and autonomic nervous functions are disturbed.

When the spinal cord is suddenly transected, a phenomenon known as *spinal shock* develops in which all cord functions including involuntary reflex responses are depressed; there is the sudden loss of all motor, sensory, reflex and autonomic responses below the site of cord injury. This occurs due to the sudden interruption of the initiating and regulatory impulses between the higher centres and the cord below the site of injury; that is, impulses are no longer being passed to or from neurones below the lesion. The result is loss of muscular tone (flaccid paralysis), an absence of reflexes and loss of sensation below the lesion. Cord reflexes for voiding and defaecation are suppressed, and retention and overflow incontinence occur. **Vasomotor tone** is lost and the blood pressure falls. Body temperature control is affected because there is no perspiration below the lesion; hyperthermia may develop. Spinal shock may subside in a few days or may persist for a much longer period. The loss of autonomic impulses and tone in the intestine may cause distension and **paralytic ileus**. Occasionally, recovery of reflex activity following spinal shock is characterized by hypersensitivity of the spinal neurones; for example, spasticity of the muscles develops and the bladder becomes hypertonic, resulting in diminished capacity and frequent reflex voiding.

The victim with injury to the spine without cord involvement retains motor and sensory functions and complains of pain at the site of the trauma and in parts innervated by that area. Later this may change; bleeding into the tissue and oedema may occur, causing swelling and compression of the cord. Initial management of spine-injured patients is on the basis of preventing potential cord damage.

The spinal cord and its tracts are not capable of regeneration, but regeneration of the nerve roots (outside the cord) can occur if the neurilemma is not severely damaged. Some recovery of function may occur in the first few weeks as oedema subsides and neurones that were compressed but not destroyed resume activity.

The paralysis that occurs with spinal cord injury may be complete or partial (paresis) and may be paraplegia or quadriplegia. If quadriplegia is complete there may be no voluntary control of function below the neck and very little potential for independence in self-care. With incomplete quadriplegia, voluntary control of selected muscles in the upper limbs may be restored and independence in many areas of self-care may be possible. Respiratory insufficiency or failure is a major concern in quadriplegia as there is usually some involvement of the nerve supply to the diaphragm and intercostal muscles (Fig. 20.21).

Care of the patient with spinal injury

Care of the spine-injured patient involves three phases: the emergency, acute and rehabilitative phases.

Emergency care at the scene of an accident

The principal problem is the potential for further cord damage to occur and the goal is therefore that the patient will suffer no further cord damage.

Paralysis
See chapter 2.3

Vasomotor tone
See chapter 4.2

Paralytic ileus
See chapter 5.1

Intervention

Spinal cord injury and permanent disability may be minimized with accurate assessment and appropriate care immediately after the accident. Injury to the spinal cord is suspected if the victim is unable to move any limbs, if numbness or peculiar sensations are present, if there is unexplained shock or if the person is unconscious after a head injury. The victim may also be having difficulty breathing if the injury is cervical. Wounds about the head or shoulders, pain, tenderness or deformity adjacent to the vertebral column also suggest spinal cord injury. If there is doubt regarding the presence of cord injury, the patient should be managed as if one were present.

Usually the spinal-cord-injured victim is conscious. The patient should be kept flat to permit free diaphragmatic breathing and should be advised to keep the head still; neck flexion or side-to-side rotation could seriously aggravate an injured cervical spine. A quick assessment is made for other injuries using the ABCD checklist (Airway, Breathing, Circulation, Disability). Airway obstruction and inadequate ventilation have first priority but, in establishing an airway or in providing assistance, extension of the neck must be avoided. If the patient is unconscious, the modified jaw thrust may be used to open the airway; two fingers are placed at the angle of the lower jaw to lift it forward. With cervical cord injury, the chest wall muscles may be paralysed and entire respiratory function is dependent on the diaphragm; respiratory assistance and suctioning may be necessary.

The patient should not be moved, except for life-saving purposes, until the Ambulance Service is present. Ambulances carry a special equipment for moving such patients with the minimum disturbance. All movements should be smooth and well coordinated. Immobilization of the head and neck using head blocks is carried out. A firm cervical collar or sand bags taped to each side of the head may be used if available.

Figure 20.21 Level of injury and extent of paralysis.

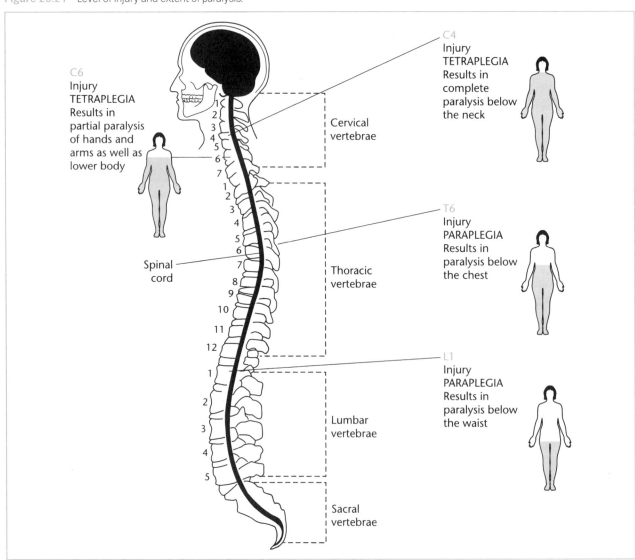

Care during the acute phase (hospital)

Assessment

1. A brief history of the accident is obtained from the victim or person who was at the site.

2. An immediate assessment is made of the vital signs and continuous monitoring established if necessary.

3. If the patient's condition permits, or a family member is available, a brief review is made of the health history so that significant factors such as allergies, pre-existing disorders and medications being taken are identified.

4. The patient is examined for other injuries and a neurological evaluation is made to identify spinal cord damage. An assessment is made of:

   a. **level of consciousness**
   b. orientation
   c. motor and sensory functions (e.g. movement of the limbs; levels of sensation)
   d. reflexes (e.g. patellar, abdominal)
   e. condition of the skin – cold or warm, moist or dry all over or above or below a certain level.

5. The patient's understanding of the situation should be ascertained together with his or her feelings.

Patient problems

- Potential for further cord injury

- Anxiety due to fear of paralysis

- Complications of actual cord injury (e.g. spinal shock, respiratory failure, urinary retention or incontinence, pressure sores).

Goals

The goals are that no further injury will occur, complications of actual injury will be avoided and the patient will talk about fears and anxieties.

Intervention

The treatment of the spine-injured patient depends on:

- **whether there is cord injury and neurological deficits or not**

- the level of the injury

- the nature of the injury (e.g. fracture fragments compressing the cord, laceration of the cord).

Glasgow Coma Scale
See chapter 2.2

Immediate efforts are directed towards sustaining life and preventing cord damage or, where it has occurred, preventing further injury. The spinal lesion is treated by immobilization of the spine. Realignment of vertebrae and relief of pressure on the cord or spinal roots may be achieved by traction. In some instances surgery (decompression laminectomy) is undertaken to relieve pressure on the cord, remove vertebral fragments that are hazardous to the cord or to realign dislocated vertebrae that do not respond to traction of hyperextension. The operation may include spinal fusion (see Table 20.9) or wiring of the spinous processes to stabilize the spine.

Table 20.9 Spinal surgical procedures

Procedure	Conditions in which used
Laminectomy Partial or complete removal of the vertebral arch by the two laminae; precedes other spinal operations to provide access to the canal	Chronic low back pain (disc problems) Spinal fracture (to remove fragments) Cord decompression Removal of a neoplasm
Discectomy Excision of an intervertebral disc	Ruptured or herniated disc Chronic low back pain
Spinal fusion Application of bone grafts to two or more adjoining vertebrae to ankylose them	Ruptured or herniated disc Relief of nerve or cord compression
Rhizotomy Division of transection of a nerve root either outside or within the spinal cord	Chronic pain
Cordotomy Division of the pain-conducting pathways (spinothalamic anterolateral tracts) in the spinal cord Percutaneous cordotomy involves the insertion of a needle (under radiographic guidance) into the spinal cord	Intractable pain (usually associated with malignant disease)

Cervical spine injury

Head blocks will be applied as a first-aid measure and should be left in place. When there is a fracture–dislocation with or without neurological deficit, skeletal traction is applied by means of tongs, a halo traction device or a halter.

Tongs are inserted into the skull at approximately the mid-lateral line, a short distance above the ears. The areas are prepared for the insertion by shaving, cleansing and the injection of a local anaesthetic. A very small incision is made in the scalp and small holes are made in the skull with a drill to accommodate the tongs. The scalp may require sutures before a dressing is applied. The sites of insertion of the tongs are inspected daily for signs of infection, the areas are cleansed and fresh sterile dressings are applied. Traction of 4.5–13.2 kg may be applied and is achieved by a rope that overlies a pulley; one end is affixed to the tongs and the other hangs free with the prescribed weight attached. The prescribed weight depends on the size of the patient and the amount of displacement. It is usually heavy at first and altered as indicated by radiography or clinical progress, and is reduced as realignment of the vertebrae or fragments occurs.

The patient may be placed on a turning bed (e.g. Egerton electrical turning and tilting bed) that is fitted with a pivoting device; this permits turning without interference to the traction. An ordinary bed with a fracture board, if necessary, beneath the mattress and the headboard removed to allow clearance for traction may be used. The head of the bed is elevated to enable the body to act as counteraction for the weights and to prevent the patient from sliding towards the head of the bed. When realignment of the vertebrae or fragments and sufficient healing are achieved, the patient is fitted with a plastic collar or neck brace to provide cervical immobilization and support, and is gradually ambulated.

The halo traction device involves the application of a metal ring to the head which is secured to the skull by the insertion of four pins (similar to the application of tongs). The sites of insertion into the skull are anterior, posterior and lateral. The ring is firmly anchored to a body cast or special vest by metal rods. This form of cervical immobilization and traction allows the patient to be ambulatory (Fig. 20.22).

If only slight traction is required, a halter-like arrangement may be used in place of the tongs. The halter is arranged to place traction under the chin and occipital area. Prolonged continuous application usually causes considerable discomfort and skin irritation for the patient as a result of the pressure and pull, especially under the chin. Careful monitoring of neurological status and breathing are essential, together with meticulous pressure care. The patient's personal hygiene is also crucial.

A great deal of psychological support is needed. It is not possible to say in the first few days after injury how much recovery will occur. The nurse should therefore be

Cervical spine
See chapter 2.2

Figure 20.22   Halo traction as used in cervical vertebral fracture. (a) Four-poster brace. (b) Halo jacket.

(a)   (b)

honest in talking to the patient and family and say it is just too soon to know the extent of possible recovery. A truthful answer is better than avoiding the question or giving false hope to the patient.

Thoracic or lumbar spinal fracture

Where there is a fracture of the spine in the thoracic or lumbar region without dislocation and compression of the spinal cord, the patient may be placed flat on a firm mattress on a bed with a firm base, or on a fracture board on an ordinary bed, or on a turning bed for several weeks. If the ordinary bed is used, specific directions are received as to whether the patient must remain on their back at all times. If turning is permitted, precautions are taken to ensure good alignment and avoidance of movement and displacement of the fragments ('log-rolling'). When there is sufficient healing, the patient is gradually ambulated. A brace, plaster jacket or firm corset may be necessary for several months to provide support and immobility of the spine.

A fracture dislocation of thoracic or lumbar vertebrae may be treated by hyperextension of the spine, which may be achieved by various methods. One method is the placing of a firm roll or sandbag across the bed under the mattress to provide the required angulation. Fracture boards are placed on the bed if it has a sprung base, and a very firm mattress is used on which a sponge rubber mattress is placed, because the patient must remain in the supine position.

Long-term care of the patient with spinal cord injury

After the initial stage of admission and stabilization, the patient faces a long road to recovery with the possibility of severe residual disability. Continuous assessment of progress is essential to monitor the effectiveness of care and to detect any of the potential complications of cord injury and immobility. Psychological care is of paramount importance in this period, together with an awareness of how the family might be affected.

Patient problems

- Alteration in breathing pattern – respiratory insufficiency due to interruption of normal innervation of the diaphragm and/or intercostal muscles

- Potential for pressure ulcers as a result of immobility and impaired tissue perfusion

- Alteration in urinary elimination – retention with overflow or incontinence, due to disturbed innervation

- Alteration in bowel elimination – distension, constipation, incontinence secondary to spinal shock and immobility

- Alteration in food and fluid intake secondary to gastrointestinal distension, anxiety and difficulty in eating caused by immobility and position

- Self-care hygiene deficits due to paralysis and enforced immobility

- Alteration in comfort – pain and spasticity

- Potential for infection

- Potential for muscle contractures, deformities, osteoporosis and thrombophlebitis

- Inability to control body temperature due to dysfunction of the autonomic nervous system

- Disturbance in sleep pattern due to impact of accident, dependency and permanent disability

- Patient and family reactions to change in patient's role, loss of mobility and independence

- Potential for injury due to paralysis, immobility, muscle spasm, loss of sensation

- Sexual dysfunction

- Lack of knowledge and depression due to loss of mobility, independence and roles.

Goals

The patient's goals are to avoid the potential problems listed above and to adapt to altered levels of functioning whilst regaining maximum independence.

Nursing intervention

Respiratory dysfunction

In the acute phase, the patient with cervical or high thoracic cord injury is at risk of respiratory failure, reduced gas exchange and ineffective airway clearance. Initially, diaphragmatic function may appear to be adequate, but during the first 48 hours, oedema develops in the area of the injury. Its progress in the patient with a cervical injury may compromise vital centres in the medulla; respiratory failure develops as well as hypotension and weakening of the pulse. Chest trauma or pre-existing respiratory disease seriously complicates respiratory function.

Endotracheal intubation or a tracheostomy and oxygen administration may be necessary. If ventilatory muscle function is not adequate to maintain blood gas levels, mechanical respiratory assistance is provided. Chest physiotherapy and increased humidity of inspired air and oxygen are provided to mobilize the secretions.

When the patient recovers sufficiently and the blood gas analyses indicate satisfactory levels, mechanical respiratory assistance is discontinued and a regimen of deep breathing and coughing is established.

The patient continues to be at risk of respiratory insufficiency and complications in the postacute phase. Abdominal muscle function may be weak or lacking, and, as a result, the cough is weak in the paraplegic and absent in the quadriplegic patient. Suction equipment should be readily available and intensive physiotherapy provided to help the patient develop an effective cough if possible, as well as to mobilize secretions. During the period during which they must remain flat while the spine heals and stabilizes, spinal-cord-injured patients are predisposed to bronchopneumonia and atelectasis.

Pressure sores
See chapter 6.1

Potential for pressure ulcers

The changes in vasomotor tone and the resulting impairment of tissue perfusion, the enforced immobility and the loss of cutaneous sensation contribute to tissue breakdown. If a pressure ulcer occurs, healing is difficult in patients with spinal cord injury and rehabilitation is delayed.

The patient needs to understand the importance of keeping the skin intact and his or her role in maintaining its integrity. After the period of immobilization to stabilize the spine, as the patient begins to assume the self-care within his or her potential, the importance of shifting of pressure is explained and the patient is taught how to change position at frequent regular intervals in bed and in a wheelchair. The patient is taught to inspect the vulnerable areas at least once daily using a mirror.

Most patients with paraplegia or quadriplegia are eventually mobilized by lightweight wheelchairs. The patient is taught transfer from bed to chair and from chair to toilet, and that at regular intervals the body-weight must be shifted. The patient learns to lift the trunk by pushing with the arms and hands on the chair arms or seat in order to relieve constant pressure on the buttocks and sacral region.

Alteration in urinary elimination

During the spinal shock, the bladder is atonic and there is retention of urine with overflow. The stasis of urine predisposes to infection and the distension may cause fissures or areas of pressure necrosis in the bladder wall.

Ureteral openings are dilated, allowing reflux of urine into the kidneys. An indwelling catheter or intermittent catheterization is introduced soon after admission to prevent overdistension of the atonic bladder. The prevention of **incontinence** also assists in protecting the skin from irritation and breakdown. If continuous catheter drainage is required, a sterile closed-drainage system is used; precautions must be strictly observed to prevent infection. Renal complications (e.g. pyelonephritis) leading to renal failure are a major cause of death in cord-injured persons. The atony of the bladder remains for a varying length of time before hyperreflexia takes over and the bladder becomes hypertonic, resulting in frequent automatic emptying of small volumes. To counteract the hypertonicity and diminished bladder capacity, an indwelling catheter is used or, if intermittent catheterization is used, the intervals are gradually increased. Catheter use is discontinued as soon as possible because of the risk of infection and a bladder training programme is initiated. The reflex emptying of the bladder and incontinence are very distressing to the patient, who may resist an adequate fluid intake with the thought that it may at least lessen the frequency of involuntary voiding. This is dangerous because it predisposes to infection and the formation of calculi. Some patients become dependent on catheter use on a permanent basis, and may have to be taught intermittent self-catheterization.

Ideally a bladder training programme should be introduced as soon as possible to avoid dependency on a catheter. The patient is taught to initiate the reflexive emptying of the bladder by the Credé manoeuvre or the Valsalva manoeuvre. With some patients, stretching of the anal sphincter by the insertion of a gloved finger into the anal canal in combination with the Valsalva manoeuvre is more effective. The bladder may not empty completely and stasis of urine predisposes to infection. Periodic catheterization may be done to determine residual volume; less than 75–100 mL is usually acceptable. A specimen of urine is submitted for analysis at regular intervals and also if the urine has an offensive odour, is cloudy or there is blood or sediment.

Alteration in bowel elimination

With spinal shock the gastrointestinal tract becomes atonic; severe distension and vomiting without effort may develop. Gastrointestinal aspiration via a nasogastric tube may become necessary until peristalsis is re-established; abdominal distension causes respiratory embarrassment by pressure on the diaphragm.

The spinal cord injury interrupts impulses from the higher centres of awareness and control. The sensation of the need to defaecate is lost and the rectal and anal sphincters function reflexly (automatic spinal cord response). Because of the immobility and dietary changes the patient experiences **constipation**, and impaction develops readily. When bowel sounds are present, a mild laxative or suppository (glycerine or bisacodyl) may be

used to evacuate the bowel at first, then, as the patient's condition improves and a more normal diet is taken, involuntary defaecation occurs. A diet high in fibre is usually necessary to prevent constipation. The diet is adjusted to the stool consistency and frequency. As soon as the patient is able to sit in a chair, training for bowel elimination by conditioned reflex begins. A regular hour for bowel elimination may be established; the morning is the normal time for most patients. The procedure involves a warm beverage, followed in 30 minutes by the insertion of a glycerine or bisacodyl (Dulcolax) suppository and stimulation by inserting a lubricated gloved finger every 10–15 minutes until defaecation occurs. Once a pattern of regular reflex evacuation has been established, the patient may find that digital stimulation alone or the use of a device to massage the anal canal may be effective.

The patient is assisted to a commode or toilet at the same time each day or every other day. Privacy should be provided. A member of the patient's family should be involved in the bowel training programme as part of the preparation for home management.

Alteration in food and fluid intake

During the initial phase oral food and fluid are withheld. Some degree of paralytic ileus develops in most spinal-cord-injured patients due to spinal shock. Fluids are administered by intravenous infusion to maintain hydration. A nasogastric tube may be inserted and aspiration established to relieve gastric and intestinal dilatation. When peristalsis is re-established, fluids are administered orally and, if tolerated, solid foods are added. A high-calorie, high-protein diet is important to combat the tendency toward a negative nitrogen balance which is commonly associated with immobility. An adequate nutritional intake also plays a role in promoting tissue healing and resistance to breakdown (e.g. pressure ulcers) and provides energy for exercises and the rehabilitative programme. Adequate dietary intake is made more difficult by the patient's positioning. Dietary supplements between meals may be necessary. Later, calorie intake may have to be reduced to prevent obesity, which complicates rehabilitation and increases the risk of complications. Bulk and roughage are necessary in the diet to promote bowel elimination.

Calcium intake (milk and milk products) may be restricted to prevent urinary calculi which may develop as calcium moves out of immobilized bones. A fluid intake of at least 3000 mL a day is encouraged to prevent concentration and stasis of urine. Grape and apple juices are preferable to citrus fruit juices; they produce an acid urine which reduces the precipitation of calcium and the formation of calculi as well as reducing the risk of infection. Organisms are less likely to grow in an acid environment.

Some cord-injured patients develop stress ulcers (gastric or duodenal). The aetiology has yet to be fully determined; hyperacidity due to histamine release following the trauma,

Incontinence
See chapter 5.4

Constipation
See chapter 5.1

Fluid balance
See chapter 2.6

or mucosal ischaemia, are among the leading theories at present. Ranitidine may be prescribed as a prophylactic measure. Dietary adjustments may be necessary to meet these patients' tolerance.

Food must be placed readily within reach and the patient encouraged to feed unaided as soon as the condition permits. Initially those with quadriplegia will require assistance with feeding until appropriate assistive devices are available. Swallowing may be difficult in the recumbent position and inhalation may occur. The patient is encouraged to take only small amounts at a time and swallow frequently. Suction equipment should be readily available in the event of inhalation.

If the partial quadriplegic patient has motor function in the triceps and biceps muscles, self-feeding may be accomplished. With flexion at the elbow and the fitting over the hand of a wide elastic band with a pocket, self-feeding may be achieved. Special utensils such as a spoon fit into the pocket.

Self-care hygiene deficits

The patient will become increasingly aware of limitations and dependency; personal care must be provided with sensitivity to the patient's feelings. It is difficult to convince the patient in the early stages that it is possible that considerable independence will eventually be regained.

In order to regain even minimal independence in self-care, the individual must be able to move about and be able to have some grasp in at least one hand. Paraplegic persons do have the distinct advantage of having the use of both hands and are capable of achieving self-care. The quadriplegic is dependent on head movements, assistive devices and care provided by others.

Alteration in comfort

The patient with a spinal cord injury may experience pain that radiates along the spinal nerves that originate at the level of injury. Spasticity of the muscles below the level of the cord injury is also a source of severe discomfort in paraplegia and quadriplegia, and may lead to contractures and deformities. The pain is severe and fatiguing and may be embarrassing at times for the patient. It may retard rehabilitation. The muscle spasms are hypersensitive reflexes that develop after spinal shock subsides. The stimulus may not even be obvious. Examples of stimuli that may initiate the spastic response include light touching of the skin, jarring of the bed, turning, cold, fatigue, a distended bladder and emotional reactions. Regular passive moving of the limbs through their range of motion is beneficial, especially when done under water. Rarely, severe painful spasticity is treated by surgery; various procedures have been used, including severing of tendons, transection of a nerve root (rhizotomy) and neurotomy (cutting of nerves).

Opioid analgesics are not used with the patient with high cervical injury because of the depressing effect on respiration.

Potential for infection

The risk of urinary and respiratory tract **infections** has already been discussed.

Potential for complications

Complications include muscle contractures, deformities, osteoporosis and thrombophlebitis.

Patients with spinal cord injury and the resulting paralysis develop muscle and tendon contractures and ankylosis of the joints unless preventive measures are observed. The shortening of the muscles and tendons may cause serious deformities that restrict rehabilitation. For example, a flexure **contracture** of the thigh at the hip joint may inhibit the patient's use of a wheelchair. Wrist drop and foot drop develop readily in paralysed limbs unless preventive measures are instituted. Immobility, muscle spasticity and poor alignment in positioning the patient are contributing factors. Preventive measures include frequent change of position and maintenance of good body alignment using sand bags, and pillows if necessary, regular passive range-of-movement exercises and a physiotherapy programme as soon as the patient's condition permits.

The health of bones normally depends on stress due to muscle pull and weight-bearing. When these are lacking, as with paralysis and prolonged immobilization, bone demineralization and osteoporosis occurs. Therefore, weight-bearing is started as soon as possible to stimulate osteoblastic activity and prevent demineralization. The head of the bed is gradually elevated as tolerated and, when safe, the patient is positioned upright on a tilt table. Weight-bearing for at least a few minutes each day may also help to prevent contractures, particularly in the hips.

Regardless of intervention, eventually atrophy of paralysed muscles does occur to some degree. This is due primarily to absence of nerve impulses to the muscle.

Thrombophlebitis is a common problem in a paralysed patient, particularly in the first 3 months following injury. Absence of the pumping action of contracting muscle and poor skeletal muscle tone which results from paralysis and immobility leads to pooling of blood in the lower viscera and extremities and a reduced venous return. This predisposes to thrombophlebitis. Localized oedema, redness, warmth, tenderness and red streaks of an extremity suggest thromphlebitis. Deep venous thrombosis may also occur.

Because of loss of sensation, pain and tenderness are not perceived. Assessment for venous thrombosis, done daily, includes calf observation, gentle palpation for calf firmness and measurement of the circumference of the thigh and calf. The tape measure is placed at the same level above and below the knee each time.

Management to prevent thrombosis includes a regular schedule of range of movement and exercises (these activities act as a mechanical pump to increase circulation), frequent change of position, elevation of the legs 15° for

Infection
See chapter 6.1

Contracture
See chapter 3.1

stated periods and the wearing of antiembolic stockings while in bed. Anticoagulant therapy (e.g. acetylsalicylic acid) may be prescribed as a prophylactic measure. Subcutaneous heparin, 5000 units twice daily, is often prescribed for the first 3 months following paraplegia.

Inability to control body temperature

This is a common problem for patients with a spinal cord injury. Dysfunction of the autonomic nervous system occurs and there is decreased ability to lose or conserve heat in the paralysed parts of the body. Room temperature is controlled to meet the patient's need because he or she is mainly dependent on environmental temperature for the avoidance of hypothermia.

Disturbance in sleep pattern

This is a common problem as a result of the psychological impact of the traumatic event and enforced immobility and dependency. The cord-injured patient may experience frightening dreams in which the accident is relived. Discomfort and the necessary frequent repositioning as well as a high level of anxiety may disrupt the patient's sleep.

Lack of adequate rest and **sleep** depletes the person's energy and endurance, which are essential for healing and rehabilitation.

Nursing care involves the provision of a quiet environment, comfort measures such as position change, warm drinks and remaining with the patient, encouraging the discussion of anxieties and feelings and to provide reassurance that he or she is not alone. Regular rest periods are scheduled to prevent exhaustion.

Body temperature
See chapter 6.1

Sleep
See chapter 2.2

Sexual dysfunction

The potential for sexual fulfilment is a major concern of the patient with permanent disability. Some patients may express this concern directly but more often concern is present long before it is expressed. If the patient brings up the topic of sexuality, a free and open discussion should be encouraged.

The cord-injured patient needs to know that meaningful and satisfying relationships are still attainable and that, even though he or she may no longer be able to function sexually in the same ways as before the injury, new ways of giving and receiving sexual satisfaction can be learned. The patient needs to understand that the sexuality of an individual involves the total person and that self-image is an important dimension in the resocialization process in disability.

The question of fertility and ability to procreate may also be raised by patients with a spinal cord injury. Male infertility is not uncommon following a cord injury because of testicular atrophy, decreased production of sperm and infrequency of ejaculation. The female with cord injury is usually able to conceive and deliver a child with few adaptations being necessary. As there is a vast body of knowledge specific to sexuality in disability, it is

appropriate to discuss other resources of information with the patient. Referral to a qualified counsellor or agency may be advisable.

Patient and family reactions

Spinal injury that results in paralysis is a very traumatic psychological experience. Suddenly, the victim is changed from an independent person to one who is dependent on others for even very personal care. Responses and adjustment to the loss of body functions usually parallel the grief reaction, with feelings of anger and despair mixing with frustration and depression.

Initially, shock and denial of reality help the victim to maintain self-control and survive. Consistent, high-quality nursing care is supportive in this phase. Gradually, as awareness develops, the patient may respond with anger and resentment. The nurse needs to listen and try to understand the patient's responses; support at this time may help to strengthen the patient's tenuous grasp of reality.

Anger may be followed by a period of despair and depression in which the patient may eat or drink very little and does not manifest any interest in rehabilitation, family or others. Close observation of reactions and comments indicate to the nurse when to encourage conversation or when presence alone is preferable to the patient. The patient may raise questions that relate to concerns such as independence, financial support and sexuality in the future. Anxiety may escalate in proportion to the unknown; anxiety depletes energy and tends to distort reality. The patient should be assured that everything possible will be done to help regain the ability to do some things unaided. Reassurance should be realistic; offering false hope must be avoided.

It will be some time before the patient begins to see things realistically and explore possibilities for the future. In this reorganization phase, learning to cope with body changes predominates. Assimilation of the changes in body image and pattern of life takes considerable time; periods of withdrawal and depression are to be expected from time to time. Such reactions are accepted but with expectation that efforts will be resumed. Thinking is directed to the positive, and as soon as possible the patient is encouraged and expected to do the things that the functional motor capacity allows. The acknowledgement of improvement and achievement helps to sustain motivation. The development of a sense of worthiness and self-esteem essential for resocialization depend greatly on the positive attitude, appreciation and reliance conveyed by professionals and significant others.

The victim's injury and the possible implications of disability are difficult for family members to accept. As well as concern for the patient, the situation may involve a complete change of lifestyle for them. They may be faced with financial hardships and a disruption of home management. Role functions change, responsibilities are shifted, and plans and goals may be shattered.

Family bonds may become greater as family members face the situation together; new strengths, capabilities and determination to cope with their problems may be revealed. In other instances, the reaction of some family members after the patient's acute phase may be resentment for the individual whose accident has altered their life. The patient is rejected and feelings of loneliness, fear and depression are increased. There may also be profound feelings of guilt if a family member was in some way responsible for the original accident.

The nurse takes time to talk with the family; they are kept informed of the patient's progress and of the therapeutic and rehabilitative programmes. Their role in supporting the patient is discussed. Time is given to discussing family problems and suggestions are made that assist them in planning and resolution.

Family and friends are encouraged to spend time with the patient to provide support and reinforce the impression that they are not rejecting the patient as useless. Encouraging and letting the patient do things unaided are emphasized. A major multidisciplinary effort will be needed to provide the long-term community care the patient needs.

Potential for injury

Limited sensation in the paralysed parts, limited mobility, muscle spasm and dependency place the paralysed patient at risk of injury and complications. It is necessary for the patient to develop the necessary strength in the unaffected parts to mobilize and control the affected parts in order to prevent complications incurred by immobilization and falls. The bones in paralysed limbs are easily fractured as a result of osteoporosis. A waist strap is used while the patient is in a chair until he or she is strong enough to control the trunk. Consistent use of wheelchair brakes during transfers is essential for safety.

Any local heat application is used judiciously; loss of cutaneous sensation predisposes to burns. The skin is inspected daily for abrasions, bruises, pressure ischaemia and irritated areas.

Rehabilitation

As soon as the patient is well enough, an active rehabilitation programme is planned and instituted. The patient and family participate in the planning and scheduling of the programme to meet their knowledge deficits and adjustments. Family members should be involved in order to support the patient and maintain consistent care. Rehabilitation begins with simple self-care activities, progressing to more complex activities as skill is achieved. Planned periods of rest and diversion are necessary to offset intensive exercises and prevent exhaustion. The family is cautioned against fostering dependence by doing things that the patient has the capacity to do or learn to do alone.

A major component of rehabilitation concerns work. Some patients may be able to manage to return to their previous employment, but many will not. Retraining may be possible and every effort should be made to allow the patient to regain meaningful employment as this will be beneficial to morale, self-concept, and also the patient's finances.

Nursing the patient treated by spinal surgery

Spinal surgery may be performed to: remove a neoplasm, a herniated or ruptured disc or bony fragments following an injury; reduce a fractured vertebra; decompress the spinal cord following an injury; relieve intractable pain or spasticity; or suppress involuntary movements.

The care following spinal surgery varies with the operation, the patient's response to it and the surgeon's preferences. For example, some patients are immobilized for weeks whereas others are ambulated a day or two after the procedure. An understanding of what was done and specific directives are necessary in planning care, especially in relation to positioning and movement. The major principles to be observed with all patients in moving and positioning are the maintenance of proper spinal alignment, the avoidance of any twisting, angulation and jerky movements of the spine and the prevention of strain on the back muscles.

Assessment

The patient's vital signs and responses are recorded as a baseline against which any changes in condition will become apparent.

When the surgery is below the thoracic region, assessment includes an evaluation of sensation and motor ability in the lower limbs. The colour and temperature of the limbs and leg and foot pulses may be checked as vascular problems may develop. If the operation was cervical or high thoracic, close observation of the person's respiratory pattern is necessary as well as sensorimotor responses of the arms. Hoarseness of the voice and ineffective cough may develop as a result of injury to the recurrent laryngeal nerve.

Wound area(s) are checked for possible haemorrhage, leakage of CSF and contamination. The patient's sensation of pain should be carefully assessed, together with the standard postoperative parameters of urine output, wound drainage, skin condition, etc.

Patient problems

- Potential for spinal injury – Even slight angulation or tension or jerky movements may injure the spine and cause nerve or cord damage.

- Potential for respiratory insufficiency due to cord and nerve compression in cervical spinal surgery, immobility and shallow respirations because of the pain.

- Pain due to oedema in the operative area, irritation and trauma of nerves at the time of operation and muscle spasm.

- Alteration in elimination pattern – **retention of urine**, **paralytic ileus**, constipation.

- Potential for wound haemorrhage or **infection**.

- Alteration in food and **fluid** intake.

- Potential impairment of **skin integrity** due to immobility and later due to the wearing of a brace or corset.

- Impairment of mobility – enforced immobility and maintenance of spinal alignment.

- Lack of knowledge – information is required to prevent recurrence of the back problem, and assistance is needed in planning the necessary adjustments in the resumption of activity and management at home.

Goals

Patient goals are similar to those set in the postoperative care of any general surgical patient. In addition, the patient should not suffer any complications related specifically to the spinal surgery.

Nursing intervention

The patient should be nursed in accordance with the same principles as a general surgical patient but also taking into account the nursing interventions specifically designed to deal with spinal problems, which were discussed earlier in this section.

Retention of urine
See chapter 5.4

Paralytic ileus
See chapter 5.1

Infection
See chapter 6.1

Fluids
See chapter 2.6

Pressure sores
See chapter 6.1

The person with a neoplasm of the nervous system

Intracranial neoplasms

Intracranial tumours may be primary or secondary (metastatic), and may occur at any age and in any part of the brain.

- *Primary* neoplasms may be benign or malignant and commonly arise from the neuroglial tissue, meninges, cerebral blood vessels, hypophysis and nerve fibres, and are named according to their tissue origin (Table 20.10). Most primary intracranial tumours are gliomas. Unlike neoplasms elsewhere in the body, primary neoplasms of the brain rarely metastasize.

- *Secondary* intracranial tumours commonly originate in the lungs or breast.

Brain tumours vary in size, location and pattern of growth. The glioblastomas are highly malignant and invasive, whereas others, such as the meningiomas, are benign and compressive. This accounts for the great variability in the development of symptoms and in the prognosis after operation. Most brain tumours in the adult tend to occur in the supratentorial compartment (above the brainstem and cerebellum).

Effects on the patient

Any intracranial neoplasm is a space-occupying lesion; as it grows, intracranial content and pressure increase within the rigid cranium. The effects of rising intracranial pressure (ICP) have already been discussed. The manifestations reflect the location: neurological deficits (sensory and/or motor) and behavioural changes appear as the tumour involves specific cerebral areas, some deficiency in mental capacity may develop and seizures may occur due to alterations in the electrical potential of cells. Hydrocephalus may develop if there is interference of the normal flow and absorption of CSF, and endocrine imbalances may occur associated with the compression or invasion of the pituitary gland.

Medical management

Investigation will involve the use of imaging techniques such as CT and MRI. Both will localize and usually identify the lesion. Contrast enhancement may be used in conjunction with CT. Prior to the availability of these specialized tests, the patient may have undergone skull radiography, EEG and isotope scanning. These are limited in that they may suggest the presence of a lesion but be unable to identify it.

Additional investigations may be indicated depending on the type of tumour. These will include endocrine studies, audiometric testing, visual field testing, chest radiography and determination of the erythrocyte sedimentation rate.

For some patients, a burr-hole biopsy may be indicated. A small piece of the tumour tissue is removed for pathological examination. The success of this technique relies greatly on the skill of the operator removing a specimen of tissue that reflects the true extent and pathology of the lesion.

Nursing the patient with a brain tumour

Caring for the person with a brain tumour can be a difficult and challenging situation for the nurse and the patient's family. The continuum of care can be divided into the care required before and during confirmation of the diagnosis, during treatment and, where applicable, during palliation.

Assessment

An initial evaluation is made and recorded of the patient's motor and sensory functions, speech ability, orientation, behavioural responses, pupillary reactions and any complaints of headache, dizziness, and tingling or numbness. It is important to obtain information about the patient's normal behaviour before the development of the tumour. Assessment is an ongoing process through successive contacts so that changes and newly developed symptoms may be recognized promptly. The nurse's recognition and recording of physical and behavioural changes may play an important role in the diagnosis and localization of the

Table 20.10   Classification of brain tumours

Tumour	Origin	Usual sites	Incidence of total	Comments
Tumours of epithelial origin				
Astrocytoma grade I	Astrocytes	Frontal lobes followed by temporal and parietal lobes	10%	Well differentiated, insidiously invasive, relatively benign
Intermediate astrocytoma grade II & III	Astrocytes	As above		Less well differentiated than grade I
Glioblastoma multiforme grade IV	Undifferentiated glial cells	As above	18%	Rapidly growing, highly malignant. Extensively invasive
Oligodendroglioma	Oligodendrocytes	Cerebral hemispheres	4%	Rare, slow growing
Ependymoma	Ependymal cells of the ventricles and aqueducts	Fourth ventricle but could be in other areas	5%	Rare, undifferentiated, slow growing. Seen in childhood and young adulthood
Optic nerve glioma	Cells of the optic nerve	Optic nerve and chiasma	4%	Occurs in young adulthood
Medulloblastoma	Undifferentiated glial cells	Cerebellum and roof of fourth ventricle	3%	Rapidly growing, malignant tumour of childhood. Development of hydrocephalus is common
Tumours of nerve sheath cells				
Schwannoma	Schwann cells	Cranial nerves VIII, V, & VII within the cerebellopontine angle	10%	Well encapsulated, slow growing, benign
Neuroma	Schwann cells	Neurilemma of nerves, e.g. VIII cranial nerve		Complex familial disorder. Occurs in young adulthood
Tumours of meningeal and related tissue				
Meningioma	Meninges	Intracranial venous sinuses	15%	Benign. Slow growing. Predilection for females
Tumours of blood vessel origin				
Haemangioblastoma	Blood vessels	Cerebellar hemisphere	2%	Slow growing. May be multiple. May be familial
Germ cell tumour				
Teratoma	Pineal parenchymal cells	Pineal gland		Rare childhood tumour
Malformative tumours				
Craniopharyngioma	Embryological remnants	Rathke's pouch	3%	
Dermoid cyst	Ectodermal	Posterior fossa		Fluid-filled cyst containing some solid material (e.g. hair)
Colloid cyst of the third ventricle	Choroid plexus	Third ventricle		Rounded cystic tumour
Vascular malformations				
Angiomas	Blood vessels	Cerebral cortex		Arterial and/or venous anomaly comprising enlarged and tortuous vessels
Angioblastoma	Angioblasts	Cerebellum		
Pituitary tumours				
Pituitary adenoma	Cells of the pituitary	Anterior lobe of the pituitary gland	8%	Benign, slow growing and well encapsulated. Classified by clinical syndrome, e.g. prolactin secreting (prolactinoma); excess growth hormone (acromegaly); ACTH-secreting (Cushing's disease)
Metastatic tumours				
Metastatic tumour		Can occur anywhere in cerebrum or cerebellum	12%	Well defined; usually multiple secondaries from breast or lung

intracranial tumour. Knowing that a space-occupying lesion is suspect, the nurse is especially alert for signs of increasing intracranial pressure. It is crucial to discuss the patient's and family's understanding of the condition in order to plan how they may be assisted and supported. Anxieties and fears, together with the patient's level of knowledge and any coping mechanisms being employed, should all be ascertained.

Patient problems

The patient faces the whole range of potential problems associated with immobility and raised ICP (see preceding sections). In addition there is the very real fear of death itself – understandably leading to severe anxiety and depression as well as seriously stressing family networks.

Goals

Patient goals revolve around avoiding the complications of immobility and raised ICP in general, and specifically in adapting to the fact that the illness may prove fatal.

Nursing intervention

Awaiting results from investigations is an extremely anxious and worrying time for the patient. The purpose of investigations is to confirm the diagnosis or identify the type of tumour, and the patient should be encouraged to discuss fears and anxieties (Amato 1991). It is important that the nurse establishes the basis of the patient's understanding of these fears and anxieties as some may be unfounded and may be alleviated.

Assessment should include observation for increasing ICP (see section on Head Injuries) and the increased likelihood of seizures. The occurrence of raised ICP and/or seizures are the events most likely to be troublesome for the patient. Each will produce potentially distressing symptoms for the patient such as severe headache, vomiting and other neurological deficits along with the anxiety and distress associated with seizures. Each patient's experience will vary according to the size, location and type of tumour, and for many in the initial stages life will continue almost as normal.

A range of interventions is available for treatment, and nursing management will depend on those selected. These may include steroids, surgery and radiotherapy.

Steroids

Steroids are often prescribed once a tumour is suspected, and routinely on diagnosis. Dexamethasone is the commonest choice. It reduces swelling around the tumour, decreasing the overall mass of the brain and therefore ICP. The effect is rapid and the patient can feel better within 24 hours, experiencing relief from headache, nausea and vomiting, and from the improvement of neurological deficits. However, side-effects arise from the use of such a powerful drug, including:

- irritation of the lining of the stomach – antacids are routinely prescribed to counteract this

- glycosuria – urine is routinely tested for glucose and ketones

- adrenal insufficiency, which will occur if medication is withdrawn suddenly.

Surgery

Biopsy, partial removal of the tumour with internal decompression, and complete removal are the surgical options. The appropriate approach is determined by the nature of the tumour and its site. In many instances this will constitute major neurosurgery entailing a lengthy operation and subsequent intensive nursing care. See Table 20.11 for further details.

Radiotherapy

Treatment may involve irradiation, either on its own or as an adjunct to surgery.

A tumour may be inoperable owing to inaccessibility or because of its type and size. It could be that surgery would involve great risk of postoperative neurological deficits. The patient's condition may be very poor and the doctor may advise the family that the condition will not improve. It then becomes necessary to reconsider the plan of care with a change in emphasis from active treatment to eventual palliation.

The person with a degenerative disorder

Commonly occurring degenerative disorders of the nervous system include Alzheimer's disease, multiple sclerosis, Parkinson's disease, myasthenia gravis and motor neurone disease. In addition, patients with AIDS will also suffer chronic neurological disease.

The diagnosis of a chronic neurological problem can affect a patient's self-esteem and feeling of confidence, as well as generating fear for the future. These feelings can be manifested as symptoms of anger, denial, powerlessness and depression. The nurse, in caring for the family and the patient, has to be aware of the difficulties in adaptation the patient may have at any given time. There are periods of stability, both emotional and physical, together with periods of increased stress when the illness exacerbates.

An explanation of the disorder and the prescribed therapy is made to the patient and family. Opportunities are provided for discussions in which they can ask questions and express their feelings and concerns. They are assisted in planning how to maintain a satisfactory lifestyle, role functions and socialization. The patient is encouraged to be independent and carry out self-care activities. Those around are advised that the patient's intellectual ability is unimpaired; it should be emphasized that he or she needs to be treated normally, to socialize and to do things unaided even though it may take much longer. The environment should be cheerful and free of haste and confusion.

Table 20.11   Care plan for patient undergoing neurosurgery

Area care	Nursing interventions	Rationale
Preoperative phase		
Physical preparation for operation	Ensure preoperative investigations are complete including appropriate blood tests. Full physical nursing assessment. Immediate preoperative checklist prior to surgery complete	Ensuring that the patient is in an optimal physical condition for surgery will reduce postoperative risks
Psychological preparation for operation	Assess patient's understanding of operation. Evaluate extent of patient's anxiety and coping mechanism in relation to undergoing surgery. Evaluate concerns that family may have. Identify and implement appropriate interventions to alleviate anxieties including the use of a preoperative teaching plan	Reduction of patient anxiety and concerns of the family will result in better recovery
Immediate and early postoperative stage		
Respiratory care	Implement interventions to avoid ineffective airway clearance including a full respiratory assessment and use of appropriate interventions such as oxygenation and suctioning. Some patients will be ventilated requiring additional care	Achievement of a patent airway and adequate ventilation will ensure optimal oxygenation of the brain thus improving outcome from surgery
Neurological status	Monitor conscious level and other neurological parameters for signs of deterioration indicating a rise in ICP. Implement measures to avoid exacerbating rises in ICP due to noxious stimuli. Assess risk of injury due to loss of consciousness or seizure activity	Early detection of complications will enable appropriate interventions to be applied to minimize risk of ill-effects
Pain	Assess for signs and symptoms of pain and initiate interventions to alleviate	Ensuring that the patient is pain free will result in comfort and reduction of anxiety
Fluid balance	Assess fluid intake and output. Administer fluids as per prescription	Achievement of the prescribed fluid balance will avoid development of cerebral oedema
Elimination	Monitor urinary output hourly. Administer catheter care (if appropriate). Avoid constipation	Ensuring optimal fluid balance will avoid development of cerebral oedema

The general *goals* of the patient and family in cases of degenerative neurological disorder are that they will:

1. have knowledge of the disease process and potential complications

2. have knowledge of the healthcare system and available support systems

3. be aware of interventions that maintain optimal functioning.

AIDS

Some 30–70% of all individuals with human immunodeficiency virus (HIV) infection will at some time during their illness develop neurological manifestations of the disease. The brain, spinal cord and peripheral nerves can all be involved in HIV infection, with the symptoms being very similar to those seen in depressive or anxiety syndromes, or they may imitate the symptoms of manic depression and schizophrenia. Opportunistic infections of the brain include viral infections such as cytomegalovirus, herpes simplex, adenovirus, varicella zoster virus and papovavirus. The most common bacterial infections include cryptococcosis and toxoplasmosis, which respond well to drug therapy, but this must be continued for the patient's lifetime.

The most frequent problem affecting the spinal cord is a condition known as *vascular myelopathy*, a degenerative condition that presents as difficulty walking, numbness in the feet and paraplegia. There is currently no treatment for this condition.

HIV can also directly invade brain tissue, resulting in a condition known as *AIDS dementia complex* (ADC) or AIDS encephalopathy. ADC has an insidious onset, with impairment in memory and concentration and subtle changes in personality being early signs. The condition may advance to motor difficulties, with ataxia being present, or to psychiatric manifestations such as psychosis or hallucinations. The patient often becomes depressed, resulting in social withdrawal and apathy. It is often difficult to differentiate between psychological symptoms of the illness and neurological changes.

AIDS
See chapter 6.2

Early and ongoing nursing assessment of neurological change is crucial. Questions relating to memory, concentration, orientation and judgement need to be asked in a safe, non-threatening environment. Safety issues must be continually examined, with the patients often requiring orientation cues and written instruction. Eyesight may be impaired by cytomegalovirus retinitis.

Alzheimer's disease

Alzheimer's disease is a presenile **dementia** of unknown aetiology and is the most common degenerative brain disorder. A history of familial incidence is considered to play a role in the development of the disease, which is incurable at present. The age of onset is between 45 and 65 years. Both males and females are equally affected. The frontal and temporal lobes are most affected but gradual progressive atrophy of the entire brain occurs. Microscopically, there is widespread loss of nerve cells.

Effects on the patient

In the progress of the disease three stages may be identified. The *first stage* lasts for 2–4 years and is characterized by subtle changes which may be dismissed as inattention or carelessness. Eventually, there are recognizable changes in personality, loss of memory for recent and remote events, apathy, loss of spontaneity and initiative, neglect of personal hygiene and appearance, and a suspiciousness of other's motives with a tendency to blame them for one's incapacities. Loss of spatial orientation is seen in the inability to put on a garment without confusion as to top and bottom and sleeve and neck. Weakness, muscular twitching or seizures may occur, and motor aphasia (the person cannot recall words he or she wishes to say) and speech slurring may become evident. Indifference to social customs and graces develops.

In the *second stage* of the disease, the changes of the first stage intensify. Disorientation is complete; emotional lability increases and there may be restlessness at night. Memory loss becomes so severe that even close friends and relatives are not recognized and the patient may not recognize himself or herself in the mirror. Movements are slow, and simple writing, reading, mathematical skills and reasoning deteriorate seriously. Other deficiencies such as inability to recognize objects by way of the senses become obvious. Motor dysfunction may progress from unsteady gait to inability to stand or walk. The person loses weight due to poor nutrition and shows no interest in meals.

In the *final stage* of the disease, movements become stereotyped, there is inability to use language, urinary and bowel incontinence, abnormal reflexes and muscular rigidity develop and, eventually, there is flexion of the lower extremities and the individual becomes bedridden and totally helpless. There is a marked tendency to grasp objects and put them to the mouth. The disease may last for several years before death occurs, often as a result of bronchopneumonia.

Dementia
See chapter 2.2

Nursing care

Assessment

The patient assessment involves paying particular attention to nutritional and fluid balance status, skin condition, general personal hygiene and appearance, and elimination patterns. The patient's level of understanding, memory and orientation are key parts of the assessment, and social and family circumstances must also be explored.

Patient problems

The patient's carers may be the focal point of nursing interventions. The age, the health and support systems of the caregivers are important considerations when a patient remains at home. The following is a list of core problems; many more individual problems are possible:

- ineffective coping because of altered cognitive functioning

- potential for injury due to loss of memory, impaired motor and cognitive functioning

- self-care deficits in relation to adequate rest, nutrition and personal hygiene

- alteration in elimination patterns – urinary and bowel incontinence

- potential for social isolation due to loss of interest, initiative and memory (friends and relatives not recognized)

- potential for complications:
  — respiratory dysfunction due to inactivity and lowered resistance to infection
  — impairment of skin integrity due to immobility, incontinence, malnutrition and injury

- inadequate knowledge.

Nursing intervention

Ineffective coping

In the early stage, the patient and particularly the family require considerable counselling. Expectations of the patient's abilities should be lowered. The patient needs to be understood and accepted as he or she is, because memory cannot be restored nor behaviour changed. A written outline of daily routines to be carried out may prove helpful. For example, if the person is to carry out a job away from home, it may be useful to refer to a written note.

Each day, the patient identifies a few essential tasks on which to focus, as coping with more than these is too difficult.

Potential for injury

The environment is kept free of hazards and stress as much as possible. As disorientation develops and body movements become increasingly more awkward, the risk of falls increases. The patient may forget that a cigarette is burning or that a gas stove has been turned on. With progressive loss of memory, the person requires close supervision. It is important that he or she carries identification in case of wandering off and becoming lost and exposed to the elements. It should be remembered that restlessness and disorientation are likely to be worse at night when sensory stimuli are minimal and there is some decrease in cerebral perfusion.

The patient can usually manage for a longer period and be capable of doing more if in the familiar surroundings of home, where an automatic routine is established.

Self-care deficits

Regular periods of rest are planned for the person: fatigue tends to aggravate the manifestations of deterioration. Some patients respond to relaxation therapy tapes. The daily food and fluid intake are noted and the patient is weighed at regular intervals. In the early stage of Alzheimer's disease, the patient gradually loses the appreciation of nutritional needs. The person becomes unable to shop and prepare food, and eventually skips meals. Prompting and assistance with meals and in-between snacks are necessary to ensure that the patient has sufficient nutrition. High-calorie foods and supplements are used when necessary. Plans are made to provide hygienic care as neglect becomes obvious. Provision is made for bathing, grooming, dressing and frequent change of washable clothing.

Alteration in elimination pattern

With progression of Alzheimer's disease, the patient develops urinary and bowel **incontinence**. A schedule for prompting the patient to go to the toilet at intervals determined by customary elimination frequency may help in avoiding incontinence. **Constipation** may be a problem due to the immobility and reduced food intake. The roughage content of the diet may be increased and a mild laxative (bulk producing or stool softener) administered. If the constipation is not recognized and corrected, faecal impaction develops readily.

Potential for social isolation

The patient tends to avoid social situations as cognitive and communicative skills diminish. Efforts should be made for exposure to human interaction and for socialization just as long as they have even the slightest meaning. Including the person in short social events and in small-group affairs could be helpful. If a daycare centre is available, the patient will be able to get out of the home and participate in structured social activity.

Potential for complications

Because of inactivity and malnutrition, the patient is predisposed to respiratory infection. An exercise programme, walking, deep breathing and coughing, adequate nutrition as well as protection from exposure to those with an infection contribute to the prevention of respiratory infection.

As the immobility, helplessness and malnutrition worsen, the patient becomes more and more predisposed to pressure ulcers. Regular bathing, careful observation and protection of vulnerable areas, repositioning at regular intervals and prompt changing of clothing or bedding following incontinence are necessary.

Inadequate knowledge

Some major adjustments in the lifestyle and relationships of the family, as well as those of the patient, are necessary as the disease advances. Planning for these at an early stage of the disorder facilitates the change process as it becomes necessary. A major effort involving social workers and various members of the community care team is needed to support the family in caring for the patient at home. Although the lifespan of the person with Alzheimer's disease cannot be protracted, the quality of the life of all concerned may be enhanced through early professional intervention, counselling and effective planning. It is helpful to introduce the family to the local branch of the Alzheimer's Society. The association provides family support through meetings, pamphlets and community referrals. The Society also provides education for the general public.

In the early stages, the family is advised of ways to help the patient maintain independence and carry on at home. The family is informed of signs of progression of the disorder and how members can best cope with increasing dependency of the patient. They are alerted to the hazards that may develop with the increasing dementia. When the affected person is no longer productive, roles and relationships must change. It is particularly difficult when a formerly responsible and productive person becomes dependent upon others for decision making and personal care. The process of adjustment is slow and requires understanding and acceptance of the patient's condition. The family's reactions may indicate the need for a referral for professional counselling.

In the later stages of the disorder, management focuses on helping the family to cope with extremely difficult situations. The family may consist of one person or several people. Anticipatory planning for institutional care has to be encouraged so that, when it becomes necessary, it is part of a rational decision-making process. The family may need considerable persuasion and support in making this decision.

Multiple sclerosis (MS, disseminated sclerosis)

Multiple sclerosis is a chronic, progressive, degenerative disease characterized by patches of demyelination throughout the brain and spinal cord. Myelin is the lipoprotein sheath surrounding the axons of the neurones and enables impulses to travel much faster along the fibre than is

Incontinence
See chapter 5.4

Constipation
See chapter 5.1

possible in unmyelinated fibres. The destruction of areas of myelin is followed by a proliferation of neuroglial cells. Scar tissue forms as hardened (sclerotic) white elevations known as plaque. Nerve fibres (axons) eventually degenerate; there is loss of impulse transmission, and focal deficits occur which in some instances may be permanent. The optic nerves and the cervical spinal cord tend to be most vulnerable to this degenerative demyelinating process in the initial episodes.

Incidence and population at risk

Multiple sclerosis has a worldwide distribution and affects 40–60 people per 100 000 population. People are twice as likely to be stricken if they live in cold, damp climates. The UK has been recognized as a high-risk zone; in northeast Scotland and Ulster, the incidence is 100 per 100 000 population, and in the Shetlands and Orkney it is 300 per 100 000. The onset of the disease is highest amongst persons aged 17–30 years, with a slightly higher incidence in women. A familial tendency has been recognized but a definite genetic pattern has not been identified.

Aetiology

The specific cause of multiple sclerosis continues to elude scientists; current evidence suggests that genetic factors, environmental factors, viruses and the individual's immune system may be collectively implicated. The view that viral infection and an immunological abnormality interact to induce the CNS damage is particularly favoured.

Effects on the patient

Multiple sclerosis is characterized by remissions and relapses. The course and the effects vary widely from one person to another and are unpredictable. Spontaneous remissions of varying lengths are common particularly in the early years of the disease, and in some instances appear to be permanent. Rarely multiple sclerosis takes a fulminating, malignant course in which a combination of cerebral brainstem and cord manifestations develops suddenly; the patient becomes comatose, there is no remission and death may occur within a few weeks.

Most patients survive more than 20 years after the initial onset and lead active productive lives for many of those years. A lesser number experience a steady progression of the disease with frequently recurring relapses leading to a chronic incapacitated state, dependency and complications.

The initial onset of symptoms of multiple sclerosis usually develops suddenly (within a day or two) but, with some, may develop slowly over several weeks. The initial onset of exacerbation usually coincides with a stressful experience such as anxiety, trauma, infection, excessive fatigue, exposure to an extreme of temperature and pregnancy.

As the location and extent of the demyelination are so variable, the clinical characteristics are also highly variable from one patient to another. They may include the following:

- extreme fatigue
- visual dysfunction (e.g. diplopia, blurring of vision, nystagmus)
- transient tingling sensations or numbness (paraesthesia) or loss of sensation
- intention tremor
- ataxia
- muscular weakness in one or both arms and legs
- paraparesis
- bladder and bowel dysfunction
- impairment of speech (scanning)
- emotional lability – alternating periods of euphoria, depression and irritability
- personality changes
- cognitive dysfunction – loss of memory and confusion.

Deficits that persist beyond 3 months are usually permanent. Weakness of the respiratory muscles and cough reflex may develop, predisposing the patient to pulmonary complications.

There is no cure for multiple sclerosis; the treatment is symptomatic and supportive, and increases in amount and complexity as the patient's disease progresses. Corticosteroids are now used for severe relapses; a dose of methylprednisolone 500 mg daily for 5 days is the accepted regimen. There is no consensus on the role of any specific dietary measures. Physiotherapy is prescribed for most patients to promote activity and independence as long as possible.

Assessment

Assessment should focus on the current neurological problems being experienced by the patient, together with the degree of insight the patient has into the illness. Fears, anxieties and other feelings such as frustration should be gently explored, together with the social and family circumstances of the patient.

Patient problems

The following is a list of the more commonly found problems associated with multiple sclerosis; it should be remembered that many other individual problems are also possible:

- Inadequate or inaccurate knowledge about the disorder, health maintenance and management of a remission.
- Alteration in self-image and fear due to the potential change in lifestyle, disability and dependence.

- Potential remissions; adjustments in activities to maintain health.

- Impaired mobility secondary to muscular weakness, fatigue, ataxia and/or paralysis.

- Potential for injury because of difficulty in walking.

- Potential sensory deficits – abnormal vision and diminished cutaneous sensation may occur.

- Alteration in pattern of elimination:
  — urinary frequency, urgency or **incontinence**
  — **Constipation**.

- Alteration in nutritional status due to loss of appetite secondary to anxiety and depression, weakened mastication and swallowing muscles, and/or inability to prepare meals.

- Self-care deficits due to muscular weakness or paralysis, immobility and depression.

- Impairment of verbal communication secondary to weakness or paralysis of the muscles involved in producing speech.

- Potential for complications:
  — impairment of skin integrity
  — **respiratory insufficiency** and infection.

Goals

The patient's goals can be summarized as avoiding the complications listed in the above problems and adapting lifestyle to the progressive deterioration in function that occurs. A key goal is to maintain maximum independence for as long as possible.

Nursing intervention

Good counselling and care may contribute to the prevention of relapses as well as help in keeping the patient active and independent for as long as possible. Hospital care usually becomes necessary during acute exacerbations or when complete dependence has been reached.

Inadequate knowledge

The patient and family are informed about multiple sclerosis, the nature of the disease, its effects, the fact that relapses of varying length occur and the potential precipitating factors in relapses. They are advised that it is not possible to predict the course of the disorder. Management is discussed in detail with emphasis on continuing former activities and gainful employment, and the necessary modifications in lifestyle to avoid factors known to contribute to a recurrence of symptoms. Important factors in the prevention of potential injuries and complications are outlined.

Community resources for assistance are made known to the patient and family. These include the Multiple Sclerosis Society, social services and community nurses. During relapses, or as the disorder progresses leaving residual disability, assistive devices (e.g. wheelchair), assistance with physical care and/or home management, financial assistance, and support and encouragement may become necessary. The local branch of the Multiple Sclerosis Society is an excellent source of information and assistance. For example, it helps in securing assistive devices, transporting patients to the physiotherapy department or clinic, and contacting other resources for assistance (e.g. social services department) if necessary. The Society also has voluntary workers who make home visits and arrange occupational and recreational programmes for patients with multiple sclerosis. If the patient's former occupation is too strenuous or stressful, vocational retraining may be appropriate so that the person can return to gainful employment during remissions.

Alteration in self-image and fears

The changes in body function and capacity and increasing loss of independence alter the patient's image of self. Feelings of uncertainty may arise because the outcomes are unclear and planning may be difficult. Roles and relationships change, counselling around sexuality may be helpful, and responsibilities shift. Sensory and motor deficits that occur with multiple sclerosis frequently lead to impaired sexual functioning, which may affect relationships. Fear of the long-term consequences of the disease, increasing dependency and the reactions of others are threatening.

Both patient and family are likely to experience the stages of grief reaction as they come to grips with the realities of the situation. Nursing care involves acceptance of their reactions, supportive understanding and open discussion of concerns. Providing information about the illness, the symptoms and the potential therapy helps to decrease the uncertainty and promote realistic expectations. Anxiety and depression on the part of the patient and family may delay the process of acceptance of the diagnosis, and counselling may be helpful. The patient and family should be allowed to make decisions and be part of the planning for the future.

Maintenance of health

In early remissions when the residual effects are likely to be minimal, the patient is encouraged to resume his or her usual pattern of life, modifying it as necessary to avoid overfatigue, emotional stress and infections as these may precipitate a relapse. Regular and adequate rest, a well balanced diet, and learning to accept what cannot be readily changed to avoid emotional stress, reduce the risk of an exacerbation.

In the case of the female patient, menstruation and fertility are unaffected but the woman is advised of the increased risk of a relapse incurred by pregnancy. In addition, delivery may be complicated by spasms of the hip adductor muscles. Contraceptive pills may aggravate symptoms of multiple sclerosis.

Incontinence
See chapter 5.4

Constipation
See chapter 5.1

Respiratory tract
See chapter 6.1

Impaired mobility

Muscle spasticity and weakness, especially in the lower limbs, is a common disabling factor in multiple sclerosis. A carefully controlled physiotherapy programme is instituted within the patient's tolerance to keep the patient active and prevent muscle **contractures** and atrophy. Exercises in a warm pool reduce the spasticity. Close observation is made for signs of excessive fatigue and a rest period should follow the exercise period.

A walking stick or crutches may be necessary to assist the patient in maintaining mobility. Walking between parallel bars may be helpful. When walking becomes impossible, a wheelchair is provided and the patient is taught to transfer from bed to chair and from chair to toilet unaided if there is sufficient strength in the arms.

Family members require instructions on how to transfer the patient from the wheelchair to the bed, and vice versa, if the patient is experiencing weakness or motor deficit in the upper limbs.

Spasticity may become a painful problem in the disabled limbs. Passive movements of the affected limbs may reduce the spasticity and prevent contractures.

Potential for injury

The patient is at risk of injury especially as walking becomes increasingly more difficult. To prevent falls, floors are kept clear of scatter rugs, stools, electrical flexes and other articles over which the patient might trip. Hand-rails in appropriate places facilitate safer mobility. Shoes that provide firm support and have non-slip soles are worn.

Potential sensory deficits

Sensory deficits such as impaired vision and diminished temperature and pressure sensations increase the patient's potential for injury. If a portion of the visual field is affected, the patient learns to turn the head in order to bring objects into the range of vision. Diplopia may be relieved by wearing an eye patch on one eye and then periodically placing it on the other eye. The patient and family are taught safety measures to prevent burns, for example control of the temperature of food and beverages as well as bath water. Areas of diminished sensation are inspected daily for irritation and injury.

Alteration in pattern of elimination

Urinary frequency and urgency are common problems for the patient with multiple sclerosis. Later, as the disease progresses, loss of sphincter control and **incontinence** develops. The patient is advised to set up a regular schedule for going to the toilet to avoid the distress caused by urgency and dribbling or incontinence. If the patient's mobility is impaired, a prompt response to the patient's request for assistance is necessary.

Some patients experience urinary retention or may not completely empty the bladder when voiding. The use of catheterization is avoided if possible because of the risk of ascending urinary tract infection. If catheterization becomes necessary, strict asepsis is observed, a high fluid intake is encouraged (3000 mL daily) and regular assessment is made for infection (temperature, culture of urine).

Constipation is a frequent problem as a result of the reduced mobility, and should be dealt with by standard methods (high-fibre diet, etc.).

Alteration in nutritional status

The patient's weight is recorded at regular intervals as the food intake is frequently reduced owing to a poor appetite which develops as a result of the patient's anxiety, immobility, weakness in mastication and swallowing, or the patient's inability to shop and prepare meals.

Well balanced meals that are easily digested are necessary; the food intake is monitored. High-calorie drinks may be necessary in order to meet the patient's requirements for energy and tissue maintenance. If the patient is overweight, a decreased caloric intake is prescribed to reduce the burden on weakened muscles.

Self-care deficits in hygiene

Nursing care includes repeated assessments of the patient's ability to complete self-care, which may become increasingly difficult as the disease progresses and care provision increases. For example, muscular weakness or paralysis of the arms may prevent the patient from cleaning the teeth and combing the hair. Food particles and mucus may accumulate in the mouth if swallowing is difficult, necessitating mouth care after each meal.

Impairment of verbal communication

The speech may progressively become slower and more difficult as muscular weakness increases, creating frustration for both the patient and carers. Referral to a speech therapist may be helpful. Nursing care includes support and reinforcement of the therapy, talking with the patient, encouraging verbal responses and acknowledging even slight achievement without, however, being patronizing.

Potential for complications

As mobility and sensory perception deteriorate, the potential for skin breakdown increases; meticulous pressure care is therefore required.

Parkinson's disease (paralysis agitans)

Parkinson's disease is a complex clinical syndrome associated with a decreased concentration of the chemical dopamine and its major metabolite. Dopamine is essential for normal neurotransmission and functioning of the basal ganglia. It is produced by the substantia nigra (black substance), a nucleus of highly pigmented cells in the midbrain which function as a part of the extrapyramidal system. Dopamine exerts an inhibitory effect on movements by opposing or lessening the stimulating effect of acetylcholine. When a deficiency of dopamine occurs,

Contractures
See chapter 3.1

Spasticity
See chapter 3.1

Incontinence
See chapter 5.4

Constipation
See chapter 5.1

tremors, rigidity, slowness and limited voluntary movement become evident.

Types, aetiology and incidence

The cause of the illness is usually unknown, although it may occasionally appear as a side-effect of some drugs (e.g. the phenothiazines).

Parkinson's disease affects one person out of 1000 in the UK, with one person in every 100 affected in the 60–70-years age group. Men and women are affected equally. There is no evidence of familial influence, nor is the disorder more prevalent in any part of the world.

Effects of the patient

The disease produces increasing physical disability as it progresses. At first, tremor and muscular rigidity develop insidiously and disappear with voluntary movement and sleep, although becoming more pronounced with fatigue and stress. The tremor initially usually develops in the fingers and thumb, producing the characteristic pill-rolling movement. The arms are adducted and semiflexed and the normal arm swing associated with walking is absent. Movements are slowed and a monotone becomes evident in the speech.

As the disease progresses the trunk and head are flexed forward, the patient may have difficulty in starting to walk and in turning, and the gait is slow and shuffling. Rigidity of the facial muscles and unblinking eyes produces a mask-like inexpressive appearance.

With further deterioration the patient becomes more stooped and when walking there is a progressive acceleration of steps, producing what is known as a *festination gait*, making stopping difficult and predisposing to falls. There is difficulty in changing position and the patient has difficulty with tasks involving finger movements.

Drooling occurs due to the decrease in automatic swallowing of saliva. Disturbances in autonomic innervation may develop; there may be excessive, or an absence of, perspiration, and disordered temperature regulation. Excessive lacrimation, ptosis and/or pupillary constriction may develop. Gastrointestinal activity may be slowed, causing constipation.

Pain and fatigue are experienced because of the continuously increased traction of muscles on their attachments. Speech becomes weak, slurred and devoid of any inflections as the muscles concerned with articulation become more involved.

In the final stages the patient becomes disabled to a greater degree because of the inability to initiate voluntary movement. Speech becomes incoherent and difficulty in mastication and swallowing develops. The respiratory volumes are reduced and the ability to cough is diminished, predisposing to respiratory complications.

Up to now, the patient's intellectual functioning is unaffected, but at this later stage dementia may become evident in some patients.

Assessment

Assessment of the patient should focus on the degree of disability and any techniques the patient may use to help cope with such disability. The effects on family and the social circumstances should be investigated, together with the patient's feelings about the condition.

Patient problems

- Inadequate or inaccurate knowledge about the parkinsonian syndrome, its characteristics, prescribed treatment and management.

- Muscular dysfunction due to impairment of **extrapyramidal** control – tremor, rigidity, slowness and lack of coordination.

- Potential for injury due to muscular dysfunction.

- Altered body image and loss of self-esteem secondary to incapacity, change in role, appearance and dependency.

- Nutritional deficit due to difficulty in eating, mastication and swallowing, anorexia and nausea caused by the prescribed medication.

- Impairment in communication – Speech difficulty secondary to the rigidity of the muscles involved in speech and reduced pulmonary volumes.

- Potential for complications:
  — respiratory complications due to respiratory muscle dysfunction, causing reduced pulmonary volumes and the inability to **cough** to remove secretions
  — break in skin due to immobility and falls
  — impairment of eye function due to diplopia or to drying and injury of the cornea caused by a reduction in blinking and moistening of the surface of the eye
  — medication reaction; medication withdrawal.

Extrapyramidal system
See chapter 2.2

Coughing
See chapter 5.3

Goals

The goals are that the patient and family will accept and adjust to the situation and the patient will maintain independence, accustomed role and a relatively normal lifestyle for as long as the condition permits.

Nursing intervention

The patient with Parkinson's disease is managed at home on a drug programme until the advanced stage of the disorder causes marked disability and dependency. The community nurse assumes the major role in assessing the patient's needs and providing the necessary counselling and guidance for the patient and family at the onset and through successive months and years. It is important that the nurse recognizes the emotional, physical and socioeconomic problems incurred by the disease. The fact that the patient's intellect is unimpaired must be kept in mind as well as a tendency to become very self-conscious, depressed and withdrawn because of the appearance and limitations enforced on the patient by the disease.

The patient is advised to contact the national Parkinson's Disease Society. Socialization in structured groups of persons with similar problems is helpful.

Difficulty in movement requires care to be taken to avoid hazards that may cause falls and also emphasizes the need for teaching about pressure care. Encouragement with a physiotherapy programme is essential to promote inability for as long as possible.

Loss of normal smooth, coordinated mobility, change in appearance, loss of the capacity for gainful employment and self-care, and loss of accustomed social interaction result in the patient's altered self-image, loss of self-esteem and depression. The patient is encouraged to express his or her feelings and to take an active role in setting realistic goals and planning management. The patient may develop an acute sense of humiliation leading to withdrawal and isolation.

The patient's strengths and potential capacity should be emphasized and independence encouraged in order that socialization and group activities may be promoted. Every effort should be made to try to encourage the patient's self-esteem.

The expertise of other professionals may be required to provide counselling, motivation, guidance and support. Involvement in the local branch of the Parkinson's Disease Society may promote acceptance and adjustment.

The quality and quantity of food taken by the patient and bodyweight are followed closely. Only a small amount of food may be taken because of fatigue and depression. The patient should be encouraged to be as independent as possible in feeding. The patient may be less self-conscious and eat more if privacy is ensured and ample time is allocated for each meal. Sensitive provision of protection for clothing at meal times is essential to preserve the patient's fragile self-esteem.

Constipation is a common occurrence because of the decreased activity, decreased food (bulk) intake and decreased fluid in the gastrointestinal tract due to an inadequate intake and the loss of saliva (drooling). The drug therapy may also contribute to the problem.

The fluid, roughage and bulk intake are increased. A stool softener or bulk-producing laxative (e.g. bisacodyl) may be necessary to prevent faecal impaction. The patient is encouraged to establish a regular time for defaecation; a raised toilet seat will make defaecation easier.

Urinary dribbling and incontinence may occur; the cause may be the inability of the patient to reach the toilet soon enough. A regular toileting schedule is arranged and the patient prompted and assisted if necessary. A commode or urinal is kept readily available for use at night.

The patient experiences the discomfort of continually contracted muscles and readily becomes fatigued. Physiotherapy, avoidance of prolonged periods in one position and planned rest periods contribute to comfort.

As a result of disturbed autonomic nervous system control, excessive perspiration may occur. Daily bathing and frequent change of clothing may be needed to promote comfort and control body odour.

The rigidity of the muscles involved in speech and the reduced pulmonary volumes that may develop interfere with the patient's enunciation and volume of speech. Deep breathing with slow exhalation, singing and speech classes in groups help to improve speech. Facial exercises such as smiling, blowing out, grimacing, eye movements and neck extension performed before a mirror may lessen facial rigidity.

The patient may experience prolonged exposure and drying of the surface of the eye due to a reduction in the normal frequency of blinking. This may lead to corneal irritation. The instillation of artificial tears may be prescribed and the patient and/or a family member is taught how to instil the solution. Diplopia may become a problem. A patch on one eye may help.

The patient is observed for any reaction to prescribed medication. Carbidopa is commonly given to promote the entrance of levodopa, the precursor of dopamine, into the brain. Long-term side-effects include memory loss, mood swings and behaviour change. Anticholinergic drugs such as benzhexol (Artane) may be used to try to reduce muscle tone, but they too have side-effects such as blurring of vision, retention of urine and palpitations. An assessment is made for positive responses as well as for undesirable side-effects, for example: Is the tremor less? Has the patient's gait improved? If side-effects develop, the doctor is notified; an adjustment in dosage may be necessary or another drug prescribed.

Sudden withdrawal of an antiparkinsonian drug or severe emotional disturbance may precipitate a reaction referred to as a *parkinsonian crisis*. This is characterized by a marked aggravation of tremors, rigidity and akinesia. Tachycardia, increased respirations, acute anxiety and diaphoresis also occur.

The reaction is a medical emergency requiring prompt treatment. Treatment includes respiratory and cardiac support, the administration of an antiparkinsonian preparation and the parenteral administration of a sedative such as phenobarbitone may be necessary.

Huntington's disease (corticostriatonigral degeneration)

This condition was first described by George Huntington, a New York physician, in 1872 as an inherited condition of chorea and dementia in a group of families on Long Island. Early in the seventeenth century many English people migrated to America for religious and political reasons. Three men from the Suffolk village of Bures landed in Boston in 1630. Some 300 years later a researcher was able to trace the transmission of many cases of Huntington's disease, via 1000 affected descendants, back to these men.

Constipation
See chapter 5.1

Inheritance

The disease is transmitted by a dominant gene which, when present, will always produce Huntington's disease. As the gene is carried on an autosome, it is an autosomal dominant disease. Both sexes are equally affected and each child of an affected parent has a 50% chance of developing the disease in later life.

Pathology

It has been shown biochemically that the concentration of γ-aminobutyric acid (GABA), an inhibitory neurotransmitter, is greatly reduced in the substantia nigra, with a resultant fall in the activity of the enzyme glutamic acid decarboxylase (GAD). It therefore appears that there is death of the nerve cells producing GABA. Experiments suggest that GABA pathways exist between the basal ganglia and the substantia nigra.

About 7 people per 100 000 population in the UK suffer from the disease, making a total of about 5000. It occurs in all racial groups. For every affected individual there are about two more who carry the abnormal gene and will later develop the disease.

Huntington's disease appearing before the age of 20 years is passed from the father in 80% of cases; in cases of very late onset the abnormal gene is more commonly transmitted by the mother. The nature, course and prognosis of the disease should be explained very carefully to the family, and they should be offered genetic counselling and encouraged to join the Association to Combat Huntington's Chorea.

Treatment and nursing care

There is little to offer the patient in the way of treatment. Phenothiazines, haloperidol or tetrabenzine may control the chorea in the preliminary stages of the disease. The patient will ultimately require long-term care. The choreic movements may make eating and drinking difficult. Swallowing can be difficult and it is important to ensure that the patient receives adequate nutrition. A high-calorie diet with frequent glucose drinks between meals is helpful. Eventually the patient will need to be tube fed. Constipation can be a problem and is dealt with using an aperient and suppositories. Speech will deteriorate to loud grunting noises which others may find distressing. Occasionally there will be outbursts of aggression arising from the sheer frustration of not being able to communicate. Devising alternative methods of communication becomes a challenge and often the carers can help with this.

The patient will eventually become totally dependent, emaciated and immobile. Limbs become rigid, producing an abnormal posture. Prevention of skin breakdown becomes a priority. Death is usually caused by exhaustion or pneumonia. The aim of care should be the relief of the symptoms as they develop to ensure that the patient maintains his or her dignity and a peaceful death. The family will also require constant support and encouragement.

Motor neurone disease (amyotrophic lateral sclerosis)

This is a progressive chronic disease in which there is a degeneration of motor neurones in the spine (anterior horn cells), brainstem and/or cortical motor areas.

The cause of motor neurone disease is unknown. The onset of the disorder occurs most often between the ages of 40 and 60 years. The muscles innervated by the affected neurones lose their ability to contract, and atrophy.

Effects on the patient

The first symptom is usually weakness of the hands and arms; finer movements are lost and articles are dropped. Twitching and hyperreflexia develop along with the spasticity and weakness of the lower limbs. As the disorder progresses, speech, swallowing and respiration are impaired as motor neurones at higher levels are involved. The diagnosis is made on the patient's symptoms and their progressive nature. Electromyographic studies are done to confirm the loss of innervation to the muscles. The course is usually progressively retrograde; rarely is there a remission.

Treatment and nursing care

There is no specific treatment for motor neurone disease. When the disease is diagnosed, the patient and family are advised by the doctor of the expected progression and fatal outcome of the disorder. They require support, opportunities to express their feelings and ask questions, explanations and assistance in planning home management. The nurse can advise them to contact the Motor Neurone Disease Society. The patient is encouraged to remain active within the potential muscular ability and every effort should be made to encourage independence despite increasing disability. It should be kept in mind that in motor neurone disease the cognitive ability remains unaffected. Obviously home management must be individualized because of the variability of symptoms and stages of the disease in patients. Progression of the disease and increasing dependency eventually necessitate the use of a wheelchair.

The speech therapist has a vital role to play in the management of swallowing and speech. He or she should be introduced to the patient early on in the illness and will monitor progression and introduce communication aids at the appropriate stages.

Dysarthria and dysphagia are very distressing features in the later stages of the illness. The patient may become very embarrassed by the speech and the constant drooling of secretions. Privacy at meal times is very important, with the patient given small meals and nourishing drinks frequently. A portable tracheal suction machine can be supplied for home use and it is important that the patient and family are taught the correct way to use it. It may become necessary in the later stages to feed the patient via a nasogastric tube, or a gastrotomy tube may be inserted under radiographic control. These are very distressing procedures to both patient and family, and much time must be taken with them to explain and teach them how to use the tubes.

Myasthenia gravis

Myasthenia gravis is not a degenerative condition but is included here because of its chronic, progressive nature. It is a neuromuscular disorder characterized by weakness and easy fatiguability of voluntary muscles due to interference with impulse condition at the neuromuscular junction.

The cause is unknown. It has been suggested that there is a deficiency of either acetylcholine or the enzyme cholinesterase. In addition, a deficiency in the number of acetylcholine-sensitive receptors in the motor endplate has been identified. There is some evidence that autoimmune and genetic factors are implicated in the disease. Abnormalities of the thymus gland and increased antibodies that react against muscle tissue elements have been identified in some patients with myasthenia gravis.

Incidence

It is not a common disorder. The incidence is highest between 20 and 30 years of age, and women are affected more frequently than men at this age. In later years, men and women are equally affected.

Effects on the patient

The onset of myasthenia gravis may be insidious with the symptoms of fatigue and weakness being associated with muscular activity. Initially, only the extrinsic ocular and levator palpebrae muscles may be involved, resulting in ptosis of the eyelids and diplopia. This may be referred to as *ocular myasthenia*. More generalized muscle involvement (generalized myasthenia) with progression of the disease produces the following manifestations:

- an expressionless appearance due to weakness of facial muscles

- difficulty with mastication and **swallowing**

- nasal voice tone that loses volume as the patient talks

- limb weakness, which becomes evident with the patient experiencing difficulty with self-care management (e.g. bathing, brushing the teeth, combing the hair)

- respiratory difficulty

- loss of control of bladder and rectal sphincters.

Muscle weakness is most noticeable at the end of the day and after exercise. Some recovery of strength is evident upon rising in the morning or following a period of rest. Mild atrophy may occur in the affected muscles and some aching may be present. Usually, sensation is unchanged.

Myasthenia gravis
See chapter 3.1

Swallowing
See chapter 5.1

There is great variability in the course of the disease; spontaneous remissions may occur. Factors that may aggravate symptoms include infection, temperature extreme, exposure to sunlight, emotional stress and physical exertion. Weakness of the diaphragm and intercostal muscles is serious; respiratory insufficiency and complications may be fatal.

Medical management

There is no known cure for myasthenia gravis. Treatment includes the administration of drugs, plasmaphaeresis and surgery. The drug most commonly used is a cholinesterase antagonist preparation such as neostigmine or pyridostigmine. Response to such a drug is used as a diagnostic test during medical investigations for myasthenia gravis. The patient is usually hospitalized and observed for reactions to the drug. If the patient does not respond to the anticholinesterase, the corticosteroid prednisone may be given for its antibody suppressant effect, on the basis that the disorder is an abnormal immune response.

Surgical therapy involves thymectomy (the removal of the thymus gland). Hyperplasia occurs in many of the patients, or a thymic tumour may be present, and removal of the gland results in a marked improvement in some and complete remission in others. Surgery is used mainly in younger patients in the early stages of the disease.

Problems and goals

The patient faces lengthy periods of remission and progressively deteriorating exacerbations of the illness. The familiar problems of progressive disability have to be faced (see preceding sections), with most of the patient's care taking place in the community.

Nursing intervention

Most patients with myasthenia gravis are managed in the home. Hospitalization may be necessary for evaluation, establishing the required medication dosage, exacerbation of symptoms, respiratory failure or myasthenic crisis. Nursing management is primarily concerned with maintenance of muscle strength and the prevention of complications especially the potentially fatal respiratory failure and muscle atrophy.

The reader is referred to preceding pages in this chapter for a discussion of the general care required.

A major potential problem unique to myasthenia gravis which may occur involves a crisis reaction to drugs. The patient who requires high doses of an anticholinesterase drug is at risk of developing a *cholinergic crisis*. This is a life-threatening reaction resulting from overmedication necessitating prompt emergency treatment. A dramatic increase in myasthenic symptoms occurs in about 1 hour, the patient experiences extreme weakness, blurred vision, nausea, vomiting, intestinal cramping, diarrhoea, increased salivation and bronchial secretions, respiratory insufficiency, bradycardia, constricted pupils and increased perspiration.

Treatment involves withholding the anticholinesterase. Endotracheal intubation, mechanical respiratory assistance and frequent suction are necessary to prevent severe respiratory failure, hypoxia and death. Atropine sulfate may be prescribed to lessen the secretions. Following the cholinergic crisis, regular dosage of the anticholinesterase is decreased.

A crisis may also develop due to undermedication, and is referred to as *myasthenic crisis*. The symptoms are similar to those that occur in a cholinergic crisis but develop 3 hours or more after taking the anticholinesterase drug. An anticholinesterase preparation is given as well as supportive treatment as indicated (e.g. respiratory assistance). Regular dosage of the anticholinesterase is increased.

The person with a paroxysmal disorder

Epilepsy (seizures)

A seizure is the manifestation of abnormal, rapid and uncontrolled neuronal electrical discharges within the brain. It is characterized by sensory, motor and autonomic disturbances, and changes in level of consciousness. The term **epilepsy** refers to a chronic disorder characterized by recurring seizures of unknown cause. In the normal brain, a certain stability exists between excitation and inhibition. When a seizure occurs, the ability to suppress abnormal neural activity may be impaired or lost, or there may be increased excitation within the neurones. The abnormal activity may occur in a small group of neurones and remain relatively localized or may spread to involve extensive areas of neurones. In some seizures, no focal origin of abnormal electrical discharges can be identified; large areas of the brain appear to be involved simultaneously.

Incidence and cause

The disorder characterized by recurring seizures and commonly referred to as epilepsy represents one of the most common neurological problems affecting individuals irrespective of geographical location, sex and race. About one person in 20 has a seizure of some type during life, and in the population at large about one in 200 has epilepsy (recurrent seizures). Most of those who develop idiopathic epilepsy do so before the age of 20 years.

Epilepsy may be idiopathic (without known cause) or symptomatic. The latter type of seizures are secondary and may be caused by almost any intracranial pathological condition and by many general systemic disorders. Symptomatic seizures may occur with increased intracranial pressure or brain damage associated with a head injury, cerebral oedema or an intracranial space-occupying lesion, haemorrhage or infection. They may be a sequel to brain injury or infection that has resulted in brain damage and

scar tissue formation. General systemic conditions in which seizures most commonly occur include hypoglycaemia, hypocalcaemia (tetany), renal insufficiency (uraemia), hypoxia, high fever (especially in children), toxaemia of pregnancy and chemical poisoning (e.g. alcohol, strychnine, amphetamine, lead, some insecticides).

There is no known specific cause of primary (idiopathic) epilepsy but an inherited predisposition to hypersensitivity and dysrhythmia of the neurones is considered to play a role.

Classification of epilepsy

Seizures are classified according to whether their onset is *focal* (partial) or *generalized*. Partial seizures are further subdivided according to whether consciousness is retained throughout the seizure (*simple* partial seizure) or impaired at some point (*complex* partial seizure). A partial seizure can progress to a generalized one.

Description of seizures

Simple partial seizures

A focus within a particular part of the brain, usually the motor strip, is irritated resulting in a disturbance in function of the affected area. Typically, a focal seizure comprises of a twitching of the thumb or side of the face. The patient does not lose consciousness. If the twitching spreads to affect other parts of the body it is referred to as a *Jacksonian seizure*. For example, the twitching may start in the thumb and then spread to affect the hand and arm, and possibly include the affected side of the body.

Complex partial seizures

These seizures, which normally originate in the temporal lobe, are usually preceded by an aura or warning. This is then followed by an episode of altered behaviour in which the patient performs a series of repeated movements. *Automatism*, in which the patient may continually rub his or her hands or pluck at the clothes, may be demonstrated. The patient may also describe a sensory experience; for example, he or she may describe a particular smell, and some describe experiencing familiarity with an unfamiliar situation (i.e. *déjà vu*).

Absence seizures

As the name implies, in an absence seizure there is a brief alteration in consciousness which onlookers often do not notice. It typically occurs in childhood and is often noticed only as the child falls further behind with school work. In complex absences, automatism, as previously described, accompanies the brief alteration in consciousness.

Myoclonic seizures

These involve sudden, repeated jerking movements of one or more of the limbs during which there is a momentary loss of consciousness. They can occur repeatedly over

Epilepsy
See chapter 2.2

a number of hours and are most frequently seen within 1 hour of waking from sleep. If standing, the person would fall to the ground.

Tonic seizures

A tonic seizure starts with a sudden loss of body posture, characteristically the arms flex and the legs extend. Loss of consciousness usually occurs and respiration may cease for a time. It may be seen as part of a tonic clonic seizure.

Tonic atonic seizures

In a tonic atonic seizure the patient experiences a tonic phase as outlined above but then experiences atony (i.e. loss of tone). It can be repeated several times, during which there is loss of consciousness.

Tonic clonic seizures

These occur in several distinct stages. First, the patient may experience an aura. This often takes the form of a strange taste in the mouth or feeling but does not occur in everyone with this type of seizure. It can act as an early warning which, once recognized by the patient, can allow them to move to a safe place. This is followed by a loss of consciousness which heralds the start of the seizure proper. Should the patient be standing, he or she will fall to the ground. The tonic phase is signalled by a stiffening of the body. The jaw closes tight shut and the patient may utter a cry as the thoracic muscles contract and air is forcefully ejected via the vocal chords. As apnoea intervenes the patient becomes cyanosed and is often incontinent of urine or faeces.

After a period of time the patient will start to breathe stertorously, accompanied by rhythmic jerking of the limbs. Frothing of the mouth occurs as a result of excessive production of saliva. The patient is usually tachycardic and sweating. Once the jerking movements begin to subside, coma supervenes. Most patients fall into a deep sleep for a number of hours and are usually amnesic once they waken, and display episodes of drowsiness and confusion.

Status epilepticus

Status epilepticus is a serious form of epilepsy in which seizures occur in such rapid succession that recovery of consciousness between the episodes does not occur. Hyperpyrexia develops, coma deepens and permanent brain damage occurs due to anoxia. Complete exhaustion and death occur, if the patient is not treated.

The most common cause of status epilepticus is considered to be abrupt discontinuation of an anticonvulsant drug. Untreated or inadequately treated seizures may also lead to this emergency condition.

In status epilepticus, intial control of the seizures is by the use of intravenous diazepam. If this and other anticonvulsant drugs fail, the patient is given muscle relaxants, intubated and ventilated.

Assessment

A tonic clonic seizure is a sudden emergency that will be over very quickly. It is important that the nurse can give a clear account of the fit to medical personnel when required, so close observation is essential.

Patient problems

- Potential for injury due to the loss of consciousness and uncontrolled strong muscular contractures.

- Lack of knowledge about the disorder, the treatment and necessary modications in lifestyle that may be necessary.

- Alteration in self-image due to anxiety and the stigma that a segment of society attaches to epilepsy.

Goals

The goals are that the patient will suffer no harm as a result of the seizure and also be aware of the needs for long-term self-care in avoiding further fits.

Nursing intervention

Potential for injury

When a patient has a seizure, the most important function is to protect the patient from injury.

During a seizure, the nurse stays with the patient; safety and the observations and recording of events are paramount. A seizure cannot be stopped once it has begun; it is self-limiting and no immediate treatment will shorten it. If the patient is in bed, the pillow is removed and the top bedding turned down so that the patient's responses can be observed. If the patient is up, and has not already fallen, he or she is eased to a semiprone position and a folded blanket or towel placed under the head to prevent injury during the clonic phase. Restrictive clothing at the neck is loosened and the immediate area cleared of anything that might contribute to injury (e.g. furniture, electric fan, lamp). No attempt is made to insert anything between the teeth as the teeth are clenched and there would be a risk of pushing the tongue into the oropharynx, obstructing the airway. In addition, injury to the teeth and soft tissue may occur; aspiration of blood or a broken tooth may become a possibility. As soon as the clonic phase begins to subside, the patient is turned on the side to promote drainage of secretions and prevent aspiration. Suction may be necessary. The patient is protected as much as possible from exposure to others.

During the seizure, the following observations are made:

- The mode of onset – Did the patient indicate an aura? Was there a cry? Is there deviation of the head and eyes; if so, to what side? In what part of the body did the initial phase start?

- Are the seizure movements localized or generalized? If generalized, are they symmetrical or asymmetrical?

- Is the patient **cyanosed**?

- Are the teeth clenched and is there frothing at the mouth?

- Is there incontinence of urine or faeces?

- How long did the seizure last?

Following the seizure the patient will be drowsy and disoriented for some time; close observation is therefore essential for the patient's safety. When the patient wakens, reorientation may be necessary as well as an explanation of the event.

In the interest of safety and the prevention of injury for self and others, the person with epilepsy may not be allowed to drive a motor vehicle, operate certain machines, or work at heights or where there is loud noise or flashing lights. The doctor may also advise the patient against swimming, climbing, riding, cycling and participation in contact sports. Decisions regarding activities are based on the type, frequency and severity of seizures and the patient's response to the prescribed drug.

Family members are taught what to do when a seizure occurs so that they can respond effectively.

Knowledge deficit

Information about the prescribed anticonvulsant drug is provided. The client and family should be alerted to the potential side-effects and are advised to get in touch with the doctor if they occur (Table 20.12). They should know that, if the drug is not tolerated, there are others that can be prescribed until optimal control of fits with minimal side-effects is achieved. It is emphasized that the drugs must be taken at the prescribed frequency, even though there are no seizures; effective blood levels of the drug must be maintained by compliance with the prescribed dosage and frequency, and alcohol should not be consumed. Drug doses must not be altered except with the

doctor's approval; the drug is prescribed on an individual basis according to the type, severity and frequency of the seizures and the individual's response. The patient is cautioned against the taking of any non-prescription drugs.

The importance of regular visits to the doctor is emphasized. Blood serum levels of the anticonvulsant drug are determined and dosage adjustment made if indicated. As a blood dyscrasia is a potential side-effect of many of the drugs used, blood cell counts, haematocrit and bleeding time are evaluated regularly.

The patient and family are requested to keep a record of seizures which includes antecedent events or any known or suspected precipitating factor(s). Information about the British Epilepsy Association may be very useful. The mutual support offered to the patient and family by groups such as this can be invaluable. A Medic Alert identification bracelet or pendant should be worn so that appropriate care can be given during a fit or an emergency. The patient should always carry the names, addresses and telephone numbers of persons to be contacted.

Alteration in self-image

Patients express anxiety and embarrassment and see themselves as being different and inferior, having to adjust to potentially disruptive seizures and dependency on medication. Acceptance of the diagnosis is difficult for the patient, who may respond with denial, anger, resentment and despair before acceptance and adaptation. Fears and anxieties that are unexpressed and unrelieved may result in ineffective coping. A thorough evaluation of the patient's attitude toward epilepsy and expectations concerning health maintenance is essential. The attitudes and expectations of family members should also be evaluated because their understanding and support is crucial to the patient's ability to adjust to his condition.

Epilepsy is not yet clearly understood and there is no known cure. Because of this, and the historical context,

Cyanosed
See chapter 5.3

Table 20.12   Principal antiepileptic drugs

Drug	Indications	Side-effects
Carbamazepine	Complex partial seizures, tonic clonic and simple partial	Dizziness, double vision, unsteadiness, nausea and vomiting
Diazepam	Status epilepticus, absence attacks and myoclonus	Sedation
Lamotrigine	Partial or generalized seizures	Mild sedation, blurred vision, ataxia, nausea and vomiting, headache, diplopia
Phenobarbital	Tonic, clonic and partial seizures	Drowsiness, unsteadiness, tolerance, habituation, withdrawal seizures
Phenytoin	Tonic clonic, simple and complex partial seizures	Drowsiness, unsteadiness, slurred speech, with prolonged use, gingival hypertrophy, acne, coarsening of facial features
Primidone	Tonic clonic and partial seizures	Drowsiness, unsteadiness, toleration, habituation, withdrawal seizures
Sodium valproate	Idiopathic generalized epilepsies	Tremor, irritability, restlessness, occasionally confusion
Vigabatrin	Partial epilepsy	Visual field defects

fear of the disorder is widespread. At one time the disorder was thought to be caused by the possession of a person by devils and, even today, myths, misunderstandings and social stigma still exist. As a result, the patient may fear rejection by peers and employers and refuse to disclose the health problem even though it would be wiser to do so. Concerns about the person's intellectual abilities, psychological stability and ability to perform efficiently on the job have been expressed by educators and employers. It is important for the nurse to be aware of potential prejudices that may be encountered by the patient and his or her family. The fact that mental capacity and abilities are as varied among people with epilepsy as in any cross-section of society and that epilepsy is not synonymous with mental handicap or psychosis requires emphasis.

Some controversy exists concerning genetic predisposition to epilepsy. It is considered by some authorities to be greatest when epilepsy develops early in childhood and when both parents suffer epilepsy. Genetic counselling may therefore be advisable for a person with epilepsy who is contemplating having children.

The person with an infection of the nervous system

There is a range of infective conditions that may affect the nervous system, for example encephalitis (infection of the brain), cerebral abscess, poliomyelitis and rabies. Fortunately these conditions are very rare, as is tetanus, a condition in which the nervous system is attacked by the exotoxins of the *Clostridium tetani* organism. Tetanus may be fatal due to effects of the exotoxin on the nerves controlling respiration – hence the importance of tetanus prophylaxis.

Meningitis

Meningitis is an acute inflammation of the pia and arachnoid meningeal membranes of the brain or spinal cord. The cause is usually a bacterium or virus. Almost any bacterium can cause meningitis, but the most common are the meningococcus, the pneumococcus and *Haemophilus influenzae*. Meningitis is frequently secondary to infection of the sinuses, ears or respiratory tract. The meningococcus can produce meningoccal septicaemia, a severe life-threatening condition associated with meningitis. This may involve a characteristic rash, shock, renal failure and intravascular coagulation, amongst other complications.

Effects on the patient

The onset of meningitis tends to be insidious when caused by a virus. The bacterial type is more sudden and acute, manifested by headache, irritability, nausea, vomiting, back pain, chills and fever and symptoms of meningeal irritation. Photophobia is a common complaint. The classical signs of meningeal irritation include neck rigidity (stiffness of the neck and severe pain with forceful

Meninges
See chapter 2.2

Nausea and
vomiting
See chapter 5.1

Fever
See chapter 6.1

flexion), positive Kernig's sign (inability to straighten the knee when the hip is flexed), and positive Brudzinski's sign (hip and knee flexion in response to forward flexion of the neck). Signs of increased intracranial pressure such as raised blood pressure, pupillary changes, changes in respiratory patterns, seizures, bradycardia, confusion, drowsiness and coma may develop. Focal neurological signs rarely occur.

The medical diagnosis of meningitis is made on the basis of clinical signs and symptoms and is confirmed by isolating the organism from the CSF. The CSF is under increased pressure, is cloudy or purulent, and has an increased leucocyte count, a high protein content and a reduced concentration of glucose. Blood, nose and throat cultures are done to assist in identifying the organism, and radiographs may be taken of the chest, skull and sinuses to detect areas of inflammation.

Meningitis requires emergency treatment, as delay may result in cerebral damage and disability or death. It includes elimination of intravenous penicillin initially and other antibiotics as appropriate after sensivity of the infecting organism has been determined. Prophylactic treatment with a 2-day course of oral rifampicin for close contacts may be ordered. There is no specific treatment for viral meningitis.

Assessment

A full assessment of the patient along the lines discussed earlier in the chapter is essential, paying particular attention to the level of consciousness and other neurological parameters.

Patient problems

A wide range of problems associated with immobility, a severe infection and a diminished level of consciousness may be encountered by the patient. They are summarized below; other individual problems may also coexist:

- Alteration in comfort due to the headache, back pain and fever.

- Potential for increased intracranial pressure secondary to the intracranial inflammatory process.

- Fluid and nutritional deficit due to **nausea**, **vomiting**, headache, **fever**, confusion and decreased awareness.

- Potential for injury due to seizures, disorientation or coma.

- Potential spread of infection to others, particularly if the causative organism is the meningococcus.

- Self-care deficits secondary to discomfort, reduced awareness, weakness or coma.

- Inadequate knowledge about management of the convalescent period and residual disabilities.

Goals

Patient goals will be the avoidance of complications and potential problems as outlined above while making a full recovery without any long-term deficits.

Nursing intervention

Much of the care required has already been discussed in this chapter; the following special points should, however, be noted.

A major problem of the patient with meningitis is discomfort due to headache, back pain, fever, photophobia and anxiety. Nursing care includes the provision of emotional support, reassurance that help is available and an explanation of all nursing activities. Irritability due to increased reaction to sensory stimuli is minimized by maintaining a cool, quiet, darkened environment, by approaching the patient gently with a soft, calm voice and by keeping communication simple and direct.

The possible spread of the patient's infection to others must be considered. The hospital infection control department is consulted; it may be necessary to use isolation procedures.

After meningitis the patient is usually debilitated and readily fatigued, and may have some residual neurological deficits. Several weeks or months may be needed for the patient's convalescence and rehabilitation. The family and patient should be forewarned of this and given support and encouragement throughout this difficult period. After the initial acute phase, a highly nutritious diet is encouraged and a regimen of range-of-movement exercises is established to prevent weakness, contractures and joint ankylosis, and to promote circulation.

Minor disabilities may resolve with time, whereas others may be residual and require detailed evaluation and an intensive rehabilitation programme. The nurse plays a role in supporting the patient and interpreting the rehabilitation programme to the family, and in assisting them to make plans for adjustments and home management.

The person with a peripheral nerve disorder

Disorders of the cranial nerves may be secondary to other diseases but a few are primary to specific nerves. The more common of these are trigeminal neuralgia and Bell's palsy. Peripheral nerve dysfunction may be incurred by direct local trauma (pressure, severance, infection and inflammation) or may be secondary to a variety of general conditions such as malnutrition, alcoholism and chemical poisoning.

Trigeminal neuralgia (tic douloureux)

Trigeminal neuralgia is a very painful disorder of the sensory fibres of the trigeminal (fifth cranial) nerve. It is characterized by recurring episodes of excruciating pain along the distribution of one or more divisions of the nerve. The attack is brief, lasting from seconds to 2 or 3 minutes. The episodes recur frequently, day or night for several weeks at a time. The onset of an episode may occur spontaneously or may coincide with touching or movement of the face or exposure to cold or a draught. The patient may relate the precipitation of pain to eating, talking, cleaning the teeth, or washing or shaving the face. The recurring incapacitating pain has been known to cause severe depression and even suicide. The cause of the neuralgia is unknown.

The patient may be treated by medication or surgery. There is no specific drug for the disorder. Anticonvulsant agents such as phenytoin or carbamazepine may suppress or shorten the painful episodes. These drugs may produce side-effects (see Table 20.12). An analgesic may be prescribed; if an opioid is used, there is the risk of addiction. Drug therapy may provide relief at first but, usually, gradually loses its effectiveness.

Injection of alcohol into the affected nerve branch may be performed to interrupt the sensory impulses and usually provides relief for several months. During this period of effectiveness, the patient has loss of sensation in the areas of distribution of the injected nerve branch.

A popular surgical measure is percutaneous radiofrequency thermocoagulation. This procedure, with the patient conscious, permits destruction of the pain sensory fibres by use of an electrode and leaves the neurones and fibres concerned with other areas and the corneal reflex intact.

Bell's palsy (peripheral facial paralysis)

Bell's palsy is a disorder of the motor component of one of the facial (seventh cranial) nerves and is characterized by loss of the ability to move the muscles on one side of the face.

The condition is most common in persons aged between 20 and 40 years. The patient may experience pain behind the ear or in the face for a day or two before the onset of paralysis. When paralysis occurs, a drawing sensation on the affected side is experienced. There is flaccidity, drooping of the mouth, drooling, flattening of the nasolabial fold, widening of the palpebral fissure and inability to close the eye completely on the affected side. There may be watering of the eye. The individual is unable to smile, whistle or grimace. The taste sensation is lost over the anterior two-thirds of the tongue on the respective side. Herpes lesions may appear on or in the corresponding ear. In 80% of the victims, muscle tone begins to return in a few weeks and movement is usually restored over a period of months.

Treatment is usually provided on an outpatient basis. It may include analgesics for discomfort due to herpes, or application of aciclovir (Zovirax) cream, a corticosteroid preparation to relieve oedema and inflammation, application of moist heat and gentle facial massage, and electrical stimulation of the facial nerve to maintain muscle tone.

Polyneuritis (multiple peripheral neuritis)

Although the term neuritis implies inflammation, it is more often applied to any neuropathy where there is dysfunction and pain of peripheral nerves from any cause. Polyneuritis is a disorder in which there is pain and impaired function along the distribution of many peripheral nerves. It is usually symmetrical and both motor and sensory disturbances occur.

Effects on the patient

The symptoms generally start in the parts innervated by the distal portions of the nerves and spread proximally. The patient first experiences pain, pins and needles, tingling and weakness in hands and feet ('glove and stocking' effect), then a progressive loss of sensation, diminished tendon reflexes and inability to perform finer movements. The areas are tender and sore when subjected to even light pressure.

The causes include toxicity, nutritional deficiencies (especially vitamin B complex), metabolic disorder and cell-mediated immunological response. In some instances the cause is not identified.

Some of the more common polyneuropathies are diabetic polyneuritis, vitamin deficiency polyneuritis associated with alcoholism, arsenic or lead polyneuritis, malnutrition polyneuritis and acute idiopathic polyneuritis (Guillain–Barré syndrome).

Guillain–Barré syndrome (acute infective polyneuropathy)

The Guillain–Barré syndrome is an inflammatory disease of the spinal nerve roots within the dural sheath, of the peripheral nerves and may also involve the cranial nerves. The loss of nerve impulse conduction that occurs is due to compression, demyelination and nerve degeneration as a result of the inflammation and oedema.

Incidence and aetiology

It may occur at any age but the incidence is greater in persons 30–40 years of age. Men and women are equally affected. The cause of the disorder is unknown but viral infection and immunological reaction are both suspect. Frequently, the patients give a history of having 'just had' an upper respiratory infection or a gastrointestinal disturbance.

Effects on the patient

The onset of Guillain–Barré syndrome is usually abrupt. Bilateral muscle weakness, beginning in the legs, may ascend to involve the trunk, arms and cranial nerves. Paraesthesia may precede the weakness. Within a few days, the weakness is followed by flaccid motor paralysis with weakness of the respiratory muscles. If the cranial nerves become involved, inability to swallow, talk or even close the eyes develops. Muscle tenderness or sensitivity of the nerves to pressure may be experienced. Autonomic changes include sinus tachycardia and hypertension in the acute phase followed by hypotension.

Guillain–Barré syndrome is life threatening due to potential respiratory and vasomotor failure if mechanical ventilation and vasopressor drugs are not promptly available. The mortality rate is estimated at 10–20%; death may result from a superimposed infection. Complete spontaneous recovery within weeks or months is usually anticipated in the survivors.

In some instances steroids may be used to counteract the inflammation. Treatment is mainly supportive and intensive nursing care along the lines discussed in this chapter is needed to help the patient survive the acute episode.

Summary

The critical importance to human functioning of the nervous system cannot be overemphasized and the features unique to this system must be borne in mind at all times. Health problems may affect a person at any age and be potentially devastating in impact, leaving major long-term deficits. The nurse's role in patient teaching is a key one in preventing head injuries, for example, while the nurse as teacher features prominently in the rehabilitation of patients after brain trauma or cerebrovascular accident. The nursing care of patients whose central nervous system has been impaired by trauma or disease is a challenging and long-term commitment in many cases, with a major contribution being made by informal carers in the home setting.

References

Acorn S (1995) Assisting families of head injured survivors through a family support programme. Journal of Advanced Nursing 21(5): 872–877.

Amatoc (1991) Malignant glioma: coping with a devastating illness. Journal of Neuroscience Nursing 23(1): 20–23.

Davies M, Lucatorto M (1994) Mannitol revisited. Journal of Neuroscience Nursing 26(3): 170–174.

Grant AM, Grinspun DR (1994) The road home from traumatic brain injury. Canadian Nurse 90(4): 22–27.

Hickey JV (1997) The clinical practice of neurological and neurosurgical nursing, 4th edn. Philadelphia: Lippincott.

Lindsay K, Bone I (1997) Neurology and neurosurgery illustrated, 3rd edn. Edinburgh: Churchill Livingstone.

Scottish Intercollegiate Guidelines Network (2000) Early management of patients with a head injury. Edinburgh: SIGN.

Annotated Further Reading

Hickey JV (1997) The clinical practice of neurological and neurosurgical nursing, 4th edn. Philadelphia: Lippincott.

An invaluable textbook covering all aspects of neuroscience nursing practice. Provides in-depth information on all the major areas of practice with a clear explanation of the underpinning skills and knowledge. Comprehensively referenced and clearly written.

Gerrero D (1998) Neuro-oncology for nurses. London: Whurr.

Useful textbook providing insightful knowledge of the multiple problems facing patients with tumours of the nervous system. Written from a multidisciplinary perspective it provides guidance on the care required by these patients.

Landstaff D & Christie J (2000) Trauma care: a team approach. Oxford: Butterworth Heinemann.

A helpful text emphasizing the team approach to the care of trauma patients. Although it deals with all types of trauma the threads woven through the book make it useful reading for nurses dealing with patients with trauma to the nervous system.

McLean C (2001) Moving and positioning patients with altered intracranial haemodynamics. Nursing in Critical Care 6(5): 239.

Helpful up-to-date article on nursing patients with raised ICP. Reviews the research previously carried out and places this in the context of modern day nursing practice.

21

Caring for the patient with a disorder of the senses

Mike Walsh

Introduction

Structure and functions of the ear

The person with a disorder of the ear

Structure and functions of the nose

The person with a disorder of the nose or nasal sinuses

Structure and functions of the eyes

The person with health problems related to vision

Summary

Introduction

The normal person is able to interpret the world and communicate with it by using five special senses. These are sight, hearing, taste, touch and smell.

The **senses** all work in a similar way: sensory receptor cells in the relevant organ are stimulated, and the sensory impulse produced is transmitted to the relevant part of the brain via the cranial or the spinal nerves. Different parts of the brain are responsible for receiving and interpreting sensory impulses from different parts of the body.

Sensory impulses for sight, hearing, taste and smell are all transmitted via the cranial nerves, whereas sensory impulses for touch are carried by general somatic afferent nerve fibres via the spinal cord to the brain. For a fuller discussion of the nervous system, refer to Chapter 20.

It can be seen from Figure 21.1 that there are many potential areas for problems to arise in the sensory pathway. The first occurs when a stimulus fails to reach the receptor cell. This happens if you have a heavy cold – even a strong smell cannot reach the sensory receptor cells for smell, which lie high up in the nose. The second potential failure is if something fails within the organ, preventing the receptor cells from functioning. For example, the receptor cells on a detached retina cannot hope to function correctly. The next possible problem area is within the transmission system of nerves that link the sensory organ with the brain. Finally, there may be problems within the brain itself, which prevent correct reception and interpretation of the incoming sensory impulses.

This chapter focuses on problems associated with the ear, nose and eye, and the care required by people with these disorders.

Figure 21.1 Problems in the sensory pathway. (a) The stimulus fails to reach the receptor cells (e.g. glue ear, heavy cold). (b) The receptor cells fail to receive the stimulus (e.g. detached retina). (c) The receptor cells fail to trigger the sensory nerve. (d) The nerve pathway is injured. (e) Brain injury or a congenital problem prevents reception of interpretation of sensory impulses.

Senses
See chapter 2.4

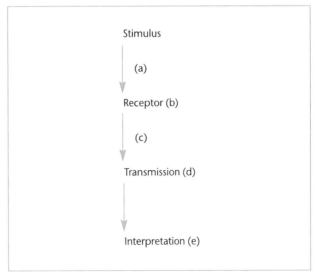

Stimulus

↓ (a)

Receptor (b)

↓ (c)

Transmission (d)

↓

Interpretation (e)

Structure and functions of the ear

The **ear** is concerned with the special sense of hearing as well as with the maintenance of equilibrium. It has three divisions: the external and middle ears for the collection and conduction of sound waves, and the inner ear, which actually serves as the receptor. The eighth cranial (auditory or acoustic) nerve provides the afferent impulse pathway of the sensory unit. Part of its fibres carry impulses to the interpretive centres for sound in the temporal lobes, and the others transmit impulses to areas of the brainstem and cerebellum associated with control of body posture.

External ear

The **outer ear** consists of the *auricle* (*pinna*) and the external auditory meatus. The auricle consists largely of cartilage and leads to the external auditory meatus. This ends at the tympanic membrane (eardrum), which separates the external and middle ears. The skin lining of the canal is covered with fine hairs near the opening and has special glands which produce a yellow waxy secretion called *cerumen* for protection against insects and dust particles. The *tympanic membrane* is a thin, semitransparent membrane covered externally with skin and internally with mucous membrane, which is continuous with that which lines the middle ear cavity. The middle layer is composed of thin elastic and fibrous tissue.

Middle ear

This portion of the ear is contained within a small cavity in the temporal bone. The cavity communicates with the nasopharynx by means of the *auditory* or *Eustachian tube*, and with the mastoid cells. The auditory tube permits the entrance of air into the **middle ear**; this equalizes the pressure on the internal surface of the eardrum with atmospheric pressure. The cavity is lined with mucous membrane which is continuous with that of the auditory tube and mastoid cells. The *mastoid cells* are small air spaces within the posterior portion of the temporal bone, just behind the middle ear.

The middle ear cavity contains three small bones called the auditory ossicles, which are movable for the purpose of transmitting sound vibrations. The first ossicle, the *malleus*, is attached to the eardrum and articulates with the second ossicle, the *incus*. The incus articulates with the third ossicle, the *stapes*, which is attached to the membranous oval window (fenestra ovalis) that leads into the inner ear. The middle ear also has two small muscles; one, the tensor tympani, is inserted on the malleus and the other, the stapedius, is inserted on the footplate of the stapes. Contraction of these muscles reduces the amplitude of the sound waves entering the middle ear and cochlea.

Inner ear (labyrinth)

The **inner ear** consists of a system of irregularly shaped cavities containing fluid and complex membranous

structures that initiate nerve impulses as a result of sound waves or change of position. The *bony (osseous) labyrinth* contains the *membranous labyrinth*, which conforms fairly closely to the shape of the bony-walled cavities, and is divided into a series of channels: the cochlea, vestibule and semicircular canals (Fig. 21.2):

■ The *cochlea* is a complex snail-shaped structure (Fig. 21.3). Auditory nerve impulses are produced by receptor cells within the organ of Corti (special cells with hair-like projections on the surface of the basilar membrane) when stimulated by vibrations of the basilar membrane (Fig. 21.4).

■ The *vestibule* lies between the cochlea and the semicircular canals. Within the cavities of the vestibule are hair-like projections and calcium carbonate concretions (*otoliths*) which respond to

Figure 21.2   The membranous labyrinth of the ear.

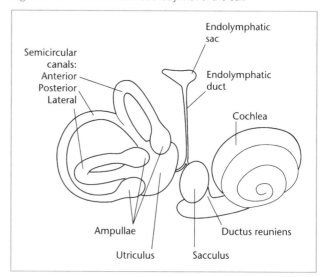

Figure 21.3   Schematic drawing of the cochlea.

Ear
See chapter 2.4

Outer ear
See chapter 2.4

Middle ear
See chapter 2.4

Inner ear
See chapter 2.4

movements of the head by giving rise to neural impulses concerned with the maintenance of equilibrium.

■ The *semicircular canals* are hollowed out of the temporal bone at right angles to each other. Each membranous semicircular canal has a dilated portion at one end, called the *ampulla*, which contains special sensory hair cells, forming the *crista acustica*, or crista ampullaris. The crista is sensitive to movement of the endolymph within the ampulla and initiates neural impulses concerned with balance and position. These are transmitted by the vestibular portion of the acoustic (eighth cranial) nerve to the central nervous system.

Auditory pathway

Sound waves passing into the external ear strike the tympanic membrane, causing it to vibrate with the same frequency as the sound waves. This in turn results in vibrations of the ossicles in the middle ear. The stapes, being attached to the oval window, causes its membrane to move in and out. The ossicles serve as amplifiers but, if the amplitude of the waves is excessive, producing excessive loudness, the vibrations may be modified by contraction of the tensor tympani and the stapedius muscles. The vibrations are transferred through the endolymph to the basilar membrane. Movements of the endolymph and basilar membrane stimulate the receptor cells of the organ of Corti, initiating neural impulses which are transmitted via nerve fibres to a ganglion in the central core of the cochlea. The axons of the ganglionic neurones form the cochlear branch of the acoustic (eighth cranial) nerve. The impulses are then transmitted through the thalami and eventually reach a cortical area of the temporal lobe (auditory centre) where they are interpreted as sound. Each ear delivers impulses to both auditory centres.

Pitch and intensity of sound

The pitch of a sound depends upon the frequency of the vibrations (number per second). The number of vibrations or cycles per second (cps) are expressed as a unit of

frequency called a hertz (Hz), which is used in measuring the pitch of sound. The fibres of the basilar membrane vary in length. It is thought that different frequencies stimulate selective areas of fibres and cells of the membrane, that is, each place on the basilar membrane is sensitive to sound waves of a certain frequency.

The intensity, or loudness, of a sound depends upon the amplitude or force of movement of the vibrations. The louder the sound, the greater is the displacement back and forth.

Physical equilibrium

When the head moves, neural impulses originate in the semicircular canals and the utricle and saccula, and are transmitted by nerve fibres that form the vestibular branch of the acoustic nerve. The vestibular nerve fibres pass to groups of neurones (vestibular nuclei) in the brainstem from which impulses may be delivered to the cerebellum, reticular formation, down the vestibulospinal tracts to motor neurones that innervate skeletal muscle, the oculomotor centre and the thalami. The principal purpose of these impulses is to orient the person in space, and to stimulate muscles in a reflex action so that he or she may assume an upright position or maintain the position that has been assumed against gravity.

The person with a disorder of the ear

The ear is concerned with the special sense of hearing and with the maintenance of equilibrium. There are several places where the mechanisms involved can be disturbed. These are shown in Figure 21.5. The principal problems for people with disorders of the ear are related to loss

Auditory pathway.
See chapter 2.4

Balance.
See chapter 2.4

Figure 21.4   Cross-section of the cochlea.

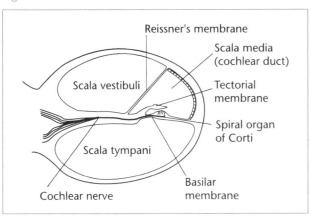

Figure 21.5   Potential hearing loss problems.

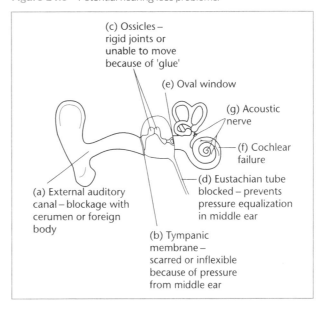

(or potential loss) of hearing. The examinations, characteristics and tests used to determine the cause and severity of hearing loss are therefore given in detail here. Any specific tests for other conditions are given in the section on common disorders of the ear.

Assessment

The aim of the assessment of a person presenting with a problem relating to hearing or equilibrium maintenance is to determine the point at which the auditory mechanism is disturbed and with what severity. Any alteration in hearing or balance has an effect on normal living which is assessed in order to document change over time and to judge the effectiveness of any treatment or aids provided.

Health history

As with any illness, the person's health history is noted, paying particular attention to previous ear disease, injuries or surgery, family history of ear problems, current and past medications that might be relevant. The details of the present disorder (including the use of any hearing aids) are noted and any relevant changes in social or psychological behaviour described.

Physical examination

The ear is inspected inside and outside. The pinna (auricle) is examined for size, position, symmetry and lesions, and the mastoid process is palpated, especially if infection of the middle ear is suspected. The entrance of the ear canal is inspected for presence of debris or pus. Examination of the inside of the auditory canal is increasingly passing into the domain of nursing with the growth of the nurse practitioner role. This should be inspected with an auriscope (otoscope) which has a magnifying lens in addition to a light. The canal is inspected for lesions, foreign bodies, and the amount and characteristics of the cerumen (wax). The tympanic membrane is viewed and the colour and tension noted (normal: light pearl-grey). It is examined for retraction or bulging, increased vascularity and perforation.

Hearing evaluation

In hearing evaluation, the examiner assesses the degree of hearing loss and establishes whether it is due to conductive or nerve impairment. Conductive deafness results from failure of the conducting mechanism to transmit sound impulses from the external ear to the inner ear fluids. Neural deafness can be a result of disease of the sensor organ (the cochlea), auditory nerve or auditory cerebral centre.

Hearing screening

A quick evaluation of hearing acuity can be made using whispered and spoken voice tests. Auditory acuity can be tested by first exhaling and then whispering softly towards one ear from a distance of 30–60 cm whilst the other ear is occluded. This is repeated for the other ear and the results are compared (Walsh et al 1999).

Tuning fork tests

These are used to differentiate the type of deafness. A tuning fork with a frequency of 512 or 1024 Hz should be used. The tests should be made in a room free of noise.

Rinne test A tuning fork of 512 Hz is struck and held 2.5–5.0 cm in front of the patient's external auditory canal. It is then placed firmly on the mastoid process and the patient is asked to state whether it is heard better by bone conduction (BC) or air conduction (AC).

A more accurate method of performing the Rinne test is to hold the tuning fork 2.5–5.0 cm in front of the external auditory meatus; the patient is asked to say when it can no longer be heard. It is then placed on the mastoid process and the patient states whether or not it can still be heard; if not, air conduction is better than bone conduction – a positive Rinne test result. Conversely if the tuning fork can be heard by bone conduction, then bone conduction is better than air conduction – a negative Rinne test result.

In the normal ear, air conduction is better than bone (i.e. positive Rinne test result).

Weber's test This test is used to assess whether there is conductive hearing loss in one ear compared to another. The tuning fork is set in vibration; the stem is held against the middle of the forehead and the patient is asked whether the sound is heard better in one ear than the other. Normally, the sound appears to be in the midline, being heard equally by both ears. If unilateral conductive deafness is present, the sound is greater in the affected ear. In lateralized, sensorineural loss of hearing (see below), the sound is heard in the normal ear.

Audiometry

More sophisticated testing of hearing loss involves audiometry. Sound is measured in decibels (dB) and the exact amount of hearing loss in decibels may be determined by the use of specialized equipment which can also measure relative loss at different frequencies. As a guide, quiet conversation is around 40 dB but sound with an intensity of 80 dB is judged unpleasant and may start to cause harm to human hearing (Smeltzer and Bare 2000).

Classification and causes of hearing loss

A hearing deficit may be congenital or acquired and may be classified as conductive, sensorineural, central or combined.

- In a *conductive hearing loss*, sound waves fail to reach the internal ear as a result of some disturbance in the external ear, middle ear or the oval window (fenestra ovalis). The person with conductive deafness tends to speak softly as he or she can hear himself or herself.

- In *sensorineural deafness*, which may also be called *nerve* or *perceptive deafness*, the disorder is located in the organ of Corti, cochlear division of the acoustic nerve, or auditory impulse pathway or centre within the brain. The person with nerve deafness cannot hear anything, so tends to shout, hoping to hear.

■ *Central hearing loss* denotes a hearing deficit resulting from disturbances within the brain, principally the auditory centre in the temporal lobe.

■ *Combined hearing loss* occurs because of impairment within both the conductive and neural auditory mechanisms.

■ *Congenital loss of hearing* may be due to a prenatal malformation or lack of development of a part of the auditory apparatus. Heredity may play a role, or it may be the result of a viral infection in the mother during the first trimester of the pregnancy, the effect of a toxic drug taken by the mother during pregnancy, hypoxia or a birth injury.

■ *Acquired impairment of hearing* may be caused by obstruction of the external auditory canal by a foreign body or impacted cerumen, infection (e.g. otitis media), a neoplasm (e.g. acoustic neuroma), an ototoxic drug (e.g. streptomycin), trauma associated with a skull fracture or excessively loud noise, or obstruction of the Eustachian tube. Degenerative changes in the auditory pathway frequently associated with the ageing process (presbycousis) may also cause acquired hearing loss.

The problems of loss of hearing depend on the degree of deficit and on the age at which it developed. In the case of a child with a congenital loss of hearing causing total deafness, all communication will need to be visual and tactile, so affecting the child's whole life and producing behavioural, socioeconomic and emotional changes for the entire family. A partial hearing loss in an adult does not have the same impact.

The clinical characteristics of loss of hearing can be described in relation to:

■ direct effects of impaired hearing (e.g. communication difficulties)

■ direct behavioural response to impaired hearing

■ indirect psychosocial response to impaired hearing.

These are described in Box 21.1.

The *goals* of nursing care are to assist the patient to:

1. preserve or maintain hearing

2. identify factors contributing to hearing loss

3. maintain or develop ability to communicate with others

4. recognize and develop strategies to counteract psychosocial changes.

Box 21.1 Clinical characteristics of loss of hearing

Direct effects

■ Failure to perceive a threatening situation

■ Failure to respond when addressed

■ Frequent requests for repetition

■ Misinterpretation

■ Changes in speech such as low volume or lack of inflection

Behavioural responses

■ Turning the head to direct the 'good' ear towards the sound

■ Strained, confused expression

■ Short attention span

■ Lack of interest

■ Irritability

■ Fatigue due to the effort of trying to hear

Psychosocial responses

■ Withdrawal from group activities (hearing is more difficult in a group)

■ Avoidance of noisy places and situations

■ Some people respond by talking continuously, to avoid the situation of someone else speaking and being unable to hear

■ Some pretend they can hear, and assume a permanent smile or responsive look, often inappropriately

■ Changes in normal activities (such as watching TV, going to the cinema, etc.) may produce anger, boredom, loneliness, etc.

Nursing intervention

Preservation of hearing

Nurses, especially those working with industrial workers and schoolchildren, have an important role in the prevention of hearing loss. The public requires education about the causes and early signs of impaired hearing and about significant preventive measures.

Good prenatal care and the avoidance of contact with persons with measles or other viral infections are important in preventing congenital deafness. Immunization against measles should be promoted. Prompt treatment of respiratory infection and infectious diseases may allay the complication of otitis media. Prompt medical treatment and follow-up are urged for persons with an ear disorder. The nurse caring for a patient receiving any of the aminoglycoside antibiotics (e.g. neomycin, gentamicin) must be alert for early signs of damage to hearing, as this is a well known dose-related side-effect of this class of drugs (British National Formulary 2001).

The danger of introducing foreign objects into the external ear canal should be emphasized to patients. Cleansing the ear with applicators or hairpins is dangerous, as accidental perforation of the eardrum may occur.

The occupational health nurse, especially in an industry in which there is prolonged, intense noise in the work environment, must be aware of the possibility of noise-induced hearing loss. Frequently the employees tend to accept noise simply as a necessary part of the occupation and do not realize that hearing damage may be developing insidiously. Gradual loss of hearing usually involves, first, failure of response to high-frequency sounds. Later, areas of the cochlea that respond to lower frequencies become damaged. In order to protect persons exposed to noise that endangers hearing, protective devices in the form of ear defenders should be provided. Employees should receive regular hearing tests and be exposed to an active educational programme.

High-intensity music such as rock music is another source of noise pollution. Public education about the effects of noise pollution and the importance of the use of ear defenders to decrease the intensity of the noise is necessary and should be directed to high-risk groups.

Advice

Suggestions of strategies that can sometimes help in interactions with someone who is hard of hearing are listed in Box 21.2.

Hearing aids

Some people with a hearing deficit may be helped by using a hearing aid, which is a small, battery-operated instrument that amplifies sounds. Aids are helpful to people who have reduced conduction of sound waves into the inner ear. Few of those with sensorineural loss of hearing receive help from hearing aids; amplification of sound does not assist with the distortion and impaired discrimination resulting from impairment of the neural elements of the auditory apparatus. Before purchasing a hearing aid, the person with a hearing deficit should be examined by a doctor for evaluation of the residual hearing and identification of the type of hearing loss. The selection of the aid is based on the patient's particular type of hearing loss. If an aid is recommended, it should be worn for a trial period to determine whether it does help.

Auditory and speech training

Auditory training is intended to help the individual utilize residual hearing effectively and improve communication skills. The process helps the patient develop good listening skills and increases his or her awareness of sounds and other clues.

Box 21.2   Suggestions to improve communication with a person who is hard of hearing

For those speaking to a person who is hard of hearing

- Use touch to attract attention

- Avoid a noisy environment

- Do not speak until you have the person's attention. The speaker's face should be in full view of the listener so that lip movement may be observed

- Determine which is the better ear and go to that side if possible

- Speak slowly, enunciate clearly and avoid raising the pitch of the voice. Increase the volume but do not shout. Guard against running words together. Use the natural form of conversation rather than broken and incomplete sentences

- Exaggerated lip movements will only confuse the listener

- If repetition is necessary, rephrase the communication if possible. Remember that vowels are heard more readily than consonants

- Always check that important communications have been understood

- Increase the use of touch to express emotion and comfort

- Patience, tact and understanding are needed. Avoid any irritation or annoyance; such reactions only discourage the listener

- Do not prolong a conversation unnecessarily

- If a hearing aid is used, give the listener time to adjust to it

- If a misinterpretation occurs, do not ridicule it or treat it as a joke

- When a person hard of hearing enters a room, make an effort to draw him or her into the group. Advise them of the topic of conversation and encourage them to participate

- If it is not possible to communicate verbally, write the message down

- If a patient is totally deaf and does not lip-read, pictures or symbols that represent objects may be helpful to orient the patient and for use during hospitalization

For those who are hard of hearing

- Look directly at the speaker (preferably in a good light), as observation of lip movements proves helpful

(Continued)

- Concentrate on the speaker

- Observe the total situation, as this may give a lead to the topic of conversation

- Acknowledge your hearing deficit; do not guess at things rather than ask for repetition

- Indicate understanding of the speaker

- Tell people you need to communicate with that you are hard of hearing

- Ask for written information where possible, or ask where you can get it

- Limit stressful situations to avoid fatigue

- If your attention is wandering, ask for a short break

- Try to develop interests that do not involve a lot of listening or verbal interaction.

Lip-reading or *speech reading* is the process of interpreting spoken words through the study of lip movements, facial expressions, body movements and gestures used in speech. Training helps the individual to use these cues consciously and effectively.

Speech training is provided to maintain existing speech skills, which deteriorate when the usual monitoring mechanism of hearing is lost. Hearing is necessary to assess loudness, clarity, tone and rate of speech. The congenitally deaf child requires a different type of programme to develop speech and language skills.

Community resources

Those who are deaf or hard of hearing and their families should be familiar with the Royal National Institute for the Deaf and Hard of Hearing. Assistance may be provided in the form of procuring medical examination and treatment, counselling as to the type of hearing aid that would be helpful, obtaining vocational training and employment, arranging for special classes (e.g. speech) and obtaining printed advice in pamphlets.

Common disorders of the ear

Impacted cerumen

The normal secretion of the external auditory canal (cerumen) may accumulate and become hard and dry. The retention may be due to abnormal narrowness of the canal, dryness of the skin or excess hair in the canal, or misguided attempts to clean the ear with cotton-wool buds. It may also be associated with the person's occupation; it is a common problem for those working in a dusty or dry environment.

Symptoms develop with the obstruction of the canal; the person may experience a sense of fullness, noises, loss of hearing, irritation or, rarely, a cough. The latter is a reflex response to stimulation of the vagus nerve. Examination of the ear with an otoscope reveals a firm yellow or dark mass.

Removal of the mass may be by irrigation with warm water. It may be necessary to soften the wax before syringing by instilling sodium bicarbonate or olive oil ear drops.

Otitis externa

This is a generalized inflammation of the external ear. The cause is frequently bacterial, but in some instances may be a fungus, or the inflammation may be associated with eczema or an allergic reaction. An infection is more likely to develop in a warm moist atmosphere or if the person swims frequently. It may be secondary to trauma inflicted by efforts to remove wax. External otitis may also be due to allergic dermatitis.

Characteristics

Pain, discharge from the external auditory meatus and tenderness are common. The patient may complain of pruritus or have raised temperature. Upon inspection the ear canal may show signs of inflammation and swelling.

Treatment

Paracetamol may be necessary for pain relief. Thorough cleansing of the ear may be sufficient to encourage recovery, although a ribbon gauze dressing soaked in a corticosteroid preparation may be necessary. If infection is present, neomycin or chloramphenicol ear drops can be prescribed.

Acute otitis media

This is an inflammation of the middle ear and is frequently a complication of an upper respiratory tract infection or an infectious disease, as in measles. Often the organisms gain access through the auditory tube and, less frequently, through a perforation in the tympanic membrane. The disorder is usually acute but may become chronic.

The initial inflammatory response causes congestion and swelling of the mucous membrane lining of the middle ear, and the cavity fills with exudate. The tympanic membrane bulges externally and, unless the infection is checked, the exudate generally becomes purulent. If the cavity is not surgically drained, the tympanic membrane may rupture spontaneously.

Characteristics

The patient with otitis media experiences a sensation of fullness in the ear and dullness of hearing at first, then severe pain, and increasing loss of hearing because of failure of the conduction of sound waves through the middle ear. The temperature and leucocyte count are raised and the patient feels generally ill. Examination of the eardrum by means of an auriscope reveals redness, hyperaemia and external bulging due to the pressure of the collection of exudate in the middle ear, or rupture and discharge in the advanced stage.

Treatment

As the causative agent is frequently viral, analgesia may be the only medication required. However, if bacteria are cultured from any discharge an appropriate systemic antibiotic is required together with analgesia. The eardrum may occasionally be surgically opened to permit drainage if the exudate is producing excessive pressure on the eardrum and there is danger of spontaneous rupture. The operative procedure is referred to as a *myringotomy*. Delayed treatment of acute otitis media may predispose to mastoiditis, chronic otitis media and permanent hearing loss.

The patient having a myringotomy receives a local anaesthetic. Fluid is aspirated from the middle ear cavity through the incision, and a culture is taken. The patient is encouraged to lie on the affected side to promote drainage. A persistent increase in temperature, pain and deep tenderness in the region of the mastoid, headache, drowsiness or disorientation is reported to the doctor. These may indicate the onset of a serious complication such as mastoiditis, meningitis or brain abscess.

Chronic otitis media

This chronic inflammatory disorder is associated with a permanent perforation of the tympanic membrane. It is usually a result of repeated episodes of acute otitis media that were not treated or were caused by virulent or antibiotic-resistant organisms. The perforation may also be the result of mechanical trauma or blast injury.

The location of the perforation is an important factor in the severity of the disease. If it is central, or at least does not involve the margin of the eardrum, the perforation is less serious and can be treated more effectively. This type of perforation is categorized as *tubotympanic*. If the perforation involves the tympanic margin in the posterior–superior area, it is called an *attic or marginal perforation*.

Characteristics

The otitis media associated with a central perforation is manifested by purulent discharge with an offensive odour. The discharge may be greatly increased during periods of acute upper respiratory infections or if water gets into the ear during bathing or swimming. Over a period of time, middle ear structures are damaged by the infection and necrosis. There is usually some impairment of hearing, which worsens during exacerbations.

Treatment

The initial treatment of the patients with a *tubotympanic perforation* is directed towards eliminating any upper respiratory tract infection as well as that in the ear. An antibiotic is administered orally or parenterally. The ear is cleansed by suction and dry mopping, followed by the instillation of an antimicrobial solution. If the exudate is excessive, it may be removed by daily aspiration by the doctor.

When the infection is cleared up, the perforated area very occasionally fills in with scar tissue. If the perforation persists, a tympanoplasty may be done to improve the patient's hearing and reduce the risk of reinfection by establishing a barrier between external and middle ears. Tympanoplastic surgery is undertaken only if infection is controlled.

In *marginal (attic) perforations* the disease involves the bony rim of the tympanic membrane and the mastoid cells as well as the middle ear structures. An invasive *cholesteatoma* may develop; this is a mass that forms in the middle ear as a result of the growth of epithelial tissue implanted in the middle ear from the collapsed parts of the eardrum when it perforates. The mass compresses middle ear structures and mastoid cells, causing necrosis and bone erosion. The presence of the cholesteatoma predisposes to the serious complications of labyrinthitis and brain abscess.

Marginal perforation and the development of a cholesteatoma are treated by radical surgery. A mastoidectomy is done, the cholesteatoma and middle ear debris are removed and reconstruction is undertaken to provide a conductive channel. The operation is done in two stages. The first operation removes the cholesteatoma and clears out the infected and necrotic tissue. The patient receives antibiotic therapy and, when the area is free of infection and there is no drainage, the reconstructive plastic surgery is undertaken.

Mastoiditis

The small spaces (air cells) in the mastoid communicate with the middle ear cavity and are lined with mucous membrane which is continuous with that of the middle ear. As a result, infection may spread readily to the mastoid in acute or chronic otitis media. The patient experiences tenderness over the mastoid process, headache and fever. Mastoid radiographs show a cloudiness in the mastoid cells.

Treatment and nursing intervention

Generally, early treatment with antibiotics checks the infection and no residual damage to hearing occurs. Rarely, if the infection is neglected or is virulent and unresponsive to the antibiotic given, bone tissue of the mastoid becomes infected, necessitating surgery. A myringotomy and a simple mastoidectomy are done. A simple mastoidectomy involves an incision behind the auricle and the removal of the diseased bone by curettage.

If the patient develops chronic otitis media and chronic mastoiditis, more extensive surgery may be undertaken.

A radical mastoidectomy involves the removal of the diseased mastoid tissue and the incus, malleus and remainder of the tympanic membrane, leaving the mastoid and middle ear as one large cavity. This operation on the middle ear results in loss of hearing.

Patients who have had surgery on the tympanic membrane should be informed that they may experience intermittent sharp pains for up to 3 weeks after operation due to the Eustachian tubes opening, allowing air to enter the middle ear (Smeltzer and Bare 2000). The external auditory canal will be packed immediately after operation and it is important that no water be allowed to enter the canal for up to 6 weeks after surgery.

The patient is observed closely for any sign of facial paralysis. Facial paralysis is a threat in mastoidectomy because of the proximity of the facial (seventh cranial) nerve to the operative site. Vertigo is another potential complication because of the proximity of the semicircular canals to the area being operated on. The patient is generally allowed up on the evening of surgery or the following morning; someone remains at first in case of dizziness and nausea which may develop as a result of labyrinth disturbance, especially following a radical mastoidectomy.

Otosclerosis

This is a chronic ear disease in which the stapes becomes immobilized because of progressive growth of bone tissue over the oval window and fixation of the stapes, interfering with the transmission of vibrations into the inner ear. Both ears are affected eventually.

The disease appears to be hereditary and has a higher incidence in females. The ability of the stapes to vibrate decreases progressively, and the loss of hearing usually becomes apparent in the teens or twenties, and during pregnancy. The person may complain of tinnitus as the deafness becomes more marked. The testing of hearing with a tuning fork reveals that the person has good bone conduction of sound but none by air.

Treatment

A hearing aid may be of some help for a period of time, but a stapedectomy has proved to be the treatment of choice at present. By means of a surgical microscope, the surgeon works through the external auditory canal and the middle ear. The stapes is removed, and a prosthesis introduced to transfer the vibrations of the incus through the oval window into the inner ear. The oval window niche is sealed using a free graft of fat or vein, and protected with Gelfoam. Only one ear is done at a time.

After operation, dizziness and nausea may be troublesome because of the disturbance of the labyrinth. A specific directive is received from the surgeon about the position in which the head is to be maintained as practices vary in different hospitals. The patient is instructed not to blow the nose to prevent air from being forced through the Eustachian tube to the middle ear. The patient is cautioned to move slowly and not to stoop over. If vertigo is experienced, ambulation may have to be delayed. The patient requires assurance that the dizziness is temporary. The patient should be observed closely for nystagmus or any sign of facial palsy.

Tinnitus

Tinnitus or ringing in the ears may be unilateral or bilateral and constant or intermittent. It may be of high or low pitch and vary in quality from a humming, buzzing, hissing, roaring, popping or pulsating sound. The sound sensation experienced by the patient is without a relevant external stimulus. It is heard only by the patient and not by others. Tinnitus is not a disease but a symptom. It may be a symptom of any abnormal condition of the ear, may be associated with deafness, or it may be drug related.

Vertigo and vestibular dysfunction

Vertigo is a disturbance of equilibrium characterized by a sensation of movement or rotation of self or of the surroundings. The patient experiences feelings of dizziness, light-headedness, falling or spinning. It may be accompanied by staggering or falling, clumsiness, nausea, vomiting or nystagmus which produces blurring of vision. Vertigo may occur suddenly, be transient in nature, or recur as with Menière's syndrome. Disorders of the labyrinth are the most common cause. Disturbances in the pathways in the central nervous system may also produce vertigo.

Disorder of the vestibular system is the most common of many possible causes of nystagmus (Haslett et al 1999). Nystagmus occurs when the systems that control eye movement are ineffective. As a result the eyes wander off target and repeated corrections are necessary to bring the eyes back on to the target object. Typically the eyes drift slowly in one direction and then move rapidly back to the correct orientation giving a to-and-fro movement.

Menière's disease or syndrome

This is a disorder of the internal ear characterized by recurrent attacks of severe vertigo, nausea, vomiting, tinnitus and a progressive loss of hearing. The cause is not known but an excess of endolymph (endolymphatic hydrops) develops, resulting in increased pressure and dilatation of the canals. Vascular spasm and allergic reaction have been suggested as possible aetiological factors. The disorder usually makes its appearance between the ages of 40 and 60 years, and occurs more often in males.

The episodes have a sudden onset, and the patient is generally prostrated by the dizziness and nausea. The duration of an attack varies from hours to days.

During an attack the patient remains in bed in a quiet environment. Cot sides may be necessary for safety because of the vertigo. An anthistamine such as cyclizine and a member of the phenothiazine group such as prochlorperazine are recommended for an acute attack (British National Formulary 2001). Hyoscine may also be used with an antihistamine and a phenothiazine in the prevention of vertigo and nausea associated with Menière's disease.

Structure and functions of the nose

The nose is concerned with the special sense of smell as well as being the first organ of the respiratory system. Any alteration to the function or structure of the nose can affect the sense of **smell**. Air breathed in through the nose is warmed, filtered and moistened before entering the lower respiratory passages and the lungs.

Nasal structure

The two anterior nares (nostrils) form the openings into the nasal cavities, which are separated from each other by the nasal septum formed of cartilage and bone (Fig. 21.6). The roof of the nose is formed by the base of the skull. The floor is formed by the roof of the mouth and is composed of the maxillary bones, the palatine bones and the soft palate. The lateral walls of the nose are formed by bone of the maxilla and the ethmoid bone. Three bony ridges – the inferior, middle and superior conchae (or turbinates) – project from the outer wall of each nasal cavity partially to divide it into three passages. At the back of the nose these passages lead to the pharynx. The interior of the nose is lined with mucous membrane. Most of this membrane is covered with minute hair-like projections called *cilia*. Moving in waves, these cilia filter the air passing through the nasal passages and sweep the debris out of the cavity, together with nasal mucus. The mucous membrane also acts to warm and moisten the inhaled air and is therefore a very vascular tissue.

The nasal cavities have connections with the middle ears by the pharyngotympanic (Eustachian) tubes, and with the eye region by the nasolacrimal ducts. The adenoids, two small areas of lymphatic tissue, can be found on the wall of the nasopharynx, behind the nose.

The olfactory region

The first cranial (olfactory) nerve provides the afferent sensory impulse pathway. The nerve endings, the olfactory receptors, are located in two pea-sized areas high in the interior of the nasal cavity.

All odorous materials give off particles of their substance and these chemical particles are carried into the nose with the inhaled air. They dissolve in the secretions of the mucous membrane and will stimulate nerve cells only when in solution. When an individual is exposed continuously to an odour, perception of the odour decreases and eventually ceases. This loss of perception affects only that specific odour. The sense of smell may be diminished or lost entirely as a result of nasal obstruction or infection or trauma to the nasal tissue or the olfactory nerve. The complete absence of the sense of smell is called *anosmia*.

Taste and smell
See chapter 2.4

Olfaction
See chapter 2.4

Figure 21.6 The nasal cavity.

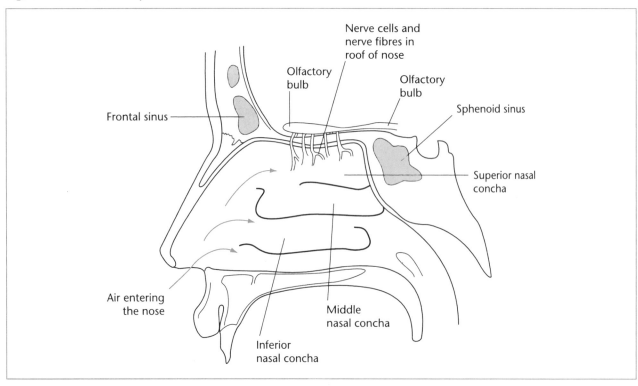

The two senses of smell and taste are inextricably linked. Taste registers only four qualities: salt, sour, bitter and sweet. Other qualities of taste depend on smell. The sense of smell may affect the appetite positively or adversely, depending on whether the smell is pleasant or unpleasant.

The paranasal sinuses

The paranasal sinuses are commonly referred to as nasal sinuses, or simply as 'the sinuses'. They are the eight cavities in the skull that are connected with the nasal cavity. They are arranged in four pairs, with members of each pair placed symmetrically on each side of the head:

- the *maxillary* sinuses in the maxillae
- the *frontal* sinuses in the frontal bone
- the *sphenoid* sinuses in the sphenoid bone behind the nasal cavity
- the *ethmoid* sinuses in the ethmoid bone behind and below the frontal sinuses.

The function of the sinuses is not clearly understood but it is thought that they may help with the warming and moistening of inhaled air and provide a resonating chamber for the voice. Being air-filled chambers, they make the skull lighter than it would otherwise be.

The sinuses, all lined with mucous membrane, are each connected with the nasal cavity; their openings into the nasal cavity are called the *ostia*. One of the functions of the nose is to drain fluids discharged from the paranasal sinuses.

The person with a disorder of the nose or nasal sinuses

Assessment

Health history

A nursing assessment of a patient with a disorder of the nose or nasal sinuses involves collecting information about any previous trauma or surgery that may have affected the anatomy of the region. Any history of previous, associated symptoms should also be recorded.

Information is obtained about the drugs being taken for the current problem, which may include inhalations and decongestants, as well as other medications.

The reason for seeking health care is identified. The manifestations, the duration and severity of the symptoms are determined.

Physical examination

The nose is examined both inside and out. The external nose is examined for asymmetry and lesions. The nostrils are examined for the presence of debris or discharge. The inside of the nasal cavity may be examined with nasal speculae and a light source for lesions and foreign bodies, and to determine the amount and characteristics of the nasal mucus. Any oedema or congestion of the mucous membranes will be noted. Air entry via each nostril is assessed by occluding the other. The patient may be asked to sniff to aid this assessment.

Common disorders of the nose and nasal sinuses

Rhinitis

Acute rhinitis is the medical term for the common cold. Most adults experience, on average, two to four attacks of acute rhinitis per year. Children may have much more frequent attacks. The mucous membranes of the nose become swollen and there is a nasal discharge. Some types are accompanied by fever, muscle aches and general discomfort with sneezing and running eyes. Breathing through the nose may become difficult or impossible. Rhinitis is often accompanied by inflammation of the throat and sinuses.

Common rhinitis is caused by a virus but may be complicated by a bacterial infection. Hay fever is another common form of rhinitis and is caused by an allergen to a particular substance. It, too, may be complicated by a superimposed bacterial infection.

The best treatment for the common cold is rest, preferably in bed, a well balanced diet and sufficient liquid intake. Mild analgesia may be taken to relieve headache or fevers. It must be remembered that the common cold is highly contagious, both by direct contact with the virus (e.g. on a handkerchief) and by droplet inhalation (transmitted when coughing or sneezing).

Epistaxis (nosebleed)

Epistaxis is usually due to the rupture of small blood vessels overlying the anterior part of the cartilaginous nasal septum. A minor nosebleed may be caused by a blow on the nose, irritation from foreign bodies (or fingers), or vigorous nose blowing. Treatment involves sitting the victim up with head tilted forward to prevent the swallowing of blood, which is a gastric irritant. Pressure should be applied to the soft portion of the nose by grasping it between the thumb and forefinger. Pressure may need to be applied for up to 15 minutes. Once the bleeding has been arrested, the person should rest quietly for an hour or so, and avoid stooping or lifting for several hours. If bleeding persists, medical help should be sought as it may be necessary to pack the nose or cauterize the bleeding vessel.

Sometimes nosebleeds have serious underlying causes such as arteriosclerosis, polyps or other growths in the nose, hypertension or vitamin deficiencies. Anyone who experiences frequent or profuse nosebleeds should therefore seek medical advice.

Surgery to the nose

Nasal surgery is indicated in a variety of conditions ranging from removal of a foreign body (usually in children) to the correction of a deviation of the nasal septum (caused by irregular growth or injury). Removal of polyps or other growths may be performed to restore normal nasal breathing, as may adenoidectomy in children. Cosmetic plastic surgery to correct disfiguring nasal anatomy is a common operation.

Any operation on the nose may result in swelling and bruising which may last for up to 6 weeks, so the success of the operation cannot be assessed immediately. The patient needs to be aware of this before the operation.

After operation the most common complication is bleeding. Excessive bleeding is indicated if the patient becomes restless, swallows repeatedly or spits up blood. Nasal packing or a splint may be left in the nose to prevent the formation of a haematoma. These are usually removed by the surgeon or at the surgeon's direction. If severe swelling or bleeding are expected, ice compresses may be used to reduce these.

Most nasal surgery results in some mild discomfort. This is partly due to the swelling and bruising but also to the presence of crusts of dried blood and mucus in the nose. The patient must be discouraged from attempting to dislodge these by nose blowing or picking. Lubricants or humidification may be used to help soften crusts, but no swabs or other objects should be inserted into the nose. Mild analgesia may be given to reduce the discomfort.

Eyes
See chapter 2.4

Sinusitis

Sinusitis is the inflammation of one or more of the paranasal sinuses. It tends to occur when an upper respiratory tract infection spreads from the nose to the sinuses but may be associated with allergies, air pollution, diving or swimming. Any alteration to normal nasal breathing, such as that caused by a deviated nasal septum or polyps, may lead to sinusitis. As the inflammation of the mucous membranes lining the sinuses increases, swelling occurs and partially or totally occludes the ostium (opening into the nasal cavity), preventing the exudate from draining. Mucus then accumulates and becomes infected, creating pressure within the sinus. Thus the symptoms of sinusitis are pain located in and around the affected sinus, headaches, nasal discharge, fever and general malaise.

Radiological confirmation of the diagnosis can be undertaken, and this helps to identify any underlying problem such as polyps or deviated septum.

The treatment of acute sinusitis is with antibiotics (amoxicillin, doxycycline or erythromycin) and decongestants, with the inhalation of steam to help encourage drainage. Analgesia is given to relieve the discomfort.

Chronic sinusitis occurs when the mucous membranes become thickened and obstruct the ostium, even when infection is not present. This prevents normal drainage from the sinus so that build-up of mucus occurs and frequent infections exacerbate the condition.

Treatment involves the identification and treatment of any underlying pathology, such as polyps or a deviated nasal septum. Changing the quality and humidity of the air in the home or workplace by using air-conditioners or filters and humidifiers may reduce the number and severity of the attacks. Failing this, drainage of the sinus may be performed surgically. Chronic sinusitis may lead to complications due to the proximity of other structures, such as the bones of the middle ear, the mastoid process and the brain, and for this reason it needs to be treated aggressively.

Disturbance in the sense of smell

While any of the above disorders can produce a disturbance or absence of the sense of smell, this condition (*anosmia*) is not uncomfortable or life threatening. The greatest impact is in the potential failure to smell burning or toxic chemicals, and the reduction in pleasure obtainable from the enjoyment of the taste and smell of foods, drinks and perfume.

Structure and functions of the eyes

Vision, like all other sensory mechanisms, requires receptors, an afferent pathway to carry the impulses into the central nervous system and an interpretive centre. The **eyes** serve as receptors which are sensitive to light rays, the pathway is formed by the optic nerves and tracts within the brain, and the interpretive centres are composed of groups of neurones localized in the cortex of the cerebral occipital lobes (visual centres). In addition, the visual apparatus includes intrinsic and extrinsic muscles which play an important role in vision. There are also several accessory structures that function to protect the eyes.

Location of the eye

Each eyeball rests in a cone-shaped cavity (the *orbit*) in the skull. The orbit is covered posteriorly by a fibrous sac lined with a smooth moist membrane which promotes smooth movement of the eye in its socket. The space between the intraorbital structures contains fatty tissue, which serves as a cushion for the eyeball.

The accessory structures include the eyelids, lacrimal system and extrinsic ocular muscles.

Eyelids (palpebrae)

The upper and lower eyelids serve as protective coverings. The space between them is referred to as the *palpebral fissure*; the angles or corners where the lids meet are known as the *inner* (medial) and *outer* (lateral) *canthi*. Each eyelid has an outer layer of skin, a layer of firm fibrous tissue (*tarsal plate*), sebaceous-like glands (*meibomian glands*) which secrete an oily substance on to the free margins of the lids, and a mucous membrane lining called the *conjunctiva*. The conjunctiva is reflected over the anterior portion of the eyeball forming the bulbar conjunctiva, and is continuous with the corneal epithelium. The secretion of the meibomian glands prevents adherence of the lids when the eyes are closed and also prevents the overflow of normal amounts of lacrimal secretion. The eyelashes emerge from the free borders of the eyelids to protect the eye from dust and perspiration.

Lacrimal system

The **lacrimal apparatus** protects the eye by continuously secreting a fluid that 'washes' over the anterior surface of the eyeball, keeping it moistened and cleansed. The system of each eye consists of a gland, ducts and a drainage system. The lacrimal gland lies in a slight depression in the outer superior portion of the orbit. The secreted fluid eventually drains through two small openings (puncta) in the medial canthus into two short canals (lacrimal canaliculi). The canals drain via the nasolacrimal duct into the nasal cavity. Increased lacrimal secretion (lacrimation) occurs in response to irritation of the conjunctiva or to certain emotions.

Extrinsic ocular muscles

Several external muscles have their origin in orbital structures and insert on the eyeball to provide movement of the eye within its socket. There are four *recti muscles* which move the eye up, down, medially and laterally, and two *oblique muscles* which provide rotation of the eye and modify the straight movements of the recti muscles. For most movements various combinations of recti and oblique muscle action are necessary.

The levator palpebrae superioris muscle inserts in the upper eyelid and is responsible for raising the upper eyelid (opening the eye).

Eyeball

The **eyeball** is spherical with a slight anterior bulge. It is composed of three layers of tissue which enclose the iris and special transparent, refracting structures. The tough, outer coat forms the *sclera* and *cornea*. Underlying and attached to the sclera is a thin, heavily pigmented, vascular coat, the *choroid*, which prevents reflection of light rays.

The *ciliary body* consists mainly of muscle tissue that holds the lens in position. The action of the ciliary muscle influences the curvature, and thus the refractive power, of the lens.

The second layer of the eyeball continues forward and inward beyond the ciliary muscle to form the iris. The *iris* is composed of circular and radial muscles and pigmented cells, and is perforated centrally, creating the opening referred to as the *pupil*. The iris, ciliary body and choroid are known as the uvea or uveal tract.

The *retina* is the innermost coat of the eyeball; it contains light-sensitive receptors that convert light into nerve impulses. There are two types of receptor cells:

- The *rods* have a lower response threshold, making them more sensitive to lower levels of illumination.
- The *cones* have a higher response threshold and, as a result, function in bright light and provide colour and detailed vision.

In the centre of the retina, a small area occurs in which the inner layers of cells are absent and only cones are concentrated. Light rays falling on this site strike the cones directly and produce the greatest visual acuity. This area is referred to as the *fovea centralis*. Near this area is a pale area called the *optic disc*, or *fundus oculi*, where the optic nerve and the central retinal vein and artery leave and enter the eyeball. The disc is a blind spot, because the area is devoid of rods and cones.

The *lens* is elastic and crystal clear, and is suspended just behind the iris by ligaments that attach to the ciliary body. Its shape varies with age; it is spherical in infancy, gradually flattening to a disc shape with age. In the elderly, the lens tends to flatten and becomes less elastic.

Divisions of the interior of the eyeball

The interior of the eyeball is divided into the anterior and posterior cavities. The *anterior cavity* is the space between the cornea and lens and is subdivided into the anterior and posterior chambers. The anterior chamber lies in front of the iris. The posterior chamber is situated behind the iris but in front of the lens. The content of the two chambers is *aqueous humour*.

The *posterior cavity* lies posterior to the lens. It is filled with the *vitreous humour*, or *vitreous body*.

Fluid system of the eye and intraocular pressure

The interior of the eyeball is filled by the aqueous and vitreous humours and the crystalline lens. The vitreous humour is a clear, jelly-like mass enclosed in a hyaloid membrane. It fills out the larger and posterior portion of the eyeball that lies behind the lens.

There is a continuous flow of aqueous humor into and out of the eye. The fluid originates from capillaries contained in processes of the ciliary body. After circulating around the posterior chamber, it flows through the pupil into the anterior chamber. From here, a small amount of the aqueous humour continuously drains into the canal of Schlemm, from which it is carried into the venous circulation. The aqueous humour carries nutrients to the lens and cornea, and removes waste products. This is necessary because both structures are avascular; the presence of blood vessels would alter their transparent nature. The production of aqueous humour and its drainage are constant in order to maintain a normal intraocular pressure, which is 16–21 mmHg. Any interference with

Lacrimal apparatus
See chapter 2.4

Eyeball
See chapter 2.4

Figure 21.7   Left and right visual fields and the visual impulse.

Visual pathways
See chapter 2.4

Optics
See chapter 2.4

Accommodation
See chapter 2.4

normal drainage of the fluid from the anterior chamber raises the pressure, leading to decreased blood supply, pain and impaired vision.

Visual impulse pathway

Impulses generated by the rods and cones synapse through several neurones and ganglions to the optic disc where they unite to form the optic nerve. At the base of the brain, the nerve fibres from the medial half of the retina of each eye cross, going to the opposite sides of the brain. The fibres from the lateral halves of the retinae do not cross but continue on to the corresponding side of the brain. This arrangement forms the *optic chiasma* (Fig. 21.7). Within the brain, visual impulses are transmitted to the visual centre in the occipital cerebral cortex, where they are interpreted as sensations of light, colour and form. Other cerebral areas are necessary for normal vision; correlation with information stored as memory has to occur in order to give meaning to what is seen.

Eye reflexes

Some fibres of each optic tract terminate in a group of neurones referred to as the *superior colliculus* in the midbrain. From here, efferent impulses originate, resulting in blinking of the eyelids, movement of the head, or dilatation or constriction of the pupil.

The pupils are normally round and of equal size. They adjust to light by constricting, and to darkness or dim light by dilating. A second reflex that may be noted is the

accommodation reflex. The normal response is constriction of the pupils as the person's gaze is shifted from a distant to a near object.

The mechanisms of focus

Several processes may be necessary to focus the light rays on the retina in order to form a clear image.

Refraction

The cornea and lens are the principal refractive media in the eye; the lens is particularly significant in that its curvature and degree of refraction can be varied by the ciliary body, according to the amount required to focus the light rays on the retina. Various errors of refraction occur that interfere with the ability of the eye to focus light rays on the retina, resulting in impaired vision.

Emmetropia implies normal refraction.

Short-sightedness, called *myopia*, is the result of light rays from an object at 6 m or more being focused at a point in front of the retina. Close objects can be seen, but distant objects are blurred. Correction may be made by use of a concave lens, which produces divergence of light rays (Fig. 21.8).

Long-sightedness (*hypermetropia*) is due to insufficient refraction and, as a result, light rays from an object at 6 m or less are focused at a point behind the retina. The person sees distant objects more clearly than close ones. Correction may be made by use of a convex lens, which focuses light rays by convergence (Fig. 21.8). In the later years of life, as part of the ageing process, the lens loses its elasticity and becomes thinner and flatter. This lessens the normal degree of refraction and the person becomes far-sighted, a refractive error referred to as *presbyopia*.

In some persons, the horizontal and vertical curvatures of the cornea are uneven, producing differences in the degree of refraction. This results in different focal points; some light rays may be focused on the retina, but others may fall short or be carried to a point beyond the retina. This type of refractive error is known as *astigmatism*.

Accommodation

This is the process by which the degree of refraction by the lens is changed in order to focus rays from objects at various distances. This is made possible by the elastic nature of the lens and the action of the ciliary muscles on the suspensory ligaments (Fig. 21.9).

Pupillary modification

The pupillary aperture is varied to control the amount of light entering the eye. For clear vision of near objects, the iris constricts the pupil of each eye to prevent divergent rays from entering. The opening is also reduced to restrict the entrance of excessively bright light, which may harm the retina. The iris constricts the pupil through parasympathetic innervation; sympathetic nervous stimulation produces dilatation of the pupil. In dim light and when

Figure 21.8 Diagram showing the use of lenses to correct common eye problems. (a) Myopia and correction by concave lens. (b) Hypermetropia and correction by convex lens.

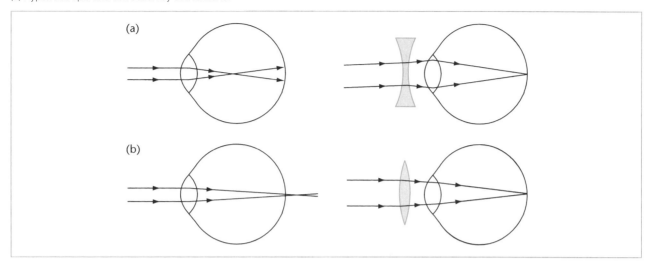

Figure 21.9 Diagram showing the ciliary body, suspensory ligaments and lens, and the changes in accommodation for (a) distant vision and (b) close vision.

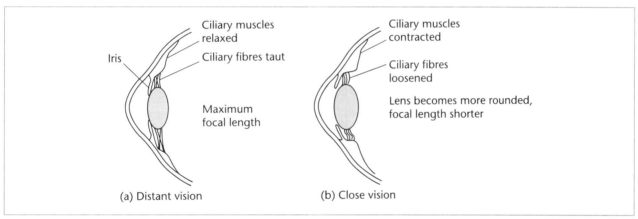

focusing on a distant, wider visual field, the iris dilates the pupil to admit more light rays.

Convergence

Although light rays from the same object(s) fall on both retinae, only single vision is experienced. This is due to light rays from the object falling on corresponding points of the two retinae. This is brought about by convergence, which involves the extrinsic muscles (recti and oblique). The movements of the two eyes must be coordinated accurately. As an object is brought closer to the eyes, convergence of their axes occurs as they turn inward. For distant objects convergence is not necessary; the eyes remain parallel. *Strabismus* (squint) is a defect that interferes with coordination of the eye movements, and the light rays do not fall on corresponding points of the two retinae. It is usually due to an abnormal extrinsic muscle, or to an undiagnosed refractive error. Two images result and the person 'sees double'; this is termed *diplopia*.

Light and dark adaptation

Light adaptation

When exposed to intense light, adaptation takes place by constriction of the pupils and lowering the eyebrows, eyelids and head; the visual purple (rhodopsin) within the rods is bleached, which reduces their sensitivity and responses.

Dark adaptation

When a person goes from a light to a dark area there is a period when nothing is seen, followed by the outlines of objects gradually becoming visible. This vision in dim light is due to an increased sensitivity of the rods as they produce a chemical pigment, visual purple or rhodopsin. Vitamin A is essential for the formation of the chemical; if it is deficient, the person experiences night blindness. At the same time that the rods increase their sensitivity, the pupils dilate to admit more light.

The person with health problems related to vision

Assessment

It is necessary, in most instances, that a thorough assessment is carried out before a diagnosis is made and, if appropriate, treatment prescribed. (*Immediate* action would be required if the patient's eye was damaged by trauma such as the accidental instillation of chemicals.) This includes a history of the patient's ocular disorder, general health and lifestyle, and an examination of the eyes. The latter involves inspection, palpation and the use of special equipment.

Health history

- *Age.* The age of the person in relation to developmental changes and effects of ageing on the eyes is important.

- *Occupation and lifestyle.* Information is obtained as to the demands for visual acuity, potential for eye injury and the use of protective devices. Sporting activity such as playing squash should be checked together with occupational hazards including the use of VDU screens.

- *Family history.* As many eye disorders are inherited, it is significant to learn of any family history of eye disorders, diabetes mellitus, cardiovascular disease and thyroid disease.

- *Past health.* Any childhood and adult illnesses, injuries and previous eye problems should be noted and the treatment and responses elicited. Ocular changes may be secondary to a disorder such as hypertension, diabetes mellitus, renal disease, hyperthyroidism and brain injury or tumour. Degenerative disease in the elderly is frequently the cause of loss of vision.

The use of corrective lenses should be ascertained together with the date of the last eye examination.

Current symptoms

The presenting complaint should be noted. Some common symptoms are listed in Box 21.3.

The PQRST symptom analysis tool may be used to assess the presenting complaint in a systematic way (see p. 258). Information concerning the nature of the complaint, duration, factors that provoke or relieve the symptom may be ascertained by use of this tool (Walsh et al 1999).

Examination of the eyes

Macroscopic examination

Tests for eye movement and measurement of visual acuity are usually performed before the examination of internal structures of the eye or tests that involve the touching of normally sensitive eye structures.

Retinal physiology
See chapter 2.4

Box 21.3   Common symptoms related to problems with vision

- Changes in visual acuity
- Blurring of vision
- Halos
- Flashes of light
- Spots before the eyes (floaters)
- Excessive lacrimation or epiphora
- Double vision (diplopia)
- Light sensitivity (photophobia)
- Night blindness
- Recurring headache
- Discomfort, burning sensation or itching of the eyes.

Initial observations of the eyes include noting: general appearance, symmetry of visual axes and physical features, any discharge and its characteristics, excessive or deficient lacrimal secretion, swelling or discoloration of extraocular structures or surrounding tissues, and the presence of a foreign body. The size and equality of the pupils are recorded. The medial canthi are examined for swelling and redness and *gently* palpated for tenderness.

The eyelids, lashes and brows are inspected for:

- redness or any discoloration
- crusting
- eversion or inversion of the lids
- complete and equal opening and closing of the lids
- swollen areas or oedema.

The areas are very gently palpated for tenderness and nodules. The colour of the conjunctiva of the lids is noted, as are any swollen or raised areas.

Assessment of extraocular muscle function

The patient sits facing the examiner, holding the head in a fixed position. The neuromuscular balance or straightness of the eyes is assessed by shining a light directly on the patient's eyes. The patient is asked to look at the light, which should be reflected in corresponding positions in the pupillary corneas. If there is deviation of one eye, asymmetrical reflection occurs.

When the light is moved, the movements of both eyes should be coordinated and symmetrical. Abnormal response may indicate paralysis of one or more extraocular muscles, muscular imbalance or injury.

Assessment of eye reflexes

Pupillary reflexes are observed in a dimly lit room by shining a light from the side on to the pupil of one eye at a time. Both pupils are observed; the normal response is constriction of both pupils when the light is shone in one. This is referred to as *consensual pupil reaction.*

The accommodation reflex is elicited by having the patient focus on a light held about 50 cm from the nose. As the light is moved toward the patient, the eyes normally converge and the pupils constrict.

Measurement of visual acuity

Visual acuity is the ability to distinguish details of objects and reflects ocular function. Each eye is tested separately; the eye not being examined is completely covered, but without any pressure being applied directly to the eye. A well-lit standard wall chart (Snellen chart) with rows of letters of gradually decreasing size is used, placed 6 m from the patient. The person is asked to read the chart through to the line of smallest letters that can be seen.

The distance from which the normal eye can read each line is known. The top line of the Snellen chart is perceived by the normal eye at 60 m, the second line at 36 m, the third at 24 m, the fourth at 18 m, the fifth at 12 m, the sixth at 9 m, the seventh at 6 m, and the eighth line at 4 m. Visual acuity is expressed as a fraction; the numerator represents the distance between the chart and the patient, and the denominator is the distance from which a person with normal vision could read the same line. Visual acuity recorded as 6/6 means normal vision. If the patient 6 m from the chart can only read the line that the normal eye could read at 12 m, the visual acuity is expressed at 6/12. The larger the denominator recorded, the poorer is the vision. In a person with severe impairment who can only see a hand moving in front of the face, the visual acuity may be recorded as HM (hand movements). If the person can distinguish only between light and dark, the recording is PL (perception of light), and if there is no light perception it is expressed as NPL (no perception of light). A recording of 3/60 or less in the better eye when wearing glasses or contact lenses indicates that the person is legally blind.

Near vision is assessed by having the individual hold a card about 32 cm from the eyes. The print on the card is sized proportionately to the 6 m.

Visual field measurement (perimetry)

A semicircular instrument, called a perimeter, which is marked in degrees, is used to determine whether the patient's visual fields are normal or restricted. Defects in the visual fields are frequently associated with intracranial lesions or damage to an optic nerve.

Estimation of the visual field may also be made by the confrontation test. An object is moved slowly from beyond the patient's peripheral vision towards the central line of vision. The patient is asked to indicate when the object first comes into view and this is compared with when it was first seen by the examiner. The difference is recorded, taking for granted the examiner's vision is normal. The test is made using lateral, upper and lower fields.

Measurement of intraocular pressure

The detection of increased intraocular pressure is important; an excessive pressure may be very painful and progressively causes permanent damage within the eye, leading to loss of vision. The pressure is measured with an instrument called a tonometer. A few drops of a local anaesthetic (e.g. tetracaine (amethocaine) 0.5–1%, oxybuprocaine 0.3%) are instilled in each eye. The tonometer is then placed on the corneal surface, causing indentation; the extent of the indentation reflects the intraocular pressure. If the pressure is high, the cornea resists indentation. The normal intraocular pressure is approximately 16–21 mmHg.

A second instrument that is now generally employed to measure the ocular tension is the applanometer. This is an electronic device that is considered to provide a more accurate measurement of the intraocular pressure.

The patient with raised intraocular pressure is at risk of serious impairment of vision due to ischaemic neuropathy.

Slit-lamp microscopy (biomicroscopy)

A more detailed examination of the internal structures of the eye can be made by the use of slit-lamp microscope. It is helpful in locating foreign bodies in the eye and identifying ulcer erosion as well as degenerative and inflammatory conditions.

Fluorescein staining

A fluorescein strip, which is a sterile strip of paper that has been impregnated with a solution of sodium flurorescein, is moistened at one end and lightly applied to the lower conjunctival sac. A single-drop, disposable dispenser may be used as an alternative. The dye flows over the eye, and abrasions and corneal ulcers readily stain a yellowish-green.

After the examination the eye is irrigated with a sterile saline solution to remove the dye.

Ophthalmoscopic examination

With an ophthalmoscope, the posterior, internal surface (fundus) of each eye is magnified 15 times and observed. The lens, vitreous body, blood vessels, retina, optic nerve and disc are viewed. To obtain a wider view, the pupil may be dilated by the instillation of a mydriatic such as tropicamide 0.5–1%. Ophthalmoscopy is valuable in the recognition of some systemic disorders, as well as in the assessment of ocular function. Nurse practitioners are increasingly carrying out opthalmoscopic examination of the eye. As a result they may detect disorders such as hypertension, renal disease or diabetes which produce characteristic changes in the eye visible only on ophthalmoscopy.

Assessment of the retina

Electroretinography may be done to record the extent of the electrical response made by the retina to light stimulation.

Gonioscopy

This involves the examination of the angle of the anterior chamber by means of an optical instrument (gonioscope).

Clinical characteristics

Impairment of vision

The development of significant signs and symptoms of impaired visual function varies greatly. The onset of changes may be insidious in some cases, but in others, the onset may occur suddenly and be acute. One or both eyes may be involved. The manifestations may be principally subjective or may be objective only, with the abnormal structure or function being noted by an observer. In some instances manifestations may be recognized without tests or the aid of instruments.

The signs and symptoms of eye disorders include the following characteristics.

Subjective manifestations

1. Difficulty in reading and seeing objects clearly, blurred vision or headaches when reading or doing close work. These symptoms may be caused by simple refractive errors or by cataract, glaucoma, inflammation of the cornea (keratitis) and ulceration leading to scarring and opacity, degenerative changes, detachment of the retina or a systemic disease such as hypertension, diabetes mellitus or arteriosclerosis.

2. Photophobia (sensitivity to light) may be associated with inflammation of the conjunctiva, cornea or iris.

3. Excessive tear flow may indicate trauma, chemical irritation, allergy, inflammation of ocular tissue or obstruction of the tear duct.

4. Dryness of the conjunctival surface due to decreased lacrimal secretion which may be due to severe dehydration or cerebral trauma or disease (e.g. rheumatoid arthritis). It is frequently a problem in an abnormally dry environment and in the elderly. Some drugs may suppress lacrimal secretion.

5. Ocular pain may be due to irritation from a foreign body, infection, inflammation of eye tissues or accessory structures, or increased intraocular pressure (glaucoma).

6. Diplopia (double vision) is most frequently experienced by patients with a head injury or cerebral disorder (e.g. brain tumour) that incurs a paralysis or functional imbalance of the extraocular muscles.

7. Spots before or floaters in the eyes, single and occasional, are common and of no clinical significance. Frequent or sudden development of numerous spots or floaters may signify an intraocular haemorrhage or threatening of the retina. In the latter, the patient may experience flashing lights followed by a clouding across the eye.

8. Scotoma or blind spot develops as a result of damage to an area of the retina or optic nerve. It may be caused by an inflammatory disease process within the eye or a degenerative disorder. If the scotoma occurs in the same area in each eye, the aetiology may be intracranial, affecting the fibres in the visual pathway.

9. Halos around lights are usually associated with increased intraocular pressure and glaucoma.

10. Extensive loss of visual acuity of 3/60 or less in the better eye with correction, or a restriction of the visual field to 20° or less, indicates blindness according to the legal definition.

Objective manifestations

1. The person is observed holding reading material or an object nearer than 30 cm to the face or beyond the distance of approximately 40 cm.

2. A strained expression or scowl may be noted when an effort to see is being made.

3. The younger person may fail to develop at a normal rate or make normal progress at school.

4. Errors are made because of misread information or directions.

5. Deviation of one eye (the visual axis of one eye differs from that of the other eye) indicates impaired extraocular muscle structure or function. The latter may be due to a disorder involving the oculomotor (third cranial) nerve.

6. Discoloration of the eyelid or surrounding tissue. Redness of the eyelids suggests infection, allergy or injury. Redness of the exposed area of the eye may be caused by conjunctival irritation by a foreign body, infection or trauma, or may be incurred by a subconjunctival haemorrhage associated with trauma, hypertension or inflammatory disease of intraocular structures. Discoloration of surrounding tissue may be the result of extravasation of blood related to an eye or facial injury.

7. Discharge (serous or purulent) or crusting may indicate infection, chemical irritation, allergy or trauma of the eyelid or eye.

8. Swelling or oedema may develop with local trauma, infection or cyst, or may be associated with renal or cardiac failure, a cerebral disorder or head injury.

9. Abnormal pupillary shape or reaction. Constriction, asymmetry or failure of normal reaction to light is most often due to some cerebral disorder or iris

collapse. A greyish white colour of the pupil suggests an opacity of the lens (cataract).

10. Exophthalmos or proptosis (prominence or bulging of the eyes) is usually caused by hyperthyroidism.

11. Ptosis or a lag in the closing of eyelid may indicate some oculomotor (third cranial) nerve involvement. The drooping of both eyelids is also characteristic of myasthenia gravis.

The person with visual impairment

In 1997, 354 153 people were registered blind or partially sighted in the UK and a total of 1 066 740 were classed as visually impaired, of whom 75% were aged 75 years or over (Royal National Institute for the Blind 2001). Visual impairment is therefore a major problem, particularly amongst elderly people. People are very dependent upon their sense of vision, as most of our knowledge of the environment is obtained through our eyes. The eyes are also used in expressing emotions. Any impairment or loss of vision is a serious threat. In many instances the ability to freely move about safely and the privilege of enjoying colour, form, depth, beauty and distance are lost. Loss of vision results in reduced sensory input and stimulation; this may lead to boredom and reduced responsiveness and disorientation to time and place on the part of the person unless stimuli by other channels (e.g. hearing and touch) are increased and the person's interest is maintained.

The nurse should appreciate the incalculable value of sight and the natural anxiety and concern of the patient when it is threatened. Reduced vision affects the patient's whole way of life – socially, physically, economically and emotionally. Effective nursing care can be planned only if the nurse has an understanding of the causes of visual impairment as this will allow the identification of appropriate goals for the individual.

Causes

Visual impairment may be due to a primary eye disorder or may be secondary to a neurological or systemic disorder. The causes include:

■ structural or functional defect in the eye or extraocular structures (e.g. malfunction of the extraocular muscles causing deviation of one or both eyes)

■ ageing (e.g. the lens becomes less spherical with age, may become opaque and the nucleus hardens)

■ infection

■ trauma – chemical or mechanical

■ new growth

■ impaired innervation of the eyes due to a neurological disorder (e.g. brain tumour or injury)

■ systemic disease (e.g. hypertension, diabetes mellitus, cardiovascular disease)

■ inadequate knowledge about the factors that contribute to the preservation of good vision (e.g. nutritional requirements, protection of eyes in potentially hazardous situations).

Goals

Patient-centred goals common to most patients with visual impairment are:

1. Vision will be preserved.

2. Factors contributing to visual impairment will be identified.

3. The patient will receive meaningful sensory input.

4. The patient will remain oriented.

5. Injury or complications will not occur.

6. If visual impairment is permanent, the patient will learn to be as self-caring as possible, retaining maximum independence.

Preservation of vision

The maintenance of vision and prevention of loss of sight includes consideration of the following.

Good general health

There is a tendency to consider vision as being independent of general health. It remains good in some serious bodily disorders, whereas others may have a serious effect on visual acuity.

Optimum diet

Vitamins A, B complex and C are considered important; a deficiency of vitamin A may cause drying and changes of the cornea and conjunctiva and a decreased production of the retinal pigment, rhodopsin, leading to night blindness. A deficiency in the vitamin B complex may predispose to retinal changes. Vitamin C plays a role in resistance to infection.

Protection of eyes

Occupational health nurses have a very important role to play in preventing eye injury by ensuring that staff wear protective goggles. Office workers also need to be aware of hazards to their eyesight resulting from inadequate lighting and overuse of VDUs.

Regular periodical eye examination

Some eye diseases and changes develop insidiously without markedly reducing vision or causing pain until they are well advanced. Regular eye examination may reveal early signs, and a serious disease may be checked before it progresses to loss of vision and blindness. If glasses are necessary, only those that have been properly prescribed should be used. Lenses are individually ground for each eye according to the testing and examination findings. Box 21.4 lists the terms used in eye examinations and to describe errors of refraction.

Care and use of glasses and contact lenses

If glasses are worn, the importance of protecting the lens from scratches and maintaining good alignment is stressed. If glasses are not straight or if the distance between the eyes and lenses is not equal, the degree of refraction is altered. Lenses in spectacles are safer if made of impact-resistant material.

When the patient receives a contact lens, detailed instructions and demonstrations are necessary. A contact lens is a thin plastic disc shaped to fit the anterior surface of the eye. The outer surface is ground to meet the patient's visual need. The patient is taught the daily procedure of putting in and removing the lens, the cleansing and care of it, and the prevention of complications. Meticulous care is necessary to prevent complications such as infection, which are painful and could ultimately cause loss of vision. Washing the hands thoroughly with soap under running water before handling the lens is emphasized. If worn in both eyes, on removal each lens is stored separately in containers marked for right and left; the correction in one may be quite different to that of the other. Directions for cleansing are provided in writing. Before applying the lenses, they are rinsed free of any chemical that may have been used for cleansing and a wetting solution may be used. Solutions must be fresh and are not reused.

The patient is advised to use the lens for brief periods at first, progressively increasing the length of time until the eye is comfortable with it. Unless the lenses are of the extended-wear type, they are removed at the end of each day; they are *not* worn during sleep. If the eye is inflamed or painful or if there is excessive lacrimal secretion (tearing), the lens is not applied. The most common complications that develop are conjunctivitis, corneal abrasion and keratitis.

Prevention of trauma

The loss of vision due to exposure to chemicals, dust, wind, glaring light or direct sun rays, and eye injury by mechanical objects (e.g. flying pieces of metal or wood), is preventable in most instances by the use of standard safety measures and devices. The use of legislated safety helmets, shatterproof goggles or shields in potentially hazardous situations should be observed. Sunglasses may be necessary to protect the eyes from ultraviolet radiation in bright sunshine (e.g. when skiing or using a sun bed). Welders should use protective eye shielding for the same reason, to avoid ultraviolet radiation causing very painful damage to the outer layers of the corneal epithelium, known as 'arc eye' (Walsh and Kent 2001). The use of adequate protective equipment as well as observance of established safety rules in sports such as squash, where there is a potential for injury, should be promoted.

Box 21.4 Terminology and abbreviations used during eye examinations

RE	Right eye
LE	Left eye
BE	Both eyes
Emmetropia	Normal vision (normal refraction)
Myopia (M)	Short-sightedness
Hypermetropia (hyperopia; H)	Long-sightedness
Presbyopia	Reduced accommodation associated with the ageing process
Astigmatism	Uneven curvature of the cornea; results in different focal points
Diplopia	Perception of two images of a single object (double vision)
Hemianopia	Loss of vision in one half of the visual field
Entropion	Turning in of the eyelid
Ectropion	Turning out of the eyelid
Ptosis	Drooping of the upper eyelid
Aphakia	Absence of the lens of an eye
Hyphaema	Haemorrhage into the anterior chamber of the eye
Hypopyon	White blood cells in the anterior chamber
Photophobia	Hypersensitivity to light
Ophthalmologist (oculist)	A doctor who specializes in the treatment of eye disorders
Optometrist	A person who examines the eyes to assess vision and prescribes corrective spectacles or lenses
Optician	A specialist who prepares spectacles or lenses according to prescription
Mydriasis	Dilatation of the pupil
Mydriatic	Drug that dilates the pupil
Miosis	Contraction of the pupil of the eye
Miotic	Drug that contracts the pupil
Proptosis (exophthalmos)	Bulging forward of the eyes
Epiphora	Excessive lacrimal secretion (tears)

Rubbing of the eyes should be avoided because of the possibility of trauma and the introduction of infection, especially if wearing contact lenses. Cautious use of sprays and caustic solutions and the wearing of protective goggles when exposed to caustic substances should be emphasized.

First aid and prompt treatment

In the event of an accident no 'eyedrops' or ointment should be instilled in the eyes. The eye should be gently irrigated with copious amounts of water which will frequently remove any foreign body. If the foreign body cannot be easily removed in this way or if there are signs of inflammation or any other disturbance in an eye, early medical treatment is required. Foreign bodies frequently end up adhering to the undersurface of the eyelid (conjunctiva) where they may be seen only by everting the eyelid. In this position they are known as subtarsal foreign bodies. If a chemical spray or irritating solution accidentally gets into the eye, immediate and extended irrigation with water or saline is recommended and urgent medical treatment sought to avoid potential ulceration and blindness.

Principles to be observed in eye-care procedures

1. The patient receives a full explanation of the procedure and is advised that it is important that the head is held steady.

2. Hands are washed thoroughly before and after doing any eye procedure.

3. Precautions are used to protect the unaffected eye from possible injury and cross-infection from one eye to another. Irrigation solution or eye drops being used in the affected eye must not be permitted to enter the unaffected eye. Similarly, dressings from the affected eye should not touch the unaffected eye. Dressings and swabs are used only once.

4. Pressure on the eyeball is avoided.

5. When irrigating the eye, the solution is directed on to the nasal side of the eyeball. The eye is gently wiped from the inner canthus to the outer canthus.

6. Solutions and drugs should always be fresh; they are dated as to preparation and expiry.

7. Frequent, regular assessment of the eye and the patient's vision is made. The eye is examined before and after each procedure; alteration in comfort, change in colour, discharge, dryness, oedema or swelling is brought to the attention of the doctor.

8. If both eyes are involved, separate sterile equipment and solutions are used for each eye. In the case of infection, the eye manifesting less inflammation and discharge is treated before the other eye. These precautions are aimed at reducing the risk of cross-infection.

9. A separate sterile eye-dropper is employed for each drug used in the eye.

10. If the eyelid does not close, precautions are necessary when handling articles such as bed-linen, towels and clothing to avoid abrasions and injury of the conjunctiva and cornea. An exposed (open) eye may become dry and susceptible to ulceration; the instillation of artificial tears may be prescribed as a prophylactic measure, as may ointment applied to the exposed conjunctiva.

11. It is important that the patient is warned of any effect the eye drops may have; some will paralyse the muscles of accommodation and cause blurring of vision.

12. Eye dressings are normally applied to protect, to absorb lacrimal secretions or exudate, or to apply pressure. The skin around the eye should always be supported gently when the dressing is removed.

13. Drops are instilled at the *lateral* aspect of the inner lower lid, with the patient looking up, so that direct corneal contact is avoided and reflex squeezing of the eye prevented.

14. In order to keep the affected eye at rest, the unaffected eye may be covered. Adaptation to light is resumed gradually; the unaffected eye may first be exposed by wearing a shield with a small central opening. This minimizes eye movement. A similar shield may also be used later on the affected eye; however, it is more usual for the patient to wear dark glasses. Extreme gentleness is used when changing a dressing or doing any treatment; caution is used to avoid pressure on the eyeball.

15. Great care should be taken to prevent the eye opening under the dressing as this can cause corneal abrasion. The dressing should be secured firmly.

Care of the visually handicapped patient

Maintenance of orientation and reduction of anxiety

Impairment and threatened loss of vision arouse considerable fear, insecurity and emotional reactions. All the implications that impaired vision may have in the present and future 'crowd in' on the patient and he or she may become panicky and lose control. Behavioural responses must be assessed frequently; with reduced or no vision, the patient (especially if elderly) may become disoriented, particularly if not in a familiar environment.

Individuals deprived of visual input become more dependent on other senses such as hearing and touch.

The understanding of the nurse as to what the patient may be experiencing, the provision of emotional support and the use of communication techniques that promote the use of other senses contribute greatly to the care of this patient.

Factors that help to reduce the patient's anxiety include the following suggestions. The patient is carefully oriented to any new environment; if confined to bed, the orientation is by a verbal description. If allowed up, the verbal description is combined with helping the person to explore the ward environment. An explanation is made of how usual daily needs will be met.

The patient is given the opportunity and encouragement to express concerns and to ask questions. The person who cannot see is spoken to while being approached and is advised who is speaking. Any treatment or investigative procedure should be well described in advance. It means a great deal to the patient to have the call-button always within reach; this means that help is always at hand. The patient should not be left alone for long periods for, although a lot of physical care may not be needed, support and contacts are still required. The nurse should take time to talk to the patient and, as required, indicate the time and describe the place and current situation and details of the environment. The patient may have visual memory from which it is possible to recall sufficiently to form a mental picture of what is being described. Some appropriate form of diversion, such as a radio and visitors to chat with or read to the patient, is encouraged to provide sensory input. Noisy, confusing situations are avoided; the visually handicapped patient is usually more sensitive to sounds and voice inflections. An effort is made to anticipate the patient's needs.

Maintenance of a safe environment

Adequate orientation and frequent observations are important to prevent accidents when the patient's vision is seriously impaired. If the patient is disoriented, it may be necessary to have someone present to ensure patient safety.

The environment must be checked carefully for any hazards for the unseeing, ambulatory person. He or she should be escorted around the area until familiar with it and encouraged to move about alone. Stools, rugs or other such articles should be removed. Furniture is not moved from its original position when possible, and doors are kept closed or wide open. The person is cautioned about nearby stairs and radiators. All members of the staff should be made aware of the individual's degree of visual handicap.

Continuous assessment

Prompt recognition of change in the eye, visual acuity and orientation is very important, as failure to do so can lead to an increase in the amount of impairment. The nurse is required to be familiar with any specific observations that are important in certain eye disorders. Generally, significant factors that should be brought promptly to the doctor's attention include increased temperature, discharge, unrelieved pain, headache, any evidence of disturbance in the unaffected eye, and signs of bleeding, infection inflammation in the anterior segment.

Positioning and activity

Patient positioning varies with different conditions and is usually indicated by the doctor. Prolonged restriction of activity is relatively rare; patients worry less and have fewer complications when allowed up as soon as possible. If the patient is required to remain in bed, lying flat with the head immobilized, the arms and lower limbs are moved through a range of motion, and active exercises of the legs are begun as soon as the doctor permits.

Eating and drinking

The patient frequently experiences anorexia due to anxiety and because of the difficulty with taking food when vision is impaired. The necessary assistance is provided and, when feeding, the food is described; only small amounts are offered to avoid choking and coughing, because coughing raises the intraocular pressure. As soon as the patient is well enough, self-care and independence are major considerations; however, assistance is withdrawn gradually, not all at once.

The position of different foods on the plate may be described using the clock analogy. Aids such as plate-guards and non-slide mats may also be useful.

Some visually handicapped patients are reluctant to socialize at mealtimes in case they cause embarrassment; the use of aids can help them overcome this. Drinks should be offered regularly and poured out if necessary; it is often difficult for the patient to do this – and they may just not drink. Aids are available to help with pouring drinks.

Communication

Verbal communication should be clear and concise and may need frequent repetition. Touch and tone are very important, as they offer a form of non-verbal and verbal reinforcement of which the patient can be aware.

Rehabilitation of the blind

There are two official categories of visual handicap in the UK:

1. *Blindness*:
   a. so blind as to be unable to perform *any* work for which eyesight is essential
   b. visual acuity of below 3/60
   c. visual acuity of 6/60 and below if there is considerable contraction of the visual field.

2. *Partial sight*: a visual acuity of 6/60 or less, the individual being substantially or permanently handicapped by defective vision. The category to which the person is assigned (according to the amount of visual impairment) dictates eligibility for help.

The patient with marked visual impairment or with total loss of vision needs a great deal of assistance in adjusting to the situation. The individual needs to realize that life still has meaning and potential. Emphasis is placed on what is possible given that the person still has visual memory of form, colour and space, and can learn that other senses may be put to greater use.

The development of independence is started as soon as possible, beginning with self-care (feeding, bathing, dressing and hair). Assistance is given with moving about the room and then from room to room, locating furniture and necessary articles by touch. The environment is organized to provide safety.

Anyone walking with a blind person allows the individual to take an arm rather than grasping the person and pushing. Writing is practised, beginning with the person's signature. Differentiation by touch is also tested and practised. The person learns to tell the time by using a specially designed watch.

Various forms of diversion and recreation are introduced (e.g. tapes/CDs of books and music). The patient is referred to the social services and the Royal National Institute for the Blind, which provide vocational training, assistance in learning Braille and in finding a job, recreation, transportation, and financial assistance when necessary. The use of the white cane is introduced and the necessary guidance given on excursions beyond the house until the person is capable of safely getting around alone. Other people may prefer the use of a guide-dog – it is a matter of personal choice.

The patient and family are advised of the financial assistance available for the registered blind or registered partially sighted, and are assisted in making application for it. The family may require help in accepting the blind patient and in organizing the home environment in the interest of safety and independence.

Common eye disorders

Refractive errors

Various errors of **refraction** occur which interfere with the ability of the eye to focus light rays on the retina, normally resulting in impaired vision. (See p. 760 for a discussion of short-sightedness, long-sightedness, presbyopia and astigmatism.)

Blepharitis

This is an inflammation of the eyelid; it is usually bilateral and affects the marginal area of the lids.

Characteristics

The patient may complain of itching or irritation. The margins of the lids are reddened and develop crusts or scales. It may be associated with seborrhoea (excessive sebaceous gland secretion) of the scalp and eyebrows or be staphylococcal in origin.

Treatment

Therapeutic measures include gentle removal of the crusts once or twice daily with warm water and the application of the prescribed antibacterial ointment; if the cause is seborrhoea, washing with an antiseborrhoeic shampoo may help.

Conjunctivitis

Inflammation of the conjunctiva may be caused by bacteria, viruses, chemicals or an allergic reaction, and may be acute or chronic. It is also the most common ocular disease worldwide (Smeltzer and Bare 2000). Sources of eye infection include foreign bodies, dust, hands, infected neighbouring structures (nose, face, sinus) or contaminated equipment or solutions used in treatment. Viral infections are a very contagious form of conjunctivitis and prompt therapeutic measures are necessary to prevent its rapid spread to other people. Infection may begin in the conjunctival lining of the eyelids and spread, or remain confined to that area.

Characteristics

The inflammation is manifested by irritation, feeling of grittiness, pain, redness, encrustations, and excessive lacrimation or serous and purulent discharge. The patient may complain of photophobia. When infection is present a culture may be made from a swab of the discharge for identification of the invading organism; this should be carried out before instilling an antimicrobial agent.

Refraction
See chapter 24

Treatment

Frequent gentle cleansing of the lid margins is necessary to prevent encrustations. Precautions must be observed to treat each eye separately so that infection is not transferred from one to the other. The patient is usually more comfortable in dim light or darkness, and dark glasses ease the discomfort in the early stages. Chloramphenicol or gentamicin ointment is usually prescribed for instillation. In an allergic reaction, an antihistamine preparation may be prescribed to relieve the irritation. The patient is advised to keep the hands away from the eyes and, if responsible for instilling medications, the patient must be cautioned to wash the hands thoroughly under running water before starting and after completing the medication procedure.

If the conjunctivitis is due to allergy, efforts are made to identify the allergen so that it can be avoided if possible; it may be airborne or transferred by the person's hands or by towels. A topical antihistamine such as antazoline or azelastine may be instilled as eye drops (British National Formulary 2001).

Hordeolum (stye)

A hordeolum, or stye, is a small abscess that develops within a marginal sebaceous gland or hair follicle of an eyelash. A small, red, swollen tender area appears. Spontaneous drainage of pus may be hastened by a topical broad-spectrum antibiotic such as chloramphenicol ointment, which should be instilled regularly.

Chalazion

A chalazion is a cyst that forms in a meibomian (sebaceous) gland. It may remain as a small, firm, painless swelling in the lid for a long period. Eventually it may become infected and irritate the palpebral conjunctiva. Application of chloramphenicol ointment is usually prescribed. Recurrence frequently necessitates a small incision for drainage and curettage.

Glaucoma

This disorder is characterized by an increase in the intraocular pressure above the normal, which causes damage to the optic disc and visual field loss. It is one of the leading causes of blindness in the world. Normal intraocular pressure is generally maintained by a balance between the production of aqueous humour by the ciliary body and its drainage from the anterior chamber via the canal of Schlemm. If an imbalance occurs between production and drainage, the pressure increases, compressing the retina and the blood vessels within the eye. Permanent optic nerve damage leading to blindness results unless there is early recognition and treatment of the disease.

Glaucoma is usually due to some interference with the outflow of aqueous humour from the anterior chamber into the canal of Schlemm. It may be classified as primary, secondary or congenital. The primary acute form may be referred to as *acute angle-closure glaucoma*; the primary chronic type is called *open-angle* or *simple chronic glaucoma*.

Secondary glaucoma may be associated with infection, inflammation, trauma or a tumour within the eye.

Open-angle (chronic) glaucoma

This chronic and more common type develops very gradually; the cause is not understood but the frequency of familial incidence points to hereditary aetiology that results in degenerative changes. It is usually bilateral and has a higher incidence in persons over the age of 35 or 40 years; this emphasizes the importance of regular eye examinations that include the measurement of intraocular pressure.

Characteristics

Because of the insidious onset of open-angle glaucoma, the central field of vision is not lost for some time. The disorder is frequently well advanced before the person seeks assistance. The visual field diminishes progressively, and the individual may become aware that something is wrong when discovering objects on either side that have been 'missed', or if halos are persistently seen around artificial lights. The condition may be discovered during a routine examination. As the condition progresses, the person may complain of some pain in the eye(s), especially in the morning on awakening. If chronic glaucoma is not recognized and treated in the early stage, the person eventually goes blind.

Treatment

In the early stages, treatment of open-angle glaucoma consists of instillation of a topical beta-blocker such as betaxolol which decreases aqueous humour production. Additionally a miotic such as pilocarpine is prescribed up to four times a day. This opens up the inefficient drainage channels in the trabecular meshwork, thereby increasing drainage of the aqueous humour. Miotics cause constriction of the pupil as a side-effect. Adrenaline (epinephrine) may also be prescribed as it reduces the rate of production of aqueous humour and increases the outflow through the trabecular meshwork (British National Formulary 2001). Laser surgery may be used to create an opening in the anterior chamber angle to improve the drainage of aqueous humour (Smeltzer and Bare 2000).

Teaching the patient with glaucoma

Because glaucoma accounts for such a large proportion of blindness, more effort has been directed toward informing the general public about the disease and the significance of early recognition. The Royal College of Ophthalmologists' web site (http://www.rcophth.ac.uk) has a series of patient education handbooks which may be downloaded covering a whole range of conditions including glaucoma.

Glaucoma cannot be cured, but blindness can be prevented by continuous use of a miotic as prescribed, by operation and by medical supervision, if it is begun early in the disease.

An important nursing responsibility is to alert the patient to activities and situations that predispose to a rise in intraocular pressure. The condition is explained to the patient and family, and emphasis is placed on the need for some precautions to prevent visual damage. Emotional and stressful situations are avoided as much as possible; the patient must learn to tolerate and live with what cannot be changed.

The patient and family must appreciate the importance of regularly scheduled visits to the ophthalmologist for measurement of the intraocular pressure and visual field and acuity testing. They are taught the correct method of instilling the prescribed miotic, and cautioned against the use of any solution or medication that is not prescribed by the doctor. An identification card or Medic Alert pendant indicating that the person suffers from glaucoma is recommended. Some job modification or change may be made by encouraging the patient to consult with the employer and occupational health department, but every effort should be made to continue employment.

Acute angle-closure glaucoma

This form of glaucoma is characterized by rapid marked increase in intraocular pressure as a result of a complete

Figure 21.10 Diagram showing how a disturbance in the balance of fluid within the eyeball increases pressure in the eye and can result in glaucoma. Solid arrow indicates normal direction of fluid movement. Broken arrow indicates abnormal movement in glaucoma.

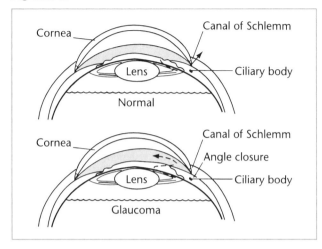

block in the outflow of the aqueous humour. The iris appears to have been pushed forward, narrowing the peripheral angle between it and the cornea (Fig. 21.10) and, with dilatation of the pupil and the concomitant thickening of the iris, the openings in the filtration angle that lead into the canal of Schlemm become occluded. The condition demands prompt emergency care because rapid compression of the retinal blood vessels develops, and destruction of the optic nerve cells and fibres occurs, with resultant loss of vision.

Characteristics

The patient with acute glaucoma experiences severe pain, nausea and vomiting, halos or rainbows around artificial lights, and blurring of vision. On examination, the pupil is seen to be dilated and fixed, and there is evidence of congestion with a marked increase in intraocular pressure. The cornea becomes oedematous losing its lustre and transparency.

Prompt treatment is necessary to reduce intraocular pressure and prevent blindness. Carbonic anhydrase inhibitors such as acetazolamide or dorzolamide are the drugs of first choice as they reduce aqueous humour production. They should be combined with a topical beta-blocker such as timolol eye-drops and an α-adrenergic agonist (e.g. apraclonidine eye-drops) for emergency management. Once intraocular pressure has been brought under control, a miotic such as pilocarpine can be given to open the closed angle (Smeltzer and Bare 2000). A quiet environment is provided and the patient is helped to relax, positioned with the head and shoulders elevated; analgesia is prescribed to relieve the pain.

If an immediate, satisfactory response to drug therapy does not occur, laser surgery is undertaken (e.g. *laser irodotomy*, where an opening is made in the iris using a laser beam).

Cataract

A cataract is a clouding of the crystalline lens, resulting in opacity. It may be classified as a *degenerative* or *developmental* (congenital or juvenile) cataract; the latter type of cataract occurs most often in infants whose mothers have a history of a viral infection (e.g. German measles) during the first trimester of pregnancy, or is associated with a genetic defect that, for example, causes an inborn error of metabolism.

The degenerative cataract has a higher incidence in persons over 50 years of age. The cause is not known; metabolic changes in the lens substance are considered to be a major factor. It is also suggested that an inherited predisposition to develop the characteristic lens changes plays a role. Degenerative cataract is frequently associated with diabetes mellitus. Opacity of the lens may also be secondary to eye trauma or to exposure to radiation or extreme heat. It may develop following prolonged use of the miotic echothiopate or a topical corticosteroid preparation.

Characteristics

The opacity develops very gradually (unless caused by trauma) and may be localized to the centre of the lens, incurring early impairment of vision, or it may start in the periphery. A cataract, even in its early stage, is readily recognized through the pupil, using an ophthalmoscope. As it matures, the examiner is not able to visualize the fundus or optic disc and the pupillary area appears grey or whitish because of the opaque lens behind it.

The loss of the normal refractive ability of the lens prevents light rays from being focused on the retina. Vision becomes blurred, objects may appear distorted and colour perception decreases. Visual loss is very gradual and is directly proportional to the degree of opacity of the lens. Cataract may be unilateral or bilateral; if bilateral, the opacity does not usually develop at the same rate in both lenses.

Treatment

Cataract is irreversible but, as loss of transparency of the lens develops, visual acuity and distant vision can usually be improved by increasing the correction of lens in the person's spectacles. Eventually, the opacity increases to the point that no light rays pass through the lens to reach the retina.

When the person's visual impairment becomes a handicap and interferes with usual lifestyle and activities, surgical treatment is undertaken. The operative procedure used may be classified as extracapsular or intracapsular cataract extraction.

In the *extracapsular extraction*, the anterior portion of the capsule and the lens content may be removed, or the procedure may involve phacoemulsification (a small incision is made in the anterior capsule and the lens content is aspirated). Phacoemulsification uses ultrasonic vibrations to fragment the lens content, which prepares it for aspiration. The extracapsular extraction leaves the posterior part of the capsule intact and the vitreous body undisturbed. If the posterior capsule of the lens has lost its transparency, a small opening (a capsulotomy) may be made in it with a laser beam several weeks or months after the initial operation.

In *intracapsular cataract extraction*, the lens is removed, complete with its capsule, usually by cryoextraction in which a probe-like instrument is introduced so that it lies against the lens and is cooled to −30 to −35°C. The lens and its capsule freeze to the probe, and are removed when the probe is withdrawn.

Following either an extracapsular or intracapsular extraction, an *intraocular lens implant* may be placed in the anterior or posterior chamber.

Usually cataract extraction is done in only one eye at a time; if both eyes are affected, they are treated (in most cases) in separate operations.

Care of a person with a progressive cataract

During the period through which the lens is progressively losing its transparency, a nurse usually has contact with the patient only at the clinic, the surgery or on home visits that are for some other purpose. However, if the patient is a nursing home resident they will be in contact with nursing staff continuously. Assessment of visual impairment should be ongoing.

Potential patient problems

■ Anxiety due to the visual impairment and fear of blindness and dependency.

■ Potential for injury.

■ Decreased mobility, usually due to a fear of moving about, especially outside the immediate familiar environment.

■ Alteration in self-image.

Anxiety

The nurse explains to the patient and family what cataracts are and reassures them that it is a common problem. They should be advised that vision can be improved by corrective lenses in glasses for a period of time and that eventually the cataract can be treated by surgery. Details should then be given about what this will entail.

Potential for injury

Advice should be given to the patient and family about adjustments within the patient's environment that may be necessary to prevent accidents. Improved lighting may help and other aids, such as stair rails, can be installed. Direct vision into sunlight and bright lights is avoided. Driving should be discussed with the patient and the advice of the ophthalmologist sought.

Decreased mobility

Because of the fear of falling, or of making errors and being unable to read signs, price tags, etc., the patient becomes reluctant to venture beyond immediate familiar environments and activity may gradually decrease. Socialization decreases. The patient should be encouraged to go out with family members and friends, not to hesitate to ask for assistance when alone, and to turn the head to obtain a direct view of an object if peripheral vision is poor. The patient and family are informed that books in large print are available in public libraries. They are also advised of the services of the local branch of the Royal National Institute for the Blind. Registration as blind or partially sighted will make certain benefits and allowances available.

Alteration in self-image

The person with loss of vision may become depressed and lose self-esteem as activity and participation progressively become restricted and dependence upon others increases. The positive aspects of life should be emphasized and accessible forms of diversion discussed. Unless there is some existing complication that contraindicates surgery, the patient is reassured that this is a temporary problem that will be relieved by the operation.

Postoperative care of patients following intraocular surgery

An operation for the treatment of cataracts is one of the most common intraocular operations. The care outlined in the following section applies to all intraocular surgery as well as that specifically for cataracts.

The period of bedrest and hospitalization following eye surgery is now reduced to a minimum, with day-case surgery becoming more common. The problems of bedrest and immobility are therefore much reduced.

The major concerns following eye surgery are potential eye injury and complications such as infection. The nursing care for each potential problem is outlined below.

Pain

The patient may experience some burning or smarting sensation which can be relieved by a mild analgesic. Severe pain, particularly if it develops suddenly, or a feeling of pressure within the eye, can be an indication of haemorrhage and so must be identified promptly and reported to the surgeon.

Potential for eye injury related to surgery

The main potential problems are intraocular haemorrhage, increased intraocular pressure and rupture of an incision line. To avoid these, the surgeon may request restrictions in activity and positioning, in which case the head may need to be supported by a nurse when transferring from trolley to bed, and when moving in bed. These restrictions must be understood by the patient and relatives.

Any increase in pressure on the eye is to be avoided. Possible causes include straining at stool, vomiting or retching, coughing, sudden movements and bending or leaning over the side of the bed. Nursing care is directed to avoid these situations, so a high-fibre diet is given, with plenty of fluids and a stool softener if necessary; antiemetics are given as necessary; the patient is shown how to cough with the mouth open, if coughing is unavoidable and instruction on permitted activity is given.

Any prescribed dressings and drugs (including eyedrops) are given and a protective eye shield may be used at night for additional protection.

Any pain that is severe or of sudden onset is reported to the surgeon.

Potential for infection

The length of time a dressing is kept on depends on the operation, the surgeon and the treatments required. Whenever a dressing is touched, strict asepsis is observed and the eye is inspected for inflammation or discharge.

Prophylactic antibiotic drops may be prescribed, with the addition of systemic therapy if infection is suspected. Any discharge is swabbed for culture and sensitivity.

Topical corticosteroids may be prescribed to reduce the effects of inflammation on intraocular structures.

Potential for injury related to sensory deprivation or disorientation

When vision is severely impaired either by the operation, swelling or dressings, or because the room is darkened, the patient will need additional care and support to reduce the fear and anxiety associated with loss of sight, even if it is only temporary.

On return from theatre, the patient will need to be oriented to location, staff and time, and this should be repeated whenever a person enters the patient's vicinity. The call button must be ready and within reach, and the patient should not be left alone for long periods; frequent communication reduces the potential for sensory deprivation.

When ambulatory, the patient is assisted until familiar with the environment. Footstools, loose rugs and other hazards should be removed, and the furniture kept in a specific position where possible. Doors should all be either kept open or kept closed.

If the patient becomes confused, sedation may be prescribed. If possible, a friend or family member should stay with the confused patient to ensure his or her safety.

Inadequate nutrition

Self-care in eating and drinking may not be possible if vision is impaired after operation. A fluid intake and output chart should be kept until a normal intake is achieved. Help should be given to pour drinks and with feeding, and appropriate foods chosen and aids used to help independence.

Nausea and vomiting should be avoided (to prevent increase in intraorbital pressure) and antiemetics given as necessary.

A high-fibre diet should be provided (to prevent straining at stool) and a stool softener given if necessary.

Inadequate knowledge of care and rehabilitation

The patient's home situation should be assessed and the patient and family assisted to make appropriate changes.

The restrictions on normal activities required to avoid an increase in intraocular pressure must be understood. These restrictions include bending over, pushing, avoidance of falls and bumps, and sexual activity. Information must be given as to how long these restrictions are likely to be needed.

The patient and/or family must understand and learn the care of the eye, eye socket or artificial eye, such as cleaning and dressing it, the instillation of drops or ointment and the avoidance of rubbing or friction on the eye. They must also be aware of the symptoms that indicate the need to contact the ward or surgeon (pain, inflammation, discharge or loss of vision).

The care and appropriate use of any glasses or contact lenses must be understood. Restrictions on reading or watching television may be imposed on the patient to avoid straining the eye, and restrictions on driving may be needed for a period prescribed by the surgeon. These need to be understood. Any further appointments or follow-up care must be given to the patient.

Specific postoperative care following cataract surgery

Spectacles and contact lenses

When the dressing is removed, dark glasses are worn because the patient may experience discomfort in the eye with exposure to light; gradual adaptation is necessary. If an intraocular lens has not been implanted at the time of the operation, the patient may be fitted with a contact lens some weeks after surgery. The lens may be of the type that has to be removed each night, or an extended-wear type that can be left in the eye for several weeks. With the latter, the patient returns to the clinic or ophthalmologist at regular intervals (approximately 90–120 days) to have the lens removed, cleansed and replaced.

When only one eye has had cataract extraction, spectacles are not useful because the thick biconvex lens that would be necessary magnifies considerably and would not produce binocular vision. When both eyes have had cataract surgery without intraocular lens implant, the patient is fitted for spectacles with thick biconvex lenses which are used for a few weeks or months before permanent glasses or contact lenses are provided. With spectacles, peripheral vision is restricted (Fig. 21.11).

Implantation of an intraocular lens at the time of the cataract extraction or at a later date is becoming more common. The advantages are the provision of greater

Infection of eye
See chapter 6.1

Figure 21.11 A view of the Bank of England used to demonstrate the effect of wearing cataract glasses. (a) Normal view. (b) Loss of peripheral vision as seen through the eyes of someone wearing cataract glasses. Only the central area is seen and this appears larger and nearer than it is, with bowed edges.

(a)

(b)

depth perception, full visual field and binocular vision (less magnification than glasses).

If glasses are to be worn, an explanation is made about the reduced peripheral vision. The patient is advised that, in order to see, he or she must learn to look straight-on; this necessitates turning the head when making a side-on peripheral observation. Because of the magnification and difference in spatial judgement, the patient is advised of the necessary precautions when using stairs and handling objects.

Complications

Complications that may occur following cataract extraction include the following:

- ■ *Haemorrhage* into the anterior chamber (hyphaema) is a serious complication that may occur in the early postoperative period. The patient experiences sharp pain in the eye and, on examination, blood can be seen in the eye. The patient is placed at rest, the head is elevated and the ophthalmologist is notified immediately. A mydriatic preparation is usually ordered to dilate the pupil and rest the eye.

- ■ *Wound rupture and iris prolapse* occurs rarely and is manifested by a misshapen iris and bulging in the incision area. It requires prompt surgical treatment to avoid serious visual impairment. Mydriatics must not be instilled if a prolapse is suspected as this can worsen the condition.

- ■ *Infection* may develop as an acute bacterial endophthalmitis leading to pain, loss of vision and inflammation. A severe infection may manifest itself as a *hypopyon* – white cells in the anterior chamber and corneal haze. It is treated by topical and parenteral antibiotics.

- *Retinal detachment* occurs rarely as a result of the formation of adhesions within the eye, usually between the retina and the vitreous (see treatment of retinal detachment below).

- *Glaucoma* may also develop as a result of adhesions forming between the iris and the cornea, blocking the filtration angle.

Detachment of the retina

Retinal detachment is separation of the pigmented epithelium of the **retina** from the layer of rods and cones; the pigmented layer remains attached to the choroid. The separation occurs as a result of tears or holes in the retina. These openings permit fluid from within the eye to leak through and accumulate in the retina, causing the separation.

The cause may be degenerative retinal changes associated with the ageing process, aphakia (absence of the lens), trauma or tumour. The trauma may be directly to the eye (e.g. penetrating foreign body) or may be associated with a head injury. Retinal detachment may occur as a complication following cataract extraction or an inflammatory intraocular disorder. There is a higher incidence in those who have myopia and are over 50 years of age. The damaged areas are usually toward the periphery of the retina but may occur in the area of the macula, causing severe visual impairment.

Characteristics

Manifestations of a detached retina appear suddenly and are preceded by flashes of light, blurred vision, floating particles in the line of vision before the sensation of a curtain coming in front of a part of the eye, restricted visual field and eventual loss of vision occurs.

Treatment

The patient is placed at rest and both eyes may be covered. A mydriatic and cycloplegic drug such as cyclopentolate hydrochloride (Mydrilate) may be prescribed for instillation to dilate the pupils and arrest accommodation by depressing ciliary action. The ophthalmologist indicates the position the patient is to assume: left or right lateral, or on the back (never prone). The position is such that the detached area of the retina will approximate the underlying layers. A sedative or tranquillizer may be prescribed to reduce the patient's fear and apprehension, and promote immobility. The patient is advised of the importance of maintaining the recommended position and of avoiding sudden movements, bending over, coughing, sneezing and rubbing the eye. The patient should be informed that assistance is close at hand and how it may be summoned.

Surgical intervention is usually undertaken fairly early. Various procedures are used, but the underlying principle is scarring of the area. As the scar tissue forms, it fills in the retinal hole and provides attachment to the underlying sclera.

Vitrectomy is fast becoming a common surgical method of treating complicated retinal detachments. The retina is reapposed to the underlying pigment epithelium by removing vitreous humour and replacing this with liquid gas or oil. This method requires strict positioning for 2–3 days after operation.

After the operation, a patch is placed over the eye for 24 hours. Dilating and antimicrobial eye-drops may then be ordered. The patient is instructed to ask for assistance when ambulating and not to bend or strain. The light in the room is kept low to decrease light sensitivity when the patch is removed and dark glasses may be worn. Because of the amount of oedema within a confined space (the orbit), pain can be a problem and may be for 6–8 weeks after the operation. A full explanation of the cause of pain and regular analgesia may be given. Analgesia to take home should also be prescribed.

Before discharge the patient is taught to instil the eye drops and is given written instructions about activity limitations. No heavy lifting or heavy work is undertaken for a period of at least 5–6 weeks. Appointments are made for follow-up care. The patient must be cautioned against bumping the head, rapid eye movements, reading and close work.

Uveitis

Inflammation due to injury or infection may develop in the uveal tract, which includes the choroid, iris and ciliary body. It may also be associated with collagen disease (e.g. rheumatoid arthritis, sarcoidosis).

Retina
See chapter 2.4

Characteristics

The eye is reddened and the patient complains of pain, photophobia and impaired vision in the affected eye. The pupil usually remains constricted.

Treatment

Treatment may include rest of the eyes, the application of heat and the administration of an antimicrobial drug if infection is suspected as being the cause. A mydriatic (e.g. atropine, cyclopentolate, tropicamide) is instilled to dilate the pupil and prevent adhesions from developing between the iris and the lens. A corticoid preparation may be given systemically and also instilled in the eye(s) to arrest the inflammatory process and scar formation; scar formation is likely to cause loss of vision.

Keratitis

This term is used for inflammation of the cornea, which is a serious condition. It may be due to infection or trauma and is likely to lead to ulceration and scarring. The affected areas lose their transparency, diminishing the light rays entering the eye.

Debilitated persons and those with vitamin A deficiency and allergies develop corneal ulceration more readily with an eye infection or trauma. The inflammation may be superficial or deep and in some instances becomes chronic.

Characteristics

Keratitis is manifested by irritation, discharge if the cause is infection, redness of the eye due to injection of the peripheral areas of the cornea by blood vessels, photophobia and lacrimation. Ulcerated areas may be identified by the instillation of fluorescein, which outlines the lesions.

Treatment

Prompt medical treatment is necessary to prevent perforation of the cornea and serious visual damage. Keratitis frequently may be prevented by early removal of foreign bodies as well as early treatment of injuries and infection.

Treatment includes rest, the use of antimicrobial drugs, the instillation of a mydriatic and the administration of systemic analgesia to relieve pain. The eyes may be covered to protect them from light and to limit eye movement. If ulcers develop and are complicated by corneal perforation, the aqueous humour escapes, the anterior chamber collapses and there may be intraocular bleeding. The patient is placed on complete bedrest, a mydriatic is instilled in the affected eye to dilate the pupil, and a pressure dressing is applied. Sometimes a soft contact lens called a protective membrane or bandage lens is applied.

If a cornea appears to be in danger of perforating, the lids may be closed over it, either by closure by tape or actually sutured shut, a tarsorrhaphy. In severe cases, surgery to the cornea (keratoplasty) may be required.

Vitreous haemorrhage

The most common cause of vitreous opacity is bleeding from adjacent papillary, retinal or ciliary vessels. With minimal bleeding the patient may be conscious of floaters or 'small black dots'; more serious bleeding causes a sudden flood of floaters and subsequent loss of visual actuity so that the patient is only able to perceive light.

The haemorrhage may be associated with trauma, retinal tears and detachment, hypertension or diabetes mellitus. Many diabetics develop diabetic retinopathy, which is a common cause of blindness; increased vascular permeability, microaneurysms and atheroma (fatty plaques in the walls of the arteries) develop in the ocular blood vessels in diabetic retinopathy. Fragile vessels in the vitreous frequently bleed.

Loss of vitreous transparency may also be caused by uveitis in which the inflammatory exudate and debris are carried into the vitreous and cause opacity.

Minor haemorrhages into the vitreous resolve fairly quickly. In more severe bleeding, which causes a serious visual impairment or where there is a loss of vitreous transparency due to other aetiological factors, a *vitrectomy* may be undertaken. This involves the removal of vitreous content and opacities with a special instrument to which there is a fibreoptic light attached. The vitreous is replaced with a liquid or gas.

Keratoconus

This is a rare degenerative disorder of the cornea that is seen in young persons, usually young men. There is a degenerative thinning and protrusion of the central cornea, usually of both eyes. Severe astigmatism develops, causing visual impairment.

An excessive amount of fluid collects posterior to the protruding cornea, and scar tissue develops as a result of the damage to tissue by stretching and rupture. The person experiences blurring of vision in the early stages but progressive changes may eventually lead to complete loss of vision. The patient may be helped at first by the wearing of hard contact lenses but may finally require keratoplasty.

Keratoplasty (cornea transplantation)

Loss of vision due to destruction of the cornea, keratoconus or loss of transparency may be corrected by a cornea transplantation. The central portion of the affected cornea is removed and replaced with a cornea obtained from a cadaver. The period between death and removal of the graft should not exceed 6–8 hours, and the transplant must be performed within 24–48 hours. Corneal tissue can now be preserved for up to 2 weeks as corneal buttons and still remain viable, which has reduced the need for the majority of patients to be sent for urgently, and this operation can now be planned for. During the interval following enucleation the donor eye is refrigerated at 4°C to minimize degenerative changes. Rejection is less of a problem with corneal transplantation than with other types of organ transplantation. It is suggested that this is due to the avascularity of the cornea. In the absence of blood vessels, donor tissue antigens do not get into the recipient's blood to initiate the formation of antibodies and sensitized lymphocytes.

Preoperative preparation

A detailed discussion of all that is involved in a keratoplasty occurs between the surgeon and the patient and family. The patient is informed that several weeks will elapse following the transplant before the results can be evaluated.

The immediate preoperative period is now a planned admission. Blood specimens are collected for the usual preoperative blood studies, and the surgeon usually prescribes the instillation of a miotic (e.g. pilocarpine 2–4%) in the affected eye to constrict the pupil so that the lens is protected during operation. Acetazolamide may be prescribed to reduce the intraocular fluid volume and tension.

Types of keratoplasty

The operative procedure may be a penetrating keratoplasty or a lamellar transplant. The *penetrating transplant* involves a full-thickness removal of the central portion of the affected cornea and replacement with an equivalent full-thickness section of the donor cornea. In a *lamellar keratoplasty*, a partial-thickness piece of the donor cornea replaces superficial layers of the recipient's cornea.

Postoperative management

The patient experiences some pain and a mild analgesic may be prescribed. The main cause of discomfort is the presence of the sutures giving a continuous 'foreign body' sensation. The sutures stay in for 3–9 months, but the eyes usually become more comfortable as the epithelium grows over the sutures.

The patient is allowed up as much as he or she wishes after recovery from the anaesthetic.

The eye is protected by a dressing. Sunglasses are worn during the day; at night a shield (usually of plastic) is applied.

Topical medications prescribed for instillation for a period of time may include, in addition to a mydriatic such as cyclopentolate (Mydrilate), a corticosteroid preparation to suppress inflammation which would reduce the clearness and transparency of the cornea. A prophylactic topical antibiotic may also be used for a few days. When instilling ointments or drops, as always, precautions are observed to avoid any pressure on the eye and having the dropper or the tube applicator touch the eye.

During the weeks and months after the transplantation, the patient may have alternating periods of optimism and discouragement. It is important for the patient to be informed before leaving the hospital that healing will be slow because a transparent cornea does not have blood vessels.

A family member and the patient receive demonstrations and instructions in the care of the eye and the instilling of medications in preparation for leaving the hospital. If a family member or the patient is not able to undertake the care safely, a referral may be made to the district nurse. The patient is followed closely by frequent visits to the clinic or surgeon.

Injury to the eye

An eye may be traumatized by a foreign body, laceration or chemical agent. The patient may experience the discomfort associated with 'something in the eye' excessive lacrimation, pain, redness and sensitivity to light. Persisting pain, loss of vision and bleeding usually manifest a serious injury. With any type of injury, contact lenses should be removed promptly.

A *foreign body* may lodge on the conjunctiva or may be embedded in the conjunctival or corneal tissue, causing inflammation and possible ulceration. In some accidents, the injury may penetrate the lens or even the retina. If a foreign body is not washed out easily, the patient is promptly referred to an ophthalmologist or accident and emergency department. Fluorescein dye may be used in the eye during the assessment to localize the foreign body. Deep metal foreign bodies may be removed with a strong electromagnet. If the foreign body has caused an abrasion or was penetrating, an antibiotic ointment is instilled and a dressing may be applied.

Lacerations of the eyeball seriously threaten vision because of the formation of scar tissue in healing and by predisposing the eye to infection. Prompt treatment and strict asepsis are very important.

Various *chemicals*, acids and alkalis (such as cement or mortar) may cause serious irritation or burns of the conjunctiva and cornea. Emergency treatment consists of washing the eye with copious amounts of water or saline. The lids must be wide open and assistance may have to be provided in order to keep the eye open during the flushing. The person should be taken to an accident and emergency department as quickly as possible where they should receive high priority in whatever triage system is in use. A local anaesthetic may be instilled to provide relief and facilitate examination of the eye(s). Both eyes are covered to limit eye movement.

Strabismus (squint)

Normally, both eyes perform an equal range of movement and assume corresponding lines of position when focusing on an object. Strabismus ('cross eyes') is characterized by the deviation of one eye from the position of the other. One eye (the normal or fixing eye) focuses directly on the object, but the other one (the deviating eye) appears to be focused on a different object or area.

The inequality in the movement of the eyes is due to an imbalance in the function of one or more extrinsic ocular muscles. The defect may result in the eye being turned medially, producing a convergent strabismus (*esotropia*). If the eye is turned laterally, the condition is referred to as divergent strabismus (*exotropia*). The result of the unequal movement and two points of focus is double vision (*diplopia*). Two images are formed on the retinae and the visual centres in the brain receive two sets of impulses, each producing a separate picture.

Strabismus may also be classified as being non-paralytic or paralytic. *Non-paralytic strabismus* (the more common) is the result of a congenital abnormality. The defect is in the central nervous system mechanism that coordinates the movements of the eyes in order to bring them into the positions that will focus the light rays from an object on corresponding areas of the two retinae. The person may be able to focus the right eye on an object of attention but the left deviates, presenting a second image.

The person with strabismus develops single vision over a period of time, seeing only what the fixing or non-deviating eye perceives by involuntarily suppressing the confusing image presented by the deviating eye. Non-paralytic strabismus is generally recognized in early childhood.

Paralytic strabismus is due to the inability of the extraocular muscles to move the eye into the position corresponding to that of the other eye. As a result the person experiences diplopia. The cause of paralytic strabismus may be a defect in the muscle itself or a disturbance in the muscle innervation. The condition may be a manifestation of a disorder within the brain or orbit that interferes with the transmission of impulses by the third (oculomotor), fourth (trochlear) or sixth (abducens) cranial nerve.

Treatment

Strabismus requires medical treatment; unfortunately, in some instances parents think it will correct itself as the child becomes older. A delay may result in permanent damage; constant suppression of the image presented by the deviating eye may lead to loss of vision in that eye (amblyopia). The form of treatment will depend on the cause and severity of the strabismus. Obviously, if it is secondary to a lesion that is interrupting nerve impulses, the primary condition is surgically treated, if possible. Strabismus in the child may be corrected by the wearing of prescribed glasses. The unaffected eye may be covered for periods to enforce the use of the deviating (or so-called 'lazy') eye. Special eye exercises may be ordered (*orthoptics*).

If the condition does not respond to these conservative forms of treatment, surgical correction may then be undertaken. The procedure may involve shortening or lengthening of one or more extrinsic eye muscles. After the operation, exercise and the wearing of glasses may still be necessary for a period of time. The patient requires continual medical supervision.

Neoplasms of the eye and accessory structures

Tumours that develop in the skin on other parts of the body may also occur on the skin of the eyelids. Neoplasms of the external structures are usually discovered in the early stages because they are visible.

Neoplasms of the eye may be benign or malignant and the latter may be primary or secondary. Secondary malignancies in the eye are rare. A biopsy is done if the neoplasm is accessible. Malignant melanoma is the most common intraocular tumour. It usually originates in the choroid, ciliary body or iris. Retinoblastoma which develops in both eyes is attributed to a genetic defect that is considered hereditary.

Early symptoms of an intraocular neoplasm depend on its location. As it enlarges and spreads, pain is experienced because of the increased intraocular pressure; retinal detachment, intraocular haemorrhage and loss of vision occur. Primary malignant tumours may be treated by radiotherapy, local excision or enucleation.

Enucleation

Enucleation is the removal of an eyeball and may be necessary because of a malignant neoplasm, deep infection, severe trauma or persisting pain in a blind eye. Rarely, an enucleation is done to remove a disfiguring blind eye.

When an eyeball is removed, the extrinsic muscles are severed close to their insertion, and may be arranged around a plastic ball to provide support and movement for an artificial eye. A plastic shell is inserted as soon as possible to maintain lid tone and prevent adhesions from developing between the layers of conjunctiva which would make the fitting of a prosthesis difficult. The prosthesis is made as soon as the incision has healed and the oedema has subsided.

The patient should not be discharged until able to clean the socket and handle the shell proficiently. A district nurse may be asked to visit.

Occasionally, the operation performed is an evisceration in which the contents of the eyeball are removed, leaving the sclera. This is more usually performed when infection is present, to prevent spread to the brain.

A more radical procedure may be necessary in malignancy or severe trauma. The operation performed is called *exenteration* and involves the removal of the eyeball and the surrounding structures. These operations can be psychologically very distressing as they alter the individual's body image. The patient should be given time to express feelings.

Sympathetic ophthalmia

After an eye injury, especially a deep penetrating one, the patient may develop panophthalmitis (inflammation of the ciliary body, choroid and iris) in the uninjured eye. This response is not understood; it has been suggested that it may be an allergic reaction to the pigment released by the damaged eye. Any redness or tearing of the uninjured eye and any complaint of photophobia, pain or loss of vision must be reported promptly. The condition may develop soon after the injury or several months or years later. Unless the inflammatory reaction is checked promptly, loss of vision results. Corticoid preparations are used locally and systemically. Rarely, the injured eye is removed to prevent sympathetic ophthalmitis from developing.

Summary

The importance of all the senses to normal human functioning and independence is apparent. The psychological trauma of any threat to a person's senses, particularly vision, hearing or touch must always be considered, whatever the setting they are in. There must be a greater awareness of the importance of good communication and education of patients threatened with the loss of one of their senses.

References

British National Formulary (2001) British National Formulary 41. London: British Medical Association/Royal Pharmaceutical Society of Great Britain.

Haslett C, Chilvers E, Hunter J, Boon N (1999) Davidson's principles and practice of medicine, 18th edn. Edinburgh: Churchill Livingstone.

Royal National Institute for the Blind (2001) Online. Available: http://rnib.org.uk

Smeltzer S, Bare B (2000) Brunner and Suddarth's textbook of medical surgical nursing, 9th edn. Philadelphia: Lippincott.

Walsh M, Kent A (2001) Accident and emergency nursing, 4th edn. Oxford: Butterworth-Heinemann.

Walsh M, Crumbie A, Reveley S (1999) Nurse practitioners; clinical skills and medical issues. Oxford: Butterworth-Heinemann.

22

Caring for the patient with a disorder of the male reproductive system

Mike Walsh

Introduction

Summary of physiology

Sexuality

Disorders of the male reproductive system

Summary

Introduction

Great attention has been paid to women's health as a subject in its own right, and men's health has been rather neglected in comparison. The men's health agenda is huge but this chapter concentrates only on the male reproductive system. You should recognize, however, that men's health encompasses issues such as cardiovascular disease, mental health, suicide risk, alcohol abuse, HIV infection, trauma and violence, all of which are more prevalent in the male half of the population. A man's self-concept and self-esteem are closely linked to his sexual health. Many individuals will have a partner whose views and feelings must also be taken into account; the partner may also have to adapt to significant changes in the patient as a result of illness and treatment.

Summary of physiology

In utero development

The adult **male reproductive system** consists of the paired testes, epididymis, vas deferens, common ejaculatory ducts, urethra, penis and scrotum. The accessory organs are the seminal vesicles, prostate gland and the bulbourethral glands (Fig. 22.1). Sex itself is determined at the time of fertilization by the inclusion of the XX chromosomal pair of the female or the XY genotype of the male. In this early period of human development, sex differentiation can be determined microscopically by the presence or absence of Barr bodies in a cell nucleus that has been taken from the embryo. As the embryo grows, an internal genital ridge develops but remains undifferentiated in either sex until the seventh week of intrauterine life.

While internal development proceeds, the external genitalia are also becoming differentiated – so much so that by the 16th week of embryological life the sex of the infant can be determined externally. At this time the testes are not present in the scrotum but are in the abdomen. As the fetal testes begin to produce testosterone, in about the seventh month of fetal life, descent occurs, and they pass through the inguinal canal and the external inguinal ring to enter the scrotum by the ninth month. After descent, the testis shows a decline in its production of testosterone until puberty. As in all processes, descent may not occur or may occur imperfectly. This may result in undescended testes.

The testes

Each lobe of the testis contains a seminiferous tubule surrounded by tissue that produces the male hormones, of which testosterone is the most prominent. At puberty, under the complex control of the hypothalamus and pituitary glands, the testes are stimulated to produce male hormones. Under the influence of these androgens, the body begins the process of puberty. The external organs of reproduction grow and develop. The distribution of body hair changes to that of the adult male. The larynx and musculoskeletal systems develop and change. Concurrently, the testes begin to produce sperm. Puberty ends with the sexual and reproductive maturity of the individual.

Spermatogenesis

Spermatogenesis begins in the seminiferous tubule and, when growth is complete, the sperm is released into the lumen of the seminiferous tubule, rapidly transported to the epididymis and thence through the duct system. Although sperm may appear to be mature at the time of

Male reproductive system
See chapter 6.3

Spermatogenesis
See chapter 6.3

Figure 22.1   The male reproductive system.

release into the tubule, they do undergo further maturation, increasing in fertility and vigour as they progress through the ducts.

Spermatogenesis is also sensitive to heat, and occurs at a temperature a few degrees lower than body temperature. It is for this reason that the testes are suspended in the scrotum, allowing the temperature of the testes to be regulated by the body.

A feedback mechanism controls the production of sperm and testosterone. The anterior pituitary gland, when stimulated by the gonadotrophin-releasing hormone (GnRH) of the hypothalamus, releases two hormones: follicle-stimulating hormone (FSH) and luteinizing hormone (LH). FSH stimulates the seminiferous tubule to begin spermatogenesis.

Luteinizing hormone stimulates the interstitial cells of the testes to produce testosterone, which maintains and completes spermatogenesis. Testosterone is necessary to complete the step from spermatocyte to fertile spermatozoa.

High levels of testosterone exert an inhibitory effect on the hypothalamus. When testosterone reaches a low level it no longer exerts this inhibitory effect and more GnRH is released, repeating the cycle.

Duct system and accessory glands

The viable sperm must be transported from the testis to the penis and thence to the female reproductive tract so that fertilization may take place. Here the duct system and the **accessory glands** play a major role. As a secretory organ, the *seminal vesicle* does not store sperm but rather produces an alkaline fluid that is rich in nutrients and prostaglandins. These nutrients provide for the sperm until fertilization. The prostaglandins are believed to aid fertilization by reacting with cervical mucus to make it more penetrable by sperm and to induce contractions in the uterus and tubes which help sperm to reach the ovum.

The *prostate gland*, which is fused to the neck of the bladder, surrounds the urethra. It develops in puberty and is easily palpable on rectal examination. During the years of sexual maturity the prostate secretes a thin, milky-looking fluid which is alkaline. This, together with the alkaline seminal vesicle secretions, reduces the acidity of seminal fluid and vaginal secretions. This is an important reproductive function, as the motility and viability of sperm are greatly reduced in an acid solution.

Further alkaline fluid is added to the semen by the *bulbourethral glands*. These paired glands lie posterior to the urethra and discharge their fluid into it when they contract at ejaculation. This fluid seems to function merely as a lubricant and fluid medium for the sperm.

Semen is an alkaline, viscous fluid varying at one ejaculation from 2 to 6 mL in quantity and containing nutrients to support the sperm. The normal sperm count is about $60–100 \times 10^6$ sperm per mL. A sperm count of below 20×10^6 per mL indicates probable infertility. The *sperm*, which are actively motile by lashing their tails, move rapidly up through the uterus into the outer third of the fallopian tube where fertilization usually takes place.

Sexuality

Sexuality is broadly defined as the becoming and being of a man or a woman. As such, adult sexuality has four major divisions, as shown in Figure 22.2.

Figure 22.2   Divisions of adult sexuality.

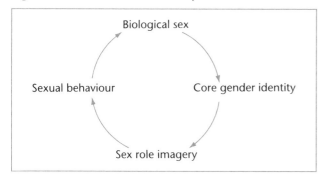

Figure 22.2   Divisions of adult sexuality.

Biological sex

Biological sex refers to the individual's physical attributes. In men this is based in the genotype XY, and includes internal and external genitalia with the corresponding underlying hormonal, neural, vascular and physical components.

Core gender identity

This refers to one's inner sense of being a man or a woman and is established early in life, usually by 3 years of age. At this age, the child knows he is a boy. In most cases the core gender identity corresponds to the physical attributes of the individual.

Sex role imagery

This refers to the learned behaviour that the particular society subscribes to its men and women. Sex or gender role imagery is complex because it includes the myriad beliefs about what is often labelled feminine or masculine by a society. It also conveys the image of appropriate sexual conduct for particular social groups. Some examples of these beliefs are: trousers are worn by men, skirts by women; women are passive, men are active. Sex role imagery represents much of the learned behaviour that influences human choice and lifestyle. Much stereotyping of human behaviour has resulted from the need for society to set up expectations by which to guide and judge sex role behaviour. These roles can be used to set the parameters of a culture's moral agenda. The learning of sex role imagery begins in infancy and continues throughout most of life. This learned behaviour, combined with personal experience, is internalized and becomes the individual's personal belief about sexuality.

Sexual behaviour

This refers to sexual expression and is the acting out of sexual feelings and beliefs. It includes a broad spectrum of human behaviour and varies from how one walks, to how and with whom one performs the sex act. For example, a person may choose to have sex with a member of the opposite sex or stay within their own sexual group, whilst a range of various sexual aids may be incorporated into sexual behaviour.

These four aspects of sexuality are interrelated and reinforcing. Biological make-up and learning promote a core gender identity which influences acceptance of specific sex roles. Sexual expression reflects biology, gender identity, sex role and behaviour.

Physiological aspects of sexual response

Human **sexual response** occurs as a result of stimulation. This varies from purely mental images such as fantasy, dreams or remembered events to stimulation received through the senses. Touch is probably the most important source of stimulation and certain areas of the body appear to be more sensitive as stimulators of sexual arousal than others. These areas vary for each individual but the penis in the man and clitoris, labia and vagina in the woman are usually the most sensitive of the areas.

Learning modifies the emotional and physiological responses to sexual stimuli. As a result of previous learning or past experience, however, similar sexual stimuli may elicit a wide range of responses.

The response is a total one, but the most noticeable changes are seen in the primary sexual organs. The sexual response cycle has been divided into four progressive phases. The phases do not differ between the sexes and depend in each sex on the same physiological mechanisms.

Male sexual response
See chapter 6.3

1. *The excitement phase*. The person becomes sexually aroused in response to any source of stimulation. This phase is quite sensitive to outside influences and, if the stimuli are interrupted or not intense enough, the excitement phase may be prolonged or aborted.

2. *The plateau phase*. Sexual tension is intensified and reaches the pre-orgasmic level. Alteration in stimuli may also cause this phase to be prolonged or to revert to the pre-plateau level of sexual arousal.

3. *Orgasm*. This is the phase of release of sexual tension and is accompanied by ejaculation. It is experienced as an involuntary subjective feeling of pleasure or relief. This feeling is concentrated in the clitoris, vagina and uterus of the woman and in the penis, prostate and seminal vesicles of the male. There is much individual variation in the intensity and duration of orgasm; generally this relates directly to the degree of sexual arousal that preceded the orgasm.

4. *The resolution phase*. Following orgasm, the individual enters the phase during which the body returns to its pre-excitement state. Within this resolution phase the male passes through the refractory period, a time during which the male cannot be restimulated to orgasm. The length of the refractory period varies with sexual episodes and may vary from a few minutes to several hours in the same individual.

Most of the observed responses during sexual excitement and resolution are due to two physiological mechanisms: vasocongestion and myotonia. *Vasocongestion* occurs as the muscular walls of the arterioles relax and expand allowing blood to rush in. This marked influx of blood into the area exceeds the ability of the veins to remove it and a period of vasocongestion occurs. *Myotonia* is increased muscle tension. During sexual activity, both smooth and skeletal muscles are affected.

Vasocongestion is triggered by a nervous impulse. Effective stimulation activates the parasympathetic nervous system and inhibits the sympathetic fibres. The parasympathetic nerve fibres cause the arterioles to relax and expand, allowing blood to rush in. Vasocongestion and penile erection result as the corpora cavernosa and corpus spongiosum become engorged with blood. It is the coordination between smooth muscle contraction and relaxation that controls the arterial and venous blood flow responsible for the erection (Vetrosky 2000). At orgasm the sympathetic fibres are stimulated, causing the bladder sphincter to close and smooth muscles in the wall of the genital ducts to contract rhythmically, producing ejaculation.

Erection of the penis may be partial but it is considered to be functionally erect if vaginal penetration can be achieved before ejaculation. The first phase of ejaculation is called emission and occurs when semen is pooled in the prostatic urethra and the man is aware of impending ejaculation. This is followed by the second stage: expulsion of semen and sperm from the penis via the urethra.

A simple reflex arc also exists in the spinal cord. With genital stimulation, erection and ejaculation will occur after the spinal cord has been severed if the area of spinal nerve damage was above the sacral and lumbar areas governing erection and ejaculation. Because pleasure is experienced via sensory input to the brain, the sexual response is not felt by the individual if the spinal cord is transected.

Disorders of the male reproductive system

Assessment

Privacy and sensitivity are essential to carry out the assessment, especially given the embarrassment that questions about sexual functioning may cause. Questions should be asked only on a need-to-know basis but should not be omitted for fear of embarrassment. The man should first be asked for his understanding of the problem and what he considers to be the chief complaint. This should be followed by checking the following:

1. Past medical history with special attention being paid to the reproductive system. Childhood should be included (e.g. undescended testicle) as well as adult life (e.g. vasectomy). Current or recent medication should be checked because the side-effects of various drugs include impairment of sexual function.

2. Any significant points in family history such as whether the man has fathered any children. If he has, this indicates he was fertile at the time and therefore probably still is.

3. Review of function to identify the cause of anxiety:
   a. any changes or disturbances in function (e.g. difficulty in passing urine – prostatic symptoms) or problems with sexual functioning which might indicate decreased libido, relationship difficulties or erectile dysfunction
   b. the presence of any symptoms of disease. If symptoms are present they are explored in order to determine their location, character, duration and severity. The common manifestations of disorders are pain, lesions, urethral discharge, itching, swelling and masses.

4. The patient's sexual roles (heterosexual or homosexual) and how the presenting health problem may affect self-concept and relationships with significant others. Other psychosocial factors such as employment and home circumstances should be explored.

The medical examination may include a general physical examination, with inspection and palpation of external genitalia. It may also include a digital rectal exam to check the size and morphology of the prostate. A careful explanation is needed together with privacy. The nurse should ensure the patient is turned on his left side with knees drawn up towards the chest. Particular care is needed in elderly men who may have arthritic hips and therefore find this a difficult position to adopt. Standing upright and leaning forward may be an easier option. The nurse should ensure the patient is safe (e.g. cot sides in situ) and provide psychological support during what can be an uncomfortable and embarrassing procedure. Asking the patient to take a deep breath and breathe out during actual insertion of the gloved finger can reduce anal spasm, making the procedure less traumatic.

Patient problems

The normal functioning of the reproductive system gives constant reassurance of a man's essential maleness. The distortion or interruption of these processes may prove very disturbing to the individual and family. The man may experience problems in relation to self-image and have fears about future sexual performance. Body parts that contribute to self-esteem and identity have a high psychological investment. The threat posed by disease or loss of these body parts depends on:

■ their meaning to the individual

■ his stage of development of body image and self

■ the reactions of the social group, including the spouse, to which the patient belongs.

The person may fear loss of reproductive function. The ability to reproduce is seen by many as a criterion of usefulness and sexuality. The loss of function may be followed by feelings of uselessness or of being only half a person. These feelings can be particularly distressing to the man with erectile dysfunction. The inability to obtain an erection may make him feel less of a man, and he may fear that his partner will see him as less a man. Indeed, in some unfortunate situations, she may. Thus, to the fear of loss of reproductive function may be added the fear of loss of a loved one. For some, the fear of loss of libido as well as sexual function may be very frightening and can cause the patient much anguish. In addition to the effects of loss of function there is also the possibility of cancer affecting the genital tract. Cancer is a word that strikes fear into most people and cancer of the testis is predominantly a cancer of younger men. This diagnosis can have a devastating psychological impact.

Most people have been culturally conditioned to the idea that some areas of the body should not be discussed, much less exposed, to examination or discussion. Such experiences may disturb the individual and produce shame that may be enhanced by lack of privacy and exposure of the body in examinations or during care. Others may feel guilt over their illness. Sexually transmitted disease and cancer arouse guilt feelings in certain individuals which may be expressed as a feeling of 'being punished for past deeds'.

You may be dealing with patients who experience anxiety and fear, shame, guilt, diminished self-esteem or re-awakened anxieties over personal identity. In addition, the long shadow of AIDS is a particular, unspoken fear for many patients.

Goals

Patient goals may include:

1. resolving dysfunctional sexual problems

2. achieving a sense of self-worth

3. being able to verbalize fears and anxieties

4. showing understanding of health problems and what medical intervention involves

5. adapting to a change in sexual role and/or function

6. being aware of and avoiding risk factors in sexual activity.

Nursing intervention

These goals may be achieved by the following nursing interventions:

- Assess the degree of threat posed by loss of function or body parts to the individual and plan, give and evaluate nursing care for that individual based on the assessment.

- Give physical nursing care that:
  — promotes feelings of dignity and self-worth by attention to personal hygiene and grooming

  — promotes the return of health, control over body functions and independence.

- Reduce fear and guilt by:
  — acknowledging and discussing feelings
  — anticipating the need for explanations and interpretations
  — clarifying and correcting misinformation about causes of illness, physiology and the consequences, if any, of treatment on present function
  — maintaining a confident, non-judgemental approach to the patient
  — assisting in acknowledging the loss, if any
  — obtaining appropriate additional sources of spiritual or emotional help for the patient
  — offering information and support for relatives.

Evaluation

Interventions are successful if behavioural changes have occurred, although these may be difficult to document in areas such as self-concept, anxiety and guilt. The patient may, for example:

- state that he feels better, less frightened or happier

- take an interest in personal appearance and renew interests in social life, which may also indicate a return to a more positive outlook toward the future

- demonstrate an understanding of the illness, treatments and any residual changes in function to the level of ability or willingness

- demonstrate a knowledge of the risk factors that may lead to a recurrence of the problem and the actions that may reduce or eliminate the risk factors, if appropriate

- discuss alterations in body function and structure with the nurse and so indicate a willingness to begin to deal with the problem or to accept it with appropriate adjustments.

Adjustment to many of these changes requires some time and complete resolution is rarely seen in hospital. Expectations of resolution and effectiveness of intervention must be realistic.

Sexual issues associated with giving nursing care

Several issues involving sexuality may arise in the course of nurse–patient interactions. They reflect the changing role of the patient and involve confusion over the meaning of nursing or patient actions. The most common arise from the intimate level of care involved in nursing and acting out sexual behaviour by the patient.

Touch

The nurse may feel uncomfortable at having to touch the genitals of patients. The patient may also experience discomfort at being cared for so intimately by the nurse.

It reinforces for many adults the dependent child-like role associated with nursing care. On the other hand, touch may be a source of great comfort to patients. Touch should be used only with permission and its purpose should be understood by both patient and nurse.

Before giving nursing care you should give an explanation of what will be done so that the patient is not surprised and has time to adjust. Your movements should be firm, purposeful and reflect a knowledge of the procedure.

Touch for the purpose of comfort is offered as seems appropriate to the situation and patient. Many patients are grateful for a hand to hold during frightening or stressful procedures or times. Other patients would be uncomfortable offered that form of comfort. A knowledge of and sensitivity to the patient assists in judging what forms of comfort are helpful to which patients.

Male erection

The erections that occur during the delivery of nursing care are most often the result of the stimulation of the spinal reflex arc. The stimulus from a full bladder or perineal care may produce this non-sexual or non-psychological erection. Should this occur during care it is important for the nurse to remain calm, acknowledge the situation and finish care. A flustered nurse who 'runs away' from the patient may increase his confusion, shame and guilt. The patient also needs to understand the nature of reflex, non-sexual erections.

Erection
See chapter 6.3

Sexual acting out

A patient may act out sexually to test sexual image, to gain control of the situation, or to attract attention. Examples of sexual acting out in this context include touching the nurse inappropriately, improper suggestions or gestures toward the nurse or self-exposure. The nurse should address the situation directly and unambiguously. The nurse–patient relationship should be defined and any misconceptions about role and function clarified. Limits are set, clearly defined and enforced. Sexual harassment from *any* source – patient or staff – is unacceptable.

The patient should be helped to explore anxiety and fears. As these are identified and appropriately dealt with, the sexual acting out usually ceases.

Variations of sexuality

Variations of sexuality can occur in each of the four areas of sexuality but most disorders are psychosexual in origin. Only a few arise from physical illness and trauma, or congenital error. Most become obvious through difficulties in sexual expression.

Variations in sexual expression are classified by object choice and sexual aim. *Object choice* refers to problems such as paedophilia, incest, animal contacts or fetishism (sexual arousal associated with inanimate objects). Variations in *sexual aim* refers to problems such as voyeurism,

exhibitionism and sado-masochism. Variations in sexual aim and object choice can be interrelated.

Gender dysphoria (transsexuality) is where the individual appears to have a gender identity at odds with his or her physical self. The person will usually cross-dress and may seek out gender realignment (sex change) therapy because of a deep need to have a body similar to the gender identity. However, transvestism (cross-dressing) itself does not indicate transsexuality. There is a whole spectrum of complex behaviours ranging from men who have a fetish about female underwear through those who like dressing fully as a woman, to those who actually wish to be women. Most transvestites are heterosexual, although some may be bisexual or gay. Transvestism might be an unusual behaviour, but it is not a health problem unless it causes significant mental distress through feelings of guilt and anxiety.

Occasionally a child reaches puberty and is then discovered to be genetically and internally different from the external genitalia. Because the child has been socialized in the sex role defined by the external genitalia, continuation in the sex assigned at birth is usually advised. It is usually more successful to alter the physical state than to attempt to reverse gender identity and several years of gender role learning. Parents of a child born with ambiguous genitalia should understand the necessity to delay sex assignment until careful physical and genetic screening indicates the true sex of the infant.

Sexual concerns

Many persons experience doubts over their inner sexual feelings. This may be more prominent in adolescence when the final development of gender identity takes place, but may recur throughout the individual's life. As sexual identity is considered to be an important component of overall identity, this may stimulate concerns over self-identity. The growing awareness that a young man is gay may cause great psychological distress and may also be the cause of bullying at school with possibly disastrous consequences. Concerns over expected performance are also prevalent in straight and gay men. The man may doubt whether he has the necessary physical attributes, experience or appeal to attract, satisfy and keep a sexual partner.

Sexual dysfunction

Sexual dysfunction in the male is most frequently associated with the inability to achieve an erection (impotence or erectile dysfunction) and to delay ejaculation until both partners achieve a sense of satisfaction (premature ejaculation). Some degree of erectile dysfunction affects 50% of men between 40 and 70 years of age, the incidence rising with age from 40% in 40-year-olds to 67% in 70-year-olds (Moskowitz 2000).

Erectile dysfunction can be the result of psychological, interpersonal or physical factors. In the large majority of cases the root cause is physical but psychological feedback mechanisms are usually at work producing a complex interplay of physical, psychological and interpersonal factors:

■ Psychological causes may be anger, depression, anxiety, ignorance, or deeper psychosexual conflicts.

■ Interpersonal factors involve conflicts with the partner or an inability to establish interpersonal relationships.

■ Physical causes include diabetes, neurological or endocrine disorders, penile problems such as abnormality of the corpora, alcohol and drug abuse, smoking, renal or liver disease or as the side-effects of drugs such as antihypertensives, antidepressants and H_2 antagonists such as cimetidine.

Diagnosis and treatment involve taking a history, physical examination and laboratory tests to ascertain the most likely cause. Many patients will not make a connection between the side-effects of their medication (e.g. antihypertensive drugs) or diseases such as diabetes and the erectile dysfunction. The nurse may have tactfully to explore these areas as part of patient teaching, and it remains a fact that some 50% of diabetic men will experience erectile dysfunction (Foster and Cole 1996).

During history taking the patient is asked whether there are any sexual complaints. This makes sexuality an acceptable topic to discuss should the patient have a problem or develop one in the future. If the patient does present with a sexual problem, it is discussed in a frank, open manner, maintaining a broad, objective attitude toward the patient's sexual beliefs and practices. The patient is not urged to disclose more information during a session than he is comfortable in revealing. The patient's sexual concerns are assessed in the context of other problems and in the context of value systems. As a general guide, the problem is more likely to be psychological in origin if the onset of erectile dysfunction is sudden, person or situation related, or there are obvious psychological problems such as severe stress or depression. If the man can still obtain a spontaneous erection – for example he has an erection during sleep – this also indicates a psychological rather than physical source of the problem. A slow onset of erectile dysfunction and any of the above physiological risk factors indicate a likely physical cause, which may be exacerbated by the psychological impact of erectile dysfunction (Foster and Cole 1996).

Treatment initially concentrates on any potentially reversible factors such as medication the patient may be taking, treating pre-existing diseases such as diabetes, lifestyle modification (recreational drug use, alcohol consumption) and relationship problems. Padma-Nathan and Forrest (2000) recommend a stepwise approach to treatment, moving on from any reversible factors to look at single interventions of which the best known is the administration of an oral erectogenic agent such as sildenafil (Viagra).

This drug is a potent inhibitor of an enzyme (phosphodiesterase 5; PDE-5) which regulates a key intracellular messenger (cyclic guanosine monophosphate; cGMP) involved in triggering smooth muscle relaxation and hence increased arterial inflow and corporeal veno-occlusion. The drug therefore works only if the patient's erectile dysfunction is caused by a disturbance in the normal blood flow involved in obtaining an erection: it is not suitable for all men. With all the recent publicity that has surrounded this drug, it is important in talking to patients and their partners to introduce an element of caution about the appropriateness of sildenafil. Other first-line therapies include counselling and the use of vacuum constriction devices, which draw blood into the penis by creating a negative pressure around it, and then applying a constrictive ring to the base of the penis.

Second-line therapy which may be used if first-line therapies do not succeed consists of intraurethral administration or intracavernosal self-injection of alprostadil, while surgical implantation of a semi-rigid or inflatable prosthesis is reserved for third-line therapy if other approaches have failed or been rejected by the patient.

Rape trauma syndrome

This condition is described in more detail on p. 808. However, since 1994 male rape has been recognized as a legal assault. Instances of reported male rape are on the increase. Benn and Siffen (1993), whilst investigating male rape victims in prison, identified power relations and undermining of the individual's gender identity as significant. A few men in the study were so affected by the experience that they had attempted suicide; the majority of others were themselves sex offenders.

Congenital anomalies of the reproductive system

Maldescent of testes

Approximately 4% of newborn males will exhibit some form of maldescent of the testes. Unilateral maldescent of testis is about four times as prevalent as bilateral maldescent. The condition is usually the result of hormonal deficiency or mechanical malfunction. The majority of testes descend during the first 3 months of extrauterine life. Many more descend at puberty under the influence of rising testosterone levels. Probably less than 1% of men remain with undescended testes following puberty. The principal sign is an inability to palpate one or both testes in the scrotal sac. *Cryptorchidism* is the term used to describe the condition in which the descent of the testis is interrupted anywhere along the normal path of descent. This is a significant risk factor for the development of testicular cancer in adult life, especially if both testes are affected.

Because histological changes are observed in the undescended testes as early as 4 years of age, treatment is initiated early to ensure maximum functioning of the testes. *Orchidopexy* (surgical placement and fixation of the testes in the scrotal sac) is the primary method of treatment and should be completed by the age of 1 year. *Hernioplasty* may also be done to repair the inguinal hernia which is often present in these cases. *Hormone therapy* in the form of GnRH alone or followed by human chorionic gonadotrophins may be given to stimulate production of testosterone in cases of bilateral undescended testes. Successful descent may occur and no other treatment is required, or partial descent may occur, frequently placing the testes in a more favourable position for surgery. Hormone therapy is less successful with unilateral conditions.

Should the condition not be diagnosed until after puberty, orchidopexy is indicated even though the man may be sterile. There are two reasons for this. First, the Leydig cells of the testes continue to produce male hormones which will sustain the secondary sex characteristics. Second, such testes have a higher incidence of malignancy than do normally positioned testes and can be more easily examined yearly for malignancy in the scrotum than in the abdomen. In unilateral conditions, the extrascrotal testis will be removed to reduce the possibility of malignancy further. This leaves the man with one functioning testis as a source of sperm and male hormones.

Fertility and infertility

These topics are discussed in full in Chapter 23. This section focuses on male aspects of fertility control.

Condom

The condom is a thin rubber sheath that is placed over the penis before intromission. It prevents pregnancy by acting as a mechanical barrier to the sperm. It is also very effective in preventing infection with a sexually transmitted disease. Proper use includes application before intromission to avoid the possibility of a pre-ejaculatory emission of semen into the vagina and careful withdrawal of the penis and condom following intercourse to be sure that some semen is not lost into the vagina or over the vulva. Some doctors advise the use of a spermicidal jelly as a lubricating agent over the condom. This provides additional safety, particularly if the condom should be defective. However, newer methods of manufacture have greatly reduced this hazard. The condom is reasonably priced and is available without prescription. This greatly increases its availability and makes it one of the most widely used methods in the world.

Some couples find the condom objectionable as a method of birth control because it may interrupt sexual foreplay; it can lessen sensation, and its effective use relies heavily on the motivation of the male. These objections can be overcome if it is used by a man who is taking a mature responsibility for his behaviour, especially in view of the risk of contracting AIDS.

Vasectomy

This simple operation can be done on an outpatient basis or at a clinic. Under local anaesthesia a small incision is made slightly to one side of each spermatic cord. The vas deferens is exposed, severed and electrocoagulated. Thus, new sperm are barred from reaching the vagina. Other sperm are still present in the tract above the ligation. For this reason a man is not considered sterile until he has had two negative sperm counts after operation.

The first sperm count is done after ten ejaculations and is repeated following a further series of ejaculations until a negative sperm count is obtained.

In the immediate postoperative period the man may expect some minor bruising and discomfort for 24–72 hours. The discomfort is relieved by a simple analgesic, rest and wearing a scrotal support. Protected intercourse is resumed when he feels comfortable to do so. Few major side-effects, either physical or emotional, are reported following the procedure.

Some cases are recorded of reconstructing the vas deferens. However, the rate of successful reconstruction is low. This is partly due to extravasation of sperm, which causes the development of sperm antibodies following vasectomy. Even though physical reconstruction of the vas deferens might be possible, the antibodies continue to destroy the sperm. Vasovasostomy (repair of the separated vas deferens) produces fertility in only 22% of men. Thus, the patient should regard a vasectomy as irreversible.

Infections of the male reproductive tract

Balanitis

Balanitis is an infection of the **glans penis**. Many different organisms may be causative. It is generally associated with poor personal hygiene in the uncircumcised male, especially if he is diabetic, but may be associated with sexually transmitted diseases. Symptoms include redness, swelling, pain and possibly a purulent discharge. The disease may be chronic and may cause the formation of adhesions and scarring.

Treatment

The infection is treated with the appropriate antibiotic following culture and sensitivity tests. Once the inflammatory process is controlled, circumcision, the excision of the **prepuce**, is advised.

On return from the operating theatre, the patient has a small petroleum jelly gauze dressing which is changed following each voiding. The patient may be taught to do this and how to care for the dressing at home.

Should bleeding occur, a pressure dressing is applied. The dressing may make voiding impossible or difficult.

Glans penis
See chapter 6.3

Prepuce
See chapter 6.3

Usually the dressing can be removed within a short period of time.

Circumcision may also be indicated as a means of dealing with the following problems.

Phimosis

Phimosis is a condition in which the preputial orifice is too small to permit retraction over the glans. It may be congenital but is most frequently a sequel to infection or trauma.

Paraphimosis

Paraphimosis occurs when a narrowed prepuce is either forced back over the glans or is gradually retracted over it. It then forms a tight, constricting band around the glans; venous return is impaired, and swelling and pain follow. The foreskin may be replaced with the aid of ice packs and lubricating gel but sometimes a general anaesthetic is needed as the condition is so painful. Occasionally the foreskin may have to be incised; a slit is made up the dorsal surface. This is usually followed by circumcision after the treatment of any infection that may have been present.

Prostatitis

Prostatitis is inflammation of the **prostate** gland and may be either acute or chronic, bacterial or non-bacterial in origin. The non-bacterial form is most common and is related to organisms such as *Chlamydia trachomatis*. The disease originates commonly as an ascending infection of the genitourinary tract, as a result of reflux of infected urine or invasion by rectal bacteria (Donovan and Nicholas 1997).

In the acute stage, fever and chills are accompanied by haematuria, frequency and dysuria. A urethral discharge may be noted. Rectal examination usually reveals an enlarged, tender, 'hot' prostate in acute cases. Infection of the seminal vesicles almost invariably accompanies prostatitis. Prostatic massage and instrumentation of the urethra are avoided to prevent possible spread of the infection to the epididymis, bladder and kidney. Exceptions are made only to relieve acute urinary retention, which may be a sequel to the enlarged prostate.

The patient is placed on bedrest. Hydration, analgesics and stool softeners are useful as supportive therapy. Appropriate antimicrobial drug therapy is prescribed in accordance with local protocols and culture and sensitivity results. The patient is in considerable pain. The nurse often sees a tense, anxious and frightened patient who needs reassurance and support. Analgesics and warm baths help to relieve the pain and bladder spasms. The irritable bladder may require special attention, and antispasmodics and bladder sedatives are frequently ordered.

In cases in which treatment is early, excellent results usually follow. However, the acute picture may become chronic. The symptoms are mild and include a low-grade fever and some bacteria and pus in the urine. Fertility and potency are not affected unless complications ensue. The chronic infection may stubbornly resist treatment. Prostatic massage every 7–14 days is done by the doctor and helps by draining the bacteria away. Sexual intercourse or masturbation accomplishes the same purpose. Daily baths also help resolve the infection.

Epididymitis

This condition is rare before puberty and involves infection of the epididymis. It may be caused by any pyogenic organism, but *Escherichia coli* and *Neisseria gonorrhoeae* are commonly implicated. It frequently follows prostatitis or may follow from an established urinary tract infection, sexually transmitted disease or be a complication of prostatectomy. Fever, malaise and chills accompany swelling and pain in the scrotum. The patient may be so uncomfortable that he may walk in a waddling fashion. Symptoms of cystitis may be present, and a painless swelling consisting of an accumulation of fluid within the scrotum often develops (hydrocele). The swelling and irritation associated with the inflammation cause congestion of the testes, which impedes the circulation of blood. Sterility follows from necrosis of the tubular epithelium and fibrosis which occludes the ducts.

The patient is placed on bedrest. The scrotum is elevated on towel rolls and ice packs may be applied. Constipation should be prevented as attempts at defaecation under these circumstances can be very painful. After the patient is ambulant, a roomy scrotal support is worn. Antibiotics and analgesics are given. Chronic epididymitis may follow an acute episode and, if the involvement is bilateral, sterility may follow.

Orchitis

Inflammation of the **testes** may follow any infectious disease or may be acquired as an ascending infection from the genital tract. Most commonly it follows mumps parotitis. The mumps virus is excreted in the urine; therefore, the spread to the testes in this case appears to be by descent. The onset is sudden, manifested by pain and swelling of the scrotum followed by fever and prostration. Urinary symptoms are usually not present. A hydrocele may develop, and the involvement may be unilateral or bilateral. Sterility probably follows death of the spermatogenic cells from ischaemia. Bedrest, scrotal support, and local applications of heat or cold are ordered. A padded athletic support may be worn continuously.

Antibiotics are used in some situations but are not of value against the mumps virus. Local infiltration of the spermatic cord with a local anaesthetic may relieve the symptoms. The prevention of mumps in the postpubertal male has some value. If a man who has not been immunized as a child against mumps or who has not previously had mumps has been in contact with the virus, gamma-globulin is usually administered.

Prostate
See chapter 6.3

Epididymitis
See chapter 6.3

Testes
See chapter 6.3

Sexually transmitted diseases

These are on the increase worldwide and groups that are most at risk are men aged 18–34 years, gay men with multiple partners, merchant seamen, armed forces personnel, frequent travellers and commercial sex workers. Men therefore make up most of the high-risk groups and are represented even in the final group in this list. The health problem of greatest concern is AIDS, which is dealt with as appropriate elsewhere in this text. Other sexually transmitted diseases are considered in this section.

Gonorrhoea

The specific organism causing gonorrhoea is *Neisseria gonorrhoeae*, which is transmitted almost exclusively by sexual intercourse. The organism dies quickly when not harboured in the human body. The incidence of gonorrhoea is a key marker for other sexually transmitted diseases, including HIV infection and is therefore closely monitored. Fenton (2000) has reported a dramatic and worrying increase in the disease during 1998–1999, which is the largest since the early 1980s when the onset of HIV/AIDS resulted in a major government public health campaign. Overall during 1998–1999 the incidence of gonorrhoea rose by 30% for heterosexual men and women, and by 10% amongst gay men. Fenton suggests that poor sexual health amongst young people, relapse to unsafe sexual behaviour such as not using condoms, and increasingly resistant strains of the organism are to blame.

Effects on the patient

Symptoms appear 2–10 days after the initial contact. In the male urethritis occurs, heralded by a purulent urethral discharge. Some itching and burning about the meatus are also present. The urethral meatus is red and oedematous. An ascending infection involving the prostate, seminal vesicles, bladder and epididymis may also occur. If adhesions develop, they may damage the urethra and duct system with consequent urethral stricture and infertility. Rectal infection is possible in gay men and is frequently asymptomatic, while infection of the pharynx may also occur due to unprotected oral–genital sex.

Diagnosis is confirmed when the gonococcus is seen microscopically in smears or cultures taken from the site of infection. If urethral discharge is slight, the first urethral washings may be used. These are obtained by collecting the first portion of a voided urine specimen. The penis is not swabbed off before collecting the specimen.

Treatment

As in all cases of sexually transmitted disease, treatment should be carried out by specialist departments of genitourinary medicine because of the need for strict confidentiality, contact tracing, counselling and adherence to antimicrobial drug protocols to combat the growth of resistant strains, the first of which was identified in 1976.

A single dose of ciprofloxacin (500 mg orally) or ofloxacin (400 mg orally) is recommended for uncomplicated cases (British National Formulary 2000).

Non-specific urethritis

Non-specific urethritis is far more common than gonorrhoea in the UK. The man complains of mild gonorrhoea-like symptoms which may become severe. It is important to rule out gonorrhoea as a cause. The infection may be due to one of several agents, but in 50% of cases is the result of a chlamydial infection. Chlamydia are a group of organisms that multiply like bacteria but do so only in the host cell, like viruses.

The infection frequently coexists with gonorrhoea but may persist as a postgonoccal urethritis following successful treatment of the gonorrhoea. This can be anxiety producing for the patient. Reassurance and teaching about the complaints are helpful in relieving anxiety.

Cultures for *Chlamydia trachomatis* are made from swabs of the anterior urethra and from first urethral washings. Doxycycline or azithromycin is the antimicrobial of choice. Sexual intercourse is contraindicated during the acute stage as it prolongs the symptoms. Repeat cultures are made to confirm the effects of treatment. The infection may progress to a chronic state or to epididymitis, prostatitis and rarely Reiter's syndrome.

Viral infection (excluding HIV)

Anogenital herpes simplex

This is a very distressing condition and the fourth most common sexually transmitted disease in the UK. The first attack leads to painful genital ulcers appearing within 7 days of infection which rupture and then form a crust. The first stage lasts for up to 12 days and recurrent, less severe, attacks occur subsequently every few months. Unfortunately up to 50% of patients may not realize they have been infected (Adler 1996).

Human papillomavirus (HPV)

HPV is the causative agent in condylomata acuminata, or genital warts. These warts may be confused with those of syphilis, but they are different: they are less flat and more cauliflower like. Perianal warts are usually confined to gay men. This viral infection was previously thought to be benign but recently HPV has been associated with several genital cancers in both men and women.

The risk factors for acquiring the virus are early age at first intercourse (less than 17 years), multiple sexual partners, a history of sexually transmitted diseases, poor personal and sexual hygiene, a sexual partner with a similar history, a history of anal intercourse, and immunosuppression or immunodeficiency for any reason. Sexual intercourse is the major method of transmission.

Those presenting with external warts are screened for other sexually transmitted diseases which, if present, are treated. The partners of infected patients should also be examined and treated if necessary. External warts are treated with podophyllin 10–25% in industrial spirit or tincture of benzoin. This caustic agent is applied with a cotton applicator and washed off in 4 hours. The surrounding skin is coated with petroleum jelly before application of the podophyllin, as this is a very irritant substance. Non-visible warts (areas of dysplasia associated with the HPV on the penis) are frequently vaporized with a carbon dioxide laser.

Hepatitis B

Hepatitis B virus (HBV) is readily transmitted between gay men but not between heterosexual couples. It is found in semen, saliva and blood. Hepatitis A and C are not, however, sexually transmitted.

Syphilis

Syphilis is a serious disease and, fortunately, is much less common than gonorrhoea. The causative organism is the spirochaete *Treponema pallidum*.

Effects on the patient

Incubation is usually 14–28 days. In most cases the disease is spread by sexual intercourse. As with the gonococcus, the spirochaete does not survive outside the host. In the untreated condition, three stages are distinguished. The stages may overlap or be widely separated.

The *primary lesion* is a small, painless chancre or ulcer. It is deep and has indurated edges. Usually, this chancre heals spontaneously, giving the false impression that the disease is cured. This primary lesion appears most commonly on the penis of the male.

The *secondary stage* is usually characterized by a rash appearing over the body. The rash is usually accompanied by malaise and fever. In a short period the rash regresses and the patient enters the latent stages. *Latency* refers to the absence of symptoms in the infected individual. Progress of the disease in the individual seems to be arrested and only rarely can others be infected in this stage.

Three outcomes are now possible:

1. The patient proceeds immediately or after a delay of 10–30 years to the third stage.

2. The disease remains latent for the rest of the person's life.

3. A spontaneous cure occurs.

In the *tertiary stage* the bones, heart and central nervous system, including the brain, can be affected. Personality disorders arise and the typical ataxic gait of tertiary syphilis appears. A large, ulcerating necrotic lesion known as a *gumma* now occurs. Rarely is it seen in the genital tract, but it may occur on the vulva or in the testes. At this stage the disease may be arrested but not reversed.

Diagnosis is made by a careful history, clinical findings, and cultures or biopsies from the lesions. Treatment is with antibiotics; penicillin is still the drug of choice.

Nursing intervention

Most patients with a sexually transmitted disease are treated on an outpatient basis; the person should be taught how to protect themselves and others. First, the nature and transmission of the disease need to be understood. No immunity develops and reinfection can occur easily. Strict personal and perineal hygiene should be observed. Handwashing following any handling of the genitalia is imperative, as the gonococcus can be readily carried to the eye, which quickly becomes infected. Blindness may ensue if treatment is not received. Sexual abuse is the cause of some cases in children.

Sexual intercourse is to be avoided until the doctor notifies the individual that the infection has been treated successfully. All equipment must be sterilized following use and dressings or swabs are disposed of in a safe way. Syphilis may be transmitted by direct contamination with living spirochaetes of a laceration. For this reason, the routine use of universal body substance precautions will also control inadvertent transmission of this disease to health professionals. Once therapy has been initiated, the patient is usually non-infectious within 48 hours.

A sexually transmitted disease may be very distressing to the patient. The patient may experience guilt feelings, and marital difficulties may arise when one partner infects the other. The disease carries a social stigma. For these reasons, confidentiality must be maintained by the nurse at all times; the issue is protected by law and the disease is reportable. Contacts must be identified and followed discreetly by the contact tracer. The contact tracer, by explaining the nature of the disease, usually obtains the patient's cooperation in identifying contacts. A great deal of tact and sensitivity is required as detailed information about sexual practices and partners needs to be obtained for the correct tests and treatment to be made available to those who need them. The interview requires privacy, reassurance of confidentiality, and is done while the patient is dressed, before the physical examination. The contact tracer should explain clearly to the patient the purpose of the questions and why they are necessary. In addition, the nurse should include sexually transmitted diseases in any lectures prepared on general health education in schools so that the population may become more aware of the signs and symptoms, the modes of transmission, and the safer sex practices needed to prevent spread of these diseases.

Safer sex guidelines

Responsible sexual conduct, based on a healthy understanding of human sexuality, should be taught at every opportunity. The definition of responsible sexual conduct varies considerably. For some, it means complete abstinence from sexual intercourse or activity until permitted by religious or cultural laws; for others, a wide range of sexual practices is accepted and practised. However, low-risk sex practices should be known to all, and some safer sex guidelines follow:

1. *Reduce the number of sexual partners.* Abstinence is safe. Adolescents and adults should be encouraged to avoid casual sexual encounters. Longer-term monogamous relationships with known sexual partners reduce the risks reducing the opportunity for exposure. Within such a long-term relationship, the latitude available for sexual practices can be broader and still be considered safe from the threat of disease.

2. *Avoid the exchange of body fluids* by:
   a. Using a condom during vaginal, anal and oral intercourse. Condoms have been shown to be effective barriers to bacterial and viral agents. Use each condom only once.
   b. Never using saliva as a lubricant. Use spermicides or water-soluble jelly.
   c. Not following or preceding anal intercourse with vaginal penetration without a change of condom.
   d. Using gentle sexual practices that avoid trauma to mucous membrane or skin.
   e. Avoiding other sexual practices such as oral–anal, oral–genital sex as it is difficult to avoid the ingestion or exchange of body fluids or organisms. Gonorrhoea, hepatitis, HIV and other viruses can be transmitted in these ways.
   f. Avoiding prolonged wet (French) kissing unless with a partner whom you consider to be safe.

Testis
See chapter 6.3

Prostate
See chapter 6.3

Other disorders of the reproductive tract

Spermatocele

A spermatocele is a cyst of the spermatic cord which contains sperm in a thin white fluid. It lies above the **testis** and is separate from it. Usually a spermatocele requires no treatment. Sometimes it may become large enough to be confused with hydrocele and to be aggravating to the patient; then it may be excised. The aetiology is unclear.

Varicocele

Varicocele is the dilatation of the venous plexus about the testis. It occurs most frequently on the left side. Its appearance on the right side may indicate that a tumour is occluding the vein above the level of the scrotum. Some testicular atrophy may occur if the circulation is impeded for long periods of time. This may result in subfertility. On palpation behind and above the testis, the doctor feels a mass of tortuous veins that empties when the patient lies down.

Treatment may consist of a scrotal support which relieves the dragging sensation. If fertility is an issue or

the condition is severe, the internal spermatic vein may be ligated. The results are usually excellent. A scrotal support may be worn for 4–5 days following surgery, as scrotal oedema may be present.

Hydrocele

A hydrocele is a collection of fluid in the tunica vaginalis. It may occur following local injury, infection or a neoplasm, and may be unilateral or bilateral. More often it is chronic and the cause is unknown. In newborn babies the cause is usually a late closure of the processus vaginalis; this frequently closes spontaneously. In some young men a chronic type exists because the processus vaginalis never closes completely, and a connection remains between the peritoneal cavity and the tunica vaginalis.

Treatment is not required unless the testis cannot be palpated to rule out abnormality, circulation to the testis is impaired, or the hydrocele becomes large, unsightly and uncomfortable. Then the hydrocele is aspirated, and a sclerosing drug may be injected. In chronic cases the tunica vaginalis is excised (hydrocelectomy). After operation the scrotum is elevated on a pillow or bridge dressing, and a pressure dressing is applied. Depending on the operation, there may or may not be a drain present in the incision. The patient must be observed for haemorrhage, which may be concealed in the hydrocele sac. When ambulatory the patient usually requires a fresh scrotal support daily. Immediately after the operation he may need a larger support than usual.

Torsion of the testis

Torsion of the testis occurs when the testis rotates within the tunica vaginalis. Often this is due to spasm of the cremaster muscle which rotates the testis in what is usually an abnormally large vaginalis. The young man experiences a sudden severe pain in the area of the testis that is unrelieved by rest or support. Because the torsion reduces the blood supply to the testis, testicular atrophy follows rapidly. Surgical intervention is required as a matter of urgency to maintain normal testicular function.

Benign hyperplasia of the prostate

It is not known why benign enlargement of the prostate gland occurs with ageing. However, it is estimated that 70% of men aged over 60 years show some signs of prostatic enlargement. Approximately half of these men will experience symptoms ranging from mild to severe (York Centre for Review and Dissemination 1995). These are due to the enlarging prostate interfering with the free flow of urine from the bladder into the urethra.

Effects on the patient

Gradually, the man may experience hesitancy in beginning the flow of urine. The stream of urine is reduced in force and size. Incomplete emptying of the bladder produces residual urine which reduces bladder capacity so that urgency and frequency result. Nocturia occurring three or more times in one night is a good indication of frequency. Often, cystitis occurs as well. In severe cases, the bladder becomes overdistended, and hypertrophy and small diverticula follow as weakened areas of bladder mucosa bulge out between the bands of muscle fibres. The back-up of urine causes hydroureter or even hydronephrosis. Over long periods of time, renal function may be impaired.

Frequently, the patient does not seek medical attention until acute retention of urine occurs. Alcohol and some medications are frequent causes. The patient is catheterized with the smallest size catheter possible and urine is slowly released from the bladder. This prevents a sudden release of pressure in the abdomen which could cause shock and haemorrhage. Shock follows the rush of blood from vital centres to fill the newly released blood vessels. This sudden filling may cause small blood vessels in the bladder mucosa to rupture. The catheter remains in place for 2–3 days, after which normal voiding patterns usually return. The patient is cautioned to avoid an excessive intake of fluid in a short period of time, as this rapidly distends the bladder, precipitating retention. He should void frequently when he has the urge to do so in order to avoid overdistension of the bladder. If followed, these instructions should help the individual to avoid acute retention. Retention may lead to frequent voiding of small amounts of overflow urine, particularly where the problem has become chronic.

Backache and sciatica may also bring the patient to the doctor, as the enlarged prostate exerts pressure on nerves.

Treatment

Watchful waiting and lifestyle modification combined with drug therapy may be sufficient to manage men with mild to moderate symptoms. Finasteride interferes with testosterone metabolism and therefore reduces the size of the prostate, improving urine flow rates and reducing symptoms. Side-effects include the development of erectile dysfunction and ejaculatory disorders. An alternative approach is through the use of alpha-blockers which relax smooth muscle in the prostate and therefore improve urine flow (e.g. alfuzosin, doxazosin). This group of drugs has significant cardiovascular side-effects and interactions with other drugs, and the patient needs careful monitoring and education about the medication. The York CRD (1995) has pointed out that there is no evidence to support the use of alternative or natural remedies in this field.

Surgery is indicated to relieve more severe symptoms and to prevent infections of the urinary tract and renal damage. If the amount of residual urine in the bladder is greater than 75–100 mL, the surgeon may feel an operation is necessary even though the symptoms are not severe. Residual urine is estimated in several ways. Immediately after voiding, a catheter may be passed and

any remaining urine is drawn off and measured. A radio-opaque contrast medium can be injected into the bladder. The man is then asked to void, and postvoiding films are made. Direct visualization of the bladder may be done by cystoscopy, and any bladder changes noted. Intravenous urography will indicate the extent of ureter and kidney involvement. Renal function tests may be ordered as well.

A period of preoperative preparation may be necessary. Education is an essential part of preoperative preparation, as for any surgical procedure.

Transurethral resection of the prostate (TURP)

This is the most frequently performed operation. The operation is carried out with a resectoscope, an instrument similar to a cystoscope but equipped with cutting and cauterizing attachments. This slender instrument is inserted up the urethra to the prostatic urethra, and the enlarged prostate is removed in pieces. The capsule remains intact. During the operation, the bladder and urethra are irrigated continuously with a sterile, isotonic, nonconductive, clear fluid. In this manner, debris and blood are washed away.

Immediately after the operation the catheter drainage is bloody. A closed irrigation system is usually initiated to prevent blockage of the catheter by any clots. The nurse must be alert for signs of haemorrhage by paying close attention to the blood pressure and pulse of the patient, and the amount of drainage. The drainage is watery and blood-tinged for 24–48 hours after operation.

The fluid used to irrigate the bladder during the operation may be absorbed, causing haemodilution. The signs and symptoms of this may be those of sodium deficiency or excessive blood volume. Complaints of headache, nausea, vomiting or muscle weakness should not be ignored by the nurse but must be reported. Hypertension, restlessness, apprehension, shortness of breath or blurred vision likewise should be reported. After the operation, 200–300 mL of normal saline may be given intravenously over 2 hours. The nurse must observe the patient for signs of pulmonary oedema.

Complaints of spasmodic, intermittent pain by the man in the suprapubic region or a constant desire to void are related to bladder spasms. In severe cases he will need medication to obtain relief. The nurse should explain bladder spasms and catheters before operation to the patient and instruct him not to try to void after surgery.

Complaints of persistent pain in the suprapubic area may be due to an overdistended bladder from a catheter that is not draining properly or from haemorrhage into the bladder. Rarely the bladder may have been perforated during the operation and blood and urine seep into the abdominal cavity. First, the nurse irrigates the catheter and patency is established. The pain should diminish proportionately; if not, other causes must be ruled out. Analgesia may be given to the patient to give pain relief during this period but analgesia alone does not provide relief from an overdistended bladder.

Because haemorrhage remains a threat, even in the later postoperative period, care is taken to prevent its occurrence. The patient is cautioned against straining to pass stool, and a light diet is usually ordered. Enemas are contraindicated during the first postoperative week.

Because of the danger of a urinary tract infection, a prophylactic antibiotic may be prescribed. The catheter is removed 3–7 days after operation and, for a short period after this, the man is usually instructed to record and measure each voiding. If difficulty in voiding is still present, the catheter may be reinserted. The nurse should watch for signs of incontinence which may follow or signs of urinary retention which may indicate a urethral stricture. Before being discharged the man should be told that an episode of bleeding may occur about the second to fourth week after surgery. In that event, he should contact his doctor. Also, he is warned to avoid any straining, heavy lifting or vigorous exercise for about 1 month after operation.

The procedure does carry potential risks. Many patients are elderly and have significant other pathology which increases the risks of anaesthesia and the other well known postoperative risks (see Ch. 10). In addition incontinence has been reported in 13% of men, difficulty with erection in 21%, and dry or retrograde ejaculation (into the bladder) in 73% (York CRD 1995). For these reasons, some surgeons prefer to carry out a less radical operation, transurethral incision of prostate (TUIP), which is suitable for men with smaller prostates and which produces fewer side-effects.

In view of the risks involved in surgery it is important that the man is allowed to explore the alternative medical management with appropriate lifestyle modifications, such as altering drinking patterns. The specialist nurse can fulfil a valuable role by having such discussions and offering support to the patient in whatever decision he comes to.

Other operative procedures

If the prostate is very large or there is evidence of malignancy, the surgeon may undertake an open operation to remove the prostate (prostatectomy). Three approaches are used, all of which carry more risk than TURP.

Suprapubic prostatectomy

A small abdominal incision is made above the pubis and directly over the bladder. The bladder is opened and, through another incision into the urethral mucosa, the prostate is excised. The prostatic capsule remains intact. Sometimes only a Penrose drain in the suprapubic incision is all that is judged necessary in the postoperative period. It is usually removed after 36 hours. If a cystostomy tube is present, it is removed 3–4 days after operation. The indwelling catheter usually stays until the incision is nearly healed. The suprapubic incision may take time to heal. Bladder spasm and leakage of urine

Prostate
See chapter 6.3

from around the cystotomy tube is a frequent difficulty for these patients.

Retropubic prostatectomy

This allows for total removal of the gland in cases of prostate cancer. Urinary results are excellent and potency may be maintained. An abdominal incision is made above the bladder. The bladder is not incised, but the surgeon dissects down between the pubis and the bladder to reach the prostate. The capsule is opened and the tissue is removed.

Perineal prostatectomy

The surgeon excises the prostate through a semicircular incision in the perineal body. The prostatic capsule is opened and the gland is removed, making this a suitable operation in cases of prostatic cancer. Incontinence and erectile dysfunction are common complications.

Carcinoma of the prostate

Carcinoma of the prostate gland is the second most common cause of death in men from malignant disease in Europe and the USA. However, far more men are likely to die *with* cancer of the prostate than *from* this disease. Selley et al (1997) cites figures showing that approximately one-third of 60-year-olds show histological evidence of the disease at autopsy, but the diagnosed prevalence amongst live 60-year-olds is only 4%. The tumour most often arises in the posterior prostatic lobe and in 85% of cases is hormone related, depending upon androgens to retain its integrity. However, the actual cause of the cancer is unknown.

The tumour causes an increase in levels of prostate-specific antigen (PSA) above the normal range of 0–4 ng/mL. However, other conditions such as benign hyperplasia of the prostate can produce the same effect, and Selley et al (1997) have reported some studies showing that between 25 and 73% of men have raised PSA levels. This creates a problem as a prostate cancer that is undetectable by any other means in its early stages shows high PSA levels (PSA-detected cancer) but a high PSA level does not necessarily mean cancer as this may be due to many other causes. As a result of this and other problems, PSA testing at present is lacking both sensitivity (the probability of identifying true positive cases with a disease) and specificity (probability of identifying true negative cases without a disease). Its use in primary care is not justified and general practitioners are urged not to use PSA testing as a means of early detection (Selley et al 1997).

Effects on the patient

The symptoms are essentially those of benign enlargement of the prostate. On rectal examination, the examiner palpates a hard nodule. As the nodule may resemble other conditions, a biopsy is often done. Transrectal ultrasonography may help in locating and staging the malignancy. Needle biopsies can now be done by putting a needle gauge into the ultrasound probe. This has greatly increased the accuracy of biopsies. The patient receives a cleansing enema before the procedure. On discharge the patient is told that blood-stained urine is to be expected for a short time.

Classification

Carcinoma of the prostate is classified into four stages, based on the results of rectal examinations, serum acid phosphatase levels, radiography of the skeleton, and metastases.

- *Stage I*, or carcinoma in situ, is often described as latent, or focal. Usually there are no symptoms.

- In *stage II* the nodule may be palpated on rectal examination and serum acid phosphatase levels are normal.

- When *stage III* is reached, the growth has spread to the seminal vesicles, the base of the bladder and outside the prostatic capsule, but no distant metastases are present. Some 75% of men have raised serum acid phosphatase levels.

- With *stage IV* carcinoma, excessive levels of serum acid phosphatase circulate in the bloodstream. Previously, the thick prostatic capsule has kept the lesion localized and prevented spread into the abdominal cavity. Now the blood and lymphatics have carried the disease to distant sites. The bones of the pelvis are most frequently affected, and raised serum alkaline phosphatase levels reflect this spread. Also, because of bone and liver involvement, severe anaemia may occur, accompanied by the other symptoms of a terminal disease.

Treatment and nursing intervention

Various treatment options have been tried over the years. Surgery may consist of radical prostatectomy by the retropubic or perineal routes, or minimally invasive TURP. Radiation therapy may be helpful in early lesions and in reducing pain from skeletal metastases in advanced cases. Alternatively hormone therapy may be tried for advanced disease, aiming to block the production of testosterone. However, the facts at present are that no treatment has been shown to cure prostate cancer, to provide an extension of life or to do the patient more good than harm. It is also true that some patients with the disease live for many years with little significant impact upon their lives, while others become very ill very quickly and die. Again, the reason for these different outcomes remains unknown (Porter 1996). As a result of this state of affairs, Selley (1997) recommends that informed patient choice should be a major consideration in deciding what treatment options to follow. The nurse has a major role to play with medical staff in facilitating informed patient choice in a clinical area such as this.

Carcinoma of the testis

Cryptorchidism or undescended testicle is the major identified risk factor for cancer of the testis. Men aged between 20 and 34 years are at greatest risk, and cancer of the testes is the most common cause of death from cancer in this age group. Approximately 1000 new cases present every year in the UK (Cancer Research Campaign 1991). As testicular cancer is usually highly chemosensitive there is a potential for a high cure rate. This is further aided by the fact that these cancers produce distinct chemical tumour markers which allow recurrence to be detected before any clinical signs (Cook 2000). When these factors are combined with the fact that the organ is palpable and early detection is therefore possible, it is desirable that all men should be taught how to examine the testes (see Box 22.1). This is especially important for men with a history of cryptorchism. Although the tumour is rare – and this should be stressed in teaching – each man should be alert to possible changes in his testes. Symptoms usually consist of a painless lump, but sometimes there may be a dull ache and a sense of heaviness or dragging in the scrotum. The man should also be alert to a testis that feels enlarged, is firm, gives the impression of heaviness and, when squeezed, fails to elicit the deep visceral pain that is usually associated with testicular pressure. Men should also be aware that there is a genetic trait in cancer of the testis.

Diagnosis and treatment of testicular cancer

Treatment involves removal of the tumour and affected testis and may be followed by radiation therapy. Cytotoxic chemotherapy may be used after operation if the patient had a teratoma or if recurrence occurs as shown by increased levels of the markers α-fetoprotein (AFP) or human chorionic gonadotrophin (HCG).

*Testis
See chapter 6.3*

Box 22.1   Procedure for testicular self-examination

- Become familiar with the normal weight, texture and consistency of your testicles by carrying out self-examination every month.

- Carry out the procedure after a bath or shower as the scrotum is then relaxed and its contents are easiest to feel.

- Roll each testicle gently between your forefinger and thumb to check that the surface is smooth and free of lumps.

- Become familiar with the feel of the epididymis which runs at the back of each testis. This is a normal part of the testis and should not be confused with a new lump.

- If you detect a lump, make an appointment at once to see your GP.

Cancer of the penis

Malignancies of the penis are essentially malignancies of the skin. The glans and prepuce are nearly always affected. The disease is less frequent among circumcised men. In populations with poor genital hygiene, frequent sex partners, low age at first intercourse and a high incidence of HPV infection, carcinoma of the penis also has a higher incidence. HPV is associated or coexists in many cases. Treatment is by excision of the affected areas or by partial or total amputation of the **penis**.

Summary

The area of men's health has been substantially neglected and the various taboos associated with sexuality have ensured that this is particularly so in the case of men's reproductive health. Nurses has a great opportunity to remedy this poor state of affairs, and low-cost interventions such as health education and allowing men to talk through the treatment options before arriving at an informed therapeutic choice can make a major contribution to improving the health of 50% of the population. There are, of course, major cultural factors such as the 'macho, laddish' image to contend with, which will change only slowly, but that is no reason for not beginning the change process. In addition the scandal of underfunding of research into clinical problems such as prostate cancer needs urgently to be addressed as a matter of public health policy. Above all, the nurse needs to be clear about his or her own sexuality and moral beliefs about sex and reproduction before addressing the needs of the patient. Empathy and sensitivity are essential for good nursing practice in this area together with a non-judgemental approach.

*Penis
See chapter 6.3*

References

Adler M (1996) ABC of sexually transmitted diseases. London: BMJ.

Benn DS, Siffen P (1993) Rape, death and resurrection: male reactions after disclosure of the secret of being a rape victim. Medicine and Law 12(12): 181–189.

British National Formulary (2000) British National Formulary, 2000. London: British Medical Association/Royal Pharmaceutical Society of Great Britain.

Cancer Research Campaign (1991) Testicular cancer UK. Factsheet 16:4. London: CRC.

Cook R (2000) Teaching and promoting testicular self examination. Nursing Standard 14(2): 48–51.

Donovan D, Nicholas P (1997) Prostatitis, diagnosis and treatment in primary care. Nurse Practitioner 22(4): 144–156.

Fenton K (2000) Increasing gonorrhoea reports; not only in London. Lancet May 27.

Foster M, Cole M (1996) Impotence. London: Martin Dunitz.

Moskowitz M (2000) The challenges of diagnosing erectile dysfunction in the primary care setting. Nurse Practitioner 25(6 Suppl): 1–3.

Padma-Nathan H, Forrest C (2000) Diagnosis and treatment of erectile dysfunction: the process of care model. Nurse Practitioner 25(6 Suppl): 4–10.

Porter M (1996) Recommendations from the first Michigan Conference on prostate cancer. Urology 48(4): 519–534.

Selley B, Donovan J, Faulkner A (1997) Diagnosis, management and screening of early localised prostate cancer. Health Technology Assessment 1(2).

Vetrosky D (2000) Anatomy and pathophysiology of erectile dysfunction. Nurse Practitioner 25(6 Suppl): 6.

York Centre for Review and Dissemination (1995) Benign prostatic hyperplasia. Effective Health Care Bulletin 2(2).

23

Caring for the patient with a female reproductive system disorder

Dolsie Allen

Introduction

Physiology of the female reproductive tract

Disorders of the female reproductive system

The woman with a disorder of the breast

Summary

Introduction

Traditionally the focus of women's health care has been directed towards their reproductive capacity and role. In the early 1900s, the average lifespan for women was approximately 50 years of age. The average female therefore spent the majority of her life fully capable of reproducing, and dying shortly thereafter from disease or infection. During the later part of the twentieth century, thanks in part to tremendous medical advances, pharmaceutical technology and disease management, women can expect to live one-third of their life in the postmenopausal phase. In a way, menopause could be considered as a fairly recently created state brought about by medical science and improved standard of living.

Comprehensive care for women needs to consider women's health experience across the lifespan from adolescence, through the reproductive years, menopause and the older years. Healthcare issues range from safer sex practices, contraception, pregnancy, domestic violence and stress management onward through the post-menopausal issues concerning osteoporosis, heart disease and improving quality of life. This chapter focuses on some of the problems that concern women across the lifespan, touching on several issues outside the traditional reproductive role.

Physiology of the female reproductive tract

In utero development

The adult female reproductive tract consists of paired ovaries, uterine tubes, a uterus and vagina (Fig. 23.1).

Externally, the labia, clitoris and Skene's and Bartholin's glands are part of the reproductive system (Fig. 23.2).

Sex is **determined** at the time of fertilization by the inclusion of the XX chromosomal pair of the female or the XY genotype of the male. As the embryo grows, an internal genital ridge develops but remains undifferentiated in either sex until the seventh week of intrauterine life. At that time, under the regulation of the Y chromosome, seminiferous tubes and Sertoli cells differentiate. At this time sex differentiation can be made morphologically because the genital ridges of the embryo have grown and evolved into a rudimentary ovary or testis depending on the sex of the cell (Fig. 23.3).

While internal development proceeds, the external genitalia also become differentiated. During this phase of development three small protuberances consist of the genital tubercle and, on either side of this tubercle, the genital swellings. The external area may be referred to collectively as the vulva, perineum or pudenda. Generally, perineum refers to the area stretching from the symphysis pubis laterally to the thighs and posteriorly to the tip of the coccyx.

The female genitalia arise from these three ridges. The tubercle becomes the clitoris, and the genital swellings develop into the labia majora and minora. As the labia meet anteriorly, they form a loose-fitting hood like a fold over the clitoris. This fold is similar to the prepuce of the male penis. Posteriorly, the labial folds fuse just before the anus.

By the 16th week of embryological life, the sex of the infant can be determined externally. In early development the ovaries are abdominal organs. As further growth takes place, the ovaries descend over the pelvic brim.

Sexual determination
See chapter 6.3

Figure 23.1   (a) Median sagittal section of the female pelvis. (b) Anterior view with some structures cut open to expose internal structure.

Prominence of first sacral vertebra
Peritoneum
Ovarian ligament
Rectovaginal pouch
Rectum
Anal canal
Perineal body
Labium major

Ureter
Fallopian tube
Ovary
Fundus of uterus
Round ligament
Cervix of uterus
Pubic symphysis
Clitoris
Labium minor
Urethra
Vagina

Opening of uterine tube
Ovarian ligament
Endometrium
Ovary
Uterine tube
Round ligament
Muscular wall of uterus
Body of uterus
Cervix
Vagina
Hymen
Labia minora
Labia majora

Physiology for Nursing Practice

Female reproductive system
See chapter 6.3

Ovary
See chapter 6.3

The **female reproductive system** functions to produce the female hormones (oestrogen and progesterone), to ripen ova for fertilization, and for intercourse to fertilize the ova. In addition, the reproductive organs incubate the human conceptus, providing it with safety and nourishment until the fetus is expelled to continue its growth and development externally.

The ovary

The **ovary** is a small almond-shaped organ lying posterior to the broad ligament of the uterus. Cross-sections of the ovary show a cortex and a medulla. The cortex, or outer layer, is composed of connective tissue and cells, among which are scattered the ova and developing follicles. Over this outer layer of the cortex is a thin layer of germinal epithelium. The medulla is composed of connective tissue containing blood vessels and smooth muscle fibres.

The fetal ovary is recognizable very early. By the fourth month of intrauterine life some cells in the ovary have differentiated sufficiently to be recognizable as primary oocytes. Initially these oocytes number in the millions, but most degenerate. At birth fewer than two million are present; at puberty there are about 300 000 and of these only 400–500 will develop to ovulation. By the menopause few primordial follicles remain, and they soon degenerate.

Figure 23.2   Female external genitalia.

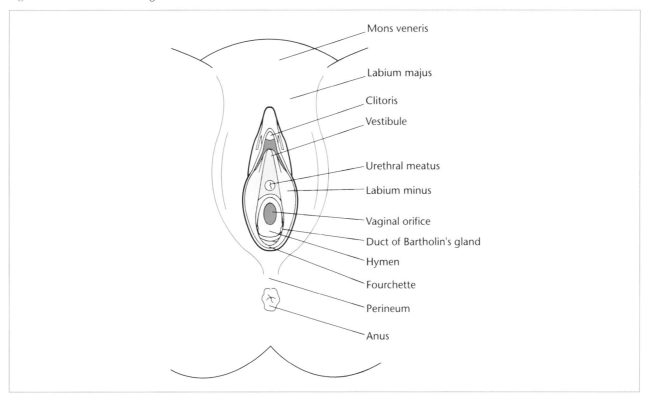

Figure 23.3   Normal sexual development in the male and female.

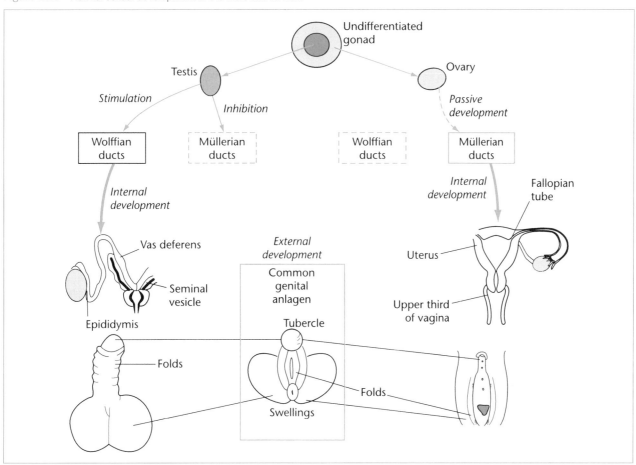

Throughout childhood some of these oocytes develop but never reach maturity and ovulate. Then, under the influence of the maturing hypothalamus, which stimulates the anterior lobe of the pituitary to produce gonadotrophins, puberty begins.

The *secondary sex characteristics* then begin to develop. First there is growth and development of the breast tissue. Pubic hairs appear and the internal and external organs of the reproduction become fully developed and functional. The vagina, under the influence of oestrogens, thickens and develops several layers of squamous epithelium. This makes it more resistant to infection. Previously the vaginal pH was neutral or alkaline; now it becomes acidic. This is largely due to Doderlein's bacillus, which oxidizes the glycogen that has been deposited in the vagina to form lactic acid. Concurrently, the ovaries are developing and menarche, or the beginning of menstruation, occurs. The age at which menses commence is decreasing, and this appears to be linked with improving nutrition (Frisch 1990, Noord and Kaakoi 1991).

As in the male, gonadotrophin-releasing hormone (GnRH) stimulates the anterior pituitary gland to release two hormones: follicle-stimulating hormone (FSH) and lutenizing hormone (LH). FSH and LH are not secreted continuously but in a pulsating manner, with the amplitude and frequency of the pulses varying with the phase of the cycle. Under this hormonal influence, *primordial follicles* in the ovary begin to develop. Each primordial follicle is composed of an oocyte and surrounding granulosa cells. As growth occurs, the oocyte or ovum enlarges and there is an increase in the number of granulosa cells. Growth is eccentric and the ovum comes to lie at one side of the group of granulosa cells. Fluid rich in oestrogens and inhibin collects between these cells and the ovum. Inhibin is produced by the granulosa cells under the

stimulation of FSH. As more inhibin is produced, it exerts an inhibiting effect on the production of FSH, causing the levels to fall. As the follicle grows, cells begin to form around it and are called *thecal cells*. These thecal cells, stimulated by the FSH and LH, produce oestrogens.

In what is known as the *proliferative phase*, many follicles in both ovaries start to ripen but usually only one follicle continues on to ovulation. The others undergo degeneration. The thecal cells surrounding these degenerated follicles continue to produce oestrogens. The mature follicle may now be termed a *Graafian follicle*, after de Graaf who first described it in 1672 (Fig. 23.4).

As the Graafian follicle approaches ovulation, it comes to lie close to the surface of the ovary. The tissue over it becomes thin and taut. Soon the follicle wall ruptures and the ovum is expelled into the abdominal cavity. The time of the rupture is designated as *ovulation* and marks the end of the preovulatory (proliferative or follicular) phase.

The ovary now embarks on the *luteal* (secretory) *phase* of its cycle. Immediately after ovulation, the wall of the follicle collapses inward and some haemorrhage may occur into this cavity. In a few hours the remaining granulosa cells hypertrophy and begin to show the characteristic yellow of the corpus luteum. These yellow granulosa cells are now called *luteal cells*. The luteal cells are stimulated to become the corpus luteum and to begin producing progesterone. Oestrogen continues to be produced as well. The corpus luteum reaches full maturity by about the ninth day after ovulation. At this time it is easily recognizable on the surface of the ovary as a raised yellow area and may constitute nearly half the volume of the ovary. Near this time the corpus luteum may receive a message that the ovum has been fertilized. If it does so, the corpus luteum is maintained and becomes known as the *corpus*

Figure 23.4   Mature Graafian follicle.

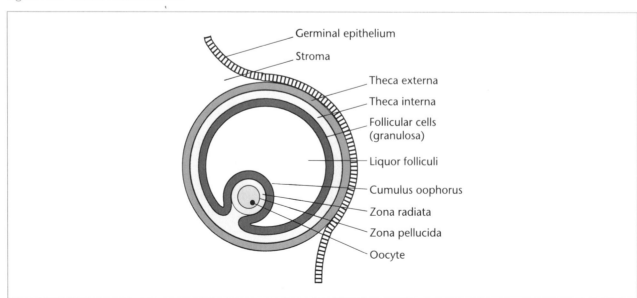

Germinal epithelium

Stroma

Theca externa

Theca interna

Follicular cells
(granulosa)

Liquor folliculi

Cumulus oophorus

Zona radiata

Zona pellucida

Oocyte

luteum of pregnancy. If fertilization does not occur, the luteal site begins to degenerate and progesterone production drops. As the site degenerates, so do the thecal cells. Oestrogen production from this source declines. The luteal site shrinks to form a small mass of whitish scar tissue on the surface of the ovary which is known as the *corpus albicans*.

Hormones and the ovarian cycle

In response to the falling oestrogen and progesterone levels, the hypothalamus signals the anterior pituitary gland to release FSH and LH. Under this stimulus the follicles begin to develop and the thecal cells produce oestrogen. The rising levels of oestrogen exert a negative feedback effect on the hypothalamus to reduce the amount of GnRH released and hence the amount of FSH and LH. The levels of FSH and LH fall slightly following the initial rise in oestrogen levels (Fig. 23.5). As oestrogen peaks, it is thought to exert a positive feedback effect on the hypothalamic–pituitary axis that results in a surge of LH and, to a lesser extent, of FSH. This surge of LH occurs about 24 hours before ovulation (Fig. 23.6).

In cycles where the LH surge does not occur or is of insufficient magnitude, ovulation fails to occur. Exactly how the LH surge affects ovulation is unclear, except that it is necessary for completion of the cycle. Follicles will grow and develop under FSH stimulation but will fail to ovulate without the surge of LH.

Ovulation occurs in a climate of falling oestrogen, LH and FSH levels and a rising progesterone level, as LH stimulates the follicular site to begin production of progesterone. As the preovulatory cycle is one of high oestrogen level, the postovulatory phase is one of high progesterone level. The other hormones continue to be produced, but at lower levels. These levels of FSH and LH are too low to stimulate the development of new follicles. The cells of the corpus luteum are organized to enlarge, proliferate, secrete and then degenerate. The surge of LH seems to be the main organizing factor for this. This stabilizes the corpus luteum and the length of the postovulatory phase of the cycle. As the 12-day-old corpus luteum degenerates and becomes a corpus albicans, the levels of progesterone and oestrogen drop, signalling the hypothalamus to begin releasing GnRH again, thereby repeating the cycle.

The uterus

The **uterus** is a thick-walled, muscular, pear-shaped organ about 7.5 cm in length in the adult virgin. It is held in position by its ligaments and by the pelvic floor. The uterus is composed of three layers:

1. an inner mucous layer, or endometrium
2. an inner muscular layer, or myometrium
3. an outer serous layer which covers the entire body of the uterus except where it is reflected up and over the bladder.

The uterus is divided into two distinct parts, the *body* and the *cervix*. The cervix projects into the vagina. The endometrial lining of the body of the uterus extends downwards, undergoing certain modifications in the cervical canal and terminating just above the external os of the cervix where it meets the stratified squamous epithelium of the vaginal wall.

Uterine cycle

The endometrium is a thin, pink membrane that is attached directly to the underlying muscle layer. It is richly supplied with blood vessels and tissue spaces. At the beginning of the new cycle it is about 0.5 mm thick. In response to the oestrogens of the preovulatory phase of the ovary, the endometrium begins to proliferate and continues to do so throughout the cycle until it reaches a peak of proliferation and secretion several days after ovulation. In this secretory stage the endometrium may be 5–6 mm in depth. In short, all is ready for implantation of the fertilized ovum, should it appear. In perfect timing the endometrium reaches its peak of development approximately 7–8 days after ovulation, or just when the fertilized ovum should appear in the uterine cavity ready for implantation.

If the ovum has been fertilized and the corpus luteum is continuing to secrete progesterone, the endometrium is maintained and implantation may occur successfully. However, should the corpus luteum not receive this message, it begins to degenerate. Oestrogen and progesterone production decline. This decline in hormone level causes the endometrium to retract and degenerate. Vasoconstriction of blood vessels occurs and the uterus becomes ischaemic. Shortly thereafter the endometrium begins to slough away and menstruation begins. The process of sloughing takes 3–7 days, with each woman usually establishing her own pattern. Menstrual flow is composed of endometrial tissue, mucus and some blood. As the tiny arterioles constrict and relax, bleeding occurs. Usually not more than 30–60 mL of blood is lost per menstrual period. This blood does not clot because of the action of fibrinolytic enzymes released into the uterine cavity during menstruation. Occasionally, a heavy menstrual loss neutralizes the available fibrinolysins and clots occur. At the completion of menstruation the endometrium has returned to its non-proliferative state. It is now ready to respond again to the rising oestrogen levels.

Ovulation

Menstrual cycle

The uterine and ovarian cycles are often referred to as the menstrual cycle. This cycle begins on day one, which is the day on which **menstruation** begins, and continues until the day before menstruation begins again. **Ovulation** occurs on or around the 14th day of a 28-day cycle. However, this is subject to many factors, and the timing

Hormones
See chapter 6.3

Uterus
See chapter 6.3

Uterine cycle
See chapter 6.3

Menstruation
See chapter 6.3

Ovulation
See chapter 6.3

Figure 23.5   Summary of menstrual cycle events. FSH, follicle-stimulating hormone; HCG, human chorionic gonadotrophin; LH, luteinizing hormone; IU, international units.

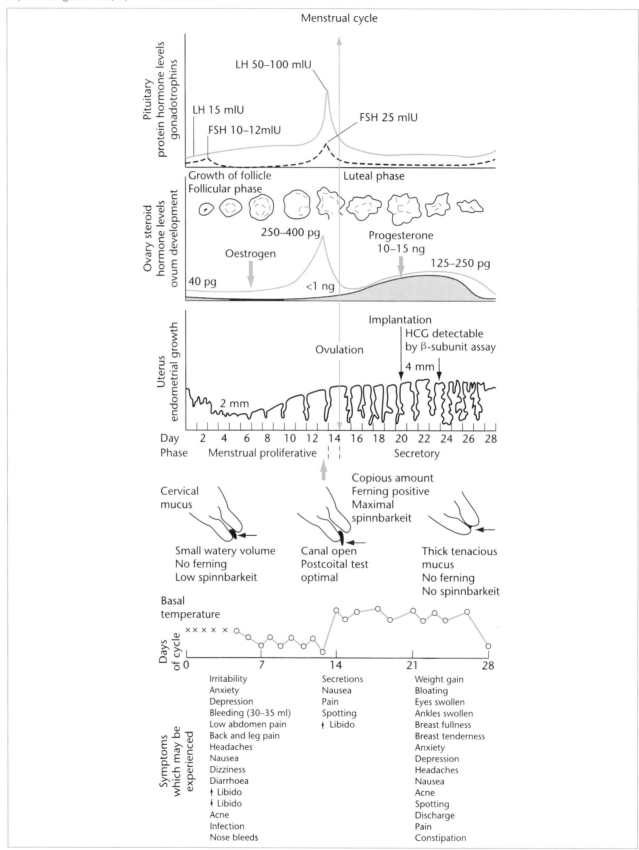

Figure 23.6   Plasma concentrations of gonadotrophins and ovarian hormones during one ovarian cycle. FSH, follicle-stimulating hormone; LH, luteinizing hormone; OHP, hydroxyprogesterone; IU, international units.

of ovulation in any one woman is a matter of considerable variation.

The menstrual cycle is divided into two independent sections: the preovulatory and postovulatory phases. The two phases are independent because the length of one does not control the length of the other. Ovulation is the dividing factor signalling the end of one phase and the beginning of the next. Not all cycles are ovulatory and it is known that women may have an anovulatory cycle and still menstruate. The precise mechanism for this phenomenon is not clearly understood. The most common explanation is that a follicle develops but there is a failure of the LH surge and the follicle degenerates. Anovulatory cycles are most common in adolescent girls in whom the first menstrual periods may be anovulatory and in women at the menopause. Follicles do not mature at the same rate each month. This produces a month-to-month variation in the timing of ovulation and the length of the preovulatory phase in any one woman. This variation in timing is evident by variation in the onset of menstruation.

The onset of menstrual flow is controlled by the corpus luteum of the ovary. Once ovulation has occurred, menstruation follows 14 days later; this time relationship is constant. Fluctuations in the length of the cycle arise in

the preovulatory phase. These events produce a natural variation in cycle length from month to month. Age is an important physical influence on cycle length in women. The menstrual pattern throughout life is divided into three zones: two of transition and a central period of increasing stability. The two transition periods (postmenarch lasting about 5–7 years, and premenopause lasting 6–8 years) are characterized by variation in cycle length.

As a girl ages, her average cycle length shortens and variation in cycle length reduces. The younger the girl when she experiences menarche, the sooner she begins to develop a more 'regular' cycle. The central period from age 20 to 40 years shows a continued reduction in variation and a shortening cycle interval. The average cycle length shortens between 0.1 and 0.18 of a day per year. Maximum stability is reached from age 35 to 39 years.

As ageing continues there is a decrease in the number of follicles that begin to develop. This results in a gradual reduction in hormone levels, particularly inhibin, with corresponding increases in circulating FSH throughout the cycle. Documentation of these high FSH levels is the first laboratory indication of the perimenopausal period. These high FSH levels induce rapid follicular development and a correspondingly shorter preovulatory phase. As the process continues there is a failure of the LH surge and anovulation follows, contributing to increasing irregularity in the **cycle** length. Eventually the ovary ceases to respond and **menopause** occurs.

Cervical, vaginal and tubal cycles

Changes may also occur in the cervix, vagina and fallopian tubes in response to stimuli from the ovary. Oestrogen prompts the endocervical glands to respond by increasing their secretions. Cervical mucus reaches its peak of production at ovulation. The consistency of the mucus changes at ovulation and becomes thinner. These changes demonstrate the timing of the body as the mucus will permit easy entry of the sperm at ovulation – the most logical time. Indeed, it appears that the cervical mucus permits passage of sperm through the cervix only at this particular time.

Changes in the vagina and fallopian tube are minimal compared with the changes in the ovary, uterus and cervix. The vaginal epithelium proliferates and reaches a peak at ovulation time. The fallopian tube secretes fluids that provide nutrients first for the ovum and then for the conceptus until implantation occurs.

Physiological aspects of sexual response

The general sexual response cycle consists of four progressive phases which are the same for both sexes. See Chapter 22, page 783 for a summary of these stages. In the female, Bartholin's glands secrete a fluid that serves to lubricate the vaginal introitus. However, the amount of mucus secreted by these vulvovaginal glands is minimal and most vaginal lubrication arises from the vaginal walls themselves. Very quickly following sexual stimulation the vaginal walls exhibit a 'sweating'-like appearance as beads of mucoid material appear throughout the rugal folds. Soon the droplets run together to form a complete coat of lubrication over the inner surface of the vagina. The cervix also appears to play a relatively minor role. This seems to be confirmed by the fact that little or no secretory activity of the cervix has been observed during sexual activity. Also, women who have undergone hysterectomy and bilateral salpingo-oophorectomy produce reasonable vaginal lubrication in response to sexual stimulation. Indeed, the same response will develop in artificially constructed vaginas, and the source of lubricating material is presumed to be the same.

The vagina also responds to sexual stimuli by enlarging. The inner two-thirds of the vagina expand and lengthen, forming a basin for the seminal pool that will form in the posterior fornix of the vagina just below the cervical os. The outer third of the vagina becomes engorged and constricted, serving to assist the vagina to form a reservoir for the semen.

An orgasm may occur as a generalized systemic feeling, with sensation localized in the clitoris, and rhythmic muscular contractions of the outer third of the vagina

and the uterus. With orgasm, pelvic engorgement of blood vessels is rapidly resolved. This causes the uterus to return to its normal position, placing the cervix near to or in the seminal pool, thus facilitating movement of sperm through the cervix.

The clitoris seems to be a unique organ in human anatomy. As the primary focus of sensual response, it appears to serve no other function. Made of fibrous tissue with two corpora cavernosa and richly innervated, it undergoes engorgement and enlargement when the female is sexually stimulated either physically or mentally. The tumescent clitoris then retracts against the symphysis pubis and becomes difficult to see or feel.

The subjective experience of orgasm is synchronous with orgasmic platform contractions and the pleasure associated with orgasm is related to their number and intensity. Following orgasm the woman enters the resolution phase. Unlike the male, a woman, if provided during this phase with sufficient further stimulation, may return to the orgasmic level.

Menopause

Around 1900, the average age at **menopause** in the UK was approximately 50 years and female life expectancy was similar. Currently, the average age of menopause has changed little as it is now approximately 51.4 years, However, mean female life expectancy has lengthened to approximately 82 years (National Statistics 2001). This means that today the average woman can expect to spend almost 30 years of her life in the postmenopausal state. The emotional, physical and medical implications of this relatively recent situation are many, and currently constitute one of the fastest growing areas of the female medical research.

Reproductive function, usually demonstrated by menses, continues until middle age. Then, at the average age of 50 years most women cease menstruating. The cessation of menstruation is perhaps the most obvious sign of menopause, or 'change of life'. This transitional period is known as the *climacteric*. The climacteric may take a few months to several years and is the result of altered ovarian function. Ovarian follicles cease to ripen. The endometrium does not respond as richly, and menstruation becomes scantier and shorter in duration. The woman may have several anovulatory cycles, just as she may have had in puberty. Eventually the menses may become irregular and finally cease. Menopause is said to complete when the woman has had no menses for 1 year. As the perimenopausal woman may ovulate erratically, family planning advice is important to her. She cannot assume she will not become pregnant until menopause is complete, after which the risks of pregnancy occurring are very slight.

Decreasing oestrogen levels stimulate gonadotrophic hormones (FSH, LH), which show a proportionate rise, but the ovary does not respond fully. The body, previously

Cycles
See chapter 6.3

Menopause
See chapter 6.3

functioning smoothly under balanced hormonal control, responds to these imbalances with 'hot flushes' in about 85% of women. A hot flush is a sudden feeling of heat in the face, neck and chest associated with patchy flushing of the skin. There is usually profuse perspiration, perhaps palpitations, a generalized feeling of heat and a sensation of acute physical discomfort. Some flushes are accompanied by nausea, dizziness and headache. A hot flush lasts for about 3 minutes. The monitoring of women having hot flushes confirms that an average temperature shift of about 2°C from core to skin occurs. The hot flush is followed by vasoconstriction and shivering as the body attempts to correct the shift in temperature from skin to core.

Hot flushes begin gradually, reach a plateau by 6–8 weeks after the last period and can occur for several years after the menopause. Hot flushes occur in parallel with LH pulses and are not coordinated with oestrogen levels. The exact mechanism is not understood but the same factors that trigger a rise in LH are also thought to trigger a hot flush. Low circulating levels of oestrogen are thought to contribute to this phenomenon. However, these symptoms are unpredictable, hence uncontrollable, and can be embarrassing, anxiety producing and sleep disturbing. Much of this may be unsettling to the woman, especially when accompanied by cessation of reproductive function and fears of advancing age. Many women accept these changes with only some minor disturbance, although most appreciate freely available sources of education and reassurance.

Hormone replacement therapy (HRT)

The principal goals in the management of the menopausal woman are threefold:

1. To maintain or improve quality of life.
2. To increase lifespan.
3. To reduce risks factors.

The benefits of HRT, although well documented (see Box 23.1), continue to remain controversial.

HRT is available in numerous combinations of oestrogen and progestogen. The administration route is equally varied: transdermal patches, subcutaneous implants, suppositories and oral administration are all possible. The latter is the least effective as absorption from the gut is direct to the hepatic system where the hormones are metabolized before achieving systemic dispersion.

To reduce the risk of osteoporosis by 50%, treatment is required for at least 5 years. In all cases treatment should be a mutual decision between the woman and her doctor. However, this is not always the case and a woman's level of knowledge may play a significant role in determining whether she receives HRT or not. The use of HRT has raised anxieties in relation to increased risks of other pathologies developing. These include thrombosis and cancer. However, the research evidence appears to suggest that risks are minimal provided there are no pre-existing diseases or contraindications from family history.

There is increasing interest and understanding of homeopathic remedies for the treatment of problems experienced during the climacteric. Some women claim relief from using these remedies. Homeopathy is particularly useful for women concerned about the systemic use of drugs, and those who object to the use of animal-based HRT preparations (National Osteoporosis Society 1993).

It should be understood that not all oestrogen production ceases at menopause. The ovaries do not appear to be inert when the woman is postmenopausal, and it is thought that they continue to excrete small amounts of hormone. This is in addition to oestrogens from the adrenal gland. Over the years oestrogen production declines further and the development of other organ changes occurs. The vulva becomes atrophic and thin as a result of reabsorption of fatty tissue. The uterus decreases in size; the endometrium becomes thin and atrophic. The vaginal epithelium thins out and is more susceptible to injury and infection. Lubrication of the vagina may require supplementation so that dyspareunia (painful sexual intercourse) does not occur. Topical oestrogen creams may relieve these symptoms.

Sexual function can continue with little change in the vast majority of postmenopausal women. The most important factors in the continuance of sexual function appear to be the opportunity for and the frequency of intercourse, so that the changes of menopause themselves do not mean this phase of a woman's life must cease. Indeed, relief from fear of pregnancy may make the experience a more enjoyable one.

Disorders of the female reproductive system

Assessment

Sensitive enquiry should be used to gain the following information:

- History of any disorders, illnesses, injury, surgery and diagnostic investigations of the reproductive system. History and character of menstruation (including menarche, last menstrual period, length of cycle,

---

Box 23.1   Documented benefits of HRT

- Relief of menopausal vasomotor symptoms
- Decreased incidence of coronary heart disease
- Reduced incidence of osteoporosis
- Reduced risk of colonic cancer
- Improved sexual function
- Longer survival rates

duration of flow, amount of flow, menopause and last cervical smear test).

- History of reproductive events including number of pregnancies and the outcome of these (abortion, premature, full-term), delivery (types), children (any stillbirth or neonatal death and cause if known), present health status, complications of pregnancy, history of infertility, and present and past use of contraception.

- Review of function to identify potential causes of anxiety:
  — any changes or disturbances in function (e.g. dysmenorrhoea, dissatisfaction with sexual functioning or birth control)
  — the presence of any symptoms of disease. If symptoms are present they are explored to determine their location, character, duration and severity. The common manifestations of disorders are: pain, lesions, discharges, itching, non-cyclical bleeding, swellings and masses.

- The patient's sexual roles and how the presenting health problems may affect self-concept and relationships with significant others.

The medical examination may include a general physical examination, with inspection and palpation of internal and external genitalia (Figs 23.7 & 23.8). The examination is personal and invades body boundaries and there is a sense of exposure, particularly during vaginal examination. For these reasons the woman having her first vaginal examination should be prepared in advance for what is involved. The examination procedure is described as she is shown the equipment. The patient undergoing a vaginal examination may have a sense of physical and emotional exposure; the nurse can help to reduce these feelings by a sensitive and supportive approach. The nurse should avoid the expression 'relax' and instead explain how to loosen the pelvic floor muscles. Most women appreciate simple explanations of what to expect as the examination progresses. One of the most critical factors in gaining a woman's confidence is to explain how you will maintain her privacy during the examination.

Patient problems

The woman with a reproductive problem presents various special concerns. Being female usually provides a woman with an inherent set of behaviours, culturally and physiologically determined, that may help to guide her actions. The normal functioning of her reproductive system can provide reassurance of her essential 'femininity'. The distortion or interruption of these processes may prove very disturbing to the woman and/or her partner. The woman may experience problems in relation to self-image and have fears about future sexual performance and attractiveness. Body parts that contribute to self-esteem and identity have a high psychological investment. The threat posed by loss of these body parts depends on:

- their meaning to the individual

- her stage of development of body image and self

- the reactions of the social group, including the spouse, to which the patient belongs.

Many people have been culturally conditioned to the idea that some areas of the body should not be discussed – much less exposed to examination. Others may feel guilt over their illness. Sexually transmitted disease, abortion and cancer arouse guilt feelings in some individuals, which may be expressed as a feeling of being punished

Figure 23.7 Internal vaginal examination demonstrating the position of the speculum and Ayre spatula used to obtain cervical cells for a smear test.

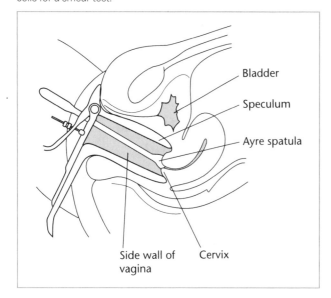

Bladder

Speculum

Ayre spatula

Side wall of vagina   Cervix

Figure 23.8 Bimanual vaginal examination.

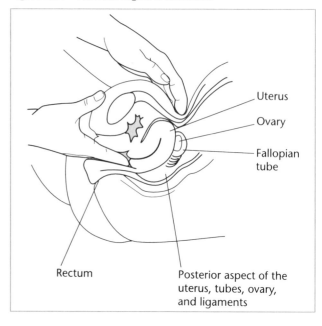

Uterus

Ovary

Fallopian tube

Rectum   Posterior aspect of the uterus, tubes, ovary, and ligaments for past deeds. You may be dealing with patients who experience anxiety and fear, shame, guilt, diminished self-esteem or reawakened anxieties over personal identity. In addition, acquired immune deficiency syndrome (AIDS) is a particular, unspoken fear for many sexually active women.

Goals

A patient's goals may include:

1. resolving dysfunctional sexual problems

2. achieving a sense of self-worth

3. being able to verbalize fears and anxieties

4. showing understanding of health problems and what medical intervention involves

5. adapting to a change in sexual role/and or function

6. being aware of and avoiding risk factors in sexual activity.

Nursing intervention

These goals may be achieved by the following nursing interventions:

1. Assess the degree of threat posed by loss of function or body parts to the woman; then plan, provide and evaluate nursing care based on that assessment.

2. Provide nursing care that promotes feelings of dignity, self-worth and attractiveness. Encourage the return of health, control over body functions and independent self-care.

3. Reduce fear and lessen potential guilt by:
   a. acknowledging and discussing feelings
   b. anticipating the need for explanations and interpretations
   c. clarifying misinformation about causes of illness and the consequences of treatment
   d. maintaining a confident, non-judgemental approach to the patient
   e. assisting in acknowledging the loss, if any
   f. obtaining appropriate additional sources of spiritual or emotional help for the patient
   g. offering information and support for relatives.

Evaluation

Interventions are successful if behavioural changes have occurred, although behavioural changes may be difficult to document in areas such as self-concept, anxiety and guilt. The patient may, for example:

- state that she feels better, less frightened or happier

- take an interest in personal appearance and renew interests in social life, which may also indicate a return to the more positive outlook toward the future

- demonstrate an understanding of the illness, treatments and any residual changes

- demonstrate a knowledge of the risk factors that may lead to a recurrence of the problem and the actions that may reduce or eliminate the risk factors

- discuss alterations in body function and structure with the nurse and so indicate a willingness to begin to deal with the problem or to accept it with appropriate adjustments.

Adjustment to many of these changes requires some time and complete resolution is rarely seen in hospital. Expectations of resolution and the effectiveness of intervention must be realistic.

Sexual issues associated with giving nursing care

Several issues involving sexuality may arise in the course of the nurse–patient interactions. They reflect the changing role of the patient and involve confusion over the meaning of nursing or patient actions. The most common arise from the intimate level of care involved in nursing and acting out sexual behaviour by the patient. Issues of touch and sexual acting out behaviour have been discussed in Chapter 22, page 785, and the same principles apply to the care of women as of men.

Variations of sexuality

Variations in sexuality can occur in several areas of sexual expression, but most differences are psychosexual in origin. Only a few disorders arise from physical illness and trauma or congenital error (see p. 786). Most variations become obvious through difficulties in sexual expression.

During middle adolescence, teenagers begin to adjust and become more comfortable with their changing bodies. The majority of adolescents proceed through this experience fairly easily, although for some it is a time of intense emotional upheaval. Sexual orientation develops during early childhood. One's gender identity is usually firmly established by the age of 2 years. Studies demonstrate that the sense of masculinity or femininity is essentially solidified by age 5 or 6 years.

Homosexual characteristics appear to surface several years before the period of adolescence. Theories about the aetiology of homosexuality include genetic, hormonal, environmental and psychological origins. The young adolescent may experience intense confusion and anxiety as he or she struggles with these personal issues. Staff must be sensitive and aware of the psychological and medical implications of homosexuality. A trusting, non-judgemental, caring attitude can provide the basis for a therapeutic relationship during this potentially sensitive time.

Sexual concerns

Many persons experience doubts over their inner feelings of being a man or a woman. This may be more prominent in adolescence when the final development of gender identity takes place, but may recur throughout the individual's life. As sexual identity is considered to be an important component of overall individuality, this may stimulate concerns over self-identity. Concerns over expected performance are also prevalent. The individual may doubt whether he or she has the necessary physical attributes, experience or appeal to attract, satisfy and keep a sexual partner.

Sexual dysfunction

In the female, sexual dysfunction may also be associated with inhibition of or a lack of response (frigidity). Some women may not become sexually excited or, if aroused, do not experience orgasm with intercourse. Women may also complain of painful intercourse (dyspareunia) or a strong contraction of the outer one-third or the vagina (vaginismus) which makes insertion of the penis extremely difficult.

Sexual dysfunction can be the result of psychological, interpersonal or physical factors:

■ Psychological causes may be anger, depression, anxiety, ignorance or deeper psychosexual conflicts.

■ Interpersonal factors involve conflicts with the partner or an inability to establish interpersonal relationships.

■ Physical causes include illness, injury or drugs.

Diagnosis and treatment involve a history, physical examination and laboratory tests to ascertain the most likely cause. During history taking the patient is asked whether there are any sexual complaints. This makes sexuality an acceptable topic to discuss should the patient have a problem or develop one in the future. If the patient does present with a sexual problem, it is discussed in a frank, open manner, maintaining a broad, objective attitude toward the patient's sexual beliefs and practices. The patient is not urged to disclose more information during a session than she is comfortable in revealing. The patient's sexual concerns are assessed in the context of other problems and in the context of value systems.

Once the nature of the problem has been identified, treatment commences. Sexual counselling operates at four levels:

1. permission
2. limited information
3. specific suggestions
4. intensive therapy.

Permission involves reassurance that the patient is normal and may continue doing what she has been doing. Limited information involves providing information specific to the patient's concern or problem. This frequently allows the patient to make appropriate changes in behaviour. These changes in behaviour usually involve the patient following a suggested course of action. This may vary from the treatment of organic disorders to the relearning of sexual behaviours, through to more in-depth education and sexual exercises. The fourth level, intensive therapy, is highly individualized therapy provided by professionals who have advanced experience and knowledge in the sex therapy field.

It is the responsibility of the nurse to create an atmosphere conducive to the identification of sexual problems. If unable to provide the appropriate intervention, the nurse should refer the patient to another professional. Nurses with the requisite knowledge and skills and who are comfortable with the subject function in levels 1 and 2, providing reassurance and knowledge of human sexual response and practice in health and illness. Nurses with appropriate postregistration education in sexual therapies may offer more specific assistance.

Rape trauma syndrome

The international statistics on sexual assault against women are extremely disturbing. At least one in every five women experiences rape or attempted rape during her lifetime.

The legal definitions of rape and sexual assault vary between legal jurisdictions. In the UK rape is legally defined in the Sexual Offences (Amendment) Act 1976 as when a man 'has unlawful sexual intercourse with a woman without her consent and at the time he knows that she does not consent to the intercourse or is reckless as to whether or not she consented to it'. By defining rape as a form of assault, the primary motivating factors of anger, aggression and need for power are acknowledged.

Sexual assault is a crisis in the life of the victim. It contains the elements of suddenness, arbitrariness and unpredictability – three factors associated with crisis and with rape. A crisis demands psychological and physical adaptation or response from the individual. Crisis is recognizable by the disruption of regular patterns of behaviour and thought that occur in the individuals involved. The degree and nature of the response will vary from one individual to another. Several key factors should be kept in mind in assessing both an individual's initial response to crisis and eventual resolution of crisis. They are:

■ how the individual perceives the incident and feelings about the incident

■ the emotional stability of the individual prior to the crisis

■ the coping skills possessed by the individual

■ the presence or absence of support systems such as family, friends and colleagues who will be available to assist the individual in the future.

The person in crisis is acutely sensitive to the responses of the individuals around them. The type of intervention a person experiences immediately after sexual assault may either aggravate the crisis or ameliorate it. As the effects of sexual assault may be long lasting if the crisis is not resolved in a positive manner, it is important that the professionals in contact with the victim attempt to alleviate the situation. The victims of such assaults have the right to expect to be treated with dignity and respect in a manner that does not take away personal control, and to receive prompt physical and emotional support.

To provide such services many areas have rape crisis centres, and some accident and emergency departments provide a rape suite. These centres ensure that the victims are treated in a knowledgeable, caring manner. All personnel associated with them should understand and be experienced in dealing with the social, emotional, legal and medical issues surrounding rape and sexual assault.

Reaction to sexual assault

In constructing a model encompassing the elements of the possible reactions to rape, Burgess and Holmstrom (1974) identified three phases of response to this form of physical and psychological trauma:

1. an acute (impact) phase
2. a recoil (adjustment) phase
3. a post-traumatic (integration) phase.

Acute phase

In the acute phase the victim presents a variety of reactions. Initially many will appear very upset; others will appear calm and controlled. The state of seeming control and calm may be an indication of the state of shock rather than the intensity of their eventual reaction. The individual may express disbelief, fear, anxiety, guilt, shame, helplessness, anger or rage. Some may be highly irritable and moody; all seem to share a fear of death, fear that the attacker will return and fear that it will happen again. Some women fear becoming pregnant and, in the present climate, there is also the added fear of AIDS. They are concerned over why it happened. Some will see their behaviour as contributing to the event; they feel guilty and worry that somehow they encouraged the attack. Occasionally society, with its biases, may support this view. The victim expresses anger toward the assailant and some may convert her anger and helplessness into depression and further guilt.

Physically these women complain of disturbances in eating and sleeping patterns, increased headaches, fatigue, gynaecological symptoms and general body pain. Socially, they are fearful and may shun going out. They have increased dependency needs and may find decision making difficult. Much anxiety may centre around the decision to press charges against the individual or to tell family, friends and colleagues because of fear of misunderstanding by family members and others of their role in the event. Sexually they may retreat from encounters and be unable to enjoy or even tolerate sexual contact for a period of time. This is further aggravated by any physical trauma they have suffered. This phase may last from a few days to a few weeks.

Recoil phase

As the victims progress from the initial shock of the acute phase, defence mechanisms emerge and most of the disturbances of that phase decrease. They return to their normal activities of work, school or home and appear outwardly composed. Most will now attribute the rape to chance or some other societal cause, but not to self. They see little need to continue professional counselling or to continue talking about the situation. This is healthy and to be expected, and should be encouraged. Most women pass into this phase. Others show a maladaptive response such as excessive self-blame, severely altered self-image, or agitation and depression. The adjustment phase can last from a few weeks to years.

Post-traumatic phase

Following the adjustment most individuals feel a need to discuss their experiences. This need is usually triggered by some event, such as an anniversary of the rape. The person may feel emotionally upset, depressed, fearful, angry and may need to talk about the experience. During this phase the person resolves feelings about the rapist and her role in the rape. She develops a new self-image that allows for the episode of rape. After this period of sorting out, the individual is free to take control of her life, accepting the feelings surrounding the assault in a more dispassionate manner. Some patients may never reach this stage.

Assessment

An accurate and precise history of the event and a physical examination are the first steps in care. Before proceeding, the doctor must obtain a signed consent form from the woman or her guardian. The consent, which must be witnessed, obtains permission to perform a complete physical and pelvic examination, and to collect the necessary specimens.

The history and physical examinations are used to assess the extent of trauma but are also used to collect evidence that may be used for forensic purposes. Because of the need to collect legal evidence there is usually a well defined protocol to follow which outlines the information to be obtained and the specimens that are to be collected. Nurses involved in accident and emergency departments must be familiar with the protocol for the assessment for rape victims applicable in their setting.

Most protocols include: a detailed history and description of the assault and the assailant; a recent sexual and menstrual history; a precise description of the physical findings; laboratory tests for infections, sperm and pregnancy; and identifying markers (e.g. hair that the attacker may have left). The woman's emotional state is also assessed and described.

Treatment

The patient receives immediate treatment appropriate to the injuries identified during examination. Follow-up care is equally important in order to prevent undesirable sequelae.

Extragenital and genital bruising and lacerations are the most common injuries suffered. Bruises are not usually evident at initial examination, but will be identified at a follow-up visit. A few patients will be more severely injured and require immediate and extensive medical and nursing care. Occasionally a patient may require a pelvic examination under anaesthesia, with suturing and repair of injury. Most patients, however, will receive treatment for trauma in the emergency department.

Victims of rape may be concerned with the risk of human immunodeficiency virus (HIV) infection. These fears should also be taken seriously. It is important that women receive prophylactic treatment for sexually transmitted infections to avoid developing pelvic inflammatory disease, which could result in subsequent infertility. The possibility of infection must not be overlooked. A referral to the department of genitourinary medicine is essential for investigation and follow-up care.

Pregnancy is a potential sequela of rape. Prophylactic treatment is instituted at the discretion of the doctor. A careful sexual, menstrual and birth control history is mandatory in assessing risk. If there is a possibility of pregnancy, the patient may receive hormone therapy (postcoital contraception) to prevent it. A combined oestrogen–progestogen preparation is used. It is given within 72 hours of unprotected intercourse and repeated once 12 hours later. The use of combined oestrogen and progestogen has fewer side-effects compared with the use of oestrogen alone. The patient is also requested to return in 6 weeks for a pregnancy test.

Psychological support

Intervention and assessment go hand in hand in the treatment of sexual assault patients. Although separated in this format, the integration of emotional support with assessment and treatment is imperative in the care of these patients. Immediate interventions should include the following:

1. Assume the patient is telling the truth.

2. Go out of your way to demonstrate concern.

3. Advise the patient not to bathe, douche or clean up in any way as this may destroy vital forensic evidence, and to seek medical attention immediately.

4. In the A&E department, give the patient as much privacy and priority as is possible.

5. Allow a supportive person to remain with the patient.

6. Do not take away personal control.

7. Be gentle in word and deed.

8. Explain clearly the reasons for all examinations and collections of specimens.

9. Assess the extent of the emotional crisis for the individual. For example: What is her manifest emotional state? Is she able to make decisions? What evidence of coping is there? What personal supports does the person have?

10. Facilitate the expression of feelings.

11. Listen supportively.

12. Explain follow-up and counselling services.

13. Give information about tests and follow-up care.

The partner and family may have a variety of emotions about the assault. Some will be supportive to the victim, others may not. Most families require help in understanding the processes of the examination and emotional reaction of the patient. They should be included in the care by the nurse.

Congenital anomalies of the reproductive system

Absence or duplication of organs

The uterus, cervix and vagina can undergo duplication or incomplete fusion. The exact incidence of such anomalies is unknown, as they are largely asymptomatic. Some may cause sterility in women or an increased risk of abortion. Rarely an organ is completely absent. Some absence (*agenesis*) or maldevelopment of tissue (*dysgenesis*) is determined genetically. *Ovarian agenesis* may be the result of an XO genotype (Turner's syndrome). The patient with this genotype may present a characteristic appearance from birth with a webbed neck, multiple anomalies, low birthweight or irregularities of the hairline. However, in others, the patient may present in adolescence because of failure of the menarche to appear. Treatment may be oestrogen replacement therapy, with $20\,\mu g$ being given every day for 3 weeks, followed by withdrawal combined with norethisterone, $5\,mg$ daily on days 12–21. Withdrawal of oestrogen permits the endometrium to slough away, thus stimulating a menstrual period. The addition of progestogen prevents endometrial hyperplasia due to oestrogen stimulation. Because the ovaries do not exist, the patient remains sterile.

Imperforate hymen

Usually this condition is not discovered until adolescence when the girl may present herself because of absence of menstrual flow. Menstruation occurs but the blood is retained behind the closed hymen. The patient may complain of crampy, lower abdominal pain occurring monthly. She may also notice dysuria, frequency and urinary retention as the growing mass of retained menstrual blood accumulates in the vagina, putting increasing pressure on the bladder and urethra. Treatment consists of a cross-shaped incision of the hymen which allows drainage of the debris. This debris is often a thick, chocolate-like material. Because of this old blood, the risk of postoperative infection is greatly increased. The nurse must pay careful attention to good aseptic technique after the operation to reduce the risk of infection further. The nurse must see that adequate drainage is maintained, frequent cleansing of the perineum occurs, and perineal dressings are changed frequently.

The hymen may also be rigid. This is usually discovered when the patient presents with a complaint of dyspareunia. In mild cases the patient will be instructed to dilate the hymen digitally, usually while sitting in a bath of warm water. If this does not succeed, vaginal dilators may be inserted by the doctor or nurse and later by the patient. In difficult cases, hymenotomy is performed.

Fertility and infertility

Control of fertility

Limiting the world population through fertility control has become a political as well as a religious and personal issue. The implications of overpopulation have usually been stated in terms of the developing nations, but have taken on a global context. In addition, contraception is considered to be a matter of personal decision: it can exercise an important liberalizing potential for the family or single person. In the light of these discussions the health professional has a responsibility to extend the knowledge and availability of contraception to anyone who requests it. With more birth control clinics available, the nurse has a major role in the control of fertility.

Nursing responsibilities

Generally, the nursing responsibilities include referral of a person to the appropriate clinic, education and interpretation. This may be taken care of in an initial interview with the person, and preferably their partner, who is seeking birth control advice. The nurse can assist the patient or couple in making a decision by presenting concise, factual information about the methods available. The woman should choose a method that will be most compatible with her personal circumstances. Most certainly this should be the one she will use and feel comfortable in using. No method of birth control is effective unless it is used constantly. This final decision is usually made with medical counsel. As the doctor reviews the patient's history, he or she may make other recommendations that will affect the person's or couple's choice.

The patient or couple will need counselling in the proper use of the method they have chosen and what to expect in the period of initial adjustment. In a simple

fashion the knowledge of an alternative emergency method should be provided as well, for it is this that may prevent a pregnancy. The patient should leave the clinic or hospital with knowledge of an alternative method. The nurse is responsible for gaining sufficient knowledge of the complex subject of contraception to be able to present factual knowledge to couples and to discuss the advantages and disadvantages of each method. In addition, the nurse will need to understand much of the emotional, social and religious aspects of contraception. A detailed presentation of family planning is beyond the scope of this work, but a brief outline of the methods follows.

Methods of contraception (Box 23.2)

Condom

The condom is a thin rubber sheath that is placed over the penis before insertion. It prevents pregnancy by acting as

---

Box 23.2

Spermicidal agents

- Foam, gels, jelly, pessaries suitable for use with barrier methods. Not adequate when used alone

Barrier methods

- Condom
- Femidom (female condom)
- Cervical cap
- Diaphragm

Hormonal contraception

- Oral contraceptive pills
- Depo-Provera injections
- Norplant system – recently discontinued, but some women may have the system in place until 2004

Intrauterine devices (IUDs)

- Mirena intrauterine system (progestogen only intrauterine contraceptive device)
- Gyne T Slimline

Surgical methods

- Tubal ligation
- Vasectomy

Emergency contraception (EC)

- Yuzpe Regime EC
- Progestogen-only EC
- IUD insertion

a mechanical barrier to the sperm. Its use is discussed on page 788. Some couples find it objectionable as a method of birth control because it may interrupt sexual foreplay, it can lessen sensation, and its effective use relies heavily on the motivation of the male. These objections can be overcome if it is used by a man who is taking a mature responsibility for his behaviour, especially in view of the risk of contracting AIDS and other sexually transmitted diseases.

Femidom (female condom)

The female condom is now available in the UK. It is pre-lubricated, but does not contain a spermicide. The female condom is available in over 35 countries and is a female-controlled barrier method for the prevention of pregnancy and sexually transmitted diseases, including HIV.

Diaphragm

The diaphragm is a thin rubber cap that is inserted into the vagina by the woman and placed over the cervical os. The cap provides a mechanical barrier to the sperm. In addition a spermicidal jelly is placed on both sides of the cap. When the diaphragm is in place, the spermicidal jelly will be in contact with the cervix and vagina. The diaphragm is not dispensed without a prescription and requires individual fittings initially, after a few months of use, and following pregnancy or miscarriage. The woman also requires careful teaching in the proper insertion and care of the diaphragm. The diaphragm is inserted manually or with an inserter which is provided. The position of a diaphragm should be checked after each insertion.

In its proper position, the diaphragm cups the cervix with the anterior side behind the pubic bone and its posterior side in the posterior fornix of the vagina. Properly positioned, it is not felt by either partner during intercourse. Removal should not take place before 6 hours following coitus to ensure completion of spermicidal action. The diaphragm can be left in place for up to 24 hours, but should then be removed for cleaning. The diaphragm is not an option for women with a latex sensitivity.

Spermicidal preparations

Spermicidal contraceptives are available in various forms including gels, creams, foams and foam tablets. These preparations are suitable for use with an additional barrier method (i.e. condom or diaphragm). These chemical agents do not give adequate protection when used alone. The spermicidal agent should remain in the vagina for at least 6 hours to be sure that all sperm are dead.

Oral contraceptives

Birth control pills are synthetic chemical hormones that resemble the female hormones of the ovary. In suppressing ovulation they mimic the action of pregnancy. The high hormone levels depress the hypothalamus, which in turn inhibits the release of pituitary gonadotrophins that stimulate ovulation. Thus, the woman is anovulatory. Protection is established as soon as the woman begins taking the pills, if she starts taking them on day 1 of the menstrual cycle.

The pills are divided into two types: the combined pill and the progestogen pill. The combined pill contains synthetic oestrogen and progesterone hormones in each pill. This pill is more effective in preventing pregnancy because it induces changes in the cervix, making the mucus thicker and more impenetrable by sperm. Also, changes occur in the endometrium that would discourage implantation should fertilization occur.

The progestogen pill, or 'mini-pill', contains a progestational agent and no oestrogen. It should not be confused with the low-dose (30 μg oestrogen) combined pill. Many of a woman's menstrual cycles while on the progestogen pill may be ovulatory. The pill depends on the effects of progestogen to produce changes in cervical mucus, the endometrium and hormonal levels to inhibit fertilization. Because of the reduced oestrogenicity of the pill, it has fewer major side-effects than the combined pill but is slightly less effective in preventing pregnancy. This makes the low-dose combined pill the pill of choice initially. The risk of pregnancy in both types of pills is minimal if taken as prescribed.

The combined pill is taken once a day for 21 days and no pill, or an inert sugar pill, is taken for the next 7 days, regardless of the woman's menstrual period. Initially the first pill is taken on the first day of the woman's menstrual period. Now the pills will regulate her menstrual cycle and she takes them as prescribed. Progestogen pills are taken every day without omission. This does make it easier for women to follow, for no timing, counting or remembering is required – other than to take the pill. Also, to maintain consistently high hormonal levels in the body, the progestogen pill should be taken at approximately the same time every day.

Withdrawal bleeding is regulated by the combined pill and occurs regularly at some time during the seven hormone-free pill days. This withdrawal bleeding simulates true menstruation. With the withdrawal of the high hormone levels, the endometrium sloughs away. However, menstruation is usually scantier and shorter, because the endometrium is thinner.

Much discussion has occurred over the possible side-effects or complications attendant on the use of oral contraceptives (Box 23.3). For many women, adjustment to oral contraceptives may take some months. During that time the woman may experience nausea, fullness and tingling in her breasts, headache, some spotting between menstrual periods, weight gain, chloasma (hyperpigmentation of localized areas of skin), acne, loss of libido or changes in vaginal discharge. On the other hand, she may feel better, have relief from menstrual cramps and have an increased libido. Sometimes changes

---

Box 23.3 Side-effects of oral contraceptives

Oestrogen

- Breakthrough bleeding
- Nausea
- Headaches
- Chloasma
- Increased vaginal discharge
- Cervical erosion
- Cystic breast changes

Progestogen

- Acne
- Depression
- Dry vagina
- Loss of libido

Oestrogen and progestogen

- Weight gain
- Post-pill amenorrhoea
- Increased breast size
- Breast tenderness

---

in dosages or in the timing of taking other pills helps. If she takes the pill with supper or lunch she may feel nauseated later.

The missed pill is cause for concern in many women. The woman should take the pill when she remembers it and take the next pill as she is accustomed to do. This may mean taking two pills in one day. Should more than one pill be missed, then the couple should use an alternative form of birth control for the remainder of that cycle. If several pills are missed, the doctor should be consulted, as the cycles may be sufficiently interrupted as to require some further regulation under medical supervision. The woman should also be taught that oral antibiotics and diarrhoea affect the rate of absorption of the pill; therefore alternative methods of contraception should be used if such problems arise.

Major complications of the pill are rare but serious. For some women the hazards of the pill are still less than the hazards of pregnancy or an abortion. Major concern revolves around the increased incidence of diseases of the circulatory system in women using the pill. The major circulatory diseases include thromboembolic disease, coronary artery disease, cerebrovascular accidents and hypertension. The risks rise with age, cigarette smoking and duration (over 5 years) of pill use. Thus the smoking

woman who has been using oral contraceptives for 5 years or more and is over 35 years of age is placing herself at considerable risk if she continues to use the pill. Such women should be counselled to give up smoking and, if unable to do so, to consider another method of birth control.

These complications have brought prolonged use of oral contraceptives into question. However, medical opinion still supports widespread use of the pill for carefully chosen women, although it may take several months for some women to find an acceptable oral preparation. Some benefits may accrue, however, for a woman who has been taking oral contraceptives. Women who have been taking the pill for longer than 1 year have lower risks of endometrial and ovarian cancer (British National Formulary 2000).

Women on a contraceptive pill should see a medical practitioner every 6 months to have their blood pressure and weight monitored, and for an assessment of their general health. Pelvic examination is carried out annually and a cervical smear test is performed at least every 3 years. Women are taught to seek prompt medical care if they experience severe or recurrent abdominal pain, chest pain and shortness of breath, severe headaches, eye problems such as blurred vision or flashing lights, or tenderness and warmth over veins in the legs.

Danger signs associated with oral contraceptives are:

- sudden severe chest pain
- sudden shortness of breath
- severe leg or calf pain
- prolonged headache
- hypertension (blood pressure above 140/100 mmHg)
- sudden vertigo, weakness or motor disturbance
- blurred vision and eye problems.

It is extremely important to note that the use of oral contraceptive agents alone in no way protects the woman from acquiring a sexually transmitted disease. Prevention of such infection through safer sexual behaviour is discussed further below.

Intrauterine device

An intrauterine device (IUD) is an object that is placed inside the uterus, where it remains and prevents pregnancy. The action is not completely understood. Some researchers believe that an IUD creates a hostile intrauterine environment either for sperm or for the fertilized ovum. Others consider that it is implantation that is prevented. The IUD ranks as a very effective method of birth control in about 80% of the women who try it. Most IUDs used today are made from a flexible plastic and are in several shapes. The addition of copper or progestogen to the IUD produces a more effective device.

The device must be inserted by a suitably trained person. It is a sterile procedure. The uterus is sounded to confirm its depth and position. Then, having threaded the IUD into the inserter, it is introduced through the cervix, and the plunger on the inserter is pressed to place the IUD. The use of the uterine sound and the skill of the person greatly reduce the risk of perforating the uterus. Uterine perforation during insertion remains a rare complication. Insertion of an IUD may be painful in the nullipara because of the tightness of the cervical os. Insertion is tolerated well by a majority of women.

Many devices are equipped with strings which hang into the vagina just below the cervix. The woman is taught to check for the presence of these strings monthly after her menstrual period. The IUD can be expelled from the uterus; this is most likely to occur during the menstrual period. Women who have never been pregnant have an increased tendency to expel the device, as do women who have previously expelled it. If the woman notices that the IUD appears to have been expelled, she should report this to the doctor so that this can be confirmed. The use of an alternative form of birth control is advisable in the interim.

Removal of the device is carried out in the clinic. A woman should be discouraged from removing her own IUD. Some are difficult to remove because of their shape. Complications of the use of an IUD include increased menstrual loss and cramping. These are the most common side-effects, and approximately 15% of women require removal of the IUD for these reasons.

Pregnancy does occur in about 3% of women using an intrauterine device. If the patient wishes to continue the pregnancy, the IUD is removed if possible. The risk of spontaneous abortion is about 50% with the IUD in place and there is an increased risk of infection. These risks vary with the type of IUD and its location in the uterine cavity.

The IUD contributes to the development of pelvic inflammatory disease (PID) in about 2% of women. If neglected, PID contributes to sterility. The only sign of this infection may be irregular intramenstrual bleeding and complaints of pain. If an infection is suspected, the IUD is removed and the infection treated. The IUD is contraindicated in women with a current pelvic infection or those at a high risk of one. Rarely an IUD can pass silently through the uterine wall into the abdominal cavity. This may be discovered when the woman cannot locate the string, becomes pregnant, or experiences abdominal or pelvic symptoms. It is removed during laparotomy.

The IUD is generally inadvisable in nulliparous women because of the increased risk of pelvic sepsis and infertility.

Intrauterine progestogen-only device

Levonorgestrel is released directly in the uterine cavity from an intrauterine system (Mirena). The effects are therefore mainly local and hormonal. The return of fertility when the system is removed is rapid and complete. Essentially, the cautions and contraindications are similar as for standard IUDs. Effectiveness continues for 5 years.

Depo-Provera

Medroxyprogesterone acetate is a long-acting progestogen given by intramuscular injection. This method of contraception can be used by women desiring short-term as well as long-term contraceptive protection. Long-term contraception is provided by repeat injections every 12 weeks. There are reports of delayed return of fertility and irregular cycles after discontinuation of treatment. There is, however, no evidence of permanent infertility associated with this contraceptive method. Heavy bleeding has been reported in patients given medroxyprogesterone acetate immediately postpartum.

Norplant

The levonorgestrel-releasing implant system (Hoechst Marion Roussel) has recently been discontinued in the UK, but some women may have the system in place until the year 2004 (British National Formulary 1999). Several problems have been associated with placement and removal of these systems. The care-provider removing these devices needs to be fully trained and experienced in the technique of removal.

Sterilization

Sterilization means the termination of reproductive capacity. As the social and emotional barriers to sterilization have altered, it has increased in popularity. When family size is complete, many couples choose sterilization as the method of birth control. In other cases, when the hazards of pregnancy are life threatening, sterilization may be strongly indicated. Removal of any or all of the major organs of reproduction in either male or female results in sterility. Generally this is considered too extreme. A simple method of mechanically barring sperm and egg from meeting is required which will neither reduce natural hormone levels nor affect sexual capacity. In men this involves the procedure known as vasectomy, which is discussed in Chapter 22.

Tubal ligation

Tubal ligation is the comparable operation to vasectomy in men. It can be done vaginally but is usually performed abdominally via a laparoscope. Under general anaesthesia two small incisions are made in the abdomen. The fallopian tube is dissected, a loop of tube is lifted up, ligated, and the tube above the ligation is either crushed with a clamp or severed. In some operations the uterine end of the tube may be turned back and embedded in the posterior wall of the uterus. Tubal coagulations, in conjunction with a laparoscopy, may also be done. The surgeon identifies the tubes through the laparoscope and then applies the heat source, which coagulates the tube. In the hands of a skilled operator the procedure is safe and associated with few side-effects.

As in the male, the tubes can be reconstructed, but the success rate is not high. Thus, the patient should see the operation as irreversible. The operation, although frequently performed as a day case, is not entirely harmless. Rare major postoperative complications are pulmonary embolism and later tubal pregnancy. In addition to the consent for operation, there is a separate consent form for sterilization which must be signed before the operation.

Rhythm method

This method requires temporary abstinence from coitus during the possible ovulation time of the woman. It is the only method of birth control that is officially sanctioned by all religions. The rationale of the method is based on several assumptions:

- that a woman is fertile only during ovulation
- that ovulation occurs once a month at a predictable time
- that the ovum can survive for approximately 24 hours
- that sperm will survive in the genital tract for 72 hours.

Placing these assumptions together, and allowing 3 days before and after ovulation for the lifespan of the sperm, we arrive at 6 days. As we know that the time of ovulation varies in any one woman, we must allow 1 or 2 days for extra safety on either side. This now gives us a fertile period of approximately 8 days' duration, falling near the middle of the menstrual cycle.

The crux of the problem is the timing of ovulation. Because no anticipatory method of timing ovulation has been discovered, we must rely on a retrospective view of the time of ovulation in any one woman. Under the influence of the rising progesterone levels following ovulation, the basal body temperature in women shows a rise. The rise will be noticeable within the first 24 hours following ovulation. The temperature remains slightly increased for the remainder of the cycle. Also, at the time of ovulation, the cervical mucus changes. There is an increase in amount and reduction in viscosity. Women can be taught to recognize and record these changes. An attempt is made to predict the time of ovulation for the woman after she has carefully recorded the dates of her menstrual periods, the mucus changes, and her temperature taken daily at a uniform time. Depending in the woman or clinic, this may be done for 3–6 months. An average is then calculated from these dates and her individual period of likely fertility should be reviewed at specified intervals. During periods of her life when ovulation is being established or re-established – postpartum, during lactation, menopause and periods of emotional stress – the method is highly unreliable. In women with very regular periods and high motivation, the method has had success. A urine testing kit is now commercially available which indicates when ovulation is due. This increases the reliability of this method.

Box 23.4 Indications for emergency contraception

- Unprotected sex
- Condom rupture
- Diaphragm displacement or misuse
- Potential pill failure
- Sexual assault

Emergency contraception (EC)

For some women or couples there is occasionally a need for emergency contraception (see Box 23.4). For more than 25 years the hormonal (Yuzpe) method has served as a suitable form of emergency contraception with an overall pregnancy rate of 3.2% when administered within 72 hours after unprotected intercourse.

This method involves taking two tablets each containing $50\,\mu g$ ethinylestradiol and $250\,\mu g$ levonorgestrel followed 12 hours later by another two tablets. The first dose must be taken within 72 hours of the unprotected intercourse in order for this method to be effective.

Side-effects are numerous and include nausea, vomiting, headache and menstrual irregularities. Vomiting can interfere significantly with the effectiveness of this method. Nausea may be lessened by the administration of $10\,mg$ domperidone with each of the two doses of EC hormones.

Progestogen only emergency contraception (POEC) is available in the UK (approved in August 1999) and is now being offered over the counter. Several research studies have shown the POEC method to be more effective, producing fewer pregnancies as well as being better tolerated by women as there are fewer side-effects (Cheng et al 1998). Levonorgestrel $750\,\mu g$ taken by mouth and repeated 12 hours later is a highly effective EC method. As with the standard Yuzpe method, the POEC needs to be initiated within 72 hours of unprotected intercourse.

Methods not recommended

The following *frequently* attempted methods of contraception *frequently* result in pregnancy. They are, therefore, not endorsed.

Douche

The vaginal douche, although not medically necessary, may occasionally be used following coitus for personal cleanliness. Some women consider the douche to be a method of birth control and are under the impression that it washes the sperm away. In fact, it may force the sperm into the uterine cavity and merely speed them on their way. It is not a method of contraception.

Breastfeeding

Under the stimulus of regular demand breastfeeding many women remain anovulatory for several months. Others quickly regain their fertility. Breastfeeding is not suggested as a form of contraception. Women who are breastfeeding should be advised to use a form of contraception that will not interfere with the physiology of lactation. Suggestions are barrier methods or progestogen-only hormonal preparations.

Coitus interruptus

This method consists of the male withdrawing his penis from the vagina before ejaculation occurs. This is a highly unreliable method as some sperm may escape before ejaculation actually occurs. Also, this method may require more control and experience than many couples possess.

Infertility

The incidence of infertility appears to be rising in the Western world, although the reasons are not yet understood. Infertility is defined as the failure to conceive after 12 months of adequate exposure without the use of contraceptives. Primary infertility refers to a couple who have never conceived. Secondary infertility refers to a couple who have had a previous pregnancy but now cannot conceive. Approximately 10% of couples prove to be infertile. Of this 10%, about 40% of the problem rests with the man, 40% with the woman and 5–10% with the couple as a unit.

Causes of infertility

The possible causes of infertility are too numerous to list. However, the major causes can be grouped under several headings. Any impairment of ovarian function that interrupts ovulation creates infertility. This may be caused by hormonal imbalances or may be due to some intrinsic defect in the ovaries themselves. The same is true of the testes, or the duct system may not be patent (see p. 782). Infections leading to adhesions are a major cause of infertility in both men and women. Malformation or displacement of reproductive organs may contribute to infertility. Infertility may arise because of unique factors particular to the union such as vaginal secretions that are not compatible with the seminal fluid, causing the sperm to die.

Assessment and diagnosis

The investigation usually begins when the couple or woman presents to the gynaecologist with a complaint of failure to conceive. By this time the problem may have become a nagging fear for both partners. Often reassurance and discussion about the problem seem to help, for many women are reported to return shortly thereafter as pregnant. A persistent infertility case will require thorough investigation. Many gynaecologists prefer to see couples together so that both partners may receive an outline and discussion of the approaches that may be used. The doctor's assessment of the possible cause of the infertility will guide the direction of the investigation. Some techniques that are used in investigating infertility are described.

Medical history and physical examination

A detailed medical history and physical examination are done for both partners. Particular attention is paid to the development of the secondary sexual characteristics and any evidence of virilizing or feminizing effects. Any history of infections and injuries involving the genitourinary tract will be noted carefully. In addition the doctor will take a marital history to gain an adequate picture of the couple's sexual pattern. The woman will be asked to give a detailed menstrual history. Before other tests are begun, infections, particularly cervicitis and prostatitis, are to be treated as they contribute to infertility. Anaemia, poor health, exhaustion, overwork, stress and other psychological situations all may be causative factors, and the doctor often tries to relieve these first if they seem of sufficient magnitude to be affecting the sexual adjustment of the couple.

Ovulation

Whether or not ovulation occurs monthly may have to be established. The patient is asked to keep a basal body temperature chart. This also helps to estimate hormonal levels. The woman is asked to come to the clinic near ovulation time. Cervical smears will be taken and tested for spinnbarkeit (ability to form a thread when cervical mucus is drawn out between two glass slides) and ferning (a fern-like pattern in dried cervical mucus). These tests help to time ovulation and the presence of oestrogens in cervical mucus respectively. If ferning appears to be unsatisfactory, the patient may be requested to return for serial vaginal smears, which give an indication of ovulation.

Plasma assays will be done to assess the levels of FSH and LH. Plasma progesterone levels are sampled 1 week after the biphasic shift in the basal body temperature graph, or day 21 in the 28-day cycle. However, levels of progesterone vary and there is doubt about the predictive value of this screening unless done sequentially. These results, together with the graphs and other test results, permit an outline of the events of the menstrual cycle that are occurring in the woman.

Urinalysis

Urine tests may be done to measure urinary oestriols and the presence and amount of 17-ketosteroids.

Endometrial biopsy

This is done to indicate whether or not a healthy endometrium is present. If it is not, then the problem may be one of failure of the fertilized ovum to achieve successful implantation. Occasionally tuberculosis and sexually transmitted diseases are discovered, and may be the cause of the infertility.

Laparoscopy

Laparoscopy allows the direct visualization of pelvic contents, an opportunity to perform ovarian biopsies, and freeing of adhesions with laser techniques if necessary. It may also be combined with hysterosalpingography. Women need to be advised about referred pain following distension of the abdomen with carbon dioxide.

Hysterosalpingography

This is the injection of a radio-opaque contrast medium into the genital tract. It serves to outline the uterine cavity and uterine tubes. The test is done in the radiography department under sterile technique. The patient is usually asked to move from side to side after the injection in order to promote spilling of the contrast medium into the abdominal cavity. This test provides information about the exact location of any abnormality.

Possible complications of tubal patency tests are pain, collapse and vomiting, which may be experienced shortly after the test is done, especially in women who were not anaesthetized. The patient should be observed for these signs for about 3 hours after the procedure. Helping the patient to assume a knee–chest position for a few minutes before standing up may prevent further discomfort. Cramps and vomiting may be more prevalent following cervical dilatation. Other complications may include exacerbation of pelvic infections, air embolism or sensitivity reactions to the contrast medium. On the other hand, both laparoscopy and hysterosalpingography may be therapeutic because they may have opened the tract. This is supported by the observation that many patients conceive with no further treatment.

Sims–Huhner postcoital test

Postcoitally, a specimen of seminal fluid from the posterior fornix of the vagina and the cervical canal is aspirated. The specimen is examined for sperm motility and the ability of sperm to survive in the vagina. The test is best performed at the time of ovulation. The patient is instructed not to douche or use lubricants for 2 days before the test. Following intercourse she remains supine, hips elevated on a pillow, for 30 minutes. Within the next 2–4 hours she comes to the fertility clinic, where the specimen is taken. A reading will assess how many live, motile sperm are in the specimen. Should sperm not be present, the investigation may be directed towards the male. Does he have sperm? If he does, why is he not capable of depositing them near the cervix? If they are dead or non-motile, the vaginal environment may be hostile to them. One such reaction is due to the stimulus a foreign protein (sperm) evokes in the woman's body. Consequently, antibodies develop. The antibodies in the female inactivate the sperm before fertilization can take place. Following a 3–6-month period of abstinence or the use of a condom by the male, circulating antibodies may be sufficiently reduced to permit sperm to live long enough to fertilize.

Cross-hostility

There may be immunological hostility between the cervical mucosa and sperm. Immunoglobulin G may be found in both men and women. The test is carried out when the postcoital test is negative. A drop of ejaculate is placed on a slide with a drop of cervical mucus. Sperm should be seen actively invading the mucus. If not, the mucus may be impenetrable for several reasons or the sperm may have low motility. If the problem is with the mucus, any infection that is present is treated and oestrogen may be given from day 1 to day 10 of the menstrual cycle to produce a more watery, penetrable mucus. Work on producing antigens from the partner's sperm or blood has been effective in desensitizing the woman to antibodies she develops in relation to her partner's sperm and genetic material.

Semen analysis

A specimen of seminal fluid is examined for volume, number, morphology and motility of sperm. Ideally, 2–5 mL of fluid should be present. The fluid should gel and then reliquify after 15–20 minutes. The sperm should number above 60 million per millilitre of ejaculate, and 60% should still show vigorous activity when examined at room temperature 2 hours after ejaculation. No more than 20% of the sperm should show abnormal forms.

The specimen is collected after a 3-day period of abstinence from coitus. It is collected in a dry, sterile jar by masturbation or coitus interruptus and is brought to the clinic for examination within 2 hours of collection. The collection jar should be kept warm by holding it against the body during transport.

If no sperm are present in the ejaculate, the patency of the duct system may be assessed by vasography. Testicular biopsy may be indicated. If the biopsy shows living sperm, then failure of the sperm to arrive in the seminal fluid may be due to a blockage in the tube. If the semen is acidic, it may result from a failure of alkaline seminal vesicle fluid to reach the prostatic fluid and neutralize the acidity of the semen. Hormone assays of FSH, LH and testosterone will also be done.

Sperm penetration assay

This test assesses whether or not sperm can penetrate a hamster egg. The sperm are washed with a buffer solution and transported to the laboratory where a test is done. Whether the sperm washed in the buffer solution have improved penetrating capacity, both in vivo and in vitro, is determined. Some sperm that cannot penetrate an ovum before being washed can do so afterwards. Even if the washed sperm do not penetrate a hamster egg, there have been cases where they have penetrated the partner's ovum. However, a penetration rate of 0% of the hamster egg is a poor prognosis for fertility. This test is a useful and rapid way to test male fertility, particularly in oligospermic men. It can be a method of treatment if washed sperm are used to fertilize the partner's ovum.

Treatment

Surgery

In both the male and female, surgery is aimed at restoring function. Adhesions may be released; the ducts are reconstructed. Cysts and tumours are removed as indicated. The nursing care is the same as that for any pelvic operative procedure.

Hormone therapy

Clomifene

This is an antioestrogenic substance that causes the hypothalamus to stimulate the pituitary to increase the output of FSH and LH. By displacing the circulating oestrogens, the hypothalamus is released from the inhibiting effects of high levels of oestrogen. In addition, clomifene may increase ovarian sensitivity to FSH and LH.

The patient must be instructed to monitor her basal body temperature carefully, as a rise in the temperature is expected with ovulation. Coitus should occur close to ovulation. Treatment may be repeated several times until pregnancy occurs or the treatment is judged ineffective. Good rates of success are recorded, although there is an increased risk of multiple pregnancy – usually twins. Clomifene is more successful when used in situations of altered function, such as amenorrhoea following oral contraceptive use. The drug does stimulate the growth of benign ovarian cysts, which usually disappear after its use.

Gonadotrophins

The gonadotrophins may be supplied artificially. Hypothalamic-releasing factors may be given to stimulate the pituitary. Human pituitary gonadotrophins made from freeze-dried human pituitaries may be administered. These are, in effect, the FSH and LH hormones. The patient receives injections of FSH to ripen a follicle and then LH to stimulate ovulation. The process is complex, necessitating close monitoring of the patient for ovulation and for overstimulation of the ovaries. Ovarian cysts follow its use, as do multiple pregnancies. Like clomifene, good pregnancy rates have been achieved.

Assisted fertility techniques

A variety of methods is used to assist fertility:

- *Artificial insemination by a donor (AID)*. This is usual where the male has been identified as sterile for whatever reason.

- *In vitro fertilization (IVF)*. The woman's ovary is hyperstimulated so that she can produce numerous ova. These are surgically removed from the ovary. The partner or donor sperm are introduced to the ova so that fertilization may occur. Once cell division is observed, some or all of the fertilized ova (blastocysts) are instilled into the uterus via the vagina. Success rates are approximately 20%, but are increasing as techniques are further developed.

- *Gamete intrafallopian tube transfer (GIFT)*. Donated ova are fertilized with sperm and, as blastocysts, are immediately instilled into the fallopian tube.

Nursing responsibilities

- To provide education in human reproduction and sex education.

- To teach the patient how to perform certain tests or treatment accurately, using clear detailed instructions. The danger of the couple 'calendar watching' and becoming obsessional about the precise timing of intercourse should be discussed. This can lead to a loss of enjoyment as sex becomes reduced to a clinical function. Ongoing failure to conceive may increase the pressure further and a vicious cycle can become established which interferes with the man's ability to perform satisfactorily (see Ch. 22 for a discussion of erectile dysfunction).

- To prepare the patient physically and emotionally for the procedure.

- To assist the patient and doctor during investigative procedures.

- To monitor the patient's physical and emotional status following treatment for the development of complications.

- To realize that the patient may come to the investigation with a sense of failure and decreased self-esteem and respond in ways that do not increase the sense of failure or that further decrease self-esteem.

- To be sensitive to the possible grief over loss of reproductive function and feelings of inadequacy.

Anyone involved with assisted reproductive techniques will be confronted with ethical dilemmas, such as the following:

- Should everyone have access to treatment which is frequently available only to those who can pay, or who are of a certain age?

- If multiple blastocysts are instilled and implant successfully, should fetal reduction follow to increase the numbers of embryos to one or two, providing them with a much increased rate of survival?

- What should become of the ova, sperm and blastocysts that are stored. Legislation and guidance are available on these issues.

Disorders of the menstrual cycle and menstruation

Mittelschmerz

Mittelschmerz is a feeling of lower abdominal pain on one side on or near ovulation time. It is thought to be caused by fluid or blood escaping from the outer ruptured follicle site and causing peritoneal irritation. It occurs in about 25% of women. Occasionally, when the right side is involved, fear of appendicitis may bring the woman to the doctor.

Premenstrual syndrome

Premenstrual syndrome (PMS) is probably experienced by most women in mild forms. However, extreme cases are seen. The symptomatology includes a feeling of fullness or heaviness in the lower abdomen, backache, painful breasts, irritability, headache, weight gain premenstrually, nervousness, depression and insomnia.

No single cause has been identified. What seems clear is that somatic and psychological symptoms exist; they occur but in varying degrees with each cycle. Among the treatments that are usually tried are birth control pills, pyridoxine (vitamin B_6), progestogen and bromocriptine. Any of these treatments may help some women. For patients suffering severe psychological symptoms, psychotherapy may be recommended, both to provide support and to distinguish between other emotional disturbances that may be present and masking premenstrual tension.

Treatment consists of taking a sympathetic and understanding approach, as the patient may be very upset by the changes of mood and behaviour that she experiences. Women are taught to chart their symptoms to reduce the unexpectedness of them and to talk about these changes with their partner and family in order to increase family understanding. Further research into the complex neuro-endocrinological relationships of the menstrual cycle is needed before all symptoms associated with the menstrual cycle can be fully understood and effectively treated.

Dysmenorrhoea

Dysmenorrhoea is defined as pain with menstruation. Two types, *primary* and *secondary* dysmenorrhoea, are commonly distinguished.

Primary dysmenorrhoea

Primary dysmenorrhoea is a spasmodic type of pain, occurring at the onset of the menstrual period and lasting from 1 to 24 hours. It is most common among young girls, beginning with the menarche and fading away around 24 years of age or after the delivery of a full-term infant. No pathology in pelvic structures is associated with this type of dysmenorrhoea. In addition to the cramps, there may be shivering, a feeling of tension, nausea, vomiting, pallor and syncope.

Prostaglandins are considered to be the cause of the increased myometrial activity and subsequent pain experienced. Excessive quantities of prostaglandins are synthesized during the breakdown of the secretory endometrium in some women. They cause increased muscular contractions and uterine ischaemia, and are also responsible for the symptoms of nausea, vomiting and pallor by their influence on smooth muscle. Other cramps are caused by clots stretching the internal os of the cervix. Dysmenorrhoea is also associated with ovulation, as anovulatory cycles are rarely accompanied by dysmenorrhoea.

Analgesics that are prostaglandin inhibitors (e.g. ibuprofen, mefenamic acid) may be prescribed together with a course of oral contraceptives. This induces anovulatory periods and may be followed by very good results. It may be diagnostic: should dysmenorrhoea continue, the doctor may look for other causes.

Nursing intervention

The school, practice or occupational nurse commonly deals with the young woman suffering from dysmenorrhoea. The patient may present herself in their office, or the nurse may be asked to interview the girl or woman who frequently misses school or work because of dysmenorrhoea. Frequent, severe dysmenorrhoea should always be investigated by the gynaecologist; it is the nurse's responsibility to suggest this to the patient and assist her in obtaining this care.

Secondary dysmenorrhoea

Secondary dysmenorrhoea is a constant type of pain which often starts 2–3 days before the period and persists well past the first day. It may continue for a day or two after the period. Pain may radiate through the abdomen into the back and down the thighs. It occurs after several years of normal painless menses and is frequently associated with pelvic pathology. The most frequent causes are endometriosis, tumours, inflammatory disease and fixed malpositions of the uterus. It is essentially a symptom of disease. Should the nurse be consulted by a woman describing these symptoms, the woman should be referred to a gynaecologist.

Abnormal bleeding patterns

Terms used to describe irregular, absent or excessive patterns of bleeding are defined in Box 23.5.

Dysfunctional uterine bleeding

True dysfunctional uterine bleeding refers to that which occurs in the presence of endocrine dysfunction rather than organic disease. It may be seen as chronic epimenorrhagia or even as an episode of acute bleeding. Some episodes of haemorrhage are caused by high levels of oestrogen in the proliferative phase of the cycle. These high levels depress the hypothalamus–pituitary complex and no ovulation occurs. Because there is no ovulation, no progesterone is produced and the endometrium remains proliferative. As oestrogen levels fall, usually after a 6–8-week period of amenorrhoea, bleeding occurs. This disorder is associated with the older woman.

Box 23.5   Abnormal bleeding patterns

■ *Amenorrhoea* – absence of menstruation; may be primary, where the periods fail to start at puberty, or secondary, where periods stop after several months or years of normal menses

■ *Menorrhagia* – excessive bleeding at the time of normal menses

■ *Polymenorrhoea* – cyclical bleeding that is normal but occurs too frequently

■ *Epimenorrhagia* – cyclical bleeding that is both excessive and too frequent

■ *Metorrhagia* – any bleeding that occurs between menstrual periods; any bleeding per vagina at any time other than normal menses is included, even if it amounts to only slight staining.

Other episodes of bleeding are related to fluctuating oestrogen levels produced by an imperfectly functioning hypothalamus–pituitary–ovary feedback mechanism. Follicles are stimulated to partial maturation: some oestrogen is produced but then the level falls, producing intermittent, irregular and possibly prolonged bleeding. The causes are related to immaturity or ageing of the feedback mechanism. In most cases treatment consists of administering oral contraceptives. They exert a regulating and inhibiting effect on the endometrium and feedback mechanism. Three to six cycles of hormonal therapy are usually required to re-establish the normal menstrual pattern.

Endometriosis

Endometriosis is the location of endometrial tissue outside the uterine cavity. The disease was first recorded in 1860, but understanding of its process is still under discussion and research. It appears to be associated with retrograde menstruation (bleeding into the peritoneal cavity via the fallopian tubes). This occurs in up to 90% of all women (Halme et al 1984). However, why it adversely affects only approximately 7% of the female population is not understood, although there may be an immunological response (Barbieri 1990).

The role of oestrogen is under scrutiny. If the disease is oestrogen dependent that explains why it is rarely found in pubescent girls or menopausal women (unless receiving oestrogen-based HRT). Oophorectomy (removal of the ovaries) has proved an effective treatment. It is significant that development of the disease in males who are receiving oestrogen hormone therapy has been reported.

The endometrial tissue can be found in the peritoneal cavity, on the broad ligaments, ovaries and in the pouch of Douglas. It responds to the menstrual cycle by proliferating and shedding in response to oestrogen and progesterone. The blood collects in small scars of bluish-black colour, usually pea sized but sometimes bigger. If the cyst ruptures, the bloody contents will promote the development of adhesions which may distort the position of the uterus and fallopian tubes, leading to infertility.

Symptoms and diagnosis

The patient may have no symptomatology, and the disease may be discovered only incidentally at abdominal surgery. More commonly, the patient complains of pain. Secondary dysmenorrhoea may appear, with pain becoming severe 1–2 days before menstruation. The pain gradually becomes worse and may be described as 'boring'. This is due to the distension and pain of the swollen, shedding areas contained within the fibrous capsule of the cysts. The patient may also complain of backache and dyspareunia of a deep nature localized in the posterior fornix of the vagina. Pain may be of an acute nature, localized in the abdomen, when a cyst ruptures. The gynaecologist may suspect endometriosis when a patient is infertile, because infertility is a common symptom of this group of patients. Sometimes the adhesions become severe enough to cause a bowel obstruction or painful micturition.

Diagnosis is frequently confirmed on bimanual examination when firm nodular lumps are felt in the adnexa. Visualizing the typical bluish nodules may be done by culdoscopy, laparoscopy or during a laparotomy. Diagnosis is confirmed by biopsy when endometrial glands and stroma are seen microscopically.

Laparoscopy

The gynaecologist may feel that direct viewing of the pelvic organs is necessary, in which case laparoscopy is used, usually as a day case. Laparoscopy provides direct visualization of the anterior aspect of the tubes and ovaries. The procedure is done under general anaesthesia and aseptic conditions.

To avoid damage and to obtain a better visualization of the abdominal and pelvic contents, the cavity is distended by the introduction of carbon dioxide. The abdominal wall is lifted by the gas above the underlying organs. The patient is tilted head downwards to about a 45° angle, shifting the abdominal contents up and away from the site of insertion of the laparoscope and from the pelvis. Through a small incision in the lower rim of the umbilicus, a trocar and cannula are inserted on an angle; the trocar is then withdrawn and the endoscope inserted. It enters the peritoneal cavity approximately half-way between the umbilicus and the symphysis pubis. The contents of the abdomen and pelvis are observed and the uterus may be manipulated from below by a clamp in the cervix. This changes angles and brings the organs into better view. At the end of the procedure the endoscope is withdrawn, the gas expressed from the abdomen through the cannula, and the incision closed with a clip or stitch that is removed in 24–48 hours.

There are few complications, but cardiac arrhythmias, collapse and death have been recorded. The patient may complain of some mild abdominal or shoulder pain following the procedure. This is usually abdominal gas, which collects beneath the diaphragm. The gas is absorbed gradually over a few days, but a change of position may help. Severe pain or signs of abdominal tenderness or tightness should be reported.

Hysteroscopy

In this technique, a fine scope is used to view the uterine cavity through the cervix. The procedure is carried out as a day case and the woman can be informed of the results and the plan of treatment on the same day, which is a major advantage.

Treatment of endometriosis

This is based on the age of the patient, her desire for more children and the severity of the disease. Pregnancy relieves the symptoms and may be advised if the couple want children. Pseudo-pregnancy may be achieved by the administration of progestogen for varying periods of time, or danazol 200–800 mg daily for 6 months. Danazol is a synthetic androgen which suppresses ovulatory function and inhibits LH and FSH synthesis and release. This produces amenorrhoea and an atrophic endometrium for the duration of therapy. Some women have intermittent spotting during therapy. When therapy is discontinued, the patient usually remains symptom-free for a period.

Treatment may be surgical and is directed at preserving reproductive function. Affected areas are ablated by laser and fixed organs are released. Infertility often ceases after operation. In very severe cases a hysterectomy may be done. Depending on the extent of cystic involvement, oophorectomy may also be performed. The symptoms usually disappear at menopause as ovarian atrophy begins and hormonal stimulation declines.

Nursing care for hysterectomy

For many women the final recourse to resolve menstrual and postmenstrual problems is to have a hysterectomy. Traditionally this has been performed via the abdomen. Whilst vaginal hysterectomies have been done for 30 years, it is only with the advent of the laparoscope that their frequency is increasing. The decision about which route relies not only on the mobility of the uterus but also the patient's social conditions at home, as discharge is likely within 3–4 days (Hancock and Scott 1993). Both routes may include a bilateral salpingo-oophorectomy (removal of the ovaries and fallopian tubes). If the woman is premenopausal, this procedure immediately induces the menopause and, because of the implications of removing the ovaries, the patient may be prescribed HRT.

On return from theatre, the patient is given intravenous fluids until she can tolerate drinks and food.

Those who have had a vaginal hysterectomy may have a vaginal pack and catheter, both of which should be removed after 24 hours. Observations of the vaginal or abdominal wound loss are essential for the detection of haemorrhage. Pelvic pain and pyrexia are indicators of pelvic haematoma, and infections are not uncommon, although they may not manifest themselves for 7–10 days. In both instances, the woman is likely to have been discharged by the time symptoms appear.

Interruptions of pregnancy

Abortion

An abortion is the cessation of a pregnancy before the 24th week of pregnancy. It may be induced or occur spontaneously, the lay term for a spontaneous abortion being a 'miscarriage'. The incidence of abortion is difficult to state accurately but between 10 and 20% of all conceptions are thought to abort. A classification of abortion is given in Figure 23.9.

Most known causes can be separated into three major groups: fetal, maternal and faulty environment. Fetal causes are often associated with chromosomal or other abnormalities that are incompatible with life. This has been considered to be as high as 40% of all causes of abortion. Maternal and environmental causes are more varied. For example, severe infection in the mother may lead to endotoxins invading the fetus, usually causing its death and later expulsion. Drugs ingested by the mother may damage the fetus directly or may damage the placenta and hence the nutrition of the fetus. Hormonal imbalances may be the cause of some abortions, especially in cases where the thyroid gland is involved. Lack of progesterone may result in a poorly developed endometrium. As a result, implantation of the fertilized ovum in the endometrium (nidation) does not occur, or does so ineffectively. Anatomical uterine defects or uterine pathology cause some abortions. Nutritional factors are linked to abortion and premature labour, for adequate nutrition of the woman plays an important role in her reproductive capacity. The emotional state of the woman is also considered a possible contributing factor. This often centres on fear, grief or emotional trauma in susceptible women. Physical trauma can also induce an abortion. This may be true of surgery performed during pregnancy.

A threatened abortion is one in which the threat to the pregnancy is slight. With care, the woman may carry the pregnancy to term. As any bleeding, however minor, per vagina is abnormal in the pregnant woman, any evidence of such bleeding is taken as a sign of threatened abortion until proven otherwise. In addition, some backache or mild intermittent lower abdominal pain may be present. If the abortion is not immediate, cramping and bleeding continue, cramps become stronger and regular, the cervix dilates and the membranes rupture.

Figure 23.9 Classification of abortion.

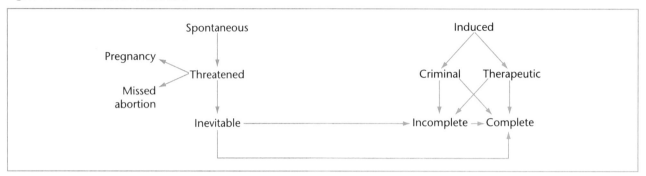

The inevitable abortion becomes the complete abortion when all products of conception are expelled. This usually occurs before the 12th week of gestation. The abortion is incomplete when some of the products of conception are retained. This is usually the placenta and membranes, and is more frequent following the 12th week, when the placenta is more firmly embedded.

A missed abortion is one in which the fetus dies and symptoms of pregnancy cease, if they had been present at all, and the products of conception are retained in the uterus. After this, the uterus is not observed to increase in size. Indeed, it begins to regress slightly as the amniotic fluid is absorbed. No fetal heart is heard. The patient remains amenorrhoeic and the breasts regress. The abortus is usually expelled spontaneously and may be retained.

A woman is considered to be a 'habitual aborter' when she aborts three or more consecutive pregnancies. The causes can be any of the causes of a single abortion but persist through several pregnancies. In addition, an incompetent cervix is frequently associated with loss of pregnancy in the second trimester. Possibly because of inherent problems in the cervix or trauma to the cervix, the cervix dilates easily and will not retain the pregnancy. Loss of the pregnancy usually occurs later, at about 16–20 weeks. Dilatation of the cervix is rapid, with little pain and bleeding. Rupture of the membranes occurs, followed by the expulsion of the fetus.

Treatment and nursing care

Threatened abortion

The treatment of threatened abortion is aimed at preserving the pregnancy. Ideally every woman should know how to recognize pregnancy and be aware that bleeding is not normal. In this case she should notify the midwife or doctor straight away.

There is a growing number of early pregnancy assessment units to which a woman with early pregnancy bleeding may be referred. This allows the woman immediate access to care, which will include ultrasonographic assessment and psychological support for herself and her partner. Admission to hospital has been significantly reduced. Bleeding usually ceases within 24–48 hours. If the cervix is seen to be closed on careful speculum examination, the pregnancy is generally thought to be safe. This examination will also reveal other causes of bleeding, such as vaginal infection or cervical erosions.

If the woman is admitted because bleeding persists, observations of vaginal blood loss are essential. All packs and clots should be saved to estimate loss, and tissue sent for histological examination. Other observations of pulse, blood pressure and temperature will be done as the woman's condition dictates.

On discharge home, the patient is instructed to take extra rest and to avoid strenuous exercise, heavy lifting or fatigue. Coitus may be restricted for a period of 2 weeks or longer. Should bleeding recur, the woman generally has access back to the pregnancy assessment unit via her general practitioner or midwife.

Missed abortion

Missed abortion is generally not diagnosed until the woman attends for review or for her first antenatal visit. She may or may not have experienced some brown vaginal loss. There may be a weak pregnancy test result that indicates only the presence of placental tissue. On enquiry the midwife or nurse may ascertain that the early symptoms of pregnancy diminished earlier than expected. Diagnosis is made by ultrasonography.

If missed abortion is confirmed, the obstetrician is faced with choice of evacuating the uterus or waiting until it is done spontaneously. Physically there is usually no pressing need, but emotionally it is very distressing to the woman and her family to know that she is carrying a dead fetus. The danger from disseminated intravascular coagulation (DIC) as a complicating factor increases if the dead fetus is retained. This occurs as some of the degenerating products of the fetus enter the maternal bloodstream. This danger appears to be the most serious about 4–6 weeks after fetal death. Coagulation studies may be done before intervention is attempted.

For these reasons the obstetrician usually intervenes approximately 2 weeks after the estimated death of the fetus. The dead fetus may be aborted by means of suction evacuation if death occurs before 12 weeks of gestation, or by prostaglandin administration if it occurs during the second trimester. The procedure is emotionally and physically exhausting for the patient. She requires much supportive nursing care. Also, the contractions are painful, and analgesia should be administered. As no danger can result to the fetus, the mother need not suffer unduly. Close observation of the patient's condition for overhydration is necessary because of the danger of administering large amounts of fluid containing synthetic oxytocin, which has an antidiuretic action. An intake and output record should be kept.

Inevitable abortion

The treatment of an inevitable abortion is similar to that of a threatened abortion. The patient is placed on bedrest. Blood is taken for estimation of haemoglobin, typing and cross-matching. The amount and character of the bleeding is observed carefully. Blood pressure and pulse may need to be taken every 10 minutes if bleeding is profuse, and the patient must be observed for other signs of shock. Any tissue or suspicious clots are saved to be examined for traces of fetus and placenta. If products of conception are retained, the uterus must be emptied. The two causes of significant bleeding are retained products of conception and spontaneous coagulation of exposed blood vessels, which may occur when the uterus fails to contract. Wherever products of conception remain, the potential for infection is high.

If the bleeding is prolonged and the woman is in severe pain, it may be that products of conception are trapped in the cervix. Immediate treatment is necessary on the ward to remove clots and products from the cervical os. The doctor will use a speculum, sponge, forceps and swabs, and will require a light to remove the trapped products. Intramuscular injection of ergometrine will help to contract the uterus to minimize the blood loss once the products have been removed.

If the situation is not life threatening, then dilatation of the cervix and evacuation to remove products of conception may be performed. Perforation of the uterus is always a possibility, so observation for interabdominal haemorrhage as well as vaginal loss should be made.

Packing of the vagina is uncommon as it can mask the degree of blood loss. Most women are allowed home once their physical condition allows, between 4 and 18 hours after operation. All products of conception are saved for histological examination.

If the abortion has been complete, the woman is treated similarly to the postpartum patient. If the patient has a Rh-negative blood group, she receives Rh_0 (anti-D immunoglobulin) to prevent the formation of antibodies in further pregnancies. A slight lochial discharge is expected and the woman must be advised upon perineal care. Depending on the state of health, she will be discharged home on the same day. To reduce the risk of infection, coitus is contraindicated until lochial discharge has ceased. This usually occurs within 2 weeks.

Incompetent cervical os

The patient who has had several abortions will receive a thorough assessment between pregnancies in an attempt to ascertain her problem. Should the cause be considered an incompetent cervical os, the obstetrician may attempt to tighten the cervix with a suture. This is usually done from 12 to 16 weeks of pregnancy. The Shirker technique consists of running a non-dissolving suture around the cervix like a drawstring or purse string.

On the return from the operating theatre, the pregnant patient is observed for signs of labour and imminent abortion. Should the abortion appear inevitable, the suture is removed and vaginal delivery follows, or the suture is retained and delivery is by caesarian section.

Emotional response to spontaneous abortion

In early abortion, the response to the loss may be surprise, disappointment, grief, guilt and anger in differing proportions depending on the meaning of the loss at that time. The woman who has had several abortions may be experiencing this loss and also the threat of the loss of ability to ever bear a live child.

Most women express surprise at the abortion. They are unprepared for the pain, loss of blood and, if recognizable or noticed, the sight of the fetus. It seems that the concept of a baby is so vague in their minds at this time that such real evidence of a fetus is unexpected. Because of the ambivalence of the first trimester, many feel guilt associated with the negative thoughts they may have had about the pregnancy or its timing. The partner too may have to readjust to his revised status.

In later abortion, the pregnancy has usually been accepted as real and the fetus becomes a baby to the majority of women. Most couples have begun to establish a relationship with the baby, and loss at this stage is usually perceived as the loss of a baby. There may be more desire to see the fetus, to know the sex and weight, and to identify the baby by name even though it may legally be an abortion. Emotional response may be more intense and appear more painful if there is no 'object' to attach the pain to. Seeing the infant or keeping a picture of the baby may assist with the grieving and the resolution of the loss for some parents. Others will not choose or require such a method of relating to the fetus.

The reactions of parents who have chosen therapeutic abortion for genetic reasons are similar to those of these parents. Guilt may be increased in some. Others are fearful of the censure and disapproval of hospital staff. Immediate nursing interventions are aimed at acknowledging the loss, accepting the feelings and wishes of the parents, and reinforcing reality. This assists in promoting the long-term goal of resolution of normal grieving, which takes a few months.

A brief review of the grieving process with the parents is helpful (see Ch. 4) so that they will understand the feelings of grief, irritability and fatigue that may come. The value of rest, sleep and exercise in coping with grieving is stressed. Unequal patterns of grieving and ways of obtaining support are discussed.

Religious rites

If the patient who aborts is Roman Catholic, the fetus can be baptized. In addition, some Protestants may feel strongly that the fetus should be baptized. The nurse may ascertain this by tactfully enquiring what the patient's wishes are. Baptism may be performed by any person, regardless of their religious beliefs. If available, a member of the clergy should be asked to perform this rite; if not, the nurse may have to baptize the fetus. Clear water must be poured over the head of the fetus while the nurse pronounces the words: 'I baptize you in the name of the Father and of the Son and of the Holy Spirit'. Other religious groups may have special rites which they wish to perform. The nurse assesses this with the parents and provides support and help.

Some late abortions may require burial, which can now be arranged with local funeral parlours and crematoriums. The arrangements may vary, but it is recognized that some parents appreciate having a place to go and continue the grieving process. Other parents may need practical assistance on how to go about this, for example referral to the appropriate chaplaincy or social work services. Follow-up support is a great value to some. This is frequently through the Miscarriage Association.

Therapeutic abortion

The past few years have seen a large increase in the number of therapeutic or induced abortions performed throughout the world, in response to the liberalization of abortion laws. It is estimated that legal abortion for social and medical reasons is now available to over half the world's population, making therapeutic abortion one of the most common medical procedures performed. This raises serious questions about poor contraceptive provision and advice, environmental factors and women's role in society.

The laws governing abortions vary from country to country. In all nations legal codes exist defining the conditions under which an abortion may be done. They outline who may do an abortion, where it may be done (in or outside the hospital), and when it may be done in relationship to the length of gestation. The law also defines the social and medical conditions that constitute cause for an abortion. In the UK, the Abortion Act 1967 gives indications and restrictions for therapeutic abortion (Box 23.6). All abortions performed outside the limits of the legal condition are illegal. In many countries, assisting a patient to procure an abortion outside the law is also punishable by law. For these reasons the nurse should be acquainted with the law pertaining to the area in which he or she practises.

Box 23.6 Indications for therapeutic abortion under the Abortion Act 1967

1. The continuance of the pregnancy would involve risk to the pregnant woman greater than if the pregnancy were terminated.

2. The continuance of the pregnancy would involve risk of injury to the physical or mental health of the pregnant woman greater than if the pregnancy were terminated.

3. The continuance of the pregnancy would involve risk of injury to the physical or mental health of the existing child(ren) of the family of the pregnant woman greater than if the pregnancy were terminated.

4. There is substantial risk that if the child were born it would suffer from such physical or mental abnormalities as to be seriously handicapped.

The restrictions

1. That one or more of the above conditions are believed to be present in the opinion of two doctors, who are acting together in good faith and in full knowledge of the facts.

2. That this opinion be notified to the Department of Health (or appropriate authority in Scotland and Northern Ireland).

3. That the operation be carried out in a NHS hospital or an approved establishment.

4. That the doctor carrying out the operation notify the Department of Health (or appropriate authority in Scotland and Northern Ireland).

5. That the consent of the woman be obtained. If the patient is under the age of 16 years, the consent of the parents is also necessary.

Early abortions

Most abortions performed before 12–14 weeks of gestation are done by suction, dilatation and curettage (D&C). If done before 8 weeks of gestation, the cervix usually does not require dilatation but it is more difficult to ensure complete evacuation of the products of conception. The procedure is most commonly done on a day-care basis. A general anaesthetic may be given but many abortions, particularly those not requiring cervical dilatation, may be done without anaesthesia or with a local anaesthetic such as a paracervical block. Some surgeons administer intravenous oxytocin (Syntocinon) before suctioning to ensure a strong firm contraction of the uterus; others do not consider this necessary.

The aspirated tissue is caught in a gauze trap to facilitate recovery for immediate inspection and for examination by the pathologist. Immediate identification of fetal tissue is important to confirm the diagnosis of an intrauterine pregnancy that has been completely evacuated. It is necessary to confirm the intrauterine pregnancy to avoid an ectopic pregnancy continuing unnoticed. Immediate inspection and, later, pathology reports may confirm a molar pregnancy which, if left undetected, would deprive the patient of important follow-up care.

Many patients experience some cramping following abortion, which is normal. The cramps are frequently gone by the the time the effects of the anaesthetic, either general or paracervical, are over, but may persist for longer. A mild analgesic may be required. The patient is then observed for a few hours more or allowed to go home with instructions, depending upon her condition.

Mifepristone (RU486) Mifepristone is an antiprogesterone agent used as a medical method of inducing abortion. A pregnancy requires progesterone to prevent uterine contraction. Abortion is induced between 36 and 48 hours using a combination of mifepristone and Gemprost under medical supervision.

Late abortions

When the pregnancy is more than 12–14 weeks a D&C becomes more difficult. Other methods must be selected by the gynaecologist, who may decide to induce labour by means of an intra-amniotic injection. The technique and preparation are similar to the paracentesis, but an amniocentesis is performed. With strict sterile technique the patient's abdomen is prepared and draped. A skin wheal is made with a local anaesthetic agent and a needle is inserted through the abdomen, into the amniotic cavity. One of several agents is injected into the uterine cavity: urea, glucose, hypertonic saline and prostaglandins have all been used. Hypertonic saline and prostaglandins seem to be used most commonly. If the drug chosen is saline, some amniotic fluid is withdrawn and replaced with an equal amount of 20% saline solution. The fetus dies and the uterus is apparently irritated and begins to contract. The contractions may need to be assisted with an oxytocic medication given intravenously.

Later pregnancies of 16–20 weeks' gestation may be terminated by the performance of a hysterotomy. This means that an incision is made into the uterus and the contents are removed. It is a miniature caesarian section. After operation the fundus must be checked for firmness and position. Lochia is observed for colour, amount and odour, as haemorrhage or infection may occur. Vulval care is carried out.

Prostaglandins may be given in an intravenous drip which is carefully regulated by an infusion pump. The dosage is started at very low levels; the responses of the patient, fetus and uterus are carefully monitored. The dose is increased gradually until the uterus is contracting satisfactorily. Labour and delivery or abortion will follow for most patients in 12–24 hours. If the stimulation is not sufficient, additional stimulation with oxytocin may be given. This is associated with an increased risk of rupture of the cervix and uterus, so the response of the contracting uterus must be monitored carefully. The patient's complaints of discomfort or pain should be heeded. The cervix may be softened by applying a topical prostaglandin preparation.

Extra-amniotic injection with prostaglandins is another common method of inducing abortion. A polyethylene tubing or Foley catheter is passed under aseptic conditions through the cervix, and directed between the uterine wall and the membranes. The bag of the Foley catheter is inflated to help retain the catheter in the uterus. The tube is attached to further tubing attached to a syringe containing the solution. The rate of infusion is controlled with an infusion pump. Small amounts are injected and the uterine response is observed. The dose is increased gradually. Abortion occurs between 12 and 24 hours later.

Nursing care

After operation the patient is nursed similarly to a patient who has had a spontaneous abortion, with a D&C to complete the process. In late abortions the patient requires more intensive nursing care. While the intra-amniotic injections are being given, the patient must be observed for reactions to the drug injected. Hypertonic saline may be absorbed into the circulatory system. To avoid this a small amount is injected, the patient's response assessed, and then the remainder injected. If saline is being absorbed intravascularly, she may complain of confusion, heat sensations, headache, tinnitus, a dry mouth and tachycardia. In this event the saline is stopped and the injection site altered. When the injection is completed, the patient awaits the beginning of contractions. To reduce the risk of infection, oxytocin is usually begun within 12 hours if uterine contractions are not adequate. The patient may express some thirst during this period of waiting. All patients who have been given saline absorb a portion of it, thus producing some electrolyte imbalance. Fluid is required and the woman should be allowed to drink.

The woman experiences labour and requires the support and care that are given to any labouring patient. This includes appropriate analgesia as the contractions are distressing. Bedrest is usually maintained after active labour begins or after the administration of an opiate. With extra-amniotic injection of prostaglandins the catheter may be expelled as the uterus contracts and the cervix dilates. Oxytocin stimulation may be required to maintain labour.

Most patients having an abortion are discharged within hours of being aborted, or within 1–2 days. They need clear discharge instructions so that they may take care of themselves in the days that follow. Each patient must be told:

■ to resume normal activities gradually

■ to expect intermittent menstrual-like discharge for the next week or two, but no heavy, bright-red bleeding

- to use sanitary pads as long as bleeding occurs; the use of tampons is inadvisable

- that some cramping may occur but should not persist or be severe

- to report any fever or unusual discomfort

- to expect a menstrual period within 4–5 weeks of the procedure; if this does not occur, it may indicate a continuing intrauterine or extrauterine pregnancy or a new pregnancy. Ovulation occurs as early as 18 days after an abortion and pregnancy is possible immediately. Birth control advice and teaching should be given to the patient as necessary

- that it is wise to limit coitus while the menstrual-like flow continues, to reduce the risk of infection

- to contact clinic immediately if any unusual signs should occur

- when she is to return for a follow-up visit

- how to obtain support and counselling after discharge as if for a spontaneous abortion.

While therapeutic abortion is now associated with low maternal morbidity and mortality rates (lower than for pregnancy in many countries), it does carry some serious risks that need to be considered. Psychiatric sequelae are rare but do occur. The main concern appears to be an increased incidence of spontaneous abortion and premature labour in women who have had a previous abortion. The risk is greatest with the older methods of dilatation and curettage, and is greater still when damage to the cervix has been documented. It is important to educate women to seek abortion as early as possible so that the need to dilate the cervix is reduced. Prevention is better than cure, and birth control should be seen as the first line of defence. Nursing has an important role to play by providing knowledge of and access to birth control to those who need it.

Criminal abortion

Criminal abortion is a dangerous procedure. Often women attempt to abort themselves by means of strong douches or instruments which they insert into the uterus. Frequently, the instrument used punctures the posterior fornix of the vagina, the cervix or perforates the uterus. The bowel may be involved should the instrument be inserted far enough. Conditions are furtive, untrained people frequently officiate, and sterility is not maintained. These patients frequently contract an infection and present a grave situation. The situation is known as a septic abortion. Infection is essentially an endometritis, which may spread to peritonitis or to septicaemia.

Ectopic pregnancy

Implantation of the fertilized ovum anywhere outside the uterine cavity is considered an ectopic pregnancy. Most frequently this occurs in the ampullary portion of the fallopian tube, but it may be ovarian, abdominal or cervical. Women with a history of one ectopic pregnancy have an increased risk of having a second one.

An ectopic pregnancy results when the passage of the zygote to the uterine cavity is impeded or slowed. Any blocking of the tube or reduction in tubal peristalsis will cause this. Previous salpingitis, tumours and hormonal imbalances may all play a part. As implantation occurs, the chorionic villi burrow into the thin tubal wall. Eventually, they burrow into a blood vessel and bleeding occurs. If the bleeding is sufficient, the fetus dies – this is the fate of most. The abortus may be retained in the tube as a tubal mole or may be extruded through the end of the fallopian tube as a tubal abortion. Occasionally, the trophoblast burrows through the wall of the tube and out into the peritoneal cavity. This is known as a ruptured tubal pregnancy and often occurs as the result of a pregnancy in the narrow isthmus of the tube. A secondary abdominal pregnancy may follow if the chorionic villi settle elsewhere in the abdominal cavity and begin to grow.

The incidence of ectopic pregnancy has been increasing throughout the Western world in the past 10–15 years. The increase seems to be due to many factors such as an increase in pelvic infection, widespread IUD use, fertility induced by ovulatory agents, reconstructive surgery of fallopian tubes, or better and earlier diagnosis. The condition is a serious one and ectopic pregnancy still contributes significantly to maternal mortality statistics.

Effects on the patient

The woman has a history of the early signs of pregnancy, including amenorrhoea usually of 6–10 weeks' duration. Soon after her first missed period she may have complaints of a localized pain on one side, probably due to distension of the tube. After that she may have sharper, intermittent pain in the same area. This may be due to strong peristaltic waves of the tube attempting to pass the embryo or abortus along the tube. At some point the patient may experience a sharp, severe pain. This is probably synchronous with separation of the embryo and some haemorrhage. The sharp pain may be followed by generalized abdominal discomfort as blood spills into the abdomen. Referred shoulder pain may occur. At this point many women present for treatment.

Diagnosis usually includes a single radioimmunoassay pregnancy test, or serial ones, ultrasonography and, if necessary, culdocentesis or laparoscopy, depending on the urgency of the presenting symptoms. Examination of patients with suspected ectopic pregnancy should be gentle as too vigorous an examination may precipitate an acute rupture before surgery can prevent it.

Acute ruptured tubal pregnancy

Sometimes the patient reports no early symptoms but experiences one episode of acute abdominal pain shortly after her missed period. This acute pain is often accompanied by vomiting and fainting. Some vaginal bleeding may be present but appears too minimal to warrant the reaction of the patient. The patient may go rapidly into shock with a drop in blood pressure, rapid weak pulse, pallor, sweating, low temperature and cold extremeties. The abdomen is distended with blood and may be tight and tender to touch. A pelvic examination of the patient may be difficult because of the exquisite tenderness. The patient presents as an emergency situation.

When the diagnosis of a ruptured tubal pregnancy is confirmed, a salpingectomy (removal of the fallopian tube) with the removal of the fetus is performed. Ectopic pregnancies in other locations are investigated in a similar fashion. Treatment is usually surgical removal of the fetus. However, abdominal pregnancies have been carried to term and have been delivered by laparotomy.

Tumours of the trophoblast

Trophoblastic tumours are a group of neoplasms that arise in the chorionic villi of the fertilized ovum during the trophoblast stage. The condition is rare in Europe and North America, occurring about once in every 2500 pregnancies. It is more prevalent in the Far East. The reason for this is not known. The tumours range from benign to malignant. Not all benign tumours become malignant, nor are all malignant tumours preceded by a benign stage.

Hydatidiform mole is an abnormal development of the chorionic villi of the conceptus. A true mole is now known to occur when the chromosomal pattern is 45,XX and the source of the chromatin material is paternal. No maternal chromatin has been lost or inactivated. The haploid sperm (23) then undergoes endo-replication. Some moles are 46,XY and these are the result of two sperm fertilizing one empty ovum. The conceptus is really an abnormal development of the placenta, which begins to develop the characteristic mole pattern about the fifth week of life.

The intermediate stages are characterized by an increased ability to invade uterine musculature and to send bloodborne deposits of trophoblast cells throughout the body. However, in some cases, the host – or pregnant woman – seems able to contain the spread of the tumour and it disappears. The intermediate stage is frequently not identified clinically but is obvious only on pathological examinations of specimens of tissue. This means that all moles must be treated as potentially malignant until demonstrated otherwise.

Effects on the patient

The patient exhibits the signs and symptoms of early pregnancy, particularly excessive vomiting. The uterus is often much larger than expected for the weeks of gestation. About the 12th week, some vaginal bleeding may occur, and this is often the first sign of some abnormality. No fetal movements are reported by the mother, and no fetal parts can be palpated. On palpation the uterus may have an elastic consistency. There is an increased incidence of pregnancy-induced hypertension, not usually expected in early pregnancy. Urine tests for the quantity of chorionic gonadotrophins excreted show very high titres that persist and do not fall as is usual in a normal pregnancy. These high levels also stimulate the formation of theca lutein cysts in the ovary. The cysts regress following abortion of the mole.

Treatment and nursing care

The patient is usually admitted to hospital and nursed as a threatened abortion until proven otherwise. All perineal pads are carefully inspected for pieces of the mole as this would be diagnostic. Thyroid function tests may be ordered, as high levels of chorionic gonadotrophins may exert a thyroid-stimulating effect.

Ultrasonography will show a distended uterus giving a 'snowflake' image, which is typical of a mole. Often the mole is partially absorbed spontaneously. Haemorrhage may be acute. Oxytocics are given to control the bleeding, and a careful and complete evacuation of the uterus is performed. Because of the danger of perforating the uterus in areas weakened by the erosion of the mole, a curette is not used. Instead, the cervix is dilated and suction equipment used to evacuate the uterine contents. After operation the patient is observed for signs of haemorrhage.

Because of the possibility of a malignancy occurring, the patient receives close follow-up care during the next 12–18 months. The first signs of recurrence of the mole or the development of a malignancy is a rising chorionic gonadotrophin level. Therefore, the urinary levels of gonadotrophin will be monitored at regular intervals. Amenorrhoea, metrorrhagia or persistent cystic ovaries may alert the gynaecologist to look for rising hormone levels. The patient is advised against pregnancy during this period, as early pregnancy also produces high chorionic gonadotrophin levels which could mask the signs. Cytotoxic drugs (such as methotrexate) are given in all intermediate cases, and may be given as prophylaxis to all women who have had a molar pregnancy.

Preparation for abdominal ultrasonography

Ultrasonography is being used increasingly in gynaecology for the localization of foreign objects in the uterus, the diagnosis of tumours of the uterus, ovary and tubes, ectopic pregnancy, and as a device to outline precise areas for irradiation. The patient suffers no discomfort save that of a full bladder during the procedure.

In preparation for an ultrasonographic scan, the woman should drink 500–750 mL of water 1 hour before the appointment. The full bladder pushes the bowel away from the uterus and tubes, permitting better penetration of the sound waves. At the same time the uterus is pushed up and away from the symphysis pubis, allowing better visualization. The full bladder also provides a water path or window through which to look – a landmark in the abdomen – as it is clearly outlined, and provides an internal reference standard for density comparisons.

Infections of the reproductive tract

Bartholinitis

Bartholinitis is an infection of the greater vestibular gland and may or may not be gonorrhoeal in origin. The infection is an ascending one, progressing up the ducts to the gland. Symptoms are usually those of an acute infection: pain, swelling, inflammation and a purulent discharge. Cellulitis of the surrounding tissues aggravates the situation, but the infection may localize and become an abscess. This is usually excised and drained. Sometimes the infection subsides, leaving the duct scarred and occluded. This may be followed by a cyst filled with the secretions of the gland, which cannot now escape. The cyst is usually a painless swelling in the lower third of the labium minus. Treatment is to excise the cyst and gland. Alternatively, a marsupialization (conversion of the duct into a pouch) of the cystic duct may be done. This leaves the functioning gland in place.

Frequent baths and/or use of a bidet are advised, as well as careful drying of the vulva and perineum. The use of a cool hairdryer is preferable to towels to reduce the risk of cross-infection.

Bartholin glands
See chapter 6.3

Pelvic inflammatory disease

Pelvic inflammatory disease (PID) has come to mean all ascending pelvic infections once they are beyond the cervix. Many organisms may be responsible for the symptoms. However, among the most frequent are *Neisseria gonorrhoeae*, *Chlamydia* and *Staphylococcus aureus*.

Effects on the patient

The typical picture is one of systemic infection with fever, chills, malaise, anorexia, nausea and vomiting. This is usually accompanied by lower abdominal pain which is either unilateral or bilateral.

In more chronic cases this pain is increased before and during menstruation. Pain is experienced on movement of the cervix. Leucorrhoea is present. With gonorrhoeal or staphylococcal infections the discharge is usually heavy and purulent. Spread of infection occurs by two main routes, although a third is possible (Fig. 23.10).

Symptoms depend on which route the infection follows. In route I, the bacteria spread along the surface of the endometrium to the fallopian tubes and into the peritoneum. The consequences of this route may be adhesions or cysts of the tube, with consequent infertility. In more advanced cases abscesses develop about the ovary or in the cul-de-sac. Infection following route II is spread mainly through the lymphatics and produces a pelvic cellulitis, in contrast to the more localized endometritis

Figure 23.10   Common routes of the spread of pelvic inflammatory disease. Route I, commonly gonococcus and staphylococcus; route II, frequently streptococcus; route III, tuberculosis, usually a descending infection from another source.

or salpingitis (infection of the fallopian tube) of route I. Thrombophlebitis may follow this cellulitis. Advanced and virulent infections admitted by either route may become systemic and may show all the signs of septicaemia.

Treatment and nursing care

The patient with an acute episode is usually admitted to hospital. The patient is placed on bedrest in a semirecumbent position to promote drainage of pus into the vagina and the cul-de-sac. Heat to the lower back and abdomen may be soothing. Analgesics and sedation may be ordered. The patient will receive antibiotics following culture and sensitivity studies. In some cases blood cultures may be obtained. A culdocentesis or colpotomy may be done to drain a pelvic abscess. Tubo-ovarian abscesses may require an abdominal approach. In cases of prolonged, debilitating infection that is resistant to conservative treatment, salpingectomy or hysterectomy may be done. In the long term, women may experience infertility from occluded fallopian tubes or fimbria, or ovaries distorted by adhesions as a result of the infection.

Toxic shock syndrome

Toxic shock syndrome is a rare systemic disease occurring as a result of the circulating toxins produced by the bacterium *Staphylococcus aureus*. The organisms produce two toxins:

- enterotoxin F, which affects the intestinal mucosa causing gastroenteritis
- exotoxin C, which is pyrogenic.

Signs and symptoms occur following the introduction of toxins into the bloodstream. The disease varies from a subclinical form to a severe septicaemia. Clinical characteristics commonly include a high fever, rash, vomiting, diarrhoea, headache, sore throat and muscle pain. Hypotension progressing to shock occurs within 48 hours

> **Box 23.7**   General instructions for the use of tampons
>
> ■ Use only one tampon at a time.
>
> ■ Use a tampon of the absorbency that will control the flow; that is, never use one of super absorbency when a regular one would do. This reduces the chance of vaginal drying with subsequent trauma and ulceration.
>
> ■ Change the tampon frequently (every 4–6 hours).
>
> ■ Do not forget a tampon; always check by finger insertion in the vagina.
>
> ■ If you suspect an infection, immediately remove the tampon and consult your doctor.

in severe cases. Laboratory results indicate renal, hepatic and haematological involvement. Diagnosis is confirmed by swabs positive for *S. aureus* taken from the patient's nose, throat, vaginal discharge and blood cultures.

The disease is associated with intravaginal tampon use but is not caused by them. A significant number of women in the severe state are menstruating and using tampons. It is related to the fact that women have *S. aureus* present in the vagina. Tampons act as a dam to vaginal flow, providing ideal conditions to bacterial growth. Some tampons were found to carry the organisms and have now been withdrawn from the market. Synthetic material tampons aggravate the situation by their greater drying effect. They may create microulcerations in the vaginal mucosa, allowing microorganisms to escape into the bloodstream.

Treatment is supportive, aimed at relieving the symptoms, and curative by eradicating the source of toxin production. If associated with tampon use, the tampons are removed and the vagina cleansed with a disinfecting solution and daily saline douches. The patient receives systemic medication to which the organisms are sensitive. These measures prevent further development of the bacteria but are ineffective against the already circulating toxins.

Box 23.7 outlines general instructions for tampon use.

Vaginal discharge

Vaginal discharge may be normal physiological discharge, which is usually clear or white, non-irritating with a pH between 3.8 and 4.2, or it may be a symptom of intravaginal pathology or infection:

■ vaginitis – inflammation of the vagina, characterized by increased vaginal discharge containing increased white blood cells

■ vaginosis – characterized by increased vaginal discharge without inflammatory cells.

Leucorrhoea

Physiological leucorrhoea is a normal whitish discharge which helps to keep the vagina moist. It is composed of endocervical secretions, leucocytes, desquamated epithelial cells and other normal flora of the vaginal tract. The pH is normally 4–5 but varies during the life cycle of the woman. At birth, the pH may be as low as 5 under the hormonal stimulus of the mother. As a child it is 6–7. At menarche the pH becomes acidic again and assumes the adult pH of 4–5. Postmenopausally, oestrogen is withdrawn, and the pH rises to 6–7 again. The quantity of the discharge also varies among women during stages of the menstrual cycle and during pregnancy. An increase is usually noticed at ovulation, during sexual stimulation and during pregnancy.

Monilial vaginitis

Monilial **vaginitis** (thrush) occurs when the vagina is invaded by the fungus *Candida albicans*. Pregnant women and diabetics are predisposed because of glycosuria and the increased glycogen present in the vagina during pregnancy. Contamination may be from the rectum. A thick, white, curdy vaginal discharge is present which frequently causes pruritus and irritation of the vulva. The vaginal walls are reddened and covered with typical white patches. When the patches are swabbed off, bleeding may occur. Diagnosis is confirmed microscopically from a vaginal smear.

The patient is instructed in perineal care and hand washing to avoid reinfection and spread of the fungus to others, especially children. Nystatin vaginally or in the form of pessaries achieves good results, and may be given to pregnant women.

Vaginitis
See chapter 6.3

Sexually transmitted diseases

The health problem of greatest concern is AIDS. This produces a range of effects on the person and has been dealt with as appropriate elsewhere in this text. Other sexually transmitted infections are considered in this section. Sexually transmitted diseases (STDs) are an increasingly serious problem, especially in the younger population. Within the UK, the number of diagnoses of gonorrhoea, genital chlamydia and genital warts has risen steadily over the past 5 years. As with previous years, rises were sharpest in teenage males and females. Risky behaviour for the acquisition of a STD is listed in Box 23.8.

Gonorrhoea diagnoses in England rose steadily from 1995 to 1999, with a total increase of 56% (from 9962 to 15 572 patients). Infection is often asymptomatic, particularly in females. Some complications include infertility and ectopic pregnancy.

Diagnoses of chlamydial infection have almost doubled since 1995: from 29 286 to 51 863 in 1999. The rise occurred in all regions and in both sexes, with the

---

Box 23.8   Risky behaviour for STDs

■ Early age of sexual intercourse

■ Multiple sexual partners

■ Sexual abuse or rape

■ Sex with a homosexual or bisexual male

■ Anal sex

■ History of previous sexually transmitted infection

■ Alcohol and drug use, intravenous drug use (self and partner)

■ Prostitution

---

sharpest increase occurring in males and females under 20 years of age. Many cases of chlamydia infection are asymptomatic and thus go undiagnosed. Long-term complications can be severe, especially for females, in whom it can lead to pelvic inflammatory disease, ectopic pregnancy and infertility.

Genital warts in England have also risen steadily. Between 1995 and 1999, diagnoses of warts in 16–19-year-old males increased by 75%. The rise in females was also greatest in 16–19-year-olds. Warts are caused by a virus, the human papillomavirus (HPV). Certain types of wart have been associated with cervical cancer.

In the UK patients with STDs are treated in specialist genitourinary medicine departments on an outpatient basis. In assessing the patient the history is crucial and should include:

■ date of last menstrual period

■ current medications

■ current symptoms including the time of onset; colour, odour, quantity and consistency of discharge; bleeding; constant or intermittent symptoms; relationship of symptoms to sexual intercourse and menses

■ associated symptoms such as fever, abdominal, pelvic or joint pain, nausea, vomiting, diarrhoea, dysuria, haematuria, genital itching, swelling, burning, ulcerations and rash

■ social history including age of first sexual activity, frequency of sexual contacts, number of sexual partners, last sexual intercourse and partners over last 3 weeks, sexual preferences, known contact with STD risk, any partner symptoms, drug use

■ past medical history including previous STD, pregnancy history, methods of contraception (oral and barrier methods), recent antibiotic use

■ personal hygiene such as tampon use, douches, sprays, menstrual towels.

Common conditions are reviewed below.

Chlamydia trachomatis

A chlamydial infection is a parasitic sexually transmitted infection of the reproductive tract. The woman may present with symptoms of increased vaginal discharge, intermenstrual spotting and vague pelvic pain. Unfortunately, the woman is often asymptomatic and the infection may go unnoticed and untreated for several years.

Chlamydia is a common cause of pelvic inflammatory disease as well as an increasing cause of infertility.

Diagnosis is confirmed via an endocervical swab for cells using a *Chlamydia*-specific antigen swab. Doxycycline 100 mg twice daily for 7 days is an effective treatment. Azithromycin, one 1-g tablet by mouth, provides an equally effective cure and significantly reduces patient error regarding compliance.

Sexual partners of the woman require treatment as well.

Gonorrhoea

The specific organism causing gonorrhoea is *Neisseria gonorhoeae*, which is transmitted almost exclusively by sexual intercourse.

Symptoms appear 3–7 days after initial contact. Infection can be transmitted to the urethra, anus and cervix, as well as the nasopharynx. As many as 50–80% of women may be asymptomatic. Early symptoms may include labia pain and swelling, and purulent vaginal drainage. Untreated gonorrhoea can produce systemic infections characterized by joint pain and generalized rash.

Diagnosis is confirmed via endocervical, pharyngeal, rectal or urethral swabs as indicated. Special Thayer–Martin cultures or DNA Genprobes are utilized.

Ceftriaxone 250 mg intramuscularly once plus azithromycin 1 g by mouth provides excellent treatment for gonorrhoea as well as the assumed concomitant *Chlamydia* infection.

Partner notification and treatment is required.

Trichomoniasis

The most common cause of vaginitis is a flagellated protozoon, known as a trichomonad. Trichomonads may be found in the large bowel and occasionally in the bladder and vestibular glands. They can be sexually transmitted and in men trichomonads may be harboured in the urethra, bladder or prostate.

The woman presents with symptoms of a heavy, greenish-yellow frothy discharge which has a foul odour. This heavy discharge may be irritating to the vulva, causing pruritus and excoriation. The vaginal mucosa is reddened and is slightly oedematous. The patient may complain of dyspareunia and, if the bladder is involved, of dysuria and frequency. As the condition becomes chronic, the woman has fewer symptoms. Diagnosis is confirmed when trichomonads are seen microscopically in a vaginal smear.

Men frequently have few symptoms. There may be some urethral itching and a slight discharge. Invasion of the bladder may produce frequency and burning on micturition. Wet smears are made of the urethral discharge, and the protozoa seen microscopically confirm the diagnosis.

Treatment is usually the oral administration of metronidazole 250 mg three times a day for 10 days. Repeat smears will then be done, and a repeat course of therapy may be necessary. During treatment a condom should be worn until both partners are considered cured. The woman may be given vaginal pessaries instead of oral therapy. A pessary is inserted morning and night daily for 4–8 weeks. This is continued throughout the menstrual period, as the menstrual flow is alkaline and provides an excellent medium for growth of the protozoa. Insertion is like that of a vaginal tampon. The patient is instructed to remain flat for about 10 minutes after insertion.

It is important to advise the patient that no alcohol is to be consumed while on metronidazole therapy as severe gastrointestinal upset will occur.

Human papillomavirus infection

Human papillomavirus (HPV) is the causative organism in condylomata acuminata or genital warts. These warts may be confused with those of syphilis, but they are different: they are less flat and more cauliflower-like. Some attain a large size. The viral infection was previously thought to be benign but recently HPV has been associated with several genital cancers in both men and women.

The infection may be silent. No visible warts are present, but a type of HPV-induced cervical dysplasia exists that is seen during colposcopy or as a result of a smear test. In a number of those cases the dysplasia may progress to cervical neoplasia or, if on the vulva or vagina, to vulvar intraepithelial neoplasia (VIN). Some 40 or more types of the virus exist, but only a few are associated with malignant changes. The virus is not thought to be carcinogenic. Some other agent may trigger it to induce malignant changes or it may simply coexist with the oncogenic agent. HPV infection is more common in women and during pregnancy but many men also have the infection. A number of babies develop laryngeal papilloma and the route of transmission is thought to be vaginal, during birth. The infection appears to go through the stages from infection with visible warts to a spontaneous regression of the warts in a significant number of women. It may then enter a latent phase.

The risk factors for acquiring the virus are early age at first intercourse (less than 17 years old), multiple sexual partners, a history of sexually transmitted disease, poor personal and sexual hygiene, a sexual partner with a similar history, a history of anal intercourse, and immunosuppression or immunodeficiency for any reason. Sexual intercourse is the major method of transmission.

Those presenting with external warts are screened for other STDs, and if present they will be treated. A colposcopic examination and smear tests will be done. The partners of infected patients should also be examined and treated if necessary. External warts are treated with podophyllin 10–25% in tincture of benzoin. This caustic agent is applied with a cotton applicator and washed off in 4 hours. The surrounding skin is coated with petroleum jelly before application of the podophyllin. It is not used on internal warts. Cervical and vaginal warts may be bathed in an 85% solution of trichloroacetic acid. This produces a stinging sensation; a vaginal discharge follows for about 1 week as the tissue sloughs away.

Non-visible warts (small flat warts on the cervix or areas of dysplasia associated with the HPV on vulva or penis) are frequently vaporized with a carbon dioxide laser. Because the virus tends to recur, treatment during pregnancy is delayed until the third trimester. This virus is a stable one and can be transmitted from specula to other patients if instruments are not properly cleaned and sterilized.

Syphilis

Effects on the patient

Incubation varies between 10 and 90 days. In most cases the disease is spread by sexual intercourse. In the untreated condition three stages are distinguished. The stages may overlap or be widely separated.

The *primary lesion* is a small, painless chancre or ulcer. It is deep and has indurated edges. Usually this chancre heals spontaneously, giving the false impression that the disease is cured. This primary lesion appears most commonly on the penis of the male. In the female, it may appear on the labia, vagina or cervix.

The *secondary stage* is usually characterized by a rash appearing over the body. This rash may be accompanied by condylomata lata on the female vulva. This is a cauliflower-like collection of flat, grey, vulvar warts. Like all lesions of syphilis, these are teaming with spirochaetes and are highly infectious. The rash is usually accompanied by malaise and fever. In a short period the rash regresses and the patient enters the latent stages. *Latency* refers to the absence of symptoms in the infected individual. Pregnant women can still infect their fetus in utero, thus demonstrating the infectiousness of the blood.

In the *tertiary stage* the bones, heart and central nervous system, including the brain, can be affected. Personality disorders arise and the typical ataxic gait of the tertiary syphilitic appears. A large, ulcerating, necrotic lesion known as a *gumma* now occurs. It is rarely seen in the genital tract, but may occur on the vulva or the testes. At this stage the disease may be arrested, but not reversed.

Diagnosis is made by a careful history, clinical findings, and cultures or biopsies from the lesions. Blood serology is also assessed. As blood serology is not positive for about 4 weeks after the onset of the disease, the early diagnosis is made from scrapings of the lesions. They can be seen on dark-field examination. These scrapings are made before antibiotic therapy is initiated so that the diagnosis can be confirmed.

Treatment

Treatment is by antibiotic; penicillin is the drug of choice. A series of injections is necessary; oral medication is not effective. The Jarisch–Herxheimer reaction is a local and systemic reaction that may occur after beginning anti-syphilitic therapy. Fever, sweating and headache appear 2–12 hours after treatment. The reaction should be differentiated from a penicillin reaction.

Genital herpes

Herpes simplex virus (HSV) enters the body via mucous membranes. After entry, the virus replicates and spreads to sensory nerves. In genital herpes, the virus travels to the dorsal root ganglion. In most cases, approximately 2–4 weeks later, the primary outbreak occurs resulting in the characteristic clinical presentation. These symptoms include multiple painful genital ulcers, headache, fever, swollen lymph nodes, fatigue and 'flu-like' symptoms. Secondary outbreaks present with similar, although less severe, symptoms.

Current primary prevention techniques do not appear to be effective as the number of new cases of genital herpes has risen steadily over the past 5 years. One of the difficulties in preventing the spread of HSV is that viral shedding, and thus transmission of the virus, can occur when the host carrier is currently asymptomatic (i.e. has no visible lesions). Condoms appear to be somewhat effective against transmission but, because lesions and viral shedding can occur over skin not covered by the condom, this protection is suspect. Despite the problems associated with safer sex practices and barrier protection, condom use must be strongly advised with each and every act of sexual intercourse.

New research involving the Disabled Infectious Single Cycle (DISC) vaccine is currently in phase II and III clinical trials. This vaccine will disable HSV replication and shows potential promise in limiting the spread of the herpes virus.

Currently, treatment involves antiviral therapy using drugs such as aciclovir 400 mg by mouth three times daily for 7–10 days for primary outbreaks. Antiviral medicines are also used for episodic and suppressive therapy. It is important to note that these drugs do not cure or prevent the spread of HSV. They are utilized simply to reduce the incidence and severity of symptoms.

Nursing intervention

Most cases of sexually transmitted disease are treated on an outpatient basis, and the person should be taught about the nature and transmission of the disease in order that they may in future protect themselves and others. No immunity develops and reinfection can occur easily. Strict personal and perineal hygiene should be observed. Hand washing following any handling of the genitalia is imperative to prevent cross-infection. For example, the

gonococcus can be readily carried to the eye, which quickly becomes infected. Blindness may ensue if treatment is not received. Women who are handling small children need to be especially careful. Sexual intercourse is to be avoided until the doctor notifies the individual that the infection has been treated successfully. All equipment must be sterilized after use, and dressings or swabs are disposed of in a safe way. Syphilis may be transmitted by direct contamination of a laceration with living spirochaetes. For this reason, the routine use of universal body substance precautions will also control inadvertent transmission of this disease to health professionals. Once therapy has been initiated, the patient is usually non-infectious within 48 hours.

Tables 23.1–23.3 summarize the physical examination findings, treatment and follow-up of patients with STDs. Box 23.9 outlines a clinical pathway for diagnosing sexually transmitted diseases.

Displacements and relaxations of the female genital organs

Retroversion and retroflexion of the uterus

The normal position of the **uterus** is one of some anteversion and anteflexion (Fig. 23.11). It is not a fixed organ. The filling of the bladder or bowel may cause a change in uterine position. On occasion the uterus assumes a retroverted or retroflexed position. When retroverted, the fundus points toward the sacrum and the cervix toward the anterior vaginal wall. Retroflexion refers to the position of the fundus of the uterus in relation to the cervix. In retroflexion the fundus bends back over the cervix (Fig. 23.11). Degrees of retroversion and retroflexion are possible, so the case may be mild or extreme.

The aetiology appears to lie in a weakness of the supporting structures which may be either congenital or acquired. The acquired weakness is frequently due to injuries during the maternity cycle. Adhesions and tumours may pull or push the uterus into this position.

The patient may complain of backache, infertility, dyspareunia or dysmenorrhoea, but she is frequently symptomless unless the situation is extreme. Backache and dysmenorrhoea are probably associated with pelvic congestion. Infertility may arise because the cervix does not reach the seminal pool. Frequently, the ovaries prolapse into the cul-de-sac and become congested and enlarged. Because of this, intercourse may be painful.

Treatment

Usually the uterus is replaced manually and a vaginal pessary is inserted to hold the uterus in place. The pessary functions by holding the cervix in a posterior position. This in turn rotates the uterus forward. When the pessary is properly in position, the patient is unaware of its presence and no difficulty is experienced on voiding or during

Uterus
See chapter 6.3

Caring for the patient with a female reproductive system disorder

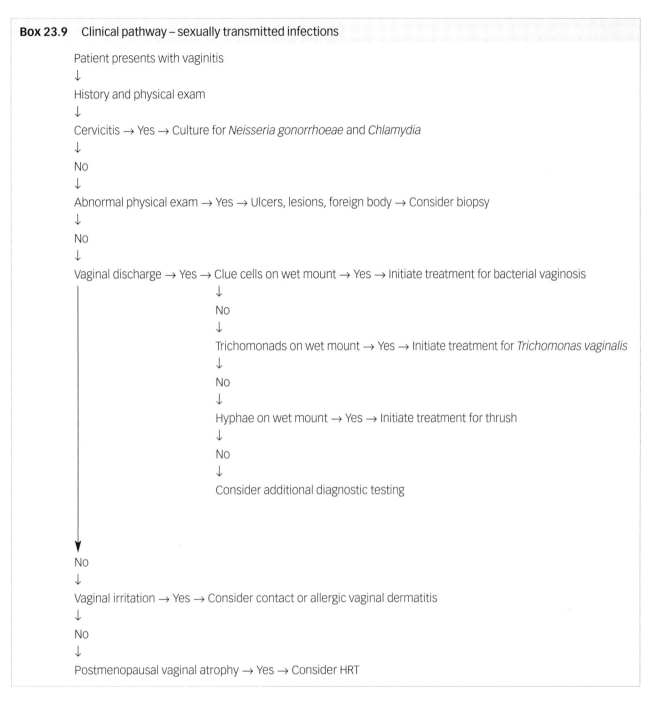

Box 23.9 Clinical pathway – sexually transmitted infections

Patient presents with vaginitis
↓
History and physical exam
↓
Cervicitis → Yes → Culture for *Neisseria gonorrhoeae* and *Chlamydia*
↓
No
↓
Abnormal physical exam → Yes → Ulcers, lesions, foreign body → Consider biopsy
↓
No
↓
Vaginal discharge → Yes → Clue cells on wet mount → Yes → Initiate treatment for bacterial vaginosis
   ↓
   No
   ↓
   Trichomonads on wet mount → Yes → Initiate treatment for *Trichomonas vaginalis*
   ↓
   No
   ↓
   Hyphae on wet mount → Yes → Initiate treatment for thrush
   ↓
   No
   ↓
   Consider additional diagnostic testing

No
↓
Vaginal irritation → Yes → Consider contact or allergic vaginal dermatitis
↓
No
↓
Postmenopausal vaginal atrophy → Yes → Consider HRT

intercourse. The gynaecologist may then give the patient a 6-week trial period without the pessary to see whether she remains free of symptoms. If not, a further trial with the pessary may be given. In other cases the uterus will be surgically suspended by shortening the round ligaments. This is done when the pessary does not correct the situation.

Prolapse, cystocele and rectocele

Uterine prolapse refers to the downward displacement of the entire organ. Prolapse (Fig. 23.12) may occur in varying degrees.

First-degree prolapse describes the condition existing when the uterus descends within the vagina. Second-degree

prolapse occurs when the cervix protrudes through the introitus. Procidentia, or third-degree prolapse, refers to the entire uterus protruding through the introitus with total inversion of the vagina.

Cystocele, urethrocele and enterocele refer to herniations or relaxations of the bladder, urethra, rectum and small bowel into the vagina (Fig. 23.13). They may occur singly or in combinations with some degree of uterine prolapse.

The single most important aetiological factor in the development of these conditions is thought to be injury at childbirth. The pelvic floor and supporting structures may be stretched and torn during the process of delivery and are

Table 23.1 Summary of physical examination findings for sexually transmitted diseases

Infection	Incubation period	Patient complaints	Clinical findings
Chlamydia trachomatis	7–21 days	Females: 80% may be asymptomatic Pelvic pain Watery, purulent drainage Postcoital bleeding Males: 50% may be asymptomatic – dysuria with scant thin, grey discharge	Mucopurulent vaginal discharge Friable cervix, positive chandelier sign Bartholinitis, salpingitis Urethritis Pelvic inflammatory disease (PID)
Neisseria gonorrhoeae	3–7 days	Females: 50% may be asymptomatic Labia pain and swelling Purulent vaginal drainage Sore throat Males: scrotal pain with creamy white urethral discharge; 10% asymptomatic	Bartholin abscess Skene abscess Purulent vaginal drainage Inflamed vulva Mucopurulent cervicitis Joint pain with rash Urethritis
Trichomonas vaginalis	7–30 days	Dysuria, vaginal pruritus Frothy green vaginal drainage Foul odour Males: 15–50% asymptomatic	'Strawberry cervix' Friable cervix Frothy, thin, green drainage Vaginal erythema Urethral discharge
Herpes simplex (HSV-2)	2–14 days (long latency period)	Painful ulcerations and vesicles, sores Dysuria, urinary retention Fever malaise Tender groin nodes	Speculum exam may be impossible Tender inguinal lymphadenopathy Multiple, clear, fluid-filled vesicles over perineal, rectal, vaginal area Crusting, ulcerations Febrile Distended suprapubic area
Human papillomavirus (HPV) Highly variable 'Genital warts' Condylomata acuminata	90 days to several years	May be asymptomatic Genital itching, burning Warty growth on genitals Bleeding warty growths Males: may partially obstruct penile meatus	Papillomatous lesions noted on vaginal areas, penis, perineal area Soft, pink, flesh coloured Cervical smear noting Koilocytes
Treponema pallidum Primary syphilis	10–90 days	Often asymptomatic Painless solitary sore noted on vaginal or oral area	Chancre non-tender with 'punched in' centre and indurated border Non-tender lyphadenopathy Chancre heals spontaneously in 3–10 weeks
Secondary syphilis	30–90 days	Warty growths on genitalia Generalized rash, especially on palms and soles of feet Headache, malaise	Genital condylomata Copper-coloured maculopapular rash Anaemia, alopecia, oral mucous patches

thereby weakened. Further relaxation results after menopause as the tissues atrophy following oestrogen withdrawal. Large intra-abdominal tumours may also place an added strain on already weakened tissue. In some rare cases, the structures seem to be congenitally weak. Diagnosis is usually confirmed by bimanual and rectal examinations. The patient will be asked to bear down, cough or strain while the doctor estimates the degree of prolapse or herniation.

Treatment and nursing care

The best treatment is prevention. Better care during pregnancy has helped to reduce the incidence of these complications. Exercises should be taught by the physiotherapist and encouraged by the nurse to all patients in the postpartum period; the same exercises may be taught to help relieve mild prolapse. These consist of alternately tightening and relaxing the gluteal and perineal muscle tone. The woman should continue to practise these exercises several times a day for several weeks.

In situations in which surgery is contraindicated, the use of pessaries may be employed. A variety is available for different degrees of prolapse. Surgical intervention is frequently necessary to correct the situation. Anterior and posterior colporrhaphy and perineorrhaphy are used to repair a cystocele and a rectocele, respectively.

Table 23.2 Summary of pharmacotherapeutics for sexually transmitted diseases

Infection	Drug of choice	Alternative choice
Chlamydia	Doxycycline 100 mg p.o. b.i.d. for 7 days or azithromycin 1 g p.o. once	Erythromycin 500 mg p.o. q.i.d. for 7 days or erythromycin 500 mg p.o. b.i.d. for 14 days
Gonorrhoea	Ceftriaxone 250 mg i.m. once *plus* doxycycline 100 mg p.o. b.i.d. for 7 days or azithromycin 1 g p.o. once	Amoxycillin 3 g once *plus* probenecid 1 g p.o. once *plus* treatment for *Chlamydia*
Trichomoniasis	Metronidazole 2 g p.o. once Counsel no alcohol during treatment	Metronidazole 200–400 mg p.o. b.i.d. for 7 days
Herpes simplex (HSV-2)	Metronidazole 2 g p.o. once or Metrogel 0.75% one application intravaginally once daily for 5 days	Clindamycin cream 2% one applicator intravaginally each evening for 7 nights or metronidazole 500 mg p.o. b.i.d. for 7 days
HPV	Podophyllin resin 15% applied weekly Allow to remain on lesions for 6 hours then wash off Protect surrounding skin Contraindicated in pregnancy, breastfeeding and children or liquid nitrogen treatments	Warticon 0.15% apply to area twice daily for 3 consecutive days Treatment may be repeated at weekly intervals Contraindicated in pregnancy, breastfeeding and children or cryosurgery
Primary syphilis	Procaine benzyl penicillin 600 000 units i.m. once daily for 10 days	Erythromycin 500 mg p.o. q.i.d. for 14 days or doxycycline 100 mg p.o. b.i.d. for 14 days
Secondary syphilis	Procaine benzyl penicillin 600 000 units i.m. once daily for 21 days	Erythromycin 500 mg p.o. q.i.d. for 21 days or doxycycline 100 mg p.o. b.i.d. for 21 days

Stress incontinence

Stress incontinence is the involuntary loss of small amounts of urine when a woman coughs, sneezes or otherwise suddenly increases the intra-abdominal pressure. It should be distinguished from urge incontinence and frequency related to abnormal detrusor function.

The urge to void and the ability of the bladder to contract are controlled by the detrusor muscle which lines the bladder wall. As the bladder fills, the detrusor muscle is stretched and nerve endings send a message of the need to void to the brain via the spinal cord. Sometimes, an irritable detrusor muscle overreacts, sending a message before the bladder is really full and contracting quite vigorously, sometimes involuntarily. The patient complains of an urgent desire to void, not always reaching the lavatory in time.

Continence is maintained at the junction of the urethra and bladder by continuous spiral muscles from the base of the bladder to the upper urethra. Assistance is also received from the muscles surrounding the urethra, as well as a tight supporting perineal floor. In the continent

woman these relationships can be demonstrated radiologically by observing that the angle between the urethra and posterior wall of the bladder is approximately 90° (Fig. 23.14a). Normally this angle is obliterated only at micturition (Fig. 23.14b), when an increased intra-abdominal pressure combines with a relaxed urethrovesical muscle and perineal floor to lower the base of the bladder. However, in stress incontinence, the slight effort of straining, coughing or sneezing is sufficient to reduce this angle, and an involuntary loss of urine occurs. This explanation is thought to describe about 90% of cases of stress incontinence. A woman may have a cystocele (Fig. 23.14c) and still be continent if the relationships demonstrated by the angle are maintained. However, many women with a cystocele also have accompanying stress incontinence.

Diagnosis is made following a physical examination and a urodynamic evaluation. A pelvic and modified neurological examination is done to diagnose any underlying pelvic or neurological disease. The urodynamic evaluation, which includes a series of tests, helps to distinguish

Stress incontinence
See chapter 5.4

Table 23.3   Summary of follow-up for patients with a STD

Infection	Clinical follow-up
Chlamydia	If no response to treatment or possibility of reinfection Gonorrhoea cultures if not done Consider test of cure 3 weeks after completion of treatment with erythromycin or amoxycillin (high rate of failure)
Gonorrhoea	Test of cure recommended at least 72 hours after treatment completed *Chlamydia* swab if not previously done
Trichomoniasis	None necessary unless symptoms persist or recur after treatment
Bacterial vaginosis	None necessary unless symptoms persist or recur after treatment
Herpes simplex (HSV-2)	As symptoms dictate Follow-up of secondary infections Suspected ocular lesions Follow-up cervical smear
HPV	Weekly for 4–8 weeks during treatment if warts recur Cervical smear every 6 months until normal
Syphilis	Serology tests for syphilis should be done at 3, 6 and 12 months Falling titre should be demonstrated if treatment adequate
Pelvic inflammatory disease (PID) Inflammatory symptoms often secondary to sexually transmitted infections	Re-evaluate outpatient therapy and symptoms within 24 hours, or sooner if symptoms worsen or fail to improve Re-examine after completion of course of medication for pelvic, bimanual exam and review of culture results

Figure 23.11   Normal position of the uterus and four different displacements.

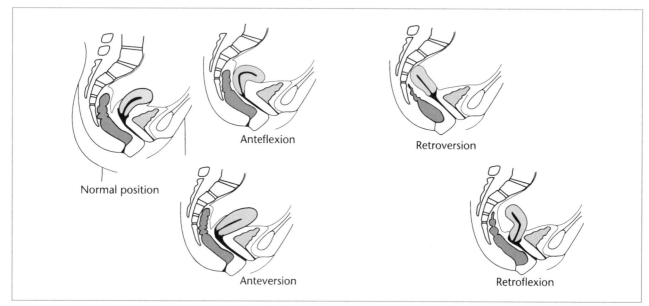

true stress incontinence from other conditions such as unstable bladder or a neurogenic disorder. The series of tests usually requires an outpatient visit. In preparation the patient is instructed not to void or take self-medication for 6–8 hours before going to the clinic. This provides a full bladder for testing and avoids drug effects on nerve conduction.

Initially the patient is instructed to void into a funnel connected to a flowmeter. This meter is an electronic device that calculates the rate at which urine flows, the

Figure 23.12 Types of uterine prolapse, from left to right: first degree; second degree; and third degree (procidentia) prolapse.

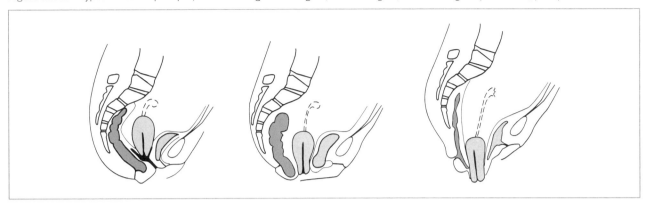

Figure 23.13 Cystocele and rectocele.

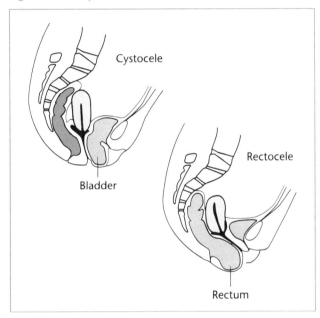

time taken to void and the volume voided. The results are printed on a graph. An abnormally high rate of flow is associated with stress incontinence. Immediately after this, the patient is catheterized for residual urine.

This test may be followed by cystometrography, which involves a catheter being passed into the bladder and a transducer into the rectum. The catheter tests for uterine contractibility and measures residual urine, while the rectal transducer measures detrusor activity. The bladder is filled with fluid, usually water, and the patient is asked to tell the operator when she feels a sense of fullness and when her bladder actually feels full. She is told to void and then asked to stop voiding. The transducer meanwhile records on a graph the changes in bladder pressure associated with these events. The operator can assess how the patient perceives and responds to these sensations and requests. Normally bladder pressure increases when voiding, as the bladder relaxes. This may be combined with a urethral pressure profile. Urethral pressure

is recorded as the catheter is slowly withdrawn at a constant rate through the urethra.

Treatment

Stress incontinence is aggravated by chronic urinary tract infections, obesity and chronic coughing. Prevention includes the education of women about stress incontinence and the aggravating factors. Any urinary and vaginal tract infections are treated; the obese patient is advised to lose weight and an appropriate diet is discussed to assist her with this. The heavy smoker is advised to reduce or stop smoking as a means of reducing coughing, and is also instructed about stop-smoking programmes designed to help in this. Mild stress incontinence and abnormal detrusor activity are treated similarly. They also frequently coexist. The woman is assisted to re-establish a normal voiding pattern and bladder control. She is usually provided with a bladder drill and exercise regimen.

Bladder drill involves routines related to voiding. The patient is instructed to void every hour by the clock whether she feels the need to or not. When she has kept herself dry in this way for 3 or 4 days, she increases the time interval between voidings by one half-hour every 3 days until she can comfortably hold urine for hours. She is instructed to drink plenty of non-stimulating fluids (e.g. caffeine-free) during the day, to drink nothing for 2 hours before going to bed, and to empty her bladder completely before going to sleep. She is also instructed to empty her bladder before and after sexual intercourse.

The *exercises* consist of always giving an extra push at the end of voiding to make sure that all urine is expelled. She is also instructed to practise tightening the buttocks and pelvic floor muscles, and to stop and start the stream of urine during micturition. The **exercises** are practised several times a day. If the patient is unsure whether or not she is practising them correctly, she can be taught to insert two fingers into the vagina and contract the vaginal muscles to grip the fingers as tightly as possible. This provides the patient with a direct measure of her progress. Once she has learned the technique, it can be practised without inserting her fingers.

Exercise
See chapter 5.4

Figure 23.14   (a) The bladder at ease; no stress incontinence. (b) The bladder during micturition. (c) Cystocele without stress incontinence.

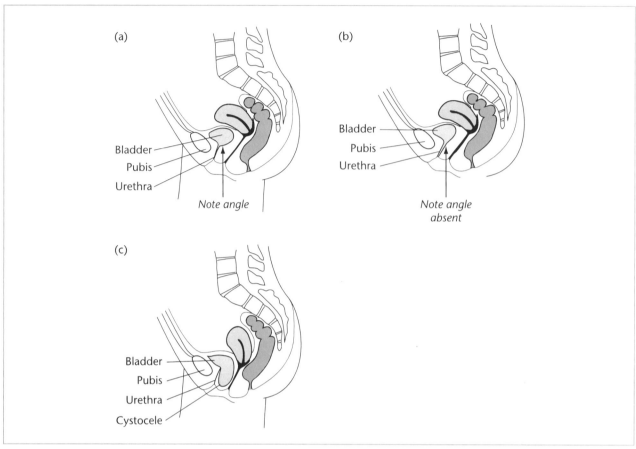

Figure 23.14   (a) The bladder at ease; no stress incontinence. (b) The bladder during micturition. (c) Cystocele without stress incontinence.

Benign and malignant disorders of the reproductive tract

Polyps

Polyps are common benign growths occurring mainly in the endometrium and **cervix**. The polyp has a characteristic smooth, shiny surface and is pink to deep red in colour. Polyps are small in size and seldom exceed more than 3 cm in length. Their aetiology is unknown. No symptoms are usually present, but occasionally postcoital bleeding occurs. Treatment is by surgical excision of cervical polyps and may be followed by dilatation and curettage to remove endometrial polyps.

Myomas of the uterus

A myoma (fibromyoma, leiomyoma) is a benign tumour of the uterus composed of myometrium and fibrous tissue. Colloquially, myomas are known as 'fibroids'. At least 25% of women over 35 years of age show some evidence of myomas. Myomas occur mainly in the uterine body. According to the position they are classified as subserous, submucous or intramural (Fig. 23.15) and may become pedunculated. A pedunculated fibroid in the uterine cavity may be referred to as a fibroid polyp. This may be extruded through the cervix and may come to lie in the vagina. Myomas in the broad ligament or cervix are rare.

Cervix
See chapter 6.3

Figure 23.15   Possible positions of uterine myomas.

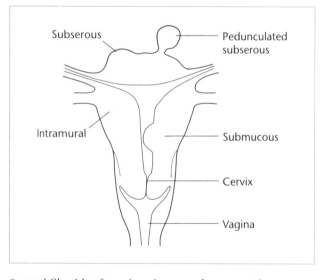

Several fibroids of varying sizes may be present in any one woman. As the fibroids become larger, their blood supply may be reduced, causing some degeneration.

Effects on the patient

Symptoms vary with the size and location of the tumour. Frequently, with small tumours, there are no symptoms. Occasionally hypermenorrhoea occurs. Pain is rarely a symptom but is associated most frequently with torsion of a pedunculated myoma. Sometimes the myoma passing through the cervix causes cramps. Dysmenorrhoea may occur as a result of mechanical interference. Large myomas can cause frequency or retention of urine. Pressure on veins, lymphatics and nerves of the pelvis may cause varicosities, unilateral or bilateral oedema of the lower extremeties, or a radiating pain through the thighs. Occasionally, these tumours may be the cause of abortion or infertility.

Treatment

Treatment depends on the age of the woman, her desire for more children and the size of the myoma. In the young woman who wants to have children, a myomectomy is usually done. This is the enucleation of the myoma, but the uterus is retained. Blood loss during the operation may be extensive if the surgeon excises multiple myomas from a large uterus which may not contract efficiently. Persistent oozing of blood may occur after operation for the same reasons. The nurse should be alert to this possibility and monitor blood pressure closely. In the young woman myomas are not a contraindication to pregnancy and usually cause no difficulty. Rarely, they may obstruct labour or cause a postpartum haemorrhage.

Tumours of the ovary

Tumours of the **ovary** are many and varied. The aetiology of most is unknown. For purposes of clarity, they are divided roughly into non-neoplasms and neoplasms.

Non-neoplasms

Non-neoplasms are usually simple cysts or collections of fluid surrounded by a thin capsule. They do not grow but expand only as more fluid accumulates. These physiological cysts are seen mainly during the reproductive years. The follicular cyst is the most common of this group. Corpus luteum cysts may occur as well.

Occasionally, the Stein–Leventhal syndrome or polycystic disease of the ovary occurs. The syndrome appears in the late teens and early twenties with variable symptoms. These may include a history of sterility, secondary amenorrhoea, hirsutism and cysts bilaterally in the ovary. The ovary shows some enlargement and presents a glistening white appearance. The system is thought to follow an endocrine imbalance, probably arising in the ovary but affecting the hypothalamus. The ovaries produce an excessive amount of androgens, which inhibit maturation of a follicle with subsequent disturbance of the ovarian–hypothalamic relationships. What triggers the imbalance is unknown. Medical treatment consists of a course of the drug clomifene, with or without gonadotrophins, to produce an LH surge and ovulation.

Neoplasms

Pseudomucinous cystadenomas are the single most common neoplasms, occurring in about 40% of patients with a neoplastic ovarian growth. They may attain the largest size of any ovarian tumour. The tumour is characterized by multiple pockets filled with a thick fluid, called pseudomucin. They may be bilateral and may become malignant.

Serous cystadenoma is the second most common neoplasm, and appears to arise from germinal epithelium. The cyst contains a serous fluid. These cysts are frequently bilateral and often become malignant.

The dermoid cyst or teratoma may be cystic or solid. When it is soft, the cyst is filled with sebaceous material, hair and ordinary skin. The solid cyst frequently contains cartilage, bone, teeth, thyroid and similar material. Rarely is the cyst malignant. It occurs most frequently in young women and may be bilateral.

Carcinoma of the ovary

Primary carcinoma of the ovary is usually the common adenocarcinoma. However, a review of ovarian growths is indicated, as almost any one of them has the potential to become malignant. The most common malignancy arises from the serous cystadenoma. Only one ovary may be affected but the other quickly follows, apparently because of the close lymphatic connections. About 5% of all cancers in the female arise in the ovary.

Effects on the patient

In its early stages the ovarian tumour is often symptomless. At regular yearly check-ups, palpation of the adnexa will reveal a mass. Often this may be the first discovery of the tumour. The symptoms result from the size of the tumour in its position. An increase in girth may be noticed but ignored. Pressure on the bladder causes frequency or a feeling of fullness. Constipation, oedema of the legs, anorexia and a full feeling in the abdomen may be present. Pain may be associated with stretching of the tissues as the tumour enlarges. Ascites may be present, accompanied by difficulty in breathing.

Ovary
See chapter 6.3

Treatment

Because of the danger of malignant growth, any ovarian mass is observed suspiciously. A rule of thumb says that any soft mass of less than 5 cm may be watched closely for 2–3 months. If no further growth occurs, then conservative treatment may be considered. Other tumours demand biopsy, and a laparotomy is indicated. After diagnosis, the surgeon strives to preserve as much ovarian function as possible. In premenopausal women benign growths (if size permits) will be enucleated and ovarian function retained. Malignant growths are treated with total hysterectomy and bilateral salpingo-oophorectomy (removal of the fallopian tubes and ovaries). Surgery is followed by chemotherapy. Unfortunately, many malignancies have metastasized before discovery of the tumour. Prognosis is poor and surgery may be only palliative. Further treatment is directed toward relieving the symptoms of the terminally ill patient. Recurrent ascites may be a problem, and frequent paracentesis may be indicated.

Complications of ovarian tumours

Torsion or twisting of the growth on its stalk frequently occurs. Circulation is impeded and necrosis may follow. The patient usually feels a sudden severe pain in the lower abdomen. Treatment is by excision of the tumour and an immediate laparotomy. The cyst may rupture. Often the 'chocolate cyst' of endometriosis ruptures and drains fluid into the abdomen. Again the patient may present with an acute abdomen.

Haemorrhage and infection occur in tumours as well. Usually they are more common in the malignant tumour. Postsurgical menopause is the result of bilateral oophorectomy. The symptoms are similar to those of regular menopause. Replacement therapy with oestrogens may begin before the patient leaves the hospital if it is not contraindicated, for example because the malignancy is aggravated by oestrogens.

Carcinoma of the cervix

Cervix
See chapter 6.3

Carcinoma of the **cervix** is a common malignancy of women. The woman who smokes, has a history of infection with certain strains of HPV, or had an early sex life with several partners is more apt to develop the disease.

Cancer of the cervix is a disease that is preceded by several earlier cervical changes (Fig. 23.16). These changes usually occur at the squamocolumnar junction of the cervix (Fig. 23.17) and initially are evident only on histological examination. They reflect a varied pattern of development. Some cases arise with no known precursor stage, whereas others appear to have gone through all the changes or any combination of them. The earlier changes may be reversible, and so do not always herald cancer. How many of these will reverse is unknown, but about 50% of women with carcinoma in situ are thought to develop invasive cancer; this development takes an average of 10 years. The cervical smear is the best method of early detection of these changes. Combined with treatment of these changes, it is largely responsible for the declining mortality rates associated with cervical cancer.

Because 5-year survival rates are excellent in cases that are discovered early, the Royal College of Nursing and the Royal College of Obstetricians and Gynaecologists both recommend that all women who are sexually active or over 25 years of age should have surgical smear tests at least every 3 years. Nurses have a role in disseminating this knowledge. However, as part of that role, it is important to provide information in relation to false-positive and false-negative results. There is evidence to suggest that women entering a cervical screening programme are unaware of the potential implications. It is imperative that nurses and doctors provide balanced information to women about the range of cervical tissue anomalies and outcomes of subsequent screening and treatment (Austoker 1994).

Effects on the patient

A small lesion develops which, in the early stages, may be confused with other cervical conditions. The early stages may be asymptomatic, but eventually some bleeding from the vagina occurs. An unusual vaginal discharge may be present and may have an offensive odour. Pain is a late symptom and is followed by weight loss, anorexia and cachexia.

Carcinoma of the cervix is divided into stages (Table 23.4):

- *Stage 0* is carcinoma in situ. There is an intact basement membrane containing the malignant cells.

- *Stage I* is invasive cancer, which means the basement membrane has been breached and the cells are invading the surrounding tissue.

- *Stages IA and IB* refer to degrees of this invasion which is still within the confines of the cervix.

Figure 23.17 Squamocolumnar junction of the cervix.

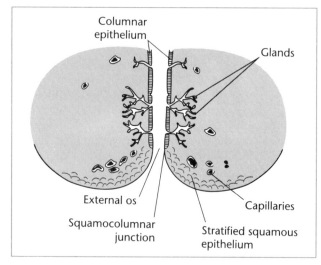

Figure 23.16 Patterns of development of cancer of the cervix.

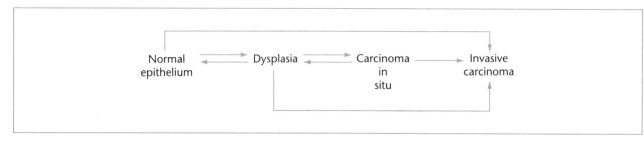

Unfortunately, about 20% of patients with stage I disease will already have spread to the lymphatics. A small lesion similar to an erosion may be present on the cervix.

■ In *stage II* the carcinoma has spread to close adjacent structures and the upper third of the vagina may be involved.

■ By *stage III* invasion has reached the pelvic walls and lower vagina.

■ *Stage IV* is marked by extensive pelvic involvement, including the bladder or bowel, and distant metastases may be present.

Treatment

Treatment is usually guided by the stage assigned to the situation by the gynaecologist. As the main method of diagnosing stage 0 carcinoma is the cervical smear test, the results of this test help to guide treatment. The smear results are organized into five classes. In classes I and II the cells are

non-malignant. Class II may have atypical cells suggestive of viral changes. Both herpesvirus and HPV are associated with atypical cervical cells. Other infections may contribute and the patient will be treated accordingly. Some of these altered cells will revert back to normal epithelium. Class III is suspicious and arouses concern. The patient is asked to have a repeat smear done in 3 months or a biopsy is performed. Classes IV and V are positive, indicating that definite changes are present that require biopsy.

Biopsy

A *punch biopsy* may be done with special punch biopsy forceps. Because of the paucity of nerve endings in the cervix, the biopsy may be done with relative comfort for the patient. She may feel something like a pinch when the biopsy is taken. A Schiller test can be performed.

Normally the cervix contains glycogen. This is depleted in areas of abnormal cell change. When Lugol's solution (iodine in potassium iodide) is swabbed on the cervix, the normal epithelium stains a dark brown. Glycogen-deficient areas are a pale colour by contrast, and these are the areas requiring biopsy; however, a much larger area of affected tissue is removed and identified by staining of the cervix. The advantages are that removing a large area of tissue for histological examination reduces the requirement to recall the woman for cone biopsy later. The procedures are done in a colposcopy clinic; whichever procedure is used, careful preparation and discussion with the woman is part of good practice.

Further treatment may be a *cone biopsy*. This is an operative procedure in which a cone-shaped segment of the central cervix is removed. The internal os remains intact (Fig. 23.18). On examination the section may contain all of the malignant area. In these cases the biopsy may be considered sufficient treatment. Preoperative and postoperative care for the patient is similar to that for other vaginal surgery, such as a D&C. The major difference is that these patients face the threat of malignant disease and may be extremely anxious. Considerable skill in providing supportive nursing is demanded of the nurse. Haemorrhage is a

Table 23.4   Grading of smear test, cervical intraepithelial neoplasma (CIN) grade and cancer stage

Smear	Class	CIN grade	Cancer stage
I	Normal cells	–	–
II	Atypical cells	–	–
IIIA	Mild dysplasia	I	–
III	Moderate dysplasia	II	–
IV	Severe, carcinoma in situ	III	0
V	Invasive, below the basement membrane	–	IA, B
–	–	–	II
–	–	–	III
–	–	–	IV

Figure 23.18   Cone biopsy of the cervix. The cone indicates the segment of cervix removed at biopsy.

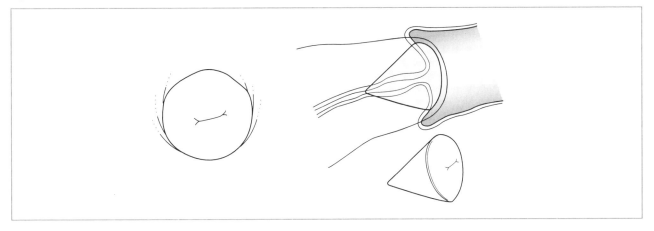

threat, and the patient should be warned of this. Bleeding from the biopsy site may occur up to 1 week after the biopsy when the patient is at home. The nurse should inform the patient of this possibility before discharge so that she will notify her doctor and not be unduly alarmed.

The biopsy results may indicate normal cells, dysplasia or invasive carcinoma. Carcinoma in situ may be treated with a cone biopsy. All carcinoma in situ must be treated to ensure prevention of invasive carcinoma. Invasive carcinoma of the cervix will be treated according to the stage in which it is classified.

Colposcopy is a method increasingly used to visualize the cervix and surrounding perineal tissues. The colposcope is an instrument that provides visualization of the cervix under a bright light and from ×10 to ×40 magnification of the field.

In cervical intraepithelial neoplasia, therapy is directed at local eradication of the lesion. Box 23.10 outlines several treatment methods and guidelines for patient teaching.

Surgery and radiation therapy

Stages IA and IB and some early stage II cases are treated by radical surgery (modified Wertheim's hysterectomy), which attempts to eliminate the cancer, and by radiation therapy. There is much debate over the optimal approach. Most seem to agree that all patients with stages III and IV are best treated by radiation and some palliative surgery. In cases where the surgeon considers that the tumour is surgically excisable, a pelvic exenteration is done. Surgery is used in cases of a radio-resistant tumour.

The patient who is having a total hysterectomy (Fig. 23.19) for carcinoma in situ will have the uterus, cervix and upper third of the vagina removed. The ovaries are conserved in most premenopausal women, but may be removed in the older woman. The patient is prepared as for abdominal surgery. After operation any vaginal discharge must be observed. Some staining may occur from the vaginal cuff. A Foley catheter may be inserted and may remain in place for 1–2 days after surgery. The nurse is alert to possible signs of hormonal imbalance following removal of the ovaries as well as signs of a urinary tract infection and thromboemboli.

In a Wertheim's hysterectomy, the uterus, ovaries, broad ligaments, surrounding tissue, upper half of the vagina and pelvic lymph nodes are removed. In a more extensive Wertheim's operation, the pelvic fascia and further lymph tissue will be removed. Before operation the patient has a cystostomy examination and her ureters are catheterized. This allows them to be identified easily during extensive pelvic dissection. The patient's vagina and cervix are painted with an iodine solution to identify any glycogen-deficient areas which would indicate further vaginal resection.

Nursing intervention

Observations are made for signs of thromboemboli after operation; the femoral areas as well as the calves are

---

Box 23.10   Cervical dysplasia: treatment and patient information guidelines

Laser surgery

- Uses carbon dioxide laser to vaporize cervical tissue and discrete vulvar lesions
- Can be done in the clinic with or without local anaesthesia
- Colposcope used during procedure allows for good visualization of the lesions and transformation zone. Precise aim and depth can be achieved
- Procedure takes an average of 20 minutes
- After treatment the patient can expect minimal vaginal bleeding and discharge
- Women's subjective experience: moderate cramps, pricking sensation
- Precautions: if bleeding is as heavy as menses, contact doctor; no vaginal insertion (tampons, intercourse, douches) for 3 weeks

Cryotherapy

- Uses cryoprobe to freeze transformation zone
- Done in the clinic, usually without local anaesthesia
- Procedure takes less than 15 minutes on average
- No bleeding but profuse watery discharge may last for up to 6 weeks
- Women's subjective experience: heat; mild-to-moderate cramps
- Precautions: as for laser surgery

Extensive laser surgery

- Indicated for extensive vaginal, vulvar, perianal lesions
- Done under general anaesthesia; usually as outpatient
- Post-treatment care: Sitz baths three or four times a day with applications of topical analgesia such as xylocaine gel
- Women usually report an improvement in vulvar pain and tenderness 5 days after surgery
- Precautions: as above and if problems with voiding or passing stool occur

Modified from Toole and Vigilante (1990).

---

examined. Early ambulation is encouraged, but does not merely mean sitting in a chair by the bedside for extended periods of time. Better venous return is achieved by having a patient lie in bed with her legs elevated to about

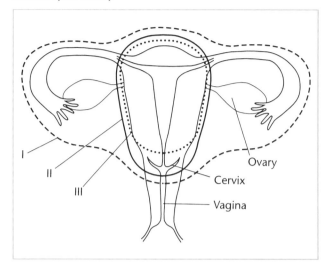

Figure 23.19   Types of hysterectomy: I, total hysterectomy with bilateral salpingo-oophorectomy; II, total hysterectomy; III, subtotal hysterectomy.

Labels on figure: Ovary, Cervix, Vagina, I, II, III

15° than by sitting for long periods of time in a chair at the bedside. Ambulation refers to movement: getting up to walk to the bathroom, getting up to eat lunch, and back to bed to rest. Leg exercises, coughing and deep breathing are important in promoting good circulation.

The postoperative adjustment to life may be difficult. Preoperative discussions with the doctor and nurse should help to prepare the patient. In pelvic exenteration, sexual function of the vagina is lost; in a Wertheim's operation it may have to be modified. Menopause may occur as oestrogen therapy is frequently contraindicated. The care of the colostomy or ileostomy must be learned and accepted. The patient will require much understanding and support from the nursing staff while the nurses gently encourage her to retain as much independence as is compatible with her situation. See Case Study 23.1.

Case Study 23.1

Sally Barlow is a 26-year-old woman with cancer of the cervix. Some 4 years ago she was treated with two caesium insertions and a 6-week course of radiotherapy to her pelvic area. She has been undergoing investigations as an outpatient for a suspected recurrence involving the rectum and has today been admitted to the ward with a view to having posterior pelvic exenteration. Sally was accompanied by Dave, her boyfriend, but he disappeared quickly saying that he would come back later in the day.

Sally's problems are related to the forthcoming operation and are prioritized to ensure she is physically and mentally prepared for this. Initially, problems 1–7 listed in Box 23.11 were Sally's main concerns. Problems 4, 5 and 6 are the most important. Problems 3 and 7 are related to the cancer and will be alleviated by the operation. Sally decided to proceed with operation and problems 1 and 2 then became priorities.

After surgery Sally was nursed in a high-dependency unit. After 24 hours she was transferred back to the ward and a reassessment was undertaken. As a result of this a revised care plan was formulated for Sally's postoperative care (Box 23.12).

By day 9 after operation Sally had made good progress and had resumed independence in all the activities of living with the exception of elimination. Two new problems (8 and 9) were identified.

Carcinoma of the endometrium

This is a frequently occurring malignancy which appears to be increasing in incidence. As it is a disease largely of older women, this increase may be due to a lengthened lifespan. Oestrogens aggravate the tumour and prolonged oestrogen therapy, especially in the premenopausal or postmenopausal woman, has been implicated as a contributing cause of endometrial cancer.

The first symptom is a painless, bloody, vaginal discharge. Between 30 and 40% of women with postmenopausal bleeding have cancer of the endometrium. Bleeding postmenopausally should therefore never be ignored but investigated immediately. A careful endometrial biopsy is usually done. The growth is usually in the fundus of the uterus, but may arise in or spread to the isthmus. The thick body of the uterus contains the growth and it metastasizes late in its growth.

Treatment is by intracavitary radiation followed by a careful total hysterectomy and bilateral salpingo-oophorectomy. Care is taken to pack the vagina or suture the cervix and tie the fallopian tubes to prevent spread by seeding from the uterus. Surgery is often followed by radiation of the vagina as well in order to reduce the risk from stray malignant cells spread during operation. Some surgeons may perform the hysterectomy first and follow this with radiation. More advanced cases are treated with combinations of external and internal radiation with surgery to relieve symptoms. Where radium is inserted, several containers attached to strings may be placed in the body of the uterus to irradiate the endometrium. Cure rates are excellent when the tumour has been discovered early.

Progesterone therapy retards the growth of the tumour and metastases. Treatment in the form of medroxyprogesterone acetate (Provera) may be started before operation.

Carcinoma of the vagina

In recent years there has been an increase in clear cell adenocarcinoma of the vagina in young girls and young women. This is a result of in utero exposure to diethylstilbestrol (DES), a synthetic non-steroidal oestrogen compound. DES was first synthesized in 1938; by 1940–1941

Box 23.11   Care plan for Sally Barlow: pelvic exenteration for cancer of the cervix

Goals	Nursing intervention
Patient problem 1: Hazards of surgery (P)	
No postoperative complications	Explain need for preoperative preparation
	Follow standard procedure including bowel preparation
Patient problem 2: Breathing problems postanaesthetic (P)	
Sally will stop smoking before operation	Explain why smoking increases risks of complications
	Help Sally set a time to stop
	Suggest Sally sets a time to stop
	Suggest alternative stress-reducing strategies
	Offer support and encouragement
	Reinforce breathing and effective coughing techniques
Patient problem 3: Discomfort associated with having bowels opened (A)	
No discomfort	Offer analgesia as prescribed
Patient problem 4: Anxiety and fear related to lack of knowledge about colostomy (A)	
Sally will be able to discuss the impact of a	Refer to specialist stoma care nurse
colostomy on her lifestyle without	Provide the opportunity for Sally to voice her specific fears
becoming tearful	Provide verbal and written information for Sally
	Arrange with ostomist of similar age if appropriate
	Sally to try wearing bag filled with water
	Mark suitable sites
Patient problem 5: Uncertainty about ability to have vaginal intercourse postsurgery (A)	
Sally will be able to state the potential outcome	Facilitate discussion with surgeons about this topic
of surgery and identify some positive coping	involving Dave according to Sally's wishes
strategies	Ensure privacy for this
	Explain to Sally and Dave the resources that exist to give them
	support and advice with sexual difficulties after surgery
Patient problem 6: Fear of surgery and death (A)	
Sally will verbally express confidence in her	Allow Sally time to express all her fears
decision to proceed with surgery	Ensure medical staff explain options fully and answer all her
	questions
	Reinforce and help Sally interpret information given
	Provide information about postoperative care
Patient problem 7: Lack of sleep (A)	
Sally will report 8 hours' sleep	Offer night sedation
	Teach relaxation techniques

(*A*) = actual; (*P*) = potential.

the drug was prescribed for women to help prevent or treat threatened spontaneous abortion, which was thought to be due to low progesterone levels. Unlike natural oestrogens, DES stimulated the body to increase the production of progesterone. The drug was withdrawn from use for this purpose in 1971. Between 1940 and 1971 many thousands of women received treatment with DES. Before its withdrawal it had been shown to be a transplacental teratogen and carcinogen, producing a wide range of congenital anomalies of the genital tract in the offspring and a rare vaginal cancer in a few daughters of such pregnancies (Box 23.13, p. 847). During organogenesis, exposure to DES affected mullerian duct tissue.

This tissue remained inappropriately or, in many women, is in the wrong place.

Time of exposure was more important than amount of exposure. Disorders following DES exposure in utero include physical anomalies, adenosis and carcinoma of the vagina. Estimates vary, but 65–95% of at-risk women have cervical and uterine anomalies and about 90% have adenosis. By contrast, the risk of developing cancer is small: perhaps 0.5% of women affected by DES exposure. There is less information concerning the sons of women treated with DES, but they appear to be at less risk of abnormalities. Perhaps 30% of 'DES sons' have testicular abnormalities. Although DES induces breast cancer in

---

Box 23.12   Revised care plan for Sally Barlow

Goals	Nursing intervention
Patient problem 1: Pain due to surgery (A)	
Sally to rate pain less than 3 on a 10-point scale	Administer analgesia via epidural infusion
	Titrate prescribed dose against pain
	Inform anaesthetist if not controlling pain
	Substitute oral analgesia as pain diminishes
	Encourage coping strategies – distraction, massage, etc.
Patient problem 2: Complications of immobility: DVT, chest infections, pressure sores (P)	
No avoidable complication	Assist Sally to change her position 2 hourly whilst in bed
	Encourage 2-hourly deep breathing and coughing when awake
	Refer to physiotherapist
	Promote mobilization by use of effective analgesia
	Ensure antiembolic stockings fit well
Patient problem 3: Dehydration (P)	
Sally to have a fluid intake of 2–3 litres in 24 hours	Monitor and care for IVI. Administer IVI fluids as prescribed
	Aspirate nasogastric tube
	Maintain fluid balance record
	Provide mouth care
	Induce oral fluids and diet as instructed by surgeon
Patient problem 4: Impaired healing due to infection (P) and previous radiotherapy (A)	
Wound will be healed in 16 days	Record vital signs 4 hourly
	Administer antibiotics as prescribed
	Abdominal wound: check dressing for any leakage on to dressing; leave intact for as long as possible
	Perineal wound: repad and redress as necessary
	Shorten drain daily after postoperative day 3
	Leave all sutures for at least 14 days
Patient problem 5: Risk of urinary tract infection (P)	
No UTI	Observe, measure and record urine output
	Ensure Sally remains in fluid balance and has an average urine output of >35 mL/hour
	Monitor temperature 4 hourly
	Maintain closed drainage system
	Vulval toilet or use of bidet p.r.n.
Patient problem 6: Alteration in elimination habits	
For Sally to manage her colostomy independently in 14 days	Check stoma for colour and evidence of retraction 4 hourly
	Measure and chart drainage
	Observe for passage of flatus and stool
	Administer medication to solidify stool as prescribed
	In conjuction with the stoma care nurse demonstrate change of appliance with full explanation
	Encourage increasing level of participation
	Encourage Sally to decide on an appliance system of her choice
Patient problem 7: Inability to perform own hygiene needs (A)	
Sally to state she is satisfied with her appearance	Give bed bath or assisted wash until Sally is independent
	Encourage Sally to wear her own clothes

(Continued)

Box 23.12 *(Continued)*

Goals	Nursing Intervention
Patient problem 8: Reluctance to assume responsibility for her stoma (A)	
Sally to touch and clean stoma within 24 hours	Support and reassure Sally
Sally to complete a bag change in 2 days	Encourage her to start participating right away in self-care by removing bag, cleaning the stoma and preparing the new bag
	To change bag with assistance tomorrow and with minimal supervision the day after
	Discuss dietary changes that may help to reduce flatus and discuss products that can reduce odour
	Discuss arrangements for coping with the stoma at home and follow-up care
Patient problem 9: Anxiety about altered body image (A)	
Sally to feel confident enough to sleep in the nude	Encourage Sally to show Dave the stoma before discharge
	Suggest interim coping strategies, e.g. wearing bag covers or a waist slip, etc.
Patient problem 10: Alteration in sexual behaviour (P)	
Sally to report a satisfying sexual relationship (long term)	Get Sally's surgeon to explain what potential for vaginal intercourse exists
	Identify potential problems with Dave and Sally and suggest alternative ways of love-making until healing is complete
	Offer follow-up support and advice
	Discuss reconstructive surgery if appropriate

(A) = actual; (P) = potential. DVT, deep vein thrombosis.
Reproduced from Walsh (1991).

---

male mice, there is no evidence at present to indicate that it does so in either sex in humans.

Treatment and nursing intervention

The regular follow-up and screening visits of those who were exposed to DES begins with the first menstrual period or at age 14 years, whichever is first. Early monitoring of the girl to detect changes at the cellular level involves regular examinations every 6 months, including cervical smears and a colposcopy examination. Cervical smears are only about 75% effective in detecting change in this condition and the cellular screening must be more rigorous and extensive. Women who have not been involved in this early screening programme present with bleeding or a suspicious lesion in the vagina.

Breasts
See chapter 6.3

The woman with a disorder of the breast

Breast cancer is the most common malignancy in women. It is currently estimated that in the UK more than 1 in 12 women will develop this disease at some time during their lives. Breast cancer statistics differ from country to country.

Early detection continues to be the mainstay of successful secondary prevention. In fact, research demonstrates there has been a reduction in the mortality rate from breast cancer since national screening was introduced in the UK in 1988. Breast problems and concerns account for a large number of consultations in general practice, family planning and well-women clinics. Nurses today stand in an excellent position to provide current practical information to these women. Although much controversy continues to surround the importance of breast self-examination, nurses can provide women with up-to-date information and act to interpret the numerous recommendations, thus allowing and empowering women to make their own health decisions regarding breast self-care.

There is so much to learn about breast screening and breast disorders that it is impossible to cover the subject in detail in a book of this nature. It is therefore suggested that the reader should refer to the further reading list and references at the end of the chapter if they need more information.

Anatomy and physiology of the breast

The breast is a glandular organ that lies over the second to sixth ribs on the chest wall. During puberty, breasts increase in size, connective tissue increases, the ducts lengthen and breast lobules are formed.

Box 23.13   Effects on children of exposure to diethylstilboestrol (DES) *in utero*

Women

Congenital anomalies

■ Cervix – hooded, ridged, ringed by fibrous tissue
   – hypoplastic

■ Uterus – abnormally shaped, small, internal adhesions, constrictions

■ Vagina – transverse ridges
   – stenosis

■ Adenosis or ectopic tissue by vagina and cervix
   – this may disappear by age 30
   – not cancer precursor but usually present when cancer occurs

Cancer of the genital tract

■ Usually clear cell adenocarcinoma

■ Most common between ages 14 and 20

■ Rare, incidence 1–40 per 1000 at-risk women

Increased reproductive difficulties secondary to abnormalities of cervix and uterus

■ Primary infertility

■ Spontaneous abortion

■ Ectopic pregnancy

■ Premature labour and delivery

Men

Congenital anomalies

■ Testis   – undescended
              – hypoplastic

■ Epididymis – benign cysts

■ Penis   – microphallus
              – urethral stenosis

Fertility problems related to:

■ Decreased sperm counts

■ Alterations in density, motility and penetrating ability of sperm

Possible increased cancer risk

■ Testicular

Figure 23.20   Sagittal section of the breast.

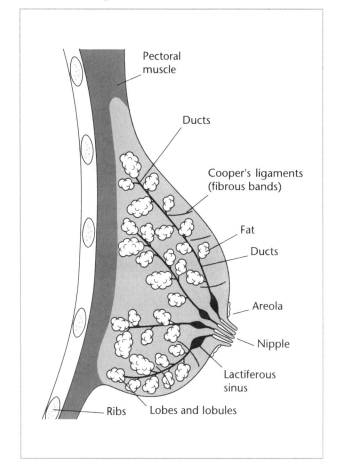

It is these that open on to the nipple for the secretion of milk. The nipple is surrounded by the areola, which may vary in colour from pinkish to dark brown. It contains small elevations known as the tubercles of Montgomery, and these help to lubricate the area during breastfeeding.

Apart from lobules and ducts, the breast contains fat and blood vessels, predominantly from branches of the internal mammary and lateral thoracic arteries. Major lymph drainage is to the axilla and internal mammary chain. The lymph drainage system is thought to be important in relation to the spread of the malignant disease. The breast tissue is held in position by Cooper's ligaments – fibrous bands that run from the fascia between the lobes to the skin and extend up towards the armpit, forming the axillary tail. Two muscles lie beneath the breast: the pectoralis major and the pectoralis minor. Breast structure varies considerably. At the time of menarche the breast begins to grow rapidly under the influence of sex hormones. Each month, when a woman approaches menstruation, the size of the breasts may fluctuate. This is in preparation for a possible pregnancy. If a pregnancy does occur, then the breast enlarges even more and the acini multiply. By the end of pregnancy the breast is almost entirely a glandular structure.

After pregnancy these changes subside and the breast becomes less glandular. As the woman grows older the

The ductal system of the breast extends from the nipple to the lobule (Fig. 23.20). There are approximately 15 to 20 ducts which open on to the nipple. From the lobule, which ends in 100 or so tiny bulbs called acini – where milk is produced – the ducts extend towards the nipple and enlarge, where they are called the lactiferous sinuses.

lobules and acini begin to decrease and fatty tissues increase. This is accelerated with the menopause.

Oestrogen and progesterone produced by the ovaries influence the initial growth and subsequent development of the breast. The proliferation and development of the mammary tissue during pregnancy is stimulated by oestrogen and progesterone produced by the corpus luteum and the placenta. Other hormones believed to be involved are prolactin and the adrenal corticosteroids. It has been surmised that the high levels of sex steroids present during pregnancy inhibit the action of prolactin on breast tissue. After separation of the placenta at delivery there is rapid fall in oestrogen and progesterone production, the inhibitory effect is lifted, and milk production is stimulated. Prolactin levels rise rapidly during breastfeeding, thus stimulating additional milk production. In the absence of breastfeeding, prolactin levels drop to a normal non-pregnant state within 7 days after delivery (DiSaia 1993).

Epidemiology and risk factors for breast cancer

In the UK, 1 in 9 women develop breast cancer. The incidence of breast cancer is ideally measured by population-based cancer registries which record all new diagnoses of cancer in a given population in a given time period (Chamberlain 1993). In the UK, 40 000 women are diagnosed with breast cancer each year, and 13 100 die each year. Eighty per cent of breast cancers occur in post-menopausal women (Breast Cancer Care 2002).

Risk factors

Family history

The most common risk factor is a history of breast cancer in a first-degree relative on the maternal side. This risk nearly doubles if the relative was pre-menopausal and almost trebles if the cancer was bilateral, or there was more than one first-degree relative who was pre-menopausal. In certain families it is clear that breast cancer is hereditary. In 40% of these families there is a mutation in a gene known as *BRCA1* located on chromosome 17 (Dixon and Sainsbury 1993). In addition a further gene, *BRCA2*, has been isolated.

Menstrual history

An early menarche before 12 years and a late menopause after the age of 55 years increases a woman's risk factors. Women who have had a premenopausal oophorectomy are at a substantially reduced risk of developing breast cancer.

Age

Age is another very important factor, with older women being at a much greater risk than younger women. The increase of risk rises steadily from the age of 40 years.

Reproductive history

Nulliparous women are at greater risk than those who have had children, but another important risk factor is a woman's age at her first full-term pregnancy. The risk of breast cancer in women who have their first child after the age of 30 years is about twice that of women who had their first child before the age of 20. Women who have their first child after the age of 35 appear to be at even higher risk than nulliparous women (Dixon and Sainsbury 1993).

Breastfeeding

Results of studies on lactation and breast cancer are confusing, although breastfeeding appears to be protective against the development of breast cancer, particularly in young women (Chilvers et al 1993). This study also demonstrated that the risk decreases with increasing duration of breastfeeding, with breastfeeding each baby for 3 months or longer giving greatest protection.

Oral contraception

Numerous case-controlled studies have been done comparing use of the oral contraceptive pill in breast cancer cases and age-matched controls. It has been established that there is no association between use of oral contraception and breast cancer amongst women in their late twenties and thirties after one or more pregnancies; moreover, oral contraception seems to have a protective effect against benign breast disease (Chamberlain 1993).

Hormone replacement therapy (HRT)

The benefits of HRT are well known, and include protection against cardiovascular disease and osteoporosis as well as an increased quality of life in women suffering from menopausal symptoms. With regard to breast cancer risk, most studies have shown a slightly increased risk in long duration of use (i.e. more than 10 years). Duration of treatment is more important than the dose used. However, it appears that if breast cancer is diagnosed in women who are already taking HRT then it will be picked up at an earlier stage, it tends to be of a lower grade and be associated with a relatively good prognosis.

Exposure to radiation

Follow-up survivors of the nuclear bombings in Japan have demonstrated an increased risk of breast cancer in those exposed. A number of other studies of women who received large doses of ionizing radiation for medical reasons have also shown an increased risk (Chamberlain 1993).

Diet, weight and alcohol

Fat consumption has been investigated and no definite conclusion can be drawn from available data, although it has been shown that obese women are at a greater risk than slim women. Alcohol has been associated with

Figure 23.21 International breast cancer rates.

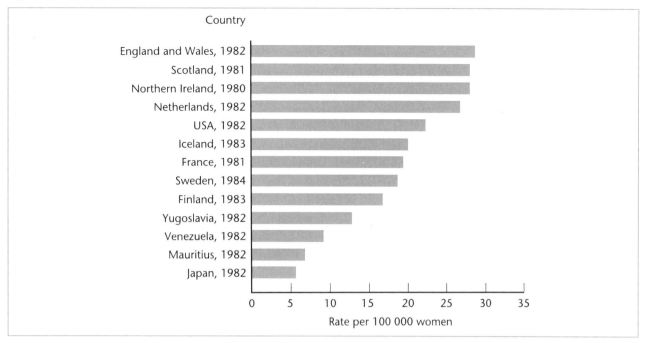

Country

Reproduced with permission from the Cancer Research Campaign's Factsheet 6 (1991) Breast Cancer.

a moderately increased risk of breast cancer, particularly in thin premenopausal women.

Geographical variations

There is a marked variation in the mortality rate from breast cancer in different countries (Fig. 23.21).

In families migrating from Japan, a low-incidence country, to the USA, a higher incidence country, studies show that second-generation women acquire the same incidence as that of the host country.

Breast cancer and men

According to Breast Cancer Care, it is estimated that 250 men developed breast cancer in 2001. This number accounted for under 1% of the new breast cancer cases diagnosed in that year and about 0.2% of all cancers in males.

Certain aspects of breast cancer in men are controversial. Some of these questions are directed towards risk factors: do men share the same risk factors as women and will men benefit from the same established treatment guidelines? Some studies suggest that breast cancer in men might be more aggressive as it appears that a higher proportion of men actually die from the disease. Many factors come into play when analysing the data, such as men are usually diagnosed later in the course of the disease. Also aggressive screening programmes are not directed toward men as they, as a whole, are not at increased risk for developing breast disease. Men do, however, share a good portion of risk factors with women. Box 23.14 lists a number of risks *specific* to men.

Box 23.14 Breast cancer risk factors specific to men

- Exposure to female hormones
- Mumps orchitis
- Undescended testes
- Hyperprolactinaemia
- Gynaecomastia
- Jewish ancestry

Clinical examination

The details of a clinical examination are presented below. This will make it easier to prepare a woman for her examination and also show the depth of knowledge required by a nurse practitioner or specialist nurse in this field. It is very important to take a detailed history before performing a clinical examination. If any of the risk factors mentioned above are present, they must be taken into account. It is important, if the woman is premenopausal, to determine the start of her last period because this may necessitate bringing her back for a further examination at a different time in the cycle as breasts are frequently tender and 'lumpy' premenstrually.

Obviously symptoms noted by the woman herself are important:

- If the patient has found a lump in her breast, has it changed in size, become larger or smaller? Is it tender?

■ Has one breast increased or decreased in size? Most women have one breast slightly larger than the other and this sometimes becomes more obvious if the patient has put on weight.

■ Has there been any nipple discharge? This is particularly significant if it occurs spontaneously. Was the discharge blood stained? Has there been any nipple change?

■ Is there any nodularity or thickening in one area? This can be just as important as a lump.

■ Has the woman noticed a dimple or crease, and what position was she in when she noticed this? For instance, was she looking down on her breasts or was she looking in the mirror, and what position were her arms in at the time? If she was looking down, the examiner should look at the breasts from the same position (i.e. from behind the patient and looking down).

Examination of the breasts should always be performed in two parts: either *looking* and then *feeling*, or vice versa. If you are looking first, the patient should sit on the side of the couch, facing you, and you should stand back to see whether there is any difference in size or shape. It is common to have one breast slightly larger than the other and the woman may be unaware of this and ask whether it means that something is wrong. She needs to be reassured, and it must be stressed that this is a common occurrence. Asking whether her bra seems to have always been slightly tighter on one side can sometimes confirm this. If not, then particular attention should be paid when examining this breast. The woman should then be asked to raise her arms above her head for you to observe any dimples or creases. She should then place her hands on her hips, push in and bring the elbows forward. At this point, it may be necessary to bend down and look at the breasts from beneath – you cannot see the lower part of most breasts without bending down. The woman should then put her hands on the side of the couch, keeping the arms straight and pushing down, and then lean forward. Again, you must bend down to observe the lower part of the breast. Women feel reassured if you always explain what you are doing and what you are looking for.

These three positions that the woman is asked to adopt – with hands raised, with hands on hips, and leaning forward – are very important when looking for a dimple or crease because they may appear in only one of the three positions. When documenting findings it is essential that, if a dimple or crease was observed, the position the woman was in is stated: for example, dimple seen only with hands on hips. If an abnormality has been noted, it is sometimes helpful to mark the area so that when physically examining the patient attention can be paid to this area with regard to identifying any nodularity, thickening or lump that may be associated with the dimple or crease that has previously been observed.

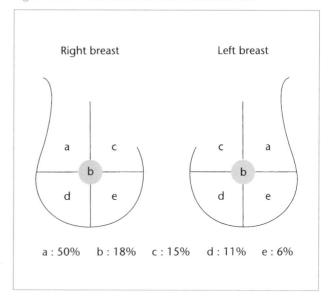

Figure 23.22   Most common sites for breast cancer.

While the woman is in the sitting position, the supraclavicular fossa can be palpated, either standing in front of the patient or from behind. The infraclavicular area can also be felt by running the hands down from the clavicle to the breast. Then the axilla should be palpated by feeling high up into the axilla with the flats of the fingers and bringing them down towards the axillary tail.

On completion of this part of the examination, the woman should be asked to lie down. Her arm should be raised above her head on the side of the breast that is to be examined first. The clinical examination should be performed with the flat of the fingers and a systematic examination carried out. If an abnormality is detected, the fingertips are used to determine the consistency, size and mobility. The clinical examination must cover the whole breast and not forget the axillary tail and beneath the nipple. After examining both breasts individually, the patient should turn on to her side in the oblique position, with her arm raised above her head. This positioning allows for a more thorough examination of the outer quadrant of the breast, particularly in the larger-breasted patient; quite often a lump that was not felt with the patient lying on her back is very obvious in this position. Figure 23.22 shows the most common sites for breast cancer.

Breast awareness and breast care advice

There has been much controversy surrounding the issue of breast self-examination. It has been stated that self-examination causes unnecessary anxiety, and that finding a lump in the breast will not necessarily alter the course of the disease. Even if it does not alter the eventual outcome, an early discovery may mean that the initial treatment need not be so aggressive.

Many women have made statements to the effect that it was nursing a close relative with breast cancer that made them anxious in the first place. Whatever the reasons, if a woman is to perform self-examination, she needs some guidance about how and when to perform it. It can be helpful to explain the basic anatomy and physiology of the breasts, so that women understand why their breasts might feel lumpy premenstrually – particularly in the upper outer quadrants.

Nowadays breast self-examination has been overtaken by the concept of 'breast awareness' which *currently* is what all healthcare professionals should be promoting in their advice to women. The difference between the two is subtle as women are still being asked to look at and feel their breasts, but not in such a ritualistic way as with breast self-examination. Women should be encouraged to become familiar with how their breasts normally look and feel, and how this can vary at different times of the month:

1. Don't feel the breasts before a period.
2. Use the flat of the fingers and not the fingertips.
3. Don't feel the breasts between thumb and forefinger.
4. Remember that nine out of ten breast lumps are *not* cancer.

There are two distinct parts to being breast aware: *looking* and *feeling*.

Looking

- Note any change in the shape of the breast, looking down and looking in the mirror.
- Note any puckering or dimpling of the skin. A crease in the skin can also be important.
- Note any change in the nipple: whether the nipple starts to go in, or points in a different direction; whether the nipple becomes reddened and perhaps moist.

Feeling

The most important aspect of feeling is for women to get to know what is normal for them, and then to notice whether there is any change from this normality. A lump in the breast should never be ignored, and any change in the way the breast normally feels should be followed up. This is why being breast aware just before a period is due is not sensible, and may give rise to unnecessary anxiety. However, women who are breast aware will appreciate that such changes are normal for them and not be alarmed at premenstrual lumpiness and tenderness.

The flat of the fingers should be used when checking the breasts, either in the bath or shower with a soapy hand, or lying on the bed using talcum powder. Starting at the 12 o'clock position, move the fingers, pressing gently down and around the outer circumference of the breast, and then in ever-decreasing circles towards the

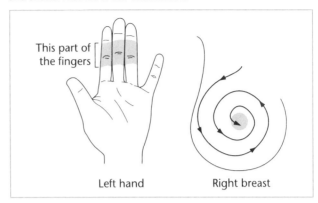

Figure 23.23 Area of fingers to be used in breast awareness and circular method of self-examination.

This part of the fingers

Left hand   Right breast

Box 23.15   Breast awareness

Women should be aware of:

- change in the breast shape or size
- any dimpling, puckering or creases in the skin
- any lump or thickening in the breast
- any alteration in the nipple – whether it starts to go in or points in a different direction
- any discharge from the nipple.

---

nipple, making sure that all areas of the breast have been examined. Finally, press gently down on the nipple (Fig. 23.23). If a woman finds anything that is different (e.g. a lump, puckering or nipple change) or is anxious or worried about her breasts, she should be advised to see her doctor for an examination (Box 23.15).

Breast care advice

Brassières

Women often complain of breast discomfort, particularly premenstrually. One of the reasons for this might be an ill-fitting bra. Women should be advised to be correctly fitted: most large department stores have experienced staff who can measure and give advice on this.

Intertrigo

A rash in the inframammary fold is common in women with large breasts and is usually due to not drying the area thoroughly after a shower or bath. Excessive perspiration may also cause a rash, and advice about wearing a cotton bra may be helpful.

Inverted nipples

Inverted nipples are very common and may be bilateral or unilateral. They should be kept clean by gently using a cotton-wool bud. Any change in nipple inversion must be reported to the general practitioner.

Breast discomfort (mastalgia)

Breast discomfort may possibly be helped by taking vitamin B_6 50 mg with one multivitamin tablet daily. Evening primrose oil or starflower oil (containing gamolenic acid) might also be helpful; the recommended dosage should be obtained from the packet. A stronger preparation of evening primrose oil (Efamast®) is available on prescription and has proved effective in helping many women with cyclical and non-cyclical mastalgia (Mansel 1994). Reducing or abstaining from caffeine may also be helpful, as may reducing salt intake in prepared food. Breast pain, of any type, is a rare symptom of breast cancer: only 7% of patients with breast cancer have mastalgia as the sole symptom.

Diagnostic investigations

Mammography (breast X-ray)

Mammography is an X-ray technique used to visualize the internal structures of the breast. The National Breast Screening Programme aims to screen asymptomatic women between the ages of 50 and 64 years by inviting them to attend for mammography. The aim of the NHS breast screening programme is to reduce mortality from breast cancer in the population of women invited to be screened.

The recommended view chosen for mammography screening is the mediolateral oblique, as this single view demonstrates the maximum amount of breast tissue. The axillary tail, pectoral muscle and inferior portion of the breast are visualized. Most abnormalities are found in the upper outer quadrant, and such a mammogram demonstrates this area clearly (Yeowell 1993). It has recently been advocated that a craniocaudal view should also be performed on the first screening visit. This view demonstrates whether abnormalities are medial, central or lateral to the nipple. Both these mammograms are obtained by the breast being compressed between two plates while the exposure is made. The procedure may be uncomfortable but should not be painful. Suspicious mammograms will prompt a recall to the screening unit, causing much anxiety to the woman, but further investigations may show nothing abnormal. It is hoped that taking two mammograms as a routine will reduce the number of recall visits and minimize stress and needless worry.

The practice nurse, as a member of the primary care team, is in an ideal setting for encouraging women in this age group to attend for screening by providing the information and counselling related to all aspects of the programme. Screening is not performed routinely in women under the age of 50 years in the UK. This is due to the poorer sensitivity of X-rays in the more dense breasts of premenopausal women, and the fact that breast cancer incidence is lower in younger women. Women over the age of 65 years are not screened routinely but can have mammography on request.

Mammographic screening of asymptomatic women may pick up small impalpable tumours and microcalcification, which may be the only indication of early disease such as ductal carcinoma in situ (DCIS). In symptomatic women it is a technique used for problem solving, although it must be remembered that 5–10% of cancers are not detected by mammography because the density of the tumour is less than that of the glandular tissue (Yeowell 1993). This can usually be resolved by clinical examination, ultrasonography and fine-needle aspiration.

Ultrasonography (sonomammography)

Breast ultrasonography is now widely accepted as a valuable adjunct to mammography and is more useful in younger women. High-frequency sound waves are beamed through the breast using a hand-held 7.5-MHz transducer. Images are built on a screen which are then frozen and a picture can be printed. The use of ultrasound in the clinical area can be very helpful for distinguishing between cystic and solid lesions. If there is any doubt with regard to the interpretation of any abnormality, the woman would be referred for detailed ultrasonographic assessment in a diagnostic imaging unit.

Ultrasonography may also be used when obtaining cells from an impalpable lesion by guided needle aspiration. The lesion is visualized on the screen and a needle is introduced into the breast. The needle is guided into the lesion by watching the screen; cells are withdrawn and sent for cytological examination. This is not a painful procedure and takes only a few minutes.

Cytological investigations (Box 23.16)

Fine-needle aspiration cytology

Fine-needle aspiration cytology (FNAC) has become an accepted diagnostic procedure in outpatient departments and specialist centres. The test should be performed only by staff trained in the procedure. The advantages of the test are that it is simple, quick and relatively painless, and in a rapid diagnostic unit results are obtained while the woman is in the clinic, thereby making further visits to obtain results unnecessary. If a diagnosis of cancer has been made, staging investigations and treatment can be discussed at that visit. If the woman is to have mammography, this should be undertaken before FNAC or cyst aspiration is performed as the oedema or small haematoma caused will obscure detail and give rise to a false-positive diagnosis. Ideally, mammography should be left for 2 weeks after FNAC if this procedure has been performed first (Tucker 1993).

Box 23.16 Cytological investigations

Nipple discharge

If a discharge is elicited by gently squeezing the nipple then it should be tested to see whether it is blood stained. A slide should be drawn gently across the nipple to obtain a smear. If two slides are obtained, one is wet-fixed with cytofixative and one is air-dried. This is because of the different staining techniques used.

Cyst aspiration

The fluid obtained from the cyst is discarded, but if the aspiration is blood stained then the contents in the syringe should be emptied into a universal container and sent for cytological examination.

Solid nodule or nodular area

Fine-needle aspiration is performed to obtain cells from the appropriate site for diagnostic purposes. It is now becoming accepted practice in younger women to leave fibroadenomas in situ once a diagnosis has been established.

Advanced Breast Biopsy Instrumentation (the ABBI system)

The ABBI system is one of the latest developments in the goal to make breast biopsy as least invasive as possible. Breast biopsy using the ABBI system has many distinct *advantages* over traditional breast biopsy procedures:

- local anaesthesia as opposed to general anaesthesia
- outpatient procedure
- small resultant scar.

Stereotactic FNAC

This is a diagnostic technique used in the X-ray department. A needle is guided into an impalpable lesion or an area of grouped microcalcification under radiographic control and cells are obtained for cytological examination. The advantage of this test is that it avoids unnecessary biopsy. However, the procedure is not available in all breast cancer centres because it requires the cytopathologist to be present and special X-ray equipment in addition to the standard mammography machine.

Tru-cut® biopsy

This test is performed when a histological diagnosis is required. Local anaesthetic is infiltrated into the skin and the breast where the core tissue is to be removed. A small incision is made in the skin and a narrow-bore cutting needle which has been inserted into a mechanical biopsy gun is then inserted through the incision and guided into the area to be sampled. A core of tissue is obtained which is then fixed in formalin. The test should not be painful, but the slight noise of the needle action should be demonstrated first so that the woman is prepared. Firm pressure should be applied over the area for a few minutes afterwards to prevent bleeding, then an occlusive dressing applied.

Problems

Complications that may occur after fine-needle aspiration, although fortunately fairly rare, include the following:

- *Haematoma or bruise*. This can occur if a large vessel is punctured during aspiration – the procedure may have to be abandoned and pressure applied. It may also occur if pressure is not applied correctly after completion of aspiration.

- *Pneumothorax*. This is a rare complication and may go undetected if the pneumothorax is small. Subtle clues, such as sharp pain, coughing or a hiss of air on withdrawing the needle without evidence of air in the syringe, may occur (NHS Breast Cancer Screening Programme 2001).

Genetic screening

It is currently recognized that many cancers have a genetic basis and that these inherited genes may predispose a patient to develop disease.

Today, many high-risk patients have the option of undergoing genetic predisposition screening. This testing cannot predict who will actually develop disease, but may provide information concerning a patient's susceptibility to disease.

Much controversy surrounds which patients should actually undergo this genetic screening. According to Newman (1998), women with a strong family history of breast cancer (i.e. four or more cases at any age) and those with a family history of both breast and ovarian cancers are best candidates for the *BRCA1* and *BRCA2* genotyping to screen for breast and ovarian cancers.

Benign breast disorders

Cysts

Cysts are basically fluid-filled sacs which are found most commonly in the 40–60 years age group. They can vary enormously in size, depending upon the amount of fluid in the sac. On clinical examination cysts may feel soft and mobile, and are often described as a lax cyst. A tense or tension cyst can feel round and hard, and clinically may resemble a carcinoma. Cysts are frequently mobile in nature and may also be bilateral.

Symptoms of tension cysts include pain and tenderness. Cysts can also fill rapidly, which of course may be very frightening to a patient, but this is something you should explain when discussing breast awareness with your patient. Cysts usually subside or disappear with the menopause unless the woman is taking hormone replacement therapy (HRT) when they may persist.

Treatment

Mammography may be performed to rule out incidental carcinoma. Ultrasonography, if available, should be performed, although occasionally the turbid contents of the cyst may produce echoes. Needle aspiration of a cyst should be performed if the cyst is causing pain, is very large, or is worrying the patient. The fluid from a cyst can vary tremendously in colour: clear, green, straw-coloured, milky chocolate coloured, or blood stained. After aspiration of the cyst, the patient should be re-examined to determine whether there is any residual mass. If so, repeat needle aspiration should be performed and the cells sent for cytological examination to check for underlying cancer.

Fibroadenomas

Fibroadenomas are the most common benign lumps in younger women and usually occur between the ages of 20 and 30 years. A fibroadenoma is a solid, fibrous nodule which is histologically composed of glandular elements and connective tissue. On clinical examination a fibroadenoma is usually well circumscribed, firm and mobile, and is often referred to as a breast mouse because of its mobility. Methods of diagnosis are clinical examination, ultrasonography and fine-needle aspiration cytology.

Fibroadenomas may increase in size, may stay the same, or may disappear. If ultrasonography is performed, a measurement can be taken, and when the patient is reassessed at a later date ultrasonography and measurement may be performed again to see whether there is any change in size. If the above tests have been performed and it has been established that the lump is indeed a fibroadenoma, the patient may be given the option of excision or observation. If the above tests are not available, excision is usually performed to exclude malignancy.

Giant fibroadenomas

When a fibroadenoma exceeds 5–6 cm in size it is referred to as a giant fibroadenoma. These are most commonly seen in adolescent and young African Caribbean women. The usual course of treatment is removal.

Mondor's disease

Caused by superficial thrombosis of a vein in the breast, Mondor's disease may present as pain with a crease in the skin. Malignancy should always be excluded but, apart from this, no treatment is necessary as the condition usually resolves within 6 months.

Tietze's syndrome

Tietze's syndrome is fairly common and occurs when the costal cartilages become enlarged, painful and tender. If it is persistent, treatment with non-steroidal anti-inflammatory drugs and/or steroid injections is effective.

Galactocele

A galactocele is a cystic lesion in women that may occur during or after pregnancy, or during breastfeeding. Treatment is by aspiration, which may have to be performed on several occasions to allow the walls of the cyst to adhere to one another, thus obliterating the space.

Duct papilloma

Duct papillomas are very common and may be single or multiple. They are caused by solitary papillary benign lesions growing in one of the main ducts close to the nipple. Presentation will be with nipple discharge, which may be serous or blood stained. Occasionally a palpable mass may be felt at the areolar margin. Treatment is usually excision of the offending duct – microductectomy.

Duct ectasia

Duct ectasia is due to dilatation of major or minor ducts within the breast which leads to the retention of secretions within them. If the secretion leaks from the duct, it may cause an inflammatory reaction.

Symptoms are nipple discharge, nipple retraction and/or a palpable mass. Investigations performed are mammography, clinical examination and FNAC and, if necessary, excision biopsy.

Lipoma

Lipomas (fatty growths) may be found in the breast and may be mistaken for cysts because, on physical examination, they are mobile and smooth. Ultrasonography and FNAC will establish a diagnosis.

Intramammary lymph nodes

Occasionally intramammary lymph nodes can be felt in the outer quadrant of the breast. On clinical examination they may feel firm and mobile. FNAC usually establishes a diagnosis.

Breast implants

Approximately 80% of silicone breast implants are placed for cosmetic purposes and about 20% for breast reconstruction after surgery. Current advice from the American College of Radiology states that adequate breast examinations can be achieved with presently available mammographic imaging techniques. With regard to breast cancer risk, no epidemiological study so far has found an increased risk of breast cancer in women with breast implants compared with those without.

Breast cancer

Breast cancer is a serious problem in the UK. One woman out of every 9 will develop breast cancer, and in 2002

40 000 women will be diagnosed with the disease. Despite the surgeons' and oncologists' best efforts, many women will die from breast cancer (Cancer Research Campaign 1991, McPherson et al 1994). Much can be done to help these women, particularly in the early stages of their diagnosis and treatment. As mentioned before, women 'at risk' can be identified and screened earlier than ever. For women who have positive diagnosis, there is a bewildering range of available treatments which can cause confusion for the woman, her family and other health professionals with whom she may wish to discuss the issues.

Types of breast cancer

Breast cancers develop from the epithelial lining cells of the terminal duct lobular unit (see Fig. 23.20). The cancer cells that remain within this structure are termed as non-invasive or in situ. Cancer cells that disseminate outside the basement membrane of the ducts and lobules are identified as invasive. It is important to define the type of cancer as this will determine the future treatment for the woman. Types of breast cancer are now defined by their growth patterns and other cellular characteristics.

Ductal carcinoma in situ

Ductal carcinoma in situ (DCIS) is characterized by a proliferation of malignant epithelial cells that remain confined to the terminal duct lobular unit. Until recently, the standard treatment for DCIS was removal of the affected breast by mastectomy. Today, mastectomy is usually considered only if the disease extends over a wide area of the breast.

Infiltrating breast cancer

Infiltrating carcinoma can escape from the structures of the breast. It has also been described as ductal or lobular carcinoma. This cancer has the potential to metastasize, or spread through the body, although it does not do so in every case. Other variants of breast cancer include Paget's disease of the breast and inflammmatory breast cancer.

Paget's disease

The incidence of this breast cancer is low, representing 0.5–3.2% of all breast cancers (Fowble et al 1991). It usually involves the nipple epidermis and the woman often presents to her general practitioner with a nipple discharge, eczema-like skin changes, nipple retraction and sometimes an underlying thickening of the breast tissue. Treatment depends on what the woman will accept and the particular surgeon's choice. Either excision of the nipple and underlying tissue with postoperative radiotherapy, or a mastectomy, is usual.

Inflammatory breast cancer

About 4% of all breast cancers are diagnosed as inflammatory. The woman presents with a breast that is swollen and red, and has skin oedema with induration of the underlying breast tissue (peau d'orange). The overall survival of these patients is particularly poor. Radiotherapy and chemotherapy are the mainstays of treatment but, if a woman's tumour responds particularly well, surgery may be added to give the woman the best possible chance of local control and survival.

Clinical staging

Before the surgeon and the woman decide on the most acceptable surgical intervention for breast cancer, the disease should be staged as accurately as possible. With information from cytology, mammography, ultrasonography and a full clinical examination, the surgeon will be able to choose the best operation for the size of lump and its location in the breast. Because breast cancer has the ability to spread via the blood vessels and the lymphatic system supplying the breast, further staging investigations may be performed according to the treatment policy of the unit (see Box 23.17).

Waiting for the outcome of bone scanning or liver ultrasonography tests can be an excruciating time for these women. It is essential that the nursing and medical staff recognize this. Support should be offered by contact with a specialist breast care nurse, giving telephone numbers of various support agencies, and by listening to the woman's hopes and fears. No assumptions should be made about how the woman is feeling at such a time. Because of initial shock she may have little opinion at all about what is happening to her, or she may have previous experience of cancer which could be positive or negative. Some breast cancers have a genetic basis and the woman may have already lost a mother or sister through the disease. Some women will wish to discuss the elements of their treatment slowly, with careful thought, before considering what comes next, whereas others are keen to know straight away what could be ahead of them.

Surgery

There is some controversy surrounding surgical options for breast cancer and there has been a considerable change of opinion over the past few years. A survey carried out in 1983 showed that mastectomy was the most commonly performed operation for breast cancer, with only 18% of surgeons undertaking conservative treatment (Gazet et al 1985). By 1989, 64% of surgeons were performing

---

Box 23.17   Clinical staging tests for breast cancer

- Blood tests (full blood count and liver function biochemistry)
- Bone scan
- Chest radiography
- Liver ultrasonography

conservative operations (Morris et al 1989). Work carried out in Milan between 1973 and 1980 comparing radical mastectomy for breast cancer with wide local excision of the disease plus an axillary lymph node dissection and radiotherapy showed clearly that there was no difference in survival between the two groups receiving different treatments, thus providing solid evidence for the effectiveness of breast-conserving surgery. The surgeon will recommend the operation that offers the best chance of successful treatment, depending on the size and location of the lump. Mastectomy is usually required if the tumour is:

- more than 4 cm in diameter
- invading the underlying muscle of the chest wall
- multifocal.

However, if the tumour can be excised without major disfigurement, which relates principally to the size of the tumour relative to the breast, the surgeon should recommend wide local excision. Surgeons may feel that by offering to preserve a woman's breast they are lessening her trauma. Offering the woman choice has been shown not to reduce the psychological morbidity (Fallowfield et al 1990). In fact, when women are given the choice of operation some do not automatically choose to retain their breast, and feel they are better off without the affected part (Wilson et al 1998). Assumptions about what the woman wants should not be made. She should be at the centre of the team involved in her care, and her needs should be taken into account at every stage of the decision making process.

The timing of surgery during the menstrual cycle

Premenopausal women have circulating unopposed oestrogen (i.e. not opposed by progesterone) between days 3 and 12 after their last menstrual period (LMP). For the rest of their cycle these hormones are low (day 0–2) or high (day 13–28). There is a small body of evidence to suggest that unopposed oestrogen at the time of surgical intervention may encourage dissemination of micrometastases (the shedding of cancer cells).

Mastectomy

A mastectomy is the surgical removal of the breast. This can mean several different operations, ranging from those that remove the breast, chest muscles and axillary lymph nodes, to an operation that only removes half the breast itself. Mastectomy may be radical, modified radical or simple (Fig. 23.24).

Radical mastectomy

This removes the breast, the pectoralis major and minor muscles, all the axillary lymph nodes, and some additional fat and skin. This procedure is also known as a Halsted mastectomy. It is an extensive operation which

Figure 23.24   Mastectomy scar.

leaves a long scar on the chest wall and a hollow chest area. The removal of all the lymph nodes may lead to arm swelling or lymphoedema, some loss of muscle power in the arm, and restricted shoulder movement. Intensive physiotherapy may be needed after operation.

Modified radical mastectomy

This removes the breast, the axillary lymph nodes and the lining of the chest wall and muscles. Sometimes the pectoralis minor muscle is removed or divided, to allow access to the axilla. Because the pectoralis major muscle is maintained, the strength of the arm is also maintained and swelling of the arm is less likely. Breast reconstruction is easier to achieve because more skin is left compared with a radical mastectomy.

Simple mastectomy

This removes only the breast. Sometimes a few of the axillary lymph nodes are removed to give an indication of whether the cancer has spread. The advantage is that the chest muscles are not removed and arm strength is not diminished. Because most of the axillary lymph nodes remain, the risk of locoregional recurrence is slightly higher than when the whole breast and axillary nodes are removed.

Quadrantectomy

A quadrantectomy removes the tumour plus a wedge of normal tissue surrounding it. Some axillary nodes are removed or 'sampled' to check for spread. This procedure is usually followed by radiation therapy to ensure equal control of the disease compared with mastectomy (Veronesi et al 1990).

Wide local excision (lumpectomy)

In a lumpectomy only the breast lump is removed and usually the whole breast is irradiated. Surgeons may also remove some of the axillary nodes. The tissue removed is examined after the operation to ensure that all the margins around the cancer are clear of the tumour. If this is not the case, the woman is strongly advised to undergo further surgery to remove the residual tumour.

Needle localization

Sometimes a breast lesion is seen on mammography but cannot be felt by palpation. Often areas of microcalcification can be seen on the X-ray film, indicating disease. This area needs to be removed for diagnostic reasons. The radiologist will be involved to locate the area for the surgeon. Using local anaesthesia, a fine guidewire is inserted into the woman's breast indicating the suspicious area. The area is also located by means of mammography. The woman is then sent to theatre with the needle in place, taped to the skin. The surgeon, using the needle and the mammograms as guidance, excises the area. The removed tissue is X-rayed while the woman is under anaesthesia to check that the affected area is totally removed. Further excision is needed if any residual disease is left behind.

Reconstructive surgery

If a woman's breast has to be removed at the surgeon's recommendation or because the woman herself wishes the breast to be removed, there can be the option of breast reconstruction. Women need to be told about their treatment options as information about the disease and its subsequent treatment can give the woman more control over a frightening situation. A breast care nurse could prove invaluable as the woman's advocate, presenting her needs and expectations regarding her treatment to the doctor concerned.

There are some contraindications to reconstructive surgery:

- if the woman has a large invasive tumour
- if there are chest wall metastases
- if there is extensive disease involvement of other body systems (distant metastases).

When discussing reconstructive surgery, it must be made clear that breast and nipple sensation will not be restored. The aim of the operation is to retain the shape and form of the breast mound, but the reconstructed breast will not be the same as the breast that has been lost.

There are several methods of reconstructing a breast. The simplest is when the surgeon working at the site of the mastectomy scar lifts muscle and fascia away from the chest wall to create a pocket for an implant. The surgeon then inserts the implant into the formed pocket and stabilizes the pocket with sutures to prevent upward or lateral movement (Soloman 1986). The implant can be silicone, or a silicone capsule filled with silicone gel (Fig. 23.25). There has been considerable controversy concerning silicone and its possible leakage causing autoimmune diseases and cancer. Implants containing saline in a silicone envelope may be used instead of solid silicone. These implants are filled with saline injected through a device attached to the implant, the filling port. The advantage of

Figure 23.25   Silicone implant.

Figure 23.26   Silicone implant with filling port.

this type of implant is that it consists largely of saline rather than potentially harmful silicone gel (Fig. 23.26).

The woman should be counselled carefully before consenting to such an operation so she knows what is involved. Photographs of the surgeon's previous work are useful to explain the operation, and information booklets or leaflets are helpful to reinforce what has been explained. The decision for such surgery needs considerable thought as there are drawbacks with these types of breast reconstruction. These include capsular contraction around the implant, flap necrosis and gel 'bleed'. There may be disparity between the colour of the transplanted skin and the woman's other breast, and the new breast may not have the same shape as the original breast.

Nursing care following surgery

Drains from the wound site are removed 24–48 hours after operation. Drains inserted into the axillary wound stay in for a few days or until the serosanguinous fluid has reduced significantly. Physiotherapy can start 24 hours after operation and the woman will be taught a selection of exercises to improve her arm movement. Often an information booklet is provided by the hospital to encourage the woman to continue the exercises whilst at home. Additional exercises are taught according to the operation and individual requirements.

Immediate postoperative complications may include the formation of a haematoma if there has been insufficient cautery of the smaller blood vessels at the time of surgery. The woman may have to return to the operating theatre for drainage of the haematoma and recautery of blood vessels. Seroma formation is always a risk after axillary surgery. Serosanguinous fluid collects beneath the wound and can be aspirated with a needle and syringe as a simple outpatient procedure. These aspirations will continue until the fluid stops collecting.

The woman should be encouraged to look at the scar whilst in hospital. The first time she looks can be an extremely traumatic moment for her, but the shock may be lessened with an understanding and supportive approach to her care. A nurse should be present when a woman looks at her scar for the first time and should encourage the woman to discuss what she is feeling about the way she looks. The woman may wish for her partner to be present, although she may want to come to terms with the scar herself before exposing herself to another person. This 'coming to terms' with her body image can be a slow and painful process, which will be helped by continuing support from the nursing team and the woman's family and friends. If the woman has had a mastectomy, she should be fitted with a soft breast form into a supportive bra or 'crop top' before she leaves the ward. This soft breast form or 'comfie' will not irritate the stitch line but will give the woman some equality of shape before she faces the outside world. An arrangement for a more permanent breast prosthesis should be made for 6–8 weeks after the operation.

Lymphoedema

Lymphoedema is caused by an excessive collection of lymph in the tissues, and can cause discomfort and pain, altered body image and a lack of mobility. There are two main categories of lymphoedema:

- *primary* – when the structure of the lymphatic system has not developed properly; it is a congenital problem

- *secondary* – when the lymphatic system is damaged by surgery, radiotherapy or by disease infiltration.

The breast is particularly well supplied with lymphatic channels which drain largely into the axillary lymph nodes. From there, lymph drains into the supraclavicular fossa and low neck.

Surgical intervention for a malignant breast lump may involve an axillary dissection. This may remove a large number of the lymph nodes, depending on the level of dissection undertaken, thereby compromising the lymphatic system. Some 15% of women are at risk of developing arm swelling after this procedure has been performed, and this risk increases to 25% if the axilla is then treated with radiotherapy (Kissin et al 1986). The woman may develop lymphoedema of the arm soon after operation, but it is more likely to develop after several months. Infection or trauma of the arm may precipitate swelling. Advice about reducing the risk of lymphoedema is given in Box 23.18.

Treatment of lymphoedema

Treatment for lymphoedema should follow the well established guidelines of the British Lymphology Interest Group. The recommendations include re-education about skin care and an explanation of why the lymph fluid is accumulating. Prompt referral to a specialist will ensure that the woman gets the right advice and education about the condition. Measurement of the limb provides a baseline for any future interventions and, when compared with the measurements of the unaffected arm, will give an indication of how swollen the arm has become. Exercises for the swollen limb to help mobilize lymph fluid will be taught and the fitting of an appropriate compression sleeve will further assist the drainage of fluid. Simple self-massage of the remaining lymphatic system can also be taught. Enabling the woman to take some

---

Box 23.18   Advice to give on reducing the risk of lymphoedema

- Avoid injections on the infected arm.

- Continue the exercises taught by the physiotherapist.

- Use gloves when gardening to avoid cuts and abrasions and the risk of local infection.

- Do not have blood pressure taken on the affected arm.

- Do not lift any heavy weights.

- Keep the skin on the arm in as good condition as possible.

- Seek medical attention promptly if the arm starts to feel tight or look swollen.

control of her condition may help to lessen the distress from this unfortunate side-effect of breast cancer and its treatment. For a chronically swollen arm, bandaging carried out daily for a prolonged period may help to reshape the limb before fitting a compression sleeve. Community nurses can take over this treatment successfully.

Management of inoperable breast cancer

If the patient presents with a locally advanced breast cancer, surgery is not the best option and primary medical treatment must be considered. A locally advanced breast cancer is defined as having the following characteristics:

- overlying, widespread oedema and/or ulceration
- chest wall fixation
- skin nodules
- disease-infiltrated axillary nodes
- an inflammatory component
- supraclavicular nodal spread.

The treatment of choice depends on the menopausal state of the woman, the extent of the disease, and the woman's wishes. Treatment will normally involve radiotherapy plus hormone manipulation, with or without chemotherapy.

Nursing care of fungating breast cancer

Some women present with locally advanced disease that has ulcerated due to infiltration of the skin of the breast. Care of lesions of this sort involves careful assessment and skilful choice of dressing.

Ulcerated lesions always grow some organisms, usually skin commensals, but sometimes pathogenic organisms may colonize the wound. Swabs should be sent for microbiological culture, and systemic or topical antibiotics given as necessary. It is usual to clean the wound with normal saline or, if it is large, it can be cleaned with a shower attachment.

Pathological staging

Clinical staging of the breast cancer takes place before operation and is based on the size of the tumour, any palpable lymph nodes and any evidence of metastatic disease. A preliminary TNM (tumour node metastasis) classification will have been assigned to the woman's disease. The pathological staging follows surgery and uses the histological details from the excised tissue.

Breast cancer cells are graded from I to III, where I is a well differentiated cell that looks very similar to the tissue from which it originated, and III is undifferentiated, retaining few of the characteristics of the cell of origin. The higher the grade, the more likely the cells are to have spread through the body, either through the lymphatic system or via the bloodstream (Fowble et al 1991). Systemic treatment is based on the size of the tumour, the

histological grade, menopausal status, age and the axillary nodal status (i.e. the number of nodes positive for cancer cells) of the patient (Richards 1991). This adjuvant treatment must be explained and discussed carefully with the woman in order to lead her gently on to the next phase of her treatment. The woman is likely to receive her definitive diagnosis and plans for future treatment whilst she is in hospital, or at her first follow-up visit. The wait can be a trying and nerve-wracking time both for her and also for her partner and family. The extent to which the axillary lymph nodes are invaded is a prognostic factor and the details of cell type will also show if the cancer is aggressive. The woman will have her cancer 'staged' according to the size of the breast cancer, the involvement of the axillary nodes and the presence of distant metastases.

Chemotherapy

Breast cancer not only has the ability to spread to the axillary nodes but also to distant sites throughout the body via the lymphatics and the bloodstream. A percentage of women who present with breast cancer will already have microscopic cancer cells in other parts of their body. If left untreated these cells would almost certainly grow into metastases despite the original breast cancer being excised. Adjuvant chemotherapy or hormone therapy will be offered to these women to prevent or delay the development of this metastatic disease. A 'meta-analysis' published in the Lancet looked at a large number of trials and showed that chemotherapy given to a woman with early breast cancer meant a longer (statistically significant) time to recurrence and a small but significant increase in the time of survival. This overview also showed that women whose biopsied lymph nodes were negative, 30% of whom develop metastases, would also benefit from adjuvant, systemic therapy (Early Breast Cancer Triallists Collaborative Group 1992). This is compelling evidence for offering some systemic treatment after surgery. A combination of chemotherapeutic drugs is usually given. Some common regimens are shown in Table 23.5.

Depending on the treatment centre, other regimens may include cyclophosphamide, doxorubicin (Adriamycin) or epirubicin. The optimal drug combination, treatment frequency and duration of chemotherapy have not yet been firmly established. Combining several drugs is thought to reduce the likelihood of drug resistance and to potentiate cell kill (DeVita et al 1993).

Adjuvant chemotherapy is usually given as an intravenous injection in an outpatient oncology clinic. The implications of receiving chemotherapy should be carefully explained to the woman. The necessity for chemotherapy and its effect in a woman's life can cause a range of feelings. Fear and anxiety about whether the cancer has spread further than the breast are common emotions. Every woman must evaluate the known side-effects of the

Table 23.5   Groups of chemotherapeutic agents

Group	Mode of action	Examples
Anthracyclines and antibiotics	Intercalate with DNA and prevent the DNA from untangling prior to replication	Doxorubicin (Adriamycin), epirubicin, miltozantrone and bleomycin
Antifolates and antimetabolites	Prevent the constituents of DNA being synthesized	Methotrexate, 5-fluorouracil
Alkylating agents and vinca alkaloids	Prevent the cell from being replicated	Cyclophosphamide, vincristine
Antimitotic agents	Prevent the cell from physically dividing (i.e. mitosis)	Vinblastine, actinomycin D
Miscellaneous	Prevent the cell from growing and dividing	Paclitaxel (Taxol)

Figure 23.27   The Hickman catheter.

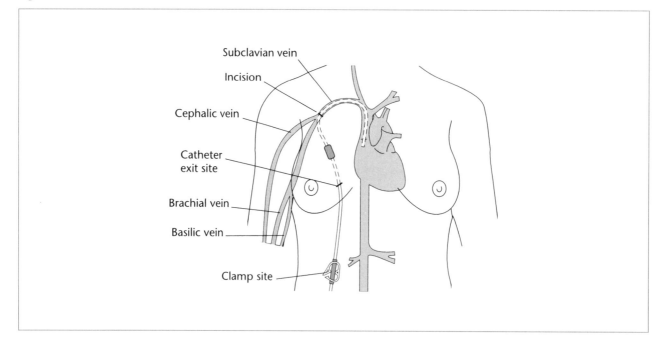

chemotherapy and discuss this with the medical and nursing team before making a decision about her treatment. Because research in this area is continually ongoing, the woman may be asked to enter a trial which could include randomization to different treatment regimens. Again, details of the trial and its consequences should be made clear to the woman before she gives consent.

Primary medical therapy

Some women may present with extensive breast tumours that are inoperable due to the extent of the disease, or because the size and location of the mass renders a mastectomy impossible. By giving these women chemotherapy or endocrine treatment first it may be possible to shrink the tumour to make surgical intervention less invasive.

Administration of chemotherapy

There is a basic principle when administering chemotherapy that the greater the dose that is administered over time, the more cells are likely to be killed (DeVita et al

1993). For this reason, some primary medical chemotherapeutic regimens are given continually from a small portable pump. One drug, often 5-fluorouracil (5-FU), is given via a Hickman line, a soft pliable tube inserted through the chest wall and tunnelled into the subclavian vein (Fig. 23.27). This line allows easy venous access for blood sampling and also ensures that prolonged (usually 6 months) administration of chemotherapy does not damage peripheral veins.

The woman will have been taught how to care for the Hickman line by the hospital team responsible for her chemotherapy treatment. General practice and community staff back-up is essential to continue this support. Infection of the exit site of the Hickman line is fairly common and this should be recognized quickly and treated with antibiotics. Prompt action will prevent further ascending infection and possible septicaemia.

Provided the site has healed completely, the woman may continue many of her physical activities, such as playing golf or tennis. It can be quite disturbing for a woman to have a Hickman line protruding from the skin of her chest. In addition, this type of drug regimen usually includes an anthracycline and platinum-based drug which, for most women, will mean some side-effects and hair loss. However, if appropriate support and careful explanation are given, and the treatment is successful in shrinking the tumour, most women cope very well (Smith and Powles 1991).

Nursing care during chemotherapy

Hair loss or alopecia

Because most adjuvant breast chemotherapy regimens tend to be hair-sparing, complete hair loss does not often occur unless a strong anthracycline is included in the regimen. Hair thinning is fairly common, though, and this can be devastating for the woman who has already lost part or all of her breast. She is struggling to maintain her self-esteem and body image anyway, so hair loss can take on an even greater significance. Support and practical advice may be invaluable to the woman at this time. Information on hair care, use of scarves and hats, and how to obtain a National Health Service wig, if required, may ease the woman's distress and should be arranged before chemotherapy is started. Hair usually starts to regrow 4–6 weeks after chemotherapy has finished.

Scalp cooling, by applying ice packs, cold caps or other methods to supercool the scalp may help to maintain the hair. By reducing the temperature of the scalp, the blood supply to the follicles is depleted, thus depriving the hair follicle of the chemotherapeutic agent. The scalp cooling is usually left on the head for 20 minutes after the chemotherapy has been given, by which time the level of the circulating chemotherapy has dropped sufficiently to not have an effect on the hair. Scalp cooling does not always work, but should be tried for any woman receiving an anthracycline as a bolus dose (Judson 1993).

Sore eyes

Antifolate and anthracycline chemotherapy often affect the conjunctiva of the eyes, causing stickiness and sometimes a dry soreness. Folinic acid given as an oral tablet may reduce the effects of an antifolate, and the use of artificial tears may provide some comfort (Goodman 1989).

Sore mouth

The mucous membrane of the mouth normally replaces itself quickly and is readily affected by chemotherapy. The woman should be advised to use a softer toothbrush to prevent unnecessary scratching of the mouth. Mouth hygiene should be encouraged and fluid input should be at least 2–2.5 litres per day. Any dental work should be completed before treatment starts or just before the next course of treatment when the blood count has recovered. Any fungal infections should be treated with nystatin or amphotericin. The woman may develop herpes simplex which must be treated promptly with aciclovir (Zovirax).

Methotrexate often causes mucositis. Mouthwashes containing a local anaesthetic (e.g. Difflam) may be soothing if mouth ulcers develop. The woman's diet should be well balanced, containing high proportions of vitamins and proteins to promote healing.

Nausea and vomiting

Because the body recognizes the chemotherapy as a toxic substance and because of increased gastric acidity, nausea and vomiting may occur. The woman is usually given antiemetic tablets to take whilst at home but these may not be sufficient or appropriate. The woman should be encouraged to report her experiences of nausea before her next treatment so that adjustments can be made to her antiemetic control as appropriate. Antiemetics that are 5-HT$_3$ antagonists may reduce nausea significantly and should be prescribed as appropriate. Because the side-effects of chemotherapy can be so traumatic, some women begin to associate attending the department with feeling sick. This anticipatory nausea may be treated prophylactically with conventional antiemetics, and sometimes anxiolytics may be useful.

Women will receive their support for chemotherapy as an outpatient and will then be encouraged to continue in their normal routine. It is essential that care and support for symptoms should be shared and continued by their general practitioner and practice nurse. The nausea caused by chemotherapy may also be eased taking small, frequent meals and eating bland food. Prolonged nausea can severely affect quality of life and considerable efforts should be made to reduce this unfortunate side-effect.

Nausea may also be eased by taking a prescribed antacid, drinking flat or fizzy drinks such as soda water, cola or lemonade, drinking ginger tea, or eating dry biscuits.

Lowered blood count

The bone marrow is constantly developing the cells that make up blood – white cells (neutrophils), red cells and platelets. The numbers of these circulating cells are reduced by chemotherapy. Depending on the chemotherapeutic agent given, the number of blood cells will usually reach a trough or nadir 8–12 days after the treatment has been administered. The number of white cells and platelets will start to recover at this point and should be at an acceptable level before the next treatment is given. The woman should be advised to contact her general practitioner or the oncology clinic if she experiences bleeding gums or a tendency to bruise – symptoms of a low platelet count. Infection, feverish chills and a high temperature could indicate a lowered white cell count and the woman must be aware of the significance of such symptoms. If the chemotherapy is particularly strong, blood levels will be determined at the predicted nadir and prophylactic antibiotics given if the white cell count is particularly low (i.e. below 2.0×10^9 per litre). For women receiving adjuvant chemotherapy, a lowered white cell count is short and recovery is predictable (Judson 1993).

Diarrhoea

This can be caused by chemotherapy damaging the gastrointestinal mucosa. Antidiarrhoeal agents may be effective. If the problem becomes prolonged, management may require the use of parenteral nutrition in addition to fluid replacement. This is unlikely with most chemotherapeutic regimens for breast cancer and would, of course, mean admission to hospital.

Lethargy

This insidious tiredness which is not eased by sleep affects most women who receive chemotherapy and increases towards the end of the usual 6 months of treatment. Some women manage to continue with their working lives, perhaps with more flexible working hours, whereas others require considerable rest and could not possibly work. No predictions should be made about how the woman might feel. The woman should be supported through this time and be reassured that her lethargy is a normal response to the treatment, although excessive tiredness could be an indication that she is not coping with her treatment or diagnosis; this needs to be addressed. The woman should be allowed to rest when tired, and family and friends should be involved to help them to understand this side-effect of chemotherapy.

Hormone therapy

The effectiveness of endocrine manipulation on breast cancers has long been known. Many newly diagnosed breast cancers and about one-third of metastatic breast cancers are responsive to hormone manipulation. The primary hormones involved are oestrogen and progesterone. Hormones are steroids that can be involved in stimulating tumour cell proliferation. They can affect tumour cells by interacting with the relevant hormone receptor within the cell's stroma and nucleus. The number of receptors can be determined by the histopathologist once some breast cancer tissue has been removed from the tumour. The presence of oestrogen and progesterone receptors (ERs and PRs) usually correlates with the clinical behaviour of the disease. The greater the number of ERs, the more likely it is that the woman's breast disease will respond to hormone therapy. There are several types of hormone therapy; the most widely used in the first instance is the drug tamoxifen.

Tamoxifen

Tamoxifen is a steroid antagonist which acts by inhibiting the action of hormones on their target issues. Tamoxifen has evolved from being a treatment for advanced metastatic disease, to being an effective adjuvant and primary therapy. Tamoxifen is taken daily at a dose of 20 mg and it is recommended that the drug be taken at a similar time each day. Side-effects include transient nausea, increased vaginal secretions and hot flushes associated with an induced menopause (Jones 1992). The British National Formulary (2000) reports a slight increase in the risk of endometrial cancer due to tamoxifen but points out that the benefits to be gained by its use far outweigh these risks. However, unusual vaginal bleeding should be reported and investigated.

Progestogens

Medroxyprogesterone acetate (MPA) is similar to the hormone progesterone, and is designed to inhibit the circulating levels of oestrogen and block progesterone receptors. The drug is taken daily in tablet form. The particular side-effects of this drug include acne, fluid retention, an irregular menstrual cycle and changes in libido. It is often given to postmenopausal women as a second-line treatment for metastatic disease.

Aromatase inhibitors

Aminoglutethimide

This drug is often used as a third-line hormone therapy for women who have already received tamoxifen and typically a progestogen. It has an antitumour activity in disseminated breast cancer, similar to a surgical adrenalectomy. It works by blocking the conversion of androgens (produced by the adrenal glands) to oestrogens in the peripheral tissues. Corticosteroid replacement therapy is also needed because one of the side-effects of aminoglutethimide is that it inhibits normal glucocorticoid production (the body's normal steroid hormones). Other side-effects include transient lethargy, nausea and muscle cramps. If these side-effects continue, the drug is stopped. Some patients develop a widespread macular rash, which generally disappears spontaneously and rarely necessitates cessation of treatment.

Ovarian ablation

In premenopausal women, the ovaries are the main source of circulating oestrogen. Three methods are used to reduce the amounts of this circulating hormone. The ovaries:

- can be removed surgically
- have their function permanently ablated by radiotherapy
- can be suppressed by chemical means.

A chemical method of suppressing the ovaries is the administration of a luteinizing hormone-releasing hormone (LHRH) agonist such as goserelin, which is administered as a depot injection into the abdominal wall on a monthly basis. Sometimes local anaesthetic is used to make the procedure more comfortable. The drug is then slowly released over the next month. The advantage of a chemical castration is that, once the drug is stopped, the effect will be reversed, which is especially pertinent to women who wish to try for a family later if their treatment is successful. These LHRH antagonists can be used as adjuvant therapy and also for the treatment of advanced disease.

Nursing care

All hormone treatments work by blocking or manipulating the normal hormone levels and so may cause many symptoms associated with menopause. These include hot flushes, vaginal dryness, tiredness, weight gain and night sweats. Clonidine has been given with limited effect to reduce some of these symptoms. Vitamin supplements such as evening primrose oil and vitamin B_{12} may also offer some relief. Menopausal symptoms need to be given as much credence as those caused by other treatments for breast cancer. The woman should be told what to expect and be allowed to discuss her feelings about such symptoms. The prospect of an early menopause can be yet another assault on a woman's body image and sexuality. Infertility may be a distressing side-effect for the woman who was planning a late pregnancy or for someone who has had problems conceiving. However, some younger women continue to menstruate whilst taking tamoxifen, albeit irregularly, and contraceptive advice should be given.

Radiotherapy

Radiotherapy is the delivery of high-energy ionizing radiation which destroys the cancer cells' ability to grow and multiply. It can be used in three ways for the treatment of breast cancer:

1. as an addition to surgery

2. as a primary treatment for a large invasive tumour

3. for recurrent disease at the original site or for systemic metastatic disease, particularly bone or brain metastases.

As an addition to surgery

The usual schedule for external-beam radiation therapy given as an adjunct to surgery is between 3 and 6 weeks. The treatment is given every week day with weekends off. It takes 10–15 minutes to set up the treatment machine for the individual patient, and then only 2–3 minutes for each 'fraction' to be given. The radiotherapist takes care to avoid the delicate structures, such as the lungs and heart. To align the radiotherapy machine, markings are drawn on the skin and a small tattoo is usually made with Indian ink to ensure that the treatment is accurately reproduced every day. The woman should be warned about the permanency of these marks during the course of radiotherapy; the small tattoo will always remain. Following a wide local excision typical radiotherapy involves treatment to the whole breast followed by a 'boost' to the bed of the tumour.

Brachytherapy

Some radiotherapy centres use radioactive implants to give follow-up radiotherapy treatment. Under anaesthesia between 4 and 25 wide-gauge hollow needles are passed through the breast tissue to where the tumour

---

> **Box 23.19** Advice to give on skin care following radiotherapy
>
> - Wear cotton or natural material next to the skin.
>
> - Do not use perfumed soaps or deodorants on the areas being treated.
>
> - Wash the area with water only and pat dry with a soft towel.
>
> - Do not wash off the markings.

---

was excised. Iridium-192 wire, a radioactive source, is then inserted into the tubes and secured firmly at each end. The wires stay in long enough to deliver the required dose of radiation, usually 2–5 days. The woman is nursed in a single lead-lined room to protect other patients, and also the nursing and medical staff, from excessive radiation exposure.

Nursing care

Some women have a marked radiation reaction on the treated area, with skin eythema, soreness, swelling of the breast and, rarely, moist desquamation or breakdown of the skin. Topical applications are to be avoided unless necessary, and then hydrocortisone 1% ointment is the only treatment of choice. Most desquamation may mean that radiotherapy is stopped until the skin recovers. Even without a marked skin reaction, general advice about skin care (see Box 23.19) will be given by the local treatment centre.

Some women find radiotherapy a depressing experience. Some of this is due to tiredness, which can continue for up to 7 weeks after the radiotherapy finishes (Graydon 1994). Women may find the daily travelling to the radiotherapy centre quite a strain. Support at home with provision of home help and childcare as appropriate is vital to ensure that the woman is able to receive the full treatment. Involvement of the general practitioner, practice and community nurses will also facilitate this treatment.

Side-effects from breast radiotherapy are local and it must be stressed that nausea and hair loss usually do not occur. The skin may darken further, changing a breast that has already had shape-altering surgery. Long-term effects may include the fibrosis of small blood vessels, causing even further discoloration.

Primary radiotherapy for a large invasive tumour

Women with large lesions which are inoperable by virtue of tumour extent or because of their general health can be managed with radiotherapy. Most radiotherapists will treat the whole breast and axilla, and the supraclavicular fossa. Intensive radiotherapy such as this can cause long-term side-effects such as fibrosis of the breast and lymphoedema (see p. 858). The prognosis for such women is particularly poor but the short term benefits of local control are thought to outweigh the morbidity of the long-term effects.

Psychological care

For the woman with newly diagnosed breast cancer, her whole world may appear to be falling apart. She may feel relatively fit and healthy but will have to face up to treatment for a disease that will at some point alter her body shape, make her feel unwell and does not carry a certainty of cure.

There may be a great disparity between what we as health professionals think the woman wishes to know or is experiencing and what she actually feels about her diagnosis. Other factors that can predispose to psychological morbidity include:

- lack of social support

- not having a regular partner

- a change in body shape, especially if the woman's breasts were an important part of her self-image

- the physical effects of having treatment

- doubts about the future.

Much can be done to recognize, ameliorate or prevent this psychological morbidity, starting from the time the woman is diagnosed with cancer. Morris et al (1977) observed that newly diagnosed women with breast cancer display five different ways of coping with the diagnosis:

1. *Denial.* The woman actively rejects the diagnosis. She 'blocks' any information given about her disease and cannot actively be involved with decisions about her treatment.

2. *Fighting spirit.* The woman has the ability to display a hopeful, questioning attitude to the disease. She appears to want to make the best of what has happened.

3. *Stoical acceptance.* Such women acknowledge the diagnosis but do not enquire any further about details. These women seem to carry on with their life without much concern for their illness.

4. *Anxious or depressed acceptance.* Such women react to knowledge of the diagnosis with excessive anxiety or depression. They ask for large amounts of information, but this information does not reassure them.

5. *Helpless or hopelessness.* These women are completely overcome by their diagnosis. Their lives are disrupted by their anxieties, so they can no longer function effectively.

It is not unusual for women who have been given their diagnosis to display one or more of these behaviours. As nurses caring for such women it is important to recognize these coping strategies and suggest therapeutic intervention such as counselling when appropriate.

Emotional support and facilitation of adjustment

To strengthen a woman's coping mechanisms she should be encouraged to ask for support. The spouse, family and friends can give practical help and emotional support, although this would involve permission from the woman herself, as not all women want their family and friends involved. Using the helpline numbers, support groups, the general practitioner, practice nurses, community nurses, Macmillan and Marie Curie nurses (if appropriate), and the breast care nurse can reinforce the woman's support network. This support should help the woman to regain some control over her life.

Information about her physical state

Most women need to understand something about their treatment. Gauging how much they want to know is difficult and requires skill. Because there is so much to know about breast cancer, and some of it is quite complex, time and sensitivity must be employed when explaining details. When first diagnosed, the woman will not be able to take in most of what she is hearing. The shock of being diagnosed as having breast cancer will be all that most women can immediately absorb. The role of the nursing team, including the breast care nurse, in reiterating what the woman has already been told is crucial in helping her to come to terms with the diagnosis.

Treatment may not only be new to the woman but she may also be asked whether she wishes to take part in a medical trial. Perhaps suprisingly, this does not appear to cause excessive stress. Provided the information given is adequate, women who allow themselves to be randomized do not suffer from any greater psychological, sexual or social problems than those who are treated outside a clinical trial (Fallowfield et al 1990). Later research by Fallowfield et al (1994) showed that the woman's need for choice is less important than her need for clear and accurate information.

Practical guide on prostheses

Helping to restore the woman's shape by giving advice on the right bras to wear, the fitting of the initial 'comfie' (soft breast form) and the fitting of the more permanent prosthesis can help the woman's return to normality. Advice on other clothing and swimwear may also facilitate recovery and the Breast Cancer Care Association (formally the Breast Care and Mastectomy Association) can be very helpful.

Female sexuality

A very important aspect of psychological care to consider when caring for the woman with breast cancer is her sexuality. Body image and sexual function are represented as a central, intellectual component of the way the woman feels about herself. The self-esteem and therefore sexuality of the woman may be severely threatened by the loss or disfigurement of the breast and changes in her body as a whole. Although sex is an important aspect of life for most women, for some their sexuality is a central part of their life, and for these women the effects of treatment for breast cancer may be devastating. Baldwin (1990) writes that society's view of the perfect woman is constantly presented through the media as usually tall, thin and with two perfectly formed breasts. The breast is a symbol of many things such as womanhood, motherhood and sexuality.

For a woman who has undergone treatment for breast cancer which is disfiguring, the difference between the reality and the 'ideal' may be a cause of great stress (Baldwin 1990). Sexuality is much more than a sexual act; it is about the quality of the human being. Individuals with a positive self-concept respect themselves and consider themselves worthwhile in a sexual sense, whereas those with a negative self-concept are often not satisfied with themselves sexually. A woman being treated for breast cancer may feel she is no longer sexually attractive, even when her partner is trying to tell her otherwise. She may fear rejection by her partner and may withdraw from a physical and close relationship. Her partner in turn may view this as a sign that she no longer wishes a physical relationship, and so misunderstanding can be perpetuated.

Many research papers look at the sexual effects of losing a breast and there is sometimes a misconception that if a woman has breast conservation her psychological trauma will be less. However, work by Rutherford (1988), who studied women undergoing a lumpectomy, highlighted the physical changes that occur. These include deformity, which may be substantial, thickening of skin and subcutaneous tissue, enlarged and pronounced pores, changes in breast contour, erythema and pain over the scar. Apart from the visual changes, the sensitivity of the breast may diminish because of radiotherapy or surgery.

The nature and quality of the woman's relationship with her primary partner and the size and nature of her support network are also important when reaffirming personal value and contributing to psychological adjustment. A woman's sexuality and her body image are about herself and the way she relates to the outside world. Such an important area of care should not be ignored by healthcare professionals when looking after the woman with breast cancer.

Metastatic disease

Breast cancer can spread to the bones, lungs, liver, brain and almost any other soft tissue. Recurrence is sometimes detected by the woman herself, with the development of pain, another lump, breathlessness or feeling unwell. It may also be detected at routine follow-up visits. Investigations for metastatic disease include routine blood tests, radiography, liver and bone scans, and perhaps the use of computed tomography (CT) or magnetic resonance imaging (MRI) to determine the nature and extent of the metastatic disease.

The aims of management of the metastatic disease are, first to palliate symptoms and, second, to reduce the development of the disease. There is no longer an expectation of cure. The timing of recurrence in relation to first presentation and the site of relapse may predict the survival of the woman. Women who have hormone-sensitive tumours and who have had a long interval between diagnosis and relapse are likely to do better than those who develop secondaries, especially in visceral sites, shortly after initial treatment (Leonard et al 1994). Some women, particularly postmenopausal patients with bone disease, may survive for many years with metastatic disease. The treatments for metastatic breast cancer are the same modalities as for the primary disease.

Radiotherapy

Radiotherapy has a very large part to play in the palliation of metastatic disease. Painful bone disease is the most common manifestation of metastatic disease, and may be treated very effectively with radiotherapy. Radiotherapy may also give considerable relief from disease in other organs (e.g. the brain) with a minimum of side-effects. Treatment may require several fractions of radiotherapy, but bony metastases in particular often respond well to a single treatment.

Hormone treatment

As described above, a variety of hormone drugs is available. Overall, the likely response rate for the first hormone treatment is about 30%. If the woman has disease that has responded to first-line hormone treatment, it is more likely that a second line of hormone treatment will be effective. With each successive hormone treatment, the probability of response diminishes.

Chemotherapy

Chemotherapy given for advanced disease has a response rate of between 40 and 60%, with the median relapse at 6–10 months (Leonard et al 1994). When treating the woman with chemotherapy, the intent should be symptom control without paying the price of excessive toxicity. The drug regimens used in metastatic disease are similar to combinations used for adjuvant therapy. Multi-agent combinations including anthracyclines have the highest response rates, but also the greatest toxicity. The choice of regimen depends on many factors.

Currently there is considerable work looking at the effectiveness of new drugs and new combinations of existing drugs. High-dose chemotherapy has been used, with promising results, but more studies are required to compare this treatment with conventional drug regimens. Careful symptom control is of paramount importance when women with metastatic disease are receiving such therapy (see section on Chemotherapy, p. 859).

Pain

Pain can be controlled with effective analgesia as well as treatment of the underlying disease with chemotherapy or radiotherapy. Pain itself can be a complex problem with many components making up the subjective experience. In a woman who has chronic pain, fear, despair, anger and anxiety can all influence what she is experiencing. When caring for such a woman an accurate measurement of the site and severity of the pain is important to understand her experience and to measure the effectiveness of any interventions. The objective of pain control should be that the woman is pain-free at night, at rest and on movement.

Pharmaceutical intervention will start with mild analgesia such as paracetamol (1 g 4 hourly) or soluble aspirin (300–600 mg 4 hourly). If the pain does not respond to this, a weak opioid analgesia will be tried (e.g. dihydrocodeine or co-proxamol). If a stronger analgesic is needed, the opioid morphine is the drug of choice. Dose requirements may start at 5–10 mg every 4 hours but may be increased to 2–3 g 4 hourly, although there is no upper limit if the patient is experiencing pain. Measurement of the woman's pain is important so that the drug dosage can be titrated against it.

Morphine can be administered as an elixir or tablet every 4 hours or as a slow-release tablet (MST) every 12 hours. Constipation is very likely to be a problem if the patient is receiving an opioid drug, and regular aperients should be prescribed as well as giving advice about taking plenty of fluid and eating fresh fruit and vegetables, and other fibre-containing foods.

Co-analgesics can be used with great effect to control pain and should be used with every category of analgesia. Non-steroidal anti-inflammatory agents may relieve bony pain or pain related to nerve compression. The use of steroids in advanced disease can also have a beneficial effect by relieving inflammation and by giving the woman a feeling of well-being. Bone pain may be helped significantly with the use of pamidronate which, when administered 2–3 weekly at a dose of 30–90 mg intravenously, inhibits bone resorption when there is infiltration of the bone by breast cancer. Carbamazepine and amitriptyline can be useful for nerve pain. The use of anxiolytics such as diazepam can reduce the psychological component of the pain as well as helping with muscle spasm.

Non-drug measures for pain relief include the use of massage, hot and cold packs, transcutaneous nerve stimulation and relaxation therapy. In an effort to relieve pain, these measures are often more acceptable to the woman than taking more medication. By providing pain relief with non-interventionist measures, the woman may feel more in control of the situation.

Metastases

Lung metastases may occur, and typically present with shortness of breath. Management involves excluding other causes of breathlessness, including benign causes such as pulmonary embolus or tuberculosis, and other malignant causes such as pleural effusion. Treatment of pulmonary metastases has to be systemic, either with chemotherapy or hormone manipulation. The prognosis is generally poor. Liver metastases carry a very poor prognosis, although chemotherapy may still help.

Brain metastases may present in a number of ways. These include symptoms of raised intracranial pressure, namely headache, vomiting, dizziness, visual disturbance and impaired intellectual function, and neurological deficits specific to the site of the disease, such as weakness or seizures. Initial treatment is the administration of steroids (to reduce brain swelling) and then whole-brain irradiation.

Pleural effusions

Many women with metastatic disease develop a pleural effusion. This collection of fluid in the pleural cavity is caused by deposits of cancer cells, and has the effect of compressing the lung. The woman usually presents with shortness of breath and possibly pain on inspiration. The usual care is to insert a catheter into the intercostal space, drain the fluid off slowly, and then instil an irritant to adhere the pleural membranes together. Many different agents have been used, but intrapleural bleomycin or tetracycline, plus a local anaesthetic, is most popular. Surgical intervention by a partial thoracotomy is sometimes used to drain off fluid and instil an adhesive substance; in a fit woman this can be a very effective way of preventing reaccumulation of the fluid (Smith and Powles 1991).

Pericardial effusion

Rarely, fluid may collect in the pericardium because of tumour infiltration. Diagnosis of this can be confirmed by ultrasonography; if tamponade is present, drainage must be carried out quickly. If fluid collects again quickly, a permanent 'window' can be surgically created in the pericardium for long-term drainage of the effusion.

Hypercalcaemia

This is a frequent complication of breast cancer and is caused by increased osteoclastic bone destruction releasing calcium into the bloodstream. Higher than normal calcium levels in the woman's bloodstream may make her feel thirsty, nauseous, disoriented, dehydrated and polyuric, and sometimes make her have an altered conscious state. These symptoms are usually reversible if the condition is diagnosed and treated quickly. Hydrating the woman with intravenous 0.9% saline usually helps but, with the addition of specific agents to help stabilize the bone, the calcium level can be kept within normal limits for longer.

Spinal cord compression

Metastatic deposits of disease within the vertebrae or dura can cause spinal cord compression. A woman who develops spinal cord compression may have symptoms of leg or arm weakness, sphincter disturbance and sensory changes. If any of these symptoms develops, the woman should be referred to her oncologist as an emergency. Treatment starts immediately, with dexamethasone 4 mg four times daily and emergency radiotherapy. Less commonly, surgical decompression is used. The better the patient's neurological status when treatment begins, the better the long-term outlook.

Carcinomatous meningitis

Metastatic involvement of the meninges may cause headache, confusion, diplopia, cranial nerve palsies and impaired sensation. The clinical diagnosis is usually confirmed with a lumbar puncture, although cancer cells are not necessarily found in the cerebrospinal fluid. The prognosis is poor; treatment can be with whole-brain radiotherapy or chemotherapy, particularly using intrathecal methotrexate.

Nursing care during this type of treatment is intensive. The woman is likely to experience hair loss, nausea and vomiting, and extreme lethargy. She may have to be barrier nursed until the bone marrow starts to regenerate. The woman will be an inpatient for a long time and, despite intensive support, a high proportion of these women suffer from neutropenic (lowered white cell count) sepsis (infection) (Ayash et al 1994).

Overview

In summarizing the care of women with breast disease, it is obvious that teamwork is an important factor in both screening and treatment. As we do not live in an ideal world, treatment is often fragmented between hospital, screening unit and home, proving emotionally traumatic for the woman and her family. The research and advances being made into the diagnosis and treatment of breast disorders mean that guidelines are constantly changing, requiring all healthcare professionals to keep up to date. The informed nurse can provide support and information, but most importantly can provide continuity of care for the woman undergoing treatment for a breast problem.

Summary

This chapter has introduced the main areas of women's health that the student will encounter in both hospital and primary care environments. Clearly it is a vast area and the nurse wishing to specialize in this field will find there is much more to learn. You need to be clear about your own sexuality and moral beliefs about sex and reproduction before you can address the needs of your patients. Empathy and sensitivity are essential for good nursing practice in this area as your patient may face some difficult moral and ethical dilemmas in seeking treatment for her health problems, often in the face of a rapidly changing healthcare environment with apparently conflicting research messages. Teamwork and a non-judgemental approach will help you to meet the needs of the patient. The nurse should be the patient's close and trusted companion at all times, as a source of health education, support and care.

References

Austoker J (1994) Screening for ovarian, prostatic and testicular cancers. British Medical Journal 309: 315–320.

Ayash LJ, Elias A, Wheeler C (1994) Double dose intensity chemotherapy with autologous marrow and peripheral blood progenitor cell support for metastatic breast cancer: a feasibility study. Journal of Clinical Oncology 12: 37–44.

Baldwin E (1990) Sexuality and breast cancer. Midwife, Health Visitor and Community Nurse 26(10).

Barbieri RL (1990) Aetiology and epidemiology of endometriosis. American Journal of Obstetrics and Gynecology 162(2): 565–567.

Breast Cancer Care (2002) Online. Available: www.breastcancercare.org.uk

British National Formulary (1999) British National Formulary. London: British Medical Association/Royal Pharmaceutical Society of Great Britain.

British National Formulary (2000) British National Formulary, no. 39, March 2000. London: British Medical Association/Royal Pharmaceutical Society.

Burgess A, Holmstorm L (1974) Rape: victims of crisis. Bowie, MD: Brady.

Cancer Research Campaign (1991) Breast cancer. Fact sheet 6.3. London: CRC.

Chamberlain J (1993) Epidemiology. In: Tucker AK, ed. Textbook of mammography, pp. 318–322. Edinburgh: Churchill Livingstone.

Cheng L, Gulmezoglu AM, Ezcurra E et al (1999) Interventions for emergency contraception. The Cochrane Library 4(2).

Chilvers CED, McPherson K, Peto J, Pike MC, Vessey MP (1993) Breast feeding and risk of breast cancer in young women. British Medical Journal 307: 17–20.

DeVita SF, Hellman S, Rosenberg SA, eds (1993) Cancer: principles and practice of oncology, 4th edn. Philadelphia: JB Lippincott.

DiSaia PJ (1993) Hormone replacement in patients with breast cancer. Cancer Supplement 71(4): 1490–1498.

Dixon M, Sainsbury R (1993) Diseases of the breast. Edinburgh: Churchill Livingstone.

Early Breast Cancer Triallists Collaborative Group (1992) Systemic treatment of early breast cancer by hormonal, cytotoxic, or immune therapy. Lancet 339: 1–15, 71–85.

Fallowfield LJ, Hall A, Maguire GP, Baum M (1990) Psychological outcomes of different treatment policies in women with early breast cancer outside a clinical trial. British Medical Journal 301: 575–580.

Fallowfield LJ, Hall A, Maguire GP, Baum M, A'hern RPA (1994) Psychological effects of being offered choice of surgery for breast cancer. British Medical Journal 309: 448–551.

Frisch RE (1990) The right weight: body fat, menarche and ovulation. In: Baillière's clinical obstetrics, pp. 419–439. London: Baillière Tindall.

Fowble B, Goodman LR, Glick JH, Rosato EF (1991) Breast cancer treatment – a comprehensive guide to management. St Louis: Mosby.

Gazet JC, Rainsbury R, Ford M, Powles T, Coombes R (1985) Survey of treatment of primary breast cancer in Great Britain. British Medical Journal 290: 1793–1795.

Goodman M (1989) Managing the side effects of chemotherapy. Seminars in Oncology Nursing 5(2 Suppl 1): 29–52.

Graydon JE (1994) Women with breast cancer: their quality of life following a course of radiation therapy. Journal of Advanced Nursing 19: 617–622.

Halme J, Hammond MG, Hulka JF et al (1984) Retrograde menstruation in healthy women and in patients with endometriosis. Obstetrics and Gynecology 64(2): 151–154.

Hancock KW, Scott JS (1993) Early discharge following vaginal hysterectomy. British Journal of Obstetrics and Gynaecology 100(3): 262–264.

Jones AL (1992) Hormonal treatment in post-menopausal breast cancer. In: Therapy express – advances in therapy, pp. 591–594. Brussels: CIBA-GEIGY Pharmaceuticals.

Judson IR (1993) Toxicology of chemotherapeutic agents. In: Andrews P, Sanger G, eds. Emesis in anticancer therapy, pp. 113–161. London: Chapman and Hall.

Kissin M, Querci Della Rovere G, Easton D, Westbury G (1986) Risk of lymphoedema following the treatment of breast cancer. British Journal of Surgery 73: 580–584.

Leonard RCF, Rodger A, Dixon JN (1994) Metastatic breast cancer. ABC of breast diseases. British Medical Journal 309: 1501–1504.

McPherson K, Steel CM, Dixon JM (1994) Breast cancer – epidemiology, risk factors and genetics. ABC of breast diseases. British Medical Journal 309: 1003–1006.

Mansel RE (1994) Breast pain. British Medical Journal 309: 866–868.

Morris J, Royle GT, Taylor I (1989) Changes in the surgical management of early breast cancer in England. Journal of the Royal Society of Medicine 82: 12–15.

Morris T, Greer H, White P (1977) Psychosocial and social adjustment to mastectomy – a 2 year follow up study. Cancer 40: 2381–2387.

National Osteoporosis Society (1993) HRT, the menopause and osteoporosis, 3rd edn. Bath: NOP.

National Statistics Official UK Statistics (2001) Online. Available: http://www.statistics.gov.uk

Newman B, Mu H, Butler LM et al (1998) Frequency of breast cancer attributable to *BRCA1* in a population based series of American women. Journal of the American Medical Association 279: 915–921.

NHS Breast Cancer Screening Programme (2001) Guidelines for non-operative diagnostic procedures and reporting in breast cancer screening. Online. Available: http://www.cancerscreening.nhs.uk

Noord PM, Hawks R (1991) The effects of wartime conditions on the 1994–5 'Dutch famine' on recalled menarchial age in participants of the DOM breast screening project. Annals of Human Biology 18(1): 52–70.

Richards MA (1991) Systemic treatment of breast cancer. Journal of the Royal Society of Health August: 141–145.

Rutherford D (1988) Assessing psychosexual needs of women experiencing lumpectomy. Cancer Nursing 11(4): 244–249.

Smith IE, Powles TJ (1991) Medical management of breast cancer. London: Martin Dunitz.

Toole K, Vigilante P (1990) Cervical dysplasia and condyloma as risks for carcinoma. Maternal–Child Nursing Journal 15: 170–175.

Tucker AK (1993) Introduction. In: Tucker AK, ed. Textbook of mammography, pp. 2–3. Edinburgh: Churchill Livingstone.

Veronesi U, Salvadori O, Luini A et al (1990) Conservative treatment of early breast cancer. Long term results of 1232 cases treated by quadrantectomy and radiotherapy. Annals of Surgery 211: 250–259.

Yeowell M (1993) In: Tucker AK, ed. Textbook of mammography, pp. 28–54. Edinburgh: Churchill Livingstone.

Further Reading

Baum M, Saunders C, Meredith S (1994) Breast cancer: a guide for every woman. Oxford: Oxford University Press.

Corwin EJ (1997) Endometriosis: pathophysiology, diagnosis, and treatment. The Nurse Practitioner 22(10): 35–37.

Davidson M (2001) Managing uterine fibroids: new approaches to treatment. Clinical Reviews 11(6): 78–87.

Devita SR, Hellman S, Rosenberg SA, eds (1993) Cancer principles and practice of oncology, 4th edn. Philadelphia: JB Lippincott.

Dixon M, Sainsbury R (1993) Diseases of the breast. Edinburgh: Churchill Livingstone.

Doughty S (2001) The postmenopausal woman: complex issues require NP touch. Advance for Nurse Practitioners 9(7): 35–39.

Fleischman C et al (1998) Guidelines for preventive health screening in women. Women's Health in Primary Care 1(5): 413–414.

Grady D, Hully SB (2001) Postmenopausal hormones and heart disease. Journal of the American College of Cardiology 38: 8–10.

Lichtman R, Papera S (1994) Gynecology: well woman care. Norwalk, CN: Appleton & Lange.

Oriel K, Schrager S (1999) Abnormal uterine bleeding: problem oriented diagnosis. American Family Physician 60: 1371–1382.

Rhodes JC, Kjerulff KH, Langenberg PW, Guzinski GM (1999) Hysterectomy and sexual functioning. Journal of the American Medical Association 282: 1934–1941.

Spencer CP, Cooper AJ, Whitehead MI (1997) Management of abnormal bleeding in women receiving hormone replacement therapy. British Medical Journal 315: 37–42.

Wells R, Tschudin V (1994) Wells' supportive therapies in healthcare. London: Ballière Tindall.

Yaffe K et al (1999) Estrogen therapy in postmenopausal women. Journal of the American Medical Association 279(9): 688.

Youngkin EQ, Davis MS (1998) Women's health: a primary care clinical guide, 2nd edn. Stamford, CN: Appleton & Lange.

Youngkin EQ, Davis MS (1998) Women's health: a primary care clinical guide. Upper Saddle River, NJ: Prentice Hall.

Young-Lewis L, Silverman J (2001) Endometriosis: supportive care is essential. Advance for Nurse Practitioners, vol 9, no. 10.

24

Caring for the patient with a disorder of the musculoskeletal system

Mike Walsh

Introduction

Structure and function of bones

Structure and function of joints

Trauma assessment

Fractures

Treatment and nursing care required for specific injuries

Injuries to joints

Amputation of a limb

Inflammatory joint disease

Degenerative joint disease

Other inflammatory joint diseases

Metabolic joint disease

Connective tissue (collagen) disease

Infective bone disease

Osteoporosis

Back pain

Osteomalacia

Paget's disease (osteitis deformans)

Bone neoplasms

Summary

Introduction

This chapter discusses the healthcare problems encountered by patients whose musculoskeletal system has experienced either disease or trauma, and describes various approaches to their nursing care.

Alteration in mobility, either temporary or permanent, is the most common consequence of interruption in bone and joint function, and obviously has a major impact upon the person's independence. Patients often represent opposite ends of the age spectrum – from young adult males through to the most elderly in society. All can suffer trauma or disease and this wide age range is only one of the factors that makes nursing orthopaedic patients such a challenging area of care. A multidisciplinary approach that fully involves the family and patient is essential if the patient is to return to the community with maximum independence.

Structure and function of bones

Bone is a rigid connective tissue consisting of bone cells, calcified collagenous intercellular substance and marrow.

Bone
See chapter 3.2

Each bone, except at joint surfaces, is covered by a tough, supportive membrane called the *periosteum*. The periosteum is firmly attached to the underlying bone by penetrating fibres, and its blood vessels give off many branches which enter the tissue to provide the essentials for growth, repair and maintenance. The inner layer of the periosteum gives rise to the osteoblasts, which function in the development and replacement of bone. The shaft of the long bones is hollow and is lined with a comparable membrane referred to as the *endosteum*. Although approximately two-thirds of bone tissue is inorganic mineral substance, which gives it the characteristic hardness and inert appearance, it is viable tissue undergoing constant metabolic processes, just as other tissues.

There are three types of bone cell:

■ *Osteoblasts* are found beneath the periosteum on the surface of growing bones and in developmental or ossification areas within the bones.

■ *Osteocytes* are matured osteoblasts that become imprisoned in small spaces by the calcification. It is believed that these regulate bone metabolism.

■ *Osteoclasts* are considered to be responsible for the breaking down and reabsorption of bone tissue.

Normally, there is a constant turnover of the mineral deposits. This continuous breaking down, reabsorption and new bone formation is necessary, because old bone becomes weak and brittle. The mineralization and strength of the bones are influenced by the amount of weight bearing and muscle pull to which the bones are subjected. Those of the active person are stronger and more resistant to stress than the bones of non-active persons. One of the complications of prolonged bedrest is the decalcification and weakening of the bones; the calcium is excreted by the kidneys and there is therefore a risk of the formation of renal calculi. In older persons the bones tend to become brittle and less resistant to stress, increasing the possibility of fractures. This is due to the general decline in cell reproduction which results in a slower rate of production of the collagenous matrix and mineralization as well as of reabsorption.

Types of bone tissue

Each bone is composed of two **types** of tissue: compact and cancellous. Outer layers consist of dense, *compact* tissue (cortical bone), and the interior is of a spongy or porous nature (*cancellous*), which contains the red bone marrow. The thickness of each type of tissue varies in different bones as well as in parts of the same bone.

In the long bones (e.g. humerus, tibia, femur), the extremities have a thin outer layer of compact tissue enclosing a larger mass of cancellous tissue (Fig. 24.1). The shaft is formed mainly of two thick layers of compact bone separated by a small amount of porous tissue. The central hollow portion of the shaft forms the medullary canal, which is filled with *yellow marrow*, consisting

largely of fat cells and blood vessels. Flat bones (e.g. skull bones, scapula, ribs) have a thicker layer of cancellous tissue lying between two relatively thin layers of compact tissue. Short and irregular bones such as those of the wrist and ankle have a thin shell of compact tissue enclosing a fair thickness of cancellous tissue.

Functions of bones and contained marrow

The bones are bound together by ligaments and collectively form the skeleton, which provides a supporting framework for the body and protection for vital structures. They assist in body movement by providing attachment for muscles and leverage for their action. The bones also serve as the body's store of calcium. If the blood calcium concentration falls below the normal level, the deficit may be met by the withdrawal of calcium from the bones. Conversely, much of the excess in the blood is deposited in bone tissue. The role of the red bone marrow in the formation of blood cells is discussed on page 373.

Development and growth of bones

The development of the bones begins early in embryonic life and is not normally completed until the late teens

Figure 24.1   Diagram of a long bone.

Bone types
See chapter 3.2

Growth
See chapter 3.2

or early twenties. They are composed of membranous connective tissue or cartilaginous tissue, which is gradually replaced by bone in the process of ossification.

The bones, which are preformed of cartilage, undergo *intracartilaginous ossification*, which involves destruction of the cartilage and its replacement by bone tissue. Osteoblasts, osteoclasts and blood vessels invade internal areas of the cartilage, setting up ossification centres around which cartilage is progressively removed and replaced by bone tissue.

In long bones (Fig. 24.1), an ossification centre appears within the shaft (*diaphysis*) and later at each end (*epiphysis*). As ossification proceeds, growth of the cartilage continues, resulting in a persisting thin strip of cartilaginous tissue between each epiphysis and the diaphysis, which is referred to as the *growth or epiphyseal plate*. The bones continue to grow as long as new cartilage develops to maintain this plate. Cessation of growth occurs when it becomes ossified, and the epiphyses are fused with the diaphysis. Bones grow in circumference by the formation of layers of bone beneath the periosteum.

Factors in bone development, growth and repair

Several factors influence the development, growth and maintenance of normal bone structure. They are summarized in Box 24.1.

Bone growth and ossification are also influenced by such hormones as the growth hormone produced by the anterior pituitary gland, thyroxine from the thyroid gland, and parathyroid hormone produced by the parathyroid glands. Bone metabolism is also affected by oestrogen, androgens and calcitonin.

In addition to these factors, the demand placed on the bones by weight bearing and muscle pull plays an important role in the shaping of bone.

Box 24.1   Factors in bone development, growth and repair

- *Calcium and phosphorus*: needed for ossification and constant formation of new bone

- *Vitamin D*: used in the absorption and utilization of minerals

- *Protein and vitamin C*: acts in formation of collagenous, fibrous, intercellular matrix in which minerals are deposited

- *Vitamin A*: essential to tissue growth

- *Somatotrophic and parathyroid hormones*: play a part in bone growth and ossification

- *Oestrogen, androgens and calcitonin*: have roles in bone metabolism

- *Weight bearing and muscle stress*: needed for maintenance of bone strength and shaping of bone

---

Structure and function of joints

A **joint** or articulation is a point of contact between bones that permits flexibility in the skeletal system and allows for movement. Joints are classified according to their structure and the kind of movement that they allow. The *structural* classification of joints is based on the kind of tissue that connects the bones and on the presence or absence of a synovial (joint) cavity, while their *functional* classification takes into account the degree of movement they permit.

Classification of joints

There are three major functional classes of joints:

1. Structurally immovable joints are classified as *fibrous*, with the bones united by fibrous connective tissue. The sutures between the bones of the skull are examples of such joints.

2. Slightly movable joints are referred to as *cartilaginous* because the bones are held together by cartilage – a strong avascular material. The inferior tibiofibular joint and the symphysis pubis (in the pelvis) are examples of slightly movable joints.

3. Freely movable joints have a space between articulating bones called the synovial or joint cavity. These joints are classified structurally as *synovial* and include the hip, knee, shoulder and elbow (Fig. 24.2). As most of the joints in the skeleton fall into this last category, they will be described in detail.

Synovial joints

Freely movable or **synovial** joints, consisting of articulating bones and the joint cavity, are enclosed in a tough fibrous capsule (the articular capsule) which is continuous

Repair
See chapter 3.2

Joints
See chapter 3.3

Synovial
See chapter 3.3

Figure 24.2   A synovial joint in frontal section.

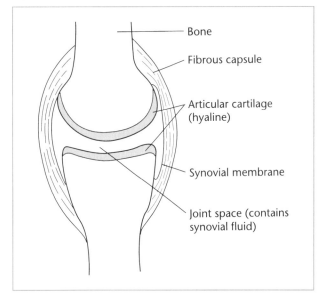

- Bone
- Fibrous capsule
- Articular cartilage (hyaline)
- Synovial membrane
- Joint space (contains synovial fluid)

with the periosteum of the bones. This arrangement serves to stabilize the joint and keep the bones in normal apposition. The joint may be further reinforced by ligaments extending from one bone to another.

The inner surface of the articular capsule is lined with synovial membrane (synovium), which secretes synovial fluid. This fluid lubricates the joint, reduces friction and provides nourishment for the articular cartilage that covers the articulating surfaces of the bones of the joint. Some freely movable joints also have flat, crescent-shaped pieces of cartilage interposed between the articulating surfaces to cushion and protect the bone surfaces. For example, in the knee joint, semilunar cartilages referred to as *menisci* are located between the condyles of the femur and tibia (Fig. 24.3). Bursae are also situated between some body parts to reduce further the friction created by various movements of the body. These sac-like structures are lined with synovial membrane.

Freely movable joints are also differentiated by the type of movement they permit. These movements are limited by several factors, including the shape of the articulating bones, the tension of the ligaments, and the arrangement and tension of muscles. Generally, these joints permit one or more of the following movements: flexion, extension, abduction, adduction, rotation, circumduction, eversion, inversion, pronation and supination (Fig. 24.4).

How movement occurs at joints

To enable **movement** to occur, each synovial joint has at least one pair of muscles surrounding it. These work together so that when one is contracting (the *agonist*) the other is relaxing (the *antagonist*). Each muscle is attached to bone by a tendon at either end. The proximal tendon is usually referred to as the *tendon of origin*; the distal tendon is referred to as the *tendon of insertion*. Thus, when the muscle on the inner aspect of the joint contracts, the distal (furthest) bone is brought nearer the body (*flexion*). To allow this movement, the muscle on the outer aspect of the joint must relax. Similarly, when the muscle on the outer aspect of the joint contracts, the joint straightens (*extension*). Examples of this are the contraction of the hamstring muscle group behind the knee which produces flexion of the knee. This can occur only if the quadriceps muscle group relaxes sufficiently to allow flexion. This 'working in pairs' is essential for smooth joint movement.

Trauma assessment

The patient who has been injured will have suffered an unpleasant experience which may well have been both frightening and painful. Whether a nurse encounters the patient in a first aid situation, an A&E unit or on the ward, these elements of psychological stress and pain should be considered carefully when assessing the patient.

Movement
See chapter 3.3

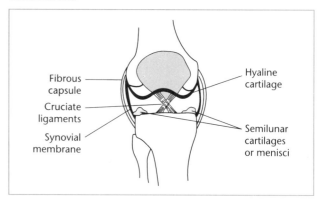

Figure 24.3   Knee joint, showing supporting ligaments and medial lateral menisci.

In all acute trauma situations the priority is to assess the 'ABCD of resuscitation', i.e. the patency of the person's *a*irway, their *b*reathing, *c*irculation and any evidence of *d*isability that might indicate cervical spine damage. This primary assessment should always precede the secondary assessment, which should then focus on pain and psychological status alongside the main injury itself. Assessment should then move on to consider the rest of the patient, checking for other less obvious injuries, unrelated but coexisting medical conditions (e.g. is the patient also diabetic?) as well as social factors. When women are assessed, the nurse should be aware of the possibility of domestic abuse which can happen to women from *any* social background.

It is important to obtain a history of the injury and the degree of force involved. Certain mechanisms of trauma produce characteristic patterns of injury; knowledge of how the accident happened will therefore focus the nurse's attention on certain possible injuries. For example, a fall on an outstretched hand in an elderly person may produce a fracture of the lower extremity of the radius (Colles' fracture) but less obviously it may produce an impacted fracture of the upper humerus.

An injured limb should be assessed gently with the minimum amount of movement because of the pain this may cause and also the risk of making the injury worse.

Pain is obviously a key sign of trauma, but is not necessarily always present or related in intensity to the severity of the injury. The cardinal sign of a fracture is localized bony tenderness, i.e. gentle pressure on the fracture site produces a painful response. In assessing a patient this is a key observation for the nurse to make.

The cardiovascular status of the limb must also be assessed as trauma may occlude the arterial blood supply leading to ischaemia, nerve damage and, in extreme cases, loss of the limb itself. The nurse must locate and mark a peripheral pulse, which should be monitored regularly. This is equally important on the ward after medical treatment such as manipulation of a displaced fracture and mobilization in a plaster cast as swelling and arterial

Figure 24.4   Joint movements.

compression within the limb may be sufficient to occlude the blood supply.

The limb should also be assessed for evidence of deformity or shortening. Dislocation of a joint will obviously lead to deformity, as may a displaced fracture. Fractures of the femoral neck region characteristically produce shortening of the injured limb by approximately 2 cm and external relation of the limb.

In assessing the injured limb for localized bony tenderness, pain, cardiovascular compromise and deformity, the nurse must not lose sight of the whole person and their psychological status. The person may be very tearful and obviously frightened, or stoically silent. Either way the person has recently had a very unpleasant and probably painful experience which may affect their life for months

and even years ahead. A wide range of thoughts and fears may be running through the injured person's head, whether it be in A&E or the ward. Quality nursing care requires these thoughts and fears be explored.

An elderly woman living alone may have suffered a fractured wrist which can usually be treated on an outpatient basis once the fracture has been reduced and immobilized in a plaster cast, but how well can that patient manage at home with her arm in plaster? Can she manage to walk safely with her Zimmer frame? What if the plaster becomes wet as a result of washing? Another common injury in elderly women is fracture of the femoral neck. The patient may be terrified of becoming a burden on relatives. She may feel her family will see this as too much of a burden and put her in a home. These are just some of the fears and anxieties that may affect a patient and which the nurse needs to try to discover if help is to be offered.

Patient assessment therefore needs to be a continual process and incorporate far more than the injured limb.

Medical investigations

Radiography is always indicated following injuries to bones and joints. Because a film is a flat surface, at least two different views of each area of interest are taken, at different angles, to provide a three-dimensional guide to structure. This is particularly important when displacement is being identified.

In the acute stage of an injury, care must be taken not to move the patient unnecessarily. Casts, immobilization devices or traction should not be removed while radiographic investigations are performed in order to prevent the risk of displacement of the fractured bone.

Although radiography is used in the A&E department, advances in imaging science allow for various other sophisticated techniques to be used subsequently, such as radioactive bone scans, computed tomography or magnetic resonance imaging.

Fractures
See chapter 3.2

Fractures

A **fracture** is a break in the continuity of a bone, separating it into two or more parts. The soft tissues in the area surrounding the fracture are also involved in the injury.

Causes

The majority of fractures are due to violence incurred by falls, blows or rotational stresses. In each case the force is in excess of the bone's resistance and may have been applied directly or indirectly. In direct violence, the fracture occurs at or near the site of the applied force. When indirect violence is the cause, the force is applied at a point remote from the site of the fracture. For example, in a fall on the outstretched hand, the stress may be transmitted to the radius, ulna, humerus or clavicle. Occasionally a fracture may be due to a sudden forceful contraction of attached muscles; this is known as an avulsion fracture.

A fracture can occur as the result of disease of the bone which has weakened its structure to the point that it can no longer withstand the normal stresses and strains of everyday life; this is known as a *pathological fracture*. Metastases, primary tumours, osteitis fibrosa cystica due to hyperparathyroidism, osteogenesis imperfecta (a congenital condition affecting the formation of osteoblasts) and osteoporosis are examples of diseased conditions of bone that may lead to spontaneous fracture. Prolonged stress may also cause a fracture in certain bones. This is known as a *stress fracture* and may, for example, affect the fibula in professional sportspeople.

Types of fracture

The types of fracture are listed in Box 24.2 and illustrated in Figure 24.5. Injury and fracture of the spine and skull are discussed in Chapter 20 as there is often serious neurological involvement.

Physiological responses

Local

A fracture is always accompanied by some degree of damage to the surrounding soft tissues. Blood vessels within the bone, the periosteum and surrounding tissues are torn, resulting in haemorrhage and then the formation of a haematoma. The periosteum at the site may be stripped away from the underlying bone tissue, interrupting the blood supply into the area and thus contributing to the death of bone cells. There may also be haemorrhage into adjacent muscles and joints and damage to ligaments, tendons and nerves. Soon after a fracture occurs the muscles in the area go into spasm, causing severe pain and possible displacement of a fragment due to tendon pull.

Box 24.2   Terms used to describe types of fracture

- *Traumatic or pathological*: traumatic is the result of violence; pathological is spontaneous or the result of disease

- *Incomplete*: break not all the way through bone (e.g. greenstick fracture in children)

- *Complete*: bone is separated into two distinct parts

- *Closed (simple)*: overlying skin is intact

- *Open (compound)*: a wound exists over the fracture establishing communication between the fracture and the outside air

- *Complicated*: fracture includes injury to adjacent structures (e.g. blood vessels, nerves or organs)

- *Comminuted*: more than one line of fracture and more than two fragments

- *Transverse*: line of fracture is at right angles to the long axis of bone

- *Spiral*: curves in spiral fashion around bone

- *Impacted*: one fragment is driven into another (cancellous bone usually involved)

- *Crush or compression*: fracture occurs in cancellous bone which is compressed beyond limits of tolerance

- *Avulsion*: a ligament or tendon under excessive stress fractures or tears away its bony attachment

- *Depressed*: a segment of cortical bone is depressed below the level of surrounding bone.

Depending on the fracture, visceral injuries may occur, which may threaten the patient's life. Examples of such injuries are rupture of the bladder by a fractured pelvis and rupture of the spleen or perforation of a lung by a fractured rib.

Systemic

The patient suffers some degree of shock which is influenced by the severity of the injury, the amount of soft tissue damage, associated disorders or multiple injuries, and the patient's age and general condition at the time of injury. A fracture of the femoral shaft results in a blood loss of approximately 1 litre and will probably lead to hypovolaemic shock, whereas a fracture of the tibia produces blood loss of approximately 500 mL. Usually a slight increase in temperature and leucocytosis occur in the first 2 or 3 days.

In addition there is also the psychological dimension to consider as different people respond in different ways to the same injury. The psychological response and degree of motivation shown by the patient may affect recovery time significantly.

Clinical characteristics of fractures and patient assessment

The following discussion is an important guide to assessment and care planning as it highlights potential and actual problems the patient may have. The symptoms of a fracture vary with its location, type, the amount of displacement of the fragments and the degree of damage to soft tissue structures (see Table 24.1). The symptoms also vary with the patient's personality and perception of the injury, coupled with the social norms experienced by the patient.

The patient or an observer usually relates a history of a fall, blow or sudden forcible movement, and the victim may actually say that he or she heard the bone break. Sudden severe pain at the site is experienced which may or may not persist. Frequently, because of injury, nerve .function is impaired and pain may be absent for a brief period following the injury. As function returns, muscle spasm in the area, as well as tissue damage, accounts for much of the pain, which becomes worse with any movement. Obvious deformity may be present as a result of

Figure 24.5 Types of fracture.

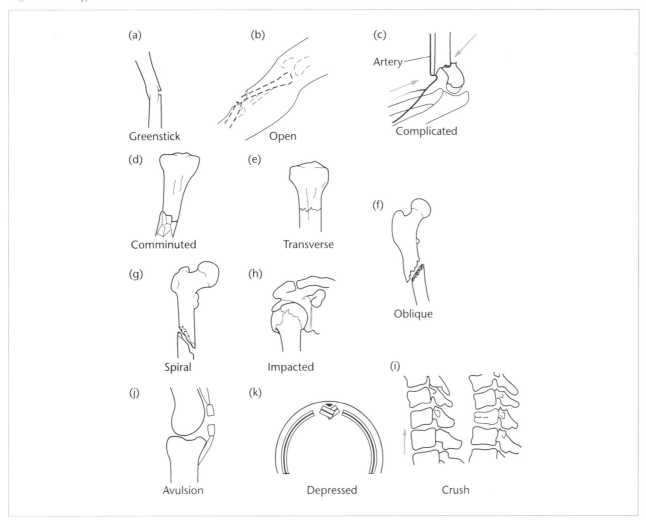

(a) Greenstick
(b) Open
(c) Artery — Complicated
(d) Comminuted
(e) Transverse
(f) Oblique
(g) Spiral
(h) Impacted
(i) Crush
(j) Avulsion
(k) Depressed

Table 24.1 Specific problems of a patient with a fracture

Patient problem	Causes
Sudden severe pain at site (may or may not persist)	Injury, impaired nerve function, muscle spasm, tissue damage
Deformity or shortening of limb	Displacement of bone fragments, muscle spasm
Impaired mobility and loss of function	Disruption of bone Nerve compression by bone fragments
Loss of circulation	Arterial compression by bone fragments
Swelling	Bleeding and/or escape of fluid into tissues; after 2–5 days area may become discoloured (ecchymosis)
Crepitation (grating sound)	Movement of bone fragments at fracture end

Healing
See chapter 3.2

displacement of the fragments, and there may be shortening of the affected limb due to contraction of attached muscles; this is particularly apparent in femoral fractures. Impaired mobility and loss of mechanical support occur, and in the case of long bones there may be obvious movement in a part that is normally rigid. Complete loss of function may result from nerve compression by displaced fragments; this is usually restored when the fracture is reduced and the fragments are placed in normal apposition and alignment. The blood supply to a limb may be severely impaired if an artery is trapped in the fracture. In severe cases the limb may be lost due to gangrene if the blood supply is not quickly restored by manipulation of the fracture to restore normal anatomy.

Crepitation (a grating sound produced by movement of the ends of the fragments) may be noted if the patient moves the part. Under no circumstances should any attempt be made to elicit crepitus because of the possibility of further serious damage to soft tissues (e.g. blood vessels and nerves), unnecessary displacement of fragments and the possible production of an open fracture. Swelling may develop rapidly over the site of the fracture because of bleeding and the escape of fluid into the tissue. After 2 or 3 days this area frequently becomes discoloured (*ecchymosis*).

In the case of the rupture of an organ by a fragment, symptoms of impaired function of the damaged organ appear. With rupture of the bladder by a fractured pelvis, extravasation of urine gradually becomes evident, and blood appears in the urine. Although rare, perforation of the intestine is associated with pelvic fracture and causes severe shock and peritonitis; the abdomen becomes distended and board-like. A serious complication of a rib fracture may be puncture of a lung. The patient

manifests severe shock, respiratory distress, coughing and haemoptysis.

Some fractures, especially those that are incomplete, impacted or of short bones, may produce few signs and symptoms. The fracture may be suspected only on the basis of the history of violence, tenderness on pressure over the site or the patient's complaint of pain upon use of the part or weight bearing on it. Again, no attempt should be made to elicit symptoms by having the person move or stand. The patient is treated as having a fracture if there is any doubt.

Diagnosis of a fracture is based on the history of the accident, physical examination of the patient and radiographs of the affected part.

Fracture healing

Bone is different from many of the specialized tissues because of its ability to regenerate and hence restore the continuity that was disrupted by the fracture. Many tissues heal by laying down non-specialized fibrous scar tissue.

Immediately after a fracture the space between the fragments and around the fracture line is filled with blood and inflammatory exudate. The haematoma and the exudate are invaded by fibroblasts and capillaries from adjacent connective tissue and blood vessels, forming granulation tissue. Simultaneously, osteoblasts proliferate, mainly from the inner surface of the periosteum (and endosteum in a long bone) and invade the granulation tissue. Calcium salts are deposited, forming a loosely woven, bone-like tissue referred to as a *callus*. This forms a 'collar' around the bone at the fracture site, giving it greater thickness than the original bone. The callus unites and helps to stabilize the fragments but is not strong enough to bear weight or withstand stress. If the blood supply is poor, or if it is disturbed by excessive mobility at the fracture site, cartilage may be formed instead of bone. As the osteoblasts increase, the callus is gradually restructured by ossification (production of a collagenous fibrous network that becomes impregnated with mineral salts) to form bone tissue. Remodelling is the final stage of fracture healing. The external bulbous bony area is remodelled by the action of osteoclasts.

In some instances, a fracture is complicated by malunion, delayed healing or non-union:

- *Malunion* implies healing of the fracture in an abnormal position. There may be angulation of the bone or overriding of the fragments which alters the shape and length of the limb. Function may be impaired. The cause is usually ineffective reduction and/or fixation during healing.

- *Delayed healing* simply implies that the fracture is not healing as rapidly as is normally expected.

- In *non-union*, the granulation tissue that formed between the fragments following the fracture is converted to dense fibrous tissue instead of normal callus and bone tissue. Causes of delayed union or non-union include too wide a gap between the fragments, the interposition of soft tissues or a foreign body between the fragments, poor blood supply to the site, loss of the initial haematoma by the escape of blood through an open wound or surgical intervention, infection of the bone, malnutrition and disease of bone (e.g. bone metastases).

General principles and methods of treatment of fractures

Emergency care

Emergency treatment of a person with a fracture usually occurs at the site where the injury took place. The patient's general condition and the extent of injuries are quickly assessed and priorities are set. Respiratory insufficiency, haemorrhage or shock may be evident and take precedence over injured bones.

The first aid treatment is very important; movement of the patient or improper handling may cause serious tissue damage and increased pain, haemorrhage and shock. If a fracture is obvious or suspected, care at the site of the accident and during transportation to a hospital is directed toward reducing pain and preventing further tissue damage, including to underlying tissues and organs, and a closed fracture becoming open. The patient should receive a minimum of handling (unless there is danger of further injury) until the emergency services arrive. Before moving the patient, the fracture site and the joint above and below are immobilized in order to reduce the risk of further damage and to relieve pain. A splint can be made from whatever is available (e.g. a board, two or three thicknesses of cardboard, a folded quilt or blanket, pillows). In the case of a board, the surface applied to the patient must be padded (towels or clothing may be used) to prevent pressure. If the limb is in an abnormal position, it is splinted in that deformed position; no attempt is made to reduce the fracture or restore the limb to a normal position. The easiest splint is the patient's own body: an uninjured leg can act as a splint for an injured leg and the trunk can splint an injured arm. Thus a lower limb may be immobilized by placing a pillow or folded blanket between the legs and tying them together. In the case of an arm, it may be secured against the trunk by bandages and a sling. If it is an open fracture, the wound is covered with the cleanest material available in order to prevent further contamination and reduce infection risks. If the bone is protruding from the wound, no attempt is made to replace it or reduce the fracture. Nothing is given by mouth in case a general anaesthetic proves necessary.

When the patient arrives at the hospital a quick assessment is made of the general condition and, if there is respiratory insufficiency or shock, appropriate treatment is instituted before the fracture receives attention. When the general condition is satisfactory, radiographs are taken of the fracture area.

The patient may be disoriented, frightened and agitated. An ongoing explanation of what is about to be done and what the patient can do best to assist in care often helps to keep the patient calm. This makes it possible to provide efficient on-the-scene care and prevent further injury.

Treatment

The treatment of a fracture usually involves reduction, fixation (immobilization) of the part, protection while the bone heals, and rehabilitation during and after the healing process to restore normal function. When possible, bone stress is utilized to increase the process of repair. The bone fragments are mechanically fixated to enable immediate use, creating stress at the fracture site which accelerates osteoblastic activity. Some fractures, such as those of distal phalanges of the fingers and toes, may heal without reduction and immobilization. However, regular analgesia will be required to maintain mobility.

Reduction

This is the procedure by which fragments are brought into their pre-injury position so that the normal shape and length of the bone are restored and union is promoted. Obviously, reduction is necessary only if there is some displacement of the fragments (Fig. 24.6). It is carried out as soon as possible. A delay makes it more difficult to obtain satisfactory alignment because of the rapid organization of the blood clot and the development of associated muscle spasm. Also, there is likely to be less tissue trauma with early reduction.

Figure 24.6 Fracture of the femoral shaft. The pull by the adductor muscles causes displacement of the fragments.

A fracture may be reduced by a number of methods, with the use of general or regional anaesthesia or an analgesic such as pethidine or papaveretum. Methods for reducing fractures include closed manipulative reduction, traction applied distal to the fracture, or open (internal) reduction. In *closed reduction*, the surgeon manipulates the fragments into position by manual traction, pressure and/or rotation. In fractures in which one fragment is overriding the other and there is considerable muscle pull, continuous *traction* may be applied to the distal fragment to bring it into apposition and maintain the alignment. This method of reduction is used most often in fractures of the femur because the pull of the strong thigh muscles tends to displace the fragments and cause overriding. The traction may be applied to the skin (skin traction) or directly to bone (skeletal traction). In some fractures, reduction can be achieved only through an *open surgical incision*.

Immobilization or fixation

Various methods are used to maintain reduction and fixate the fragments. They may be categorized as external fixation, external skeletal fixation, skin or skeletal traction, or internal fixation. The method used depends upon the particular bone (e.g. location – short, long or flat), the type of fracture and the muscles involved.

External fixation

This is most commonly achieved by enclosing the part in a cast (Box 24.3). A *plaster cast* is most widely used and is made by the application and moulding of moist plaster of Paris bandages to the affected part. As the water evaporates from the bandages, the plaster hardens and the application becomes rigid. This takes more than 24 hours to set fully. An alternative is to use fibreglass, synthetic casting materials which set fully in 30 minutes, and are much lighter and stronger.

Before either cast is applied, the skin is cleansed and examined for any contusions or abrasions. The part is

---

Box 24.3   Types of cast

■ *Plaster*: a cylinder that encases a fractured limb

■ *Walking*: a weight-bearing wooden heel and sole (rocker) is incorporated into the cast

■ *Body* (*jacket*): applied to the trunk

■ *Spica* (*shoulder/hip*): applied to the trunk and shoulder or hip

■ *Bivalve*: moulded to trunk or limb and cut down each side when dry. Held in place with Velcro or bandages

■ *Splint*: plaster of Paris, metal, fibreglass thermoplastic or polyurethane material moulded to support the affected limb.

---

then enclosed in stockinette for skin protection. Extra padding is used over bony prominences or to fill in spaces that might weaken the cast. It is also applied when swelling is anticipated.

A *walking cast* may be applied with stable fractures of the tibia and fibula. A 'rocker' or sole plate incorporated in the base of the plaster enables the patient to be weight bearing. A *bivalve* cast may be removed for brief periods to allow skin or wound care or other treatment; however, this is rarely used for fracture prior to callus formation because of the danger of loss of position. When swelling of the limb is expected, for example in a recent injury, a plaster back slab may be applied rather than a cylindrical cast. This is made by the application of slabs of plaster of Paris to the posterior of the limb; the slabs are then secured in position with cotton bandages. The rationale is that, if necessary, the cotton bandages can be easily split to prevent circulatory and neurological impairment.

External skeletal fixation

With this method of treatment the bone fragments are held in alignment by skeletal pins. Two or more pins are inserted into each fragment either side of the fracture and the fracture is reduced. The pins are then held in proper relation to one another by an external support which either runs parallel to the bone or is circular around the limb. External skeletal fixation may be used in the treatment of fractures associated with extensive damage to the soft tissues where traction is not suitable and internal fixation would carry a high risk of introduction of foreign material into the wound. It may also be used in the management of infected fractures, in multiple fractures (to allow the treatment of other fractures by traction) and in pelvic fractures with disruption of the symphysis pubis. The technique can also be used to correct deformity, lengthen limbs and in the arthrodesis of infected joints after unsuccessful arthroplasty (Sims 1999). External skeletal fixation is designed to hold the fracture without a plaster cast until union, and allow access to any wounds. The disadvantages are the risks of pin-track infections, the loosening of the pins and delayed union, as external callus formation may be suppressed by tissue trauma and rigid immobilization of the fracture. The incidence of pin-site infection is common. Sims and Saleh (2000) found that, in a series of 248 patients who had external fixators applied, 71% developed infection at the pin sites. In 13 cases the pin had to be removed or local surgical curettage had to be performed as the infection was so severe.

Traction

Traction (which may also be employed to correct a deformity, relieve pressure on a spinal nerve or prevent a contracture deformity in cases in which there is muscle spasm) is most commonly used to reduce and maintain reduction in fractures of the limbs by overcoming the effects of gravity and muscle pull. It involves the application of a force along the long axis of the bone distal to the fracture. For this force to be effective, a force in the opposite direction is required (countertraction). Countertraction is necessary and is usually provided by elevating the foot of the bed in the case of a lower limb; the weight of the body on the incline supplies the required countertraction. Traction is used much less frequently as both internal and external fixation techniques have become more widespread and the importance of early mobilization has increased.

An important use of traction is to overcome the deforming muscle pull that is associated with fractures of long bones such as the shaft of femur. This is needed in emergency care environments such as A&E. A fracture of the femur is accompanied by marked displacement of the fragments due to the contracture of the very strong muscles of the thigh and hip. The adductor muscles produce a lateral bowing (see Fig. 24.6). Fixed traction is commonly applied via the traditional Thomas' splint or one of the more modern telescopic versions (Walsh and Kent 2001).

Fixed traction This is traction between two fixed points; for example, a lower limb is supported in a Thomas' splint, which is a metal splint with a medial and lateral bar and a leather-covered ring which surrounds the thigh at the groin. Traction is exerted by either skin extension tapes tied to the distal end of the splint or by passing a pin through the tibia and pulling directly on the bone. Countertraction is obtained by the thrust of the ring against the ischial tuberosity (Fig. 24.7).

Balanced traction In balanced or sliding traction there must also be two opposing forces (traction and

Figure 24.7   (a) Fixed traction using skin traction and a Thomas' splint. (b) Fixed traction using a skeletal pin and a Thomas' splint.

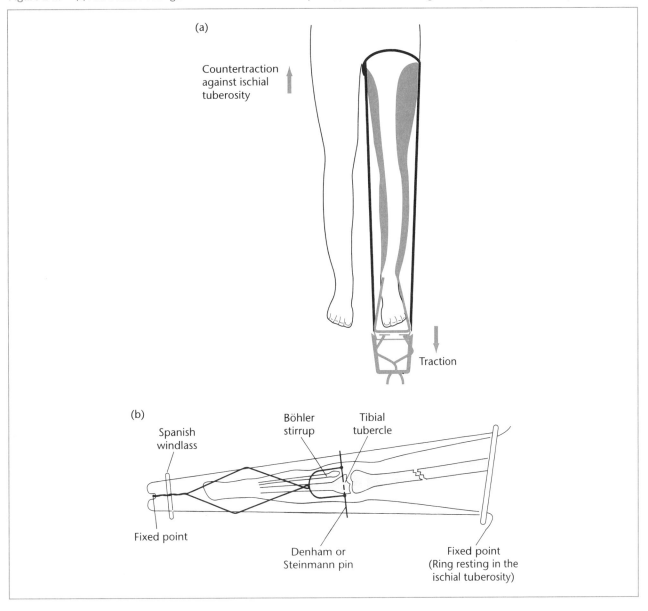

countertraction). The forces are balanced and mobile, allowing the patient to move about the bed without disturbing the desired line of pull. Traction is applied by the use of a weight and pulley system. A cord passes over the pulley to the weights and is attached at the proximal end to skin extensions in skin traction, or to a skeletal pin which passes through the patient's bone in skeletal traction. Countertraction is obtained by elevation of the foot of the bed. Gravity, together with the patient's bodyweight, provides the required countertraction (Figs 24.8 & 24.9).

Skin traction This is established by application of adhesive or non-adhesive tapes to the medial and lateral surfaces of the limb. These are secured by a firm encircling

Figure 24.8 Balanced (sliding) traction. Note elevation of foot of bed uses patient's own bodyweight as countertraction.

Figure 24.9 Suspension of the Thomas' splint.

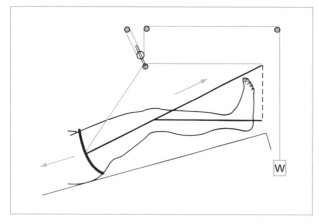

Figure 24.10 Skin traction of a lower limb.

crêpe or elasticated bandage (Fig. 24.10). The bandage must not be applied tightly around the limb as this may cause skin or vascular complications. The use of skin traction has declined over the past 10 years except in the care of children with femoral fractures.

Skeletal traction This is achieved by the insertion of a metal wire (Kirschner wire) or pin (e.g. Steinmann or Denham pin) through the bone distal to the fracture. By this means traction is applied directly to the skeleton. A special traction stirrup or U loop is fastened to the protruding wire or pin (Fig. 24.11); cord is attached to this which leads to a weight and pulley system. Countertraction is obtained by gravity and the patient's bodyweight on an inclined bed. The limb in traction is then usually suspended off the bed surface.

Various arrangements are used in applying traction to the lower limb. The most frequently used are Buck's traction (or extension), Hamilton Russell traction, Perkin's traction, and balanced skeletal traction with a Thomas' splint and knee flexion piece. Bryant's, or Gallow's, traction is used only for very young children and involves suspending both legs from an overhead bar, lifting the buttocks clear of the cot mattress.

Buck's traction This involves simple skin traction (Fig. 24.12). The leg is supported on a soft pillow to keep the heel clear of the bed. Particular care is taken to avoid pressure from tight bandaging over the fibula head to prevent compression of the peroneal nerve which lies close to the surface. Damage to the nerve could result in interference with normal ankle movement. Countertraction is obtained by elevating the foot of the bed. It is used for undisplaced fractures of the acetabulum, for the correction of minor fixed flexion deformities of the hip or knee, and following relocation of a dislocated hip or total hip replacement. Bilateral Buck's traction may be used for the treatment of a prolapsed intervertebral disc.

Hamilton Russell traction This has been used mainly in the preoperative treatment of a fracture of the neck of a femur. However, a major review of the research evidence by Parker and Handoll (2000) found no evidence that traction offers any benefit to the patient and continued use of this approach is not evidence based. Vertical traction is applied at the knee; at the same time a horizontal force is exerted on the tibia and fibula (Fig. 24.13). It is a straight Buck's traction with weights attached to the footplate or spreader bar, and a vertical pull from a sling under the patient's leg just above the knee.

Perkin's traction This involves balanced skeletal traction without any form of external splintage. Active movements of the limb are commenced as soon as possible. Perkin's traction can be used in the management of fractures of the femur from the trochanteric region distally (Fig. 24.14). A split bed in which the distal one-third of the mattress and base of the bed can be removed is used when the patient has a fracture of the femur managed by Perkin's traction, as this facilitates flexion of the knee.

Balanced skeletal traction   This is commonly used with a half- or full-ring Thomas' splint and with a Pearson's knee flexion piece to obtain reduction of a fracture of a shaft of a femur and to maintain reduction until union occurs.

Firm cotton slings are secured to the upper part of the Thomas' splint to support the thigh and to the Pearson's knee flexion piece to support the leg. The Thomas' splint extends from the groin to beyond the foot in line with the femur. The knee is in 10–20° of flexion to control rotation and prevent stretching of the posterior knee capsule and ligaments, and subsequent joint instability. Some provision may be made to support the foot to prevent footdrop.

Figure 24.11   Skeletal traction may be applied by (a) a Kirschner wire and traction stirrup; (b) a Steinmann pin and traction stirrup; or (c) a Steinmann pin and Böhler stirrup.

Figure 24.12   Buck's traction.

Figure 24.13   Hamilton Russell traction. Forces A + B = C, which is counterbalanced by the patient's bodyweight (D).

Figure 24.14   Perkin's traction.

The skeletal traction is usually applied to the proximal area of the tibia. The pull is exerted in line with the femur by means of a traction cord attached to the bow or stirrup that is fitted to the protruding ends of the pin that passes through the bone. The traction cord passes over a pulley and suspends a weight. The proximal and distal ends of the splint are suspended by separate cords, pulleys and weights. Countertraction is obtained by elevating the foot of the bed. When the patient moves up or down in the bed the splint moves as well, and traction is maintained. The patient has greater freedom of movement and is usually more comfortable in this system of traction. It also has the advantage of allowing a certain amount of movement in adjacent joints.

Internal fixation

Some fractures require internal surgical reduction and fixation. Various types of internal fixation devices are used. These include stainless steel or vitallium wire, screws, plates, rods, and pins and bone grafts. They may be secured to the sides of the bone, placed through the fragments or passed through the intramedullary cavity of the bone. Internal fixation may be reinforced after the wound is closed by the application of a cast or splint. However, new devices of such strength and design are being made that external splintage is not always required, thus allowing immediate joint freedom, early weight bearing and short-term hospitalization. This system of fracture fixation has been developed by the Association for the Study of Internal Fixation (ASIF or AO).

Special internal fixation devices are used to immobilize the fragments in a hip fracture or fracture of the femoral neck. Three-flanged nails (Smith–Petersen pins or nails; Fig. 24.15), a Neufeld nail or a McLaughlin nail and plate, or a compression hip screw may be used (Fig. 24.16). In patients with an intracapsular fracture through the neck of the femur there is a risk of avascular necrosis of the femoral head (death of bone due to lack of blood supply); in these cases a hemiarthroplasty is performed by replacing the head of the femur with a metallic prosthesis. (A discussion of hip fracture can be found later in this chapter.)

Following any method of reduction and fixation a post-operative/reduction radiograph is vital to ensure that the position is maintained. Radiographs are then taken periodically to determine that healing is occurring and the bone fragments remain in the correct alignment.

Open (compound) fractures

The patient with an open fracture requires special treatment as soon after the accident as possible. The site is potentially infected and there is usually a greater amount of soft tissue damage and destruction. Infection and necrosis impede bone union and may result in serious disability. An initial wound assessment takes place in A&E as soon as possible. The wound will be irrigated to remove gross contamination and dressed with saline and iodine soaks. Intravenous opioid analgesia is essential (usually morphine) and the limb should be kept immobile with frequent checks on the foot pulse to ensure there is no neurovascular damage. The patient will be a high priority for theatre, where the surgeon will explore and debride the wound (the removal of foreign material and excision of dead tissue). The repair of severed or torn tendons or nerves may be necessary. The fracture is reduced and then immobilized. If there has been gross contamination, the wound may be packed and left open until the danger of infection is past. Drains are inserted in the wound (e.g. Redivac drainage system). Antibiotic therapy may be prescribed.

Before administration of the anaesthetic, it is determined whether the patient has had previous immunization for tetanus. If so, a booster dose of tetanus toxoid may be ordered. If not, human tetanus immunoglobulin is given.

Care of the patient in a cast

The care of the patient following the application of a cast requires the following considerations.

Drying of the cast

Complete drying of a plaster cast following its application may take several hours or days, depending on the material used, its thickness and the temperature, humidity and circulation of the air. During this period, support of the cast and handling are very important, because the cast is vulnerable to pressure and cracking which could alter its shape and cause indentations that result in undue pressure on an area of the body or make it ineffective. When the part must be lifted, it is supported on the palms of the hands to avoid making indentations by the fingertips. In the case of a body or long leg cast, firm support along the line of the cast is ensured. Pillows with plastic or rubber undercovers are placed under the part encased in plaster so that the cast is not subjected to pressure by the firm mattress. As it is moulded to the contours of the part to which is is applied, support by an extra pillow or folded flannelette sheet may be necessary under such regions as the lumbar or popliteal area.

Drying is promoted by exposure to dry, warm, circulating air which evaporates the moisture from the cast. The bedding is arranged so that the cast is left uncovered. If it is a large or body cast, two or three persons work together to turn the patient and pillows are used to avoid strain on any part of the plaster. A moist cast has a dull grey appearance but, when dry, it appears white and shiny. Casts made from materials other than plaster of Paris usually dry more quickly. A study of the instructions that come with these materials will explain the drying time.

Weight bearing on a walking cast is begun when the cast is thoroughly dry. If plaster of Paris has been used, this is usually after 48 hours.

Patient problems

Unless the patient experiences complications or requires surgery, the plaster cast will be applied in the A&E department. This greatly reduces the time the nurse has to assess the patient and/or family for their response to, or understanding of, the injury and the care required. Rapid assessment and intervention is necessary.

It is important to assess whether there are any skin lesions (e.g. wounds, pre-existing skin conditions) as these will be enclosed in the cast, possibly for several weeks, leading to the risk of tissue necrosis, suppuration or infection. Swelling should be assessed carefully because of the risk of neurovascular compromise if the limb becomes compressed within the cast. It is important

Figure 24.15   (a) Smith–Petersen nail; (b) Jewett nail plate; (c) dynamic hip screw; (d) hip prosthesis (Thompson).

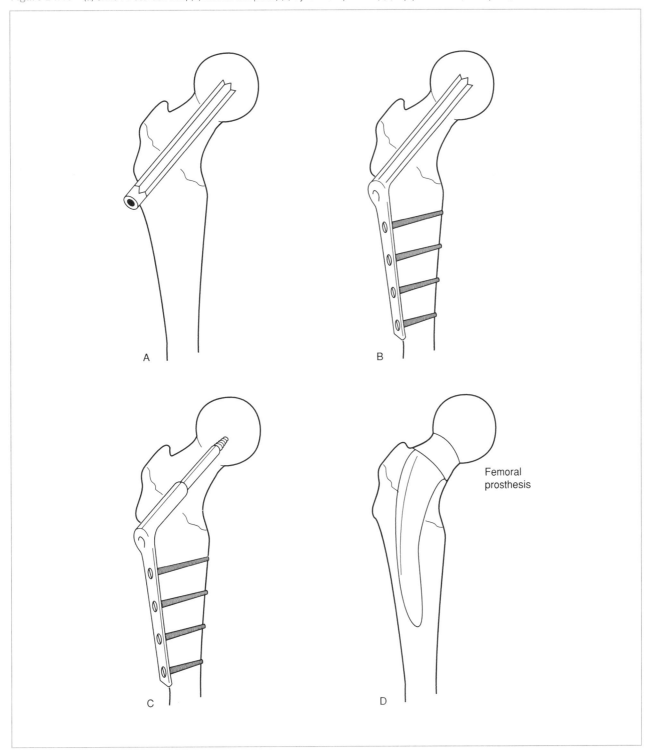

to check that any jewellery has been removed; a ring, for example, could act as a tourniquet around the finger if severe swelling develops.

Apart from such physical factors the nurse should assess the patient's level of comprehension of what is

Figure 24.16   Compression (dynamic) hip screw for trochanteric fracture.

happening. After discharge from A&E the patient will be responsible for the self-care of the cast and fracture. This requires understanding of teaching about swelling and circulation, the condition of the cast, pain control, etc. The nurse needs to assess the patient's grasp of language and intellectual functioning in order to ensure that teaching is delivered in an effective and appropriate way.

The social consequences of injury have already been raised and the nurse has a responsibility to assess whether the patient will have any significant social problems as a result of having a limb in a cast. This is particularly true of groups such as the elderly or lone parents who may find coping alone very difficult in these circumstances.

Table 24.2 gives a summary of some of the principal health problems that assessment may reveal for the patient with a limb in a cast.

Nursing management

Assessment and monitoring of the cast

Assessment of an inpatient with a cast involves neuro-vascular evaluation of the affected limb every 30 minutes for the first 4 hours and then every 4 hours for several days. The affected extremity is compared with the uninjured one for alterations in colour, temperature, sensation, movement and swelling. Any blanching or the presence of a bluish colour indicates an interruption in circulation to the part. Touching the toes or fingers will identify

Table 24.2   Principal problems for the patient with a limb in a cast

Patient problems	Goals
1. Potential problem of further injury related to pressure on soft tissue, nerves or arteries	The patient will: 1. Understand the importance of the absence of pain and feeling of pressure, irritation or loss of sensation in the affected limb 2. Have normal temperature and colour in the fingers or toes 3. Demonstrate movement of the fingers or toes 4. Show no sign of skin breakdown
2. Immobilization due to limitation of movement by the cast	The patient will: 1. Demonstrate a safe method of walking, and the use of aids such as crutches and walking sticks when these are being used 2. Demonstrate a safe method of transferring from bed to chair or chair to chair when walking is restricted
3. Potential problem of lack of knowledge due to changes in self-care	The patient and/or family will be able to: 1. Describe the care of the cast 2. List risk factors related to potential for further injury or damage to the cast 3. Describe the action to undertake if the cast becomes loose 4. Describe the activities the person may engage in 5. Identify the outpatient clinic for follow-up treatment and where emergency care can be received

temperature differences; pressure applied to these extremities will elicit from the patient any differences in sensation; patients should be asked to demonstrate movement of fingers or toes. Pain assessment is ongoing.

The nurse checks the cast with the palm of the hand for any warm or soft areas. Areas of discoloration or changes in discoloured areas are looked for. A musty smell will be present if infection has occurred, so any odour should be noted as part of the nurse's assessment. As odour is a late sign, infection may be suspected before a musty smell is detected due to localized pain, raised temperature, etc. When an opening (window) has been made in a cast to allow for treatment of an incision or wound, the section is removed regularly to assess the status of the wound and surrounding skin. The skin next to the edges of the cast should also be inspected for signs of rubbing, soreness, etc., especially if a resin cast is used.

The mood of the patient should also be assessed; younger patients in particular may become bored and frustrated at their lack of activity.

Nursing intervention

To alleviate and prevent further swelling, the affected limb is elevated above the level of the heart. This is achieved by the use of pillows, and elevating the foot of the bed when a leg is affected. To elevate the arm, a draw sheet (or towel) may be used by folding the sheet in half and placing the flexed elbow on the fold with the fingers towards the sheet ends. Several large safety pins are carefully inserted on either side of the arm and the sheet ends are pinned over an intravenous stand which suports the weight of the arm. Ideally the hand should be well above the elbow and the elbow off the bed to promote drainage of tissue and reduce swelling. Once the oedema has gone, normal positioning may resume.

If the patient is going home from A&E, detailed printed instructions, reinforced verbally, should be given on care of the cast and limb. Swelling in an injured arm is prevented by the use of a high arm sling. When the lower limb is injured, it should always be elevated above heart level to prevent swelling, when the patient is sitting down.

Care must be taken to avoid getting a plaster cast wet as it will disintegrate with resultant loss of immobilization and fracture position. The cast can be protected when bathing or in inclement weather by plastic bags or some other waterproof material which is sealed around the edges of the cast to prevent moisture from seeping under it. Casts of other materials may be allowed to become wet but saturation should be avoided.

To prevent skin irritation, exposed edges of a cast may be padded by folding the stockinette from under the cast over the top and bottom edges of the cast. The use of powder or lotion under a cast should be avoided as these tend to cake and cause more irritation. The patient should be cautioned against inserting objects such as knitting needles under the cast to try to relieve irritation as this may lead to serious skin breakdown and infection.

Patients with leg casts may be taught to use elbow crutches. The nurse will walk with the patient initially to ensure safety. Walking casts should be protected with a boot or other covering.

The patient and/or family are taught to assess the cast and affected limb, the care of the cast and where to report any alterations in sensation, comfort or signs of drainage. Activities that may be undertaken should be discussed and reasons given for any restrictions.

Removal of the cast

When the cast is taken off, the rigid support to joints that have been immobilized for a considerable period of time is removed. The patient is likely to be discouraged by the stiffness, instability and weakness encountered and requires reassurance that with exercise and progressive use function will be restored.

The cast is removed by special cast cutters or a plaster saw. As this may be frightening, the nurse describes the equipment and the process to the person before removal begins. The limb must be handled gently and with support under the joints. The skin is bathed gently, and an application of oil or lanolin is made to soften the accumulation of dry, scaly skin. Vigorous rubbing is discouraged to avoid skin irritation and abrasions.

Rehabilitation

A regimen of passive and active exercises and massage is established to restore joint and muscle function. Weight bearing and activities are gradually resumed. When the cast is removed and the limb becomes dependent, oedema and swelling are likely to occur. The patient is advised to elevate the limb when sitting and lying, and elasticated tubular bandage (Tubigrip) may be applied when walking to control the oedema, which gradually becomes less troublesome as muscle tone improves and there is increasing activity.

Care of the patient with external skeletal fixation

Preoperative preparation

The length of time that elapses between the time of injury and surgery varies and is dependent on the patient's general state of health and associated injuries. Forms of treatment, such as traction, may be employed temporarily to immobilize the fracture before operation. The care of the patient in the A&E department and following admission to the ward includes observations of vital signs to detect signs of haemorrhage and shock, and observations of colour, temperature, sensation, movement of digits and pulse are made of the injured limb to detect impaired circulation or nerve damage; any abnormal signs are reported to the doctor immediately. Pain as a result of the injury and potential for infection as a result of an open wound are specific problems that need to be addressed between arrival in A&E and transfer to the operating theatre. Analgesics as ordered are administered to alleviate pain. Wounds and surrounding skin are cleansed according to the preference of the surgeon and covered with an antiseptic soak and sterile dressings. This reduces the risk of infection and, by keeping the tissue moist, improves its viability, thereby promoting post-operative wound healing.

The operation is explained to the patient and the external skeletal fixation system is described as it is essential that the patient has a realistic understanding of what the limb will look like after return from the operating theatre (Sims 1999). This will help to alleviate some of the problems that could otherwise occur after oper-ation, associated with altered body image. The nurse should be available to the patient and encourage free discussion of fears and anxieties concerning treatment and recovery.

Postoperative care

The general principles of postoperative care are applicable (see Ch. 10). If an external skeletal fixation system has been applied to a fractured limb, the limb *must* be elevated to help reduce swelling.

In addition to the problems usually experienced after operation, the patient with external fixation has an added potential problem of infection at the pin sites. The nurse checks the external fixation system daily to ensure that the clamps and nuts are tight. This routine is explained to the patient so he or she understands that it is an expected procedure. The pin sites are observed for bleeding or leakage of exudate; they should be dry approximately 48 hours after surgery. Most trauma units have their own protocols for care of pin sites – these should be observed. Pain, tenderness, erythema, swelling and increased skin temperature at a pin site must lead the nurse to suspect pin-site infection. Any of these clinical features must be reported to the doctor, and a wound swab should be taken and sent for microscopy, culture and sensitivity. Antibiotic therapy is prescribed and the pin may be removed. Any loosening of a pin must also be reported as this increases the risk of pin-track infection; the offending pin is usually removed. Any exposed pin tips must be covered by metal or plastic caps or corks to prevent damage by the sharp-ended pin to the other limb or body or to the nursing staff.

The patient usually requires a strong analgesic at regular intervals during the first 48 hours following surgery. If severe or moderate pain persists after this time, the surgeon must be informed as it may be an indication of infection. The patient is usually confined to bed until bone and skin healing is progressing satisfactorily. Exercises of all joints, including those of the affected limb, are commenced as soon as possible to maintain muscle tone, strength and mass, and to maintain joint movements. The patient with a lower limb fracture is at

high risk of the formation of deep vein thrombosis. Foot and leg exercises are commenced on the day after the application of the fixation device and observations are made to detect any signs of this complication.

Some patients may be upset on seeing their injured limb and the fixation system. The nurse needs to show patience and understanding, and should encourage the patient to express any anxieties and fears. By encouraging the patient to participate in the planning of care and to take an interest in the care of the fixation system and the rehabilitation programme, the nurse may assist the patient in coming to terms with an altered body image.

The patient with a lower limb fracture is taught to mobilize with the aid of crutches; weight bearing on the affected limb is not permitted because of the risk of refracture and bone displacement until callus formation is detected by radiography. Once callus has formed, the patient may be taught to bear weight partially through the affected limb.

The external skeletal fixation device is removed once fracture union has occurred, as diagnosed by radiography. After removal of the fixation system (from a lower limb) the patient is generally not permitted to bear weight fully for a further 2 weeks.

Care of the patient in traction

Assessment

The ongoing nature of assessment is well illustrated in the case of a patient on traction where several weeks may elapse before the traction is discontinued.

Of particular importance is the patient's skin condition due to the high risk of **pressure sore** development. Regular monitoring is therefore essential along with the pin sites to detect any early signs of tissue breakdown or infection. The use of a pressure sore risk calculator such as the Norton or Waterlow scale is strongly recommended.

The patient's normal bowel habits and diet should be assessed due to the risks of **constipation** associated with inactivity. Constipation should be detected early by frequent monitoring rather than at the late stage where the patient is impacted. Hospitalization, immobility and frequent use of opioid analgesics predisposes to constipation and in older patients an accompanying detrimental effect on mental state.

Micturition is difficult in traction, particularly for female patients. Any previous history of retention or incontinence needs to be noted and ongoing assessment of urinary output is essential to prevent the risk of retention developing.

The patient's hobbies and interests should be explored as inactivity and boredom can quickly become major problems. Worries about work, income, housing and family, to name but a few social factors, may develop and the nurse therefore needs to assess how the patient feels about these important areas.

Pressure sores
See chapter 6.1

Constipation
See chapter 5.1

Micturition
See chapter 5.4

Table 24.3 Principal potential problems for the patient in traction

Potential patient problem	Goals
1. Infection at the pin site	The patient will not develop an infection at the pin sites
2. General muscle wasting due to immobility	The patient will not suffer muscle wasting in the uninjured limb and it will be minimal in the injured limb
3. Skin breakdown due to traction and immobility	The patient will not suffer any break in skin due to traction or immobility
4. Constipation due to immobility	The patient will be able to defaecate normally without feeling discomfort or requiring artificial stimuli
5. Urinary retention	The patient will be able to empty the bladder in comfort when the need is felt
6. Boredom and depression due to enforced immobility	The patient will develop ways of coping with the inevitable boredom and will be able to express any negative feelings that might occur

Patient problems

The nurse plans the care of the patient in traction to prevent the potential problems listed in Table 24.3.

Nursing intervention

Infection at the pin sites

See care of pin sites (p. 886). While the pins are in place they should remain static and the patient pain free. On removal, there should be no sign of infection and the pin sites should heal within a week.

General muscle wasting due to immobility

The following steps should be taken to minimize this problem:

- Encourage the patient to be as self-caring as possible within the confines of the traction. This will promote the use of various muscle groups, particularly in the upper body, and may be more appealing to the patient than simply 'doing the exercises'.

- Teach the patient to lift himself or herself up the bed on to a bedpan using an overhead monkey pole. This will strengthen the muscles of the arms and chest, which will help the patient to use crutches once mobilizing commences. It also helps to prevent skin breakdown due to friction caused by dragging on the sheets.

- Commence a physiotherapy programme to ensure all muscle groups are put through a range of activities daily. The physiotherapist can identify muscles that are particularly at risk of atrophy and teach the patient the required specific exercises. The nurses and physiotherapist should work together with the patient to ensure the patient understands the exercises and the nurse can supervise them in the physiotherapist's absence. The aim is that, when the traction is removed, the patient's general musculature will be in good condition with minimal evidence of muscle wasting, enabling mobilization to commence.

Skin breakdown due to traction and immobility

Pressure sores are not inevitable and can be prevented. Frequent inspection of all vulnerable **skin** areas should be carried out for the first 48 hours

- *Under the ring of the Thomas' splint*. When this is first applied the skin is at special risk as the thigh may continue to swell and the circulation in the skin becomes compromised. By gently moving the skin under the ring the nurse can see the skin and also relieve any pressure. It is essential that all the skin under the ring is inspected. The patient may find this uncomfortable and unnecessary, and clear explanations are required beforehand. The use of padding under the ring is to be discouraged as it only creates pressure in other areas. If the ring appears to be getting tighter and the skin is in danger, the doctor should be informed and bolt cutters obtained in case the ring needs to be split and removed.

- *In the popliteal area where slings may rub and the skin is vulnerable*. When a Pearson knee flexion piece is used, the knee will be partly flexed which increases the likelihood of rubbing. The skin should be protected from the rough sling by padding.

- *Over the head of fibula*. Here the skin and peroneal nerve are at risk of pressure from the side of the splint. This is a particular problem if the leg falls into external rotation and rolls outward, resting on the side arm of the Thomas' splint. The patient's leg should be positioned in such a way that it rests centrally and any rotation is corrected by small pads. The use of a foot piece may also correct this malalignment.

- *Over the Achilles tendon*. This is superficial and frequently damaged by pressure from the edge of the last sling. If a foot piece is not used and the heel is left free to hang over the edge of the last sling (thus avoiding the heel rubbing), the area that is then at most risk is the skin over the Achilles tendon. If a sore develops

Immobility
See chapter 3.1

Skin assessment
See chapter 6.1

the resultant injury to the Achilles tendon may mean further hospitalization and immobilization long after the original injury has healed.

■ *The back of the heel of the injured leg*. This should be free of the bed; if it is found to be lying on the bed, the balance weight suspending the Thomas' splint needs increasing, thus elevating the leg (helping to reduce swelling), making it easier for the patient to move and lifting the heel free.

■ *The back of the heel of the uninjured leg*. This is subject to friction on the bedding, particularly while the patient is learning to lift himself or herself free of the bed. If counterpanes are traditionally used at the bottom of traction beds they should be removed because they are very rough. Occasionally the use of sheepskin bootees may be called for but these are of use only if they are put on when the traction is first applied and if they are maintained in the correct position.

■ *Buttocks and sacrum*. These areas are at risk due to friction caused by the patient not being lifted properly or not lifting themselves properly. Shearing forces caused by the movement of muscle and bone under the skin may destroy the microcirculation to the skin and reduce the skin's viability. Unrelieved pressure is also a cause of skin breakdown in these areas. When patients are on traction it is very difficult to change their position so that their buttocks and sacrum are free from pressure. Simply asking the patient to lift themselves free of the bed for a short while and then replacing themselves in a slightly different position will help. Specialized mattresses such as Pegasus or Nimbus may be used. The potential need should be recognized on admission and the patient either admitted on to the mattress or transferred on to it from theatre.

■ *Elbows*. Even in young patients elbows become quite sore from their use as 'body props'. To prevent this occurring, patients must be well supported by pillows in a position that is comfortable but allows them access to locker, books, etc.

After 48 hours the skin will still need to be inspected in all these areas at least twice a day. However, there should be much more patient involvement, with the patient being told exactly what to look for in the early signs of skin breakdown. For some patients, 48 hours is too early even to start to take on this responsibility, but many patients are ready and will take a much more active interest in their progress if given this responsibility in these early days.

Constipation due to immobility

The following interventions should be applied to prevent problems with defaecation:

■ Dehydration must be avoided; a fluid intake goal of 2 litres a day may be set. If the general condition

does not allow for this, an intravenous infusion may be required. If the patient is dehydrated in the first 24–48 hours, the faeces will become hard and painful to pass. This will make the patient reluctant to use a bedpan.

■ The patient must be given some privacy – somewhere where nobody else will be aware of the noises and odours that may result in attempts to defaecate.

■ Although hospital food is supposed to be high in fibre, the patient might be encouraged to ask any friends or family who visit to bring in fruit, fruit juice or bran-based breakfast cereals, especially in the first few days when the problem of constipation appears to be at its worst.

■ The nurse should ensure that using a bedpan is not a painful experience. Ideally analgesia should be kept at an appropriate level from admission so that the patient will not equate moving with pain. If a patient is having difficulty opening the bowels, pain experienced due to being transferred to a bedpan will only make matters worse; the situation may be eased by the use of a slipper bedpan.

Urinary retention

The following interventions should reduce the risk of urinary retention and infection.

■ Male patients find the position they have to adopt (lying on their back with the foot of the bed elevated) much more difficult to cope with than females. The man should be regularly offered a urinal and told about the need to pass urine. The nurse will need to give constant explanations about the importance of emptying the bladder, why he may be finding it more difficult than he expects, and how it should not result in a wet bed. (However, if it does, the patient will need to be reassured that the problem can be overcome.) In exceptional circumstances the doctor may agree to lowering the foot of the bed to see whether that helps the patient to adopt a better position. However, as this may alter the fracture position, it should not be undertaken without written instructions. Occasionally the use of a sedative such as diazepam may be used to relax the patient, facilitating the passing of urine in these unnatural circumstances.

■ Catheterization should be seen as the last resort and the catheter should be removed straightaway. After a few days, passing urine usually becomes less of a problem, but the patient needs to be reminded to continue drinking to prevent dehydration and the renal complications of calculi and urinary tract infections.

Constipation
See chapter 5.1

Retention
See chapter 5.4

Boredom and depression due to enforced immobility

To reduce the boredom of traction, the following interventions can be used:

- Ensure the patient has sufficient diversions such as books, radio, television, etc. to hand. These may help the patient to keep in touch with usual interests and activities.

- The nurse should spend time listening to the patient and concentrate on what the patient is trying to say. It sometimes takes time and practised skills by the nurse to produce a situation where the patient is ready to talk about what is really bothering him or her.

- The nurse must recognize that there are times when it is more appropriate to call in other professionals, such as a social worker, counsellor or minister of religion. Simpson (1987) described the 'traction intolerance syndrome' in which patients fiddle with their traction, become threatening or abusive, and are subject to large mood swings. In this situation he suggests the need for referral to a psychiatrist to help the patient recognize the seriousness of his (it usually occurs in men) injury and the consequences of not following advice.

Convalescence and rehabilitation

Patients may from time to time feel depressed and unhappy but progress may be aided by the free expression of needs and fears. When the traction is removed, the patient will probably be surprised and depressed by the weakness, joint stiffness and joint instability in the limb. Before being allowed up, the head of the bed is elevated so the patient may adjust to having the head and trunk in an upright position after being flat and in the countertraction position for so long. The elevation is gradual; otherwise faintness may be experienced.

Appropriate passive, active and resistive exercises of the affected limb are introduced. These may be planned and supervised by a physiotherapist, but the nurse must be familiar with the plan so that the necessary assistance is provided when the therapist is not at the bedside. In the case of a lower limb, arm and shoulder exercises are continued to strengthen the upper limbs in preparation for the use of a walking frame or crutches. When weight bearing is permitted, the person begins to relearn to walk using a walking frame, crutches or a walking stick. Firm, low-heeled, walking shoes, preferably with a non-skid rubber heel, should be worn.

The patient may need prompting to maintain an erect posture (avoid bending forward) and to increase the degree of flexion of the thigh and leg when raising a foot off the floor to take a step in order to overcome the tendency to shuffle. Most patients require a good deal of encouragement and reassurance from the nurse. Physical

assistance and support are withdrawn gradually, but the nurse remains with the patient when getting in and out of bed or a chair until it is evident that he or she can safely manage alone.

A home assessment may be carried out before discharge to determine what barriers to access and mobility may exist and whether there is someone who will be at home to assist the patient. If the patient experiences difficulties with self-care or mobilizing, a referral may be made to the primary health team so that assistance and supervision will be available. Resumption of the former occupation and activities will depend on progress in relation to mobility and independence.

The patient should know the date, time and place of appointments for follow-up examinations.

Care of the patient with internal (surgical) fixation

Preoperative care

A person requiring internal fixation may need care for several complicating health problems. When the person has suffered fractures of the shaft of femur or pelvis hypovolaemic shock is likely. This should be treated in the A&E department by the use of plasma expanding agents and blood transfusion. By the time the patient is transferred to theatre the condition should be stabilized and the patient pronounced fit for anaesthesia.

How soon after injury the internal fixation occurs depends on factors such as the patient's general condition, the type of fracture, the position of the bone ends and the surgeon's preferences.

During the preoperative period, some temporary form of immobilization is applied to prevent the situation worsening. The injured limb should be handled as little as possible but the patient will need to use a bedpan and pressure area care, so some form of external splintage may be used, such as a vacuum splint, backslab or sandbags. Hamilton Russell traction may be applied if there is a fracture in the femoral neck region. Analgesia will need to be given and its effect monitored.

When elderly patients are awaiting surgery the nurse must be aware of the psychological effects of the strange environment, the accident, pain, journey to hospital, and perhaps several hours of lying in the A&E department looking at the ceiling. The use of reality orientation should be employed to remind the patient exactly where he or she is, what has happened, and what is going to happen in the near future in order to prevent anxiety and confusion.

Before surgery most patients will have an intravenous infusion started to correct any evidence of dehydration and provide a drug route. Blood should be taken for biochemical analysis, grouping and cross-match should a transfusion be needed. A fluid balance chart should be started at the same time and all intake and output recorded. The patient's urine should be tested as soon as possible to detect any abnormalities such as bleeding into the urinary tract, particularly in patients who may have incurred even apparently minor pelvic injuries. Patients will need electrocardiography (ECG) if this was not done in the A&E department in order to ensure their cardiovascular system is fit for general anaesthesia and the stresses of surgery.

Postoperative care

Following internal fixation of fractures the general principles of postoperative care are applicable, with the following additions.

Where surgery is performed on a limb it should be elevated as soon as the patient is back in bed. If a plaster cast has been applied, the patient's extremities should be examined for colour, sensation, warmth and movement every 30 minutes to ensure there is no compromise of the circulation. The digits should be compared with those on the uninjured side and if any difference is observed the nurse in charge should be informed immediately. Sometimes the situation can be relieved by elevating the limb higher, thus reducing the swelling, but more often than not the plaster will need to be split to allow some 'give'. If a backslab has been applied the cotton bandages will need cutting down to skin, especially if there has been some haemorrhage, as blood-soaked bandages are notoriously harsh: they do not 'give' and may act as a tourniquet. Any blood staining on a plaster should be outlined after the first couple of hours so that continued bleeding can be monitored.

Where a plaster cast has not been applied, the circulation to and sensation of the limb distal to the operative site should be monitored to ensure no damage was incurred during the operation or before surgery while the limb was splinted.

All wound drains should be inspected regularly and changed as required. The amount of drainage should be entered on the patient's fluid balance chart. Drains are removed when they have stopped draining, usually after 48 hours.

The patient may be allowed out of bed but, in the case of surgery on a lower extremity, is not usually permitted to bear any weight on it for several days or weeks. He or she may be allowed the use of a wheelchair and is gradually introduced to the use of crutches. When sitting, provision is made for elevation and support of the affected limb. Precautions against pressure sores and slumping posture are necessary when the patient is allowed up in a chair for long periods. Skin care is provided at regular intervals and patients are taught to shift the weight frequently so that no one area is subjected to continuous pressure. Adjustments may also be necessary to avoid prolonged pressure on the popliteal area of the unaffected, dependent leg and to prevent forward sagging of the shoulders.

Exercises of the affected part are started as soon as the surgeon permits. They may be limited to isometric contractions for a period, followed by the gradual introduction of passive and active movements and resistive exercises. In the case of a lower extremity, weight bearing is not introduced until radiography indicates satisfactory healing. The overambitious patient is cautioned not to attempt standing or walking without the assistance of a physiotherapist or nurse. The patient should have a firm, non-skid pair of shoes and be assisted first to stand. The physiotherapist or nurse stands facing the patient and places the hands to the sides of the patient's lower chest. The patient is encouraged to stand erect, knees extended and head up. When sure of balancing in the upright position, the patient is then assisted with the next step, which may be the use of crutches, a walking frame or simply walking with only the assistance of one person. Support is given to the affected side.

Treatment and nursing care required for specific injuries

Below, a brief summary is provided of the more common injuries, their treatment and the nursing care required.

Fractures of the neck of femur

Fracture of the neck of femur occurs more often in elderly women, due in part to hormonal changes and the effect this has on bone reabsorption, leading to osteoporosis (McClung 1999). Osteoporosis is discussed in more depth later in this chapter (see p. 919). There are two categories of fractures involving the femoral neck region (Fig. 24.17):

- *Intracapsular fractures* occur through the joint and capsule and include subcapital fractures, transcervical fractures and impacted fractures at the base of the neck of femur.

- *Extracapsular fractures* may pass through either the greater or lesser trochanter or the intertrochanteric area. These are called intertrochanteric fractures.

Assessment

The initial assessment in A&E should focus on how much pain the patient is experiencing and, apart from gently examining the affected leg (which classically is shortened and externally rotated), the nurse should assess the rest of the patient for other injuries sustained at the same time. Such are the effects of ageing that the nurse should also be alert to other pathological processes that may exist at the same time. It is important therefore to screen for hypothermia (especially in winter), diabetes (possibly undiagnosed) or any signs of cardiovascular disorder. Such information is essential for correct triage and nursing care in A&E.

Other important information concerns the patient's general condition, whether he or she looks well cared for

Figure 24.17   Intracapsular and extracapsular fractures of the neck of femur.

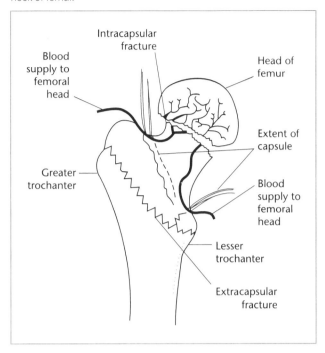

or neglected, and the state of the skin. This is a group of patients at high risk for pressure sore development. Many departments now have a fast track policy aimed at admitting elderly patients with fractures of the neck of femur to a ward bed within 1 hour in recognition of the special problems faced by this group of patients, such as pressure sore development (Morley 1998). Vital information about home circumstances is available from the ambulance crew in A&E that may not be available to the ward staff. The patient's orientation and understanding of the situation should also be assessed as confusion may develop speedily.

While the surgeon may carry out a technically correct repair to the fracture site, the patient's long-term prognosis may depend far more on skilled nursing care to prevent complications such as pressure sores, constipation, chest infections or confusion, and on the resolution of social problems.

The patient's nutritional status should be assessed. In a study of 63 patients following femoral fractures, Patterson et al (1992) found 59% with moderate to severe protein depletion. These patients were found to have a higher incidence of postoperative complications ranging from delayed wound healing to a decreased survival rate.

The principles outlined above, of assessing not only the obvious injury but also the rest of the patient, of checking for coexisting health problems, assessing the patient's psychological status and exploring social factors, apply equally to all types of injury.

General principles of treatment

Surgical reduction and fixation of the joint is the treatment of choice. The research evidence offers no support for the continued traditional use of Hamilton Russell traction before operation (Parker and Handoll 2000). A variety of metal nails, plates and screws may be used for internal fixation (see Figs 24.15 & 24.16).

Intracapsular fractures are highly likely to damage the blood supply to the head of the femur if there is any displacement at the fracture site (see Fig. 24.17). If there is no displacement and it is thought the head will survive, two screws such as Garden screws are inserted in a relatively simple operation. However, if there is any displacement the femoral head will need to be removed and replaced with a prosthesis such as Thompson's or an Austin Moore. In extracapsular fractures, head viability is not a problem and a fixation device such as a dynamic hip screw or nail and plate is used to hold the fragments. Older patients with coexisting medical problems may not be fit for a general anaesthetic but, such is the importance of early operation to prevent all the complications of immobility that could arise, that surgery is performed under spinal anaesthesia if necessary (Marcangelo 2000).

After 48 hours, following a check radiograph and the removal of any wound drains (provided they have stopped draining), the patient should be able to mobilize. The amount of weight bearing allowed depends on the severity of the fracture, the precision with which the bone fragments are held by the fixation, and the ability of the patient to understand how much weight can be taken by the injured leg.

Nursing care for patients who have had a prosthesis inserted is much the same as that following a total hip replacement. The principle governing care is that the hip is in danger of dislocating if it is allowed to flex more than 45° or if it adducts and the injured leg crosses the good one. Patients are therefore nursed with their legs in abduction, with a frame or two pillows between them, and are not allowed to sit upright either in bed or in a chair.

Good pain control is essential and patient-controlled analgesia (PCA) is used if the patient is able to manage a PCA pump. Apart from the continuing risk of pressure sore development, other major potential postoperative complications include dehydration, constipation, confusion and deep venous thrombosis.

A multidisciplinary rehabilitation process should begin immediately after operation so that the patient has the best chance of maximum recovery (Marcangelo 2000). Many patients however remain institutionalized after this injury, being unable to regain independence. A major Canadian study found that increased risk of institutionalization was directly related to poor mental functioning in hospital and that the risk was 4 times greater in men than women (Cree 2000). This latter finding is an example of the influence of social factors on health. The study also found that each increase in age by 10 years was associated with an increased risk of institutionalization by a factor of 2.5.

Much interest has centred on the use of multidisciplinary care pathways in this group of patients. A recently reported Australian study by Choong et al (2000) is therefore of interest. These researchers compared the progress of 55 patients who were on a pathway with 56 who were not. There were no significant differences between the groups (e.g. mean age 84 and 82 respectively) but the pathway group had a mean total length of stay of 6.6 days compared with 8 days for the control group. This suggests that an integrated care pathway approach has contributed to reducing inpatient stay by 21%. Commenting on this research Swanson et al (2000) noted that those patients who benefited most from the pathway approach were the most frail and elderly. However, as they observed, community services have to be fully involved in coping with the accelerated throughput of such elderly patients that may result from pathway use.

Fractures of the shaft of femur

The causes of and the group of patients associated with this type of fracture differ considerably from those suffering a fractured neck of femur. It is caused by high-energy trauma, frequently a road traffic accident, and often involves men in the 16–35-years age group.

Anatomically these fractures range from the subtrochanteric region in the proximal third of the femur, through midshaft fractures, to supracondylar fractures in the distal third. The fractures are often spiral, with at least three fragments, due to a twisting injury, but direct trauma usually results in the more manageable transverse fracture.

Shock
See chapter 4.2

Complications

The major complications which may result from fractures of the shaft of femur are the following:

- *Hypovolaemic **shock***. Even when there is no obvious sign of haemorrhage a litre of blood can be contained within the thigh from a fracture of the shaft of femur.

- *Damage to the femoral artery,* often a tear from a sharp bone fragment.

- *Damage to the femoral nerve*, again from a sharp fragment.

- Following an open comminuted fracture, *loss of bone fragment* at the scene of the accident. This will lead to a shortening of the limb. Occasionally the fragment may be found and used in the treatment.

- *Fat emboli*. There are two theories behind the explanation of the development of fat emboli following fracture of the shaft of femur: (1) that trauma causes disruption of the veins and fat cells in the bone allowing fat into the circulation, and (2) that catecholamine release due to the stress of trauma mobilizes lipids from adipose tissue which then become fat droplets. In the lung these droplets

are converted to free fatty acids which are toxic to lung tissue and disrupt alveolar function. Small globules of fat may become enmeshed in the capillary network around the alveoli and prevent small amounts of gaseous exchange occurring; however, if large blood vessels in the pulmonary system are obstructed, the result will be fatal. The signs and symptoms of fat embolism occur between 12 and 72 hours after injury and consist principally of a decrease in level of consciousness, increased respiratory and pulse rate, pyrexia and a fall in the concentration of oxygen in arterial blood. Greaves et al (1997) recommend early fracture stabilization and vigorous treatment to prevent hypoxia and hypovolaemic shock as the best way to prevent fat embolism.

Treatment

The treatment for fractured shaft of femur depends on the severity and position of the fracture and how well callus formation takes place. In most cases the patient is nursed in skeletal traction for the first 2–3 weeks until callus is seen on radiography and the fracture is in an acceptable position. As most patients fall into a relatively young age group there is a need to obtain as good an anatomical result as possible; otherwise there may be considerable stress on the weight-bearing joints in the future. This could eventually lead to an early onset of secondary osteoarthritis.

The alternative treatments following callus formation are as follows:

1. Remain on traction until fracture has united.

2. Intramedullary nailing using a Küntscher or AO nail. An intramedullary nail acts as an internal splint and is inserted the length of the femur along the medullary canal. A piece of the nail is usually left protruding from the greater trochanter but under the skin to allow easy access for its removal 12–18 months later.

Once the wound drains have been removed and the check radiograph shows a satisfactory position, the patient is usually allowed to commence mobilizing either partially or non-weight bearing using crutches. The patient will require a programme of exercises, particularly static exercising of the quadriceps, to ensure the retention or building up of the quadriceps muscles. The physiotherapist will also gradually introduce knee flexion, although this may be limited in the early stages of rehabilitation.

Once the patient is confident on crutches he or she may be discharged, although an appointment will be required for the removal of stitches and follow-up in the outpatient department. Before discharge patients should be reminded that, if the leg suddenly becomes painful or swollen or the wound becomes red and inflamed, they should telephone the orthopaedic outpatient clinic (giving the name of the consultant concerned) or, if out of clinic hours, attend the casualty department. All internal fixation carries a risk of infection which should be treated aggressively at the first indication.

3. Femoral cast brace may be applied 2–6 weeks after fracture. The main aims of such a brace are to encourage bone healing and prevent knee stiffness by early weight bearing and mobilization. The cast is usually made of synthetic resins, which are light and dry very quickly, and is applied in two sections – the thigh section and the lower leg section – by specially trained technicians. The two sections are joined by a pair of hinges. The position of the hinge is crucial to avoid undue stress on the patient's knee. The patient will require considerable help at the first attempts at weight bearing but should be able to be discharged within a few days of application of the brace.

Fractures of the tibia

Tibial fractures are classified according to whether they are open or closed, their position, and the degree of displacement at the fracture site. Fractures of the fibula are not considered separately as the treatment is usually in association with that of the tibia. Isolated fractures of the fibula with no tibial involvement are relatively minor and are treated in the A&E department.

Tibial plateau fracture

Although this frequently appears to be a minor fracture, its position within the knee joint and its effect on future knee function mean that it is treated aggressively and every endeavour is made to retain and/or restore good anatomical position of the articular cartilage.

One of the overriding principles of treatment is the maintenance of knee movement. If the fracture is depressed, the patient will require elevation of the fragment under general anaesthesia to restore the joint surface. Any displacement of the fracture will require internal fixation using a buttress plate, screws or bone graft in combination. After operation the patient is nursed on a continuous passive movement (CPM) machine. This machine (frequently used following total knee replacements) can be set to specific degrees of flexion and speed of movement. For the first few days the amount of flexion should be very small while the wound is healing and the swelling starts to subside. This may be gradually increased with time and within the patient's pain threshold. The nursing staff must be aware of the need to maintain a constant level of analgesia as the machine is moving the patient's knee 24 hours a day.

Patients with undisplaced tibial plateau fractures will be placed on the CPM machine after a period of Hamilton Russell traction. The nurse must be able to explain the need for 24-hour movement to the patient.

Because the patient's leg is held in the machine quite firmly, it is crucial that the skin is examined every day for any sign of redness or breaks.

Once healing is beginning to take place and there is knee flexion of at least 45°, a femoral cast brace will be applied and the patient may be up, weight bearing. Because the patient's weight is transferred through the upper component, the hinges and the lower leg piece of the brace, there is no danger that the fragment will become depressed.

Tibial shaft fractures

These fractures vary from the undisplaced, closed fracture which is treated with an above-knee plaster of Paris cast in the A&E department, to the open, grossly contaminated, displaced comminuted fracture seen following a severe road traffic accident. As tibial fractures, particularly in the middle to lower third, have a reputation for poor healing, if the fracture is open the problem of infection has to be considered very quickly. The problem of soft tissue swelling and fracture shape frequently make the use of plaster of Paris unacceptable. The alternatives in regular use are intramedullary nailing, external fixators, which allow nursing access to any wounds while holding the fracture position, open reduction and internal fixation using a compression plate.

Specific patient problems

The specific problems that patients with these fractures may develop include the following:

- *Gross infection.* The patient will require diligent observation of temperature, pulse and respiration 4 hourly until all the wounds are healed.

- *Poor healing rate.* A close observation of pedal pulses must be made to ensure adequate perfusion of the lower leg. Excessive soft tissue damage may produce swelling, leading to compartment syndrome in which the muscle fasciae of the three compartments in the lower leg come under intense pressure, eventually compromising the major arteries. This situation requires prompt action; usually fasciotomies are performed in theatre to relieve the pressure and restore an adequate blood supply.

- *Knee and ankle stiffness.* The physiotherapist and the nurse are responsible for ensuring that the patient's range of movements in these joints are kept at an optimum. Ankle stiffness will add considerably to the patient's mobilization problems when the fracture is united.

- *Problems from the pin sites.* These were discussed above (see p. 886).

Fractures of the malleoli

These are usually the result of a twisting injury from stepping on to uneven ground. To understand the mechanism

infection
See chapter 6.1

of the injury the nurse needs to know the anatomy of the ankle joint (Fig. 24.18). The talus is held in a box-like structure, with three sides provided by the lateral malleolus of the fibula and the medial and posterior malleoli of the tibia. If the leg is held straight and the foot forced to twist, the displacement of the talus may break off one, two or three of the malleoli. These fractures are referred to as a bimalleolar or trimalleolar fractures.

As the fracture is frequently displaced, patients are usually admitted for open reduction and internal fixation. The internal fixation is often performed using a plate and screws on one side and a malleolar screw on the other. If a diastasis has occurred in which the inferior tibiofibular joint has been displaced, a diastasis screw, which crosses from one bone to the other, will be used. The patient is non-weight bearing following this procedure as the normal movement at the inferior tibiofibular joint when weight bearing is prevented and there will be unnecessary stress on the diastasis screw and the surrounding bone. This can lead to further bone damage at the ankle.

Specific patient problems

The specific problems following surgery to the ankle are the following:

- *Risk of infection.* The patient may have two wounds so the risk of infection is doubled. If the fracture was open, the chances of infection are also increased. If it was initially a closed fracture, it has now effectively been converted to an open fracture.

- *Circulatory compromise* due to swelling. On return to the ward the patient's leg should be elevated well above the level of the heart. Circulatory observations should be performed half-hourly for at least the first 12 hours; these should include pedal pulses if

Infection
See chapter 6.1

possible. Some surgeons use plaster of Paris following internal fixation, especially in severe fractures where it is considered that the fixation is less than perfect. Sometimes the patient will simply have wool and a crêpe bandage around the wounds. If there is a plaster cast it should be split to allow for swelling.

- *Wound drains,* which require attention to ensure their patency is maintained. These should be changed as required until the wound(s) stop draining. Any drainage stains on the plaster should be outlined 4 hourly so that loss can be monitored.

Fractures of the calcaneum

These fractures are the result of jumping or falling from a height and landing on the feet. The calcaneum is frequently crushed, with many fragments. Traditionally the treatment has been high elevation and ice packs to reduce the tremendous swelling that can result. However, more recently the use of internal fixation has been introduced.

Specific patient problems

This injury is often seen following an unsuccessful attempt to commit suicide. The result is that the patient has both the physical discomfort of two very painful heels and the emotional trauma of still being alive and facing the problems that prompted the suicide attempt, and also having to face the world in the knowledge of the failure of the attempt. The nurse must be able to care for such patients with empathy, being non-judgemental and recognizing the need to bring in other professionals and take their advice on care.

Ankle stiffness is a common problem. As soon as the swelling starts to subside, the physiotherapist and nurse must outline a programme to improve the patient's ankle movement. At first this may be mainly passive movement but will gradually progress to include more active exercises.

Fractures of the pelvis

Fractures involving the posterior sacroiliac region are associated with the highest morbidity and mortality rates, whereas those affecting the pubic rami appear to be painful but do not carry many dangers. Because of the difficulty in making exact diagnoses in some parts of the pelvis, the patient may require a CT scan to augment the radiographs. As the function of the pelvis is to protect key internal organs, when it is fractured there is a high risk of damage to the bowel, bladder and urethra. Also in danger are the abdominal aorta and internal iliac arteries.

In displaced, open and complicated fractures the patient usually requires open reduction and application of an external fixation device. Some parts of the pelvis may also be fixed with a small plate and screws. This can be performed only once the general condition has been stabilized and any bleeding blood vessels repaired.

Figure 24.18 The anatomy of the ankle joint.

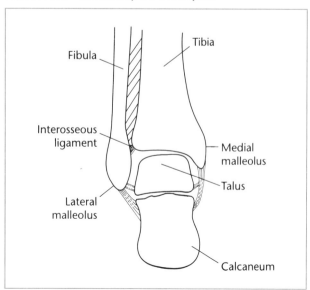

Undisplaced fractures, such as those sustained by the elderly when they fall and 'sit down', resulting in fractures of the pubic rami, are treated by a short period of bedrest, analgesia and early mobilization. Often there is little visible damage, but after 2–3 days the bruising starts to show and the whole of the perineum may turn purple.

Injuries resulting in diastasis at the symphysis pubis may be treated by nursing the patient on slings that cross over the front of the pelvis, pulling the pelvis into shape.

Specific patient problems

The following problems commonly affect patients with fractures of the pelvis:

- *Pin sites.* The care required for these is slightly different as very often there are more than one inserted in adjacent bone. Instead of a puncture in the skin there may be a slash of 2–4 cm which will require regular dressings to prevent infection.

- *Bladder and/or urethral involvement.* All urine passed should be tested for haematuria for at least 24 hours or until it has been clear for 24 hours. A suprapubic catheter may be inserted to keep the bladder empty until it has healed and the risk of chemical peritonitis has subsided.

- *Bowel involvement.* Rupture of any part of the intestinal tract introduces the risk of peritonitis from spillage of the bowel contents into the peritoneum. Signs such as abdominal pain, pyrexia and shock indicate this complication may have occurred.

- *Implications for childbearing in females.* In females of child-bearing age, injuries to the pelvis carry with them the risk of creating the inability to carry a fetus to full term. Thus every effort must be made to restore the anatomical position of the pelvis. The situation must be discussed with the patient, who should be examined by an obstetrician. This would be an opportunity for these problems to be aired and may provide the patient with some comfort.

- *Neurological problems.* These mainly affect the sacral plexus and the sciatic nerve. Such damage is recognized by absent plantar flexion and ankle jerk. However, the damage is usually only a temporary result of bruising and stretching of the nerves rather than any more permanent damage.

Fractures of the *acetabulum* are usually caused by indirect violence and have their own problems. The head of the femur needs to be held out of the acetabulum by traction to allow healing to take place. A major worry is the development of secondary arthritis in the hip joint, especially in a young patient. Many patients who require total hip replacement in their forties have a history of severe trauma to the hip in their twenties and thirties.

Fractures of the neck of humerus

Most of the fractures of the neck of humerus occur at the surgical rather than the anatomical neck. They are caused by falling on an outstretched hand or on the side. Impacted fractures are treated symptomatically, using the support of a collar and cuff sling until the pain starts to subside, and then encouraging movement. For slightly displaced fractures the arm should also be supported in a collar and cuff sling. Movement should be introduced gradually; this is often limited and follow-up physiotherapy is usually required.

Grossly displaced fractures of the neck of humerus require open reduction and internal fixation using a Rush pin and/or AO plate and screws.

Specific patient problems

Patients with undisplaced or minimally displaced fractures are treated in the A&E department. More serious fractures may result in any of the following problems:

- *Injury to the brachial plexus.* As well as circulatory observations, sensation and motor function of the affected hand should be observed because stretching of the nerve plexus at the time of the accident or during operation may occur. Usually this is only temporary; nevertheless it must be monitored in case it is of a more serious nature.

- *Avascular necrosis of head of humerus.* This is not common and tends to occur in fractures of the anatomical neck.

- *Arterial obstruction.* Occasionally a displaced bone fragment may cause occlusion of the axillary artery. This usually resolves following reduction of the fracture. Circulatory observations of the hand (including a radial pulse) must be performed half-hourly for at least the first 12 hours after operation.

- *Maintenance of the position of the hand and arm after surgery.* The patient may have a collar and cuff sling, with or without a body bandage, after operation. The nurse should ensure both are comfortable, not rubbing, and are providing the support required.

- *Joint stiffness.* This is a particular problem with the elderly and, left untreated, quickly leads to loss of independence even when the fracture has united. The importance of performing exercises prescribed by the physiotherapist cannot be overemphasized.

Fractures of the shaft of humerus

Humoral fractures may be the result of indirect violence such as falling on an outstretched hand, or direct violence such as falling on the side. They may be open or closed fractures, although open fractures are mainly found in those involving the middle third of the humerus. Conservative treatment of such fractures involves reduction of the fracture under sedation or general anaesthesia (if necessary) and the application of a hanging 'U' slab. The patient will require a broad arm sling under the clothes for support. If an above-elbow plaster is applied with the elbow at right angles, a collar and cuff sling should be applied as the weight of the plaster is designed to act as traction on the fractured shaft. Occasionally internal fixation using an intramedullary nail or plate may be performed.

Specific patient problems

The following problems may occur:

- *Radial nerve palsy*. This is recognized by a drop wrist and sensory loss on the back of the hand between the thumb and index finger.

- *Non-union due to loss of position*. To prevent this the nurse must be vigilant in ensuring that the correct sling is worn and that it is providing the correct support. This may be difficult if the patient is unable to get out of bed and sit upright. Careful explanations of the rationale for care should be given to the patient and repeated as frequently as necessary.

Fractures of the wrist

Colles fractures are probably one of the most common fractures the nurse is likely to encounter. Most are dealt with in the A&E department. They are usually the result of falling on an outstretched hand, particularly in the elderly. The displacement of the radius leads to the 'dinner fork' deformity when the wrist is viewed laterally. Following reduction of the fracture, usually under intravenous regional anaesthesia (Bier's block), a below-elbow back-slab is applied. This is completed when the medical staff are sure that the inevitable swelling is receding and that finger movement is good, usually up to a week later.

Specific patient problems

The following problems may occur after a Colles fracture:

- *Stiffness and swelling of the fingers*. All jewellery, including wedding rings, should be removed as soon after the accident as possible. Finger exercises should be taught, and a leaflet with a description of the exercises and information on who to contact if the fingers suddenly swell or movement becomes more difficult should be supplied.

- *Carpal tunnel syndrome*. This is caused by median nerve compression in the wrist and is recognized by paraesthesia over the anterior aspect of the thumb, index and second finger, and half the ring finger. Surgical decompression is required.

- *Loss of independence*. As this fracture frequently occurs in the elderly, the nurse must ensure that the patient will be able to manage alone or has someone to help.

For many old people, adapting to changes in circumstances takes a long time and 'young' hospital staff are in danger of dismissing the difficulty that such patients encounter in coping with relatively minor fractures.

Smith's fractures are often described as reverse Colles fractures. They are caused by falling on the flexed wrist; radiography confirms the anterior displacement of the distal fragment. Unlike most Colles fractures, it is difficult to maintain a good position after reducing a Smith's fracture; therefore internal fixation using a buttress plate is usually required.

The foregoing is not an exhaustive list of fractures but highlights some of the more common fractures a nurse is likely to encounter. For a more detailed account of fracture care, the reader should consult a specialist text.

Injuries to joints

Injuries to joints may range from a mild sprain to complete dislocation with associated fractures. The overall aim of care is to allow the joint surface time to recover, in order to reduce the likelihood of secondary osteoarthritis, while keeping the patient as active as possible to overcome muscle wasting around the joint which may lead to permanent joint instability.

Shoulder dislocation

In this injury the shoulder is usually dislocated anteriorly. In the 18–35-years age group it is usually due to a sports or motorcycle accident in which the individual is thrown and lands on an outstretched hand and the body rotates above the hand. It is also quite common in the elderly, usually following a more minor injury due to the lax musculature of the shoulder joint in this age group.

As soon as the injury has been confirmed by radiography, the shoulder should be reduced as the longer it is left the harder it is to relocate the humoral head. One approach is to give the patient intramuscular analgesia and lie him or her prone on a trolley with the affected arm hanging free over the side. Spontaneous reduction may occur due to gravitational traction and the muscle relaxant effect of the analgesia. However, some patients will find this position suffocating and very difficult to maintain. Alternative techniques, such as Kocher's or the Hippocratic method to reduce the dislocation, are usually successful if combined with intravenous diazepam and an opioid analgesic. Occasionally general anaesthesia is required.

In younger patients, postreduction care includes the application of a body bandage (including the forearm) to prevent abduction and external rotation. Both these movements predispose to recurrence, which is about 50% in this age group. If recurrence becomes a problem the patient may eventually require a surgical repair.

In the elderly recurrence is not such a problem but there is a high risk of stiffness leading to loss of independence; thus mobilization of the shoulder may begin after a week.

Specific patient problems

Axillary nerve palsy This may be tested for in the A&E department by a pin-prick test over the outer aspect of the shoulder. The condition may be severe enough for the patient to lose deltoid function and, although it is usually temporary, months of physiotherapy may be necessary for full recovery.

Rotator cuff tear The head of the humerus is held in place in the glenoid cavity of the scapula by the tendons of the shoulder joint muscles which fuse and form the rotator cuff. The cuff inserts at points around the greater and lesser tuberosities of the humerus. If it is torn, the most common problem is in abducting the arm. The condition may be helped by physiotherapy but a repair of the tear may eventually be required.

Loss of independence Use of the shoulder is essential to perform many aspects of self-care. Ability to perform self-care must be assessed in all patients.

Hip dislocation

This injury may range from incomplete dislocation (subluxation), when the head of the femur is partly out of the acetabulum, to complete dislocation, when the femoral head is lying behind the acetabulum (posterior dislocation). Once the hip has been reduced the joint should be rested, usually on skin traction and then 'free in bed' for several weeks, before weight bearing can take place.

Meniscal injuries in the knee

These injuries usually occur in young people who engage in sports and are the result of rotational stress on the flexed, weight-bearing knee. The extent of the tear may vary from being small and undisplaced to one in which the whole of the meniscus is involved and displaced to such an extent there is complete loss of joint function. Arthroscopy may confirm diagnosis and a partial meniscectomy may be performed via the arthroscope. The aim of treatment is to leave as much of the meniscus intact as possible.

A major postoperative problem is instability of the knee joint following quadriceps wasting. Static quadriceps exercises are necessary to overcome muscle wasting in the thigh. The physiotherapist will organize an exercise programme but the nurse needs to be able to reinforce the necessity of practising the exercises and ensure they are being performed correctly for maximum benefit.

Soft tissue injury of the ankle

These injuries occur most commonly following inversion injuries, damaging the lateral ligament. The patient complains of pain and swelling over the lateral malleolus, although the radiographs are normal. Following mild sprains the patient requires support of the ankle, such as double Tubigrip, and should be advised to rest at home with high elevation of the ankle to reduce the swelling. If weight bearing is painful, a pair of crutches should be provided.

In more serious injuries where the lateral ligament is completely torn the patient will require complete immobilization in a below-knee weight-bearing plaster.

Specific patient problems

Specific problems include the following:

- *Loss of independence*. Some patients will need to be admitted overnight, even following relatively minor injuries, until they are safe to mobilize on crutches. This, of course, is particularly true of the elderly individual who lives alone.

- *Circulatory compromise* due to swelling.

- In the long term, *ankle instability* may be the result of this injury and the patient will require surgery to reconstruct a stable joint.

Amputation of a limb

The incidence of amputation of part of a limb increases sharply in people aged over 55 years as a result of peripheral vascular disease (PVD). Amputation of a limb is a very mutilating procedure and an extremely devastating experience for the individual. However, it frequently provides relief from severe intractable pain due to PVD or osteomyelitis and allows a significant improvement in mobility.

In those for whom an amputation is a necessity, the loss of the limb has become less obvious and less disabling nowadays as a result of improved prostheses and rehabilitation programmes.

Reasons for amputation

An amputation is performed to preserve the patient's life or may be undertaken to improve function and usefulness. Conditions that necessitate amputation include:

1. insufficient blood supply to the part (PVD) and resulting gangrene

2. severe, uncontrollable infection such as gas gangrene (*Clostridium perfringens* infection) or chronic osteomyelitis in which there is marked bone destruction

3. malignant neoplasm (e.g. osteosarcoma)

4. an injury that has resulted in irreparable crushing of the limb or laceration of arteries and nerves

5. a handicapping deformity (e.g. flail limb).

Level and types of amputation

Occasionally an amputation is an emergency surgical procedure performed because of irreparable traumatic damage to a part. But, when possible, the level of the amputation is decided before operation so that the patient may be informed of the anticipated extent of the loss. The decision as to the level is based on achieving:

- complete removal of the diseased tissue

- viable tissue and an adequate blood supply to the remaining part of the limb

- a stump that will allow for a satisfactory fitting and functional movement of a prosthesis.

Adequate soft tissues (skin, subcutaneous tissue and muscle) are preserved so that the end of the bone is well padded and covered. If possible, the stump should be the optimum length for adequate leverage on the prosthesis. Too long a stump may interfere with the function of the prosthesis joint below. In amputation of the lower extremity the knee joint is maintained, if at all possible, because mobility and agility are acquired more readily. The prosthesis for the above-knee amputation limits the person, especially if elderly, because of the high energy demands for locomotion.

Two types of operative procedures are used:

1. In the *closed* or *flap type* of procedure, fascia, probably muscle, and full-thickness skin flaps are brought over the end of the bone. In a below-knee or a Syme's amputation, the posterior flap is usually longer, with the suture line situated on the anterior aspect of the stump. This arrangement prevents direct pressure on the scar by the prosthesis in weight bearing.

2. A *guillotine* or *open amputation* is reserved for emergency cases in which the limb has been severely traumatized and contaminated, or in which an infection such as gas gangrene has already developed. The skin and other soft tissues are severed at the same level as the bone. The wound is left open to promote adequate drainage and closed later when infection has been brought under control. Traction may be applied to the skin while it remains open to prevent retraction of the soft tissues.

Traumatic amputation implies the loss of a whole or part of a limb in an accident. This is frequently a life-threatening situation because of the concomitant haemorrhage. A second problem incurred by such circumstances is contamination of the wound. Immediate emergency care is directed toward arrest of the bleeding and getting the person to where blood replacement may be instituted. Precautions are taken to handle and transport the amputated part with the patient carefully, because efforts may be made to reattach the separated unit.

Disarticulation is the term used when the amputation is at the level of a joint.

Preoperative nursing intervention

Psychological preparation

When the amputation is an elective procedure, the surgeon, nurse and the rehabilitation team work together to inform the patient and family of the need for the operation and the level at which the limb will be removed and what functional restoration can be anticipated. When the patient is first advised of the loss of a part of the body, regardless of how functionally insignificant, the information is still likely to be a shock, causing considerable emotional disturbance. The patient's body image and independence are seriously threatened and encouragement is needed to talk freely about fears and anxieties. Good nurse–patient communication is essential both before and after operation to help the patient resolve these fears and adapt to a change in body image. Reactions vary among patients, depending on culture, personality, life situation and the impact loss of a limb is perceived as having on the individual's social circumstances.

The patient and family receive explanations of how the problems associated with the loss of a limb may be handled through a planned rehabilitation programme. The knowledge that the interest and assistance of specialists in this area are available may help the patient to develop a positive attitude toward overcoming the handicap. Opportunities are provided for questions and discussions about what is likely to take place before and after the operation. The patient may derive support from a visit by someone who has had a similar amputation and has been successfully rehabilitated.

Physical preparation

Normal preoperative preparation is required as for any major operation, but in addition exercises are introduced that will facilitate postoperative mobilization and rehabilitation. These include active exercises of the unaffected limbs to prevent loss of muscular strength. If the use of walking aids is anticipated, arm strengthening exercises using weight-lifting and push-ups may be introduced to strengthen the shoulder and arm muscles. Overprotection of an affected lower limb usually results in continuous flexion of the hip and knee joints, leading to contractures. This is discouraged by lying the patient in a prone position several times a day.

Postoperative nursing care

Assessment

The blood pressure, pulse and respirations are recorded, colour noted and the stump examined at frequent, regular intervals for the first 48 hours for early signs of shock and haemorrhage. The patient is observed for psychological distress following the amputation. Even though he or she was prepared for and consented to the operation, the actual loss of the body part may cause severe depression. The nurse is also alert for any indications of infection such as pyrexia, raised pulse, increased pain, erythema and wound discharge.

Patient problems

Potential patient problems following an amputation are listed in Table 24.4.

Nursing intervention

Promotion of healing

The stump is usually enclosed in a thick soft dressing and elasticated bandages. When a soft dressing is used, any blood staining is reported immediately. If serous drainage soaks through the dressing, it is promptly reinforced and pressure is applied until the bleeding is brought under control, if necessary by the surgeon. Continuous closed wound suction drainage may be established to prevent haematoma formation. The wound dressing, provided it is comfortable, is generally left undisturbed until the wound drain is removed, thus reducing the risk of introduction of infection. The wound drain is removed 2–4 days after operation and the sutures are left in place for 10–12 days for an above-knee amputation and 3–4 weeks for a below-knee wound, in order to ensure firm **healing**.

Unless the surgeon instructs otherwise, the patient should lie in a supine position with the stump resting flat on the bed. Following an amputation above the knee, the patient must be guarded against shortening of the hip flexors and abductors. In an amputation below the knee, the patient is encouraged to maintain extension of the knee to avoid contracture of the hamstrings (posterior thigh muscles).

The patient or a member of the family is taught the care of the stump and the correct application of the bandage. The stump is bathed as necessary with a mild soap and rinsed and dried thoroughly. Lanolin may be applied if the skin is dry and flaky. The patient is taught to inspect the stump twice daily, using a mirror, for redness, swelling, irritation and calluses. If any symptoms develop, weight bearing on the stump is avoided and the doctor or clinic consulted. Stump bandaging is resumed if the prosthesis is not worn during this time. Certain activities may be ordered that apply pressure to the stump in preparation for the use of a prosthesis and weight bearing. Contact is first made with something quite soft and, as tolerance is developed, the firmness and resistance of the contact surface and pressure are increased progressively. If the patient complains of muscular spasms and discomfort, massage to the stump may provide relief. Figure 24.19 illustrates points the patient is taught 'not

Wound healing
See chapter 6.1

Table 24.4   Identification of patients' problems following amputation

Problem	Causative factors	Goals
1. Failure of wound to heal	Infection Poor blood supply Haematoma formation	The wound will heal without any complications
2. Potential for injury	Surgical construction of a residual limb (stump) Altered balance Possible disorientation in the postoperative period Phantom limb phenomenon	1. To achieve a residual limb that will support activity with a prosthesis 2. Physical injury will not occur
3. Discomfort or pain	Surgical intervention Phantom pain phenomenon	1. Patient will be pain free 2. To understand and minimize the experience of phantom sensations
4. Disturbance in body image	Amputation of a body part	1. To express feelings about the loss of a body part 2. To attain an acceptable level of social and physical functioning
5. Nutritional intake lower than body requirements	Surgery and anaesthesia	To maintain nutritional and fluid balance
6. Impaired mobility	Surgery and loss of a body part	1. Complications of immobility will not occur 2. To increase physical activity and ambulation
7. Inadequate knowledge about care of the residual limb and prosthesis, application and use of the prosthesis, and follow-up care	Lack of information, skill and resources	1. To develop self-care skills 2. To develop a plan for follow-up health management

Figure 24.19 Positions to be avoided by lower-extremity amputee during the immediate postoperative period.

Pain
See chapter 2.3

Fluid balance
See chapter 2.6

to do' with the stump in order to prevent injury and promote healing.

Prevention of physical injury

The most common cause of falls is that the patient forgets momentarily that he or she has only one leg. The patient may experience the sensation that the limb is still present; this phenomenon is known as *phantom limb*. The majority of amputees experience this phenomenon, which is strongest immediately after surgery. Awareness that it is a common experience following amputation helps to decrease the patient's anxiety.

Control of pain

An opioid analgesic is usually required by the patient at regular intervals during the first 48 hours after surgery. Persistent **pain** 24–72 hours after operation may indicate haematoma formation. This must be reported to the surgeon immediately, as breakdown of the wound could occur if the haematoma is not evacuated. If pain occurs later in the postoperative recovery period it may be due to wound infection. If infection is suspected the wound is inspected, a wound swab is taken for microscopy, culture and sensitivity, and the relevant antibiotic is prescribed. Some patients experience pain which is interpreted as originating in the portion of the limb that has been removed. This is referred to as *phantom pain*. It varies in

severity and may be temporary, but if it persists treatment in the form of local nerve blocks in the stump, transcutaneous nerve stimulation, ultrasound or relaxation training may be tried. No single method of treatment has shown itself to be consistently successful.

Adjustment to altered body image

Acknowledgement by the nurse of the patient's feelings of depression, anger and frustration, and provision of opportunities for the patient and family members to discuss feelings, help the patient to accept the situation. An understanding of the meaning of the loss is necessary for the health professional to provide constructive support. The nurse and other healthcare workers may set expectations that the patient will increase mobilization, socialization and self-care activities. The patient may feel very differently, however. Support and encouragement are therefore essential. Early mobilization and patient participation in decision making promote the development of a more positive attitude. A temporary prosthesis is worn as soon as possible so the patient experiences an empty sleeve or empty trouser leg only briefly. The permanent prosthesis is fitted within a few weeks for most patients. As the patient's functional capacity increases, feelings of self-worth and tolerance of the change in body image may begin to emerge. Friends and relatives are encouraged to visit and opportunities for the patient to go home for an evening or weekend are created whenever possible.

Involvement of members of the rehabilitation team prior to surgery and during the postoperative period enables them to provide information about the expectations for functional restoration, to develop plans for rehabilitation and to establish a trusting relationship with the patient and family. Rehabilitation centres usually provide both individual and group sessions to allow patients to share experiences, gain support, and learn new and effective coping strategies.

The patient is encouraged to discuss with the limb-fitter how the artificial limb will look, as well as function. Help is provided in selecting shoes, trousers, skirts, shirts and blouses to promote a favourable and acceptable appearance.

Psychological and social adjustment is generally a longer process than is the relearning of physical functioning.

Maintenance of fluid and nutritional status

Intravenous **fluid** may be necessary during the first 24–48 hours to maintain an adequate intake. Oral fluids are given freely, and the patient progresses to a regular diet as soon as it is tolerated. An explanation is made, if necessary, of the importance of adequate nutrition in maintaining and promoting muscular strength for the exercises that will assist in rehabilitation.

Promotion of mobility

An hourly routine of coughing and deep breathing and frequent change of position are necessary until the patient is allowed up and becomes sufficiently active, to prevent limited ventilation and circulatory stasis.

As soon as the patient is well enough, a daily regimen of exercises is introduced to maintain and promote the muscular strength and joint mobility that are needed for rehabilitation. The tone of the trunk muscles, as well as that of the limb muscles, receives attention because adjustments and compensation are necessary for the amputee to maintain balance. If the leg has been amputated above the knee, the hip extensors and adductors play an important role in remobilization, as hip flexion and abduction deformity may occur. The patient should be taught active stump exercises to maintain and improve joint mobility and muscle strength. To prevent flexion contracture of the hip, the patient lies in the prone position for a minimum of 30 minutes two to three times a day. The stump should not be propped up on a pillow for the same reason. If the leg has been amputated below the knee, particular attention is given to quadriceps exercises. Following the amputation of an arm, the shoulder muscles of that limb are exercised to prevent adduction and rounding of the shoulder.

The patient is allowed out of bed as soon as possible. Assistance must be available until he or she can maintain balance and is able to manoeuvre safely. In the case of a lower limb, the patient first learns to stand and gain balance, to transfer safely from bed to chair and from wheelchair to toilet. When fitted with a temporary prosthesis (pylon) the patient mobilizes using a walking aid such as a stick. A walking frame is generally not recommended as there is a risk of the patient falling backwards. Crutches should not be used as they hinder the patient in learning how to weight-bear. To ensure the patient is able to walk safely with walking sticks, he or she is first taught to walk between parallel bars, one hand holding a bar and the other a stick. The patient progresses to walking with the aid of two sticks and then with one stick, held in the opposite hand to the amputation, before the permanent prosthesis is fitted.

When the stump has shrunk sufficiently and is conditioned, measurements are taken and a permanent prosthesis is made.

When learning to use a permanent lower limb prosthesis, the patient uses one or two walking sticks for support. When a satisfactory stable gait has been achieved, the patient is encouraged to discontinue the use of a stick. All of this takes considerable time and perseverance; the amputee will require encouragement and support from family and those working with him or her in rehabilitation.

Inadequate knowledge

After an amputation, the patient and their family are taught to care for the stump and to inspect it several times daily for oedema, redness, drainage or breaks in the skin, and to note any changes in sensation or tenderness. When the prosthesis is fitted, they are taught how to care

for it, to assess for proper fit, what to do if the fit alters and when to return to the limb-fitter for reassessment. The physiotherapist helps the patient to develop a plan for continuing the exercise and activity programme at home. The nurse helps the patient and family plan how they may incorporate the recommended healthcare measures and activity programme into the daily routine of the patient. Referrals to a community nurse or resettlement officer are made as indicated. Arrangements are made for follow-up visits to the surgeon's clinic in the outpatient department. Phantom limb pain should be discussed further with the patient as this may persist many years after amputation and be very distressing.

Evaluation

Expected outcomes

1. The skin over the stump is clean, dry and intact.

2. The patient indicates understanding of the phenomena of phantom limb and phantom pain, if present.

3. The patient and family are able to express feelings regarding the loss of a body part and the change in body image.

4. The patient is able to apply the prosthesis and wear it with comfort.

5. The patient follows the planned exercise regimen to maintain and/or increase muscle tone and strength and joint function in all limbs.

6. The patient moves about safely.

7. Suitable bodyweight to aid mobilization is maintained or achieved.

8. The patient is able to assess the condition of the skin over the stump.

9. The patient knows how to contact the limb-fitting centre should problems occur.

10. The family takes part in the rehabilitation programme and is able to give assistance to the patient if required.

Inflammatory joint disease

Rheumatoid arthritis

Rheumatoid arthritis is a chronic systemic disease that occurs worldwide. There is an element of genetic susceptibility in the disease, which is then induced by a 'triggering factor' that causes a pathological autoimmune reaction. In effect the body mistakes the synovial lining of **joints** for a foreign antigen, leading to a chronic and destructive **inflammatory response** (Byrne 1999). Antibodies called rheumatoid factors are found in the blood of 70–80% of persons with rheumatoid arthritis. These antibodies interact with antigens in various

Joints
See chapter 3.3

Inflammatory
response
See chapter 6.1

connective tissues, but the reaction is greatest in the synovium of **synovial joints**.

The disease is a major health problem and is the most common form of chronic inflammatory joint disease. The age of onset is most commonly between 30 and 50 years of age, and women are affected about three times more often than men (Springhouse Corporation 1998).

Pathophysiology

There is some evidence that microvascular injury and mild proliferation of synovial lining cells are the initial events in rheumatoid arthritis. Leading contenders for the role of triggering factors include viral gene products, degraded bacterial cell wall peptidoglycans, and bacterial or viral antigens (Haslett et al 1999). The normal synovium becomes swollen and inflamed (synovitis) and eventually extends into the joint space. The process is reversible in the early stage, and the joint may be left undamaged and functional. As the inflammation continues the synovium proliferates and, with the fibrin of the inflammatory exudate, forms a thick spreading membrane of granulation tissue known as a *pannus*. It spreads over the joint surfaces, gradually eroding the cartilage, and may even destroy the denuded bone surfaces. A radiograph may show rarefaction of the ends of the involved **bones**. Instability and irritation of the joint may cause muscle contraction with a resulting flexion or extension deformity or partial dislocation (subluxation) of the joint.

Fibrous scar tissue and adhesions develop between the opposing joint surfaces, leading to fibrous ankylosis of the joint, which becomes fixed and immobile. The exposed, roughened ends of bone tissue may eventually proliferate bone cells into the joint cavity, resulting in calcification and bony ankylosis.

The patient with rheumatoid arthritis may also have diffuse involvement of non-articular connective tissues. Degenerative lesions of the collagen component of the connective tissue may develop in muscles, tendons, blood vessels, pleura, heart or lungs.

Synovial joints
See chapter 3.3

Bone
See chapter 3.2

Clinical characteristics

The onset is usually insidious: the person experiences a period of general fatigue and non-specific illness. Pain, swelling and morning stiffness of several peripheral joints is the typical beginning of the disease. The small joints of the hands or feet, or the wrists, elbows or knees, are generally the first to be involved. The disease develops symmetrically and, as it progresses, the affected joints become swollen, painful, red and increasingly difficult to move. Their range of motion is reduced. The overlying skin may take on a stretched, smooth, glossy appearance.

Muscle weakness and spasm are common in the early stages and are frequently followed by marked muscular atrophy. Unless early treatment is instituted, progressive joint tissue destruction and deformities develop,

leading to permanent disability. Subluxation and flexion contractures occur. Deformities commonly seen include hyperextension of the distal phalanges, flexion contracture or ulnar deviation of the fingers due to metacarpal–phalangeal joint involvement and flexion contraction of the wrists, knees and hips. Subcutaneous nodules (*rheumatoid nodules*) appear principally on extensor surfaces or areas subjected to pressure. These are composed mainly of fibrinoid material (degenerative tissue cells) and granulation tissue.

General constitutional disturbances are manifested; the patient is pale and looks ill; anorexia, loss of weight, fatigue and depression may develop. Low-grade fever, tachycardia, anaemia and a mild leucocytosis may also be present. Later, leucopenia may develop. The widespread effects of the disease on the whole person are summarized in Box 24.4. The erythrocyte sedimentation rate is usually raised and, later in the disease, a blood examination may reveal the presence of the rheumatoid factor. When rheumatoid arthritis develops in children, it may be referred to as *Still's disease* or more commonly *juvenile chronic arthritis*. In addition to the symptoms mentioned for adults, children usually have some enlargement of the lymph nodes (lymphadenopathy).

Classification

The disorder may be classified according to the pathological changes (clinical stages) and the loss of functional capacity (functional classification) (see Table 24.5).

Box 24.4   Major extra-articular features

- Anaemia
- Weight loss, fatigue, fever
- Lymphadenopathy
- Oedema
- Nodules
- Osteoporosis, bursitis and tenosynovitis
- Muscle wasting
- Episcleritis
- Keratoconjunctivitis
- Entrapment neuropathy (e.g. cervical cord compression)
- Nailfold vasculitis
- Peripheral sensory neuropathy
- Splenomegaly
- Cardiac complications (e.g. pericarditis, endocarditis)
- Pleural complications (e.g. effusions, bronchiolitis)

Table 24.5 Classification of rheumatoid arthritis

By clinical stages		By functional classification	
Stage	Manifestations	Class	Manifestations
1 (early)	No evidence of joint destruction or osteoporosis	1	No loss of functional capacity
2 (moderate)	Evidence of some destruction of cartilage and probably of subchondral bone. No deformity but full range of motion may be limited. Adjacent muscle atrophy present	2	Able to carry out usual activities despite some discomfort and limited joint mobility
3 (severe)	Cartilage and bone destruction quite evident. Muscle atrophy and joint deformities such as hyperextension, flexion contracture, ulnar deviation and subluxation present	3	Functional capacity impaired; occupational and self-care activities quite limited
4 (terminal)	Criteria of stage 3 plus fibrous or bony ankylosis present	4	Confined to a wheelchair or bed; not able to carry out self-care. Dependent

Nursing assessment

As rheumatoid arthritis is a systemic disease with a range of signs and symptoms that impact on all aspects of daily life, an extensive nursing *history* should be obtained that explores the following areas:

■ current local and systemic effects on the patient

■ self-care abilities

■ coping responses to the disease

■ knowledge of the disease and its management.

Reliable and valid assessment tools such as the Arthritis Impact Measurement Scale may be useful as a guide to data collection.

A further assessment scheme used to assess the patient's pain in various joints is the Ritchie Articular Index. The nurse applies digital pressure to a list of joints commonly affected in rheumatoid arthritis. The patient is asked to rate the pain on a scale of 0 = no pain to 3 = patient winces and withdraws joint. A total score is then calculated and an index achieved (Arthur 1994).

Symptoms

The nurse should explore all symptoms the patient is experiencing to obtain some understanding of the extent of the disease. A plan of care can be determined only when the extent of the physical effects the disease has on the patient has been determined together with the psychological consequences. The nurse should determine which joints are involved and obtain a description of the severity, duration, precipitating, aggravating and relieving factors of the common problems: pain, swelling, stiffness and impaired movement. The systemic symptoms of generalized weakness, fatigue, listlessness, anorexia and weight loss should also be explored and enquiry made about the presence of extra-articular symptoms including subcutaneous nodules, sensory loss in one or more of the extremities and dryness of the eyes.

Self-care abilities

Depending on the number and extent of symptoms present, the patient may be able to continue to perform self-care independently or may be completely dependent on others. The ability to walk and use the hands should be assessed along with general mobility. Determine from the patient what activities can be performed and how important each activity is to the patient. Continuing to perform personal hygiene is generally very important to the patient, and giving up household chores may be equally distressing as it represents a loss of independence.

Coping responses

Coping with the pain, stiffness and decreased mobility of rheumatoid arthritis is often overwhelming. Like other chronic illnesses, the symptoms disrupt everyday life, the medical treatment is acknowledged as being only partly effective and the therapeutic regimen further disrupts day-to-day patterns of living (Ryan 1999). Equally distressing is the uncertainty about when remissions and exacerbations may occur. The loss of self-care ability coupled with the physical effects of the disease described above can lead to the patient being depressed or very anxious and fearful for the future. The psychological effects of the illness need to be sensitively explored along with the possible social consequences if the nurse is to be able to plan care for all the patient's needs.

Shaul (1995) has described several stages associated with rheumatoid arthritis that the patient passes through. Initially there is *becoming aware,* which is followed by *learning to live with it.* Eventually the person achieves a stage of *mastery* when they are setting realistic goals for themselves, asking for help from others and using resources to their best advantage. As Ryan (1999) has observed, the nurse's involvement with the patient will vary according to where the patient is on this coping journey. When the patient has achieved mastery, maintaining contact may be all that is required; however, in the earlier stages a great deal of support and teaching is necessary.

For many women with rheumatoid arthritis pregnancy brings a relief of all symptoms (Richardson 1992). However, following the birth of a baby the symptoms will return to their pre-pregnant level within 8 months.

Knowledge of the disease and its management

In order to maximize independence the patient must participate in ongoing care and this requires knowledge of the disease process and the treatment regimen. The nurse should determine the patient's knowledge base, interest level, ability to learn and degree of physical comfort. Teaching sessions must be based on a thorough assessment of the patient and their level of understanding.

Physical assessment

Individual joints or groups of joints and their surrounding tissues are observed, palpated and their range of motion determined. Joints are inspected for swelling, redness, physical deformity, discoloration, scars or discharge. The adjoining muscles are observed for signs of atrophy. Each joint is compared with the corresponding joint for symmetry and degree of change. Painful joints are supported by the examiner's hands, and movements are performed gently and slowly. Illustrations of the human body may be used to record joint assessment and provide an overview of involved joints (Fig. 24.20). A goniometer, which measures angles, may be used to measure degrees of movement of a joint. For example, the normal range of flexion of an elbow is 135–150°, and tension 0–5°; hip abduction varies from 45 to 50°, with

Figure 24.20   Illustration for use in joint assessment.

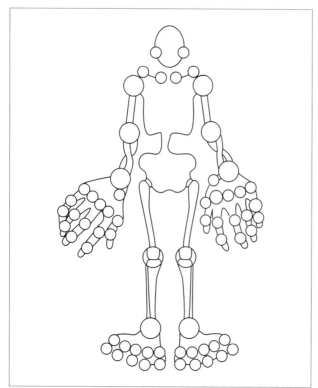

hip adduction being approximately 20–30°. Some decrease in mobility of joints occurs with age.

Diagnostic procedures

Radiographs are made of the joint(s) and may include *arthrography*, in which a radio-opaque contrast medium is injected into the joint cavity so that the soft tissue components may be visualized. This is generally done with investigation of a knee. The procedure takes 30–45 minutes. No special post-test precautions are necessary and the patient should be reassured that the contrast substance will be reabsorbed systemically and joint swelling will subside. Other imaging techniques such as CT or ultrasonography may be used to assess the progress of the disease.

Aspiration of synovial fluid may be performed to obtain a specimen for laboratory examination for the presence of blood, pus, organisms, sodium urate crystals or malignant cells. A local anaesthetic is used and strict asepsis must be observed although use of sterile gloves and draping are not necessarily routine. A large-bore needle is inserted into the joint space to aspirate a fluid specimen. The synovial fluid of a patient with rheumatoid arthritis may be cloudy or have a greenish hue, and will have a raised leucocyte level.

Arthroscopy may be done to examine a joint by direct vision. This procedure is used most often in knee disorders. The doctor is able to visualize and assess the synovium, articular surfaces, menisci and ligaments, and a biopsy of synovial tissue may also be taken. The examination is performed in the operating theatre under strict aseptic conditions. A large-bore needle is introduced into the joint following anaesthesia and normal saline is introduced to 'fill out' the cavity. The arthroscope is then introduced. After the examination the puncture area is sealed and a compression bandage applied. Activity is usually limited for approximately 3 days. Arthroscopic examination of the patient with rheumatoid arthritis reveals cartilage destruction with fibrous scar formation. Synovial villi appear swollen, thick and pale.

Laboratory *blood and serum tests* that may be used in investigation of rheumatoid arthritis and other disorders include the following:

1. Erythrocyte and leucocyte counts.

2. Determination of haemoglobin, erythrocyte sedimentation rate (ESR), serum alkaline phosphatase, calcium and phosphorus concentrations and blood uric acid level.

3. Examination for rheumatoid (Rh) factors, antinuclear antibodies (ANAs), lupus erythematosus cells (LE prep), anti-DNA and complement fixation.

The blood cell counts, haemoglobin and ESR are used to determine the presence of anaemia, infection or tissue destruction. The serum phosphatase level is raised in malignant disease, as is the ESR. The phosphorus and calcium concentrations are significant in bone disease, and the blood uric acid level is increased in gout. The presence of rheumatoid factors and autoimmune antibodies in serum occurs in 85% of people with late-stage rheumatoid arthritis.

The *latex fixation test* is used most commonly to identify rheumatoid factor immunoglobulin (Ig) G. Antinuclear antibodies and lupus erythematosus cells are usually present in patients with acute, active, systemic lupus erythematosus. The anti-DNA test detects antibodies that react with DNA and is considered a specific test for systemic lupus erythematosus.

Patient problems

Assessment of the patient with rheumatoid arthritis often reveals some or all of the following problems:

- *reduced physical mobility* related to inflammation and deformity of joints, muscle weakness and atrophy, and limitation in range of motion of joints

- *activity intolerance* related to disease process and to prescribed treatments

- *pain* related to the disease process and accentuated by movement

- *reduction in self-care activities* related to decrease in activity and to lack of knowledge

- *depression* related to pain and decreased mobility

- *inadequate nutrition*

- *lack of knowledge* about rheumatoid arthritis.

Goals

The goals derive from the identified problems and generally include:

1. Maintain or increase mobility and activity tolerance.

2. Obtain relief of pain and discomfort.

3. Perform self-care in daily living.

4. Achieve an optimal nutritional intake.

5. Achieve or maintain a positive mood state.

The overall goal is to achieve a maximum state of wellness within the limitations imposed by a chronic and potentially disabling health problem. Criteria for evaluation of goal attainment should be negotiated with the patient. The nurse uses assessment skills in determining the extent to which each goal is achieved. Criteria may include any of the following:

- Demonstrates stable or improved joint mobility.

- Demonstrates an optimal level of functional mobility.

- Performs therapeutic measures to minimize further impairment of joint function.

- Controls pain through appropriate use of treatment measures including medications.

- Maintains a satisfactory level of independence.

- Consumes a well balanced diet.

- Demonstrates a satisfactory level of psychosocial health.

Nursing intervention

Rheumatoid arthritis is a disease for which there is no cure but one in which control is possible by the use of a variety of measures developed and implemented in teamwork between the patient, nurse, doctor, physiotherapist, occupational therapist and other healthcare workers. The patient plays a critical role in the management of rheumatoid arthritis and the attainment of the goals of therapy. As arthritis is a disease characterized by remissions and exacerbations, the patient must be able to adjust management appropriately, including rest, exercise and medications. This requires that the patient learn to make and implement appropriate decisions, and this is possible only if the patient is well informed. Arthritis patient education has been effective in changing knowledge, behaviours, psychosocial status and health status. The most successful programmes use an interactive approach that emphasizes an understanding of the disease and the development of a daily routine of self-management activities. Education that includes coping strategies, problem-solving approaches to common problems, and endurance exercise should supplement the more traditional areas of focus such as joint protection and range-of-motion exercises.

Following a study of 22 families in which one adult had severe or very severe rheumatoid arthritis for at least 5 years, le Gallez (1993) made the following observations. Although the effect of rheumatoid arthritis could be seen on all members of the family, the degree of disability was not crucial. What was important was the ability of the patient to adapt to the limitations of the disease. One-third of those involved in the study felt that rheumatoid arthritis had threatened their marriage. The inability to work had a major impact on the male participants of le Gallez's study and led to their feelings of uselessness and inadequacy. When looking at the effect on sex and sexuality, le Gallez found that the couples were often at variance with each other over the effect the disease had on their sex lives.

There is an identified need for education and counselling to prepare patients with rheumatoid arthritis for the effect it will have on their family relationships.

Maintain or increase mobility and activity tolerance

Maintenance of joint mobility and the promotion of optimal joint function and activity tolerance are achieved through a combination of planned rest and exercise, and by protecting the joints from unnecessary stress. Planning and implementation of care requires cooperation between the nurse, physiotherapist and occupational therapist, doctor, patient and family.

Rest

Rest is necessary as it helps to control fatigue, inflammation and pain. The patient with limitation of joint function expends excessive energy in movement. Bedrest may be prescribed for a brief period during acute episodes of the disease when many joints are acutely inflamed and when systemic symptoms such as fever, anaemia and severe fatigue are present. Body positioning is important to prevent contractures and deformity during periods of bedrest and during sleep.

The patient should rest and sleep in a position as nearly anatomical as possible, that is with knees and elbows fully extended and with the neck and wrists in a near-neutral position. Pillows may be placed under the full length of the legs to maintain extension of the leg when the patient is supine, but never under a painful knee or elbow as this contributes to the development of contractures.

When an acute episode of the disease has passed, patients are encouraged to continue to have several rest periods daily and to alternate periods of activity with periods of rest. Patients must be convinced that rest is as important a part of their treatment regimen as medications, exercise and splinting, and must be assisted to develop a balanced programme of rest and exercise. Relaxation techniques may also be used by the patient to promote body relaxation and decrease emotional stress.

Joint rest may involve the use of splints to support and protect involved joints. The type of splint that may be applied depends on the purpose to be achieved (Fig. 24.21). Resting splints are used to immobilize inflamed and painful joints and are worn continuously during periods of acute inflammation. They are removed for short intervals for essential activities such as eating and cleansing of the skin. During chronic or inactive phases of joint disease, rest splints are worn only at night. Functional splints are designed to stabilize and support a joint during activity. Corrective or dynamic splints are used to immobilize an involved joint, realign soft tissues, or

Figure 24.21   Different types of splint. (a)–(e) Resting splints to immobilize joints. (f) Example of a functional splint used to stabilize and support joint during activity. (g) A corrective (dynamic) splint used to immobilize an involved joint, realign soft tissue or correct contractures or deformities.

correct contractures or deformities. Splints are usually made of a lightweight thermoplastic material that is pliable when heated. They are moulded to the affected part and held in place with Velcro straps. The patient's skin is protected from the splint by a layer of cloth material. The protective layer is either placed on the patient (e.g. a tube stocking) or incorporated into the splint. Splints may be used on the fingers, hands, wrists, knees or ankles. Cervical collars may be used to restrict movement of the head and neck, and thus protect the extremely vulnerable joint between the first and second cervical vertebrae.

Patients and family members should learn how to apply the splint and how to prevent any side-effects such as skin breakdown. A demonstration should be given to illustrate the pressure points that are created if the splint is not a proper fit or is not applied correctly. The patient is taught to inspect the skin under the splint for redness and tenderness each time it is removed. Splints may need to be replaced following acute illness, when the oedema has abated, and at regular intervals when used for a long time.

Heat and cold applications

This is usually the responsibility of the physiotherapy department. At home the community nurse and physiotherapist assist the patient with heat and cold applications. Moist heat is considered more effective than dry heat and may be applied in the form of a warm bath or shower, or paraffin wax immersion, which consists of the application of several layers of melted paraffin wax to the affected extremity (Springhouse Corporation 1998). The extremity is then wrapped in plastic to retain the heat.

Dry heat may be applied in the form of hot water bottles wrapped in towels, electric heating pads or infrared lamps. Short-wave diathermy and ultrasound equipment provide deep (dry) heat and should be applied by a physiotherapist. Deep heat application is usually contraindicated for acutely inflamed joints. Whatever form of heat is used, precautions must be used against burning the skin over the affected joints.

Applications of cold in the form of ice packs may be more or equally as effective as heat in relieving discomfort and spasm for some patients and are particularly useful in acute exacerbations (Springhouse Corporation 1998). Cold may be applied as an ice water bath to the affected body part, or as a plastic bag pack applied directly to the joint. Cold applications should be removed when numbness has been achieved (generally not more than 15–20 minutes), and the skin should be dried thoroughly after treatment. Cold should not be used if the patient has impaired circulation. Selection of either heat or cold is usually based on patient preference and perceived effectiveness of the modality in relieving pain and spasm.

Exercise

General exercise and therapeutic exercises contribute to the maintenance and promotion of joint function. An individualized exercise programme is designed by the physiotherapist in consultation with the patient, nurse and medical staff. Patients are told the purpose and importance of exercise in the management of their disease. Although the exercise programme is supervised by a physiotherapist or nurse when it is first begun, it is eventually performed by the patient as independently as possible. Support, including family members, can provide encouragement and assistance to the patient as the exercise programme is incorporated into daily living. Patients are encouraged to report excessive fatigue or increased pain associated with the performance of their exercises so that the programme can be modified.

Any exercise programme includes a *range-of-motion* component. Normally, each joint is capable of a certain range of movement. In a joint disorder, that range of movement may become limited and the muscle fibres shorten. Range-of-movement exercises involve the movement of a limb or part through its maximal potential range of movement to maintain or increase joint function. They may be passive, active or active assisted. Active range of motion involves movements that are performed by the patient unassisted. Active assisted exercises involve movements initiated by the patient that require some assistance in taking the joint through its available range of motion. These exercises should become as important a part of self-care as brushing teeth or bathing. They are most easily accomplished after initial morning stiffness has subsided or shortly after application of moist heat.

In passive exercise a person other than the patient moves each limb or part through its maximum potential range of movement. This may be necessary for an apprehensive patient or one who is unable to move the limbs. The exercise regimen also includes isometric or isotonic exercises, designed to maintain muscle strength and maintain or promote joint mobility. Isometric (static) exercises involve alternating maximum contraction and relaxation of muscles without movement of the respective part and joint. In isotonic exercise (dynamic) there is active contraction and shortening of muscles to produce movement with a minimal force of contraction. Isotonic exercise should be avoided if the joint is inflamed because pain will be increased and the inflammatory process may increase.

Patients with rheumatoid arthritis exhibit greatly reduced muscle strength, aerobic capacity and physical performance compared with age-matched controls. Patients are encouraged to participate in specially designed long-term fitness and cardiovascular conditioning programmes during periods of remission.

Surgical procedures

Various surgical procedures may be used with arthritic patients to facilitate joint function and mobility, to retard disease progress or to correct a deformity. These procedures and the nursing care of the patient are described in the section on osteoarthritis (see p. 912).

Obtain relief of pain and discomfort

The **pain** associated with rheumatoid arthritis is variable in intensity and aggravated by movement. Although the amount of pain does not always correlate with the degree of inflammation present, it generally corresponds to the pattern of joint involvement. Pain is further caused by muscle spasm that develops adjacent to affected joints. Patients should be advised that the therapies for maintenance of joint function are also useful in the relief of pain. Rest, splinting, the use of heat and cold applications, and the continuation of muscle-strengthening exercises all help to prevent and relieve pain. The patient can be helped to identify those activities that aggravate and relieve pain, and take action to improve pain control.

Drug therapy with one or more classes of pharmacological agents has a vital role in the management of rheumatoid arthritis and the associated pain (see Fig. 24.22 for the 'pyramid approach' to drug therapy).

Drug therapy

Non-steroidal anti-inflammatory agents (NSAIDs) provide the first line of therapy in rheumatoid arthritis. Their main purpose is to relieve joint pain and inflammation. Aspirin is the obvious choice but has to be taken in large doses to be effective. The drug has numerous side-effects that must be monitored by the patient and the nurse, including gastrointestinal disturbance, tinnitus and loss of auditory acuity particularly in the elderly. For these reasons, aspirin is being used less frequently (Byrne 1999).

Other NSAIDs are used in preference to aspirin but they too have their side-effects, such as digestive tract disturbance, dizziness, anaemia and fluid retention in people with heart disease. Patients with asthma should not use NSAIDs because of the risk of a hypersensitivity reaction leading to bronchospasm. Commonly used NSAIDs

include ibuprofen and indometacin. The serious nature of the side-effects caused by NSAIDs has led to much research into a new generation of drugs which will have the beneficial effects of NSAIDs but without their harmful side-effects. Love (2000) reports that the first such drug, rofecoxib (Vioxx), to be licensed for use is promising, and looks to be a substantially cheaper option, although long-term effects are yet to be evaluated. The drug is still prone to the long list of interactions associated with NSAIDs and is contraindicated in cases of impaired renal function, inflammatory bowel disease and severe congestive heart failure (British National Formulary 2000).

If the pain and discomfort continue or if there is evidence of gastric erosions, second-line drugs including gold or antimalarials are added to the drug therapy. Collectively they are known as disease-modifying antirheumatic drugs, or DMARDs. They have the capacity to alter the course of the disease but are used in conjunction with NSAIDs because they exert only minimal anti-inflammatory effects.

Gold compounds are preferred because of substantial evidence of their efficacy. When a preparation of *gold salts* such as sodium aurothiomalate (Myocrisin) is given, the patient is observed closely for signs of toxic reactions. The initial dose is small to test the patient for adverse reactions. Reactions that may be seen include stomatitis (inflammation of the oral mucous membrane), dermatitis, renal damage and bone marrow depression leading to severe anaemia, leucopenia (agranulocytosis) and thrombocytopenia. Gold therapy usually involves an intramuscular injection given each week for a period of 4–6 months. Most responses occur during the first 16 weeks of treatment. Once a response has been obtained, maintenance therapy should be continued. Urine analysis and blood cell counts are done weekly, and the patient is checked for possible signs or symptoms of adverse side-effects.

The *antimalarial drugs* such as chloroquine (Avloclor, Nivaquine) and hydroxychloroquine (Plaquenil) may be prescribed over a period of several months for some patients. Toxic effects that may develop include skin eruptions, headache, anorexia, nausea, vomiting, and auditory or visual disturbances. Frequent blood cell counts are done because occasionally bone marrow depression occurs, and frequent eye examinations are required to check for keratopathy which is reversible or a serious irreversible retinopathy.

Adrenal corticosteroids are now usually reserved for patients whose rheumatoid arthritis is rapidly progressing, is very painful and has not responded to therapeutic courses of other antirheumatic drugs. Examples of oral preparations used are prednisone, prednisolone and hydrocortisone. The dosage is individualized and kept to a minimum because of the unfavourable side-effects that may develop. It is important that the patient understands the drug will be given for only a limited period.

Pain
See chapter 2.3

Figure 24.22   Treatment pyramid for rheumatoid arthritis.

Intra-articular agents, corticosteroids for acute episodes

Mechanical; orthopaedic

Experimental drugs/procedures; other cytotoxics

↑

Penicillamine, methotrexate, azathioprine

↑

Antimalarials, gold

↑

Education, rest, exercise; social services; salicylates or other salicylates, NSAIDs

The dosage is gradually reduced and then completely withdrawn. Adverse side-effects that are likely to develop with overdosage or prolonged therapy include reduced lymphocyte and antibody production, leading to increased susceptibility to infection, sodium and water retention, excessive potassium excretion, mood swings or euphoria, restlessness or overactivity, hyperglycaemia and glucosuria, fullness or rounding of the face (moon face), and growth of hair on the face in the case of a female. The patient who has experienced increased appetite, a marked sense of well-being and some remission of the disease while receiving a corticosteroid may feel quite depressed and let down when the drug is withdrawn, and will require considerable emotional support from the nurse.

Immunosuppressive drugs such as azathioprine (Imuran) and cyclophosphamide (Endoxana) have been used to treat the patient with rheumatoid arthritis, using the rationale that the cause is an antigen–antibody reaction. These drugs are prescribed for patients who are unresponsive to any of the drugs mentioned previously in this section. Ciclosporin has become more widespread in its use in recent years, and the cytotoxic drug methotrexate is also used.

The suppression of leucocyte and antibody formation makes the patient very susceptible to infection. The rheumatoid arthritic patient is frequently debilitated and already has a lowered resistance. Precautions are necessary to avoid exposure to infection; recognition of early symptoms is reported promptly so that an antibiotic may be prescribed. The patient should be fully informed of the major side-effects that can occur with these drugs. Combination therapy of two or more DMARDs is frequently used and the patient will need a great deal of support from the nurse in order to manage the side-effects that occur and stay with the drug regimen that has been prescribed (Byrne 1999).

Carry out daily self-care

Activities that previously seemed simple and were taken for granted become difficult and time consuming for the patient with rheumatoid arthritis. Often there are some activities that are of particular importance to the patient, whether related to personal hygiene, housekeeping or social and recreational life. The nurse can help the patient identify key areas and encourage performance of self-care in these areas. The importance of alternating periods of rest with periods of activity should be reinforced. Self-help devices should be provided to maximize independence. The occupational therapist has an important role in providing such aids, and the nurse reinforces their importance and usefulness.

Box 24.5 lists general guidelines that help a patient to protect a damaged, inflamed or painful joint from further injury. The patient learns new ways to perform activities to decrease stress on affected joints. Conditions and unnecessary movements which cause pain and discomfort are avoided and the person learns to perform tasks with the least effort and greatest efficiency to minimize joint stress.

Family members must be included in any discussion of self-care, as they must allow the patient to achieve maximum independence. This may be difficult for those who feel that 'doing for' the patient is helpful. Instead, they should encourage the patient to perform activities alone or with help as requested. They need to be aware of the additional time and patience required to allow the patient to achieve various activities that appear simple.

Achieve an optimal nutritional intake

Nutritional problems including anorexia, weight loss and anaemia frequently accompany rheumatoid arthritis. A well balanced diet, similar to that essential to the health of all persons, is recommended for the arthritic patient. The total calorie intake may require some adjustment with a view to achieving or maintaining the person's normal weight. Obesity increases the strain on joints and may also reduce motivation to exercise.

Breakfast should be easily available and simple to prepare to accommodate the patient's morning stiffness. Eating utensils may be adapted to help the patient. Padded handles on cutlery make them easier to grip; hand supports on cutlery eliminate the need for fine finger movements; special handles on cups and glasses are easier and safer in handling; suction cups stop dishes from sliding; and high edges on dishware prevent food from spilling.

Achieve or maintain a positive mood state

Rheumatoid arthritis may be accompanied by a number of significant losses, both physical (e.g. loss of mobility) and psychosocial (e.g. loss of perceived control, loss of role, loss of relationships). Some patients manage these losses without significant threat to their psychological

---

Box 24.5 Guidelines for joint protection

- Maintain good posture and body alignment at all times
- Change position frequently
- Use the largest muscles and strongest joints available for any task
- Distribute weight of objects over several joints
- Perform activities slowly and smoothly
- Limit repetitive movements
- Minimize use of swollen, painful joints
- Stop activity when pain occurs
- Space activities to provide frequent rest periods
- Use assistive devices in the environment to eliminate unnecessary stress.

well-being, whereas others exhibit evidence of decreased psychosocial health, including symptoms of anxiety, depression and a withdrawal from others (Ryan 1999). Psychosocial health in patients with rheumatoid arthritis is influenced by many factors, including level of perceived support from others and a sense of helplessness toward the disease. The severity of impairment and disability is not a major factor in the mood state of rheumatoid arthritic patients. The nurse has an important role in assisting the patient to achieve and maintain a positive mood state, despite having rheumatoid arthritis. Since emotional and instrumental support from family and friends influences response to illness, the nurse needs to determine with the patient who makes up the patient's social network and who provides the most valuable support. If the patient receives limited support, the nurse can work with the patient to identify alternative sources of support such as self-help groups and home care agencies.

Helping the patient to learn management of the disease is essential. This decreases the feelings of helplessness and hopelessness that the patient may experience and influences the psychological health of the patient. The nurse and other health team members must continue to support the patient and family as they learn about the disease. As this encouragement and support must continue in the community, referral to appropriate community agencies should be made.

Joint dysfunction
See chapter 3.3

Nursing intervention also involves helping the patient to identify feelings about the illness and what it means. By identifying how he or she copes in certain situations, the patient develops insight into his or her behaviour and looks at the consequences of that behaviour and the alternatives open. Is social interaction worth the cost of occasional embarrassment and/or excessive fatigue? Hiding problems and trying to keep up with others drain the patient's energy, but asking for help may reinforce fears of being dependent. Hope may be a positive factor that motivates the patient to comply with therapy and learn to control symptoms. The patient and family need opportunities to discuss such ideas to help in making decisions about what is best for the patient. Family members and friends also need the opportunity to express their feelings and develop understanding of the patient's illness, limitations and potentials, and how to respond to the daily fluctuations in the patient's behaviour.

Preparation for discharge

Specific actions are required to prepare the patient for discharge from hospital in addition to the actions taken throughout a patient's hospitalization. The quality of life of the patient with rheumatoid arthritis following discharge depends largely on the severity of the patient's disease and whether or not the pathological process in the joints is arrested. Obviously, if the disease is severe and more and more joints are progressively involved, the patient is less likely to be well enough to return to a former occupation and will require a more active and

closely supervised care programme. Many patients are well enough to go to work and adjust their daily life to provide for extra rest as well as continuance of a daily physical exercise regimen. A period of vocational training or assessment by the Disablement Resettlement Officer (DRO) may be necessary before the arthritic patient can be re-employed.

If the patient is sufficiently handicapped to require physical care, a referral will be made to the community nurse. The community nurse and the occupational therapist can be of assistance in assessing the home situation and making recommendations for adjustments that will simplify the care of the patient and increase mobility and independence.

The patient and family should be acquainted with the societies and organizations that are concerned with rheumatic disease and with publications that may be helpful. Transport is frequently a problem for the person with arthritis. If the patient is required to go regularly for physiotherapy as an outpatient or to a rehabilitation unit, hospital transport may need to be organized.

Degenerative joint disease

Osteoarthritis

Osteoarthritis is a common chronic joint disorder characterized by degenerative changes in articular cartilage and marginal bony overgrowth. The disorder affects both men and women, but has a higher incidence in women over the age of 55 years. The prevalence of the disease increases with age. At age 65 years, 25% of people have symptoms of osteoarthritis and in 80% of the population arthritic changes are visible on radiographic examination. Disease of the hips is far more common in Caucasians than those of African–Caribbean or Chinese ethnic groups (Haslett et al 1999).

Primary osteoarthritis refers to the development of the disease as a result of ageing, whereas secondary osteoarthritis describes a situation where some localizing factor has contributed to the problem (Walsh et al 1999). The placement of stress on joints is implicated in the development of secondary osteoarthritis regardless of age, so that previous joint trauma, athletics, obesity and strenuous labour are all considered factors in the development of the disease. The importance of obesity is shown by the estimate that for every extra 5 kg in weight, a woman over 50 increases her chances of developing osteoarthritis of the knee by 30% (Spector 1996). Genetic factors are important in certain presentations of the disease.

Pathophysiology

The pathology of osteoarthritis is associated with biochemical and inflammatory changes that occur in response to ongoing stress on affected joints. The cartilage on the articular ends of the bones becomes thin and worn, and gradually breaks down, leaving the denuded bone exposed. The reaction of the denuded bone is manifested in outgrowths of bone from the joint margins, resulting in thickening of the ends of the bones and protruding ridges and spurs (osteophytes) which impair joint movement. Spurs may break off and become loose in the joint, causing further impairment of movement and more pain.

The weight-bearing joints, such as the hip and knee, and the interphalangeal joints of the fingers are most frequently the site of degenerative joint disease. It may occur in a single joint or may involve several.

Clinical characteristics

The clinical manifestations of the disease include soreness and an aching, poorly localized pain that occurs with use of the involved joint(s) and is relieved by rest. As the disease progresses, pain occurs even at rest. Joint stiffness is most pronounced in the morning and after periods of activity during the day, and usually lasts for less than 30 minutes. The patient complains of stiffness, soreness and pain in the affected joint(s). Crepitation may be felt or heard on movement. The range of motion becomes increasingly limited because of pain, muscle spasm and the bony outgrowths. Joint enlargement and instability develop, and the joint feels hard and irregular. Bony outgrowths on the dorsal surface of affected interphalangeal joints give the knuckles a knobbly or gnarled appearance. Systemic manifestations do not occur.

Nursing assessment

Pain, stiffness and decreased mobility should be assessed. The nurse should ask the patient what makes the symptom better or worse, where the symptom is located, the onset, frequency and duration of each symptom, and how the symptom rates on a scale of 0–10, with 10 being the worst. Assess how much each symptom interferes with the ability to perform self-care and work-related activities and what changes the patient has made in usual daily life. Equally important is an evaluation of the emotional response of the patient to the disease. Some patients feel helpless and hopeless because of the limitations imposed by the disease, whereas others continue to enjoy life despite having osteoarthritis.

The patient's gait, movement and ability to walk are observed. All joints are assessed with particular attention to those that are most troublesome. Detail on the assessment of joints and surrounding structures is presented in the section on rheumatoid arthritis. It is important to gather data in this way not only to identify problem areas where nursing intervention is required, but also as a baseline against which to measure progress. A pain rating scale of 1–10, for example, allows careful pain control while a progressively reducing stiffness rating allows both patient and nurse to see progress. This can act as a powerful reinforcer for the patient, encouraging maximum

participation in a plan of therapy. Assessment should therefore be an ongoing activity rather than a one-off activity performed on admission.

Patient problems

Assessment of the patient with osteoarthritis often identifies one or all of the following health problems:

■ *pain* due to the disease process and accentuated by activity

■ *impaired physical mobility* related to limitations in the range of motion of joints

■ *reduced self-care* ability due to decreased activity

■ *mood alteration* related to discomfort and reduced mobility.

Overall goals for patients with osteoarthritis include achieving optimal physical mobility, relief of pain and discomfort, and attaining realistic levels of independence and hopefulness for the future. Medical and surgical interventions are important components of treatment, as are physiotherapy and occupational therapy. Most patients are treated conservatively but if the pain becomes intractable and the disability severe surgery is indicated.

The nurse has a role in the total care of the patient, including the coordination of the various patient services. The nurse and patient work together to identify patient-centred goals; these may include:

1. a demonstration of optimal physical mobility

2. relief of pain

3. a satisfactory level of independence

4. a satisfactory level of psychosocial health.

Nursing intervention

Achieving optimal physical mobility

Appropriate exercises are prescribed to maintain muscle tone and movement and to promote good alignment and joint stability. The patient is encouraged to be posture-conscious and to review regular daily activities and posture. Work should be interspersed with short intervals of rest, and unnecessary walking, climbing stairs, lifting and bending should be eliminated. A fitted corset may be helpful to immobilize and provide support in the case of degenerative changes in the spine. A firm mattress is recommended to promote good alignment and support for the affected joints.

Relief of pain

Patients with osteoarthritis are encouraged to use the same measures for **pain** relief and joint protection as outlined for the patient with rheumatoid arthritis: application of heat and cold; splinting; use of assistive devices; rest alternating with activity; and the maintenance of an exercise programme.

Pain
See chapter 2.3

Medications used in treating the patient with osteoarthritis are prescribed primarily to control pain. They include analgesic agents, initially paracetamol, and the non-steroidal anti-inflammatory agents described in the section on rheumatoid arthritis. As no medications are known that halt the disease process of osteoarthritis, medications such as gold compounds and hydroxychloroquine are generally not prescribed for patients with osteoarthritis.

Local corticosteroids injected into the affected joint provide short-term relief. A recent innovation has been the intra-articular injection of hyaluronic acid in patients who have not responded to simple analgesics and other conservative therapies. Hyaluronic acid is a disaccharide that is necessary for the functional integrity of healthy cartilage and extracellular matrix. It is responsible for the viscous and elastic properties of synovial fluid. Joint sodium hyaluronate and hylan G-F 20 are slow-acting drugs that contain various fractions of hyaluronic acid and which, when injected together at weekly intervals, reduce pain and increase mobility, particularly of the knee joint (Leslie 1999). Ultimately joint surgery is indicated for pain and disability that is unrelieved by conservative measures.

As the disease progresses, nursing care in the community is directed towards the promotion of maximum independence through patient education and self-care programmes until such time as surgery is available.

Surgical treatment

When an arthritic or deformed joint causes intractable pain and severe disability, surgical intervention may be undertaken. The operative procedures used are osteotomy, arthrodesis or total replacement arthroplasty.

Osteotomy is the reshaping of the bone by cutting or curettement. This operation is used mainly on young patients with osteoarthritis whose range of motion is still good but whose pain requires surgical relief.

Arthrodesis is the surgical fusion of a joint, which results in loss of joint movement. It is done to provide relief from pain or to correct joint instability. In this operation, the articular cartilage is removed and bone grafts are implanted across the joint surface. Arthrodesis is rarely used now in the management of knee or hip osteoarthritis but is considered in the treatment of severe osteoarthritis of the cervical spine.

An *arthroplasty* is a reconstructive procedure that may entail replacement of part of the joint or of the whole joint with a prosthesis. It is done to relieve pain and permit patient mobility.

Total hip replacement

Total hip arthroplasty is performed on approximately 40 000 patients per year in the UK (Hill and Davies 2000) and involves surgical replacement of both articulating surfaces of the joint.

The femoral head and neck are removed. The cartilage is removed from the acetabulum and a polyethylene cup is fitted into the socket. Surgical bone cement may be used to secure the plastic cup to the surface of the acetabulum, or a porous, non-cemented prosthesis may be used. The head and neck of the femur are then replaced with a metal prosthesis consisting of a spherical head and stem (Fig. 24.23). The latter is implanted and cemented into the proximal portion of the femoral shaft. The ball part of the prosthesis is fitted into the acetabulum and tested for a range of motions to make sure it does not dislocate on movement.

It is important that the nurse caring for the patient is familiar with the postsurgical position to be maintained

Figure 24.23   (a) Total hip arthroplasty prosthesis. (b) Knee replacement prosthesis.

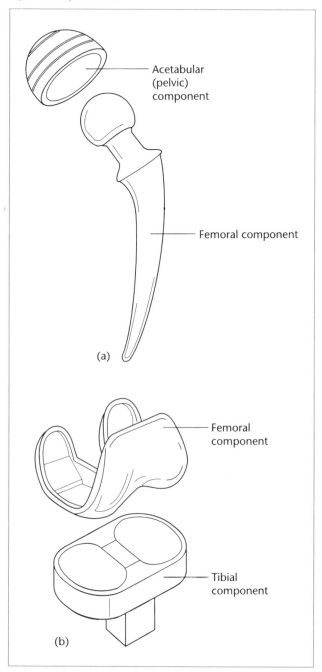

and when movement may be resumed in order that the prosthesis does not dislocate accidentally. If surgical cement is not used, the period of immobility is longer. When the wound is closed, a closed drainage system is established to promote drainage of accumulating secretions. Until adduction movements are judged safe by the surgeon, the limb should be kept in abduction.

Preoperative care

Preadmission assessment is increasingly being carried out by nurse practitioners using advanced skills to determine the fitness of the patient for operation. This avoids admitting patients and then cancelling the operation because they are unfit for general anaesthesia. A great deal of patient education and preparation, together with discharge planning, can take place in such a preadmission clinic setting. The patient's psychological assessment should include examining how realistic the person is being about the benefits of surgery in order that unrealistic expectations may be dealt with appropriately. Family and social factors should also be explored.

The patient must also be told what to expect after operation and how to help in the rehabilitation process. The importance of abduction of the hip is explained and techniques to maintain abduction demonstrated. These may include the use of abduction splints, wedge pillows, or two or three pillows between the legs. The limits of hip flexion should be explained (45–60°). An overhead bed frame or pulley can be used to demonstrate how the patient can move about the bed after the operation.

The patient requires instruction in and practice of postoperative exercises. Specific exercises include quadriceps and gluteal contractions, and plantar and dorsiflexion of the toes and ankles are essential to maintain function and aid circulation. Blood is typed and cross-matched and made available for blood replacement during and after operation, if necessary.

During the preoperative period an anticoagulant may be prescribed. The anticoagulant is administered to reduce the risk of thrombophlebitis and ensuing embolism, and to promote microcirculation in the operative site.

Postoperative care

In the immediate postoperative assessment the nurse monitors carefully for the complications and sequelae of any operation, including the state of the wound, pain, shock and haemorrhage.

Patient-centred *goals* include:

1. Hip is maintained in correct anatomical position.

2. Prescribed exercise plan is followed in hospital and plan for exercise after discharge is described.

3. The patient is free of pain.

4. Infection is prevented in the postoperative period.

5. Satisfactory cardiovascular, neurovascular and respiratory function is maintained.

6. Anxiety related to surgery is avoided or reduced.

7. Mobility is restored to the affected joint.

Preventing dislocation of the hip prosthesis Nursing actions to maintain the prosthesis in position include positioning of the patient in bed, assistance with early ambulation, and instructions for physical mobility at home. The patient returns from surgery supine and will have abductor splints or pillows in place to keep the hip in abduction and maintain neutral rotation. Acute flexion of the hip must be avoided because of the risk of dislocation. Indications of dislocation, including severe hip pain, shortening of the affected extremity, a firm palpable mass in the operative area and rotation of the hip, should be reported immediately. Two nurses are generally required when turning the patient. One nurse supports the limb, maintaining the abducted position, while the second person turns the patient to the unaffected side. Pillows are placed anteriorly and posteriorly to provide support in the side-lying position. Alternatively a device such as Immoturn may be used to facilitate turning a patient while maintaining hip abduction.

King (1994) explored the views of orthopaedic surgeons regarding their preference in the way patients are turned following replacement. The crucial factor appeared to be the surgical approach used and the nurse should be aware of differences between an anteriolateral and a posterior approach. King also suggested that patients should practise rolling before operation and that all patients should have an individualized care plan.

Infection
See chapter 6.1

A limited range of movement and slow flexion of the hip are introduced and gradually increased under the supervision of the nurse or physiotherapist. The patient is usually assisted from bed on the first postoperative day but this varies with the individual surgeon. Patients are instructed to avoid flexing the hip joint more than 90° when moving from bed to chair or wheelchair.

The patient is assessed for weight bearing and, if appropriate, crutches should be used for weight support. Walking is started using crutches or a walking frame. The patient usually remains in hospital for 5–10 days.

Preventing infection **Infection** is disastrous in arthroplasty as it results in destruction of bone and failure of the prosthesis to stabilize and fuse. The routine use of closed (Redivac) drainage systems is increasingly being questioned as studies have failed to show any obvious benefits (Hill and Davies 2000). Strict asepsis is essential in wound care and in the emptying of a drainage system. The appearance of the wound and the colour and amount of drainage should be assessed for any signs of infection so that they can be detected and reported. Close observations for other signs of infection are also made, including raised temperature and pulse, complaints of pain and pressure in the affected hip, or general malaise.

Preventing thromboembolism Patients undergoing arthroplasty are at high risk for thromboembolism, owing to a possible combination of advanced age, immobility and conditions conducive to venous stasis. Pulmonary embolism is the most common cause of death after arthroplasty, and low molecular weight heparin therapy appears to be the most effective drug regimen in the prevention of deep venous thrombosis and pulmonary embolism (Hill and Davies 2000). The effectiveness of anticoagulant therapy is increased if it is combined with exercise (taught before operation) and graded pressure antiembolic stockings. Careful monitoring is conducted for indications of thromboembolism, such as calf oedema, tenderness or redness.

Reducing pain The patient normally experiences **pain** following arthroplasty. Pain should be assessed and analgesia provided regularly to control the pain, promote early ambulation and enable the patient to receive adequate rest. Patient-controlled analgesia (PCA) is particularly suitable for this group of patients. Other pain-relieving techniques such as a change in position may also be helpful in maximizing the comfort of the patient. Extreme pain that does not respond to prescribed analgesia should be evaluated carefully and reported to the surgeon as it may indicate a complication such as dislocation of the prosthesis.

Reducing anxiety and maximizing function Patients experience anxiety over many aspects of the operation. Concerns should be assessed and dealt with on an individual basis. Generally, all patients express concern over commencement of activity and ambulation. Having experienced so much pain and instability when walking before the operation, the patient is likely to require repeated reassurance that walking is now possible without discomfort or damage to the new joint. The patient needs much support, both physical and emotional, in the early phase of ambulation. The support is withdrawn very gradually when the patient has sufficient control to be safe and displays confidence.

Another area of potential anxiety concerns the return to sexual activity. Counselling should be offered to all patients, regardless of their age. The patient should refrain from intercourse for about 6 weeks after operation to avoid extreme hip flexion or adduction that could lead to dislocation of the prosthesis. Healing of the internal capsule takes about 6 weeks, after which sexual intercourse can be resumed.

Preparation for discharge To prepare for going home and becoming as independent as possible, the patient gradually takes over self-care and receives instructions for home care. It is likely that the more control exerted by the patient with respect to rehabilitation and recovery, the better the outcome will be. Patients should be taught not to flex the hip by more than 90° and to avoid extremes of other movements of the hip. They should avoid lying on the affected side for at least 2 months. Legs should not be crossed and low, soft chairs should be avoided. A high, firm chair with arms is recommended, along with a raised toilet seat in the bathroom. The importance of continuing the exercises and walking is stressed, while excessive bending, heavy lifting and jogging are discouraged. Support stockings are helpful until no swelling remains in the legs or feet. This information should be reviewed verbally with the patient and written instructions given at discharge.

A referral to the community staff is appropriate to reinforce hospital teaching and to provide support to the patient and family as full activity is resumed. A home visit with the occupational therapist before discharge is helpful to assess the situation and for suggestions of any adaptations that would promote the patient's independence and safety.

Knee replacement

Total knee joint prostheses consist of two components: a tibial component and a complex femoral component with a channel in which the patella moves. These artificial joints allow for flexion and extension movement of the knee. The prostheses are secured by bone cement or by bony ingrowths through a porous base. Some devices combine the two methods to obtain firmer fixation to bone. A more recent development has been that of the unicompartmental or 'sledge' arthroplasty. In this operation either the medial or the lateral femoral condyle is replaced, together with the corresponding tibial articulating surface. The operation is performed in the relatively early stages of osteoarthritis of the knee and often offers the patient several years of pain-free mobility before a total knee replacement is performed.

Before operation the patient is taught and practises quadriceps, hamstring and gluteal setting exercises to maintain optimum strength. These exercises are performed 4 hourly. The patient is also taught to transfer from bed to chair and may practise with a Zimmer frame or crutches before operation.

After surgery, during the first 24–48 hours, a drain is left in place in the wound to promote drainage. The closed drainage system is checked regularly to ensure it is draining and is not clogged. Postoperative knee exercises are started early. These may be facilitated by the use of a continuous passive movement (CPM) machine from the operation to several days afterwards. This machine may also be employed for patients who are having problems improving their knee flexion with orthodox physiotherapy.

Care of the patient following total knee replacement is similar to that after total hip replacement.

Evaluation

Nursing care of the patient with osteoarthritis is effective if the patient is able to achieve a maximum level of self-care while controlling pain and discomfort. For patients undergoing surgical intervention, the nursing care has been effective if complications of surgery are avoided (or detected and treated promptly) and the patient regains a

Pain
See chapter 2.3

satisfactory level of mobility and independence. Osteo-arthritis can be controlled with the ongoing collaboration of the patient, family and the healthcare team.

Other inflammatory joint diseases

Ankylosing spondylitis

This is a chronic disorder characterized by inflammation and ensuing ankylosis of the sacroiliac joints and spinal articulations. The pathological process is similar to that seen in rheumatoid arthritis, but there is a greater tendency toward calcification. In most instances the disease remains confined to the joints cited above but occasionally does spread to peripheral joints.

The highest incidence is in the second and third decade of life with a male : female ratio of approximately 4 :1 (Haslett et al 1999). It is also recognized that underdiagnosis in females is high, mainly due to the lack of knowledge about female incidence and reluctance to perform pelvic radiography. The asymmetrical inflammatory arthritis of hips and knees, which is the early presenting problem in women years before the onset of any back problem, only adds to the difficulty of 'labelling the problem'. The cause is unknown, but heredity is suspected of having a role, because a large majority of those afflicted have a family history of some form of inflammatory arthritis.

Clinical characteristics

The onset of this disease is usually insidious; the patient first complains of stiffness in the back in the morning or following a period of inactivity. Progressively, this becomes more noticeable; limitation in the range of spinal flexion develops, chest expansion is reduced, and there is low back pain radiating to the buttocks and thighs along the sciatic nerve pathways. General systemic symptoms are usually absent or are limited to unusual fatigue and probably some weight loss.

Laboratory examinations indicate an increase in the erythrocyte sedimentation rate, but in most cases rheumatoid factor is absent. Recently it has been recognized that the histocompatibility antigen HLA-B27 is present in 90% of these patients; this has become a confirming diagnostic of ankylosing spondylitis. Leucocytosis and anaemia may be present and the protein concentration of the cerebrospinal fluid is frequently increased.

Remissions and exacerbations of the acute disease are common. In most advanced stages, some patients develop some peripheral rheumatoid arthritis. A few develop circulatory complications due to aortitis and aortic valvular insufficiency. Uveitis (inflammation of the iris, ciliary body and choroid of the eye) is also seen in about 25% of the patients.

Progressive involvement of spinal segments may continue over a period of years and eventually leave the patient with practically the whole spine firmly ankylosed, producing what may be referred to as a poker back or poker spine. Rarely, osteospondylitis has an abrupt, acute onset and spreads rapidly through the lumbar, thoracic and cervical segments, leaving the patient with a poker spine in a relatively short period.

Nursing assessment

A patient with this condition may be admitted for review and stabilization. It is important to assess mobility, pain levels and the possible side-effects of long-term non-steroidal anti-inflammatory drug (NSAID) therapy such as gastric disturbance. The patient's social circumstances should be assessed as these may have a profound effect upon mood and self-concept. The condition may be seriously affecting the person's ability to work or may have led to loss of employment. The inability to be involved in favourite recreations or sports, or even to play with children, may contribute to a depressed mood state, while self-concept may be severely damaged.

During the inpatient period medical staff will be reviewing the patient's condition, drug regimen, etc., and there will also be an intensive physiotherapy review. The nurse should be sensitive to the person's psychological and social problems in order that the person may achieve maximum benefit from the hospitalization and return home with a positive, but realistic, view of the future based upon an effective mix of physical therapy, psychological support and patient teaching.

Nursing care

In general terms goals for the patient with ankylosing spondylitis include the relief of pain (usually with NSAIDs), maintenance of good spinal alignment and preservation of maximum spinal function.

Rest and good posture at all times are extremely important so that ankylosis of the affected joints occurs while they are in the normal neutral position, thus preventing deformity and handicap. The patient is advised of the need for constant attention to good posture when up, with emphasis on contraction of the buttock and lower abdominal muscles and keeping the chest up, shoulders back and head erect. In some instances, the patient is fitted with a back brace to maintain optimal alignment of the affected joints. A fracture board and a firm mattress are placed on the bed, and it is suggested that the patient does not use a pillow or, if necessary, only a very small one. The patient is advised to sleep straight and flat on the back or in the prone position to discourage possible flexion of the spine.

A daily physical exercise programme is prescribed with the objective of strengthening the muscles that help to support the spine, maintain good alignment and promote the patient's functional capacity. As ankylosis of the costovertebral joints may occur and reduce the ventilatory capacity, breathing exercises are also included in the suggested exercise regimen.

Heavy lifting and activities that place strain upon the back are restricted. The patient assists in determining the level of tolerance of physical activity; activity that produces pain or exhaustion should be avoided, and additional rest is important.

In some cases hip arthroplasty may be needed to assist with mobility and pain relief, and to prevent subsequent spinal deformities.

Metabolic joint disease

Gout

Gout is a disorder of uric acid metabolism, characterized by recurring episodes of acute inflammation, pain and swelling in a joint. Any joint may be affected, but those of the foot are more susceptible; the condition usually develops first in the great toe. Gout occurs more commonly in men and is rarely seen in females except for post-menopausal women on diuretics (Springhouse Corporation 1998).

The disorder is caused by an excessive concentration of uric acid in the plasma (hyperuricaemia) which may be brought about by an overproduction or faulty disposal by the kidneys. Urate crystals may be precipitated and deposited within joint tissues, setting up irritation and a local inflammatory response. The small masses of crystals, which are called *tophi*, may also form in cartilage, the kidneys or soft tissues in other areas of the body.

Secondary gout may develop in disorders such as blood dyscrasias in which there is a marked breakdown of cellular nucleic acid. When the urate crystals are deposited in joints and produce inflammation, the condition may be referred to as *gouty arthritis*.

Collagen
See chapter 6.1

Clinical characteristics

Acute episodes are characterized by the sudden onset of excruciating pain in the affected joint, usually the base of the big toe, with the hind foot or hand joints the next most frequent. It becomes very tender, red, hot and swollen. Veins in the area stand out because of congestion and distension. The patient may also experience anorexia, headache, fever and constipation. The blood uric acid concentration is raised (normal 0.18–0.42 mmol/L). Subcutaneous tophi are frequently apparent in the ears or over joints or knuckles. Precipitations of urates may occur in kidney tissue, leading to impaired renal function. In some patients, the excessive concentration of uric acid results in the formation of kidney stones.

The acute attack usually subsides in a few days, and in the early stages of the disease the joint returns to normal. Remissions may gradually become shorter, and the disease may become chronic. More joints become involved, and there are irreversible changes, leading to deformity and loss of function.

Nursing assessment

Patients with gout are usually admitted to hospital only for a severe acute exacerbation. Assessment should include checking the principal vital signs, monitoring pain levels and mobility. As in the case of ankylosing spondylitis, it is important to find out how the condition is affecting the person's everyday life in terms of work, family relationships, recreation, etc. Much unhappiness may result if these areas are adversely affected, which may in turn affect patient compliance with therapy. It may be very beneficial for the patient to use the time in hospital to talk freely and frankly about such worries and anxieties.

The nurse in the community may also encounter a patient with gout if the urate crystal deposits lead to tissue breakdown and the formation of open lesions requiring dressing.

Nursing care

During an attack of gout, the patient may be placed on bedrest and the affected part immobilized. Drug therapy is promptly instituted. Apart from NSAIDs, the preparation used most commonly is colchicine, which may be administered orally or intravenously. If given intravenously, precautions are taken to avoid any of the drug being deposited in the subcutaneous or extravascular tissues because of its local irritating effect. Side-effects include nausea, vomiting, abdominal discomfort and diarrhoea. The drug generally relieves the pain fairly quickly but does not lower the hyperuricaemia.

A fluid intake of 2500–3000 mL is encouraged to promote dilution and renal elimination of the uric acid. This minimum daily intake should be continued during remissions.

The patient is instructed to limit foods high in purines such as organ meats (liver, kidneys), shellfish, sardines and meat extracts, and also to limit the intake of alcoholic beverages. As it is more difficult for uric acid crystals to precipitate as urate crystals in alkaline urine, alkaline-producing foods are encouraged, such as milk, potatoes and citrus fruits.

Prevention of acute episodes may be achieved by drugs that lower serum urate levels. Allopurinol is very effective as it interferes with the production of uric acid, while probenecid promotes the urinary excretion of uric acid and lowers the serum uric acid level by inhibiting renal tubular reabsorption.

Connective tissue (collagen) disease

Systemic lupus erythematosus (SLE) (disseminated lupus erythematosus)

This disorder is a multisystem disease that is characterized by diffuse inflammation and biochemical and structural changes in the **collagen** fibres of connective tissues in organs and tissues throughout the body. The root of the problem is a severe disturbance of immune regulation.

Systemic lupus erythematosus is an autoimmune disorder characterized by antibodies that develop against cells' nuclear components. A sensitivity to the individual's own DNA develops and the antigen–antibody complexes damage the vasculature, structure and functions of tissues and organs. Several factors are suspected of having a role in precipitating the onset or an acute exacerbation of the disease; these include exposure to the sun's rays, emotional stress, infection and drugs (e.g. sulfonamide, penicillin, procainamide, isoniazid). The incidence is increasing and many patients are diagnosed with mild forms of lupus. The 15-year survival rate for patients with mild disease is over 90%. Prognosis depends on the age of the patient (it is usually more severe in children; in the elderly it may be mild and respond well to treatment), severity of the disease, the organs affected, and the patient's response to treatment and ability to participate in the treatment plan.

Clinical characteristics

The disease may begin at any age in either sex, but is seen most often in young women between the ages of 20 and 30 years. It has a female : male incidence of 9 : 1. It also affects black and oriental women more than caucasians (Dieppe et al 1991). The signs and symptoms, especially at the onset, vary greatly from one person to another, depending upon the systems and organs involved. Those most commonly seen include fever, general malaise, excessive fatigue, weakness, anorexia, weight loss and joint pain. An erythematous rash may be evident on the face, neck and/or extremities. The lesions on the face typically spread over the nose and cheeks to form a butterfly pattern. Angioneurotic oedema with burning or itchy sensations, areas of hyperpigmentation, mucosal ulceration and alopecia may develop. (*Angioneurotic oedema* is the temporary appearance of large oedematous areas in the skin or mucous membrane due to a disturbance in the innervation of the vasomotor system.)

In the systemic type of lupus erythematosus, generalized lymphadenopathy occurs. The patient may complain of impaired vision as a result of corneal involvement and retinopathy. Raynaud's phenomenon may be troublesome, especially if the patient is exposed to even slight cold. As the disease progresses, serious visceral involvement and ensuing dysfunction are likely to develop. Impaired pulmonary, cardiovascular and kidney functions are common. Central nervous system involvement is also common.

The erythrocyte sedimentation rate is raised and anaemia is a frequent development. The presence of the lupus erythematosus cell factor and other antinuclear antibodies in the serum facilitates diagnosis. The haematocrit falls and thrombocytopenia may be manifested in petechiae and purpura.

Nursing assessment

The patient with SLE is likely to be encountered in hospital either as a result of an acute exacerbation or on admission for joint replacement surgery. However, it should be remembered that the patient may have been admitted for other reasons not directly related to this condition, a consideration that applies to all the types of condition discussed in this chapter.

If the patient has been admitted with an acute exacerbation of SLE the nursing assessment must be comprehensive yet tailored to individual needs, as the disorder can affect the patient in many different ways. Multisystem involvement is possible. The person who has been admitted for joint replacement surgery requires careful assessment to ensure they are fit enough for the anaesthetic and the stress of surgery, in addition to the normal assessment required for a patient undergoing joint replacement surgery.

Nursing care

The care of the patient is mainly supportive and symptomatic; at present, no therapy is considered curative. In remissions, the patient is advised against exposure to sunlight, infection and excessive fatigue which are thought to predispose or precipitate an exacerbation of the disease process. Lotions may be used to screen out the ultraviolet sun rays when the person has to be exposed. Cold should be avoided because of the vascular reaction (Raynaud's disease).

Medications that may be prescribed include NSAIDs to control fever and joint involvement, and an antimalarial drug such as hydroxychloroquine (Plaquenil) for skin and joint involvement. If the condition is unresponsive to NSAIDs an adrenocorticosteroid preparation may be considered. The latter is used for the more severe stage of SLE when there is renal, central nervous system, cardiovascular and haematopoietic involvement. The steroid drug is given in relatively large doses during an acute exacerbation, and then gradually reduced to a maintenance dose or withdrawn completely. If hydroxychloroquine is given, frequent ophthalmological examinations are necessary because the drug may precipitate retinopathy. Cyclophosphamide (Endoxana) or azathioprine (Imuran) may be used when the patient with severe disease is unresponsive to the more conservative drugs. Aspirin may be given if there are thrombotic problems.

Dialysis may be necessary when the disease attacks the kidneys. Infection is treated promptly with antibiotics. Emotional stress should be minimized and fatigue avoided. Plasma exchange and immunosupressive drug therapy are reserved for advanced cases.

SLE is a serious chronic disease that is unpredictable in nature. The patient experiences remissions and exacerbations. Nursing intervention focuses on assisting the patient to manage the disease and adapt his or her lifestyle to altered functional level. Emphasis is placed on the patient's strengths and the positive aspects of functional ability. The patient is helped to identify factors that precipitate flare-ups or exacerbation of symptoms and to create an environment free of stress. A daily routine is planned to provide adequate rest.

The following points are emphasized in teaching patients and their families about the disease and self-management:

1. Knowledge of the disease process, its management, and signs and symptoms of disease activity.

2. Actions, dosage and possible side-effects of the prescribed drug(s) and adjustment of medication dosage in response to symptom changes.

3. The importance of carrying an identification card if the patient is receiving corticosteroid therapy.

4. Awareness of expected weight gains with corticosteroid therapy and measures to minimize and cope with the weight gain.

5. The necessity for regular medical supervision so that tissue changes can be detected early by laboratory tests and prompt adjustment made in drug therapy to help control tissue damage.

6. The importance of prompt identification of infection and the action to take when infection develops.

7. The importance of regular rest, sleep and good nutrition.

8. Methods of decreasing physical and emotional stress.

9. Knowledge of community resources including self-help groups.

10. Avoidance of overexposure to sunlight.

Systemic sclerosis and related scleroderma syndromes

This is a chronic disorder in which the collagen component of the skin undergoes degenerative changes and becomes sclerotic. The dermal changes and contraction produce deformities and restricted movement. The pathological sclerosing process may spread to viscera, causing systemic disturbances and organ dysfunction similar to those that may occur in systemic lupus erythematosus. The rate of progress varies with patients: some survive for many years, whereas the disease may prove fatal to others within a few months.

Infective bone disease

Osteomyelitis

When bone tissue becomes infected, the condition is known as osteomyelitis. The pathogenic organisms may be introduced directly through an open fracture or from infected contiguous tissue, but are more commonly carried by the blood to the bone from a distant primary focus such as boils (furuncles), an abscessed tooth or infected tonsils. When the infection is bloodborne, the condition is referred to as *haematogenous osteomyelitis*. The most common bacterial offender is *Staphylococcus aureus*, but the disease may also result from the invasion of streptococci, pneumococci or other strains of staphylococci.

Growing bone is more susceptible to haematogenous osteomyelitis and, as a result, the incidence is highest in children and adolescents. The infection usually develops in long bones at the diaphyseal side of the growth plate. In adults the pelvis and vertebrae are more often affected. The bone marrow is affected first. Unless it is checked at the onset, the inflammatory process forms a purulent exudate that collects in the minute canals and spaces of the bone tissue. The pressure of the exudate builds up because of the resistant, rigid bone and compresses the blood vessels, causing thrombosis and occlusion. The accumulation under pressure eventually breaks through the cortex of the bone into the subperiosteal space. The periosteum at that site becomes elevated and stripped from the bone, interrupting the blood vessels that lead into the bone. Interference with the blood supply results in an area of dead bone tissue, which is called a *sequestrum*. The periosteum may rupture, and the infection may then extend into the adjacent soft tissues, forming a sinus tract that discharges on to the skin surface. Small sequestra, separated from the living bone tissue, may escape with the exudate through the sinus.

The infection may destroy the growth plate (epiphyseal plate), leading to reduced growth of the limb, or it may extend into the adjacent joint with ensuing permanent loss of joint function. The periosteum initiates the formation of new bone tissue around the affected area. The new tissue is called the *involucrum* (a covering or sheath, such as contains the sequestrum of a necrosed bone) and may enclose and trap sequestra and infecting organisms. These organisms continue to grow in the confined area and the osteomyelitis becomes chronic, characterized by recurring abscess formation and sequestration. Chronicity is more likely to occur in non-traumatic osteomyelitis.

Patient problems

The actual and potential problems of acute osteomyelitis include the following:

■ severe pain in the affected limb (caused by the pressure of accumulating exudate and bone destruction) aggravated by even slight movement

■ protection of the limb by avoiding weight bearing, any movement and flexion of the adjoining joints

■ tenderness and swelling of the affected part; a draining sinus may develop over the involved area

■ restlessness and irritability

■ nausea and vomiting

■ radiographs show destructive bone changes and periosteal elevation after 1–2 weeks.

Nursing assessment

The patient admitted with this condition after trauma has usually been affected over a lengthy period involving significant loss of mobility and function together with chronic pain. A careful assessment of the patient's social and psychological state is essential if nursing care is to address the patient's main problems, while pain assessment is also of prime importance. A patient who is self-employed may, for example, face bankruptcy as a result of a prolonged period of inactivity and frequent hospitalizations, while the chronic nature of the pain and apparent lack of progress in resolving the condition may severely affect the person's morale. The patient may be aware that in some cases the only way of resolving the condition is amputation.

If the condition is acute, it usually involves adolescents. The nurse needs to pay particular attention to vital signs as the patient may be very febrile and toxic in the initial stages; pain should also be assessed carefully. The developmental stage of the person should be considered together with the family situation as this can have a significant bearing upon nursing care.

Nursing care

Antimicrobial drug therapy and rest in the early stage of osteomyelitis may bring the infection under control with minimal bone damage and before a sinus is formed. In more advanced cases, surgery may be necessary to provide drainage to relieve the pressure within the bone and periosteum and to remove dead bone tissue.

Efforts are made to identify the infecting organism by making cultures of the blood, nose and throat secretions and discharge from any skin lesions (e.g. boils). If a positive culture is obtained, sensitivity tests may then be done to determine the most effective antibiotic therapy.

Large doses of antibiotics are given, usually by parenteral channels. Antibiotic therapy is begun after culture and sensitivity tests. Effective oral antibiotic therapy has been achieved only recently. Clindamycin is recommended for Gram-positive staphylococcal osteomyelitis, although it has serious toxic effects such as antibiotic-induced colitis (British National Formulary 2000). Ciprofloxacin has been shown to be effective in treating Gram-negative bacillary osteomyelitis when treatment extends from 4 to 6 weeks or longer. In some cases, when the acute phase of the illness is over, the patient may be discharged and continue therapy at home.

Large doses of antibiotics may be given parenterally over several weeks (usually a minimum of 4 weeks). If the response is favourable and the infective process controlled, antimicrobial therapy is generally continued for several weeks to ensure destruction of the organisms.

The patient is placed at rest, and the affected limb is handled very gently. It is positioned and supported to prevent contractures and deformities. A splint may be used to immobilize the adjacent joint, or skin traction may be applied if a lower limb is affected. Careful monitoring of pressure areas and rigorous pressure care are essential. A well balanced high-calorie diet is needed to help cope with the metabolic demands of what is a serious infective process.

If surgical drainage or a sequestrectomy is performed, the wound is packed and allowed to heal by granulation from within towards the surface. Antibiotic or sulfonamide preparations may be introduced locally into the wound. The dressing is changed often enough to keep the wound clean and to prevent the development of an offensive odour that may become very distressing to the patient and those in his or her environment. Precautions must be taken to observe aseptic technique when dressing or treating the wound to prevent the introduction of secondary infection and the transmission of the patient's infection to others.

When the patient is allowed up, protection must be afforded against falls and injury to the limb. The loss of bone substance may weaken the bone structure, predisposing it to fracture when subjected to even slight injury or pressure. In the case of a lower extremity, weight bearing may be contraindicated for many weeks while new bone tissue is being formed. The patient may then have to be taught to use crutches and may be discharged from the hospital, but is likely to require guidance and supervision for a considerable period of time.

Osteoporosis

Osteoporosis
See chapter 3.2

Osteoporosis is a disease that results from an imbalance between calcium reabsorption and bone formation. This results in an overall loss of bone mass and increases the risk of fracture, often with little trauma. Women suffer more from this problem than men as there is accelerated loss of bone mass due to deficiency in oestrogen after the menopause. Burden and Allsworth (1999) cite extensive evidence to show that, in the UK alone during the 1990s, osteoporosis contributed to approximately 60 000 fractures of the upper femur, 50 000 wrist fractures and 40 000 veretebral fractures per year, largely in postmenopausal women.

Primary osteoporosis is age related or postmenopausal in origin but is genetically influenced. Satisfactory levels of calcium intake and exercise during adolescence also play a major part in building up bone mass and hence reducing the risk of primary osteoporosis in later life. Smoking, alcohol abuse and anorexia nervosa contribute to a reduction in bone mass. Men may also develop osteoporosis and factors such as lack of exercise and inadequate diet during adolescence will have a similarly detrimental effect on bone mass. Secondary osteoporosis occurs as a result of either another disease process or drug therapy (e.g. corticosteroid treatment).

Bone mass is investigated using a dual-energy X-ray densiometer machine which measures X-ray absorption, hence the term DEXA scanning. A scan of the spine takes only 10 minutes, and of the hip region even less.

Bone mineral density (BMD) as measured by DEXA scanning is used to define the degree of osteoporosis. However, whole-population screening for osteoporosis is not carried out at present (Burden and Allsworth 1999).

Nursing assessment

Osteoporosis is a condition that is likely to be present in many elderly patients, particularly women, although it is not usually the prime cause of admission. The nurse therefore needs to be aware of the likely existence of this condition in assessing elderly patients, whatever other health problems they may have.

Clinical characteristics

Actual and potential problems may include the following:

- Fractures of any bone but most commonly of the vertebrae between T10 and L2, the femoral neck region and the wrist. Fractures may be complete or impacted (see Box 24.2).

- Pain, localized or radiating, and tenderness.

- Muscle spasm.

- Loss of normal lumbar curve and progressive development of kyphosis (curvature of the spine) due to collapsed vertebrae.

The presence of these problems leads to decreased mobility, which exacerbates the condition, and interferes with normal self-care.

Nursing care

Calcitonin
See chapter 2.6

As treatment for osteoporosis cannot reverse the condition, it is directed at arresting or slowing the rate of calcium reabsorption, reducing discomfort and maintaining a satisfactory lifestyle. These goals are addressed through medication, diet and exercise. Health promotion has a major role in preventing the condition, especially in younger people.

Medication

Hormone replacement therapy (HRT) restores levels of oestrogen to premenopausal levels and therefore slows bone loss and maintains bone levels in most women. Progestogens should also be given to women who have a uterus in order to avoid the risk of cancer of the endometrium which is real because of the stimulatory effect of oestrogen on the endometrium. There is also a slightly increased risk of breast cancer in women taking HRT which increases as the length of time on HRT increases (British National Formulary 2000). Women on HRT should therefore be taught breast self-awareness (see Ch. 23). Some women find the side-effects of HRT are such that they discontinue therapy.

Calcitonin helps to regulate bone turnover and may be used to help women who are at high risk of osteoporosis and for whom HRT is unsuitable. It can also help to relieve pain after a vertebral fracture.

Vitamin D is necessary for the use of calcium in building bone mass. It may be prescribed in a range of preparations such as ergocalciferol (calciferol, vitamin D_2).

Biphosphonate drugs are used in an attempt to prevent osteoclasts from carrying out their normal function. Osteoclasts are bone cells whose main purpose is to reabsorb bone. Cyclical etidronate is given in a 90-day course to women with established osteoporosis, along with calcium supplements. Alendronate is the other main drug in this group, and has contributed to building significant bone mass at key skeletal sites. Studies in the USA have shown a 50% reduction in fractures of the hip, wrist and spine over a 3-year period in elderly women with osteoporosis and previous vertebral fractures after use of alendronate (McClung 1999).

Diet

Diet therapy stresses the importance of the intake of foods high in calcium, supplementary vitamin D and protein, and of fluid intake, and the monitoring of the types of foods chosen to accomplish this.

Exercise

Regular weight-bearing exercise (e.g. dancing, walking, keep fit) places bone under stress, and they respond by becoming stronger. Three 20-minute exercise sessions per week are recommended. The general beneficial effects of exercise are added to the skeletal benefits.

Health promotion

Nurses should be aware that women are more likely to suffer from osteoporosis than men. Nurses have a responsibility to teach health habits related to a lifestyle believed to assist in the prevention of osteoporosis. The target group is premenopausal women, but all women may benefit from such teaching. After assessing the patient for the risk factors discussed above, a teaching plan should be developed that covers diet, exercise and any medication the person may be taking, and is directed towards the reduction of any risk factors identified. Dietary advice should cover the importance of a well balanced diet, high in calcium and low in animal fats. Vitamin D supplements may also be recommended. The fact that excessive intake of alcohol and caffeine can accelerate the onset of osteoporosis is stressed.

An older person who is given the diagnosis of osteoporosis may be very frightened and anxious. Depression, sleep disturbance, apathy and a loss of self-esteem may ensue (McClung 1999). These feelings have to be brought out into the open and worked through if the nurse is to support the patient and allow him or her to take a positive and healthy approach to the later years of life.

Back pain

Back pain is a common and serious health problem in the UK which, in 1998, is estimated to have cost the UK

£1632 million (York CRD 2000). Back pain may have a mechanical cause located at the articulation of one vertebra with another and involving degeneration of the intervertebral disc. The interaction of the diseased disc with surrounding tissues gives rise to the pain. This may be by pressing on a nerve root or involvement of surrounding ligaments and joint facets. Non-mechanical causes include bad posture, poor lifting technique, unequal leg length, secondary malignant growths that have metastasized from cancer of the breast or prostate, and other degenerative diseases of the spine (Walsh et al 1999).

Early treatment in primary care should focus on pain relief with the use of simple analgesia and NSAIDs, maintaining activity and physiotherapy. Chronic disability due to back pain is usually associated with serious psychological and sociological problems, so it is essential to try to maintain a positive approach on the part of the patient. Otherwise the person becomes increasingly dependent upon others, anxious, and experiences disturbed family relationships associated with these factors, plus sleep disturbance, reduced self-esteem and interpersonal friction (Austin 2000).

Current guidelines stress that advice to continue ordinary activity may provide equivalent or even faster symptomatic recovery from acute back pain and lead to less chronic disability and time off work. Bedrest should not be recommended as a treatment for low back pain. Drug therapy with NSAIDs and/or benzodiazepines is effective in relieving the symptoms of an acute attack, but both groups of drugs have side-effects that should be monitored. Physiotherapy is very effective in helping patients with chronic low back pain and all patients benefit from a multidisciplinary approach to treatment (York CRD 2000).

Osteomalacia

Osteomalacia is an adult disorder comparable to rickets in children and, for this reason, it is occasionally referred to as adult rickets. It is characterized by an insufficient plasma concentration of calcium and inorganic phosphate for normal calcification of bone tissue.

Osteomalacia may be the result of an insufficient amount of calcium reaching the plasma or an excessive urinary excretion of the mineral. The deficiency of calcium may be due to a lack of calcium-containing foods in the diet or insufficient absorption of the mineral from the intestine caused by steatorrhoea or prolonged diarrhoea. Vitamin D is necessary for normal absorption of calcium and its deposition in bone tissue; therefore a diet deficient in vitamin D will lead to osteomalacia. This condition may also occur during pregnancy if the woman does not receive additional calcium to meet the increased demand incurred by the developing fetus. Excessive urinary excretion of calcium is usually the result of acidosis associated with renal failure or of renal tubular damage and malfunction.

Actual and potential *problems* may include:

- softening and weakening of bone
- tenderness and aching
- deformity of the long bones
- loss of weight and muscular strength
- tetany.

The *treatment* consists mainly of the administration of calcium, phosphorus and vitamin D. If the serum calcium concentration is markedly low, calcium (e.g. calcium gluconate 10%) may be given intravenously.

Paget's disease (osteitis deformans)

Paget's disease is a chronic disorder of bone remodelling. Localized areas of bone show abnormally rapid reabsorption due to osteoclasts and subsequent replacement with abnormal new bone that is prone to deformity and fracture. The disease may be limited to one area or occur in several parts of the skeleton. The pelvis and femur are most commonly affected. The cause is not well understood although viral particles have been found in affected bone (Lewis et al 1999).

Bone pain is the most common symptom associated with skeletal deformity, pathological fractures and symptoms of nerve compression. Rarely, malignant degeneration of the bone may occur leading to sarcoma in about 1% of cases. It is most commonly found in persons over 50 years of age, but may affect younger persons as well. Men are slightly more likely to contract this disease than women and the disease is mostly seen in caucasians.

Nursing care

When the disease is asymptomatic and weight-bearing bones are not involved, no treatment is necessary. Treatment and nursing intervention are supportive and directed toward alleviating presenting symptoms with the use of NSAIDs. In more advanced cases calcitonin is frequently used. Biphosphonates are, however, the drug of choice (see p. 920). The objective of this treatment is to control the metabolic action of the disease, reduce the rate of bone turnover and ease pain. Patients are advised to eat a diet high in calcium and protein, with vitamin C and D supplements. An individualized exercise programme is taught and the person is encouraged to follow it unless symptoms recur.

Bone neoplasms

Primary and secondary neoplasms may develop in bone tissue. Primary new growths may be benign or malignant; secondary bone neoplasms are metastases from malignant disease in another area of the body and have a much higher incidence than primary bone neoplasms.

Osteomalacia
See chapter 3.2

Paget's disease
See chapter 3.1

Most primary bone neoplasms develop in children and adults younger than 40 years. They may be classified by the type of cell from which they originate, whether they are benign or malignant, and whether the tissue response is osteolytic or reactive. The neoplasm may cause a breakdown of the bone structure with loss of calcium from the tissue; this type of reaction is referred to as *osteolytic*. The response of bone tissue to some types of neoplastic cells is the formation of dense bone tissue around the lesion, which may be referred to as a *nidus*. This type of process is called *reactive bone formation*.

The more common primary bone neoplasms are listed in Table 24.6.

Clinical characteristics

Neoplasms of bones may be asymptomatic for a period of time and may be discovered only when the person has radiography for some other reason (e.g. sustained injury) or has a pathological fracture. Persistent pain, progressively increasing in severity, and limitation of activity of the affected part are common characteristics. Local tenderness, swelling and warmth may be present. If the neoplasm is malignant, systemic symptoms such as weight loss and anaemia develop. Diagnosis is made by bone scan as this is more sensitive than radiography, although this may also be performed.

Benign bone neoplasms are treated by excision or curettage. The bone structure may have to be reinforced following the removal of the lesion by filling in the space with bone chips or small grafts. Treatment of primary malignant neoplasms involves a combination of surgery and chemotherapy. Radical excision is done if the lesion is accessible or, in the case of an extremity, the limb is amputated.

Table 24.6   Common primary bone neoplasms

Cell of origin	Neoplasm	Benign or malignant	Comments
Osteocyte	Osteoid osteoma	Benign	Small, reactive lesion. Femur and tibia common sites. Especially painful at night. Treatment involves surgical removal
	Osteochondroma	Benign	Most common benign bone neoplasm; a hamartoma[a] consisting of bony outgrowth with a cartilage cap. Distal end of femur, proximal end of tibia and proximal end of humerus are common sites. Symptoms depend upon impingement on surrounding tissues
	Osteogenic sarcoma (osteosarcoma)	Malignant (rapid spread)	Destroys medullary and cortical bone tissue. Usually develops in end of long bone; almost 50% involve the knee joint. Severe pain and tenderness; area may be hot and swollen. Treatment consists of amputation and chemotherapy, or chemotherapy and endoprosthetic replacement
	Osteoclastoma	Benign – may become malignant	Develops most often in epiphyseal region of femur, tibia or humerus of young adults. Rarefaction of bone occurs. It causes pain, swelling and rarely pathological fracture. Treated by curettage or by resection of the bone and replacement with a bone graft. If malignant, the limb is amputated, or chemotherapy and endoprosthetic replacement
Chondrocyte	Endochondroma	Benign	Growth of tumour cells of the hyaline cartilage may cause a pathological fracture. Treatment is by curettage
	Chondroblastoma	Benign	Develops toward end of adolescence. Common sites are femur, tibia and humerus. Highest incidence in males. Causes pain and swelling in epiphyseal area. Treatment is curettage and bone grafts
	Chondrosarcoma	Malignant (slower spread than osteosarcoma)	Age group most often affected 30–60 years. Common sites are scapula, pelvis, humerus and femur. Treatment involves radical excision, amputation, or chemotherapy and endoprosthetic replacement
Fibrocyte	Non-osteogenic fibroma	Benign	Most common site is end of diaphysis of long bone. If asymptomatic, it may be left untreated. If painful, it is excised
	Fibrosarcoma	Malignant	Rare. Usually in adults. Treated by amputation if in a limb or chemotherapy plus endoprosthetic replacement
Uncertain; reticulocyte suggested	Ewing's tumour or sarcoma	Malignant	May involve ilia, ribs, vertebrae and shafts of long bones. Begins in marrow cavity and gradually erodes the bone tissue. Manifestations include severe pain, swelling, fever and leucocytosis. Treatment is combination of irradiation, chemotherapy and surgery, including endoprosthetic replacement

[a] A hamartoma is a benign tumour formed by an overgrowth of normal mature cells characteristic of the area.

The use of custom-made joints and of bone replacement has preserved the mobility of many patients. Suitable cases may be those where there is no diffuse spread of the tumour into surrounding secondary deposits. Extending prostheses have been developed in the past decade. They can be used in the tibia, femur and humerus of the growing child or adolescent.

Treatment of the patient with skeletal metastases depends principally on the origin of the primary malignant disease. Chemotherapy, hormones and/or irradiation may be used. Irradiation may be used to reduce the severity of the pain experienced by the patient. Analgesics are prescribed to keep the patient comfortable; a small dose is used at first, but usually has to be increased as the condition worsens and the patient develops a tolerance for the drug.

Nursing intervention

Nursing care is directed toward symptom management, psychosocial support, and patient and family teaching.

The most common patient problems include pain, nausea and vomiting caused by the treatment of the disease, anxiety and fear. Above all the patient will have a major knowledge deficit about the condition and be in need of teaching and education if informed decisions about treatment options are to be made.

Pain

Specific points for assessment include the presence, location and degree of **pain**. It is important to determine the exact location of pain in order to learn whether new areas of the skeleton are involved, particularly in metastatic bone cancer.

The *goal* is that the patient will be as free from pain as possible. Alleviation of pain may best be achieved through regular scheduling of optimum doses of opioids with follow-up assessment of the effectiveness of each dose. Time-scheduled medication should prevent patients from experiencing pain. If this is not the result for any individual, the medication regimen should be reassessed with the patient and doctor and necessary changes made.

Potential for nausea and vomiting

The *goal* is that the patient should be free from nausea and should not vomit. The patient should be closely assessed for **nausea and vomiting** as they have many causes and should not be quickly attributed to any particular one; radiation therapy, additive hormones, opioids and hypercalcaemia may all contribute. Effective intervention to prevent nausea is possible only when the cause has been identified.

Lack of knowledge

Patient and family teaching includes issues related to treatment options and signs and symptoms of further advancing disease, including early indications of spinal cord compression and hypercalcaemia. Family members are taught basic care techniques in order to care for the patient at home. These include positioning, bathing, skin care, assisting the person in ambulation, and safety measures. The nurse also assists the patient and family in understanding the need for a diet high in calories, fibre and fluids. Support from community nursing services is essential.

Anxiety and fear

The *goal* is that the patient may adapt to the disease in a positive way. The psychosocial needs of patients with bone neoplasms and their families are most severe when the neoplasm is malignant, particularly as a malignant neoplasm is usually metastatic. Supportive care in the form of guided questioning, attentive listening, use of touch and information giving is provided. If this proves insufficient, referral for more intensive support should be made.

Summary

Disease and trauma affecting bones and joints may have a short-term limited effect or may result in the patient suffering years of chronic pain with occasional acute episodes. Hospital admission is often during the acute stages of the disease and the nurse must be aware of the patient's normal coping strategies.

In caring for patients with orthopaedic conditions nurses may develop long-term relationships with them. Individuals with a chronic condition will frequently return to the same ward or unit when they need hospitalization. There is a great scope in this situation for the patient's care to be discussed with the family and multidisciplinary team. For example, the work of the physiotherapist is closely linked to that of the occupational therapist and they both need the cooperation of the family at home for their ideas to be continued in the community. It is the patient's quality of life in the long term that must be of paramount importance. This may require specialist advice for chronic pain counselling, the involvement of social services and support groups for both the patient and/or the relatives in addition to a wide range of therapeutic interventions. The ageing population of the UK means that orthopaedic and trauma services will have increasing demands placed upon them in the future. These demands require new ways of working both in terms of expanded nursing roles, better multidisciplinary teamwork and increasingly coordinated care between hospital and primary care teams.

Pain
See chapter 2.3

Nausea and vomiting
See chapter 5.1

References

Arthur V (1994) Nursing care of patients with rheumatoid arthritis. British Journal of Nursing 3(7): 325–330.

Austin J (2000) Early management of patients with back pain. Professional Nurse 15(6): 399–403.

British National Formulary (2000) British National Formulary. London: British Medical Association/Royal Pharmaceutical Society of Great Britain.

Burden J, Allsworth A (1999) Osteoporosis: do we take it seriously? Journal of Orthopaedic Nursing Suppl 1, 9–14.

Byrne J (1999) Rheumatology part 2: the role of medication. Professional Nurse 14(5): 355–358.

Choong P, Langford A, Dowsey M, Santamaria N (2000) Clinical pathway for fractured neck of femur: a prospective controlled study. Medical Journal of Australia 172: 423–426.

Cree M (2000) Mortality and institutionalisation following hip fracture. Journal of the American Geriatric Society 48(3): 283–288.

Dieppe P, Cooper C, Kirwan J, McGill N (1991) Arthritis and Rheumatism. London: Gower.

Haslett C, Chilvers E, Hunter J, Boon N (1999) Davidson's principles and practice of medicine, 18th edn. Edinburgh: Churchill Livingstone.

Hill N, Davies P (2000) Nursing care of total joint replacement. Journal of Orthopaedic Nursing 4: 41–45.

King L (1994) Safe handling of hip replacement patients. Nursing Standard 8(47): 31–35.

le Gallez P (1993) Rheumatoid arthritis: effects on the family. Nursing Standard 7(39): 30–34.

Leslie M (1999) Hyaluronic acid treatment for osteoarthritis of the knee. Nurse Practitioner 24(7): 38–48.

Lewis T, Tesh A, Lyles K (1999) Caring for the patient with Paget's disease of the bone. Nurse Practitioner 24(7): 50–65.

Love C (2000) A review of the nursing care when using the new generation drugs COX2 selective in osteoarthritis and rheumatoid disease. Journal of Orthopaedic Nursing 4: 112–114.

Marcangelo C (2000) Surgery and acute care following hip fracture. Nursing Times 96(9): 47–48.

McClung B (1999) Using osteoporosis management to reduce fractures in elderly women. Nurse Practitioner 24(3): 26–47.

Morley J (1998) The case for fast tracking fractured neck of femur patients. Journal of Orthopaedic Nursing 2(2): 91–94.

Parker M, Handoll H (2000) Pre-operative traction for fractures of the proximal femur (Cochrane review). The Cochrane Library, issue 3.

Patterson BM, Cornell CN, Carbone B et al (1992) Protein depletion and metabolic stress in elderly patients who have a fracture of the hip. Journal of Bone and Joint Surgery 74A: 251–256.

Richardson E (1992) Rheumatoid arthritis in pregnancy. Nursing Standard 6(45): 25–28.

Ryan S (1999) Rheumatology part 4: psychosocial issues. Professional Nurse 14(7): 509–512.

Shaul M (1995) From early twinges to mastery: the process of adjustment in rheumatoid arthritis. Arthritis Care and Research 8(4): 290–297.

Simpson M (1987) Psychiatric problems on an orthopaedic ward and the traction intolerance syndrome. Nursing RSA Verpleging 2(8): 14–15.

Sims M (1999) External fixation: part 1. Journal of Orthopaedic Nursing 3: 203–209.

Sims M, Saleh M (2000) External fixation – the incidence of pin site infection: a prospective audit. Journal of Orthopaedic Nursing 4: 59–63.

Spector T (1996) Epidemiology of rheumatic diseases. In: Snaith M, ed. ABC of rheumatology. London: BMJ.

Springhouse Corporation (1998) Handbook of medical surgical nursing, 2nd edn. Springhouse, PA: Springhouse Corporation.

Swanson C, Yelland C, Day G (2000) Clinical pathways and fractured neck of femur. Medical Journal of Australia 172: 415–416.

Walsh M, Kent A (2001) Accident and emergency nursing, 4th edn. Oxford: Butterworth Heinemann.

Walsh M, Crumbie A, Reveley S (1999) Nurse practitioners: clinical skills and professional issues. Oxford: Butterworth Heinemann.

York CRD (2000) Acute and chronic low back pain. Effective Health Care Bulletin 6(5).

25

Caring for the patient with a skin or wound care need

Mark Collier

Introduction

Pressure ulcers

Burn injuries

General skin conditions

Summary

Introduction

Health problems involving the **skin** vary from minor to catastrophic. Nurses require a wide range of skills to provide not only the necessary physical care but also much needed psychological support.

A preventive approach to the maintenance of skin integrity combined with specific education can be of greater benefit to a person than a delayed, reactive one. For example, the prevention of skin cancers by educating people about the hazards of overexposure to the sun is a far more desirable goal than successful treatment. Today's better educated healthcare consumers increasingly expect to be involved in their own care. They are also more conscious of the need for information related to health promotion.

A typical cross-section of the skin is shown in Figure 25.1a, and the outermost layer, the *epidermis*, is shown in more detail in Figure 25.1b. The epidermis is avascular but is supported by the dermis, a region of the skin that has a rich blood and nerve supply. It is important to remember, especially when assessing patients for signs of damage to the skin such as pressure ulceration, that as an organ the skin covers a surface area of over 2 square metres (Collier 1994).

Cells responsible for the regeneration of skin are produced in the basal (germinating) layer of the epithelium and then gradually move through the other layers to the surface. As they ascend, they progressively undergo degenerative changes. The nuclei disintegrate, the cell substance changes to a water-repellent, waxy, protein-like substance called *keratin*, and the cells become flat. They are continuously reproduced in the basal layer and cast off from the surface. The cells that are shed disintegrate, leaving their keratin on the surface; this keratin helps to protect the skin.

The thickness of the epidermis varies in different areas of the body from a minimum of 0.07 mm to 0.12 mm in depth. It is thickest on the soles of the feet and palms of the hands, and thinnest on the lips and eyelids. This provides maximum 'wear and tear' qualities for areas of maximum stress. Imparting physical strength to the skin and potential wounds remains, however, the role of the dermis.

The *dermis*, consisting of fibrous and elastic connective tissue, contains many blood and lymphatic vessels, nerves and their end-organs, sebaceous and sweat glands, ducts and hair follicles.

Lying between the epidermal germinating layer and the dermis are the melanocytes, which produce the pigment melanin and deliver it to the epidermal cells. The amount of pigment is determined mainly by the person's genetic inheritance. The activity of the pigment-producing cells may also be influenced by melanocyte-stimulating hormone (MSH), which is released by the anterior pituitary and by exposure to sunlight and friction.

The subcutaneous fatty tissue functions as a heat insulator, a cushion against mechanical pressure and an energy store. The subcutaneous tissue is distributed in varying thicknesses over the entire body surface. The thickness of the skin overall is therefore dependent upon regional anatomy and is also influenced by an individual's sex and age.

The cutaneous sebaceous glands secrete an oily substance (sebum) which reaches the skin surface via the hair follicles. Glands are plentiful in the face and scalp but are absent in the palmar and plantar aspects of the hands and feet. The secretion prevents drying of the hair and skin and helps to keep the skin soft and pliable. Blackheads are discoloured accumulations of sebum in hair follicles and frequently provide a medium for organisms, causing pimples or the condition acne. Sebaceous gland activity

Skin
See chapter 6.1

Skin structure
See chapter 6.1

Figure 25.1   (a) Cross-section of the skin. (b) Cell layers of the epidermis.

(a)

Hair
Sebaceous gland
Sweat gland
Epidermis
Superficial vascular plexus
Capillary
Hair root
Nerve
Blood vessels
Dermis
Subcutaneous fat
Subcutaneous tissue

(b)

Cornified (keratinized) layers of dead cells (thickness variable)
Clear layer
Granular layer
Prickle cell layer
Germinal or basal layer

increases at puberty and decreases in later life due to the influence of gonadal hormones on the output of sebum.

The skin protects the internal structures from injury, acts as a barrier to keep vital fluids and chemicals from leaking out, and prevents invasion of organisms. Its protective functions are enhanced by the water-repellent, waxy nature of the surface cells.

The abundance of sensory receptors and afferent and efferent nerves in the skin function in the sensations of touch, pressure, pain and temperature. These sensations serve as an important protective mechanism for the body and also convey impulses that contribute information about the external environment. For example, through touch we can appreciate shape, composition and texture.

The skin plays an important role in regulating body temperature by varying the calibre of its blood vessels and the activity of the sweat glands. The fluid sweat lying on the surface of the skin cools the body by the process of evaporation. Sweat contains traces of albumin and urea; therefore sweating helps to remove these waste products from the body.

A hair is a cylinder of keratinized cells. Distribution of hair over the body varies with human groups, and with age and sex within each group. Hair serves primarily psychological functions.

The absorptive function of the skin is limited mainly to the absorption of ultraviolet rays from the sun or special lamps; it then converts sterol substances in the skin to vitamin D. A few drugs, which may be included in ointments or lotions, may be absorbed in small amounts.

The dermis and subcutaneous tissue may act as a storage area for water and fat. For instance, when an excess of water is retained in the body, the accumulation in these tissues becomes evident as oedema. The subcutaneous tissue serves as one of the main fat depots and acts as a pad over muscle and bone, cushioning them from mechanical forces.

The sebaceous glands protect the skin from moisture and prevent desiccation. With advancing years, they become less active as a result of the decreased production of hormones, and the skin becomes dry.

Owing to its high proportion of collagen bundles and elastin fibres, the dermis provides mechanical strength and serves to anchor the epidermis to the basal layer of the dermis. The epidermis and its various appendages receive nourishment and support from the dermis. With age, degenerative changes occur in the elastic tissue and collagenous component of fibrous tissue, and the skin becomes wrinkled. Frequently, areas of melanocytes produce more pigment, and 'brown spots' characteristic of ageing skin appear.

From the above introduction it is apparent that the skin plays an essential role in the maintenance of health. It is also a key component of our self-concept and hence is of fundamental importance in maintaining psychological health. This chapter reviews some of the most common health problems related to the skin that the nurse may encounter.

Pressure ulcers

A **pressure ulcer**, formerly referred to as pressure sore, bedsore or decubitus ulcer, is a localized area of tissue damage leading to ulceration of the skin due to the effects of prolonged pressure in combination with a number of other variables (Collier 1995, EUPAP 1997).

Pressure sores.
See chapter 6.1

Continual pressure for as little as 20 minutes is sufficient (Livesley 1992), while other contributory factors may be intrinsic or extrinsic in nature (Collier 1999c). Without immediate intervention the situation deteriorates as the ulcer enlarges, possibly involving deeper structures. The lesion may become infected and lead to the death of the patient in extreme cases. Good preventive measures remove the need for any treatment as the problem simply does not occur.

The nurse plays a major role in the prevention and management of pressure ulcers and in assisting individuals and families to acquire the necessary knowledge and skill to promote, maintain and restore skin integrity.

Risk factors

The principal factor in pressure ulcer development is excessive tissue pressure that prevents the normal supply of blood to the affected area. The normal mean capillary blood pressure is between 12 and 32 mmHg; therefore, pressure in excess of 30 mmHg will render tissue ischaemic and liable to damage and death (Burman 1993). By comparison, lying on a hard floor generates surface interface pressures (SIPs) of 240 mmHg on the sacrum, whereas a standard hospital mattress produces a SIP between 21 and 71 mmHg (Agate 1985). The severity of damage depends upon the length of time for which the tissue is exposed to excess pressures; immobility is therefore a key factor contributing to pressure ulcer formation – a point that has been highlighted at great length in the literature (Bliss 1993, Collier 1999b). In addition, the way in which this pressure (compression) is transmitted through tissues to the underlying skeletal anatomy also determines the extent of damage that may be assessed, either initially or at a later stage. This explains why a sinus or cavity may later appear under what initially appeared to be a superficial defect.

Three other main factors contribute to tissue breakdown: friction, shearing forces and tissue maceration (Lockyer-Stevens 1994). Other contributory factors include the age of the patient – 66% of pressure ulcers occur in patients aged over 70 years (Reid and Morison 1994) – poor nutrition, loss of subcutaneous fat, incontinence, drug therapy and systemic illness such as diabetes mellitus or arteriosclerosis (Morison 2001). Impairments in cognitive and perceptual function also play a key role in pressure ulcer development as the patient is unable to practise self-care in preventing skin breakdown.

In summary, the key to pressure ulcer development is immobility and prolonged unrelieved pressure; however, the situation can be made worse, or to some extent mitigated, by the presence or absence of the other factors mentioned above.

Estimates concerning the cost to the NHS of pressure ulcers have been reported as between £60 million and £321 million per annum (Department of Health 1992, 1993). Direct and indirect treatment costs incurred for a patient with a pressure ulcer that has damaged all layers of the skin have been estimated at £26 000 (Hibbs 1990). This figure has since been updated to £40 000 following analysis of treatment costs for a number of patients at a large teaching hospital in the UK (Collier 1999c). Prevention of pressure ulcers is therefore highly desirable and the need to continue to improve upon the present situation was highlighted by the *Health of the Nation* document, which set a target of reducing pressure ulcer prevalence by between 5 and 10% over time (DoH 1992).

Reid and Morison (1994) reviewed the extensive literature on the prevalence of pressure ulcers in the hospital population and summarized the rate as lying between 6 and 14%. Recent surveys have given higher figures, reflecting the changing nature of the hospital population. O'Dea (1993), for example, found a rate of 18.6% in a sample of over 3000 patients. However, certain groups of patients are at much greater risk, particularly elderly patients with a fracture of the upper femur (Versluysen 1986). It is important not to confuse prevalence (the number of pressure ulcers at any one time) with incidence, which refers to the number of patients developing pressure ulcers over a period of time such as their total in patient stay.

It is acknowledged that often many risk factors are present in elderly patients with fractures of the proximal femur; however, the situation may be compounded by delays and lengthy periods of time spent on trolleys in A&E, X-ray departments and theatres. A study by Mullineaux (1993) showed that, using the Norton scale, 77% of a sample of such patients when assessed in A&E was at risk of developing pressure ulcers. Despite a triage system, the mean time spent on a hard A&E trolley was 2.5 hours and a third of these patients spent between 3 and 6 hours on such a trolley. During this time they were immobile and no pressure-relieving devices were available.

Versluysen's work (1986) found that A&E trolleys in use at that time generated mean sacral pressures of 54 and 56 mmHg, whilst the heel area had mean pressures of 182 and 154 mmHg, depending upon the trolley used. Ward beds produced mean sacral pressures of 34 and 41 mmHg and heel pressures of 96 and 136 mmHg. Operating table pressures were some 50% higher than ward beds. The development of pressure ulcers is therefore hardly surprising if patients have to lie for lengthy periods on such surfaces without pressure-reducing or relieving equipment (Kenney and Rithalia 1999).

At risk from pressure sores
See chapter 6.1

The person at risk of developing pressure ulcers

Assessment

Assessment of the person at **risk** for the development of pressure ulcers includes identification of the contributing factors. Extrinsic factors are those that cause pressure, shearing and/or trauma to the skin as well as the presence of prolonged moisture. Intrinsic factors include the individual's age, nutritional and circulatory status, degree of mobility and dependence, continence, sensory and mental awareness, and degree of alertness. All these factors need to be assessed accurately.

A series of risk assessment tools has been developed, of which the forerunner was the *Norton scale* (Norton et al 1975) (Box 25.1). The maximum score that may be allocated to any individual is 20 (one score from each category); patients with high scores are least likely to develop a breakdown of their skin, while those with lower scores are at greater risk. Goldstone and Goldstone (1982) investigated the predictive ability of the Norton score. They concluded that it was a reliable guide to the incidence of pressure sores but that it tended to overpredict which persons would develop lesions. The physical and incontinence scores were found to be the most discriminatory.

Other scales have been devised, of which the best known in the UK is the *Waterlow scale* (Box 25.2), which adds extra dimensions to the basic Norton scale. When using the Waterlow scale it is important to remember that a low score indicates that the patient is less at risk of developing a pressure ulcer than a patient whose assessment has indicated a high score. Barratt (1987) reviewed these scales alongside the Norton scale and stressed that, while there is insufficient research evidence to favour one against the other, the use of risk scales is to be encouraged as an objective measure of pressure sore risk, an objective that has been further emphasized by the DoH (2001) as a result of its benchmarking process. Further testing is needed to increase the usefulness of these scales in clinical practice for the identification of persons at risk and the prevention of pressure ulcer development. Before any risk assessment scale is used in a clinical setting it is important that all practitioners understand the origins of the scale, as well as the applicability, validity and reliability of the identified risk factors being assessed (Flanagan 1993). Norton's scale was developed for use in a care of the elderly setting; the validity of

---

Box 25.1   The Norton scale for identifying the patient at risk of developing pressure ulcers

A General physical condition		B Mental state		C Activity		D Mobility		E Incontinence	
Good	4	Alert	4	Ambulant	4	Full	4	Not	4
Fair	3	Apathetic	3	Walk with help	3	Slightly limited	3	Occasionally	3
Poor	2	Confused	2	Chairbound	2	Very limited	2	Usually urinary	2
Very bad	1	Stuporous	1	Bedfast	1	Immobile	1	Double	1

From Norton et al (1975).

Box 25.2   The Waterlow pressure sore risk assessment

Build/weight for height		Visual skin type		Continence		Mobility		Sex Age		Appetite	
Average	0	Healthy	0	Complete	0	Fully mobile	0	Male	1	Average	0
Above average	2	Tissue paper	1	Occasionally	1	Restricted/	1	Female	2	Poor	1
Below average	3	Dry	1	incontinent		difficult		14–49	1	Anorexic	2
		Oedematous	1	Catheter/	2	Restless/	2	50–64	2		
		Clammy	1	incontinent		fidgety		65–75	3		
		Discolour	2	of faeces		Apathetic	3	75–80	4		
		Broken/spot	3	Doubly incontinent	3	Inert/traction	4	81+	5		

Special risk factors:

1 Poor nutrition, e.g. terminal cachexia	8	
2 Sensory deprivation, e.g. diabetes, paraplegia, cerebrovascular accident	5	Assessment value
3 High-dose anti-inflammatory or steroids in use	3	At risk 10
4 Smoking 10+ per day	1	High risk 15
5 Orthopaedic surgery/fracture below waist	3	Very high risk 20

Reproduced by kind permission of *Nursing Times*, where this scale first appeared in an article on 18 February 1987.

Figure 25.2   Risk areas for pressure sores. (a) Supine position. (b) Side-lying position.

Back of head
Scapula
Sacrum
Heels
(a)

Toe   Ankle   Knee   Hip   Shoulder
Heel   Ear
(b)

---

its application to younger patients is therefore open to challenge.

Figure 25.2 illustrates the areas receiving greatest pressure in different body positions and therefore at most risk.

Bodyweight also influences the areas receiving greatest pressure. In the underweight individual, areas are more vulnerable in both the lying and sitting positions. In obese individuals pressure is redistributed over larger areas. Casts, braces and underlying tubing are additional causes of pressure; the skin under these areas should be inspected regularly.

The skin over each pressure point should be examined carefully at frequent, regular intervals for redness, swelling, warmth, flaking and erosion.

The goal for the individual at risk for the development of pressure ulcers is to maintain the integrity of the skin.

Pressure ulcer prevention: nursing intervention

Strategies and actions to promote skin integrity and to **prevent** the development of pressure ulcers are important aspects of the individual's healthcare that fall into the realm of nursing.

All individuals at risk of pressure ulcer development should be assessed for the degree of risk and identification of the specific factors (DoH 2001, Royal College of Nursing 2001). Assessments should be carried out on admission to the hospital or nursing home, during community visits and whenever the person's health status changes. It should be remembered that it takes only a few hours for pressure ulcers to develop (Goode et al 1992).

Box 25.3 lists the principles for nursing intervention directed at *maintaining skin integrity* and *preventing pressure*

Box 25.3   Principles of nursing intervention to maintain skin integrity and prevent pressure ulcer development

- Assess individual(s) for risk factors
- Ensure regular changes of position to relieve pressure on 'at-risk' areas 2 hourly, or more frequently if indicated by patient's condition
- Maintain cleanliness and hygiene
- Prevent mechanical, physical and chemical injury
- Ensure adequate nutrition and hydration
- Promote control of incontinence
- Ensure good body alignment and proper positioning
- Utilize devices to redistribute pressure over at-risk anatomical areas
- Inspect the skin at regular intervals during any 24-hour period
- Promote mental alertness and orientation
- Educate the individual, family and caregivers in skin care measures.

---

ulcer development. Specific nursing interventions include the following measures:

1. Promote ambulation and range-of-motion activities.

2. Have the patient change position frequently. If the patient is immobile, change his or her position at least every 2–4 hours throughout the day and night, dependent upon the support surface they are resting on and according to an established schedule. If redness is noted and persistent (Collier 1999a), increase the frequency of the turning schedule.

3. Provide regular bathing and good perineal care twice daily and immediately after incontinence; keep skin dry but avoid friction and rubbing with towels. Many topical applications that are claimed to prevent pressure ulcers are of no value and some may actually be harmful (Walsh and Ford 1989, Redfearn 1991, Collier 1995).

4. Establish a programme to control or manage incontinence.

5. Encourage consistent intake of a nutritionally balanced diet with adequate fluid intake.

6. Use special pressure-redistributing equipment, which will either alternate the area of the body under pressure or redistribute body pressure more evenly over a larger surface area of the body. The former consists of alternating pressure or newer

Prevention
See chapter 6.1

more expensive low air loss, patient support systems. Both of these, however, can be referred to generically as dynamic patient support systems. Low air loss systems have more evidence in the form of randomized controlled trials (RCTs) to support their use and appear to be more effective than alternating pressure systems for the prevention of pressure ulceration (Redfearn 1991). They work by moulding themselves to the contours of the patient's body and redistributing pressure away from the high-risk areas.

7. Keep sheets dry and free of wrinkles and crumbs. Flannelette sheets or pads provide protection from any underlying plastic or rubber covers.

8. Use devices to support specific pressure areas, such as foam pads, gel flotation pads, natural not artificial sheepskins, and splints or pads over heels and elbows to reduce the effects of *friction* forces on vulnerable areas and thereby prevent epidermal damage. The use of water-filled gloves should be discouraged as Lockyer-Stevens (1993) has shown that they generate higher pressures than simply leaving the patient's heels on the mattress.

9. Use a footboard or cradle to prevent pressure on toes.

10. Provide space between the footboard and mattress for heels when the patient is lying supine, or the anterior part of the foot when lying in the prone position.

11. Use pillows and trochanter rolls in positioning the patient to maintain good body alignment and to relieve pressure on known risk areas (see Fig. 25.2).

12. Keep connectors, tubes, pins and clamps from under the patient's body.

13. Avoid shearing forces caused by the patient sliding or slumping down the bed.

14. Those caring for the individual should keep their nails trimmed and remove rings, watches or other jewellery that might scratch or injure the patient during turning or care activities.

15. Teach people to inspect their skin regularly using a long-handled mirror.

16. Avoid the use of bedpans when possible for persons with sensory loss and paralysis. If the use of a bedpan is unavoidable, a slipper pan should be used.

17. Avoid the use of tight straps on urinary drainage leg-bags.

18. Take steps to prevent at-risk patients from lying for lengthy periods on hospital trolleys without any pressure-relieving devices.

Evaluation

Strategies to promote skin integrity and to prevent the development of pressure ulcers are effective if the person's skin remains clean, dry and intact. If skin breakdown does occur, the nurse reassesses the total situation and determines whether the original goal was realistic or whether the person's status or situation has changed. Although the prevention of pressure ulcers is desirable, it must be recognized that this is not always possible (Waterlow 1985).

A quality assurance programme with defined standards for the care of persons at risk of skin breakdown provides a means for nurses to monitor the effectiveness of their practice. Information obtained from auditing health records is analysed by the nurses involved to identify areas of strength and weakness. The nurses define the standards they expect to achieve in preventing pressure ulcer development in their patients, and develop and implement remedial actions to reinforce positive patient behaviours and minimize negative behaviours.

The person with a developed pressure ulcer

Assessment

The area may appear blanched and cool at first, followed by redness, warmth and a breakdown of the skin. As the necrotic tissue is sloughed off, an open, moist, inflamed excavation (ulcer) develops which is open to infection and is slow to heal by granulation.

The pressure ulcer area is examined closely to determine the extent and depth of tissue involvement and must be described accurately. The size of the lesion is monitored either by measuring in centimetres or by tracing its outline on a transparent film at weekly intervals to assess healing. Several grading systems have been devised to classify pressure sores. An example of one basic system is given in Box 25.4 and Figure 25.3, but it must be remembered that a number of classification systems are in current clinical use and this can cause some confusion.

The lesion is examined for inflammation, bleeding, sloughing, infection and fibrous scar tissue formation. The area surrounding the lesion is inspected for discoloration, oedema and inflammation which may signify extension of tissue damage.

Pressure ulcers may develop in underlying tissue as a result of internal pressure exerted by the bony prominences on the deep tissues adjacent to the bone. Such deep tissue necrosis may occur without any initial signs of damage to the overlying skin. Subsequently there is an area of swelling and tension and the skin becomes shiny and/or cyanosed. Erythema and a sinus develop at a later stage.

Box 25.4 A basic classification of pressure ulcers

Grade I

Involvement of epidermis with some extension into the dermal layer, producing redness, induration, warmth and slight erosion of the epidermis. The reddened area blanches to the touch.

Grade II

Involvement of the epidermis and dermis with extension into the subcutaneous layer. The shallow ulceration shows induration, redness and heat, and does not blanch to the touch.

Grade III

Involvement of epidermis and subcutaneous layers with extension down to and including muscle. The ulceration is deep, may be foul smelling with a necrotic base and undermining of tissue. The borders are hyperpigmented.

Grade IV

The ulcer involves all layers of the skin, the underlying muscles and communicates with bone or joint. The ulcer is deep; the tissue is necrotic and may be foul smelling. Undermining is extensive. Borders are darkly pigmented.

Figure 25.3   Classification of pressure ulcers. See Box 25.4.

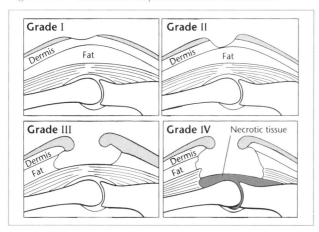

The person with a pressure ulcer is at risk of developing further lesions, so vulnerable areas should be inspected at least every 2–4 hours or when the patient's position is changed. Nursing care for the individual is designed, whenever possible, to restore skin and tissue integrity and to prevent further skin breakdown.

Established pressure ulcer: nursing intervention

The number and variety of therapeutic measures and topical preparations used in the management of pressure ulcers indicate an urgent need for further controlled research studies. Multiple patient variables contribute to the complexity of the problem. Nursing intervention for a patient with a pressure ulcer has to be individualized, and is based on a detailed assessment of the patient as well as of the pressure ulcer; the general condition is important as well as the grade of the pressure sore. Consistency in carrying out the treatment plan is essential.

The measures cited for the preventive care in the preceding pages are still applicable. Further considerations include:

- adequate nutritional intake
- measures to correct existing health problems
- the use of mechanical devices
- care of the lesion
- physical activity
- the control of injurious factors in the environment
- surgical intervention.

Adequate nutritional intake

Nutritional status and dietary intake have been shown to be associated with the presence and healing of pressure ulcers (McLaren and Green 2001). Studies have been reported that patients with exuding ulcers have lower serum albumin levels, probably due to the loss of plasma proteins in exudate from pressure ulcers, particularly full-thickness lesions (McLaren 1992). A high-protein, high-vitamin diet is therefore important to combat the tendency toward a negative nitrogen balance and to provide the essentials for healing and continued tissue resistance.

The objectives of nutritional support for the patient may be summarized as follows:

- to improve Body Mass Index (BMI)
- to maintain optimal bodyweight
- to optimize healing potential
- to prevent further tissue breakdown.

Control of existing health problems

Optimal control of health problems is essential to promote healing as well as to prevent a break in the skin. Management of these problems requires the cooperative efforts of the patient, doctor, nurse and other individuals caring for the patient – a multidisciplinary approach.

Mechanical devices

The mechanical devices used in the prevention and treatment of pressure ulcers may be divided into three categories:

1. Those designed to support specific pressure areas of the body such as heels, sacrum, buttocks or elbows. These devices include gel flotation pads, natural sheepskins, splints and air-filled wheelchair cushions.

2. Those designed to aid in turning and moving a patient, such as turning frames, rotating beds and hydraulic lifts.

3. Those designed to support the entire body surface by minimizing or equalizing pressure. These can include static pressure-reducing mattresses as well as dynamic alternating pressure mattresses and low air loss beds, which are individually pressurized according to the person's height and weight, and air-fluidized beds.

Low air loss and air-fluidized flotation treatment strategies have been shown to be more effective than conventional therapy for hospitalized patients with large pressure ulcers (Allman et al 1987). Turning and positioning of patients is often easier with these beds. Wounds can be kept moist or dryness can be promoted, depending upon the direction of air flow to the area. These devices supplement rather than replace the administration of excellent basic skin care and nutritional support.

Wound care and care of a pressure ulcer

A pressure ulcer is a wound and the principles of **wound healing** therefore apply to managing and treating an established pressure ulcer (Collier 1996). The essential components of an ideal wound dressing, according to Turner (1982), are that it should:

Wound healing
See chapter 6.1

Criteria for wound healing
See chapter 6.1

- maintain a high level of humidity at the wound surface

- remove excess exudate and toxic compounds produced in the wound

- allow gaseous exchange

- prevent the wound surface chilling

- form an inpenetrable barrier to bacteria

- be free from particles and toxic wound debris

- be able to be changed easily without causing damage to underlying tissue.

The first procedure to be carried out with an established pressure ulcer is the removal of dead and infected material (*debridement*), which may be undertaken surgically, chemically or via a process of autolysis. Surgical debridement may range from the nurse removing small areas of necrotic tissue with a scalpel and forceps to a full-scale operation under general anaesthesia. Chemical debridement was traditionally carried out with hypochlorite agents such as Eusol. However, extensive research evidence has suggested that these agents are harmful and their use should be discontinued (Walsh and Ford 1989, Redfearn 1991). Swabbing the dead tissue with antiseptic lotions is also of little value, and is possibly harmful. For cleansing purposes, normal saline is perfectly adequate, harmless and much cheaper.

Modern wound management materials that are effective include the use of proteolytic enzymes, such as Varidase, which can be applied to the necrotic area. Varidase liquefies dead tissue, thereby desloughing the wound and allowing healing to commence. The other types of desloughing agent recommended for use are the dextranomer bead preparations, such as Debrisan. These beads absorb wound exudate and bacteria and are very effective in desloughing pressure ulcers and other wounds. They should be changed once they have become saturated. In addition, hydrogels such as Intrasite are often used as desloughing agents. They are made up mainly of water, and by rehydration of the tissues and the maintenance of a moist wound healing environment assist the process of autolysis. Other commonly used agents include Iodosorb, which consists of microbeads of cadoxemer iodine (modified starch gel containing iodine 0.9%), and calcium alginate fibre dressings such as Sorbsan.

The use of an 'occlusive' dressing is also necessary during the desloughing phase and subsequently while healing occurs. This must conform to the requirements set out above by Turner (1982) and therefore there is no place for ordinary gauze as it allows drying of the wound and fibres of gauze may become incorporated in the wound with the result that dressing removal is very traumatic (Thomas 1990). A range of modern interactive wound management products suitable for the management of pressure ulcers is identified in Box 25.5.

Thomas (1990) and Redfearn (1991) offer an excellent discussion of the various modern types of wound management product (dressings) on offer. The range of new dressing materials can be both bewildering and appear to be an expensive option. Nurses must therefore have rational, cost-effective and evidence-based guidelines for their practice, whether for the management of pressure ulcers or any other wounds.

In dealing with chronic wounds such as pressure ulcers, it is important to remember the observation of Gilchrist (1994), who pointed out that in chronic wounds the presence of bacteria is not uncommon. Wounds may be contaminated but with no sign of multiplication or host reaction; it is only when there is multiplication and a reaction as shown by signs such as localized heat, increased pain, increased exudate and discharge, or cellulitis that it is appropriate to talk about infection. Gilchrist goes on to stress that to deal with a wound infection, topical antibiotics and other applications are inappropriate: only systemic antibiotics will be effective. Nurses can therefore waste a great deal of time debating the fine points of applications and dressings to infected wounds. The dressing in this scenario merely helps to clean the wound up, prevents further contamination, and facilitates a moist wound healing environment. This in turn facilitates pressure ulcer healing by the patient's own resources, which may be supplemented by

Box 25.5 Dressings suitable for use on pressure ulcers

Alginates

Alginates are made from seaweed and may be composed of galuronic acid or mannuronic acid, or both, with the proportions of these determining the gel-forming properties of the final fibre. Examples are Sorbsan and Algisite M. Alginates with a high proportion of galuronic acid produce firmer fibres, adding strength and shape retention to the dressing material as well as absorption.

Film membranes

Typically, these are transparent thin polyurethene films with adhesive properties, which are also vapour permeable, waterproof and extensile. Opsite and Tegaderm are commonly used examples. They are best used on superficial sterile wounds such as operation sites and superficial pressure sores.

Foam dressings

These are most suitable for pressure ulcers producing large volumes of exudate. They are made using advanced polymer technology and therefore combine both hydrophilic and hydrophobic properties in varying proportions, depending on the product selected. They are available in both flat sheet (Allevyn and Lyofoam) and cavity filler forms (Allevyn Cavity and Cavi-Care).

Hydrogels

Hydrogels come in two basic forms, sheets (Gelliperm) and gels (Intrasite, Granugel, Nu-Gel). The sheets comprise polysaccharide agarose cross-linked with polyacrylamide. Gels have a high water content, as previously discussed, and assist the process of autolysis.

Hydrocolloids

These act on a similar principle to the particulates and alginates in that they interact with wound moisture to form a gel; however, they also have occlusive properties. Granuflex, Comfeel and Tegasorb are common examples where the hydrocolloid layer, consisting of a mixture of pectins, gelatines, sodium caboxymethylcellulose and elastomers, is bonded on to a plastic foam layer with an outer plastic impermeable film. These types of dressing may be left in place for up to 5–7 days.

Particulates

These are occlusive dressings that interact with moisture in the wound to form a paste or gel. Examples are Debrisan and Iodosorb; they are particularly useful for dealing with contaminated and recurrently infected wounds.

antibiotics and other steps to deal with underlying pathology such as pressure reduction/relief or compression bandaging to relieve venous congestion in venous leg ulcers (Moffatt and O'Hare 1995).

Physical activity

Pressure on the area is relieved as much as possible by having the patient change position frequently. If unable to turn unaided, the patient is turned every 2 hours throughout the day and night. It is important to remember, however, that 2-hourly turning regimens should never be considered absolute and the frequency may need to varied as the patient's condition either improves or deteriorates, or as a change of patient support surface is indicated. When moving or transferring a patient, precautions are observed to prevent further damage to the skin; the patient is gently lifted clear of the bed or chair, using appropriate aids such as mechanical hoists, to avoid dragging and shearing forces.

Patient activity is encouraged; it stimulates metabolism as well as the circulation. A programme of regular exercises adapted to the person's ability to participate actively is established as soon as possible.

Control of environmental factors

A frequent assessment is made of the person's environment for possible sources of pressure and injury to skin. Again, the reader is referred to the measures cited in the prevention of a pressure ulcer. The bedding, wheelchair, bedpan or commode, clothing and appliances such as a prosthesis and drainage tubes or bags are examples of factors in the patient's environment that could be a source of pressure or injury.

Surgical treatment

Minor surgical debridement of a pressure ulcer may be undertaken on the ward to remove mobile slough and necrotic tissue. Overgranulation of an ulcer may require removal of some of the excess tissue with scissors. Grade III and IV ulcers may require surgical excision and repair by skin flaps in the operating theatre.

Selection of the treatment and nursing care for the patient with a pressure ulcer should be a cooperative effort by all members caring for the patient and should take into consideration the patient's needs, overall status and resources. For example, if frequent dressing changes cause discomfort for the patient (Hollinworth and Collier 2000), consideration should be given to a treatment regimen that involves interactive wound management materials and requires dressing changes less frequently. A variety of interventions are usually required; selection is based on evaluation of the effectiveness of care and assessment of the individual patient, including the amount of pain and discomfort caused by the pressure ulcer.

Patient and family education

The learning needs of the patient and family are assessed on an ongoing basis and they should be fully involved in the management of the patient's pressure ulcer. They are taught to identify risk factors and to plan and carry out measures to prevent further skin breakdown. If the patient is in the community or returning home before healing is complete, the patient, family and caregivers are taught the skills necessary to carry out the skin care regimen. They are also advised to make lifestyle changes to promote adequate nutrition, rest and activity.

Evaluation

The evaluation of nursing interventions designed to treat an individual's pressure ulcer(s) includes documented evidence that healing is occurring. The dimensions of the lesions are decreased, exudate is reduced or absent, and healthy granulation tissue is present. When healing is complete, the area will be clean, dry and intact. Related outcomes include the absence of discomfort, and appropriate and realistic improvements in nutritional status, mobility and incontinence.

If documentation indicates that the pressure ulcer is the same or that deterioration has occurred, the patient's status and the identified treatment objectives (goals for care), as well as the suitability of the strategies used, are re-evaluated.

In a previous review of pressure ulcer treatment Walsh and Ford (1989) stated that much care is meaningless ritual that is of little value and may be of positive harm. Time has moved on since then, but the need for rational, evidence-based pressure care – not ritual and tradition – remains.

Burn injuries

Burn and scald injuries may constitute major trauma. For most of the population who experience a burn or scald, even in a mild form, there is some understanding of how painful and distressing this type of injury may be. A burn injury affects not only the skin but every aspect of the patient's life – psychologically, physically and socially. These effects may last a lifetime. Even those with less serious injuries may find their quality of life affected due to pain, wound management and fear of disfigurement, albeit for a shorter period. Therefore, it is essential that treatment of a burn patient be delivered by a multidisciplinary team approach, where no single health professional is more important than another. Every year more than 100 000 people need to visit hospitals because they are injured as a result of a burn or scald (Department of Trade and Industry 1999). Many burn patients may have other pre-existing health or social problems which complicate their burn injury. The most severe require intensive care nursing, including ventilatory support or haemofiltration due to renal failure, and all need expert nursing care.

Causes

Causes of burn injuries include:

- *scalds* – moist heat such as boiling water, steam or hot liquid at more than 66°C

- *dry heat* – direct contact with a flame or hot object; may also be associated with a flash or friction injury

- *friction* – contact with a moving wheel, rope, wire or road surface

- *radiation* – overexposure to sun and radiant heat sources (e.g. tanning lamps)

- *chemical* – acids (sulfuric, nitric, hydrofluoric, hydrochloric), alkalis (caustic soda, oven cleaners) and cement

- *electrical* – direct passage of current through the body, and lightning injuries.

Related factors

A high proportion of burn injuries occur as a result of carelessness, a lack of knowledge and resources, or personal feelings of invulnerability. Whilst the mortality rate from burn injury in children of relatively well-off families is decreasing, it is actually increasing amongst the poorest families in society (Walsh and Kent 2001). The age of the person is an important factor in the type and severity of the burn. Scalds are the most common cause of burn injury in the toddler, for example, and the impact of any given burn injury is more severe in children and the elderly than in other adults.

Prevention of burn injuries

Burn injuries may be prevented by basic safety precautions. Immediate first aid measures will also minimize the complications resulting from a burn injury. Health promotion activities planned for the population at greatest risk such as the elderly, children and their parents, and those with epilepsy, should involve joint collaboration with local fire brigades. They are an excellent means for nurses to disseminate health promotion messages to the public. Posters in waiting rooms of general practitioners' surgeries or A&E departments are another useful means of getting the message across. Such messages may inform individuals about home safety tips, fire and burn prevention strategies, and give important information on first aid.

Inpatient education focuses on different areas and should include praise for appropriate actions taken and emphasize any good first aid techniques demonstrated. Sensitive and well timed discussions with patients can focus on prevention of burn injury, re-emphasizing first aid advice and home safety tips. The nurse must be alert to the person's readiness to learn about this topic. Experience with burn survivor support groups has indicated that, following their recovery, people who have sustained a burn injury, regardless of the cause and circumstances, in most instances become avid fire and burn prevention advocates. Their support can and should be mobilized through prevention programmes.

Professionals have to battle with the common problem associated with most trauma prevention activities: the 'it will never happen to me' phenomenon. Increased interaction between the public and burn survivor organizations, together with straightforward written material, helps to decrease the sense of personal invulnerability – but at an acknowledged slow pace.

Education, however, is not the sole answer. National legislation and industrial awareness are necessary to make our world a safer place for adults and children. Many experiences have demonstrated that if a child, for example, were put in the same or similar situation again they would do the same thing, with the same result – a burn or scald injury. Further legislation on children's and adults' flame-retardant sleepwear, banning cigarette smoking, smoke detector installation, use of short flexicords for electrical appliances, and hot water heater temperature regulation are all needed.

Characteristics of burn injuries

The *severity* of a burn injury is determined by five factors:

1. surface area of body burned

2. depth of tissue damage

3. age of patient

4. past medical history

5. part of body burned.

However, it should be remembered that the severity of the injury is not necessarily related to its depth. Severity will be dependent upon whether the injury is classed as complex or non-complex; the age of the patient; the site, mechanism and nature of the injury; presence of associated inhalation injury; the size of the injury; and the presence of any existing conditions and other associated injuries.

Surface area

The most accurate estimation of the proportion of body surface burned may be based on the Lund and Browder chart (1944) (Fig. 25.4). The chart assigns a certain percentage to various parts of the body and includes a table indicating the adjustments necessary for different ages, as the head and trunk represent relatively larger proportions of body surface in children. Copies of these charts should be kept available in the emergency department or intensive care unit so that the burned areas can be mapped out when the patient is examined and the percentage estimated.

If the Lund and Browder chart is not available, a quick approximate estimate of the percentage of body surface burned may be made using the Rule of Nines (Walsh and

Figure 25.4   The Lund and Browder burn chart.

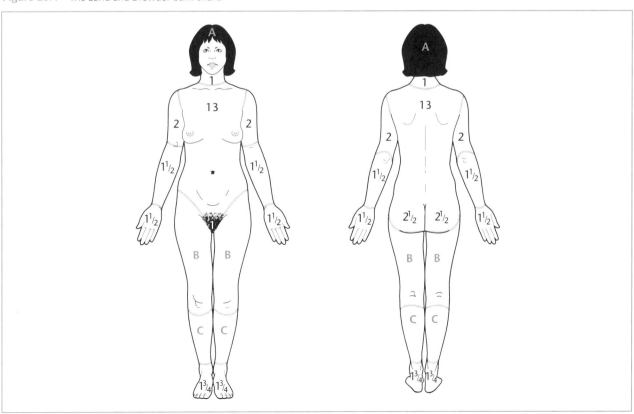

Kent 2001). The Rule of Nines, unlike the Lund and Browder chart, is useful for adult patients only and should not be used for children under the age of 15 years. The body is divided into areas, each of which represents 9% as follows:

The whole of the upper limb	9%
A thigh	9%
A leg (below the knee)	9%
The anterior chest	9%
The posterior chest	9%
The abdomen	9%
The lower half of the back (lumbar and sacral regions)	9%
The head and neck	9%
The perineum	1%

When neither of the above assessment charts is available, or when the injured area is relatively small, the palmar surface of the patient's hand can be used to approximate the extent of injury, as this has been identified as being equal to 1% of the patient's total body surface area (TBSA) (Fowler 1999). This assessment technique may also prove to be useful when the burnt areas are scattered over the patient's body.

The TBSA affected by the burn is very closely associated with the incidence of inhalation injury and mortality. According to Walsh and Kent (2001) a major burn requiring immediate IV resuscitation is defined as 15% or more TBSA in adults and as 10% or more TBSA in those either under 10 or over 50 years of age (only full- or partial-thickness burns are counted; see below). Burns of less than 10% TBSA in adults and 5% in children may be managed on an outpatient basis, but the patient may require hospitalization for social or medical reasons.

Depth

The depth of burn wound is primarily due to the *temperature* of the burning agent and the *duration* of contact or exposure. However, in assessing the wound accurately many factors have to be considered including heat source, mechanism of injury, the patient's age, the location of the burn and the wound characteristics. Burn depth is classified as superficial, superficial partial-thickness, deep partial-thickness (deep dermal) or full-thickness (Table 25.1). Superficial burns, such as those that result from sunburn and lead to simple erythema of the skin, are not generally taken into consideration when assessing the area of burns.

A *full-thickness* burn is characterized by the destruction of the full thickness of the skin and its appendages. Underlying tissues such as the subcutaneous fat, muscles, tendons and bone may also be burned. The skin's re-epithelializing cells are located throughout the dermis and along the dermal appendages, such as the shafts of the hair follicles and the sweat glands. Therefore, when the dermis is damaged, spontaneous regeneration and replacement of the skin is not possible. The area may be slowly filled in with granulation tissue and fibrous scar tissue, proliferated from marginal or underlying connective tissue. To avoid the contracture disability that occurs with the fibrous scar tissue, the area may be covered with a skin graft.

Table 25.1 Summary of burn characteristics

Depth	Tissues involved	Usual cause	Characteristics	Pain	Healing
Superificial	Epithelium Epidermis	Sunburn, cooking steam	Dry, no blisters, pink/red, blanches with pressure	Present	5 days approx. No obvious scarring
Superficial partial-thickness	Epidermis Minimal dermis	Flash flame, weak chemicals or hot liquid	Moist, pink or red mottled, blisters Some blanching	Very painful	10–21 days approx. Slight scarring May appear very red for approx. 6 weeks, then hypopigmented or hyperpigmented depending on amount of remaining intact melanocytes
Deep dermal partial thickness	Epidermis Dermis but epidermal-lined Sweat glands, hair follicles survive	Flame, hot liquids, solids	Few blisters, red with white patches	Sensitive to pressure	6 weeks or more Hypertrophic scarring Skin graft early to maximize healing and scar formation and to prevent contractures
Full thickness	As above plus subcutaneous fat and deeper tissues if chemical or electrical injury	Sustained flame, hot liquids or solids, chemicals, electricity	Leathery, cracked, avascular, pale white, brown or charred	Little pain	Cannot self-regenerate, skin grafts needed Scar will be influenced by genetic predisposition and grafting techniques used

After Burgess (1991).

Age

Very young children and adults aged over 50 years have higher mortality and morbidity rates associated with burn injury. The mortality rate increases sharply with advancing age; Wilmhurst (1992) has cited data showing that on average in the 5–34 years age group a 71% burn gives a 50% chance of survival, whilst for those aged over 75 years the area of burn associated with a 50% chance of survival falls to only 20%.

Pathophysiological effects of burns

A burn injury involving 10% TBSA in children and 15% TBSA in adults may significantly alter the body's cardiovascular function, the result of which is commonly called 'burn shock'. Patients with these types of injury require fluid replacement therapy – known as fluid resuscitation. The result of a significant burn injury is insufficient blood flow through the body to maintain adequate perfusion at the capillary level. This hypovolaemia is a result of both the fluid losses through the burn wound and the movement of intravascular fluid into the interstitial spaces due to the increased permeability and dilatation of the capillaries in the burnt area. The result of this shift of protein-rich fluid out of the vascular compartment leads to the formation of blisters and **oedema**. There is also a substantial loss of sodium associated with burn oedema. Large volumes of the fluid, which is similar in composition to plasma, may seep into the tissues. Some is carried away via the lymphatics, but they cannot usually cope with the total volume leading to an accumulation of fluid in the tissues. The loss of blood proteins with the fluid and the ensuing reduction in the intravascular colloidal osmotic pressure also promote oedema. As a consequence oedema also occurs in non-burned tissue, resulting in generalized oedema. **Oedema of the lungs** from this cause may be life threatening, even in the absence of any respiratory injury. In a full-thickness burn the fluid loss is extensive, and in areas of greater vascularization, such as the face, the oedema and swelling may be very severe.

In response to the massive inflammatory reaction postburn, there is an increased release of catecholamines. The intravascular volume is reduced, the blood pressure falls, the cardiac output may be decreased by as much as 30–50% (in burns greater than 40%, the decrease occurs within 15–30 minutes of the injury), and the blood flow through the tissues is reduced. **Hypovolaemic shock** develops rapidly unless there is adequate fluid replacement.

An 8–10% decrease in the number of red blood cells occurs, especially in deep burns, due to trapping and heat injury of the blood cells in the skin capillaries at the time of the injury. Often red cells, including transfused cells, may also be destroyed in the immediate postburn period; blood transfusion may be delayed for at least 48 hours. Normal red blood cell production may also be reduced because of depression of the bone marrow.

Inhalation of smoke and chemical fumes may seriously impair ventilatory function; irritation of the mucosa may cause laryngeal oedema and airway obstruction, or pulmonary oedema and severe respiratory insufficiency.

The urinary output is decreased as a result of the decreased intravascular volume and subsequent hypotension. If the blood supply is markedly reduced in the shock phase, renal tubular damage may also result. A reliable indicator of a good prognosis is the maintenance of **urine output** at a rate of at least 0.5 mL per kg per hour in adults. This indicates adequate renal perfusion. When there is massive red blood cell destruction, large quantities of haemoglobin are released. These blood pigments may block the renal tubules, causing renal shutdown. Another cause of **renal failure** in the burn-injured patient is the breakdown of protein from damaged tissue, especially muscle, and the release of these products (e.g. myoglobin) into the renal tubules.

The appearance of brownish-black urine indicates the presence of free haemoglobin and/or myoglobin; this is an ominous sign that requires urgent action to achieve diuresis.

In severe burns gastrointestinal peristalsis is depressed; **nausea**, **vomiting** and abdominal distension may occur. Haematemesis or melaena may develop, indicating the presence of stress ulcers.

Electrolyte imbalances develop because of the burn oedema, loss of fluid through the open wound, impaired renal function due to shock, and excessive release of potassium by the damaged tissue cells and erythrocytes. These disturbances are exacerbated by the release of aldosterone from the adrenal cortex in response to the renin–angiotensin pathway (see Ch. 19). This results in sodium and hence water retention by the kidneys (if they are functioning satisfactorily) and potassium excretion. The adrenocortical hyperactivity also accelerates protein catabolism, resulting in a negative nitrogen balance. Immunologically, after a major burn, the patient is compromised, which may have serious consequences, particularly for a patient with an established human immunodeficiency virus (HIV) infection. All burn wounds are colonized with bacteria. Once the bacterial counts become high and infectious organisms enter the lymphatic system, the patient may develop septicaemia. Sepsis is the largest single cause of death in burns patients (Ward 1992). Multisystem organ failure, often secondary to sepsis, is a serious and frequently fatal consequence of septicaemia.

The layer of burned tissues may form a dry, charred, coagulated surface, called an *eschar*, or a soft, moist non-coagulated area. **Inflammation** and oedema develop at the wound margins and below the layers of dead tissue. Many small blood vessels below the devitalized tissue may be thrombosed, promoting further cellular destruction. The decomposition of dead tissue and sloughing

Oedema
See chapter 4.2

Pulmonary oedema
See chapter 4.2

Shock
See chapter 4.2

Oliguria
See chapter 5.4

Acute renal failure
See chapter 5.4

Nausea and vomiting
See chapter 5.1

Inflammation
See chapter 6.1

produce a favourable culture medium for organisms and the development of serious infection.

Assessment

Assessment of the person with a burn injury is a collaborative function between the nurse and physician. A significant factor that has helped to reduce the mortality rate associated with major trauma, including burns, has been the introduction and implementation of protocols that are part of the Advanced Trauma Life Support (ATLS) course and other similar courses that are available for healthcare professionals throughout the world. The protocols identify three major stages of patient care. The first, known as the 'primary survey' is intended to find all the immediate life-threatening conditions and to initiate resuscitation of the same. The second, called the 'secondary survey', is undertaken immediately after the primary survey and its aim is to identify all the patient's injuries, no matter how trivial. Finally, the third stage of patient management is the stage of definitive care, for example when the patient goes to theatre, intensive care or the burns unit (Bradley and Collier 1994). In the ideal situation the burnt patient should initially be assessed in an appropriate environment, such as an A&E department or burns unit, in order that the assessor has the knowledge and ability to distinguish between pertinent issues relevant to either or both paediatric and adult patients.

Physical examination

An assessment of the ABCD of trauma management should follow as soon as possible after admission. Although an assessment of the individual's airway, breathing patterns, circulation and cervical spine immobilization will have been performed at the accident scene by paramedics, A&E staff must carry out such an assessment immediately the patient arrives in A&E. The patient should also be assessed for vital signs, pain, shock and concomitant injuries.

The potential for airway obstruction and an ineffective breathing pattern is a primary concern. The airway should be checked for patency, the patient's vital signs and level of consciousness monitored and recorded, and the presence or absence of inhalation injury determined. If the patient is experiencing respiratory distress, the nurse may play an important role in calming the individual and providing support while interventions take place to restore an adequate airway.

Signs and symptoms of smoke inhalation include burns to the head and neck, singed nasal hairs, darkened oral and nasal membranes, carbonaceous sputum, stridor, a history of being burned in an enclosed space, and exposure to flame. Following an assessment of the status of the cervical spine, a laryngoscope and/or fibreoptic bronchoscope may be inserted in the airway to determine the extent of any inhalation injury and subsequent risk of impaired **gas exchange**. The nurse can provide much

needed emotional support to the burned individual during these diagnostic tests.

Circulation to burned and unburned areas should also be assessed and noted. Altered tissue perfusion may occur with the oedema as a result of hypovolaemic shock and constriction of blood vessels in circumferential burns. If the nurse cannot feel the pulses, Doppler ultrasonography should be used to determine their presence or absence.

The previously mentioned severity factors of extent and depth of burn and the part of the body burned are included in the physical assessment.

After removal of all constricting items, such as jewellery, belts and remaining clothing, the burn wounds can be inspected more closely. The extent of the burn may be determined by filling in a Brund and Lowder form. This exercise should be performed by more than one person (e.g. doctor and nurse) to ensure accuracy. Hypovolaemic shock is likely if the extent of the burn is greater than 15% of the TBSA, making fluid replacement a top priority.

The depth of the burn may be determined using criteria such as those described in Table 25.3. It may take several days of ongoing assessment before an exact determination of depth can be made. Burns can also become deeper if the burning process continues, if infection develops and/or if the wound is allowed to dry out.

The location of the individual's burns needs to be assessed and noted (e.g. the face, hands, feet and perineum). These particular areas pose specific functional and aesthetic challenges that should be identified early postburn.

The burned individual's renal and gastrointestinal function also needs to be assessed. The nurse can pass a urinary catheter and assess the quantity and quality of the urine produced. Laboratory data such as a complete urinalysis and haemoglobinuria provide further objective information. Determining the presence or absence of bowel sounds, the insertion of a nasogastric tube and the assessment of gastric contents should also be performed by the nurse or the doctor.

The burned individual's pain level must be assessed continually and the request made for an analgesic and perhaps an anxiolytic to relieve pain and decrease anxiety. Initially analgesic therapy should be administered via the intravenous route to ensure the desired outcome.

Once the patient has been transferred or admitted to a burn treatment unit, physical parameters need to be monitored on a consistent basis to note changes in the patient's physical status.

Health history

As soon as it is appropriate, the nursing staff should introduce themselves to the patient or their family or other relatives. This will enable practitioners to collect data about the accident, past medical history, existence of any known allergies and medications the patient may be

Blood pressure measurement
See chapter 4.2

Glasgow coma scale
See chapter 2.2

Gas exchange
See chapter 5.3

currently taking as well as to answer any questions that the patient or family may have.

Psychosocial concerns and developmental factors

These include an assessment of the individual's age, sex, ethnic origin, cultural background, usual coping mechanisms and responses to stress, responses to previous hospitalizations or illnesses, and interactions between the patient, family and significant others. Other factors such as financial implications of the injury, acceptance (adaptation to altered body image), and changes in roles and responsibilities need to be assessed at a later date.

Patient and family knowledge

It is important to assess the patient's and family's perception of the burned individual's health status, potential for rapid and fluctuating changes in that status, the educational level, readiness and willingness to learn, ability to comprehend what is being said and potential for non-compliance with treatment.

While the physical examination is taking place, someone from the healthcare team should be providing the family or significant others with information and emotional support. The burned individual should also be made aware of what is, and will be, taking place during the hospitalization and that loved ones are being kept fully informed. To assist with this process, documentary and photographic material may be used over time to demonstrate the progress being made.

Health problems common to the person with a burn injury

Impaired skin and tissue integrity is the major health problem experienced by the individual in relation to the burn injury. The restoration of skin and tissue integrity is a major nursing concern. Much of what has been discussed in the previous sections of this chapter regarding this patient problem will apply to the individual with burns. Nursing care will be discussed in relation to the seven phases of recovery: *rescue, resuscitate, retrieve, resurface, reconstruct, rehabilitate* and *review*. Associated health problems common to persons with burns will be discussed in relation to each highlighted phase.

Rescue, resuscitate, retrieve and resurface phases

Care during these initial phases is directed towards ensuring that the individual receives prompt, knowledgeable and appropriate first aid and initial medical and nursing care to enhance their chances of survival. The following key points require urgent attention:

- The patient should have a patent airway.
- The patient's wounds must be protected.

- Further injury and contamination of wound(s) should not occur.
- The patient's pain should be controlled and relieved.
- Prescribed treatment for hypovolaemic shock needs to be implemented immediately.
- The patient should be able to talk about concerns and feelings of anxiety.
- The patient and family should be able to verbalize awareness of the patient's status and care.

Care during the rescue, resuscitate and retrieve period includes first aid at the site of the injury and the initial medical and nursing care. This initial care is directed toward establishing and maintaining an airway, if necessary, reversing hypovolaemic shock, and cleansing and assessing the severity of the burned areas. These phases may last for 2–7 days.

Nursing intervention

First aid

Initial steps to be taken at the accident scene are listed in Box 25.6.

The overall *aim* of burn first aid is to stop the burning process. With flame burns, the words 'Stop – Drop – Roll – Cool' apply. Running fans the flames and increases the severity of the injury. Immediate cooling of the burn wound is the next priority. Water is usually accessible. The burned area must be held or immersed under cool running water, or cool moistened towels or compresses can be applied. Burn blisters should be left untouched in the first aid situation as they help protect the wound from contamination. Cooling reduces pain and decreases the effect of

---

Box 25.6 First aid at the accident scene for the burned patient

1. Stop the burning process.

2. Maintain airway – resuscitation measures may be necessary.

3. Assess for other injuries.

4. Flush the burn with copious amounts of cold water, except for electrical injuries, facial burns and burns involving certain chemical agents such as metallic sodium, potassium and calcium, as these react violently with aqueous solutions (Fowler 1999).

5. Protect wounds from further trauma.

6. Provide emotional support – have someone remain with patient. Explain that assistance will be available.

7. Transport the patient to where medical care can be obtained.

heat transmission through the tissues. Ice is avoided because of the sudden vasoconstriction that it produces. Hypothermia is a potential complication which can be decreased by the use of sheets and then blankets over the patient and adjusting the temperature of the cooling agent.

Once the burning process has been stopped, the ABCs of burn trauma management become crucial.

Oils, ointments, lotions and other preparations *should not* be applied, and no attempt should be made to remove clothing that is adherent. The burn area is covered with a moist, sterile or clean material to exclude air (which stimulates pain) and to reduce contamination. Cling film is an excellent first aid dressing. Non-burned areas are covered with warm, dry covers. While awaiting transportation, the patient is kept at rest. A minimal amount of movement and handling is important.

In the case of chemical burns, the area is washed with generous amounts of water for at least 20 minutes or until the pain is lessened. The patient's clothing and any contact lenses are removed, because they may contain some of the chemical substance. Caregivers should also protect themselves from any residual chemical. Neutralizers are no longer indicated as they produce an undesirable thermal reaction with the acid or alkali.

The patient with severe burns is conscious unless other injuries interfere with awareness. Simple explanations of what is being done should be provided and repeated frequently. The presence of a nurse can be very supportive and helps to reduce the considerable amount of anxiety and fear experienced by the patient.

Most superficial burns involving approximately *less than* 10% of TBSA may be treated at home or in the review clinic attached to an A&E department, but only after a full and thorough initial assessment has been undertaken. Systemic effects in such cases are usually minimal and are not generally considered sufficiently significant to require hospitalization.

Outpatient management

It is essential that nursing staff ensure the patient will be able to manage at home before discharge from the A&E department is arranged. Attention should be paid to ensuring the wound is securely dressed and the patient has adequate analgesia. The patient should be encouraged to return to the department before their next appointment if they are worried about the state of their injury (Walsh and Kent 2001).

In certain circumstances non-debrided wounds may be managed on an outpatient basis; however, this decision will depend upon discussions between several members of the multidisciplinary team.

Treatment of the severely burned patient on admission

An immediate *assessment* of the patient's general condition is made before attention is directed to the burn

Oxygen therapy
See chapter 5.3

Box 25.7 Treatment of the severely burned patient on admission

1. Maintain an airway and administer oxygen if necessary.
2. Assess severity of injuries and degree of shock.
3. Initiate fluid replacement – establish an intravenous line.
4. Control pain.
5. Insert a nasogastric tube.
6. Insert an indwelling catheter.
7. Provide emotional support.
8. Provide initial wound care.
9. Initiate protective isolation measures.
10. Administer tetanus prophylaxis.

---

wound (Box 25.7). A history as to how the burn was sustained is obtained from the patient or the accompanying person; this may indicate the need to search for other injuries. The burn patient is usually sufficiently alert to provide information; if drowsy, confused or comatose, other disorders or injuries are suspected (e.g. hypoxia, head injury, cerebral aneurysm or stroke).

Potential for airway obstruction

Damage to the respiratory tract and respiratory insufficiency demands prompt attention. Respiratory impairment is frequently associated with burns of the face or neck, and may be the result of the inhalation of smoke, a gaseous chemical or flames. If an inhalation injury is suspected, 100% oxygen should be given through a non-rebreathing mask. This rule applies even when the patient is known to have chronic airways disease as adjustments can be made easily in the very small number of patients who deteriorate as a result of this action (Ferguson 1990). To assess ventilatory function, observe respiratory effects and listen for inspiratory wheezes, check odour of breath (a smoky or chemical odour may be detected which indicates inhalation of smoke or fumes), listen for hoarseness and examine any sputum for blood and carbon particles.

Humidified oxygen is generally administered and suctioning may be helpful to clear the airway of secretions. Intubation may be performed if respiratory embarrassment increases. If there is marked insufficiency, a mechanical ventilator may be used in conjunction with the endotracheal tube. Frequent estimations of the blood gases and expiratory or tidal volume may be done. In addition, a chest radiograph should be taken to establish baseline lung findings and ensure proper placement of invasive tubes and lines.

Respiratory insufficiency may develop later in circumferential or severe chest burns due to the firm, unyielding eschar that forms around the trunk preventing normal chest expansion and hence severely limiting lung ventilation. The doctor may have to make several incisions in the eschar to relieve the thoracic restriction. This is known as *escharotomy* and may also be performed wherever there is constriction and circumferential burns such as full-thickness limb burns to prevent neurovascular compromise from the tourniquet-like effect of the eschar. After the initial assessment and treatment, the patient is required to breathe deeply and to cough hourly to avoid the risk of chest infection.

When satisfactory ventilation is established, attention is directed toward fluid therapy and assessment of the extent and severity of the burn and any other injuries.

Hypovolaemic shock

The control of **shock** resulting from the loss of intravascular volume in a severe burn is dependent upon prompt, adequate fluid replacement. The extent and depth of burn and the patient's age and health status determine the need for fluid therapy. Burns greater than 15% of the total body surface area in adults require intravenous therapy. A reliable intravenous route is established by the insertion of two large intravenous catheters, preferably through unburned tissue. The intravascular fluid shift commences immediately after burning but signs of shock may not appear for a few hours. In the A&E department fluid replacement is based on ATLS guidelines which use crystalloids. Note that colloids should be used with caution in patients with inhalation injury and that the choice of a fluid resuscitation formula is based upon crystalloid or colloid depending upon the attending doctor's and the institution's burn care protocol. In the initial resuscitation stage a plasma substitute such as Haemaccel or Gelofusine may be used to expand the circulation but human albumin solution (4.5%) is needed subsequently to restore plasma volumes. Other fluids that may be used include Ringer's solution to correct electrolyte imbalances (particularly sodium) and fluid loss.

The volume, composition and rate of flow of the intravenous fluids are based on the percentage body surface burned, the weight of the patient, the hourly urinary output, arterial blood pressure, haematocrit and serum electrolyte concentrations, especially potassium and sodium. An adult may require as much as 500–1000 mL per hour intravenously to maintain a minimum acceptable urinary output of 30–60 mL per hour. Close monitoring and frequent adjustment of the intravenous flow rate is essential. If oral fluids are permitted, the amounts ingested are recorded accurately.

Generally, after the first 24–36 hours fluid extravasation into the tissues lessens and the intravascular volume tends to stabilize gradually. This physiological phenomenon of fluid remobilization signals the end of the emergent period of care. Nursing documentation of intake and output continues to be an essential part of the patient

assessment. The intravenous fluid therapy is gradually reduced and may be discontinued when laboratory studies indicate satisfactory concentrations, when the patient is able to take adequate amounts of fluid orally, or their urinary output has increased. Close observation is needed for signs of circulatory overload, because much of the fluid in the interstitial spaces is reabsorbed into the intravascular compartment as capillary integrity is re-established. Overloading of the circulatory system may be manifested by a urinary output greater than 100 mL per hour within the first 48 hours, pulmonary oedema, a central venous pressure in excess of 13 cmH$_2$O and a weak pulse. If renal function is satisfactory, the excessive amount is controlled by diuresis.

An indwelling catheter is passed as soon as the patient requiring fluid resuscitation therapy is admitted so that the hourly urinary output may be noted. This serves as a guide in determining intravenous fluid requirement and also provides information about the patient's general circulatory status and renal function (acute renal failure is possible after burn injury). A bolus of a diuretic with mannitol (100–200 mL i.v.) may be ordered in the immediate phase of care for electrical burns where there is a high incidence of haemoglobinuria and myoglobinuria. The catheter is removed as soon as the patient's condition is stable and shock is reversed, as the indwelling catheter predisposes to bladder infection and loss of bladder tone.

The patient is observed closely during the early post-burn period for signs of shock and continually to monitor their response to treatment – a nursing responsibility. The **blood pressure**, pulse and **level of consciousness** are noted every 15–30 minutes and the urinary output and quality is noted continually, documented hourly, or as the condition of the patient dictates. A diminishing intravascular volume and subsequent circulatory failure may be reflected by a fall in blood pressure, weak pulse, abnormal drowsiness, disorientation and a urinary output of less than 30 mL per hour.

Frequent haemoglobin and haematocrit determinations are made; abnormal increases indicate haemoconcentration due to loss of intravascular fluid into the tissues. After 6 or 7 days a deficiency of erythrocytes and haemoglobin may indicate the need for a blood transfusion. Blood transfusions may be given anyway if escharotomies have been performed. As a consequence of hypovolaemic shock, a nasogastric tube needs to be inserted to relieve gastric dilatation and the patient is given nothing by mouth until bowel sounds return. H$_2$ blockers such as ranitidine (to prevent peptic ulceration), antacids, and enteral or parenteral feeds may also be indicated. Serum protein and electrolyte concentrations are also determined frequently; these help in selecting the type of intravenous solutions required.

An accurate record of the fluid intake (oral and intravenous) and output is of paramount importance. The patient is weighed on a regular basis – usually on admission

Shock
See chapter 4.2

Blood pressure
measurement
See chapter 4.2

Glasgow coma scale
See chapter 2.2

and at the time of every dressing change (naked). A gain is manifested at first because of the increased extracellular fluid and the intravascular infusion. Then a marked weight loss accompanies the diuresis that corresponds with the recovery from shock. Much of the fluid that escaped into the interstitial spaces is reabsorbed into the blood vessels. During this period, the patient is observed for any signs of overhydration. If the intravenous infusion is continued at the previous rate of administration at this time the vascular system may become overloaded, placing an excessive demand on the heart and causing pulmonary oedema. The reabsorption of the tissue fluid can usually be recognized by a marked increase in the urinary output.

In summary, as well as the nursing responsibilities that have been outlined above, a successful patient outcome is also dependent upon how all the members of the multi-disciplinary team care for the severely burnt patient. For example, the anaesthetist and surgeons are responsible for the patient's airway, fluid management, and early excision of tissues and grafting. Rehabilitation starts from the time of admission; the physiotherapist is essential for maintaining passive limb movements and the occupational therapist is required to start making splints (to prevent contractures) as soon as the patient arrives. Both a minister of religion and a counsellor should be available to support the relatives of critically ill patients.

After this initial period of management the nurse must remain alert for an increase in temperature, rapid pulse, odour and discharge from the burned area, as this may indicate the onset or presence of infection.

The patient's position, especially that of the burned parts of the body, is checked frequently during the day and night for optimal alignment. Flexion contracture may develop very quickly and preclude restoration of function.

Pain
See chapter 2.3

Pain

Pain assessment is a highly individualized and subjective process. Analgesics are administered to decrease pain, and anxiolytics are used to decrease the emotional overtones of the trauma. Many burns units successfully use a pain-control regimen based on continual opiate infusion, delivered by one of the many regulating devices now available. Patient-controlled analgesia (PCA) devices, although encouraged as soon as the patient is able to understand the principles of administration, are usually reserved for use in the later stages of management and postgrafting stage. The intravenous route is always preferred because the circulatory disturbances and oedema previously discussed reduce absorption via alternative routes.

Pain assessment and intervention are ongoing, varying from patient to patient and from day to day in the same patient. The patient's subjective response is the best indicator of the efficacy of a chosen strategy. The nurse's role in pain assessment and management is even more crucial when the patient is ventilated and/or comatose or confused. Particular attention must be paid to providing pain relief while changing dressings, and the use of Entonox gas is recommended. For more information on pain management, see Chapter 7.

Anxiety

Following a severe burn, the patient and family experience considerable emotional disturbance. As with any severe stress, the reactions and adaptive mechanisms may vary markedly from one person to another, depending mainly on the particular situation and past experiences of each person. Factors that generate fear and anxiety in both the patient and family include the actual threat to life, permanent incapacity and disfigurement, the prolonged period of treatment necessitating dependence as well as separation, and the uncertain future. Feelings of guilt may be lurking near the surface, particularly in the parents of a child who has suffered burn injury. A sensitive approach by the nurse is therefore essential.

The nurse should encourage the patient and family to discuss their concerns and fears. It is important that they are kept informed of all activities and why certain procedures and actions are being carried out. Repetition of information is necessary as the patient and family will be anxious and experiencing varied and rapidly changing phenomena, over which they perceive minimal, if any, control. Questions such as 'Will I be scarred for life?' should be given the honest answer 'Yes – but we cannot predict to what extent or how you will eventually look', and the patient should be encouraged to express fears and anxieties as the nurse explores the patient's self-concept.

Wound care

The aim of wound care in burns is to:

- maintain a clean, moist wound environment
- promote patient comfort
- offer protection from infection or further trauma
- facilitate optimal activity and function (Fowler 1999).

Before a dressing is applied, burned areas must be gently but thoroughly cleansed with warmed sterile normal saline solution, sterile water or warmed tap water dependent upon local policy. Burned tissue (eschar) may be removed (debrided) carefully, with sterile scissors and forceps, in order to reveal the presence of healthy tissue, and burn blisters may or may not be deroofed again according to local policy. An example of a dressing guide is shown in Table 25.2. Following a minor burn, the patient should return to the outpatient department or clinic to have the dressing(s) changed every 3–4 days, or more frequently if it is disrupted or if breakthrough

Table 25.2   Dressing minor burn wounds

Layer of dressing	Rationale
Flamazine cream (silver sulfadiazene)	Antibacterial cream prevents infection of wound
Non-adherent dressing pads (e.g. Melolin, Release) are usually used over skin grafts (ideally not as a primary contact layer) *or* wound contact material such as Mepitel	Prevents damage to new tissue when dressing removed. Makes dressing changes less painful
Thick gauze pad	Absorbs wound exudates
Tubular bandage for limb(s) (e.g. Tubigrip or Tubifast); may be supplemented by traditional crêpe bandages	Holds dressing securely in place

The choice of subsequent dressing materials should be based on the characteristics of the dressing and Turner's criteria as previously discussed.

drainage occurs. With facial burns appropriate wound care may need to be performed two or three times a day.

Evaluation of the person following these initial phases of management

The care provided to the person with a severe burn injury during these initial phases is multifaceted and should demonstrate collaboration among first aid workers, paramedics, nurses in A&E and special burns units, doctors, physiotherapists and other health professionals.

The criteria listed in Box 25.8 may be used to evaluate the effectiveness of nursing care during this 'immediate' phase.

Resurface and reconstruct phases

Sepsis is the principal cause of death in patients who die from burn injuries. *Pneumonia* and *cardiovascular, respiratory, gastrointestinal* and *renal system failures* are the other main causes of death. Complications tend to be the rule rather than the exception for individuals with severe burns. Experience of patients with burn injuries indicates the need to take a proactive approach to their care to try to prevent complications.

There are two primary patient *goals* in the intermediate phase for individuals with burns: (1) healing and closure of the burn wound; and (2) coping with physical and psychosocial complications that cannot be avoided. Through effective management of the first goal, many of the complications can be avoided or kept to a minimum.

The success of care can be measured using the criteria listed in Box 25.9.

Nursing intervention

Infection risk

It is important to remember that nearly all burns patients wounds will be colonized (presence of organisms without an associated host reaction); however, the presence of

---

Box 25.8   Criteria used to evaluate the effectiveness of nursing care during the initial four phases of recovery from burn injury

1. The patient's airway is patent.

2. The patient's breathing pattern is effective.

3. Fluid balance is being maintained.

4. Initial wound assessment has been completed.

5. Initial wound care protocols have been initiated.

6. Pain and discomfort are controlled.

7. The patient and family are able to describe what has happened and the patient's status and progress.

8. The patient and family acknowledge receiving emotional support relevant to the emergency situation.

---

infection (presence of organisms with an associated host reaction) may be reduced by the use of several measures. Avoiding or minimizing **infection** involves appropriate use of topical antimicrobial agents, primarily silver sulfadiazine (Flamazine), support for the patient's immune mechanisms, rapid elimination of reservoirs for potential infection and prevention of the transfer of infection.

Fresh frozen plasma may be administered to support the patient's weakened immune system. Strict, aseptic technique is used when inserting invasive lines and when applying sterile dressings. If the patient has dressings in place, standard infection control measures and protective isolation will be undertaken when the patient is first admitted. Infection control measures also focus on the safe handling of all body substances and fluids as potential sources of infection.

Everything in the patient's room is considered a source of contamination to him or her. Hospital personnel serve

Infection
See chapter 6.1

Wonld healing
See chapter 6.1

as potential vectors in the transmission of organisms between patients. The nurse wears a protective isolation gown when rendering physical care to the patient. The importance of handwashing guidelines and strict adherence to them must be stressed.

Septicaemia can develop at any stage until complete wound coverage is achieved. It may have a sudden onset, with rigors and a rapid increase in temperature, or it may develop gradually over 2–3 days. Septicaemia is characterized by high fever that may fluctuate, rapid pulse, drowsiness and disorientation. Paralytic ileus is a common concomitant. Oozing from the burn wounds or the appearance of purulent exudate or petechiae require wound swabs for microbiology. Blood cultures are necessary for a definitive diagnosis. *Staphylococcus aureus*, haemolytic streptococcus and *Pseudomonas aeruginosa* are common causes of septicaemia.

Nursing interventions for the patient whose wound(s) has shown organisms on culture and is at risk for or has become septic include: careful and continuous monitoring for the early signs of impending sepsis; the administration of antibiotics; assistance with the insertion of invasive lines for more sophisticated diagnostic monitoring; and scrupulous wound and skin care. If a patient does develop a resistant organism, strict isolation procedures are implemented and enforced at all times. Regardless of the type of isolation employed, however,

the most definitive answer to the problem of infection and resultant complications due to burns lies with coverage of the burn wound.

Wound healing and skin grafts

Various forms of local treatment are used to prevent further wound contamination and tissue destruction, to suppress the growth of bacteria in the area, and to promote separation of the devitalized tissue and its replacement with skin. Initially, the burn is cleansed of dirt, foreign substances and detached epithelium, using non-filamented gauze and a mild soapy solution, water or normal saline. Loose, sloughing skin and debris are removed with sterile forceps and the skin may be removed from blisters. The cleansing must be *very gentle* to avoid damage of exposed viable tissue and the area is rinsed with generous amounts of water or saline.

Burn wounds are generally treated using either the open method or the closed method. In the *open method*, used almost exclusively for the management of facial burns, the wound remains exposed. A thin layer (2–4 mm) of topical antimicrobial ointment may be applied over the wound surface. The exposure results in drying and the formation of a protective coagulum of serum. A cradle is used over the patient to support a sterile sheet and blanket to reduce body heat loss. If infection develops under the coagulum, it is removed and baths and topical antimicrobials used.

With the *closed method*, a dressing may be left intact for 1–7 days. The burned areas may be covered with a topical antimicrobial preparation and non-adherent dressing. The topical applications commonly used include silver sulfadiazine (Flamazine) or povidone–iodine (Betadine). The choice and frequency of dressing varies among institutions, and also according to the condition of the burn wound. Flexibility with the wound management approach is very important in burn care (Box 25.10).

If a patient has a circumferential burn on a limb, close observations are made for signs of interference with the circulation as a result of the constricting effect of the dry, shrinking eschar. If signs of constriction appear, the eschar is surgically divided immediately under aseptic conditions (escharotomy). If the wound is deep enough, fasciotomies may also be performed.

Choice of dressings used will be dependent upon assessment of the burn and a multidisciplinary protocol that should highlight wound management materials to be considered including the rationale for their use. Considerations should include those that promote a moist wound healing environment, optimize the patient's healing potential, alleviate pain, enhance debridement, permit immobilization or mobilization (as desired at the time), preserve function and provide the patient with the least amount of psychological stress.

In a partial-thickness burn, healing (i.e. re-epithelialization) occurs under the coagulum, which gradually separates. When a full-thickness burn is sustained, the non-viable tissue changes in 3–5 days to a hard, tough black layer (eschar). The eschar eventually sloughs off, liquefies and detaches from the viable tissue. There may be considerable drainage before there is complete separation. The wound will not granulate until the eschar has been sloughed off, so treatment in wound care is directed towards the promotion of this process. Alternatively, the wound may be debrided surgically. As the eschar is removed (by slough or debridement) granulation tissue consisting of fibroblasts and capillaries is gradually formed. If the granulation tissue is allowed to mature to fibrous scar tissue, the natural shortening of the collagenous fibres results in contracture of the area and possible deformity or loss of function, depending upon the location. Some marginal growth of epithelium may take place but, unless the burn is very small, this is usually insignificant.

Wounds that are full thickness in nature do not have the capacity for self-healing. These patients have their wounds surgically excised and *skin grafts* placed to provide permanent coverage. The patient's general condition and the size of the burn area determine whether the grafting will require several stages. Priority is given to areas where scarring and contraction produce loss of movement and marked deformity. The grafts may be laid or sutured or stapled, depending on their thickness. They are dressed with a pressure dressing or may be left exposed. If the grafts are around or over a joint surface, a splint or plaster cast may be applied to immobilize the part.

Split-thickness grafts may also be applied to deep partial-thickness burns as they produce a much better scar with improved wear and tear tolerance.

The only graft that is permanent is the *autograft*. As the name implies, the skin is taken from an unburned part of the patient's body (the *donor site*) and placed over the debrided granulation tissue. No tissue rejection is experienced but 100% graft take is not guaranteed with every procedure. If there are not sufficient donor sites available, a temporary skin covering may be used.

Temporary synthetic dressings are available when it is necessary to gain time for the patient awaiting further grafting. Such products include Tegaderm and Opsite.

During the past decade, selected patients with major burns and with no available donor sites have been managed with autologous epidermal skin cultures or a bilayer 'artificial' skin covering with dermal components. In addition, cadaver skin and skin substitutes such as Integra are becoming more widely available and accepted, offering further hope for future burn survivors.

Donor sites are usually covered with a protective inner dressing at operation. After one to several days following surgery, depending on the unit protocol, the outer dressings are removed and the wound redressed once daily. Great care must be taken with donor sites because they increase the open body surface area and put the patient at greater risk of infection. The donor sites can be reharvested in about 10 days, once they have healed, providing the patient with the opportunity to have several grafts taken from the same place. Donor sites can be very painful wounds.

Patient teaching related to skin grafts

The nurse who is involved in all stages of wound healing plays a very important role with respect to patient and family teaching and support around this crucial aspect of burn care, as do other members of the multidisciplinary team. When the patient learns that skin grafts are needed, he or she may become apprehensive or have unrealistic expectations regarding graft 'take' and the final appearance. Initially the nurse may re-emphasize what the surgeon tells the patient, with the physiotherapist and occupational therapist also discussing grafts. This support and teaching continue until the wound and scars have fully matured, which may take several years.

Oedema
See chapter 4.2

Positioning and exercises

The patient is generally turned every 2–3 hours to prevent respiratory congestion and circulatory stasis. If the back is burned, care is facilitated if the patient is nursed on an alternating pressure, low air loss or air-fluidized patient support system, dependent upon the acceptance of the bed to the patient. Because of the **oedema**, burned extremities are elevated on pillows or other form of support during the initial phase. Frequent attention is paid to body alignment; flexion contractures, outward rotation of thighs and footdrop must be prevented.

Splints may be applied for immobilization to promote healing and to prevent contracture and deformity. The splint used must fit the contour of the part to which it is applied and be secured well enough to provide stability but not cause pressure or interfere with circulation.

Burned parts that involve joints are moved through their range of motion as soon as possible. Early skin grafting permits the patient to be mobile earlier and prevents contractures. The patient in a bath is encouraged to exercise while soaking. As healing occurs, the activity programme is progressively increased to preserve normal range of motion and function.

Nutrition

In addition to fluid therapy, nutrition plays an important role in the recovery of the burned patient. In the initial shock period in severe burns intravenous fluids mainly sustain the patient. Intravenous fluids such as dextrose are given to sustain metabolic water demands in addition to fluid resuscitation, and then this will be titrated against the enteral and dextrose input. The initial hypovolaemic **shock** produces depression of gastric motility. Once oral fluid intake can be resumed it is progressively increased through soft foods, to a full normal diet.

The patient develops a negative nitrogen balance as a result of tissue catabolism which increases susceptibility to infection and debilitation and delays healing. A high-calorie, high-protein and high-vitamin diet is recommended to provide the essentials for tissue repair and the production of antibodies and blood cells.

Supplements of protein concentrates may be added to fluids or given through a fine-bore nasogastric tube. Adequate assistance should be provided so that taking meals does not require too great an effort for the patient. A close check is made of their daily intake and their weight should also be recorded regularly.

Evaluation

Shock
See chapter 4.2

After the initial and intermediate periods of care following a severe burn injury, the criteria outlined in Boxes 25.9 & 25.10 may be used to evaluate care. During this intermediate period of care, the nurse assumes both independent and collaborative responsibilities for the assessment and management of the patient's wounds, for the identification of patient and family concerns and anxieties, and for teaching the patient and family about the wound and overall plan of care.

Rehabilitation and review phases

Rehabilitation of the burned patient is fostered throughout by means of positive communication with the patient and their family, in order to prepare them for the resumption of their lives, and through the earlier stages by conscientious attention to good body alignment, the prevention of infection and contractures, and the maintenance of joint and limb mobility as much as possible. After recovery from the burn, considerable reconstructive surgery and retraining may be required before the patient can resume independent and self-supportive functioning. Rehabilitation is a lengthy process for many, and they and their families may require social guidance and financial assistance as well as psychological support throughout. Retraining for a different occupation may be necessary. In some instances the patient finds it very difficult to resume social contacts and to take his or her place in society because of scarring and gross disfigurement.

The *goals* for the person are: (1) to achieve maximum function and optimal reconstruction, and (2) to achieve

> **Box 25.11**   Criteria for evaluation of care during rehabilitative and review phases
>
> - Absence of infection
> - Intact skin
> - Range of movement exercises and functional movement in involved joints
> - A plan to continue the prescribed exercise programme
> - A diet plan to obtain adequate protein, vitamins, minerals and calories
> - Understanding of prescribed skin care routine
> - Independence in personal care
> - Return to social activities
> - Return to employment or plans for job retraining
> - Plans for continuing health care.

an acceptable quality of life. The achievement of these goals may be measured by the criteria outlined in Box 25.11.

Nursing intervention

Skin and tissue integrity

Healed burns must be kept well moisturized because the sebaceous glands are unable to secrete sufficient lubricating oils. Frequent applications of mild, non-perfumed, water-based moisturizers are recommended; oil-based lotions may block pores and do not penetrate into the dermis. When out in the sun, the patient must be reminded to wear sunblock and clothing/hat to prevent sunburn and hyperpigmentation.

All wounds heal by the process of contraction. Burn patients must be made aware of the possibility that the splints and other corrective devices they may have been utilizing since the day of admission (in essence, day 1 is when rehabilitation begins) may not bring about a miraculous or 'good as new' result. Further corrective surgery may be needed to release the contracture and insert a skin graft.

Hypertrophic scarring is another result of healing from a burn injury. Some individuals have a greater propensity for scarring than others. The burns team may frequently be unable to give definite answers regarding the need or duration of use of pressure garments or devices for pressure therapy. Counselling should also include information on skin care and cosmetic camouflage. Further surgery may be necessary for these patients, but in the future – for it takes approximately 2 years for the pressure to exert its maximal effect and for the burn scar to mature fully. It is important that, when counselling these patients, the nurse emphasizes that these timeframes are estimations and that every patient responds to therapy in a unique manner. A good rule is to be cautiously optimistic, to repeat a number of times and to document what the patient and family have been told.

Compliance with positioning and exercises may be a difficult challenge for the burn survivor. Patient education and support from burns team members can be very helpful in meeting these challenges in a positive manner. In addition, the patient is encouraged to undertake more responsibility for self-care. The occupational therapist and nursing staff need to encourage the patient to perform self-care activities, such as personal hygiene, dressing and participating in recreational activities. In order not to lose valuable function, rehabilitation activities must be attended to with much energy by all concerned.

Changes in coping mechanisms

As the burned individual prepares to leave the protective environment of the burns unit, numerous feelings may be experienced. The nursing staff, who have formed a unique and trusting bond with surviving patients and families, should be sensitive to and encourage the need for the patient to verbalize concerns and questions. The burned person may experience feelings of uncertainty, fear and anxiety about what lies ahead. This is linked to decreased confidence due to lengthy dependence on hospital staff, impaired physical mobility and learning to re-enter society, potentially with an altered body image and decreased sense of self-esteem. Nervousness about returning home after a prolonged absence and concerns about resumption of previous roles and responsibilities may also be experienced.

It is important to make the person aware that these concerns are very normal for the burn survivor at the same stage of recovery. Knowing that one is not alone can be very comforting. Introduction to previously discharged patients and members of a burns support group, if available, can be a helpful pre-discharge strategy.

Family members generally experience anxiety because they are now assuming the caretaker role once held by burns team members. They may have many questions about their loved one's physical care and emotional readjustment. They may express concerns about how to support the burned individual emotionally as he or she adjusts to being at home, re-enters society and begins to socialize with friends and be seen in the community by strangers and contemplates what the future may bring. Families may have concerns about their own reactions to the burn survivor and should receive support and advice in this regard. Both the patient and family members will experience challenges upon the return home. Coping strategies must either be developed or previous positive strategies reinforced and applied to this particular situation.

A comprehensive discharge teaching programme should begin as soon as possible before discharge.

Important topics to discuss include skin care, emotional reactions to returning home, adjusting to alterations in appearance and mobility, coping with discomfort (itchiness and pain), nutrition, rehabilitation needs, family readjustment, and continuity of care (i.e. home care, burns clinic and rehabilitation department visits). The information conveyed and the opportunity to talk with nursing staff and other burns team members are both valuable means to support individual and family coping.

Both the individual and the family need to know that nursing staff are anxious to provide support, answer questions, assist in problem solving and conflict resolution, and offer a reassuring pat on the back for the courage and perseverance displayed during a very traumatic time. This supportive and informative presence can do much to assist in the individual's efforts at reaching the optimal level of physical and emotional recovery; in other words, establishing a 'new normal' pattern of living, incorporating the adaptations necessitated by the burn injury with positive activities from the past.

Evaluation

Box 25.11 contains the key criteria that may be used to evaluate care in this final phase of treatment.

Summary

In recent years a better understanding and delivery of nutritional support, anaesthesia, the provision of enhanced intensive care facilities and skin replacements have all contributed to improved outcomes for patients who suffer from burns injuries, whether major or minor. None the less, the importance of evidence-based nursing interventions cannot be stressed enough. Burns nursing is one of the few specialties where practitioners have the opportunity to nurse a patient from the critical stage of their hospital admission, through the continuing care and rehabilitation phases of management up until the patient's discharge home.

General skin conditions

Promotion and maintenance of healthy skin

Issues that should be addressed concerning the promotion and maintenance of healthy skin include the following.

Cleansing Obviously this is essential for healthy skin. There are a number of products available to care for the wide variety of skin types – dry, normal, oily, combination. Cleanliness is the first step in achieving and maintaining healthy skin.

Moisturizing The skin can become dry due to moisture loss through the use of inappropriate cleansing agents, illness, trauma or exposure to sun, wind, pollution and hot water. Patients should be advised to use water-based moisturizers to replenish that which has been lost and for the maintenance of healthy, intact skin, which is the body's primary barrier against infection.

Noting changes in the skin's appearance Nurses should teach the individual to look for any changes in colour, texture or appearance of the skin and changes in moles or other skin lesions. If changes are noted, the person should consult a healthcare professional immediately.

Avoiding exposure to ultraviolet radiation People are becoming increasingly aware of the dangers associated with exposing the skin to the sun and other sources of ultraviolet radiation (e.g. tanning lamps and beds). The increasing incidence of skin cancer is a cause for alarm, and individuals, health professionals and manufacturers alike are advocating the education of consumers regarding the use of protective practices. These include the use of sunscreens and blocks, decreased time in the sun and the wearing of protective clothing, such as a wide-brimmed hat and a shirt.

In the UK the incidence of malignant melanoma of the skin increased by 6% per annum between 1979 and 1986, and this rate of increase has accelerated since 1986 so much so that, by 1994, the incidence had almost doubled from 1979 levels. There is a proportionately greater increase amongst males and those aged 20–39 years. There is therefore a need for urgent health education about the dangers of overexposure to direct sunlight, particularly amongst young males.

Diet Good nutrition is an essential component in the promotion and maintenance of healthy skin.

Annual physical examinations To encourage healthy patterns of skin care and to detect any changes that may have gone unnoticed by the individual, the nurse should advise each person to visit their practice nurse or nurse practitioner to have an annual examination. This also provides an excellent opportunity for general health education about a range of issues.

Skin assessment
See chapter 6.1

Assessment

Health history

Skin problems cannot be examined 'in isolation'; information about the patient's total health may reveal very significant diagnostic factors and influence the therapeutic plan. Although skin disorders may present with a striking appearance, it is important to obtain a good history before examining the patient (Walsh et al 1999). In taking the patient's health history, particular attention is given to eliciting information about:

- any previous skin disorders, their nature, the patient's age, the season of the year at which they occurred and the treatment

- any known allergy or drug reactions

- drugs being taken, and for what reason

- known food(s), fluid(s) or contact substances (e.g. soap, certain material) that worsen the condition

- substances that are brought in contact with the skin throughout daily activities (e.g. cosmetics, chemicals at work)

- dietary habits

- recreational customs (including use of tobacco, alcohol and other drugs) or hobbies

- family history, especially in relation to skin disorders, allergy and systemic disease

- emotional stress resulting from job, interpersonal relations and other situations are identified. Stress and anxiety may influence the severity of skin disorders and the patient's responses to treatment.

Walsh et al (1999) have shown how the PQRST tool (see p. 258) may be used for symptom analysis in skin disorders:

- *provocation and palliation* – what brings on, exacerbates or relieves the problem?

- *quality* – the appearance of the skin lesions, sensation (itching, sore, etc.), bleeding, discharge, etc.

- *region and radiation* – the area affected and whether this has spread

- *severity* – this should include changes in the severity of skin lesions and how they affect the person's life

- *time* – how long the patient has had the problem and whether it varies over time.

Physical examination

The history taking is followed by an examination of the skin. This involves touching, feeling and observing the person's skin. A good light and warm room are essential and the skin must be clean. Care is taken to prevent unnecessary exposure of the patient and to respect dignity by closing curtains or doors and protecting the patient with a gown or sheet.

A general **survey of the skin** is undertaken noting *colour* (redness, pallor, cyanosis, yellowness or brownness), *vascularity* (any evidence of bruising or bleeding), *moisture* (dryness, sweating, oiliness), *temperature, texture* (roughness and smoothness), *thickness* and *turgor* (the rate at which the skin returns into place when a section is pinched and lifted).

Lesions are inspected and the nature of the lesion is established and its characteristics recorded according to size, shape, colour and whether it has a dry or wet surface. It should be noted if an odour is associated with the affected areas. The entire skin surface of the body is examined to determine the general condition of the total skin in addition to the distribution and grouping of the affected areas. The latter is of assistance in diagnosis as certain disorders are known to develop more commonly in certain areas. For example, acne, impetigo, contact dermatitis, herpes simplex and discoid lupus erythematosus develop most commonly on the face. The oral mucosa is usually included in an examination of the entire skin. The fingernails and toenails are observed and palpated for colour, shape and the presence of lesions. The quantity, texture and distribution of hair is also noted. A more advanced account of the examination of the skin may be found in Walsh et al (1999).

Diagnostic tests

The diagnosis of many skin lesions can be made through a process of physical examination and history taking. If the lesions are moist or discharging, a swab of the exudate may be obtained for culture. If the affected areas are dry or scaly, scrapings may be taken for cytological examination and/or culture. Other laboratory tests may be done, such as leucocyte and thrombocyte counts, examination for the lupus erythematosus (LE) cell, anti-D test for systemic lupus erythematosus (SLE) and **erythrocyte sedimentation rate** determination. A biopsy of a lesion may be done if malignancy is suspected or if the lesion is long-standing and obscure in nature. If the condition is dermatitis, patch intracutaneous (prick) tests may be done during a remission to identify the allergen or substance to which the person is sensitive. The substances are either administered intracutaneously or applied to the skin on the back and observed at intervals over 48 hours. If positive, the reaction is manifested by inflammation and papules or vesicles.

Although the skin lesions prompted the patient to seek medical assistance, the disorder may have internal or systemic components. This may necessitate other investigative procedures, such as urinalysis, radiography, pulmonary function tests or further blood studies.

Risk factors

Health problems involving the skin are related to the presence of one or more risk factors:

1. *Internal factors* – alterations in nutrition, metabolism, circulation, sensation, immune system, mental status, skin turgor, pigmentation, body fat and moisture, thickness and texture of the skin, the presence of infection, and actions of medications

2. *External or environmental factors* – mechanical forces including pressure and shearing, chemical substances, radiation, temperature extremes, moisture and physical immobilization

3. *Systemic disorders* such as:
   a. malnutrition (e.g. nutritional deficiency, obesity)
   b. metabolic disorder (e.g. **diabetes** mellitus, hypothyroidism or hyperthyroidism)

c. cardiovascular disease

d. neurological disorders that impair sensation and cause immobility (e.g. **cerebral haemorrhage**, brain tumour, spinal cord injury, multiple sclerosis)

e. severe infection and **fever**

f. debilitation (such as occurs in cancer and anaemia).

4. *Skin characteristics*:
   a. thickness and texture of the skin vary in different areas of the body and are influenced by the person's genetic code and age
   b. turgor – dehydration and **oedema** reduce the resistance of the skin.

5. *Age* – the **older person's** skin is drier, less elastic and less turgid, predisposing it to breakdown when subjected to pressure or other mechanical forces or irritants.

Manifestations of skin disorder

Lesions

Various changes in areas of the skin may occur, and the exact nature of these is important in diagnosis and treatment.

Primary lesions

Characteristic primary lesions in which the skin is usually intact include the following (Peters and Watts 1998):

■ *erythema* – an area in which the blood vessels become dilated, causing redness, warmth and increased tension of the skin

■ *macule* – a flat non-palpable lesion less than 1 cm in diameter

■ *papule* – a small elevated macule that may or may not be discoloured.

■ *vesicle* – an elevated area that contains clear serous fluid

■ *pustule* – similar to a vesicle, elevated and superficial but filled with purulent fluid

■ *nodule* – an elevated firm palpable lesion, more than 0.5 cm in diameter and extending deeper into the dermis than a papule

■ *wheal* – a localized, elevated, irregularly shaped area of cutaneous oedema, which is red at the margins with a blanched centre

■ *bulla* – an elevation larger than 1 cm of superficial skin layers containing serous or purulent fluid

■ *comedo (blackhead)* – a plug of sebum and keratin within a hair follicle

Erythrocyte sedimentation rate
See chapter 4.1

Diabetes
See chapter 2.6

Cerebrovascular accident
See chapter 2.2

Fever
See chapter 6.1

Oedema
See chapter 4.2

Ageing
See chapter 6.1

- *telangiectasia* – a lesion composed of a group of small blood vessels that are abnormally dilated

- *plaque* – a patch on the skin or mucous membrane.

Secondary lesions

These develop as a result of a break in the skin and destruction of cells. They include:

- *crust (scab)* – a rough, dry area formed by the coagulation and drying of plasma and exudate over a primary lesion

- *scales* – thin, flat, minute plates of dried epidermal cells that have not completely undergone the normal keratinization process before being separated. Desquamation is the term that refers to the separation of scales or patches of cells

- *fissure* – a split or crack in the surface, extending through the epidermal layers and possibly into the dermis. If it extends into the dermis, bleeding occurs. This type of lesion is most likely to occur in a natural skin or surface crease such as those located over knuckles, at the angles of the mouth, in the groin, between the buttocks and behind the ears

- *erosion (excoriation)* – loss of the epidermis producing a superficial, reddened, weeping lesion as a result of trauma or the prolonged presence of 'toxins' on the skin

- *ulcer* – a denuded area of irregular size and shape extending into the dermis or subcutaneous tissue from, or to, the epidermis due to necrosis of superficial tissue

- *lichenification* – thickening and hardening of skin as a result of continued irritation

- *atrophy* – the skin is thin and wrinkled, resembling tissue paper. Atrophy is seen with ageing

- *corn, callus* – an excessive thickness of the epidermis caused by chronic pressure and/or friction. In the case of a corn, the hyperkeratosis is sharply circumscribed

- *leucoplakia* – a white plaque seen most commonly on the lips or mucous membranes of the oral cavity or tongue. About 10% of patients subsequently develop carcinoma in the lesions

- *scar* – an area of fibrous tissue replacing tissue destroyed by trauma or disease

- *hypertrophic scars* – Normally a scar becomes paler and flatter as it matures. Hypertrophic scars become increasingly raised, red and itchy for several months after injury, due to excessive formation of fibrous tissue within the scar. The scar is then classified as hypertrophic. Over the next few years these scars usually flatten and lose their vascularity, thus becoming paler. The hypertrophy is confined to the site of injury. If these scars are excised there is some tendency for the hypertrophy to recur. It may be very difficult to determine whether a scar is hypertrophic or keloid (see below)

- *keloids* – Histologically keloids are similar to hypertrophic scars, but keloids behave differently. Fibrous tissue formation is sometimes so excessive that the keloid has the appearance of a tumour, and the initial injury producing the keloid may be so small as to appear insignificant, for example ear piercing or an insect bite. Unlike hypertrophic scars, the keloid extends into surrounding uninjured skin and persists for many years. There is a high tendency for recurrence after excision. The incidence of keloid is highest in negroid skins. It appears that tension within a scar encourages hypertrophy and keloid formation; therefore, redistribution of the tension by use of elastic pressure garments usually produces some improvement in scar quality.

Pruritus

Generalized or localized itching is a common complaint in skin disorders. It may be associated with an internal disorder, such as diabetes mellitus or obstructive jaundice. Excessive dryness due to overbathing, a dry atmosphere and the ageing process can also cause pruritus. Emotional distress may play an important role in the development and control of this disturbing symptom. The patient is hard-pressed to refrain from scratching, which further irritates the area and is frequently responsible for fissures, abrasions and subsequent secondary infection.

Urticaria

Urticaria is a skin disorder characterized by itching wheals of varying size, which may develop rapidly and become widespread. The reaction consists of dilatation and increased permeability of the capillaries and arteriolar dilatation. The combination of these is referred to as the **triple response**.

A severe and possibly life-threatening form of the disorder is known as angioneurotic oedema of the skin and mucous membranes. The lesions frequently disappear in a few hours when the blood vessels return to normal. General malaise and fever may also develop if the urticaria is widespread. The most common cause of angioneurotic oedema is a severe allergic reaction to a drug, food or insect bite.

Pain

The pain associated with skin lesions may be described as prickly or burning. Chemical, mechanical or pressure irritation of the cutaneous sensory nerves, actual cellular damage or exposure of the nerve endings due to tissue destruction and erosion may cause it.

Triple response
See chapter 6.1

Redness

Erythema or redness of the skin indicates vasodilatation and hyperaemia in the area. Erythematous lesions are initially macular but frequently become papular because of the oedema or developing exudate in the affected tissues.

Swelling

A puffy swollen area of the skin is usually due to localized oedema, resulting from increased permeability of the capillaries, or to localized inflammatory reaction.

Systemic disturbances

The skin reflects the individual's general physical and emotional status. Skin lesions are frequently manifestations of a systemic disorder (e.g. measles, systemic lupus erythematosus), or a systemic or emotional disturbance may be secondary to primary skin lesions. A raised temperature is likely to be present if the skin disorder involves infection.

Health problems common to individuals with skin disorder

Each individual has to cope with varying physiological problems, depending upon the nature of the disorder. The nurse can explain the nature of the disorder to the patient and the rationale behind local skin or wound care, systemic therapy and nutritional support. The patient can then be encouraged to participate in as much of the care as is realistic.

Along with the physiological sequelae, there are individual psychological responses. Emotional support and health teaching are important nursing functions in assisting the individual to understand and learn to cope with health problems affecting the skin in a positive manner.

General principles of care for persons with skin disorder

The extent of the skin involvement as well as the nature of the condition determines whether or not the patient continues activities, is ambulatory and is treated at home. The patient's reaction to the disease also influences the plan of care and progress. The following are general considerations that will require adaptation and modification according to the individual.

Psychological support

The person is likely to be sensitive about the condition. Many are self-conscious about their appearance, worry constantly and tend to withdraw, believing that a skin disease carries a stigma. The disease may be such that it persists over a long period, interfering with the individual's ability to work or go out socially. Many skin diseases are aggravated by emotional stress. The understanding nurse helps the patient to identify any emotional factors that may contribute to the skin condition and carefully assesses his or her own responses to the person. Expression of revulsion at the patient's appearance adds to the distress. The nurse should make a conscious effort to touch the person's skin, thus reassuring him or her that the appearance and texture of the skin are both accepted. The patient is advised whether or not the disorder is contagious, and there should be no hesitation on the part of the nurse to touch the affected parts when giving care. In accordance with institutional infection control guidelines and the introduction of universal and body substance precautions, gloves may be indicated. The rationale should be explained calmly and matter-of-factly to the patient so as not to add to the psychological distress. An effort is made to convey an appreciation of the patient's feelings, to make the patient aware that he or she is accepted and to provide the necessary support and care which will help to reduce anxiety.

Local care

A common skin problem that receives little medical attention is that associated with the area beneath the breasts. Research by McMahon and Buckeldee (1992) indicated a lack of any consensus amongst nurses regarding the correct treatment of skin lesions in this area. For example, as many nurses advocated the application of talcum powder as stated that it should not be applied (18% each in a sample of 115 nurses). A wide range of adverse effects upon patients was identified by some nurses, while 17.4% of the sample stated there were no effects at all. Given that from zero up to 15 different approaches to treatment were listed by some respondents in this research, this is clearly an area of nursing practice prone to ritual and urgently needing research and rationalization.

Cleansing of the skin covering any area of the body should be determined on an individual basis for each patient. In some instances the application of soap and water may be contraindicated, and an alternative method of cleansing is necessary. For example, cleansing the skin with a vegetable oil may be necessary. If soap is permitted, it should be mildly alkaline and used very sparingly. A soft flannel is preferable, and the surface is washed lightly and gently to avoid injury and erythema. If there are open, discharging lesions, sterile gauze or a disposable absorbent cloth may be used. If the skin is dry, it may also be advisable to limit bathing to once or twice a week.

Special local or general therapeutic baths may be prescribed. These may be used to relieve itching, remove scales or crusts, or apply medications as well as for cleansing purposes. Caution is used against having the water or solution hot: a temperature higher than 35–38°C is likely to be too hot for the sensitive areas. Also, higher temperatures are likely to promote hyperaemia and itching. The patient is usually encouraged to remain in the bath for 10–20 minutes, and an attendant remains with the patient or close by, depending on condition and age. After bathing, excessive rubbing to dry the skin is avoided. Skin should be dabbed dry gently with a towel.

Fingernails are kept short and clean, and the patient is advised to refrain from scratching due to the threat of skin damage and infection.

Moist compresses Wet dressings may be applied over wet, exuding lesions, especially if they are open and discharging. The compresses are generally left uncovered and dry out very quickly, necessitating frequent changing or resoaking. Buxton (1993) recommends the addition of 0.1% potassium permanganate solution to the soak if there is any sign of infection. The prescribed solution is usually used at room temperature. Wet dressings are not usually applied to dry or scaly lesions; an ointment or creamy lotion is more appropriate.

Cold applications Application of cold dressings can cause vasoconstriction and decrease skin sensitivity and itching.

Clothing Woollens and other irritating clothing are avoided. Loose-fitting 100% cotton is best. Maintaining a cool environment can enhance the effectiveness of this strategy, when possible.

Topical applications

Many different drug preparations are used in treating skin diseases. Topical applications may be in powder, lotion, oil, cream, paste or ointment form. They may be classified according to their effect:

- *Antipruritic preparations* are applied to relieve itching. Examples are calamine lotion, corticosteroid cream or ointment, and antihistamines.

- *Keratolytic agents* soften and remove scales and the horny layer. An example is salicylic acid ointment.

- *Antieczematous agents* are applied to relieve itching and remove the vesicular drainage. Examples are corticosteroid lotion or spray and coal tar solution.

- *Keratoplastic preparations* stimulate the epidermis, increasing its thickness. An example is a weak salicylic (1–2%) acid ointment.

- *Antimicrobial agents* destroy or inhibit the reproduction of bacteria and fungi. Examples are antibiotic ointments such as neomycin and gentamicin.

- Zinc undecylenate is a common *antifungal agent*.

- *Antiparasitic preparations* destroy or inhibit parasites. Examples are benzyl benzoate lotion and gamma benzene hexachloride.

- *Emollients* are used to soften the skin. Examples commonly used are lanolin, petroleum jelly and Alpha Keri bath oil. Agents that contain lanolin and/or mineral oil, in moderate to large quantities, do not offer moisturizing properties and should not be used as such.

Frequently, topical preparations are a combination of two or more agents that have been selected for their specific effect.

Assessment

After each cleansing and before each local therapeutic application, the lesions are examined carefully. Any increase or spread, or change in size, colour or appearance, is noted. The nurse is constantly alert for factors in the individual's environment (e.g. contacts, diet, drugs) with which exacerbations of the condition may be associated.

The person with angioneurotic oedema may have intercutaneous patch or scratch sensitivity tests done to identify the offending substance. In the case of severe respiratory involvement, the patient experiences respiratory distress secondary to laryngeal obstruction. Total obstruction of the airway may ensue with alarming speed. If laryngeal stridor is present, the patient should be prepared immediately for emergency laryngostomy or tracheostomy. Prompt action is necessary. A corticosteroid preparation such as hydrocortisone is given intravenously; this usually reverses the reaction rapidly. However, as soon as it is suspected that the airway is or will be compromised, the doctor should attempt to intubate the patient. When a patient is in respiratory distress, the nurse plays a very important role by calming and being with the patient throughout.

Physical agents

Ultraviolet rays may be prescribed in the treatment of psoriasis, acne and seborrhoeic dermatitis. Irradiation is used if the lesion is malignant. Electrosurgery or cautery may be employed in the removal of warts, leucoplakia and seborrhoeic or senile keratoses (areas of horny thickening of epidermis).

Systemic therapy

If the skin disorder is secondary to a systemic disease, treatment is directed principally toward the primary condition.

Systemic drugs

The treatment of primary skin disorders may include the administration of systemic drugs. The choice of drug depends on the nature of the disorder and the patient's general health and response to the condition. An oral corticosteroid (e.g. prednisolone) is frequently prescribed in dermatitis, urticaria and pemphigus. If the skin lesions are infected, an oral antibiotic (e.g. tetracycline) may be prescribed and given. An antihistamine such as chlorphenamine (chlorpheniramine) maleate (Piriton) may be used in urticaria. If the patient is very agitated and distressed, a sedative may be necessary. However, long-term use of antihistamines and sedatives is to be avoided. Through patient education, the nurse can emphasize the role of non-pharmacological approaches. Adrenaline (epinephrine) 1 : 1000 may be ordered subcutaneously if the urticaria is widespread and causing considerable irritation. Vitamins may be given to improve the patient's appetite, general condition and resistance. Consultation with the pharmacy and infectious disease services is very helpful from a patient management perspective and for the discharge teaching these patients require.

Concern about the condition and fear of disfigurement and rejection as well as itching may result in a considerable loss of sleep for the patient. A sedative may be necessary to provide rest, which plays an important part in the patient's recovery. In the event of a significant degree of depression, psychiatric services may be appropriate for the patient.

Nutrition

Attention is paid to the nutritional status and to whether the patient is taking sufficient food. Frequently severe anorexia is a problem with the dermatological patient because of the skin irritation experienced, as well as the emotional disturbance. Dressings, ointments, lotions or similar applications on the hands may make self-care in feeding difficult. A creative occupational therapist and nurse should be able to assist in choosing appropriate assistive devices if problems with feeding occur. Continuity of such practices in hospital and following discharge are essential if such strategies are to bring about long-term gain.

Patient education

Nurses have a key role in advising the patient and family members of the day-to-day care required and precautionary measures applicable to the prevention of an exacerbation of any skin. Verbal and written directions are given about the local applications and taking of medicinal preparations. For example, adrenocorticosteroid preparations in the form of an ointment or cream are used topically to suppress inflammation and reduce sensitivity of the tissues. The patient must be cautioned to apply the corticoid preparation sparingly. If compresses or therapeutic baths are to be continued, specific details of the preparation, temperature and application are outlined and demonstrated if necessary.

Discharge planning

In the recovery phase, nurses can also help to boost the person's self-esteem and prepare for greater independence by assisting him or her to cope with an altered sense of self-esteem. The need to consider changing employment should be discussed with the patient, and the occupational therapist and social worker may be consulted to discuss retraining facilities if appropriate.

Documentation

Nursing documentation in the form of a 'wound documentation tool' is helpful in the assessment, planning, implementation and evaluation of care strategies. Sections for subjective and objective data, treatments given and an assessment of their effectiveness, together with the progress of the skin disorder, are very helpful and appropriate in the nursing record.

Common skin disorders

Patient assessment

In assessing patients suffering from skin diseases it is necessary to assess the whole patient, not just the state of the patient's skin. The extent of the skin disorder should be recorded accurately in order that progress can be monitored and possible allergic substances recorded.

The patient's view of his or her condition should be determined, together with any coping mechanisms used. The patient's self-concept should be explored along with how the illness is affecting everyday life. Other psychosocial factors such as developmental status and family relationships should be explored.

Some common conditions and their causes are now considered, together with patient goals and specific nursing care.

Dermatitis or eczema

These two terms are synonymous and refer to an inflammatory disease of the skin that is very common and, according to the cause, may be referred to as *irritant contact dermatitis* or *allergic contact dermatitis*. In the former case previous sensitization by exposure is not necessary, unlike the latter. A less common form is referred to as *exfoliative dermatitis*. If mucosal involvement is present, it is referred to as *toxic epidermal necrolysis syndrome* (TENS), a form of erythema multiforme.

Risk factors

- Contact with an irritant substance such as strong soaps and some acids/alkalis.

- Contact of hypersensitive or allergic skin with an agent such as cosmetics, hair dye, nickel, rubber or cement.

- Exfoliation due to drug therapy, such as antibiotics or anticonvulsants and infectious agents such as *Mycoplasma pneumoniae* and herpes simplex virus.

Characteristics

- Development of an erythematous area with small papular development 2–4 days after contact, then progression to vesicles.

- Vesicles may rupture and discharge contents, followed by crusting and scaling.

- Denuded areas may ooze a serous discharge and then be covered by regenerated epidermis.

- Itchiness and burning leading to scratching, which may result in infected lesions.

- With TENS, virtual universal erythema desquamation, peeling and itching of the skin and loss of hair; malaise, fever, headache and sore throat may precede lesions; extensive sloughing of epidermis (positive Nikolsky's sign); involvement of mucous membranes also evident.

Patient goals

The patient will recover from the contact dermatitis with a minimum of scarring and mucosal damage. The patient will maintain or achieve a positive body image and sense of self-esteem, and will demonstrate relaxation techniques to reduce emotional exacerbations.

Nursing intervention

- Local applications of cold, wet compresses, bland, unmedicated lotions or thinly applied steroid-based creams.

- If extensive, therapeutic baths may be helpful. Explain rationale to the patient.

- Antibiotic ointment may be applied if there is an infection. Advise the patient regarding use.

- Advise the patient to avoid scratching and keep nails short and clean. Mittens may be helpful with children.

- Advise the patient of correct use of corticosteroid (e.g. prednisolone) for reduction of tissue response and inflammation, particularly topical steroids, and antipruritic agents (e.g. diphenhydramine) for itchiness. Topical steroids are very helpful but can have serious side-effects such as skin atrophy if used incorrectly, reddening of the skin due to fixed vasodilatation, perioral dermatitis and the masking of infection (Bowman 1994).

- Educate patient regarding stress reduction techniques.

- With TENS, early recognition, immediate debridement and coverage with biological and/or biosynthetic dressings are essential; excellent respiratory care (i.e. incentive spirometry), postural drainage, suctioning, chest physiotherapy, and intubation or ventilation if necessary.

- Lubrication of ocular mucous membranes and use of a glass rod to remove conjunctival discharge.

- Provide the patient and family with psychosocial support.

- Arrange for follow-up care.

Psoriasis

Risk factors

- Family history: if one parent has psoriasis, 25% of their children will (Buxton 1993).

- Onset common during adolescence.

- Association with rheumatoid arthritis, since raised uric acid level is present in some patients.

- May be precipitated by trauma, infections and psychological stress.

Characteristics

- Chronic inflammations of the skin that produce dry scaly lesions, exacerbations and remissions.

- Dull, red, papular lesions form.

- Silvery white, waxy scales accumulate in layers, with epidermal replacement every 4 days (normal rate is every 28 days); therefore, skin's normal protective layers are not able to form.

- Lesions may increase in size, coalesce and form large scaly plaques. Typically lesions do not itch.

- Small, pinpoint bleeding areas are found when the plaque is removed.

- Nail involvement: pitting, discoloration and separation from thick, hard and dry underlying tissue.

- Onset may be gradual or sudden.

- Duration may be lengthy or short lived.

Patient goals

The patient will recover from the psoriasis with a minimum of scarring; the patient will maintain or achieve a positive body image and sense of self-esteem.

Nursing intervention

- Teach the individual regarding the rationale and limitations of treatments – to reduce scaling and itchiness, not to cure the condition.

- Provide psychosocial support to individual and family, particularly about living with a chronic illness, and assist with the development of adaptive techniques as necessary.

- Apply and instruct the patient regarding various treatments – local applications, baths and exposure to ultraviolet rays.

- Topical applications may include pastes, ointments or creams, including salicylic acid, coal-tar derivatives or dithranol.

- Caution individual about the use of topical and systemic corticosteroids.

- Instruct the patient to soak in prescribed bath for 20–30 minutes and to scrub off scales gently. Daily shampooing may be necessary if the scalp is affected.

- If ultraviolet light therapy is used, teach the individual about the wearing of dark glasses during treatment and to begin at exposures of 1-minute duration, to be gradually increased under medical supervision.

■ If dithranol paste is used, instruct the patient on the importance of protecting unaffected skin with petroleum jelly.

■ Provide support to the patient as occlusive dressings, plastic bags, vinyl suits and shower caps may be necessary for these time-consuming and aesthetically unappealing treatments.

■ Explain to the individual and family that topically applied agents will suppress epidermopoiesis, whereas tar therapies retard and inhibit rapid growth of psoriatic tissue.

■ Reinforce the symptomatic management versus the cure nature of therapies.

■ If appropriate, gently touch the patient's arm or hand in a gesture of acceptance, not revulsion or fear, of the sight of the skin lesions.

■ Encourage the family to accept the individual's condition and not to be fearful that it is contagious or infectious.

■ Encourage adequate rest, a balanced nutritional diet and prevention of skin irritations and infections.

■ Arrange for follow-up care.

Parasitic infestations

Pediculosis (lice)

Risk factors

■ Poor hygiene.

■ Intimate or casual contact with an infected person.

Characteristics

■ Appearance of eggs (nits) or lice on body, head and/or pubic areas; may also be found on seams of clothing.

■ Haemorrhagic points may be noted, along with hyperaemia, linear scratches and a slight degree of eczema.

■ Thickened, dry, scaly darkly pigmented patches noted with long-term infestation.

Assessment

■ *Health history* – present social situation, i.e. access to bathing facilities; contact with an infected individual, clothing or bedlinen.

■ *Physical examination* – visually assess the involved areas in a well-lit room. Include the neck, thighs and trunk. Pubic lice and head lice can be found on hair shafts.

■ *Psychosocial concerns and developmental factors* – assess changes in patient or other interaction due to the

contagious nature of the condition. Identify the patient's social situation, i.e. living conditions, health practices, non-compliance with healthcare treatments.

■ *Patient and family knowledge* – identify their perceptions of health status, disease condition and relationship to health practices and contacts with infected individuals, education level, readiness and willingness to learn.

Patient goals

The patient will have no evidence of pediculosis infestation and will learn preventive healthcare practices to avoid reinfestation and transmission to other people during the treatment period.

Nursing intervention

■ Teach the patient and family regarding the cause, nature and prevention of pediculosis.

■ *Body lice*:
— instruct individual and family to launder clothing to destroy lice and nits
— check family for infestation
— administer antipruritic, systemic antibiotic and topical corticosteroid applications as ordered
— teach patient to look for evidence of rickettsial disease (lice serve as vectors).

■ *Head lice*:
— cleanse hair vigorously with gamma benzene hexachloride shampoos followed by a combing with a vinegar-soaked fine-toothed comb; repeat in 24 hours
— disinfect combs and brushes with shampoo
— instruct patient and family to wash all bedlinen
— check family members for infestation and treat as necessary.

■ *Pubic lice*:
— as above for head lice
— check sexual contacts for infestation and treat as necessary
— discuss the possibility of coexisting sexually transmitted disease.

■ Establish a realistic plan of care including follow-up for the individual and others involved.

Scabies

Risk factors

■ Contact with the parasite *Sarcoptes scabiei* (itch mite).

Characteristics

■ Appearance of greyish-white, slightly elevated, zigzag lines on skin.

■ Secondary lesions develop in form of vesicles or papules, pustules and encrustations.

Assessment

- *Health history* – contact with an infected person or scabies mite (via an alternative vector).

- *Physical examination* – visual assessment of involved site in a well-lit room; common sites include flexor surfaces of the wrist, palms, between the fingers and toes, groin and areolae of the breasts; in addition to lines on skin and secondary lesions, individuals complain of severe itchiness.

- *Psychosocial concerns and developmental factors* – identify changes in patient and other interaction due to the infectious nature of the condition; social situation, i.e. living conditions, health practices.

- *Patient and family knowledge* – perception of health status, disease condition and relationship to health practices and contacts with infected individuals; education level, readiness and willingness to learn.

Patient goals

The patient will have no evidence of scabies infestation and will learn preventive healthcare practices to avoid reinfestation and transmission to other people during the treatment period.

Nursing intervention

- Teach the patient and family about the cause, nature and prevention of scabies.

- Instruct the patient to take a hot bath and vigorously scrub open infested burrows.

- Apply a preparation such as benzyl benzoate emulsion or 0.5% malathion cream.

- Advise the individual to repeat bath and ointment application once again, usually the next morning.

- Advise the individual and family to wash bedlinen and clothing in boiling water or to press with a very hot iron.

- Examine all close contacts of the individual for scabies and treat if necessary.

- Establish a realistic plan of care, including follow-up for the individual and others involved.

Skin cancer

Risk factors

- Long periods of exposure to sunlight, radiation, chronic irritation (e.g. scars of poor quality that frequently break down), and long-standing contact with chemicals (e.g. oil, tar and paraffin).

- Light skin complexion, Celtic family background.

Health-seeking behaviours related to the prevention of skin cancer

Skin cancers can be prevented. Some 95% of skin cancers are curable, if diagnosed and treated early. Health promotion programmes and the encouragement of health-seeking behaviours are therefore important for nurses to stress to the public.

Educational points to reinforce with individuals include:

- The avoidance of unnecessary sun exposure, especially between 10.00 and 14.00 hours when the ultraviolet rays are strongest.

- The application of sunscreens and/or sunblocks with high levels of *para*-aminobenzoic acid (PABA) whenever exposure to the sun is unavoidable. PABA-free lotions are available for people who are allergic to it.

- The wearing of protective clothing, i.e. long-sleeved shirts and broad-brimmed hats, but to recognize that sunscreens and blocks are still necessary.

- The treatment of moles if they are particularly prone to repeated friction and irritation.

- An awareness of indicators of potential malignancy, i.e. an increase in size, ulceration, bleeding or serous exudate from a mole or other skin lesion.

Characteristics

- Changes in moles or other skin lesions that may at first appear innocuous; changes include an increase in size, ulceration, bleeding, serous exudate, and brownish, scaly thickening of the dermis (*Bowen's disease*).

- Sores that do not heal and become enlarged; a small nodule that is waxy in appearance with a rolled, translucent border with plaque formation (*basal cell carcinoma*), often grey or yellow in colour.

- Open sores, nodular lesions, long-standing scars that repeatedly break down (*squamous cell carcinoma*).

- Pigmented lesions arising from an existing mole that has changed in size and/or colour (*malignant melanoma*).

- *Kaposi's sarcoma (KS)*, a malignancy of lymphatic endothelial cell origin which presents as moderately infiltrated reddish-brown plaques located on the trunk of the body and face is a complication of HIV infection. KS lesions have particular affinity for the tip of the nose, necessitating body image adjustments for the individual. Radiotherapy is useful in treating some KS lesions, being particularly useful for short-term cosmetic effect and pain management. When KS lesions are found systemically, in either the gastrointestinal tract or the lungs, chemotherapy such as α-interferon or etoposide may be useful.

Individuals with HIV infection are also susceptible to attacks from viruses such as herpes simplex and varicella-zoster which may cause painful, deep and destructive ulcers in a variety of different locations. Topical or intravenous aciclovir may be used if these conditions are diagnosed in early stages. Many people are also prone to seborrhoeic eczema and may develop severe widespread dermatitis in late HIV disease, which may respond to cortisone preparations.

Assessment

- *Health history* – age, history of sun exposure, knowledge of changes in moles or skin lesions, occupation, recent changes in general health status (to rule out metastases), family history of cancer, in particular skin cancer.

- *Physical examination* – visually assess the involved areas in a well-lit room. Common sites include exposed areas, especially of the upper extremities and of the face – lower lip, nose, ears and forehead.

- *Psychosocial concerns* – anxiety, fear once the word 'cancer' is mentioned, patient and family interaction, coping abilities.

- *Patient and family knowledge* – perception of health status and skin cancer; level of understanding.

Patient goals

The patient will recover from the skin cancer, will have a minimum of scarring and learn preventive healthcare practices to avoid or detect recurrences. If the cancer has metastasized rapidly and extensively, the goals will include acceptance or adjustment to cancer treatment and/or palliative care measures.

Nursing intervention

- Provide the patient and family with psychosocial support once the diagnosis of skin cancer has been confirmed.

- Inform the patient and family about the causes, treatments and outcomes of the particular type of skin cancer.

- *Basal cell and squamous cell carcinoma* – discuss with the patient, in collaboration with the attending physician, what the treatment options are and what the individual wishes to do. Options may include surgery, radiation therapy or chemical destruction of the tumour.

- *Malignant melanomas* – prepare the individual educationally and psychologically for surgery to remove the tumour. Warn the patient that future surgery may be necessary to remove surrounding lymph nodes.

- Encourage the individual to engage in regular visual assessments for changes in moles or the appearance of lesions to the skin. If found, encourage him or her to seek medical help immediately.

- Reinforce the important role of prevention and the high cure rate with early detection.

- Capitalize on society's growing awareness of the alarming increase in skin cancer rates by encouraging the use of health promotion and disease prevention strategies.

- Arrange for follow-up care.

Summary

This chapter discusses the important role that the skin plays in maintaining overall health and well-being. The skin fulfils a multitude of functions, many of which we are unaware of until something threatens to alter or impair its integrity. The consequences of an insult to the skin's integrity may be relatively minor, or may be devastating and life threatening. The person with impairment of skin integrity must cope with changes in self-image as well as with minor or major disruptions to physiological functioning.

The nurse plays a key role in the prevention, assessment, planning, administration and evaluation of care strategies to manage potential and actual impairment of skin integrity. Patient and family education is a vital function of the nurse as a primary caregiver and one of those closest to the individual and family.

The care of persons with impaired skin integrity can be challenging and calls upon many facets of the nursing role. The nurse must be knowledgeable about the structure and function of the skin, measures to maintain skin integrity and promote healing and tissue repair, and the impact of changes in body image on the individual and family.

Critical incident

Mr Jones, an 80-year-old retired coal-miner, is about to be discharged from the acute care setting in which you work, having been treated for a left fractured neck of femur with a hemiarthroplasty that was inserted under spinal anaesthesia. His injury was sustained in the garden at home when he stumbled on uneven ground as he was returning from church one Sunday with his wife.

Mr Jones' wife – his childhood sweetheart – is herself frail and is registered blind, although she is able to differentiate objects in good light. Together they are a very independent couple who, although they have a willing supportive family (their oldest daughter lives in the next village), have indicated to you that they want no

(Continued)

Critical incident (*Continued*)

district nurse visits in the immediate future following Mr Jones' discharge.

Although Mr Jones' mobility is currently improving steadily (he still requires the use of a Zimmer frame), he spends long periods of time in a chair or in his bed, depending on the time of day. His appetite in hospital has been deemed adequate. At the time of his discharge, the skin on Mr Jones' sacral area appeared continually red and the final Waterlow score recorded in the hospital was 18. Previous history included chronic bronchitis and atopic eczema. At home Mr and Mrs Jones will be sleeping in the divan bed that they were given as a golden wedding present from the family.

Reflection

■ What factors might increase Mr Jones' risk of developing pressure ulcers, at the time of his discharge from hospital? Highlight any research that could underpin your rationale for the factors identified.

■ Highlight the relevance of the Waterlow risk assessment score identified here, and identify how this score should be interpreted in a clinical setting. Identify potential care interventions that could be indicated following the assessment and recording of a Waterlow score of 18, taking account of other information contained within this critical incident.

■ Reflect on a patient whom you may have nursed in the recent past – who is not too dissimilar to Mr Jones – and, having read this chapter, discuss with a colleague the care you gave that patient (or indicated should be given), highlighting any identified differences between the two patients.

See Appendix 2 for guidelines on reflection.

References

Agate J (1985) Pressure sores. In: Pathy M, ed. Principles and practice of geriatric medicine. London: Wiley.

Allman R, Walker J, Hart M et al (1987) Air-fluidized beds of conventional therapy for pressure sores. Annals of International Medicine 107(5): 641–648.

Barratt E (1987) Putting risk calculators in their place. Nursing Times 83(7): 65–68.

Bliss M (1993) Aetiology of pressure sores. Clinical Gerontology 3: 379–397.

Bowman J (1994) More than skin deep. Nursing Times 90(23): 43–46.

Bradley D, Collier M (1994) Principles of trauma and the treatment of traumatic wounds. Educational Leaflet 2(3). Huntingdon, UK: Wound Care Society.

Burgess C (1991) Initial management of the patient with extensive burn injury. Critical Care Nursing Clinics of North America 3(2): 167.

Burman P (1993) Using pressure measurements to evaluate different technologies. Decubitus 6(3): 38–42.

Buxton P (1993) ABC of dermatology, 2nd edn. London: British Medical Association.

Collier M (1994) Anatomy of the skin and the natural healing process. Educational Leaflet 2(1). Huntingdon, UK: Wound Care Society.

Collier M (1995) Pressure sore prevention and development. Educational Leaflet 3(1). Huntingdon, UK: Wound Care Society.

Collier M (1996) The principles of optimum wound management. Continuing Education Series. Nursing Standard 10: 47–52.

Collier M (1999a) Blanching and non-blanching hyperaemia. Journal of Wound Care 8(2): 63–64.

Collier M (1999b) Fundamental concepts. In: Journal of Wound Care. Resource file – mattresses and beds, Part 1, pp. 1–8. London: EMAP.

Collier M (1999c) Pressure ulcer development and principles for prevention In: Glover D, Miller M, eds. Wound management: theory and practice, pp. 84–95. London: EMAP.

Department of Health (1992) The health of the nation. London: HMSO.

Department of Health (1993) Pressure sores: a key quality indicator. London: HMSO.

Department of Health (2001) The essence of care: patient focused benchmarking for health care practitioners. London: HMSO.

Department of Trade and Industry (1999) Burns and scalds in the home – report. London: HMSO.

EUPAP (1997) Proceedings of the first European Pressure Ulcer Advisory Panel Conference. Oxford: EUPAP.

Ferguson A (1990) A systematic approach to trauma relief. Professional Nurse November: 82–90.

Flanagan M (1993) Pressure sore risk assessment scales. Journal of Wound Care 2(3): 162–167.

Fowler A (1999) Burns. In: Glover D, Miller M, eds. Wound management: theory and practice, pp. 48–60. London: EMAP.

Gilchrist B (1994) Treating bacterial wound infection. Nursing Times 90(50): 55–58.

Goldstone L, Goldstone J (1982) The Norton score – an early warning of pressure sores? Journal of Advanced Nursing 7(4): 419–426.

Goode H, Burns E, Walker B (1992) Vitamin C depletion and pressure sores in elderly patients with femoral neck fractures. British Medical Journal 305: 925–926.

Hibbs P (1990) The economics of pressure sores. In: Bader D, ed. Pressure sores; clinical practice and scientific approach, pp. 35–42. London: Macmillan.

Hollinworth H, Collier M (2000) Nurses' views about pain and trauma at dressing changes: results of a national survey. Journal of Wound Care 9(8): 369–373.

Kenney L, Rithalia S (1999) Technical aspects of support surfaces. In: Journal of Wound Care. Resource file – mattresses and beds, Part 2, pp. 1–8. London: EMAP.

Livesley B (1992) Aetiology of pressure sores – pressure. Proceedings of the Tissue Viability Conference in Bath. Salisbury: Tissue Viability Society.

Lockyer-Stevens N (1993) The use of water filled gloves to prevent decubitus ulcers on heels. Journal of Wound Care 2(5): 282–287.

Lockyer-Stevens N (1994) A developing information base for purchasing decisions. Professional Nurse 9(8): 534–542.

Lund C, Browder N (1944) The estimation of area of burns. Surgery, Gynecology and Obstetrics 79: 353–360.

McLaren S, Green S (2001) Nutritional factors in the aetiology, development and healing of pressure ulcers. In: Morison M, ed. The prevention and treatment of pressure ulcers, pp. 195–215. Edinburgh: Mosby.

McMahon R, Buckeldee J (1992) Skin problems beneath the breasts of in-patients: the knowledge, opinions and practice of nurses. Journal of Advanced Nursing 17: 1243–1250.

Moffatt C, O'Hare L (1995) Venous leg ulceration: treatment by high compression bandaging. Ostomy/Wound Management 41(4): 16–25.

McLaren S (1992) Nutrition and wound healing. In: Proceedings of the Second European Conference on Advances in Wound Management, pp. 67–78. London: EMAP Health Care.

Morison M, ed. (2001) The prevention and treatment of pressure ulcers. Edinburgh: Mosby.

Mullineaux J (1993) Cutting the delay reduces risk. Professional Nurse 9(1): 22–30.

Norton D, McLaren R, Exton-Smith A (1975) An investigation of geriatric nursing problems in hospital. Edinburgh: Churchill Livingstone.

O'Dea K (1993) Prevalence of pressure damage in hospital patients in the UK. Journal of Wound Care 2(4): 221–225.

Peters J, Watts J (1998) Accurate assessment of skin conditions. Practice Nurse 15(9): 525–530.

Redfearn S (1991) Nursing elderly people, 2nd edn. Edinburgh: Churchill Livingstone.

Reid J, Morison M (1994) Classification of pressure sore severity. Nursing Times 90(20): 46–50.

Royal College of Nursing (2001) Risk assessment and prevention of pressure ulcers. London: RCN.

Thomas S (1990) Wound management and dressings. London: Pharmaceutical Press.

Turner T (1982) Which dressing and why? Wound care series no. 11. Nursing Times 78(29): 41–44.

Versluysen M (1986) How elderly patients with femoral fractures develop pressure sores. British Medical Journal 292: 1311–1313.

Walsh M, Ford P (1989) Nursing rituals: research and rational action. Oxford: Heinemann.

Walsh M, Kent A (2001) A&E nursing, 4th edn. Oxford: Heinemann.

Walsh M, Crumbie A, Reveley S (1999) Nurse practitioners; clinical skills and professional issues. Oxford: Butterworth Heinemann.

Ward C (1992) Infection in burn patients. In: Rylah L, ed. Critical care of the burned patient. Cambridge: Cambridge University Press.

Waterlow J (1985) A risk assessment card. Nursing Times 89(27): 49–51.

Wilmhurst A (1992) Prognosis of the burn injury. In: Rylah L, ed. Critical care of the burned patient. Cambridge: Cambridge University Press.

Further Reading

Collier M (1999) Blanching and non-blanching hyperaemia. Journal of Wound Care 8(2) 63–64.

A review article that discusses both the seminal research that underpins the concepts of blanching and non-blanching hyperaemia as well as highlighting the practical interpretation of the concepts in the clinical setting. Assessment issues are also discussed in addition to the care interventions that, it could be argued, should be initiated in response to the recognition of these important concepts.

Flanagan M (1997) Wound management. Edinburgh: Churchill Livingstone.

Part of the Access to Clinical Education (ACE) Series, this book consists of several chapters that cover all issues and underlying principles related to the assessment, management and evaluation of patients with a variety of wounds, including burns. Throughout the publication there are numerous opportunities for the reader to participate in self-assessment exercises (feedback is identified) and in addition a number of key journal articles are reproduced within the text as 'readers'.

Fowler A (1999) Burns. In: Glover D, Miller M, eds. Wound management: theory and practice, pp. 48–60. London: EMAP.

A chapter within an excellent introductory text covering a number of important tissue viability issues. This chapter looks at the assessment and management of patients with burn injuries, both major and minor, and highlights the importance of correct burn assessment, classification and patient management within a holistic care framework.

Morison M, ed. (2001) The prevention and treatment of pressure ulcers. Edinburgh: Mosby.

An invaluable reference source for all practitioners and other professionals allied to medicine who care for patients at risk of developing pressure ulcers. Written by a team of internationally acknowledged experts, each chapter contains self-assessment questions and activities, and to conclude there is a section containing advanced case studies that allow the reader to reflect on the many complex issues.

Peters J, Watts J (1998) Accurate assessment of skin conditions. Practice Nurse 15(9): 525–530.

An excellent review article that incorporates practical definitions of a number of related terms before highlighting both assessment and management issues for a number of skin conditions. Additionally a number of 'common' skin irritants are highlighted and a range of topical treatments discussed. The writers, to their credit, manage to introduce a number of complex concepts in a easy to understand (reader friendly) manner.

Royal College of Nursing (2001) Risk assessment and prevention of pressure ulcers. London: RCN.

This technical report and appendices produced by the Royal College of Nursing form the basis of the clinical guideline on pressure ulcer risk assessment and prevention circulated by the National Institute for Clinical Excellence (NICE) in April 2001. There are a number of recommendations highlighted within the document, with the strength of evidence that supports each identified from a continuum (1 = best evidence (e.g. randomized controlled trial) and 3 = 'expert' opinion only). A number of important references are highlighted which cover the vast range of issues related to the prevention of pressure ulcer development.

26 Caring for the patient with substance misuse

Steve Morgan and Tara O'Neill

Introduction

Definitions and descriptions of terminology

Alcohol

Tobacco

Commonly abused illicit drugs

Multidisciplinary working and service structures

Assessment

Treatment interventions

Suicide

Deliberate self-harm

Summary

Introduction

The ever-increasing health, social and economic costs related to drinking alcohol, smoking tobacco and the use of illicit drugs have become a major public health concern. They are important contributing factors in most areas of medical and mental health problems. Indeed, substance misuse remains the largest cause of preventable morbidity and mortality in the UK, and targeted intervention is required to reduce the high costs (Department of Health 1998). Although specialist drug and alcohol services are established to work with substance misusers, it would be both unrealistic and inappropriate to expect them to respond alone to the challenge of prevention and health promotion in this field.

Scale of the problem

The harm associated with the misuse of alcohol constitutes a major public health problem in both developed and developing countries. World Health Organization (WHO) statistics record around 750 000 alcohol-related deaths each year. Alcohol-related diseases and injuries account for 3–4% of the annual global burden of disease and injury (WHO 1996). According to WHO estimates, there are more than one billion (1.1×10^9) smokers in the world – about one-third of the global population aged 15 years and above. Globally, approximately 47% of men and 12% of women smoke.

Reliable estimates of the extent and prevalence of illicit drug consumption are difficult to obtain, because users of these substances are unlikely to report on an illegal activity or give truthful responses for fear of reprisals. Despite these difficulties, it is estimated that approximately 15 million people worldwide incur a significant risk to their health as a result of using psychoactive substances. It is further estimated that one-third of these users inject drugs, and many believe this figure to be an underestimate. Recent figures suggest that drug injection is responsible for between 100 000 and 200 000 deaths per year worldwide (WHO 1996).

Scope and remit of this chapter

In this chapter we will attempt to outline the descriptions, effects and possible interventions associated with a range of commonly misused substances.

Definitions and descriptions of terminology

Substance use This is used to denote both use and misuse (experimental, recreational, dependent and problematic use). It is a catch-all term that describes the use of substances – drug, alcohol or other – to alter an individual's psychological state.

Problematic use This is generally accepted to include physical, social, psychological and/or legal problems related to intoxication, excessive consumption or dependence resulting from use of substances.

Drug abuse or misuse This describes the use of any drug, whether legal or illegal, for a medical or recreational purpose when other alternatives are available, practical or warranted, or when drug use endangers either the user or others with whom he or she may interact. The concept of drug abuse can be viewed as a social construct. The acceptability of using a drug may change in any given society at any given time and will generally be context driven. An example of this could be the growing public acceptance of the use of cannabis as an analgesic in chronic conditions such as cancer, where cannabis is increasingly viewed as an acceptable alternative to prescribed pain relief despite its illegality. However, members of the public still generally view users of cannabis for recreational purposes with suspicion. In this case, the concept of illegality is pushed to the fore, thus denoting cannabis use within the recreational domain as abuse or misuse.

Dependence This is the state in which the use of a substance is necessary for either physical or psychological well-being.

Physical dependence This results from the extended use of drugs such as tranquillizers, heroin and alcohol (i.e. drugs that alter body chemistry). When experiencing physical dependency the individual will require repeated doses of the drug to maintain normal function. Ceasing to use the drug results in symptoms of physical withdrawal.

Psychological dependence This is more common than physical dependency and may occur with any type of drug. People may use the drug experience as a way of coping with their world, or as a way of maintaining feelings of well-being. The individual will feel that they cannot cope without drugs, although they may not be physically dependent. Individuals can be psychologically dependent on almost anything, such as chocolate or gambling.

Addiction Donovan and Marlatt (1988) define addiction as follows:

- The individual chooses to maintain the addictive behaviour even when other, more gratifying, sources of reinforcement are present.

- Dependence on the behaviour or experience, on either a physiological or psychological level, that may lead to withdrawal discomfort when the individual is prevented from engaging in the behaviour.

- Increasing high need for a given experience or behaviour representing a form of tolerance.

- Perceiving the need for the experience or a powerfully strong desire in the form of a 'craving' on both a physiological and cognitive level.

- The power of the addiction promotes a tendency for rapid reinstatement of the behaviour pattern following a period of non-involvement with it.

Tolerance As an individual takes more of a substance the body adapts to tolerate increased amounts. More of the drug is needed to sustain the desired effect, i.e. the body has a progressively decreasing responsiveness to the drug.

Cross-tolerance In this condition tolerance to one drug results in a lessened response to another drug.

Withdrawal symptoms These are the symptoms that can result from stopping long-term use of certain drugs, notably opiates such as heroin, benzodiazepines such as diazepam, and also alcohol. Physical effects may include shaking and flu-like symptoms, and will depend on the drug being withdrawn. Examples of the effects of withdrawal from nicotine are irritability, frustration, anger, difficulty concentrating, restlessness, decreased heart rate, and increased appetite or weight gain. Withdrawal from the moderate use of alcohol can cause cravings, irritability and frustration. Withdrawal from high levels of alcohol use may result in *delirium tremens*. This syndrome incorporates tremors with hallucinations, psychomotor agitation, confusion and disorientation, sleep disorders and other associated discomforts, and lasts for several days after alcohol withdrawal.

A biopsychosocial explanation for substance misuse

A number of different theories have been formulated over time to attempt to explain why people abuse drugs and alcohol. These fall broadly into four main categories: moral, biological, psychological and social.

Moral

Moral theories tend to focus on the individual, who is viewed as weak or having a poor character. Interventions associated with moral theories focus the responsibility for change on the individual, and treatment emphasizes deterrence and punishment. An example of a moral intervention would be the incarceration of a drug user for possession of their drug of choice with the hope that they would come to the realization that drug use is bad and leads to negative consequences.

Biological

Biological theories incorporate disease models of substance misuse and genetics. Substance misuse is sometimes also viewed as a primary mental disorder. Treatment is focused around abstinence to halt progression of the disease. Biological approaches tend to remove the focus from the individual's power and responsibility to change, laying the responsibility firmly on medically based interventions. Treatment will vary but may be targeted initially with prescribed medication to break the cycle of drug use, with the overarching principle that once the individual reaches abstinence from their drug of choice medical interventions can be discontinued. An example of a biologically based intervention would be the substitute prescribing of methadone to treat heroin dependence.

Psychological

A readily applied psychological theory of substance misuse is social learning theory. Substance misuse is viewed as a learned behavioural disorder. Interventions associated with psychological explanations focus on the individual's ability to learn more adaptive behaviour as an alternative to substance misuse. This may involve learning new behaviours or substituting known behaviours in place of the substance. An example of this approach might be an individual who drinks to relieve feelings of stress or anxiety, i.e. the function of the drinking is to relax rather than enjoyment of the alcohol per se. The individual may benefit from attending a stress management course focusing on relaxation techniques – the relaxation techniques being an ultimately less damaging coping strategy for stress management than alcohol use.

Social

Social theories view substance misuse as a means for the individual to cope with their environment and social situation. Interventions therefore focus on helping the individual improve their social functioning either by modifying the way they engage with their environment or by changing the environment itself. An example of this approach might be the individual who uses amfetamines on a regular basis when going to the pub. A social approach would focus on why the drug use occurs in that particular environment and look at ways of modifying it. Is it that amfetamine use only happens in the pub; if so, change the meeting place (i.e. modify the environment). Or is it that the dealer frequents that pub, so access to amfetamines is more readily available; thus treatment might be focused towards teaching the individual effective refusal skills (i.e. modifying the way the individual engages with the environment).

Rather than focus on one particular theory as explanation, clinically it is generally more relevant to combine the different theories according to the individual's expressed need. Thus, substance misuse problems are viewed not merely as a function of the person's self, but as the result of a complex interaction between biological, psychological and social dimensions. The reasons why any individual uses substances will be unique to that individual, and it is important when trying to help the person that a full understanding of the biopsychosocial dimensions is reached before treatment is planned. A number of examples of precipitating and maintaining factors of substance misuse are:

- curiosity
- rites of passage
- pleasure
- experimentation
- relief of underlying distress
- self-adventure
- spiritual meaning or loss of faith
- immediate satisfaction.

Alcohol

The Health Education Authority recommends the limits shown in Box 26.1 for sensible drinking. These have been drawn up for adults, and it should be assumed that limits for young people are lower.

These limits were established in December 1995, following a Department of Health (DoH) review of the previously held limits of no more than 21 units per week for men and 14 units per week for women. This reflected a desire to shift from weekly to daily units of consumption. In 1996 an Office of National Statistics General Household Survey (DoH 1998) found 28% of men and 14% of women to be exceeding the old sensible limits. For men this had remained stable over the years, but it represented a steady increase for women. Proportions of over-the-limit drinkers are higher in the younger age groups (Institute of Alcohol Studies 1997–2000).

Box 26.2 provides a quick guide to calculating units of alcohol.

The ONS Health Survey also outlined that, at any one time, the drinking levels of the adult population of

---

Box 26.1 Health Education Authority recommendations for sensible drinking

Males

- Between 3 and 4 units/daily, or less, constitutes no significant risk to health
- Regularly drinking 4 units or more per day constitutes an increasing health risk

Females

- Between 2 and 3 units/daily or less, constitutes no significant risk to health
- Regularly drinking 3 units or more per day constitutes an increasing health risk

From Clancey (1997).

Box 26.2   Calculating units of alcohol

One unit of alcohol = half a pint of ordinary strength
                          lager, beer or cider (3.5% ABV)

                       = one small glass of wine (9% ABV)

                       = one single pub measure of
                          spirit (40% ABV)

The exact number of units in a particular drink can be
calculated by multiplying the volume of the drink
(number of milliliters; mL) by the % ABV (alcohol
by volume) and dividing it by 1000. For example,
the number of units in an alcoholic lemonade
(e.g. Hooch) of 330 mL with a 4.7% ABV is:

$$330 \times 4.7/1000 = 1.5 \text{ units}$$

From Clancey (1997).

Table 26.1   Drinking levels for the adult population of
England in 1996 (data from DoH 1998, with permission)

	Men	Women	Total
Non-drinkers	1 300 000	2 390 000	3 690 000
Light drinkers (men up to 10 units/week; women up to 7 units/week)	8 019 000	11 750 000	19 769 000
Moderate drinkers (men 11–21 units/week; women 8–14 units/week)	3 916 000	3 187 000	7 103 000
Over the sensible limit (men over 21 units/week; women over 14 units/week)	5 594 000	2 589 000	8 183 000

England are approximately as shown in Table 26.1. Of
the 8 million or so people exceeding the sensible limits,
around 1 700 000 are drinking at 'definitely harmful'
levels of more than 50 units per week for men and more
than 35 units per week for women. On the basis of the
main surveys conducted for the Government during the
1990s, at any one time there are probably around 2 million people in the UK experiencing symptoms of alcohol
dependence, the male : female ratio being around 3 : 1
(Institute of Alcohol Studies 1997–2000).

Effects on health and social well-being

There are three components of drinking behaviour associated with medical and/or social problems: intoxication,
regular heavy consumption and alcohol dependence (alcoholism). Examples of such problems are:

■ *intoxication*:
  — drunken driving
  — alcohol poisoning
  — accidents
  — violence.

■ *regular heavy consumption*:
  — health problems
  — financial problems
  — family difficulties
  — absenteeism from work.

■ *alcohol dependence*:
  — psychological problems
  — health problems
  — family difficulties
  — problems of withdrawal.

Alcohol-related problems are often believed to occur
predominantly among 'alcoholics' and problem drinkers.
Whilst they do experience some of the most severe problems, in terms of the total impact on society as a whole, it
appears that most of the problems are contributed or experienced by regular heavy drinkers who are not and may
never become 'alcoholics', combined with the results of
intoxication experienced by a wide range of drinkers. This
paradox occurs because there are so many more of them in
the population, collectively contributing the larger share of
the total amount of harm, especially in relation to the
social problems related to alcohol consumption.

Table 26.2 summarizes the medical complications of
excess alcohol.

Alcohol is generally found to be a significant factor in:

■ hospital admissions

■ road traffic deaths

■ industrial accidents

■ accidental drowning

■ homicide

■ suicide

■ domestic violence

■ marital breakdown

■ absenteeism from work

■ child abuse.

Alcohol and the family

In 1997 Alcohol Concern estimated that there are likely to
be one million children in Britain living with a parent
whose drinking has reached harmful levels (Institute of
Alcohol Studies 1997–2000). A paper published by the
Institute of Alcohol Studies (IAS) shows that the children of problem-drinking parents have high rates of
health, behavioural and emotional problems such as tru-
ancy and poor school performance, antisocial behaviour
and delinquency, difficulty in forming relationships, and
psychiatric problems including depression. They are also
at increased risk themselves of abusing alcohol or other
drugs in later life (IAS 1997–2000).

Table 26.2 Medical complications of excess alcohol

System or organ	Clinical findings	System or organ	Clinical findings
Nervous system	Acute intoxication ■ blackouts Persistent brain damage ■ Wernicke's encephalopathy ■ Korsakoff's syndrome ■ cerebellar degeneration ■ dementia Cerebrovascular disease ■ strokes, especially in the young ■ subarachnoid haemorrhage ■ subdural haemotoma after head injury Withdrawal symptoms ■ tremor ■ hallucinations ■ fits Nerve and muscle damage ■ weakness ■ paralysis ■ burning sensation in hands and feet	**Respiratory system**	Fractured rib due to trauma Pneumonia from inhalation of vomit Overproduction of cortisol leading to obesity, acne, increased facial hair and high blood pressure Condition mimicking overactivity of the thyroid with loss of weight, anxiety, palpitations, sweating and tremor Severe fall in blood sugar level, sometimes leading to coma Intense facial flushing in many diabetics taking the antidiabetic drug chlorpropamide
Liver	Infiltration of liver with fat Alcoholic hepatitis Cirrhosis and eventual liver failure Liver cancer	**Reproductive system**	In men, loss of libido, reduced potency, shrinkage in size of testes and penis, reduced or absent sperm formation and so infertility In women, sexual difficulties, menstrual irregularities, and shrinkage of breasts and external genitalia
Gastrointestinal system	Reflux of acid into oesophagus Tearing and occasional rupture of oesophagus Cancer of oesophagus Gastritis Aggravation and impaired healing of peptic ulcers, diarrhoea and impaired absorption of food Chronic inflammation of the pancreas leading in some to diabetes and malabsorption of food	**Occupation and accidents**	Impaired work performance Increased risk and severity of accidents
Nutrition	Malnutrition from reduced intake of food, toxic effects of alcohol on intestine, and impaired metabolism, leading to weight loss Obesity, particularly in early stages of heavy drinking	**Fetus, child and family**	Damage to fetus and fetal alcohol syndrome Acute intoxication in young children produces hypothermia, low blood sugar levels, depressed respiration Effect on physical development and behaviour of child through heavy drinking by parents Interaction of alcohol with medicinal substances
Heart and circulatory system	Abnormal rhythms High blood pressure Chronic heart muscle damage leading to heart failure		Increased likelihood of unwanted effects of drugs Reduced effectiveness of medicines

From Royal College of Physicians (1987), with permission.

Alcohol and women

In recent decades it seems that the gap between men and women has narrowed, at least to some extent, in relation to both alcohol consumption and alcohol problems. Recent reports estimate that 2% of women aged 16–64 years report symptoms of alcohol dependence (compared with 7.5% of men). Some 5% of women who are more than occasional drinkers are 'problem drinkers' (psychological and/or physical dependence). This is an estimated 746 962 female problem drinkers (compared with 1 443 378 men; 9%); 13% of women are drinking more than 14 units per week, and 2% over the definitely harmful level of 35 units per week (IAS 1997–2000).

Many of the adverse effects of alcohol consumption are common to women and men, but some are more specific or acute for women (IAS 1997–2000):

- Social problems seem to be similar at any level of drinking.

- Women suffer some physical problems at lower levels of drinking than men.

- Women attain higher blood alcohol concentrations than men, even when allowing for differences in bodyweight.

- Women have a proportionately higher fat : water ratio and are less able to dilute alcohol in the body.

- Women are more prone to liver damage.

- Alcohol is linked to an increased risk of breast cancer.

- Some women report being more affected by alcohol when ovulating or when premenstrual because it takes longer for the alcohol to be metabolized.

- Oral contraception delays the absorption of alcohol into the bloodstream, and some women take longer to become intoxicated on this count.

- Moderate to heavy drinking may cause infertility.

- Alcohol consumption in pregnancy may occasionally result in damage to the fetus.

- Women may particularly become the victims of other people's drinking (e.g. sexual assault and rape).

Factors that predispose some women to develop problems in relation to alcohol include (IAS 1997–2000):

- family background of heavy drinking
- a history of sexual abuse
- low self-esteem
- traumatic life events
- association with eating disorders
- strain of sustaining multiple roles
- conflicts over female social roles.

Ageing
See chapter 1.3

Alcohol and young people

It was not until the 1960s that pubs and drinking became an integral part of the youth scene. By the 1980s, those aged 18–24 years had become the heaviest drinkers in the population, and the group least likely to abstain. This change has been accompanied by a decline in the age of onset of regular drinking.

A survey of 15–16-year-olds found that UK teenagers came at or near the top of the international league for binge drinking, drunkenness and the experience of alcohol problems (IAS 1997–2000):

- 21% of UK teenagers reported individual problems from their own drinking (reduced performance at school)

- 22% reported relationship problems (quarrels or arguments)

- 15% reported sexual problems (unwanted sexual experience or unprotected sex)

- 12% reported delinquency problems (scuffles or fights).

Alcohol and the elderly

Three types of elderly drinkers may be identified:

1. early onset or 'survivors' – a continuing problem that developed earlier in life

2. late onset or 'reactors' – often in response to traumatic life events

3. intermittent or binge drinkers.

People in categories 2 and 3 are thought to have a high chance of managing their alcohol problem if they have access to counselling and general support.

Tolerance to alcohol is significantly lowered in the elderly because of physical changes (IAS 1997–2000):

- a fall in the ratio of body water to fat, with less water for the alcohol to be diluted in

- decreased hepatic blood flow, so the liver receives more damage

- inefficiency of liver enzymes, so alcohol is not being broken down as efficiently

- altered responsiveness of the brain, with the alcohol having a faster effect.

Ageing tends to be associated with a growing burden of disease, and prolonged heavy drinking is itself a cause of health problems such as liver disease, raised blood pressure and some forms of cancer. Alcohol may also lead to an increased likelihood of falls, incontinence, cognitive impairment, hypothermia and self-neglect. These sorts of problems may be regarded merely as signs of ageing, by both health professionals and family members. The Royal College of Physicians (1987) suggested that as many as 60% of elderly people admitted to hospital because of confusion, repeated falls at home, recurrent chest infections and heart failure may have unrecognized alcohol problems.

Alcohol misuse can also be obscured by non-specific health problems such as gastrointestinal problems and insomnia, or misdiagnosed as dementia or depression. Health professionals may recognize and diagnose the secondary medical problem, but fail to combat the possible primary cause.

General practitioners are generally the first point of contact for elderly people, but some doctors may fail to diagnose alcohol misuse in a population where there are other urgent medical matters, and some believe that it may be better for the individual to continue their established pattern of drinking as altering it could be harmful. Elderly patients may show reluctance at disclosing their alcohol intake, and relatives may wish to hide the evidence of misuse of alcohol and deny existence of the problem. Appropriate screening measures are necessary to identify alcohol or other substance misuse among the elderly – and these measures need to be ongoing. It has been suggested that a full history of alcohol use should be taken at regular intervals, including questions about amounts taken in tea and coffee, which patients may regard as being irrelevant.

Treatment and counselling of older people needs to be based on assessment and matching of each person's needs to the range of treatment and services available. Emphasis needs to be placed on non-drinking social activities such as day centres and clubs in the context of the person's life circumstances and social support network. It may be necessary to work on redefining a social or family support mechanism. Some specialists argue that there is a need for specific treatment programmes designed for older people, as the likelihood of success would be higher than when older people are treated within a mixed-age client group.

Tobacco

In a vast number of countries, smoking typically begins in adolescence. Evidence suggests that the longer a person delays the onset of smoking the less likely they are to take up the habit. Therefore, it is vital that intensive efforts be made to encourage young non-smokers to stay smoke-free (WHO 1996).

The process of graduation from first use to addiction may take months or even years. In fact, initial experiences with tobacco are sometimes negative, and social pressure and other factors are required to maintain exposure until the addiction develops. Tolerance to nicotine appears to be acquired over time, and experienced smokers can accept doses of nicotine that would make non-smokers ill (WHO 1996).

Effects on health and social well-being

Nicotine has been clearly recognized as addictive, and tobacco dependence has been classified as a mental and behavioural disorder according to the WHO's International Classification of Diseases, version 10 (ICD-10). All tobacco products contain substantial amounts of nicotine. Nicotine is absorbed readily from tobacco smoke in the lungs, and from smokeless tobacco in the mouth or nose. Nicotine is a powerful pharmacological agent that acts in a variety of ways at different sites in the body. After reaching the bloodstream, nicotine enters the brain, interacts with specific **receptors** in brain tissue, and initiates metabolic and electrical activity in the brain (WHO 1996).

Smoking is estimated to have caused around 3 million deaths a year worldwide in the early 1990s, and the death toll is steadily increasing. Unless current trends are reversed, that figure is expected to rise to 10 million deaths per year by the 2020s or early 2030s, with 70% of those deaths occurring in developing countries. The chief uncertainty is not whether these deaths will occur, but exactly when. Of all the diseases causally associated with smoking, lung cancer is the most well known. However, smoking causes more deaths from diseases other than lung cancer. In 1995, there were 514 000 smoking-caused lung cancer deaths in developed countries, compared with 625 000 smoking-related deaths from heart and other vascular diseases (WHO 1996).

The potential for behavioural and pharmacological treatment of the addicted tobacco user and the problems of withdrawal should be recognized. Although 75–85% of smokers (where this has been measured), want to quit and about a third have made at least three serious attempts, less than half of smokers succeed in stopping permanently before the age of 60 years. Nicotine dependence is clearly a major barrier to successful cessation. Therefore, smoking control policies should contain activities both to strengthen smokers' motivation to quit (health education, public information, price policies, smoke-free policies, behavioural treatment) and to reduce dependence-related difficulties for smokers to quit (behavioural and pharmacological treatment) (WHO 1996).

To achieve successful cessation of smoking on a very large scale, special 'cessation programmes' are far from enough. All health professionals, including doctors, nurses and pharmacists, should be given both basic and in-service training so that they are capable of providing advice and/or treatment for tobacco dependence.

Nicotinic receptors
*See chapters
2.1 & 2.5*

Commonly abused illicit drugs

This section of the chapter describes the key characteristics of commonly abused drugs. It is not a definitive guide to all drugs abused, but will give a summary of those that you will commonly come across in nursing practice. It will be structured into three main categories:

1. stimulant
2. depressant
3. hallucinogen.

It is important to bear in mind that drugs will be assigned to the category that describes their main effect. Some drugs cross over categories depending on, amongst other factors, the quantity they are taken in and the route of ingestion, i.e. the same drug (e.g. cannabis) may have a different subjective effect when smoked (depressant) than when swallowed (hallucinogen).

The groupings of drugs into stimulant, depressant and hallucinogen categories has been used in preference to the categorizations of 'hard' and 'soft' drugs. The terms 'hard' and 'soft' are not based on any description of effect and imply that some drugs are less harmful to all individuals.

Drugs produce a spectrum of effects, which will be perceived differently both across and within individuals. In some individuals 'soft' drugs such as cannabis can have a devastating effect on their ability to function. Conversely, some individuals manage to continue to function and maintain their everyday lives despite reliance on 'hard' drugs such as heroin and methadone.

The terms stimulant, depressant and hallucinogen describe the drugs' primary effects. They also indicate to us the possible effects when individuals simultaneously use drugs from two different categories (e.g. cancelling out the effect of a stimulant by using a depressant on top) or use two different drugs from the same category (e.g. the dangers of mixing two types of depressant – the increased risk of depressing the central nervous system, leading to unconsciousness and cardiac arrest).

Descriptive categories of commonly abused drugs

Classification Under the Misuse of Drugs Act 1971,'controlled drugs' are subdivided into three categories (Class A, B and C). The penalties received by individuals for illegal use of these drugs are defined by their category and the nature of the offence (i.e. possession, intent to supply, or supply):

- *Class A* – e.g. heroin, methadone, cocaine, ecstasy, cannabis oil, magic mushrooms (when prepared for consumption). Class A carries the highest penalties.

- *Class B* – e.g. amfetamine, methylamfetamine, cannabis resin and herb, barbiturate-based tranquillizers. Any Class B drug prepared for injection automatically becomes Class A.

- *Class C* – e.g. benzodiazepines (diazepam, temazepam, etc.) when not supplied by prescription from a physician; anabolic steroids.

Form and appearance What forms the drug commonly takes and how it looks.

Street names It is important to note that street names change across time and across region. The street names described here represent a sample of possibilities but it is worth checking with your local drug service to elicit up-to-date names.

Monetary cost Costs vary across time and across geographical regions. Knowing the approximate cost of the drug is useful in practice. Patients may often be unable to give you a reliable measure of how much of a drug they are using on a daily or a weekly basis, but they will probably be able to tell you how much they are spending on drugs during that period. By knowing the approximate cost of the drug for your region, you can work out with the patient how much of the drug they are using on a daily or weekly basis. Your local specialist drug service is the best source of up-to-date costs.

Method of use How the drug is commonly taken. The same drug can be treated and taken in a number of ways. The way the drug is taken affects the strength and often the nature of the effect that the user experiences from it. This is due to the speed and concentration of the drug permeating the blood–brain barrier. For example, smoking cocaine powder with tobacco weakens the effect of the drug, as much of the drug is lost to the air in smoke. In this case the amount ingested through this method is fairly minimal. Sniffing (snorting) cocaine intranasally means that the majority of the powder goes into the body and taken into the bloodstream through the capillaries in the nose; thus the effect is quicker and more intense than smoking the drug. However, the process is somewhat slowed by the amount of time the drug takes to be absorbed through the small capillaries in the nose into the bloodstream. Dissolving cocaine powder in water and injecting it directly into the vein ensures maximum take-up of the drug into the body. The drug goes directly into the bloodstream, thus permeating the blood–brain barrier at a higher concentration more quickly, maximizing the drug's effect and causing the user to experience a far faster and more intense 'high'.

Short-term use The effects of using the drug over the short term. This generally describes the sort of effect the user is aspiring to when using the drug. This section also covers unwanted side-effects of short-term use.

Long-term use Use over a longer period generally decreases the subjective 'positive' effects of the drug, making way for more negative effects. It is during this period with certain drugs that physical dependence may be a problem. In the case of drugs not associated with physical dependence, problems associated with psychological dependence may come to the fore.

Stimulants

Amfetamine

Classification Class B, unless prepared for injection, then Class A.

Forms and appearance There are three basic types of amfetamine: racemic amfetamines, dextroamfetamines and methylamfetamines. Amfetamine sold on the street today is generally illicitly manufactured amfetamine sulfate powder (which may be formed into tablets) rather than amfetamine diverted from legitimate sources. Production is relatively simple. Methylamfetamine is the most potent of the three types but has virtually disappeared from the streets since stocks were limited to hospitals.

Street names Sold under a variety of names: Speed, Billy, Whizz, Sulfate, Buzz.

Method of use Amfetamine powder can be sniffed (snorted), swallowed, dissolved in water and injected, or smoked with cannabis and/or tobacco.

Associated equipment Straws, needles, syringes, metal foil, rolled-up bank notes.

Effects of use Amfetamines act much like the body's natural adrenaline does in the face of stress, by arousing and activating the user. **Heart rate** and **breathing** speed up, pupils widen and appetite decreases. The user feels more alert, energetic, confident, cheerful, and less tired and bored. Higher doses induce feelings of intense exhilaration, rapid flow of ideas and feelings of greatly increased physical and mental capacity. Use of the drug may cause sleeplessness and increased aggression.

For some users the predominant feeling elicited by using amfetamine may be anxiety, irritability and restlessness, particularly as the body's energy stores become depleted. High doses, especially if repeated over a few days, can cause delirium, panic, hallucinations and feelings of persecution ('amfetamine psychosis') which should gradually disappear as the drug is eliminated from the body.

The effects of a single dose last about 3–4 hours and leave the user feeling tired; it may take a couple of days for the body to recover fully, even after small doses.

Possible adverse effects Amfetamine use may lead to lethargy, fatigue, depression, irritability, panic, dry mouth, diarrhoea and increased urination, an increase in blood pressure with increased risk of stroke. Long-term use or a 'run' of use will lead the user feeling depressed, lethargic and ravenously hungry, as amfetamines postpone fatigue, sleep and hunger. The mood-elevating aspects of amfetamine can lead to psychological dependence. Physical dependence is rare, but in frequent users tolerance may develop to the stimulant effect of amfetamine, so users have a tendency to increase the dose. With increased doses toxic effects may develop, including delusions, hallucinations and feelings of paranoia. Fatal overdose is possible, particularly with inexperienced users.

Cocaine

Classification Class A.

Forms and appearance Cocaine hydrochloride, white crystalline powder, occasionally in paste form.

Street names Coke, charlie, snow.

Methods of use Usually sniffed (snorted) or rubbed on the gums, but may be mixed with water and injected. The paste form may be smoked in a pipe.

Associated equipment Rolled-up bank notes, shiny surface such as a mirror, straws, pipes, needles and syringes.

Effects of use As with amfetamine, the drug activates the body's fight or flight mechanism, acting like adrenaline, causing the heart to beat faster and the body to speed up generally. It gives a sense of heightened awareness, euphoria, increased confidence, of being affable and chatty, an energy rush and agitation, and feelings of power.

Possible adverse effects Users may experience lethargy, fatigue, paranoia, panic, depression, irritability and weight loss (over prolonged periods of use). Cocaine use may also lead to delusions and aggression. Regular use by snorting can damage the nasal passages. Like any injected substance, cocaine use can lead to skin ulcers or collapsed veins at the injection sites. Use may lead to both physical and psychological dependence. Heavy long-term users may experience paranoid psychosis, although this may also occur in some individuals with relatively low levels of use.

Ecstasy (3,4-methylenedioxymethamfetamine; MDMA)

Classification Class A.

Forms and appearance Capsules and tablet form in a variety of shapes, colours and sizes. Also available as an off-white powder.

Street names E, pills, Erics, XTC, love doves, disco biscuits.

Associated equipment None.

Method of use Will generally be swallowed, but can also be snorted in powder form or by emptying contents of capsules.

Effects of use Users experience increased energy, loss of inhibitions, feelings of euphoria and loss of appetite. Less positive aspects may include dry mouth and throat and muscle cramps. Objectively, facial grimacing and increased sweating may be observed. It should be noted that a lot of ecstasy purchased contains very little or no MDMA; rather, it is a combination in variable concentrations of LSD, amfetamine and ketamine. This obviously has implications for the effects experienced by the user, which are highly variable. Thus, a user reporting that they have ingested ecstasy may present with hallucinations more commonly associated with the ingestion of a hallucinogen such as LSD. It is therefore important in assessment to ask the user what they have taken, but also to enquire after the subjective effects. Do not assume that individuals presenting after ingestion of ecstasy will always present with the effects documented above. There is no method of buyers exercising quality control in the drugs market!

Possible adverse effects The user may experience nausea and vomiting, dehydration, raised blood pressure, overheating (hyperthermia), convulsions and sudden death, through heart attack or brain haemorrhage. In the aftermath of the drug the user may feel fatigue and depression.

Crack cocaine

Classification Class A.

Forms and appearance Crack is a much stronger form of cocaine consisting of small crystals. It is produced by 'washing up' cocaine hydrochloride with ammonia or baking soda. The crystals are of varying sizes, shapes and colours, ranging from waxy white to pinkish yellow and clear yellow.

Heart rate
See chapter 4.2

Respiration
See chapter 5.3

Street names Rock, crack, stone, nuggets, freebase, wash.

Associated equipment Crack pipe, perforated can, metal foil, Rizla papers, tobacco and cannabis mix (smoked as a 'spliff'; see section on cannabis).

Method of use Smoked from pipe.

Effects of use Euphoria and indifference to fatigue.

Possible adverse effects Depression, fatigue, lethargy, irritability, anxiety and severe paranoia. The user may develop a psychosis accompanied by bizarre and often violent behaviour. Increased risks of lung damage due to harsh effects of smoking. Psychological and physical dependence is common.

Alkyl nitrites

Classification Not classified under the Act, although amyl-nitrite is classified as a pharmacy medicine.

Forms and appearance Clear, yellow, volatile and flammable liquids (essentially solvents). The two most common are amyl nitrite and butyl nitrite. The main medical use of amyl nitrites is as an antidote to cyanide poisoning.

Street names Poppers, and by brand name, e.g. TNT, Rush, Rock Hard.

Associated equipment Small bottle approximately the size of a Tippex bottle.

Method of use Sniffed in short bursts.

Effects of use After inhalation the effects are almost instantaneous. The user experiences a 'rush' as blood vessels dilate, heartbeat quickens and blood rushes to the brain. The person may experience a pounding headache, dizziness, flushed face and neck, and 'light-headedness'. The drug is sold freely in sex shops with the claim that it enhances sexual pleasure, prolonging the sensation of orgasm and preventing premature ejaculation. It may, however, impede erection in some male users.

Possible adverse effects Irregular heartbeat, rise in blood pressure and strain on the heart. Increased health concerns if injecting, associated with sharing of injecting equipment.

Depressants

Cannabis

Classification Class B.

Forms and appearance Three main types predominate. Herbal cannabis is a greenish-brown dried plant material. These include Skunk and Sinsemilla. Cannabis resin comes in various colours and shapes in dried and compressed blocks. Cannabis oil is thick and ranges in colour from dark green to brown. It has a distinctive smell like rotting vegetation.

Street names Hash, draw, puff, blow, dope, herb, weed.

Associated equipment Rizla papers, home-made pipes, cling-film wraps.

Method of use Most commonly smoked but can be swallowed raw, added to cooking or made into a drink.

Effects of use Relaxation, light intoxication, giggles, increased appetite (the munchies) increased talkativeness and heightened senses. Skunk, which is intensively grown in special circumstances to increase its strength, has a much quicker onset of effects. Users of skunk have reported elation, profound relaxation, alteration of time and perception, and mild hallucinations. As with many drugs, the mood of the person may determine the effects experienced. First-time users of cannabis may feel very little effect from the drug, and may have to learn what effects to look for.

Possible adverse effects Controversy continues over whether long-term use of cannabis causes lasting damage to physical or mental health. There is still little conclusive evidence either way. However, users may experience inability to concentrate, clumsiness and 'red eye'. Objectively they may appear drunk. Due to inhalation through smoking either with or without tobacco there may be potential for bronchial problems and cancer. Users may experience short-term memory loss and demotivation. Withdrawal effects such as anxiety, panic, restlessness and disturbed sleep patterns have also been noted.

Heroin

Classification Class A.

Forms and appearance Brown-pink or off-white powder. Naturally occurring substance derived from the opium poppy.

Street names H, skag, smack, junk.

Associated equipment Needles, syringes and tin foil.

Method of use Can be injected, smoked ('chasing the dragon'), snorted or taken orally.

Effects of use Comfort, warmth, euphoria, emotional detachment and pain relief. The drug's effect lasts for 3–6 hours.

Possible adverse effects Heroin, like all opiates, depresses the central nervous system, thus lowering breathing and heart rate. Initially users may experience nausea and vomiting. Users may also suffer from severe constipation. There are a number of well publicized problems associated with intravenous drug use such as the development of abscesses on injecting sites, sharing needles leading to a greatly increased incidence of HIV and hepatitis infection. High incidence of physical and psychological dependence. Opiate use may interfere with women's menstrual cycle but will not necessarily stop her from becoming pregnant.

Methadone

Classification Class A, unless individually prescribed.

Forms and appearance Clear injectable ampoules, small white tablets, brown, orange or green linctus.

Street names 'Script', juice, red rock, doll, linctus.

Associated equipment Medicine bottles, needles and syringes.

Method of use Methadone is a synthetic opiate used as a heroin substitute and prescribed to those engaging in a heroin detoxification or treatment package. It also has a street value and is regularly sold on the drugs market. It is usually swallowed in syrup form but can also be prescribed as tablets. Doctors have, however, been advised by the Department of Health to not prescribe it in tablet form, as tablets are worth more on the illicit market, increasing the likelihood that it will be sold on. Methadone can also be taken in an injectable form.

Effects of use Methadone has a less intense but longer lasting effect than heroin. Users experience relaxation, bodily warmth and suppression of the withdrawal effects of heroin dependency that lasts for up to 24 hours.

Possible adverse effects Users may experience bouts of sweating, disruption to the menstrual cycle, constipation, nausea, itching and tiredness, physical and psychological dependence.

Benzodiazepines

Classification Class C. Supply without prescription is illegal, but it is not illegal to possess benzodiazepines in medicinal form without a prescription, with the exception of temazepam. Benzodiazepines include diazepam (Valium), chlordiazepoxide (Librium), nitrazepam (Mogadon), Nobrium, lorazepam (Ativan), temazepam, flurazepam (Dalmane) and flunitrazepam (Rohypnol).

Forms and appearance Commonly prescribed tranquillizers and hypnotics, the benzodiazepines are in tablet and capsule form in various colours, shapes and sizes.

Street names Benzos, jellies, goosies, temazzies, tranx, pills.

Associated equipment Needles and syringes.

Method of use Swallowed or melted down or crushed for injection.

Effects of use Light intoxication, drowsiness, headache, confusion, ataxia. May be used by stimulant users to 'come down' or sleep after a prolonged period of stimulant use. May also be used by injecting opiate users when their drug of choice is unavailable or they cannot afford it. Benzodiazepines may also be used to augment the effect of other depressant drugs such as alcohol or heroin.

Possible adverse effects Users may experience a 'hangover' effect after use. In high doses aggression, violent mood swings, deep depression, liver damage, lethargy and bizarre sexual behaviour may occur. Physical and psychological dependence is common.

GHB (gamma hydroxybutyrate)

Classification GHB is classed as a medicine, so possession is not an offence, but unauthorized manufacture and distribution could be an offence under the Medicines Act.

Forms and appearance GHB was developed in the USA as an anaesthetic and is used as a premedication to promote sleep before surgery. It has sedative rather than painkilling effects. It is a colourless, odourless liquid that is sold in small bottles or capsule form.

Street names GBH, liquid E, liquid X.

Associated equipment GHB bottles.

Method of use Swallowed.

Effects of use As GHB is sold in liquid form, it is impossible to tell how concentrated the liquid is: a bottle could contain 3 g of the drug, quite a mild dose, or up to 20 g – a very high dose. At low doses the drug induces euphoria and loss of inhibitions. At higher doses, however, euphoria gives way to powerful sedative effects along with hallucinations, muscular tremors and facial grimacing. The effects of the drug are experienced between 10 minutes and 1 hour after ingestion, and are reported to last for up to a day.

Possible adverse effects Users may experience nausea, vomiting, disorientation, muscular pain, depression, fatigue, convulsions, coma, respiratory collapse and death.

Ketamine

Classification Ketamine is not controlled under the Misuse of Drugs Act, so possession is not an offence; however, unauthorized supply is illegal.

Forms and appearance Tablets, capsules or as a soluble crystalline powder, or in its liquid pharmaceutical form for injecting.

Street names K, Special K, Vitamin K, kit kat.

Associated equipment Straws, rolled-up notes, needles and syringes.

Method of use Swallowed, snorted or injected.

Effects of use Users experience euphoria in an initial 'rush', intense hallucinations and feelings of depersonalization.

Possible adverse effects Users may experience fatigue, cramps, severe depression, vomiting, irritability, violent reactions, flashbacks similar to those experienced with LSD, heart failure.

Solvents

Classification Not controlled under the Act, although it is against the law to sell solvents to known or suspected young solvent misusers.

Forms and appearance Solvents are commercial products.

Street names Glue, gas, can, cog.

Method of use Sprayed directly into the mouth or inhaled from a bag, handkerchief or rag.

Effects of use The user experiences intense intoxication, loss of balance, and auditory and visual hallucinations. Solvents are a manufactured product that generally have a depressant effect on the central nervous system, although in some individuals they may have a stimulant effect. Effects can be heightened by increasing the concentration of the vapour by sniffing from a plastic bag held at the mouth or nose, or in some instances placed over the head, which is extremely dangerous for obvious reasons. It is also equally dangerous to spray the chemicals directly into the mouth.

Possible adverse effects There is a danger of accidents whilst intoxicated or hallucinating. Loss of short-term memory and cognitive skills, personality changes, kidney damage, liver and bowel disorders, and acute brain damage. There is a danger of sudden death. Solvents cause more deaths than any other recreational drugs – apart from alcohol and tobacco.

Barbiturates

Classification Class B. Barbiturates are known as hypno-sedatives. In lower doses they have a calming effect and in higher dose act as sleeping pills.

Forms and appearance Tablet or capsule form in various sizes and colours.

Street names Barbs, downers, sleepers.

Associated equipment Needles and syringes.

Method of use May be swallowed. Barbiturates do not tend to be popular with younger recreational drug users. They tend to be abused by 'heavy end' dependent drug users. Barbiturates can also be dissolved in water and injected into the vein.

Effects of use Barbiturates provide temporary relief from fears, tensions and anxiety. The user may appear drunk. Effects are considerably increased when combined with alcohol and other drugs, and can last for up to 16 hours.

Possible adverse effects Sudden withdrawal from very high doses may be fatal. If there are no complications, withdrawal effects generally subside within a week. Heavy users are susceptible to bronchitis and pneumonia (because the cough reflex is depressed), hypothermia and accidental overdose (as the drugs can cause confusion and tolerance effects). Most of the adverse effects are increased when if the drug is injected.

Hallucinogens

LSD (lysergic acid diethylamide)

Classification Class A.

Forms and appearance $0.5\,cm^2$ blotters of paper, usually printed with a design from popular culture such as cartoon characters. More rarely, very small tablets and, rarer still, powder form.

Street names Acid, trips, micros, tabs, dots.

Associated equipment None.

Method of use Swallowed or dissolved on the tongue.

Effects of use LSD is a powerful hallucinogen. Hallucinations may be visual, auditory or tactile. They can range from being very pleasant to extremely unpleasant. This may be influenced by the mood of the user before ingestion. The person's sense of time appears to change, and things take on a new perspective. Effects last between 8 and 12 hours.

Possible adverse effects Reoccurrence of hallucination many weeks or months after stopping the drug (referred to as 'flashbacks'). Accidents whilst hallucinating; users may believe they have powers above their ability, for example that they can fly. Use may precipitate latent psychiatric disorders.

Magic mushrooms

Classification The mushrooms are not illegal but their active ingredients psilocin and psilocybin are controlled Class A drugs. It is therefore illegal to boil, crush or make a 'preparation or other product' containing the active ingredients.

Forms and appearance There are several varieties that are all very different in appearance. Identification may be difficult, and mistakes are easily made.

Street names Shrooms, mushies.

Associated equipment None.

Method of use Swallowed, raw, cooked or boiled.

Effects of use The effects of magic mushrooms are similar to those of a mild LSD experience. Variability in effect due to user's mood: euphoria, high spirits and well-being, bouts of giggling, visual and auditory hallucinations.

Possible adverse effects Dizziness, nausea, possibility of stimulating latent psychiatric disorders. Accidental ingestion of poisonous mushroom by mistake.

What if I haven't a clue about the drug a patient is talking about?

If, during assessment or care, a patient discloses use of drugs that are not described in this section, there are a number of different sources to contact for information on the effects of the drug. It is easy to feel deskilled in these circumstances, but accessible information is available in a variety of places. Your local health promotion unit should be able to provide information produced by national organizations such as Lifeline or Release. These organizations provide booklets and pamphlets that are readily accessible to both professionals and the general public.

You should also be careful not to fall into the common trap of assuming that because a patient uses certain drugs they have a sound knowledge of the long-term effects of drug use. Drug use is generally focused on short-term gains and clients may often find it difficult to project into the future concerning their use. It is good practice to give the patient as much information about the drugs they are using as possible. The use of pamphlets such as those developed by Lifeline provides an opportunity to give patients objective information without appearing patronizing or pushy. You should also give patients the opportunity to discuss the contents of the leaflet with you wherever possible, to ensure they fully understand the information presented in the leaflet. In these circumstances it is important to be aware of the address of your local drug service, in order to be able to direct the patient there should they require more specialist information or help.

Multidisciplinary working and service structures

With the continued rise of substance misuse in the general population, it is inevitable that nurses will increasingly find they are providing care to individuals with substance misuse problems. Nurses can have a number of pivotal roles when working with individuals with these complex difficulties. This work may occur at the primary care, secondary care or tertiary care level.

A number of the key roles nurses can take are:

- engaging, assessing and appropriately referring on if there is a perceived level of significant harm related to substance use
- screening and early recognition
- harm minimization and prevention
- health promotion and education
- advice and support to the individual
- promotion of risk awareness in relation to substance misuse
- advice and support to the family
- counselling
- ongoing support in the community to individuals on maintenance or withdrawal programmes
- crisis intervention
- shared care
- acting as a key player in policy developments
- use as a consultant and resource for colleagues.

The extent to which each of these roles will be taken on by a nurse is dependent on the context of the service they are working in and their level of experience and interest in working with this client group. However, it should be acknowledged that a number of these roles are core business for any nurse, whatever setting they are working in, namely:

- screening and recognition of substance misuse problems
- promotion of risk awareness to substance-misusing individuals, including basic harm minimization strategies
- ability to engage, assess and refer on to the appropriate agency, according to the individual's expressed need.

The support of an individual with entrenched substance misuse problems often requires a multidisciplinary approach, rather than a response by an individual clinician. A multidisciplinary response takes account of the complexity and difficulties surrounding substance misuse.

For example, an individual with an enduring heroin habit may require support and advice on harm minimization techniques that can be provided by the general nurse. However, he or she may also require a methadone prescription for maintenance or reduction of the use, which will involve a prescribing physician, such as a general practitioner or specialist psychiatrist. The patient could also require the skills of a social worker for a community care assessment, for inpatient detoxification services or housing issues. He or she may have had contact with the criminal justice system, and therefore need to see a probation officer, and might also be seeing a counsellor for mental health-related issues.

As you can see, individuals can quickly develop their own multidisciplinary 'team' around them to meet their complex needs. In some areas, individuals such as this will be referred on to a specialist drug team. In other cases, which may among other reasons be due to the client's reluctance to engage with the specialist team, or because a specialist team approach is not available in that area, care may be coordinated at a primary or secondary care level. In these cases, communication between each of the workers associated with the individual is imperative. This is where the service model of shared care originates.

Shared care

The Department of Health (1995) defines shared care as:

> The joint participation of specialists and GPs (and other agencies where appropriate) in the planned delivery of care for patients with a drug misuse problem, informed by an enhanced information exchange beyond routine discharge and referral letters. It may involve the day to day management by the GP of the patient's medical needs in relation to his or her drug misuse. Such arrangements would make explicit which clinician was responsible for different

aspects of the patient's treatment and care. These may include prescribing substitute drugs in appropriate circumstances.

A recent policy document on guidelines for clinical management of drug misuse and dependence produced by the DoH (1999a, p. 10) highlighted a number of factors, of particular relevance to drug misusers which highlighted the need to firm up the process of shared care:

■ Shared care aims to deliver a flexible service, based on individual need, utilising the differing skills of a number of health professionals in the most effective manner.

■ The general shift towards a better balance of primary and secondary healthcare provision, with the emphasis being placed on a primary care led NHS.

■ An increasing preference by drug misusers to receive care in a primary care setting in the community wherever possible.

■ Expansion of the primary healthcare team to include a wide range of specialist mental health staff, including community psychiatric nurses, clinical psychologists, and specialist drug and alcohol workers.

■ The increasing number of young drug misusers whose natural first point of contact is their family GP.

The document further comments that shared care should not be limited solely to those drug users who require substitute prescribing, but should aim to include interventions to support and aid drug misusers who wish to give up but do not need substitute prescribing. It should also include specific treatment interventions such as counselling and other therapeutic input, and also interventions carried out between general practice and voluntary drug agencies.

Shared care arrangements already exist in all parts of the UK. However, the success of shared care in any given area will depend heavily on good communication, trust and understanding between all the services involved and the evolution of shared protocols to meet regional needs.

Primary care

Over 90% of the population enjoy an occasional drink, one-third of all adults smoke tobacco, minor tranquillizer use is estimated to be in the thousands, and at least 6% of the population are believed to take an illegal drug. About two-thirds of patients consult their general practitioner at least once a year, and more than 90% at least every 5 years. Therefore, nurses working in primary healthcare teams will directly or indirectly come into contact with substance misuse. The importance of screening at this stage lies in the fact that many people accessing primary care may not present with an obvious substance misuse problem. The nurse's knowledge and clinical skills in relation to drugs, solvents and alcohol, and to the risks and consequences of their use, may be the basis for effective interventions with patients, families and communities (Clancey 1997).

A number of opportunities present for screening in primary care settings:

■ prenatal checks

■ child and adolescent check-ups

■ well woman clinics

■ family planning clinics

■ well men clinics

■ new patient registrations

■ specialist clinics (e.g. asthma, diabetes)

■ routine primary care visits.

These opportunities are reinforced by factors such as the flexibility of surgery hours, giving more accessibility for consultations, and the reduced stigma of labelling, whereby some people perceive specialist services to be only for 'addicts'. However, the perception of obstacles still impedes some people from seeking help:

■ poor previous experiences with health and social care agencies

■ treatment of substance misuse being seen as a specialist, rather than primary care, function

■ judgemental attitudes towards substance misuse

■ being refused treatment and appropriate support

■ fear that prescribed medication for other conditions may be stopped

■ potential breaches of confidentiality, e.g. to other family members or employers.

Accident and emergency

Nurses working in A&E departments, and increasing numbers of minor injuries units, will be well aware of the problems caused by acutely intoxicated people: verbal aggression, physical violence, demanding and uncooperative behaviour. However, the real picture is also one of many people presenting whose alcohol or drug problems go unnoticed.

A national survey of A&E departments by Waller et al (1998) found that:

■ alcohol is an important factor in about 10 000 attendances a year at the average A&E department

■ few departments have detection procedures or intervention practices in place

■ little training or specialist information is routinely available

■ literature identifies that brief interventions have been effective in reducing alcohol consumption by up to 25–30% in excessive drinkers in primary care and hospital wards

- potential for effective intervention in A&E is unclear

- staff perceive considerable barriers to the adoption of a preventive role

- attitudes towards improving the response to alcohol-related problems are mostly positive (especially among nurses).

A&E provides a main interface between primary care and specialist secondary care services, presenting important opportunities for early detection, prevention, appropriate assessment and intervention, and referral to the appropriate sources of help and support.

For many patients A&E may be the only place they present to health services. Consequently, the opportunity to screen, intervene and refer on should not be lost. People may present to A&E with a range of symptoms from mild to life-threatening, and full assessment is vitally important.

The following conditions may mimic drug or alcohol use intoxication, and are frequently encountered in the A&E setting:

- early signs of cerebrovascular accident

- head trauma

- neurological disorders

- shock due to injuries

- confusion due to hypoglycaemia

- infection

- side-effects of prescribed medication

- acute schizophrenia.

Dual diagnosis (substance misuse and severe mental illness)

There is a high incidence of crossover between psychiatric disorders and substance misuse. A number of research studies have found that approximately one-third of heavy drinkers have associated mental health problems, and one-half of dependent drug users have mental health problems of varying severity (DoH 1999a).

There have also been several studies indicating that individuals in contact with mental health services have increased rates of alcohol and drug problems, with upwards of one-third reporting such difficulties (Menezes et al 1996). Individuals with these complex needs also tend to be over represented in the prison and homeless populations.

Service structures for this group in the UK are in their infancy. Individuals with these difficulties often rely on a number of services, which requires good communication and high levels of coordination. Studies from the USA suggest that integrated services – where the individual receives help for both their mental health problems and their substance misuse difficulties from the same

team – show better results than parallel or concurrent service structures (Gournay et al 1997, Manley 1998).

Although there are specialist integrated services for those with a 'dual diagnosis' under development in the UK, it is unlikely that specialist teams will serve all such individuals.

Assessment

Good assessment is essential to high-quality continuing care of any individual who misuses substances. For the nurse assessment can take place on three levels:

1. triage – for emergency screening

2. screening

3. in-depth assessment.

Aims of assessment

- Treatment of any emergency or acute problem.

- Confirmation that the individual is taking alcohol and/or drugs (history, examination and urine analysis).

- Assessment of the degree of dependence.

- Identification of any complications of alcohol or drug misuse, and assessment of risk behaviour.

- Identification of other medical, social or mental health problems.

- Provision of advice on harm minimization including, if appropriate, access to sterile injecting equipment, testing for hepatitis, HIV and immunization against hepatitis B.

- Determination of the individual's expectations of treatment and the degree of motivation to change.

- Assessment of the most appropriate level of expertise required to manage the individual (primary care, specialist team, etc.).

- Determination of the need for substitute medication (DoH 1999a).

Triage assessment

Triage assessment is a short assessment, typically lasting only a few minutes and carried out by specially trained nurses. Triage is practised in situations requiring a quick response to emergencies such as A&E departments or telephone help-lines, and sometimes other primary care settings. The aim of triage is to establish the degree of emergency for the presenting individual, to determine whether they need immediate intervention or a longer, more specialized, assessment. The aim of triage could be described as a system designed to treat any emergency or acute problem whilst filtering out problems that can be assessed or treated over time.

Screening

Screening is an essential part of the assessment process. This part of the assessment should be covered as a matter of course for any individual presenting to health services. It involves a low level of assessment, with generally unobtrusive questioning to establish whether the individual might have problems with substances. A well validated example is the CAGE tool which is used extensively by nurse practitioners and practice nurses to screen for alcohol-related problems. The tool uses four simple questions:

Cutdown: Ever felt the need to cut down?

Annoyed: Ever felt annoyed by criticism of your drinking?

Guilty: Ever had guilty feelings about your drinking?

Eye-opener: Ever felt the need for a drink to get you started in the morning?

If the person answers yes to any of these questions, this indicates there is a problem (Mayfield et al 1974). Used in a non-judgemental way this sort of questioning can give people a chance to disclose any 'use' that may have been causing them concern.

Screening should be carried out in a safe, confidential environment, with sensitivity towards the individual's, the family's, or the community's race, culture, gender, sexuality, religion and age (Clancey 1997). It is also of paramount importance that you are clear about your own attitudes towards these issues, in order that you enable all individuals to obtain equal access to services (Clancey and Coyne 1997).

If the results of the screening procedure highlight any issues in need of further consideration, the nurse might take one of the following routes:

1. discussion with or referral to a specialist worker or team

2. brief intervention advice with follow-up

3. in-depth assessment and specialist follow-up.

In-depth assessment

An in-depth assessment of substance misuse should cover at least the following areas:

- reason for presenting to the service

- past substance use

- current substance use (over the past 4 weeks)

- history of injecting and risk of hepatitis and HIV

- medical history

- psychiatric history

- forensic history

- social history

HIV
See chapter 6.2

- past contact with treatment services

- other, for example substance misuse in spouse or family members.

The following areas should also be subject to examination:

- assessment of motivation

- assessment of general health

- assessment of mental health

- assessment of social and family situation.

The following special investigations may also be carried out to aid an in-depth assessment:

- haematological – such as testing for **HIV** antibody (before any test of this sort full informed consent should be received from the individual), liver function tests, blood alcohol levels

- urine toxicology

- breathalyser

- physical examination – e.g. gait, track marks, abscesses, injection sites, skin pallor, pupil size, irritability, drowsiness, smell of breath, hair analysis.

Barriers to effective assessment include (Clancey 1998):

- fear of professional judgement

- fear of being refused treatment

- belief that disclosure of substance use is not appropriate in a particular setting (e.g. A&E)

- poor previous experiences

- fear of 'loss of control'

- difficulty staying in the waiting area due to withdrawal symptoms

- fear of information being placed on medical records

- concern about the family being informed

- concern about police and other agencies being informed

- fear of being labelled 'drug user' or 'alcoholic'

- nurse's experience and confidence

- lack of information about specialist agencies or services

- negative attitudes towards drug and alcohol users

- appropriate skills.

Assessment is not merely for assessment's sake, but should form the basis on which to build a care plan that adequately meets the individual's needs. During the care planning stage the nurse should help the individual to explore and clarify his or her aims and objectives with regard to substance use. Care planning should always take into account the individual's motivation to change and also the outcomes the individual perceives as desirable. The assessment process should also enable the nurse to identify where the individual's care needs would best be met, for example in the primary care setting or in a specialist service.

Treatment interventions

Reducing alcohol problems

There is no single solution to reducing alcohol-related harm. What is required is a comprehensive range of strategies, that can address the many causes and dimensions of alcohol problems. These may include (WHO 1996):

- controls on price and availability
- minimum age for purchasing alcohol
- legislative measures to curb driving while under the influence of alcohol
- restrictions on the promotion, marketing and advertising of alcohol
- public education and awareness programmes
- primary healthcare and community-based interventions.

In the UK, at a national level, because of the known link between total national consumption and the amount of alcohol-related harm, reducing alcohol problems means reducing the total consumption of alcohol. There is also a need to impact upon patterns of consumption and social attitudes to drinking and drunkenness, e.g. drinking and driving.

At the individual level, people who are already experiencing alcohol problems or who are in danger of doing so need to be encouraged to eliminate the risk by stopping drinking, or to reduce it by cutting down. Depending on the severity of the problems, this could involve getting help from a treatment agency or a process of self-help. People who are alcohol dependent are advised to seek specialist help. Either way, individuals need to make a firm decision to give up or cut down, and then look for ways of maintaining their resolve over time. This is likely to involve (IAS 1997–2000):

- recognizing and understanding the harm experienced as a result of drinking
- understanding the functions that alcohol was performing (psychological, social), so as to be able to find alternatives
- identify high-risk times and situations, so as to be able to learn to cope with them in another way, or avoid them.

Aims of treatment for drug misuse

Substance misuse treatment, as befits its complex nature, aims to fulfil a number of individual and social needs. Treatment aims are summarized in Box 26.3.

> **Box 26.3** Treatment aims for substance misuse
>
> - Reduction of the use of illicit or non-prescribed drugs by the individual
> - Assist the individual to remain healthy, until, with appropriate care and support, they can achieve a drug-free life
> - Deal with the problems related to substance misuse
> - Reduce the duration of episodes of substance misuse
> - Reduce the dangers associated with substance misuse, particularly the risk of HIV, hepatitis B and C, and other bloodborne infections from injecting and sharing injecting paraphernalia
> - Reduce the chance of future relapse to substance misuse
> - Reduce the need for criminal activity to finance substance misuse
> - Reduce the risk of prescribed drugs being diverted on to the illegal market
> - Stabilize the individual, where appropriate, on substitute medication, to alleviate withdrawal symptoms
> - Improve overall personal, social and family well-being.
>
> Adapted from DoH 1999a.

As previously discussed, no single model can provide us with a full explanation of drug misuse or addiction. Donovan and Marlatt (1988) eloquently describe this in their attempt to draw together a definition that covers all aspects of addiction, not just to alcohol and drugs. They define an addiction as 'a complex, progressive behaviour pattern having biological, psychological, sociological and behavioural components'. The pattern differs from others because of the individual's overwhelming pathological involvement in or attachment to it, and because of his or her reduced ability to exert control over it despite its negative impact on physical, psychological and social functioning. Thus interventions need to be targeted to take account of each of these factors. Every individual will have his or her own unique profile of how each of the factors interrelate, and the aim of a good care plan would be to target each of these factors according to individual need. This further highlights the importance of a thorough and well-structured assessment, as without this a key area maintaining drug and alcohol use may be overlooked.

There are many variations of therapeutic approach that can be used with individuals misusing substances. This section aims to give an overview of some of the common interventions used in clinical practice in the substance misuse field. The interventions are linked to a common model of behaviour change, to highlight how efficacy of intervention may be impeded or increased depending on how ready the individual is, on a psychological level, to maintain that change.

Prochaska and DiClemente (1982) model of behaviour change.

This model was developed in an attempt to make sense of the processes individuals go through in making changes to their behaviour. It provides a good structure to think about changing drug (including tobacco) and alcohol using behaviours as, not only can the stage the patient is at on a cognitive level be mapped, but the model also give some guidance on the interventions the patient may be able to respond to and make use of at any given time. The model follows a number of stages:

1. Pre-contemplation
2. Contemplation
3. Determination
4. Action
5. Maintenance.

Each of these stages is explained below.

Pre-contemplation stage This is the period prior to the individual recognizing the need to change. People around them may have highlighted that they think there may be a problem, but the person concerned does not recognize it.

Contemplation stage The individual recognizes that there is a problem and begins to consider doing something about it.

Determination stage The individual begins to think through how they can effect change.

Action stage The individual attempts to change behaviour, either through his or her own efforts, or by seeking treatment.

Maintenance stage The individual seeks to maintain the change.

It is important to note that the model is circular in approach rather than linear. This acknowledges that effecting change is difficult and not a direct process. Individuals may journey around the circle any number of times before effecting behaviour change. They may fall out of the stages at any point. When this happens during the active change stage or the maintenance stage it is called relapse. Individuals who experience relapse may then enter back into the circle at any given point. Individuals will also reside in each of the stages for varying lengths of time; for example, they may stay in contemplation for years and then a significant event might occur that focuses them into thinking about how to change.

How does the model of behaviour change fit with intervention?

Substance-using individuals will go round this cycle autonomously, without treatment. Things will happen in their lives that will make them think about their use, and spur decisions to attempt to change their behaviour. Some people will be successful on their own in this; for example, the birth of a child means a couple can no longer attend clubs, so their use of ecstasy is discontinued. But for others, who may be physically or psychologically dependent on the substance, or be in a context where social factors may make it difficult to change, outside help may be required.

The model works as an aid to guide both the clinician and the user toward which interventions would be most useful at a given time. For example, individuals who have been referred to drug services via the probation service may not feel that they have a problem with drug use. They would be in the Pre-contemplation stage of the model. They might then benefit from an approach such as motivational interviewing (Miller and Rollnick 1991), which would work towards moving them on to look at their drug or alcohol use in a less positive light. They would not generally, however, benefit from an intervention such as relapse prevention at this stage, as they have not yet acknowledged that they have a problem. An intervention such as relapse prevention would be targeted mainly around the Maintenance stage.

A sample of clinical interventions used with substance misusers

Medical interventions

Medical interventions tend to be focused on the detoxification or maintenance of substance users who are physically dependent on their substances. The major treatment groups for medical interventions are people using heroin, benzodiazepines and alcohol. There is also a limited amount of medical intervention for people with dependency on stimulant drugs.

Why prescribe substitute drugs?

Prescribing is the responsibility of the prescribing doctor, whether this is the individual's general practitioner or a specialist doctor in a drug treatment facility. Prescribing medication as an alternative to the individual's drug of choice may fulfil a number of different functions, some of which are listed below:

- Offer an opportunity to stabilize drug intake and lifestyle whilst breaking with previous illicit drug use and associated unhealthy behaviours.

- Reduce or prevent withdrawal symptoms (see Box 26.4).

- Promote the process of change in drug taking (giving the person a 'clean' start).

- Promote the process of change in risk-taking behaviours (e.g. moving to oral methadone from injecting heroin reduces the risk of hepatitis and HIV infection).

- Helping to maintain contact and offer the individual an opportunity to gain support in working towards change.

The prescription of substitute drugs can fulfil two main functions: withdrawal and detoxification. Some individuals can withdraw from their drug of choice without substitute medication. This might require outside support and changes in the individual's lifestyle and environment. They may be using a drug on which they are not physically dependent, or they may have the support and be prepared to endure the effects of withdrawal in order to become drug free in as short a space of time as possible.

For others, who may have a history of serious withdrawal complications, for example alcohol withdrawal epileptic fits, or a number of failed attempts at self-detoxification or other problems such as lack of social support, substitute prescribing may be necessary. Substitute prescribing for withdrawal gives the user the opportunity to withdraw from their drug in a controlled manner. This is achieved by titration of the substitute drug (for example methadone as a substitute for heroin) to the user's current level of use of the illicit drug. The level is then reduced in a controlled manner over an agreed period of time. Withdrawal symptoms should therefore be prevented by careful titration of dose and careful management by both the prescribing doctor and the user. Theoretically, detoxification in this way can be slow (possibly over a period of months in the community) or quick (over a period of days or weeks in an inpatient facility).

Withdrawal symptoms are not unified phenomena and differ according to such factors as the pharmacological profile of the individual and the half-life of the drug. The severity of the withdrawal symptoms is not clearly or directly related to the quantity of drugs previously consumed, thus withdrawal cannot be quantified directly. It is therefore probably best to assume that any drug that has been consumed heavily for a significant period of time may give rise to withdrawal effects in the user. This can apply to cocaine, amfetamines and also cannabis, as well as alcohol and the opioid drugs such as heroin and methadone. Box 26.4 gives an example of symptoms and signs of opiate withdrawal.

Detoxification programmes will generally prove to be successful only if the individual is motivated to remain drug-free. Therefore the individual will generally be in the Action and Maintenance stage of the cycle of change (Prochaska and DiClemente 1982). Controlled use is problematic, as tolerance will quickly develop, leading to redevelopment of old patterns of use. There is also a danger of unintentional suicide, particularly with opioid drugs, as the detoxified body will have low tolerance of the old drug of choice, particularly at pretreatment dosage levels. Thus reverting back to the same quantity of drug may result in fatal overdose, owing to the body's low tolerance.

Medical regimens such as detoxification should not be applied in isolation. As we know, substance misuse is a complex biopsychosocial phenomenon, and as such requires a raft of supporting interventions. The newly detoxified individual will need additional support around how to stay drug-free, particularly returning to the very context where drug use was maintained. Concurrent approaches such as relapse prevention and counselling are essential to such a treatment package.

Maintenance prescribing

Substitute prescribing can be used to maintain the individual on a level so that withdrawal does not begin, thus allowing the person to carry out normal tasks of daily living (e.g. manage to keep their job). Methadone maintenance programmes have been shown to be effective in reducing all of the following factors: injecting behaviour, illicit opiate use, criminal activity and costs to society (Marsch 1998). Maintenance programmes may be used for patients who take longer to work towards abstinence. It is a useful intervention particularly with patients in the Contemplation stage, giving them space and time away from pursuing their addiction to think through the life changes they want to achieve.

Withdrawal profile and substituted drug for opiates

- Untreated heroin withdrawal typically reaches its peak 36–72 hours after the last dose. Symptoms usually subside after 5 days.

- Untreated methadone withdrawal typically reaches its peak between 4 to 6 days after the last dose. Symptoms do not usually subside for 10–12 days.

Box 26.4   Signs and symptoms of opiate withdrawal

- Sweating
- Lachrymation and rhinorrhea
- Yawning
- Feeling hot and cold
- Anorexia and abdominal cramps
- Nausea, vomiting and diarrhoea
- Tremor
- Insomnia and restlessness
- Generalized aches and pains
- Tachycardia, hypertension
- Gooseflesh
- Dilated pupils
- Increased bowel sounds.

Motivational interviewing

Motivational interviewing is a key therapeutic technique when working with individuals who abuse substances. It is particularly useful as a means of engaging and working with individuals in the primary stages of change, notably Pre-contemplation, Contemplation and the Determination–Action stage. It is based on the work of Miller and Rollnick (1991) and is readily compatible with the cycle of change model.

Motivational interviewing adopts the tenet that motivation is not something that an individual *has*, but rather is something that an individual *does*. It recognizes that individuals, in general, are ambivalent to the change process. It is not, therefore, until something happens to tip the balance that individuals work towards change. For example, a person may have spent many years smoking. They may be well aware of the significant health risks involved, but these seem far removed and they enjoy smoking. Therefore they are fairly ambivalent about changing their behaviour and giving up. They may attempt to give up on 1 January every year, but their motivation to change is not significant enough and they may quickly return to the 'weed'. At this point the positives and negatives of smoking are fairly equally balanced for the individual. When visiting their general practitioner they may discover that they have a tumour of some kind, and have to go for tests to see whether it is cancerous or benign. They may link this to smoking – and suddenly the negatives outweigh the positives. This may move the individual from the Pre-contemplation or Contemplation stage of the model to the Determination and Action stages, where they begin actively to formulate plans on how to give up.

Motivational interviewing seeks to tap into this process of behaviour change by working with individuals in stages of Pre-contemplation and Contemplation to speed up their movement round the cycle. By allowing the individuals space and time to come up with their own list of positive and negative aspects of the behaviour, the process brings to the fore discrepancies and highlights disparities. Its primary aim is to aid individuals to come to their own conclusions about the need to change their substance use; consequently this technique may be as helpful in smoking cessation work as in helping people to give up alcohol and other drugs. There are four main principles of motivational interviewing which are highlighted below.

Express empathy

This involves the nurse reflecting back what they have heard, the use of good 'active' listening skills, paying attention to things such as eye contact, facial expression and body orientation. The therapist attempts to understand the client's 'world', while suspending advice, judgement and questioning.

Develop discrepancy

This involves a process of exploration of the individual's personal goals, prompting him or her to consider the steps that would be needed to achieve the goals. The individual is asked to highlight any possible consequences of substance use. Reflective listening is used selectively to reinforce the individual's recognition that substance abuse interferes with goal attainment.

Avoid arguments

It is better to 'roll with resistance' rather than oppose it. Exploration of resistance is far more useful as arguments tend to strengthen, not weaken, the individual's beliefs and convictions. You should avoid supplying the reasons for behaviour change: individuals should state these themselves. Ambivalence to change should be viewed as 'normal', not pathological.

Support self-efficacy

The therapist should express confidence that change is possible. It is important to instil hope, whilst acknowledging past frustrations. It is also useful to explore how the individual has experienced other successes in the past.

Relapse prevention

Relapse prevention is a cognitive behavioural intervention based on the theoretical model of relapse proposed by Marlatt and Gordon (1985). The basis of the approach is encouraging the individual to use self-management strategies aimed at enhancing maintenance of a change in behaviour, once that change has been achieved. Wanigaratne et al (1990, p. 2) sum up the approach as 'a self-control programme that combines behavioural skills training, cognitive interventions and life-style change procedures'.

Addictive behaviours are seen as 'over-learned habits' – certain behaviours that have become a way of coping and that the individual can change. Instead of focusing on avoidance, the therapist as educator seeks to help the client learn different ways of coping with stressful situations.

Relapse prevention work is located in the Maintenance stage of the cycle of change model. However, it is useful if a number of skills associated with avoiding relapse are practised during sessions with the individual's keyworker or therapist prior to the Maintenance stage. This will give the client a sense of achievement over some of the skills needed to prevent relapse.

Wanigaratne et al (1990) highlight the following goals and lifestyle changes that would take place during a maintenance (relapse prevention) programme:

- To equip the client with the skills to identify, anticipate and avoid or cope with high-risk situations.

- If a slip or lapse into old patterns of substance use does occur, to equip the individual with the skills and strategies to avoid it becoming a full-blown relapse.

- To increase the individual's sense of self-efficacy.

- To identify sources of stress in lifestyle.

- To identify and change unhealthy habit patterns.

- To discover and take up positive activities.

- To learn more effective time management, to fill up the time left from ceasing to use substances.

- To arrive at a 'moderate' or 'balanced' lifestyle.

Relapse prevention work can be carried out in outpatient appointments, as part of an aftercare and follow-up package.

The importance of timed intervention

It is impossible to overstress the importance of the interventions in substance misuse being linked directly to the stage of change of the client, if they are to be effective. In substance misuse, where there is evidence of significant physical dependence, the initial phase of treatment may involve 'detoxification' in an inpatient or community setting (principles of which are described above). These interventions may be physical or psychological, or both.

In substance misuse, where 'detoxification' is not deemed necessary, the initial phase of treatment should involve a clear decision about what the goals are, and what changes need to be made. Motivational interviewing techniques are ideal for working with an individual during this stage. This may involve the individual aiming for abstinence or aiming to cut down on their intake (control).

The initial stage of treatment will comprise assessment and some form of therapeutic technique (e.g. motivational interviewing). With clients who are aiming for abstinence, relapse prevention work is best carried out during the Maintenance phase, i.e. once they have stopped using their substances.

For individuals whose goal is control rather than abstinence, relapse prevention techniques can be used soon after they have made the decision to change their behaviour, thereby equipping them with the means to alter both the ways they think about substances and their lifestyle patterns to make it more likely that change will be adhered to.

Relapse prevention may also be an appropriate intervention if an individual has made a 'slip' during a successful period of maintenance. Individuals need regular reviews and support to maintain the change in their behaviour, and any intervention should have a good period of follow-up attached to it.

Self-help groups

Self-help groups have an important role in the maintenance of a drug- or alcohol-free lifestyle once treatment has ended. They may also be used as an adjunct to treatment or as a treatment regimen in their own right. Self-help groups such as Narcotics Anonymous (NA) and Alcoholics Anonymous (AA) aim to help the substance misuser become or remain abstinent. AA and NA are based on a 12-step approach through which a limited number of objectives is set. The approach aims gradually to build up the individual's refusal skills and sense of self-efficacy by initially getting the individual to pledge to give up their substance(s) of choice for just 1 day. (A shorter time period may be involved if 1 day appears too difficult.) From that, the length of time is extended. The groups provide daily support that the individual can key into, wherever they are. They also provide a buddy system from existing members. As with any treatment approach, it may be highly successful for some individuals but not for others. Good practice would dictate that, for all individuals with drug or alcohol problems, their awareness is raised to the location of any available, relevant self-help groups in their area.

Health promotion and education

Nursing staff should be ideally placed to offer advice on health promotion and education, in any work settings. The aim is to achieve 'prevention' or 'early intervention' through clear information. Ways you might achieve this could be (Clancey 1997):

- an environment conducive to health promotion (e.g. poster displays)

- contact with local and national health promotion units

- providing information leaflets, with clear explanations

- advice and support, for example on local self-help groups for individuals and/or families or significant others

- advice on legal issues, for instance contact with the Citizens' Advice Bureau

- advice on health hazards of injecting (e.g. abscesses, scepticaemia, thrombophlebitis, hepatitis B and C, HIV).

Simple information may involve discussing some of the steps outlined in Box 26.5.

Health promotion is also about challenging the many misconceptions that surround substance misuse. In the case of drug taking, the following messages need to be promoted, alongside active measures to reduce the level of drug use:

- All young people do not take drugs.

- All drug takers are not addicts.

- All drugs do not kill.

- All drug takers do not commit crime.

- Illegal drugs are not the unique preserve of people from particular social or ethnic backgrounds.

Box 26.5   Advice on alcohol, tobacco and drug use

Advice on reducing alcohol use

- Drink more slowly

- Avoid buying rounds

- Set a specific amount of money for each time you go out drinking

- Alternate alcoholic drinks with non-alcoholic drinks

- Encourage a friend or relative to cut down as well

- Have one or two alcohol-free days during a week

- Think of positive health reasons for cutting down

Advice on minimizing harmful tobacco use

- Set a goal of stopping smoking

- Set a stop date – gradual reductions do not work because the fewer cigarettes take on more powerful meaning

- Find replacement activities

- Discuss nicotine replacement therapy (e.g. gum, patches).

Advice on minimizing harmful drug use

- Not sharing injection equipment (e.g. needles, syringes, spoons, filters or water for mixing drugs)

- Avoid getting too hot when using drugs such as ecstasy

- Avoid using alone

- Try to socialize with non-drug-using friends

- Find alternative non-drug-using activities

- Seek professional support and counselling

- Acquire basic training in resuscitation methods in the event of a drug-using friend collapsing.

From Clancey (1998).

- The majority of people in the UK do not take, nor have they ever taken, an illegal substance.

- The majority of those who have are experimenters or casual users.

- The majority of illegal drug users do so for 'recreational purposes'.

- The minority of illegal drug users become addicts – between 100 000 and 200 000.

Suicide

There is no doubt that substance misuse is inextricably linked with the increased incidence of suicide and suicide attempts. A form of substance misuse may all too frequently be the chosen method of suicide. Also, self-medication of a primary psychiatric disorder or a medical condition may lead to increased impulsivity and poor judgement, and thus may enhance the potential for accidental suicide risk. In the UK, the leading source of information on suicide is the National Confidential Inquiry into Suicide and Homicide (DoH 1999b). It reports approximately 5000 suicides occurring annually in England and Wales. Some 24% of individuals who committed suicide had been in contact with mental health services in the year before their death (this represents more than 1000 cases per year). Of these, there were high rates of alcohol and drug misuse, with 17% misusing both alcohol and drugs.

A drop in suicide rates is a major government target (DoH 1994, 1999c), yet until now there has been little evidence of it being addressed. Appleby (1997, p. 193) suggests: 'A century of suicide research has confirmed the main influence to be social ... But evidence of effectiveness of clinical services in reducing suicides is lacking ... Making clinical practice safer is desirable and achievable, and strategies to protect at risk individuals are worthwhile; whether or not suicide rates are seen to fall as a result is a separate and more complex issue'. If we also see substance misuse as being a significant social phenomenon, then its improved identification and management may have a positive effect on reducing the number of suicides.

Definitions

Some of the broader definitions have linked suicide with degrees of self-harm (the latter is considered more specifically below). Morgan (1998, p. 12) offers the following definition: 'The inflicting of damage or injury to self, with an intention of relieving extreme tension or distress, or drawing attention to a need for help, or causing death'. This broad category of risk includes suicidal behaviours with a planned intent, suicidal behaviours as a call for help, attention through cutting or mutilation, and abusing or addictive behaviours with the intention of inflicting harm or injury.

More specific definitions of suicide focus on the final outcome. Appleby (1997) sees suicide not as a single event, but more as an endpoint of a series of events. Vaughan (1995, p. 16) states it is 'the act of killing oneself in the context of despair, rather than self-sacrifice or altruism'. This simple definition links the emotional state to the final action.

Risk factors

Risk factors are characteristics of people that are used to attempt to predict the degree of risk for individuals. Effective suicide assessment involves the use of these risk factors to attempt to understand the risk to a particular individual, in the context of his or her own environment

Box 26.6   Risk factors for suicide

Personal characteristics

- Gender component (more females attempt, more males succeed)
- Age-related component (higher rates with increasing age)
- Cultural components (e.g. Asian women, young males)
- Marital status or disruption (higher in single, widowed, separated, divorced people)
- Employment status (higher in unemployed people)
- Family history of suicide increases risk potential
- Social network development (higher in socially isolated people)
- Recent adverse life events

Health characteristics

- Terminal illness
- Major physical illness or disability
- Psychiatric diagnosis
- Previous history of suicide attempts
- *Alcohol or drug misuse*
- Time of hospital discharge
- Persistent sleep disruption

Characteristics of plan

- Definite statements of planned intent
- Degree of irreversibility of plan
- Absence of proximity of others (in stated plan)
- Preparation (e.g. hoarding tablets, settling financial affairs)
- Perceived absence of, or unwillingness to use, support systems

Intangibles

- Strength of emotional ties to significant others; expressing real or perceived feelings of worthlessness in the eyes of others will increase the potential risk
- Trust in the clinician – the working relationship may form a significant bond to provide some source of hope in an otherwise hopeless situation
- Likely effectiveness of treatment – this will depend on the individual's previous experiences of prescribed treatment interventions, or openness to persuasion about the potential benefits of different ideas
- Potential transference and countertransference – depending on feelings released in either service user or practitioner, through unconscious links to previous experiences.

From Morgan (1998).

at this particular moment. Williams and Morgan (1994) have suggested that they are correlates and associations, not necessarily direct causes of suicide. They are more effective in predicting risk in the long term than in the immediate future.

The most significant variables across the literature and research for suicide risk factors have been summarized by Morgan (1998); See Box 26.6.

The incidence of substance misuse, as a characteristic risk factor in suicide, features prominently in the research and literature. The expression of suicidal ideas was the strongest predictor of suicide; however, some people indicated their risk in less direct ways, for instance through increased alcohol intake (Appleby 1997).

Alcohol and drug abuse increase the risk of death by suicide dramatically, and are second only to depressive illness as a contributory factor in suicidal behaviour. It has been found, for example, that chronic alcoholics have a 70–80 times greater risk of suicide in the 5 years following discharge from inpatient treatment than the rest of the population. Moreover, post-mortem studies have shown that almost half the men and one-fifth of the women had taken alcohol a few hours before the actual act of suicide. Alcohol is likely to produce a depression of mood, which in itself is a major factor in suicide. In addition, alcohol tends to reduce inhibition and releases aggressive behaviour in some individuals and thus may prompt precipitate action in those who otherwise would refrain from such behaviour (Vaughan 1995).

The *Safer Services* report (DoH 1999b), focusing on suicides in the mental health population, found the commonest drugs used in overdose were those prescribed to treat mental disorder (psychotropic drugs); suicides who had previously harmed themselves were more likely to commit suicide with psychotropic drugs. The commonest diagnoses were depression, schizophrenia, personality disorder, and alcohol or drug dependence. Around half also had a second (co-morbid) diagnosis, indicating more complex treatment needs.

Alarmingly, suicide rates for the 15–24 years age group have risen 75% since 1982 (DoH 1994). Although it is difficult to identify clear reasons for this, the considerable social and economic changes in society may have contributed. Vaughan (1995) suggests that amongst the most notable of them are alcohol and drugs. The link appears well established, as over the past 20 years the misuse of these substances has increased dramatically, particularly in young men. Volatile substance abuse (e.g. glue and lighter fuel sniffing) has also increased greatly, especially in males under the age of 20 years.

Risk-mitigating factors

Assessment of suicide risk based on risk factors alone fails to recognize a balance between risk factors and protective factors. People with high scores on risk factors may be mitigated by a counterbalance of protection against each. Similarly, a stable condition may become high risk if the individual's care is reduced (Appleby 1997).

Assessment

We cannot be effective without acquiring skills at recognizing suicide risk at interview. From the first encounter, we need to engender an alliance based on hope. Caution is advised in the use of the risk factor research because the assessment needs to be individualized, using the research as a secondary check to back up the clinical assessment. Any use of weightings or rating scales should carefully reflect the person's own context – reducing a person to a series of numbers will never accurately reflect their real experience.

When meeting a client there are a number of clues that may indicate the presence of depression or abnormal distress, both of which heighten the risk of suicidal behaviour. Careful observation is required to ensure that such signs are not missed, and a quick ABC test should be applied (Vaughan 1995):

A *Appearance* – evidence of self neglect in a normally well groomed person should not go unnoticed; conversely, some people will maintain a 'front' by not allowing their appearance to give away important clues to inner feelings.

B *Body language* – dejection, characterized by loss of spring in step, laboured gait, retarded body movements.

C *Content of speech* – negative attitudes towards the future, no point in planning ahead, general lack of concern, no prospect of future improvements.

A profile of risk can be built up by gathering detailed accurate information as indicated in Box 26.7.

The assessment of suicide is fraught with problems. Some that may be encountered are:

- deliberate denial of suicide risk by the patient
- variable degrees of risk, linked to ever-changing circumstances
- false improvement
- lack of trust by the patient in services
- staff feeling 'manipulated' by the expression of suicidal intent

---

> **Box 26.7   Profile of suicide risk**
>
> *Family background and support*
> - Deprivation in childhood
> - Broken family
> - Family history of suicide
> - Lack of support from current family
>
> *Personality*
> - Antisocial, aggressive and impulsive behaviour
> - Difficulties in personal relationships
> - Criminal record
>
> *Psychiatric illness*
> - Depression
> - Schizophrenia
> - Previous outpatient or inpatient treatment
> - Current symptoms
>
> *Physical illness*
> - Chronic pain
> - Terminal illness
> - Insomnia
> - Epilepsy
> - Abuse of alcohol or drugs
>
> *Previous suicide attempt*
> - Number of previous attempts
> - Circumstances of each incident
> - Degree of suicide intent
> - Outcome
>
> *Current problems*
> - Unemployment
> - Financial problems
> - Isolation
> - Bereavement
> - Loss
> - Loneliness
>
> Reproduced with permission from Vaughan (1995).

- staff or patients avoiding the difficult, and potentially traumatic, issue
- dealing with feelings of anger, resentment and lack of cooperation.

This is a difficult area that may result in fatal consequences, so staff need to attempt to assess the likelihood of a serious suicide attempt (see Box 26.8).

Box 26.8　Assessment of lethality

Plans

- Has the person made any?
- How well formulated are they?
- For how long has the person had them?
- How often does the person think about them?
- How realistic are the plans?

Method

- How lethal is the method chosen?
- Is the method chosen irreversible?
- What does the person know about this method?
- Do the person have access to this method?

Discovery

- How likely is the person to be discovered?
- Has the person made active plans to avoid discovery?

Past history

- Has the person attempted suicide before?
- What were the details and circumstances of the previous attempt?
- Are there current similarities in circumstances?
- Is there a family or significant other history?

From Gianfrancesco (1999), with permission.

Interventions

If the nurse is concerned about a potential suicide risk in a patient, the mental health services and the patient's general practitioner should be involved immediately, whatever the situation. If the nurse finds him- or herself with a crisis situation in which a patient is threatening immediate suicide or actually attempting suicide, the key points to consider are:

- Do I attempt to take control to save the person?

- What can I realistically do in the circumstances?

- Making the patient fully aware of the consequences of his or her actions, stating that there are certain things that are impossible for you to do.

- Acknowledge that sometimes, despite the best efforts of staff, patients do kill themselves on hospital wards and in other care environments.

The nurse always owes the patient a duty of care and, in the case of a suicidal patient, this includes (Morgan 1998):

- performing professional responsibilities to an accepted standard

- considering all the options with relevant others, where permissible by time and accessibility

- clearly documenting discussions, decisions and interventions

- being explicit about what is possible and what is clearly impossible in the light of:
  — time
  — place
  — available resources
  — expectations.

Case Study 26.1 outlines care plan interventions that might be instituted for a patient with alcohol problems and a history of suicide attempts.

Case Study 26.1

Tom is a 47-year-old man who lives alone in a ground-floor one-bedroom flat. His father and younger sister both live close by and he has regular contact with them when he is sober. They are afraid to visit when Tom is drunk, partly because of his aggressive behaviour and partly because of the other people who congregate at his flat (who are suspected of using alcohol and drugs).

Psychiatric history

Tom is known to local inpatient psychiatric services through 12 hospital admissions over the past 15 years. He has had diagnoses of manic depression and psychotic depressions recorded over this period of time. Most of these admissions record Tom in a depressed and/or agitated state, expressing suicidal ideas. His psychotic symptoms are predominantly in the form of persecutory voices telling him he is worthless, that he is a curse on people he comes into contact with and that he should kill himself. He has made three serious attempts on his own life, including drinking car battery acid, attempted self electrocution and stabbing himself in the stomach with a carving knife. Tom settles quickly on each hospital admission as he reinstates his prescribed medication and ceases to use the alcohol. On occasions, he absconds briefly from the ward, and returns inebriated. He has frequently become lost to contact with community services, through non-attendance at outpatient clinics. Tom's family suggest they are the only people who contact him at home when he is out of hospital.

Substance misuse history

Tom has reported using alcohol from his teenage years and throughout his working life, but it seems to have become a problem for him only since he became unemployed and in contact with psychiatric services. He mainly uses cheap ciders and strong lagers, and when drinking may begin early in the morning when a range of 'friends' visit. Tom smokes about 40 cigarettes a day, denies using any illicit drugs, but does suggest that his visitors use a lot of cannabis.

Assessment

The initiation of an assertive outreach team has enabled some intermittent contact with Tom at his home. He readily engages in discussion when sober. He is accepting of the role prescribed medication plays in keeping away distressing suicidal thoughts, and admits to becoming very forgetful about his tablets when drunk (he is unable to take depot injections because of a previous adverse physical reaction to them during an early hospital admission). Tom says he becomes bored very quickly, which is why he easily reverts to the friends who visit him and engage in substance misuse. People in this social network actively discourage him from taking prescribed medication and encourage him to withdraw amounts from a savings account he built up many years ago.

Care plan interventions

1. Assertive outreach team to engage a working relationship with Tom in the short term through daily, but relatively short, home visits.

2. Establish Tom's use of a dosett box for his oral medication, clearly separating his daily doses (one box holds a week's supply of tablets, refilled weekly by staff of the team).

3. Frequent discussions with Tom about the established pattern of becoming suicidal, to identify and monitor the early warning signs with him.

4. Support family members, by offering education about the psychiatric condition and direct effects of the substance abuse on Tom's suicidal thoughts; also offer them a quick telephone contact when they have concerns about his condition.

5. Actively discuss Tom's interests and talents, and investigate potential options for meaningful activity that may loosen his reliance on current damaging social contacts.

6. Develop a crisis plan for the possible actions if Tom loses contact with the team, or his family express fears of deterioration and/or negative social influences.

Deliberate self-harm

'Self-injurious behaviour', 'self-destructive behaviour', 'deliberate self-harm', 'self-mutilation', 'self-abuse' are clinical labels used to describe actions by a person towards herself or himself that result in physical harm to the body. Self-injury ranges from mild or superficial effects, to permanent physical damage, to life-threatening dangers. The nurse will encounter patients who have self-harmed in A&E and on overnight short-stay wards, usually after self-poisoning.

Types of self harming include:

- cutting
- burning
- scalding
- head banging
- hair pulling
- ligatures around the neck
- scratching
- swallowing objects
- punching
- inserting objects
- overdosing.

Estimates of the prevalence of self-harm vary between 0.4% and more than 10% of the population. Given the prevalence, however, self-harm is still generally misunderstood. Self-injury is often labelled as 'attention seeking' or attempted suicide, and when people who harm themselves come into contact with health and social care agencies they often feel that the treatment they receive exacerbates rather than relieves their distress (Pacitti 1998).

The true figures for people self-injuring are not known. Some people will self-injure in the privacy of their own home and never share their distress. Self-injury is often linked to suicide and the term 'para-suicide' is sometimes used to label the behaviour. Most people who self-injure do not wish to commit suicide. Rather, they want to find some tangible way of relieving their emotional pain and distress. Individuals who harm themselves frequently describe a history of physical or sexual abuse in childhood. Hidden within a shame-bound family system, abusive events are kept secret from outside the family, and are often denied within the family as well. Self-injury can often be an outward, visible signal from the self-injuring person to himself or herself and/or others about the internalized pain of the victimization (North West Self Injury Group 1996).

Myths and fantasies surrounding self-injury (North West Self Injury Group 1996, Pembroke et al 1998):

- self-injury is a sign of madness or deep mental disturbance
- people who self-injure are trying to kill themselves
- the severity of the injury represents the severity of the condition
- if it's not an artery they don't mean it
- people who injure themselves are a danger to others

- self-injury is about attention seeking
- self-injury is used to manipulate others
- self-injury is just a habit to be stopped
- people who self-injure enjoy or do not feel physical pain
- it is masochism.

Self-injury and suicide have an intimate relationship, but they are different. Every individual has their own motivations and mix of self-injuring and suicidal feelings:

- self-injury often represents the prevention of a suicidal period
- self-injury may be one way of averting suicide
- self-injury may be a survival strategy
- self injury frequently represents the least possible amount of damage and represents extreme self-restraint.

Many people who commit deliberate self-harm repeat the act at some time: 15–25% are readmitted to hospital within 12 months, the first 3 months being the most risky time. The more social and personal problems that are present, the greater the likelihood of the suicidal behaviour being repeated. Unfortunately each repetition increases the chances of unintentional suicide and many such people have undoubtedly died unintentionally through misjudgement or bad luck, and are recorded under the suicide statistics.

Moreover, there is a subgroup of individuals who chronically repeat their self-harming behaviour and who pose an enormous challenge for the helping agencies. They tend to differ from the repetition group in that they consist of those with much more severe personality problems, criminal records, and abuse of alcohol and drugs. Their lifestyle tends to be rather disorganized with frequent visits to psychiatric hospital, court appearances, prison sentences, etc. They may also have a history of violence to others or property (Vaughan 1995).

Assessment

Bluglass and Horton (1974) offer a simple checklist for predicting short-term risk of further suicide attempts after an episode of deliberate self-harm:

- sociopathy
- problems with the use of alcohol
- previous inpatient psychiatric treatment
- previous outpatient psychiatric treatment
- previous deliberate self-harm resulting in hospital admission
- not living with a relative.

One point is scored for each characteristic present. It was found that the range of probability of repetition is 5% for a score of zero, up to 48% for a score of 5 or 6. Clearly such measures make decisions about future management and support a little easier, although of course they are by no means foolproof.

Intervention

A study into A&E staff attitudes to self-harm found a number of common characteristics (Hemmings 1999):

- ambivalence
- judgement
- punitive
- taboos.

Murray (1998) suggests that the challenging behaviour we sometimes encounter in those who self-harm is usually a defence against other people's judgements. Most of these individuals need nothing more than the kind of care that any injured person would expect. While there will be debate over areas of safe practice, cooperation creates trust and allows the individual and the clinician to explore the pain together verbally. Although the behaviour may be seen as an observable manifestation of a person's pain, it is really a consequence of their intervention against that pain, and not a symptom of it. For nurses to be able to help with the problems that underlie self-harm they must first learn to recognize this difference. In the past, nurses were encouraged to ignore or suppress these values when dealing with the distress of individuals who self-harm. This has led to professionals applying unnatural standards in their interactions with patients. Pacitti (1998) suggests that basic human qualities rather than clinical techniques are most effective, particularly when dealing with people who have these sorts of difficulties.

Summary

This chapter has reviewed the effects of alcohol, tobacco and other drug use on health, and offered insights into the assessment and management of these conditions. Nurses working in general hospitals or primary care will spend a great deal of their time caring for people whose health problems stem from the use of drugs, both legal and illegal. The subject is therefore the business of all nurses, not just mental health nurses or nurses working in specialist treatment centres. Whether it be the school nurse, practice nurse, nurse practitioner or A&E nurse, to name but a few, all nurses have a role to play in reducing the harmful effects of drugs in common use today. The principles outlined in this chapter for assessment and for helping people reduce or cease altogether their drug use are valid whether applied by a practice nurse to smoking cessation clinics in primary care or by specialist nurses in a drug detoxification and treatment centre.

Critical incident

You are a psychiatric liaison nurse in a busy district general hospital A&E department. On your return from 2 weeks' annual leave your first consultation is with a 27-year-old woman brought in by her husband with their two children (8 and 4 years old). You already have messages that she has been brought to A&E on four previous occasions during the last fortnight.

She is once again alcohol intoxicated, has reopened wounds on her forearms, upper arms and abdomen, initially self-inflicted with a cheese-knife. She tells you that she smokes 30 cigarettes a day and occasionally smokes cannabis when her husband is out at work. She has a previous psychiatric history, with two suicide attempts on the ward shortly after admission to the psychiatric unit.

Her Muslim husband and the family's GP are requesting a psychiatric admission. On each recent presentation she has been kept overnight on the A&E observation ward, and discharged home the following day. She strongly suggests she does not need medication and will only use it to overdose if her home circumstances become too intense.

Reflection

■ What is your assessment of the problems presented within the scope of this case scenario?

■ What role do you think substance abuse may be contributing to these problems?

■ What reasons may this woman have for using the substances mentioned?

■ What treatment interventions and support options may be available to use in this situation?

See Appendix 2 for guidelines on reflection.

References

Appleby L (1997) Assessment of suicide risk. Psychiatric Bulletin 21: 193–194.

Bluglass D, Horton J (1974) A scale for predicting subsequent suicidal behaviour. British Journal of Psychiatry 124: 573–578.

Clancey C, ed. (1997) Substance use: guidance on good clinical practice for nurses, midwives and health visitors working within primary health care teams. London: Association of Nurses in Substance Abuse.

Clancey C (1998) Substance use: working within accident and emergency. London: Association of Nurses in Substance Abuse.

Clancey C, Coyne P (1997) Specialist assessment in a multidisciplinary setting. In: Rassool H, Gafoor M, eds. Addiction nursing: perspectives on professional and clinical practice. Cheltenham: Stanley Thornes.

Department of Health (1994) 'The health of the nation' key area handbook: mental illness, 2nd edn. London: The Stationery Office.

Department of Health (1995) Reviewed shared care arrangements for drug misusers. London: The Stationery Office.

Department of Health (1998) Our healthier nation. London: The Stationery Office.

Department of Health The Scottish Office Department of Health, Welsh Office, Department of Health and Social Services, Northern Ireland (1999a) Drug Misuse and dependence– guidelines on clinical management. London: The Stationery Office.

Department of Health (1999b) Safer services: national confidential inquiry into suicide and homicide by people with mental illness. London: The Stationery Office.

Department of Health (1999c) National service framework for mental health: modern standards and service models. London: The Stationery Office.

Donovan DM, Marlatt GA (1988) Assessment of addictive behaviours. New York: Guilford Press.

Gianfrancesco P (1999) Suicide risk. Presentation at a practitioner workshop, for South Islington Crisis Response Team, St Pancras Hospital, London, 21 April 1999.

Gournay K, Sandford T, Johnson G et al (1997) Dual diagnosis of severe mental health problems and substance abuse/dependence: a major priority for mental health nursing. Journal of Psychiatric and Mental Health Nursing 4: 1–7.

Hemmings A (1999) Attitudes to deliberate self harm among staff in an accident and emergency team. Mental Health Care 2(9): 300–302.

Institute of Alcohol Studies (1997–2000). IAS factsheets. London: IAS.

Manley D (1998) Dual diagnosis: approaches to the treatment of people with dual mental health and drug abuse problems. Mental Health Care 1(6): 190–192.

Marlatt GA, Gordon JR (1985). Relapse prevention: maintenance strategies in the treatment of addictive behaviours. New York: Guilford Press.

Marsch LA (1998) The efficacy of methadone maintenance interventions in reducing illicit opiate use, HIV risk behaviour and criminality: a meta analysis. Addiction 93: 515–532.

Mayfield D, McLead G, Hall P (1974) The CAGE questionnaire. American Journal of Psychiatry 131: 1121.

Menezes PR, Johnson S, Thornicroft G et al (1996) Drug and alcohol problems among individuals with severe mental illness in South London. British Journal of Psychiatry 168: 612–619.

Miller WR, Rollnick S (1991) Motivational interviewing. New York: Guilford Press.

Morgan S (1998) Assessing and managing risk – a practitioner handbook. Brighton: Pavilion Publishing.

Murray I (1998) At the cutting edge. Nursing Times 94(27): 36–37.

North West Self Injury Group (1996) Self injury: a resource pack. Liverpool: Mind/Ashworth Hospital Authority.

Pacitti R (1998) Damage limitation. Nursing Times 94(27): 39.

Pembroke L, Smith A, National Self Harm Network (1998) Information pack on self injury. London: National Self Harm Network.

Prochaska JO, DiClemente CC (1982) Transtheoretical therapy: toward a more integrative model of change. Psychotherapy Theory, Research and Practice 19: 276–288.

Royal College of Physicians (1987) A great and growing evil – the medical consequences of alcohol abuse. London: Royal College of Physicians.

Stephens S (1999) Treating the addicted nurse. Mental Health Care 2(9): 310–313.

Vaughan PJ (1995) Suicide prevention, 2nd edn. Birmingham: Pepar.

Waller S, Thom B, Harris S et al (1998) Perceptions of alcohol related attendances in accident & emergency departments in England: a national survey. Alcohol and Alcoholism 33(4): 354–361.

Wanigaratne S, Wallace W, Pullin J et al (1990) Relapse prevention for addictive behaviours; a manual for therapists. Oxford: Blackwell.

Williams R, Morgan HG, eds (1994) Suicide prevention: the challenge confronted. NHS Advisory Service, Thematic Review. London: HMSO.

World Health Organization (1996) WHO Factsheet N127: Trends in substance use and associated problems. Genevo: WHO.

Further Reading

Association of Nurses in Substance Abuse (1997) Working within primary health care teams. London: ANSA.

Association of Nurses in Substance Abuse (1997) Working with children and young people. London: ANSA.

Association of Nurses in Substance Abuse (1997) Working with alcohol and drug users. London: ANSA.

Association of Nurses in Substance Abuse (1998) Working within accident and emergency. London: ANSA.

These ANSA booklets provide a good basic introduction to drug and alcohol assessment and management for nurses working in generic services. Highly recommended. Publications can be obtained from: Pinpoint Communications, 12 Skenen Road, Kingston upon Thames KT2 5AF, UK. Tel: 020 8547 1810.

Department of Health (1999) Drug misuse and dependence – guidelines on clinical management. London: DoH.

Sets practice in the context of recent policy guidance for those working with individuals with dependent drug problems.

Department of Health (2001) Safety first: five-year report of the confidential inquiry into suicide and homicide by people with mental illness. London: DoH.

Summary report giving substance misuse figures as a primary factor in recorded suicides and homicides. This summary covers the findings and recommendations for action from the leading UK research in this area.

Morgan S (2000) Risk-making or risk-taking? Openmind 101: 16–17.

Risk assessment and risk management have become essential components of effective work with people misusing drug or alcohol. This article explores the dangers of promoting too restrictive an approach to risk management and outlines the importance of engaging with individuals on their terms.

Tyler A (1986) Street drugs: London: Coronet.

A good and easily readable text on different drugs that may be encountered in everyday practice. The book is not written from a predominantly medical position but looks at the effects of certain common drugs and places the drugs within their social, historical and political context.

Shock, cardiac arrest and resuscitation guidelines

Shock

This term is used loosely by the lay person but in medical and nursing care refers to a distinct physical syndrome characterized by inadequate perfusion of tissues and organs. This sets in motion a chain of events associated with inadequate tissue oxygen supply and leads to organ dysfunction, then failure and finally the death of the person unless there is rapid intervention.

Types of shock

There are three main categories of shock: distributive, cardiogenic and hypovolaemic.

Distributive shock

In this type of shock, widespread vasodilatation leads to a collapse of the circulation. The three main types of distributive shock are:

- *Anaphylactic shock*. This is due to a massive allergic reaction to an antigen to which the person has already been sensitized. Massive vasodilatation occurs and the blood volume is reduced due to increased vascular permeability resulting in loss of plasma to the extravascular tissues. Profound hypotension and collapse rapidly occur, together with bronchospasm and laryngeal oedema.

- *Septic shock*. Bacterial endotoxins (frequently from Gram-negative bacteria) can trigger an immune response that sets in motion a chain of events leading, amongst other things, to increased vascular permeability, vasodilatation and reduced peripheral vascular resistance (i.e. circulatory collapse and shock). The patient initially shows evidence of sepsis with increased cardiac output, hyperthermia and vasodilatation before the hypodynamic, cold, collapsed terminal phase.

- *Neurogenic shock*. If the sympathetic constrictor tone in vascular smooth muscle is lost the result is vasodilatation. Blood pools in the venous system reducing the volume of blood returning to the heart which in turn reduces cardiac output. The combination of these two effects is a dramatic collapse in blood pressure and shock. This may be a temporary response to a noxious sight resulting in fainting or it may be of a more long-term nature in spinal cord injury.

Cardiogenic shock

Cardiogenic shock is caused by failure of the left ventricle of the heart to maintain an adequate output. This is frequently associated with a myocardial infarction. The body may be able to compensate for a short period but shock can rapidly intervene, especially if the patient has myocardial ischaemia.

Hypovolaemic shock

The most common situation is a loss of fluid from the circulatory system due to major bleeding or severe burn injury. Alternatively there may be a shift of fluid from blood vessels to the interstitial or intracellular spaces as described above in distributive shock. In either case there is reduced venous return to the heart which in turn leads to falling cardiac output and shock.

Progression of shock

Whatever the cause of the shock, it is possible to discern three stages, called the *compensatory*, *progressive* and *irreversible* stages.

Compensation mechanisms include the secretion of adrenaline (epinephrine) and noradrenaline (norepinephrine) to increase peripheral resistance, blood pressure and cardiac contractility. The renin–angiotensin–aldosterone system initiated by the kidneys conserves water and sodium and also causes vasoconstriction. As a result of these mechanisms a person may, for example, be able to maintain a normal blood pressure for some time, despite serious injury.

If these compensation mechanisms begin to fail, however, the person enters the progressive stage and cardiac output falls leading to the development of tissue hypoxia. Systolic blood pressure typically falls to below 90 mmHg. Cells begin to function on anaerobic metabolism in response to tissue hypoxia leading to the build up of lactic acid and acidosis which further inhibits myocardial function. Tissue hypoxia also leads to vasodilatation and increased capillary permeability. Eventually permanent damage to organs occurs as the patient enters the irreversible stage leading to circulatory and respiratory failure, and finally a stage at which death is inevitable.

Recognition of shock

The changes described above explain the classic picture of hypotension and tachycardia. The patient's skin is cold and clammy and the respiratory rate is raised. Respirations become progressively more shallow as shock develops, and become slower in the terminal phase. Cerebral underperfusion leads to irritability and restlessness initially, progressing to drowsiness and finally unconsciousness in the irreversible stages of shock. Shock may lead to acute renal failure; urinary output

Figure A1.1   Anaphylactic reactions: treatment for adults in the community. ALS, advanced life support; CPR, cardiopulmonary resuscitation.

Consider diagnosis of anaphylaxis when compatible history of severe allergic-type reaction with respiratory difficulty and/or hypotension especially if skin changes present

Call ambulance, suggesting diagnosis[1]

Stridor, wheeze, respiratory distress or clinical signs of shock[2]

Lie patient flat with legs raised (unless respiratory distress increased)

Adrenaline (epinephrine)[3] 1:1000 solution 0.5 ml (500 µg) i.m.[4]

Repeat in 5 minutes if no clinical improvement. Remember urgency of hospital transfer

1. Ambulance will be equipped with oxygen, salbutamol and fluids which may be used as adjunctive therapy.
2. If profound shock judged to be immediately life threatening give CPR/ALS if necessary.
3. Half doses of adrenaline (epinephrine) may be safer for patients on amitriptyline, imipramine or beta-blocker.
4. If adults are treated with an Epipen, the 300 µg will usually be sufficient.
    A second dose may be required, but this should be considered ONLY if the patient's condition continues to deteriorate 5 minutes after the first dose.
    NB: Remember the urgency of hospital transfer.

From Resuscitation Council (2001).

therefore needs to be monitored closely. Poor urine output is due to renal underperfusion and indicates the development of shock. The average-sized adult should have a minimum urine output of 30 mL/h. Complete anuria is a grave sign indicating that shock may have entered the irreversible stage.

Treatment of shock

Treatment depends upon the cause. However, as the root of the problem is tissue hypoxia, administration of a high concentration of oxygen is essential in all cases, whatever the cause. Key points are summarized below, but obviously in such seriously ill patients a great deal of intensive medical and nursing care is required. The reader is referred to the appropriate chapters in this book for further information.

Anaphylactic shock

The current UK Resuscitation Council (2001) guidelines for immediate treatment of anaphylactic shock are given in Figures A1.1 (community situation) and A1.2 (hospital). This is a sudden life-threatening event and the nurse must keep calm, act swiftly and provide psychological support for both patient and other family members. Persons who are known to have a serious allergy problem carry an Epipen, which is a preassembled syringe that delivers an intramuscular injection of 300 µg of adrenaline (epinephrine) in one dose. Junior Epipen devices deliver half the dose and are carried by children.

Septic shock

Specific management consists of antimicrobial therapy to try to eliminate the causative pathogen and intravenous fluids to restore the circulating volume. Hyperpyrexia is a particular problem requiring nursing intervention. Supplemental nutrition is essential to help the patient combat the infective organism and meet the increased metabolic requirements of sepsis (typically 4000 kcal per day). Prevention of septic shock is, of course, the ideal treatment, and this emphasizes the need for basic measures to prevent cross-infection of patients and good aseptic technique for all invasive procedures at all times. Hyperpyrexia is a particular problem requiring nursing intervention.

Figure A1.2   Anaphylactic reactions: treatment for adults by first medical responders..

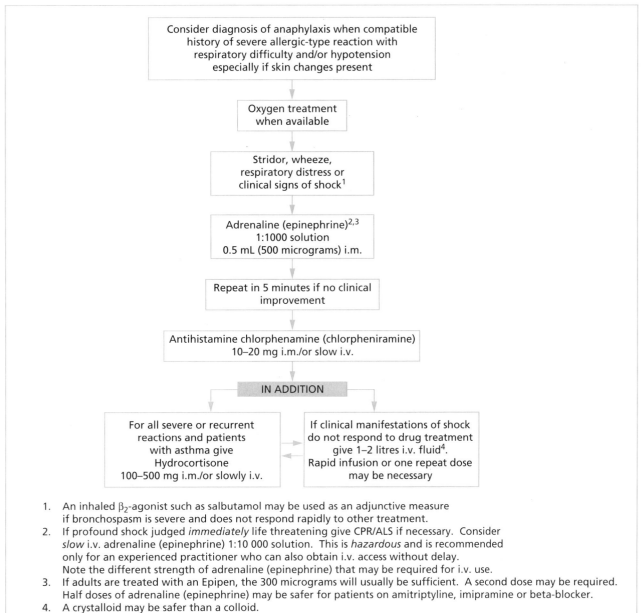

1. An inhaled β₂-agonist such as salbutamol may be used as an adjunctive measure
    if bronchospasm is severe and does not respond rapidly to other treatment.
2. If profound shock judged *immediately* life threatening give CPR/ALS if necessary. Consider
    slow i.v. adrenaline (epinephrine) 1:10 000 solution. This is *hazardous* and is recommended
    only for an experienced practitioner who can also obtain i.v. access without delay.
    Note the different strength of adrenaline (epinephrine) that may be required for i.v. use.
3. If adults are treated with an Epipen, the 300 micrograms will usually be sufficient. A second dose may be required.
    Half doses of adrenaline (epinephrine) may be safer for patients on amitriptyline, imipramine or beta-blocker.
4. A crystalloid may be safer than a colloid.

From Resuscitation Council (2001).

Neurogenic shock

Neurogenic shock associated with a simple faint is rapidly self-correcting. However, the other likely cause is spinal cord injury and here there is no specific treatment that can restore spinal cord function. Treatment is therefore supportive and geared to preventing further harm to the spinal cord by correct immobilization and the prevention of long-term complications.

Cardiogenic shock

The fundamental problem is that the heart (left ventricle) can no longer cope with the demands made upon it. Treatment is directed towards preventing further damage to the myocardium by increasing its oxygen supply,

assisting the myocardium by increasing its contractility and reducing the work the heart has to perform by reducing ventricular afterload. Administration of a high concentration of oxygen is therefore essential, while vasoactive medication will assist in achieving the other two goals. Dobutamine and dopamine are the most commonly used cardiac stimulants to treat cardiogenic shock and will increase cardiac output. The dosage of dopamine is critical, because if given in doses of over 5 μg per kg per min it will cause vasoconstriction and may exacerbate heart failure. Effective opioid analgesia should also be given intravenously if the patient is experiencing chest pain associated with a myocardial infarction. Psychological support is essential as the patient is likely to be very stressed and frightened.

Hypovolaemic shock

Treatment is aimed at restoring the lost volume of intravenous fluid and expanding the circulation to its normal level. However, the intravenous fluids used must be capable of remaining within the circulation to be effective. Frequently used solutions in emergency resuscitation (e.g. A&E) are Gelofusine (a gelatine-based solution) or dextran (70 or 40), another fluid with very large dextran molecules that are retained in the circulation. Burn victims will have lost large amounts of plasma; after initial A&E resuscitation they should therefore be treated with plasma or plasma protein fractions containing large amounts of albumin together with electrolyte replacement therapy. Effective pain control and psychological support are essential in trauma victims at all times. Elevation of the lower limbs will also help venous return and is of value in resuscitation.

Cardiac arrest

When the heart ceases effective function, the patient is described as being in cardiac arrest. This may due to *ventricular fibrillation* (chaotic electrical activity producing no output), *asystole* (no electrical activity) or *electromechanical dissociation* (electrocardiographic (ECG) complexes are present but they fail to produce any effective cardiac muscle contractions). See Chapter 12 for a further detailed discussion. In all cases the patient loses consciousness immediately, and without rapid intervention will almost certainly die. Serious brain damage will occur within 3 minutes due to lack of oxygen reaching the brain and the chances of resuscitating the patient decline rapidly with each passing minute of inaction.

The nurse may encounter a patient who collapses with cardiac arrest either outside a healthcare facility (usually when off duty) or when on duty. Two sets of guidelines have been prepared by the European Resuscitation Council to cover these two situations, known as Adult Basic Life Support (ABLS) (Handley et al 2001) and Adult Advanced Life Support (AALS) (De Latorre et al 2001). The ABLS guidelines are designed for the lay rescuer and are therefore suitable for the off-duty nurse or a situation where no equipment is available. The AALS guidelines assume that resuscitation equipment is available and that professional staff are on scene who know how to use it.

Adult basic life support guidelines

The most recent set of guidelines (produced in 2000) include some changes to pre-existing guidelines. Some people may not be aware of these changes. The two most important changes are: (1) that lay rescuers are no longer required to spend time looking for a carotid pulse as this has been found to be too time consuming; and (2) that the ratio of chest compressions to ventilations is now set at 15 : 2 for both one- and two-person cardiopulmonary resuscitation (CPR). The sequence of actions is described in Box A1.1 and summarized in Figure A1.3.

Box A1.1   Sequence of actions for Adult Basic Life Support

The following is the agreed sequence of actions that constitute the European Resuscitation Council Guidelines 2000 for Adult Basic Life Support. In this context an adult is considered to be a person aged 8 years or over. In the text, use of the masculine includes the feminine.

1. *Ensure safety of rescuer and victim.*

2. *Check the victim and see if he responds:*
   - Gently shake his shoulders and ask loudly: 'Are you all right?'

3A. *If he responds by answering or moving:*
   - Leave him in the position in which you find him (provided he is not in further danger), check his condition and get help if needed
   - Send someone for help or, if you are on your own, leave the victim and go for help yourself
   - Reassess him regularly.

3B. *If he does <u>not</u> respond:*
   - Shout for help
   - Unless you can assess him fully in the position you find him, turn the victim on to his back and then open the airway:
     — Place your hand on his forehead and gently tilt his head back keeping your thumb and index finger free to close his nose if rescue breathing is required
     — Remove any visible obstruction from the victim's mouth, including dislodged dentures, but leave well fitting dentures in place
     — With your fingertip(s) under the point of the victim's chin, lift the chin to open the airway

   Try to avoid head tilt if trauma (injury) to the neck is suspected.

4. *Keeping the airway open, look, listen and feel for normal breathing (more than an occasional gasp or weak attempts at breathing):*
   — Look for chest movement
   — Listen at the victim's mouth for breath sounds
   — Feel for air on your cheek
   - Look, listen, and feel for not more than **10 s** to determine if the victim is breathing normally.

5A. *If he <u>is</u> breathing normally:*
   - Turn him into the recovery position (*see below*)
   - Send someone for help or, if you are on your own, leave the victim and go for help yourself
   - Check for continued breathing.

(Continued)

Box A1.1 (continued)

5B. *If he is not breathing, or is only making occasional gasps or weak attempts at breathing:*

- Send someone for help or, if you are on your own, leave the victim and go for help; return and start rescue breathing as below
- Turn the victim onto his back if he is not already in this position
- Give two **slow, effective** rescue breaths, each of which makes the chest rise and fall:
  — Ensure head tilt and chin lift
  — Pinch the soft part of his nose closed with the index finger and thumb of your hand on his forehead
  — Open his mouth a little, but maintain chin lift
  — Take a deep breath to fill your lungs with oxygen, and place your lips around his mouth, making sure that you have a good seal
  — Blow steadily into his mouth whilst watching his chest; take about 2 s to make his chest rise as in normal breathing
  — Maintaining head tilt and chin lift, take your mouth away from the victim and watch for his chest to fall as air comes out
- Take another breath and repeat the sequence as above to give two effective rescue breaths in all
- If you have difficulty achieving an effective breath:
  — Recheck the victim's mouth and remove any obstruction
  — Recheck that there is adequate head tilt and chin lift
  — Make up to five attempts in all to achieve two effective breaths
  — Even if unsuccessful, move on to check the circulation.

6. *Check the victim for signs of a circulation:*

- Look, listen and feel for normal breathing, coughing, or movement by the victim
- **Only if you have been trained to do so**, check the carotid pulse
- Take **no more than 10 s** to do this.

7A. *If you are confident that you have detected signs of a circulation:*

- Continue rescue breathing until the victim starts breathing on his own
- About every ten breaths (or about every minute) recheck for signs of a circulation; take no more than 10 s each time
- If the victim starts to breathe normally on his own but remains unconscious, turn him into

the recovery position. Be ready to turn him onto his back and re-start rescue breathing if he stops breathing.

7B. *If there are no signs of a circulation, or you are at all unsure start chest compressions:*

- With your hand that is nearest to the victim's feet, locate the lower half of the sternum (breastbone):
  — Using your index and middle fingers, identify the lower rib edge nearest to you. Keeping your fingers together, slide them upwards to the point where the ribs join the sternum. With your middle finger on this point, place your index finger on the sternum itself
  — Slide the heel of your other hand down the sternum until it reaches your index finger; this should be the middle of the lower half of the sternum
  — Place the heel of the other hand on top of the first
  — Extend or interlock the fingers of both hands and lift them to ensure that pressure is not applied over the victim's ribs. Do not apply any pressure over the upper abdomen or bottom tip of the sternum
  — Position yourself vertically above the victim's chest and, with your arms straight, press down on the sternum to depress it between 4 and 5 cm
  — Release all the pressure without losing contact between the hand and sternum, then repeat at a rate of about 100 times per min (a little less than two compressions per second); it may be helpful to count out aloud. Compression and release should take an equal amount of time
- Combine rescue breathing and compressions:
  — After 15 compressions tilt the head, lift the chin and give two effective breaths
  — Return your hands without delay to the correct position on the sternum and give 15 further compressions, continuing compressions and breaths in a ratio of 15 : 2
  — Only stop to recheck for signs of a circulation if the victim makes a movement or takes a spontaneous breath; otherwise resuscitation should not be interrupted.

8. *Continue resuscitation until:*

- Qualified help arrives and takes over.
- The victim shows signs of recovery.
- You become exhausted.

From Handley et al (2001).

Figure A1.3   Adult Basic Life Support.

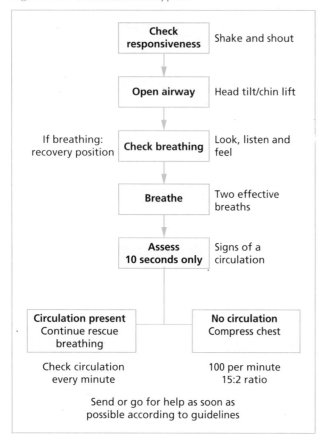

From Resuscitation Council (2001).

Figure A1.4   Management of choking in adults. BLS, basic life support.

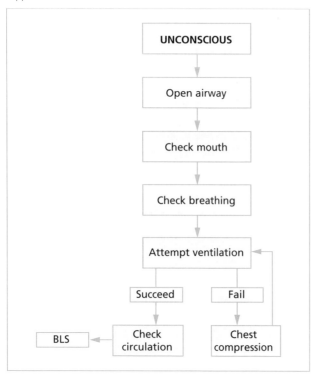

Reproduced with permission from Handley et al (2001).

Guidance is also given on the patient who is choking (Fig. A1.4), with the recommendation that backslapping (five sharp thumps between the shoulder blades) be administered if coughing fails to clear the obstruction. Should five thumps between the shoulder blades not work, then abdominal thrusts (the Heimlich manoeuvre) should be used. In the event of breathing ceasing altogether, Figure A1.4 indicates the actions to follow. It is vital to get help as soon as possible.

Adult advanced life support guidelines

A common situation is that a patient collapses or is found collapsed somewhere in the hospital or health centre. Cardiac arrest should be assumed if the patient is collapsed, unresponsive, showing no respiratory effort and has no carotid pulse. No more than 10 s should be spent in coming to this conclusion and time should not be wasted searching for a carotid pulse if one cannot be located within a few seconds.

The nurse should initiate AALS immediately after raising the alarm. This can be greatly expedited with the use of an oral airway and a self-inflating bag delivering 100% oxygen until such time as the resuscitation team arrives and can intubate the patient. The sooner the patient can be defibrillated, the greater the chance of recovery, assuming the person has a shockable rhythm. Seconds therefore count, and every effort should be made to ensure that registered nurses can use defibrillators. The steps to follow are set out in Box A1.2 and summarized in Figure A1.5.

Box A1.2   Sequence of actions for Adult Advanced Life Support

1.   *Precordial thump, if appropriate*

If the cardiac arrest is witnessed or monitored, a precordial thump may be given before a defibrillator is attached. This is unlikely to be successful more than 30 s into the arrest.

2.   *Establish basic life support, if appropriate*

Basic life support should be started if there is any delay in obtaining a defibrillator, but must not delay attempted defibrillation. The priority is to avoid any delay between the onset of cardiac arrest and attempted defibrillation.

Use adjuncts for airway control and ventilation, provide positive pressure ventilation with a high inspired oxygen concentration, preferably 100%.

3.   *Attach a defibrillator–monitor*

Monitor the cardiac rhythm:

  ■ Place the defibrillator paddles or self-adhesive electrode pads on the chest wall; one just below the right clavicle, the other at the left mid-axillary line.

(Continued)

Box A1.2 (*Continued*)

- Place monitoring electrodes on the limbs or trunk but well away from the defibrillation sites. To avoid delaying the first shock, the initial rhythm may be assessed through the defibrillation pads or electrodes. After a shock has been delivered there is a possibility of spurious asystole being displayed if monitoring is continued through paddles and gel pads. If a non-shockable rhythm is displayed via paddles and gel pads after the first or second shocks, monitoring leads should be attached, and the rhythm confirmed.

4. *Assess rhythm (± check for pulse)*

Check for signs of a circulation, including the carotid pulse, but only if the ECG waveform is compatible with cardiac output.

- Take no more than 10 s

Assess the rhythm on the monitor as being:
— A shockable rhythm: Ventricular fibrillation (VF) or pulseless ventricular tachycardia (VT).
— A non-shockable rhythm: Asystole or Pulseless Electrical Activity (PEA).

5A. *VF/VT*

(a) Ensure that everybody is clear of the patient. Place the defibrillator paddles on the chest wall.

Use up to three sequential shocks, if required, of 200, 200 and 360 J with a monophasic defibrillator, observing the ECG trace after each shock for any changes in the rhythm. Use appropriate alternative levels with a biphasic defibrillator.

The aim should be to administer up to three initial shocks, if required, in less than 1 min.

(b) If VF/VT persists after three shocks, perform 1 min of CPR (15 : 2).

(c) During CPR:
Consider and correct reversible causes.
If not already:
Check electrodes, paddle position and contact.
Secure and verify the airway, administer oxygen, obtain i.v. access.
(Once the trachea has been intubated, chest compressions at a rate of 100 min^{-1} should continue uninterrupted, with ventilations performed at about 12 min^{-1} asynchronously)

- Give 1 mg adrenaline (epinephrine) i.v.

If venous access has not been established consider giving 2–3 mg adrenaline (epinephrine) via the tracheal tube in a 1 : 10 000 solution.

- The interval between the third and fourth shocks should not be more than 1 min.
(d) Reassess the rhythm on the monitor.

Check for signs of a circulation, including the carotid pulse, but only if the ECG waveform is compatible with cardiac output.

(e) If the rhythm is non-VF/VT, follow the right-sided path of the algorithm [*see Fig. A1.5*].
(f) If VF/VT persists:

Consider amiodarone in VF/VT refractory to three initial shocks.

Attempt defibrillation with three further shocks at 360 J with a monophasic defibrillator or an equivalent energy for an alternative waveform defibrillator.

- Give 1 mg adrenaline (epinephrine) i.v.

The process of rhythm reassessment, delivery of three shocks and 1 min of CPR will take 2–3 min. One mg of adrenaline is given in each loop every 3 min.

Repeat the cycle of three shocks and 1 min of CPR until defibrillation is achieved.

(g) Each period of 1 min of CPR offers a new opportunity to check electrode/paddle positions and contact, secure and verify the airway, administer oxygen, obtain i.v. access, if not already done.

- Consider the use of other medications (e.g., buffers).

5B. *Non VF/VT – asystole, pulseless electrical activity*

(a) Check for signs of a circulation, including the carotid pulse.
(b) Perform, or restart, 3 min of CPR (15 : 2), if the patient is in cardiac arrest.

NB: If the non-VF/VT rhythm occurs after defibrillation, perform only 1 min of CPR before reassessing the rhythm and giving any drugs.

(c) During CPR:

Consider and correct reversible causes. If not already:
Check electrodes, paddle position and contact
Secure and verify the airway, administer oxygen, obtain i.v. access.

(Once the trachea has been intubated, chest compressions should continue uninterrupted, with ventilations performed at 12 min^{-1} asynchronously)

- Give 1 mg adrenaline (epinephrine) i.v.

If venous access has not been established, consider giving 2–3 mg adrenaline (epinephrine) via the tracheal tube in 1 : 10 000 solution.

(Continued)

Box A1.2 *(Continued)*

(d) Reassess the rhythm after 3 min of CPR.

Check for signs of a circulation, including the carotid pulse, but only if the ECG waveform is compatible with cardiac output.

(e) If VF/VT, follow the left-sided path of the algorithm [*see Fig. A1.5*].

(f) If non-VF/VT, perform 3 min of CPR (15 : 2).
- Give 1 mg adrenaline (epinephrine) i.v.

As the process will take 3 min, 1 mg of adrenaline (epinephrine) is given in each loop every 3 min.

(g) Each period of 3 min of CPR offers a new opportunity to check electrode/paddle positions and contact, secure and verify the airway, administer oxygen, obtain i.v. access, if not already done.

(h) Consider the use of other medications (atropine, buffers) and pacing.

6. *Consider the use of other measures (medications and pacing)*
   (a) *Antiarrhythmics*

There is incomplete evidence to make firm recommendation on the use of any antiarrhythmic drug.

Amiodarone is the first choice in patients with VF/VT refractory to initial shocks. The initial dose is 300 mg diluted in 20 mL 5% dextrose given as an i.v. bolus. An additional 150 mg of amiodarone may be considered if VF/VT recurs.

Consider the use of amiodarone after three shocks, but do not delay subsequent shocks.

   (b) *Buffers*

Consider giving sodium bicarbonate (50 mL of an 8.4% solution) or an alternative buffer to correct a severe metabolic acidosis (pH <7.1). When blood analysis is not possible, it is reasonable to consider sodium bicarbonate or an alternative buffer after 20–25 min of cardiac arrest.

   (c) *Atropine*

A single dose of 3 mg of atropine, given as an i.v. bolus, should be considered for asystole and pulseless electrical activity (rate <60 beats min^{-1}).

   (d) *Pacing*

Pacing may play a valuable role in patients with extreme bradyarrhythmias, but its value in asystole has not been established, except in cases of trifascicular block where P waves are seen.

7. *Consider/treat reversible causes*

In any cardiac arrest patient, potential causes or aggravating factors for which specific treatment exists should be considered:

Hypoxia
Hypovolaemia
Hyper/hypokalaemia
Hypothermia

Tension pneumothorax
Tamponade
Toxic/therapeutic disturbances
Thromboemboli

8. *Advanced life support procedures*
   (a) *Secure a definitive airway*

Attempt tracheal intubation. When undertaken by experienced personnel, tracheal intubation remains the optimal procedure.

The laryngeal mask airway (LMA) or Combitube are acceptable alternatives to tracheal intubation when the healthcare providers have little experience with tracheal intubation and are well trained in the use of LMA and/or Combitube.

Verify the position of the tracheal tube or the LMA or Combitube at regular intervals.

   (b) *Establish ventilation*

Ventilate the patient's lungs with 100% oxygen using a self-inflating bag with a reservoir or an automatic resuscitator.

   (c) *Establish vascular access*

The central veins are the optimal route for delivering drugs rapidly into central circulation. However, these routes require special training and may have complications, some of which are potentially life-threatening. Peripheral venous cannulation is often quicker, easier, and safer to perform. Drugs administered by this route should be followed by a flush of 10–20 mL 0.9% saline. When venous access is not available, (adrenaline, atropine, and lidocaine only) may be given in the relevant tube. In this case, use higher doses (2–3 times) and dilute the drug in 10 mL of sterile water (or use the contents of appropriate prefilled syringes).

From De Latorre et al (2001).

Figure A1.5   Adult Advanced Life Support. BLS, basic life support; CPR, cardiopulmonary resuscitation; VF, ventricular fibrillation; VT, ventricular tachycardia.

Reproduced with permission from De Latorre et al (2001).

References and Further Reading

British National Formulary (2001) British National Formulary, no. 41. London: British Medical Association/Royal Pharmaceutical Society of Great Britain.

De Latorre F, Nolan J, Robertson C et al (2001) European Resuscitation Council Guidelines 2000 for Adult Advanced Life Support. Resuscitation 48: 211–221.

Handley A, Monsieurs K, Bossaert L (2001) European Resuscitation Council Guidelines 2000 for Adult Basic Life Support. Resuscitation 48: 199–205.

Haslett C, Chilvers E, Hunter J, Boon N (1999) Davidson's principles and practice of medicine, 18th edn. Edinburgh: Churchill Livingstone.

Resuscitation Council UK (2001) Update on the emergency medical treatment of anaphylactic reactions for first medical responders and community nurses. Resuscitation 48: 239–241.

Smeltzer S, Bare B (2000) Brunner and Suddarth's textbook of medical–surgical nursing. Philadelphia: Lippincott.

Springhouse Corporation (2000) Handbook of pathophysiology. Springhouse, PA: Springhouse Corporation.

The most up to date guidance on resuscitation can be obtained by logging on to the European Resuscitation Council website: http://www.erc.edu

Learning by reflection

You are recommended to use the following framework to help you reflect upon each critical incident given in the book. You can also use this framework to reflect upon and learn from experiences in clinical practice. It involves a staged approach to analysing each incident and is derived from the work of Boud et al (1985), Johns (1994) and Neary (2000).

Step 1: Go back to the experience itself

Describe what happened in some detail but be sure you are describing what actually happened, not what you think might have happened or should have happened. Ask yourself how the experience made you feel and check with yourself what you actually did (or what the nurse actually did in the examples given in this book). You are aiming for an overview of the event itself.

Step 2: Concentrate on the feelings involved

How do you think the nurse or patient felt in the examples given here? How do you personally feel about the examples? Be honest about the negative feelings as well as the more socially desirable positive feelings which are easier to acknowledge and work with.

Step 3: Rework the events

Go back over what happened, think about the feelings that the events generated and link them back to the events. Consider what specific events generated particular feelings, be they positive or negative. Start to think about alternative courses of action that the nurse (or yourself) might have taken and what different outcomes they may have produced.

Step 4: Learn from the experience

This starts by asking how you now feel about the experience and how you might have dealt better with the situation. In short, what lessons have you drawn from the experience? These need not always be negative as it may be that you see a member of staff handle something really well or you yourself deal with a difficult situation successfully. Think about why things worked out well and what lessons you can take forward to future similar situations where you can apply the same approach. Learn from positive events as well as negative situations where things went badly.

Reflection should lead you to consider different options in future, to think more widely and perhaps to clarify things where previously you were unsure. It may lead you to go and look something up in the library or on the internet and discover new knowledge. You have to be big enough to realize when you were wrong and learn from those mistakes. Ultimately, reflection should lead you to do things differently. Reflection turns experience into learning.

References

Boud D, Keogh R, Walker D (1985) Reflection: turning experience into learning. London: Kogan Page.

Johns C (1994) Nuances of reflection. Journal of Clinical Nursing 3(2): 71–75.

Neary M (2000) Teaching, assessing and evaluation for clinical competence. Cheltenham: Stanley Thornes.

Index

A-delta fibres 111
Abdominal distension
  intestinal obstruction 486
  postoperative care 184
Abdominal pain 441–2
  appendicitis 476
  intestinal obstruction 486
  pancreatitis
    acute 530, 532
    chronic 533
  peritonitis 477
Abdominal paracentesis 522–3
Abdominal reflex 669
Abdominal rigidity 443
Abdominal thrusts (Heimlich manoeuvre) 369, 996
Abducens (VI) nerve assessment 679
Ablative cancer surgery 203
Abnormal uterine bleeding 819, 820
ABO blood group 378
  blood donations typing 425
  blood transfusion 425
    incompatible 429
  kidney transplantation 637, 638
Abortion 821–6
  causes 821
  classification 822
  criminal 826
  definition 821
  emotional response 823–4
  habitual 822
  inevitable 822, 823
  management 822–3
  missed 822–3
  religious rites 824
  septic 826
  therapeutic 824–6
  threatened 821, 822
Abortion Act (1967) 824
Absence seizures 739
Absorption, gastrointestinal 441
ABVD chemotherapy 406
Acarbose 575
Accelerated idioventricular rhythms 297
Acceptance 63, 235
Accessory muscles 337–8
Accessory (XI) nerve assessment 679
Accommodation 679, 760
  reflex 760
    assessment 763
Accountability 4, 5, 9, 13, 21
Acetabular fracture 895
Acetazolamide 771
Acetylcholine 676
  neuromuscular transmission 677
Acheson Report 45
Achlorohydria 457
Aciclovir 743, 832
Acid–base balance, renal function 612, 614
  disorders 619–20
Acne 952
Acquired immune deficiency syndrome (AIDS) see HIV infection/AIDS
Acromegaly 600–1
Activated partial thromboplastin time (APTT) 328, 421
Active listening 35–6

Activity intolerance
  anaemia 392, 393
  cardiovascular disease 274–5
    arterial occlusive disease 324
    heart failure 312–13
  chronic obstructive airway disease 348, 350
  chronic renal failure 635
  osteoarthritis 911
  respiratory disorders 338
  rheumatoid arthritis 905
Activity theory, elderly people 50
Acupuncture 118
Addiction 962
Addisonian crisis (acute corticoid deficiency) 606
Addison's disease (adrenocortical insufficiency) 604–7
  management 605–7
Adenohypophysis see Anterior pituitary
Adenoids 756
  enlargement 368
Adenosine 297
Adenosine triphosphate (ATP) 538
Adenovirus 729
Adherence see Compliance
Adipose tissue 538, 539
Administration of drugs 95–7
  group protocols 96
  nurse's key roles 96
  routes 100–2
    local 99–100
Adrenal cortex 566
  disorders 604–8
Adrenal gland surgery 608–9
Adrenal glands 565–6
Adrenal medulla 566, 675
  disorders 608
Adrenal sex hormones 566
Adrenaline (epinephrine) 539, 566, 675
  anaphylaxis management 429
  excess see Phaeochromocytoma
  local anaesthetic agent combinations 174
Adrenoceptor subtypes 104
Adrenocortical insufficiency see Addisonian crisis; Addison's disease
Adrenocorticoids 566
Adrenocorticotrophic hormone (ACTH) 562, 564, 566
Adult respiratory distress syndrome (ARDS) 360, 361
Advance directives 309
Advanced Breast Biopsy Instrumentation (ABBI) system 853
Advanced life support 264, 308, 996–9
Advanced Trauma Life Support (ATLS), burn injuries 938
Adventitious breath sounds 339
Adverse drug effects 107–8
Advocacy for suddenly bereaved 67
Afferent (sensory) neurone 666
Afterload 252
Ageing 47–51
  biological/physiological aspects 47–9
  cardiovascular risk 255
  causes 47
  degenerative joint disease 910

influence on clinical investigation results 152
  psychological changes 49
  skin changes 926
  sociological perspectives 49–51
  see also Elderly people
Ageism 43, 46
Ageusia 224
Agnosia 678, 693
Agonist muscle 872
Agonist receptor activity 103
Agrochemicals exposure 397
AIDS dementia complex 729
Air-fluidized beds 932
Airway assessment 335
Airway management
  cardiopulmonary resuscitation 307
  head injury 711–12
  spinal cord injury 718
  trauma assessment 872
Airway obstruction 335, 368–9
  artificial airway 361–7
  burn injuries 938, 940–1
  cancer patients 234
  respiratory failure 360, 361
  thyroid surgery postoperative care 595
Alanine aminotransferase (ALT) 510
Albumin 372, 373
  preparations for transfusion 427
Albuminuria 619
Alcohol consumption 514–17, 961, 963–7
  cardiovascular risk impact 257
  case study 516–17
  cirrhosis 521–2
  gastritis 452
  hypertension 321
  intake assessment 515
  mouth cancer 445
  peptic ulcer 453
  problem drinking 39, 964
    carbohydrate-deficient transferrin test (CDT) 511
    elderly people 966–7
    impact on families 964–5
    interventions 977
    withdrawal symptoms 962
    women 965–6
    young people 966
  related health problems 515, 965
    empowering management approach 516
  sensible drinking recommendations 514, 515, 963
  suicide association 983
  units of alcohol calculation 963, 964
Alcoholics Anonymous (AA) 981
Aldosterone 320, 566, 614
Alendronate 920
Alfentanil 119–20
Alfuzosin 792
Alienation 90
Alkaline phosphatase 510
Alkaloids 204
Alkyl nitrites 970
Alkylating agents 204, 397
Allergic conjunctivitis 769
Allergic contact dermatitis 953

Allergic drug reactions 108, 136
  chemotherapeutic agents 233
Allergic purpura 420
Allergic reactions 323, 376
  preoperative history-taking 168
  transfusion reactions 429
  see also Anaphylaxis
Allergy alert bracelet 168
Allogenic bone marrow transplantation
    216
Allogenic stem cell transplantation 402–3
  aplastic anaemia 402
Allograft (homograft) 637
Alloimmune haemolytic anaemia 386
Allopurinol 233, 395, 409, 916
Alopecia *see* Hair loss
Alpha-glucosidase inhibitors 575
Alpha-thalassaemia 387–8
Alprostadil 787
Aluminium hydroxide 455, 598
Alveolar hypoventilation 360
Alveoli 333
Alzheimer's disease 6, 728, 730–1
Ambiguous genitalia 786
Ambu bag 365
Ambulation, postoperative 187, 188, 189
Ambulatory chemotherapy 208
Ambulatory electrocardiography (Holter
    technique) 264–5
Ambulatory electromyography 684
Amfetamine 739, 968–9
Amino acids 539, 541
  essential 540, 541
  renal handling 613
Aminoglutethimide 862
Aminoglycosides 133
  nephrotoxicity 622
  ototoxicity 752
Amiodarone 297, 301
Amitryptiline 233, 866
Ammonia serum levels
  liver function assessment 511
  toxicity 514
Amoebic dysentery 126
Amoebic liver abscess 527
Amoxycillin 455
Amphotericin 444
Amputation 897–901
  closed (flap type) 898
  disarticulation 898
  indications 897–8
  information for patient 901
  level 898
  mobility following 900–1
    with prosthesis 901
  nursing management 899–901
  open (guillotine) 898
  pain relief 900
  phantom limb 900, 901
  postoperative care 898–9
  preoperative preparation 898
  psychosocial adaptation 900
  stump healing promotion 899–900
  traumatic 898
Amyl nitrite 970
Amylase 437, 439, 440
  serum level 510, 531
Amyotrophic lateral sclerosis *see* Motor
    neurone disease
Anabolism 538
Anaemia 380–94
  abnormal erythrocyte destruction
      (haemolytic) 386–91
  activity limitation 392, 393
  blood loss-related 383, 384, 385–6

cancer patients 208, 221
causes 382
chemotherapy side effect 208, 398
clinical manifestations 382, 383
definition 380
erythropoiesis abnormalities 382–5
gastric resection patients 464
haemoglobin levels 337
history-taking 392
information for patient 394
mental disturbance 392, 393
nursing management 391–4
pain relief 392, 393
physical examination 392
preoperative preparation 169
renal failure 620
skin/mucosal tissue care 392, 393
Anaesthesia 173–6
  general 173
  informed consent 169
  regional 173
  respiratory function 178, 179
Anaesthetic agents 174–5
  regional anaesthesia 175
Anaesthetic nurse 176
Anaesthetist 176
Anal sphincters 437
Analgesic ladder 119, 230, 231
Analgesics 118–20
  cancer pain 230–2
  chest pain 276
Anaphylaxis
  chemotherapeutic agents 233
  shock 991
    treatment 992, 993
  transfusion reactions 429
Androgens
  adrenal cortex 566
  bone effects 871
Anger 37–8
  arterial blood pressure 253
  body image alteration response 71
  cancer patients 237, 239
  chronic illness 89
  grief reaction 61, 63, 235
  staff safety issues 38
Angina pectoris 254, 262, 285–8
  activity management 286
  case study 288
  immediate care 286
  intra-aortic balloon pump 288
  medication 286, 287
  percutaneous transluminal coronary
      angioplasty (PTCA) 286–8
  Prinzmetal 285
  risk factor modification 286
  stable 285
  unstable 285
Angiography
  arterial occlusive disease 324
  cardiopulmonary 266–7
  cerebral 685
  renal vessels 617–18
Angioneurotic oedema 917, 950, 952
Angiotensin converting enzyme (ACE)
      inhibitors 273, 292, 293, 312
  diabetes mellitus 570, 579
Angiotensin II 320, 566
Angle-closure glaucoma, acute 770–1
Aniline dyes 196, 656
Animal reservoirs of infection 136
Ankle brachial pressure 324
Ankle instability 897
Ankle soft tissue injury 897
Ankylosing spondylitis 915–16

Ann Arbor classification (lymphoma
    staging) 405, 406
Anorexia 545
  cancer patient 225, 239, 240
    chemotherapy side effect 399, 400
    radiotherapy side effect 214
  cardiovascular disease 262, 274, 311
  endocrine disorders 568
  gastrointestinal disorders 442
  renal function impairment 620, 627
Anorexia nervosa 551
Anosmia 756, 758
Antacids 104, 448, 455, 474
Antagonist muscle 872
Antagonist receptor activity 103
Antazoline 769
Anterior communicating artery 672
Anterior pituitary (adenohypophysis)
    562–4
  hormones 562, 599
    functions 562, 563, 564
  hypothalamic hormone regulation 562
Antiangina medication 286, 287
Antiarrhythmic agents 306
Antibiotics 101
  bacterial resistance 132, 133
  cytotoxic agents 204
  diarrhoea 467, 468
  infectious illness 132, 133
  infective endocarditis 284
  inflammatory bowel disease 481
  osteomyelitis 919
  resistance 134
  sensitivity testing 159
  topical preparations 952
Antibodies 129, 141
  diagnostic procedures 131
  titre 131
  see also Immunoglobulin
Anticholinergics
  acute pancreatitis 531, 532
  Parkinson's disease 736
  preoperative 171
  urinary incontinence 648
Anticholinesterases 738, 739
Anticipatory grief 60, 63, 450
Anticoagulants
  arterial occlusive disease 324–5
  atrial fibrillation 301
  cardiovascular disease 279
  deep vein thrombosis 189, 328
  haemorrhagic complications 420–1
  monitoring 324, 328, 421
  myocardial infarction 292, 293
  stroke 686, 687
Anticonvulsants 474
  epilepsy 741
  trigeminal neuralgia (tic douloureux) 743
Antidiuretic hormone (ADH) 564, 710
  hypersecretion 603
  hyposecretion 602
  urine concentration regulation 613
  variceal bleeding management 524
Antieczematous agents 952
Antiemetics 101, 102, 460
  morphine therapy initiation 233
  postoperative nausea/vomiting 184
  radiotherapy side effects 214
Antifungal topical preparations 952
Antigen–antibody interaction 129
Antigens 127
  diagnostic procedures 131
Antihelminthics 99
Antihistamines 952
Antihypertensives 318, 321

Anti-inflammatory analgesic drugs 118
Antilymphocyte globulin 402
Antimalarial drugs 908
Antimetabolites 204
Antinuclear antibodies (ANAs) 904
Antiparasitic topical preparations 952
Antiplatelet drugs 292
Antipruritic agents 952
Antipsychotic drugs
   co-analgesic actions 233
   intramuscular slow release preparations 101
Antithymocyte globulin 402
Antithyroid drugs 592
Antituberculous drugs 352–3
Antiulcer agents 99, 455
Anuria 618, 619, 628
   acute renal failure 622
Anus 437
Anxiety
   acute renal failure 626
   advanced cancer patient 240
   arterial blood pressure 253
   burn injuries 939, 942
   cancer patients 237–8, 239
      recurrence fears 241–2
   cardiovascular disease 277
   chest pain 277
   clinical investigations 153, 154
   communication skills 38
   heart failure 311
   intracranial surgery 713
   measurement tools 290
   musculoskeletal trauma 873–4
   myocardial infarction 290
   oesophageal surgery 450
   pain experience impact 114–15
   postoperative care 184, 190
   preoperative preparation 165–7
   state 114
   trait 114
Aortic aneurysm 322, 447
   dissection 322
Aortic atresia 282
Aortic regurgitation 315
Aortic stenosis 281, 283
Aortic valve 249
Aphasia 678
   motor (expressive; Broca's) 678
   sensory 678
   stroke patients 693, 694, 695
Apheresis 395, 396
Aplastic anaemia 385, 401–2, 417
Apoptosis 196
Appearance 31
   cardiovascular system assessment 259–60
   nutritional status assessment 546
Appendicectomy 477, 478
Appendicitis 476–7
Appendix 437
Appetite 545
   endocrine disorders 568
   see also Anorexia
Approved (non-proprietary; generic) medicines 97
Apraclonidine 771
Apraxia 678, 693
Aqueous humour 759
Arachnoid mater 669
Aromatase inhibitors 862
Aromatherapy 54
Arousal 682
Arterial blood pressure 253
   cardiovascular system assessment 260–1

Arterial bypass grafting 325
Arterial disorders 322–6
Arterial occlusive disease
   acute occlusion 322–3
   anticoagulants 324–5
   chronic 323
      exercise 325–6
      positioning 325
      protection from cold 326
      skin care 325
      smoking cessation 326
   diagnosis 324
   signs/symptoms in extremities 323
   surgical management 325
Arteries 250
Arterioles 250
Arteriosclerosis 323
Arteriosclerosis obliterans 323
Arteriovenous fistula
   haemodialysis access 631–2
   patient education 634
   postoperative care 633
Arthritis Impact Measurement Scale 903
Arthrodesis 912
Arthrography 904
Arthroplasty *see* Joint replacement surgery
Arthroscopy 904
Articular cartilage 872
Artificial airway 361–7
Artificial heart valves 315
   microangiopathic haemolytic anaemia 386
Artificial insemination by donor (AID) 818
Artificial saliva 447
Artificial skin 945
Artificial urethral sphincter 650
Asbestos 196, 199
Ascites 510
   abdominal paracentesis 522–3
   liver disease 514, 522
   peritoneovenous shunt 523
L-asparaginase 233
Aspartate aminotransferase (AST)
   liver function assessment 510
   myocardial infarction 291
Aspergillus 410
Aspiration of gastric contents 342
   chronic respiratory failure 361
   postoperative patient 181, 189
Aspiration pneumonia 342
Aspirin 324, 325, 417, 866, 908, 917
   fever management 133
   myocardial infarction 292
   pain management 118
   warfarin interaction 102
Assessment
   care planning 10–11
   elderly people 51–3
   starting interview 34–5
   see also Investigations
Assisted fertility techniques 818
Association tracts 671
Asterixis 514
Asthma 82, 90, 345–7
   acute attack 346
   clinical features 347
   management 99, 346–7
      peak flow expiratory rate (PFER) monitoring 346, 347
      primary care 84, 86
      prophylaxis 346
      severe attack 347, 348, 349
      teaching about drug therapy 351–2
   prevalence 345
   register of patients 84

Astigmatism 760
Asystole 307
Ataxia telangiectasia 397
Ataxic gait 680
Atelectasis 335, 369
   postoperative 181, 188
Atenolol 102
Atherosclerosis 285
   arterial occlusion 322, 323
   cerebral 686
      thrombosis/embolism 687
   diabetes mellitus 570
Athetoid movements 677, 680
Atorvastatin 256
Atria 248
Atrial arrhythmias 293, 296
Atrial ectopic beats 298
Atrial fibrillation 300, 301, 307
Atrial flutter 299, 301, 307
Atrial septal defect 280–1
Atrioventricular block
   complete 293, 303
   first degree 302
   second degree 293, 302–3
Atrioventricular node 249, 251
Atrioventricular valves 248
Atrophic skin 950
Atropine 171, 298, 302, 303
Audiometry 750
Audit
   aims 85
   criteria 86
   cycle 85
   data collection 86
   improvements planning/implementation 87
   methods 86
   presentation of results 87
   primary care management of chronic illness 85–7
   review 87
   selection of team 85–6
   selection of topic 85
   standards 86
      performance comparisons 86–7
Auditory (Eustacian) tube 748
Auditory nerve (VIII) 748, 749
   assessment 679
Auditory ossicles 748
Auditory pathway 749
Auditory training 752
Auricle (pinna) 748
Auriscope (otoscope) 750
Autoclaves 139
Autografts (skin) 945
Autoimmune disease 129, 136
Autoimmune haemolytic anaemia 386
Autoimmune thyroid disease (Hashimoto's thyroiditis) 588
Autologous blood transfusion 430–1
Autologous bone marrow transplantation 216
Autologous epidermal skin culture 945
Autologous stem cell transplantation 402
   acute leukaemia 400
Automatism 739
Autonomic nervous system 665, 675–6
   chemical mediators 675–6
Autonomic neuropathy 570
Autonomy 5, 13, 18
   moral conduct principles 13, 25
   nurse practitioner role 9
   patient-centred education 18
   of suddenly bereaved 66

Axillary nerve palsy 897
Axon 666
Azathioprine 136, 640, 909, 917
Azelatine 769
Azithromycin 790, 830

B lymphocytes 129, 375, 376
    memory cells 129, 375
Babinski reflex 682
Bacillary dysentery 467
Bacilli 125
Back pain 920–1
Backslaps 996
Bacteraemia 130
Bacteria 125–6
    capsule 126
    Gram staining 158
    peptidoglycan cell wall 125
    toxins 126
Bacterial food poisoning 466–7
Bacterial overgrowth 473
Bacterial samples
    culture 159
    sensitivity 159
    specimen collection 158
Bactericidal substances 127
Bag-mask device 307
Balance (equilibrium) 748, 749
    following limb amputation 901
    testing 680
Balanced traction 879–80, 881
Balanitis 788–9
Balloon tamponade 523–4
Barbiturates 107
    misuse 968, 972
Bargaining, grief reaction 63, 235
Barium studies
    inflammatory bowel disease 480–1
    small intestinal cancer 488
Barotrauma 367
Barr body 781
Barrel chest 337
Barrett's oesophagus 448
Barriers to infection 127
Bartholinitis 828
Bartholin's glands 804
Basal cell carcinoma 956, 957
Basal ganglii (nuclei) 671
Basic life support 307–8, 994–5, 996
Basic metabolic rate 538
Basophils 375, 376
Baths, therapeutic 951–2
Batten's disease 216
Beclometasone 99
Bed exercises, postoperative 186
Bedrest
    bone effects 870
    heart failure 271, 312
    osteomyelitis 919
    rheumatoid arthritis 906
Behavioural change 18
    barriers in chronic illness 89–90
    cardiovascular risk modification 254–5
    patient teaching process 24–5
    stages of change model 23–4, 978
        substance misuse interventions 978, 981
    weight reduction programme 549
Behavioural interventions, urinary incontinence 648–9
Bell's palsy (peripheral facial paralysis) 743
Bence Jones protein 409
Beneficence 13, 25
Benign idiopathic neutropenia 396

Benign prostatic hyperplasia 651–2, 792–4
    treatment 792
        surgical procedures 792–4
        urinary symptoms 792–3
Benign tumours 197–8
Benzene 196, 199, 397
Benzhexol 736
Benzodiazepines 171, 921
    misuse 968, 971
    tolerance 103
    withdrawal symptoms 962
Benzylpenicillin 101, 105
Bereavement 59–73
    breaking bad news 68
    help to find immediate resources 68
    Lindemann's characteristics of bereaved 61
    sudden death see Sudden death
    viewing body 66–7
    see also Grief; Loss
Berry aneurysm 688
Beta₂ agonists 99
    asthma management 346
Beta human chorionic gonadotrophin (β-hCG) 201
Beta-blockers
    arrhythmias 297, 301, 303
    glaucoma 770, 771
    heart failure 273, 312
    myocardial infarction 291
Beta-thalassaemia major 387
Beta-thalassaemia minor 387
Betaxolol 770
Biceps reflex 669
Biguanides 474, 575
Bile 439, 440, 507
    functions 508
    production/excretion 508
        regulation 440
    reflux 453
Bile ducts 507, 508–9
Bile pigments 508
Bile salts 508
Biliary colic 513
Biliary drug excretion 105
Biliary function tests 510–11
Biliary tract disorders 507–34
    clinical features 512–14
    history-taking 509–10
    imaging investigations 511–12
    laboratory investigations 510–11
    malabsorption 473
    nursing care 525–30
        obstruction 529
    physical examination 510
    terminology 528
Bilirubin
    serum level 510
    urinary levels 511
Billroth I gastrectomy 456
Billroth II gastrectomy 456
Bioavailability 101
Biofeedback, urinary incontinence management 649
Biography 51, 52
Biological response modifier therapy 217–19
Biological sex 783
Biomedical model of health 14
Biopsy, cancer diagnosis 200–1, 202
Biorhythms, influence on clinical investigation results 152
Biot's breathing pattern 336
Biphasic intermittent positive airway pressure (BIPAP) 368

Bisphosphonates 233, 409, 598, 920, 921
Bivalve cast 878
Black Report 15, 17
Blackhead (comedo) 949
Bladder 614
    micturition process 615
Bladder injury 655
Bladder irrigation 658
Bladder surgery 657–60
    postoperative care 658–60
        bladder drainage 658
        patient education 659–60
    preoperative preparation 657–8
Bladder training 648, 837
    spinal cord injury 722
Bladder tumour 656–7
    risk factors 656
Blalock–Taussig shunt 282
Bleeding time 417
Bleomycin 233, 406, 866
Blepharitis 769
Blindness 768
    see also Visual impairment
Blink reflex 760
Blood 371–9
    composition 372
    pH 373
Blood cells 372, 373
Blood coagulation 377–8
    disorders 417–23
        coagulation factor deficiencies 418–22
        liver disease 513
        renal disease 620–1
    laboratory tests 382
Blood disorders (dyscrasias) 379
    bone marrow examination 380
    erythrocytes 380–96
    history-taking 379–80
    investigations 380, 381, 382
    leucocytes 396–416
    physical assessment 380
    platelets 417
Blood flow, drug absorption effects 99
Blood gas analysis
    normal values 340
    respiratory disorders 340–1
Blood glucose 152, 372, 511, 567
    insulin actions 567
    monitoring in diabetes mellitus 579–80
Blood groups 378–9
    blood donations typing 423, 425
Blood loss, anaemia 383, 384, 385–6
Blood pressure 253
    cardiovascular disease 261
    cardiovascular system assessment 260–1
    measurement technique 260
    myocardial infarction 289
    postoperative monitoring 181
    renal function impairment 620
    see also Hypertension
Blood tests 156
    factors influencing values 157
    technique 156–7
Blood–brain barrier 98, 102, 672
Blood/blood product preparations 425–7
Blood/blood products transfusion 385, 386, 423, 425–31
    acute leukaemia 398–9
    adverse reactions see Transfusion reactions
    autologous blood 430–1
    cross-match 425
    documentation 428
    donation 423, 425
        blood collection/storage 427–8

indications 423
infection transmission 425
nursing responsibilities 427–8
patient refusal 430
procedure 428
quality control measures 423, 425
sickle cell disease 389
surgical patient 184–5
variceal bleeding 525
Bloom's syndrome 397
Body fluid exposure management 138
Body image
alteration 69
burn injuries 946–7
cancer patients 236–7
case study 69–70
loss response 70–1, 236, 237
urinary diversion 662
eating behaviour relationship 545
Body language 35, 36
Body lice 955
Body mass index (BMI) 543
calculation 547
Body mass, influence on clinical
investigation results 152
Body temperature regulation 926
spinal cord injury 724
Bone 869–71
ageing changes 47, 48, 919
cancellous 870
compact 870
development 870–1
growth 871
hyperparathyroidism-related
decalcification 598
infective disease 918–19
turnover 870
factors influencing 871
Bone marrow 129, 371, 870
depression
chemotherapy side effect 208
nursing care 221, 222–3
radiotherapy side effects 211, 213
examination 380
haematopoiesis 373
stem cells 373
Bone marrow transplantation
acute leukaemia 400
cancer 215–17
chronic myeloid leukaemia 401
donor bone marrow sources 216
engraftment period 217
peripheral blood stem cell transplants 217
Bone mass determination 919–20
Bone mineral density 920
Bone neoplasms 921–3
clinical features 922–3
metastatic disease 923
osteolytic lesions 922
primary 922
reactive bone formation 922
Borborygmi 443
Bowel elimination
immunocompromised patient 412
infectious illness 132, 133
postoperative care 185–6
regularization 470, 472
Bowel preparation, preoperative 170
Bowen's disease 956
Bowman's capsule 611
Brachial plexus 675
Brachytherapy 210
breast cancer 863
nursing care 214–15, 216
patient preparation/education 215

Bradycardia 293, 296, 298
Bradykinin 112
Bradypnoea 336
Brain 670–1
blood supply 671–2
blood–brain barrier 672
ventricles 672–3
Brain injury 699
Brain tumour 726
classification 727
investigations 726
nursing care 726, 728
treatment 728
neurosurgery 728, 729
Brainstem 671
Brainstem lesions 703
Brassières 851
BRCA1 196, 202, 848
BRCA2 196, 203, 848
Breaking bad news 68, 162
Breast 846–8
axillary tail 847
ductal system 847
lymph drainage system 847
Breast awareness 851
Breast cancer 846, 854–67
chemotherapy 859–62
complications 861–2
clinical examination 849–50
clinical staging 855, 859
diagnostic investigations 852–3
epidemiology 848
geographical variation 849
familial predisposition 196, 848
fungating lesions 859
grading 859
hormone therapy 862
menopausal symptoms 863
hormone-dependence 196
infiltrating 855
inflammatory 855
information for patient 14, 864
inoperable 859
men 849
metastatic disease 865–7
clinical features 866–7
pain control 865–6
treatment 865
needle localization 857
ovarian ablation 862
psychological care 864
radiotherapy 863–4
risk factors 848–9
sexuality following 864–5
surgery 855–9
lymphoedema 858–9
postoperative care 858
prostheses advice 864
reconstructive 857–8
timing during menstrual cycle 856
types 855
Breast care advice 851–2
Breast cysts 853–4
Breast discomfort (mastalgia) 852
Breast disorders 846–67
benign 853–4
diagnostic investigations 852–3
genetic screening 853
skin beneath breasts 951
Breast fibroadenoma 854
Breast implants 854, 857
Breast lipoma 854
Breast self-examination 846, 850–1
Breastfeeding 848
contraception 815–16

Breath sounds 338–9
Breathing
assessment 335
burn injuries 938
cardiopulmonary resuscitation 307
immediate postoperative care 181
trauma assessment 872
Breathing exercises
postoperative care 188
gastric surgery 463
preoperative instruction 166, 167, 168
Breathing pattern 336
chronic obstructive airway disease
347–8, 350
Breathing retraining 350
Breathlessness (dyspnoea) 336
anaemia 393
cancer patients 227, 234, 240
cardiovascular disease 262
chronic obstructive pulmonary disease
348
heart failure 272, 273, 310
myocardial infarction 289
renal function impairment 620
respiratory disorders 335, 338
Bretylium 298
British National Formulary (BNF) 97
Broad complex tachycardia 297–8
Broca's area 671
Broca's (motor; expressive) aphasia 678
Bronchi 333
Bronchial angiography 340
Bronchial biopsy 341
Bronchial breath sounds 338
Bronchial obstruction 369
Bronchioles 333
Bronchitis, chronic 345
Bronchodilators
asthma 346
chronic obstructive airway disease 350
patient teaching 351
respiratory failure 361
Brudzinski's sign 689
Bruise (echymosis) 422
Buccal administration route 101
Buck's traction 880, 881
Buerger's disease (thromboangiitis
obliterans) 323
Bulbourethral glands 782
Bulimia nervosa 442, 551
Bulla 949
Bundle branch block 302
Bundle branches 249, 251
Bundle of His 249, 251
Burn injuries 934–47
airway obstruction 938, 940–1
assessment 938–9
burn characteristics 936
causes 934
complications 943
depth 936, 938
discharge preparations 947
escharotomy 941
exercise 945
first aid 939–40
fluid balance 937, 941–2
healed skin care 946
history-taking 938–9
hypertrophic scarring 946
hypovolaemic shock 937, 941–2, 948
immediate treatment 938, 940
infection risk 943–4
information needs 939, 942
inhalation injury 936, 938
nutrition 946

Burn injuries (*contd*)
  pain relief 938, 942
  pathophysiological effects 937–8
  physical examination 938
  positioning 945
  prevention 934–5
  rehabilitation 946–7
  rescue, resuscitate, retrieve, resurface
      approach 939, 943
  severity determinants 935
      age 937
  skin grafts 944–5
  social factors 934
  surface area estimation 935–6, 938
  wound care 942–3
  wound healing 944–5
Burr-hole 713

C fibres 111
Cachexia 225
Caecum 437
CAGE questionnaire 515, 976
Calcaneal fracture 894
Calciferol 920
Calcitonin 233, 565, 871, 920, 921
Calcitriol 612
Calcium
  acute pancreatitis 531
  bone metabolism 870
  hormonal control 565
  malabsorption 474
      gastric resection patients 464
Call/recall systems 84
Callus, skin 950
Cancer 6, 195–242
  advanced 239–41
      spiritual issues 240–1
      symptom control 239
  anorexia/weight loss 214, 225, 239, 240
  biological response modifier therapy
      217–19
  bone marrow depression 208, 211, 213,
      221
  bone marrow transplantation 215–17
  breathlessness 227, 234, 240
  cachexia 225
  causative factors 196–7
  chemotherapy 203–8
  complementary therapies 219–20
  constipation 208, 225, 232–3, 239, 240
  coping processes 235–9
      body image changes 236–7
      information needs 235–6
      psychosocial/emotional responses
          237–9
      sexual function 236
  diagnosis 200–1
  diarrhoea 208, 211, 214, 226
  early detection (secondary prevention)
      199–200
  fatigue 214, 226, 227
  grading 201–2
  grief response 235
  hair loss (alopecia) 208, 211, 213, 226
  hormone-dependence 196
  implantation (seeding) 197
  incidence 198–9
  inherited predisposition 196
  invasion 197
  lymphatic involvement 197
  malignant nature 197–8
  micrometastases 198
  mucositis (stomatitis) 208, 211, 213, 221,
      223–4
  nature of disease 195

  nausea/vomiting 208, 211, 214, 221, 223,
      233, 239, 240
  nursing care 221–34
  oncological emergencies 233–4
  openness about dying 235
  pain *see* Cancer pain
  prevalence 199
  radiotherapy 208–15
  regional spread/metastasis 197–8
  rehabilitation 241
  risk factor reduction (primary
      prevention) 199
  somatic disorders 196
  staging 202
  stress associations 197
  surgery 202–3
      ablative 203
      curative 202
      incisional/excisional biopsy 202
      nursing care 203
      palliative 203
      prophylactic 202–3
      reconstructive 203
  survivorship 241–2
  taste alteration 224–5
  tumour markers 201
Cancer antigen 125 (CA-125) 201
Cancer pain 228–33, 237, 240
  acute 228, 230
  advanced cancer 239
  aetiology 228
  assessment 228
  breast cancer metastatic disease 865–6
  chronic 228, 230
      continuous analgesia 231
  complexity of experience 228
  drug treatment 230–2, 239, 866
      analgesic ladder 230, 231
      co-analgesics 231–2, 866
      dose titration 231
      opioid side effects management 232–3
      principles of opioid therapy 230–1
  measurement 229
      flow sheet 229, 230
  non-pharmacologic relief methods 232
  pain history 228, 229
  types of pain 228
Candida albicans 223, 410, 444, 500, 829
Candidiasis (moniliasis)
  cancer patients 223
  diabetes mellitus 569
  oral thrush 444
  peristomal skin infection 500
  vagititis 829
Cannabis 967, 968, 970
Canthi, inner/outer 758
Capillaries 250
Capillary refill time 260
Capsule 126
Carbamazepine 743, 866
Carbidopa 736
Carbimazole 592
Carbohydrate 540
  dietary intake 168–9
      recommendations 543
  digestion 437, 440
  metabolism 538
      insulin actions 567
      liver 508, 538
Carbohydrate-deficient transferrin test
      (CDT) 511
Carbon dioxide retention 360
Carbon dioxide transport 373
Carbon tetrachloride 521, 622
Carboxypeptidase 439

Carcinogenesis 195–6
  chemical agents 196
  dietary factors 196
  initiation stage 195–6
  physical factors 196
  progression stage 196
  viruses 196–7
Carcinomatous meningitis 867
Cardiac arrest 307, 994–9
  advanced life support 308, 996–9
  basic life support 307–8, 994–5, 996
Cardiac arrhythmias 296–307
  electrophysiological studies 268–9
  management 304–7
  myocardial infarction 291, 292–3
  postoperative 182
Cardiac bed 272, 313
Cardiac catheterization 267
  electrophysiological studies 268
Cardiac cycle 251–2
Cardiac output 252
  impairment *see* Heart failure
Cardiac pacing 296, 304–5
  complete atrioventricular block 303
  environmental electrical hazards 305
  modes 304–5
  nursing care 305
  positions 304
  temporary/permanent 304
Cardiac rehabilitation 293–4
Cardiac reserve 252
Cardiac sphincter (lower oesophageal
      sphincter) 436
Cardiac surgery 314–18
  cardiopulmonary bypass 314
  complications 315, 317–18
  ischaemic heart disease 314–15
  off-pump 314
  patient education 318
  postoperative care 315, 316–17
  postoperative pain 318
  preoperative care 315
Cardiogenic shock 991
  treatment 993
Cardiomyopathies 282–3
Cardioplegia 314
Cardiopulmonary angiography 266–7
  complications 267, 268
  informed consent 267
  normal haemodynamic values 267
  nurse's role 267–8
Cardiopulmonary bypass 314
  complications 314
Cardiopulmonary resuscitation 307–9,
      994–8
  advanced life support 308, 996–9
  basic life support 307–8, 994–5, 996
  decision to withhold treatment
      (inappropriate CPR) 308–9
  post-resuscitation care 308
  presence of relatives 309
Cardiovascular disease 6, 247–329
  activity intolerance 274–5
  assessment 258
  chest pain 275–7
  classification 279–80
  diagnostic investigations
      blood tests 263
      invasive 266–9
      non-invasive 263–6
  history-taking 258–9
  lifestyle modification 270–1, 278–9
  patient characteristics 269–71
  patient education 278–9
  physical examination 259–63

prevention 254–8
signs/symptoms 261–3
terminal disease 271
Cardiovascular risk factors 254–8
cerebral atherosclerosis 686
COMA report dietary recommendations 543, 544
determinants of high-risk behaviour 257–8
diabetes mellitus 570
hypertension 318
modifiable 255–8, 286
cardiac rehabilitation 293
non-modifiable 255
obesity 547
Cardioversion 306–7
atrial fibrillation 301
atrial flutter 301
Care concept 7, 13
components of caring 29–30
importance of communication 29
Care delivery 9–12
Care planning 10–12
assessment 10–11
evaluation 12
goal setting 11–12
implementation 12
problem identification 11
Caring for people 77
Carotid arteries 672
Doppler ultrasound assessment 683
Carotid artery bruit 686
Carrier state 130
Cartilaginous joints 871
Case studies
acute leukaemia 400
acute pancreatitis 531
alcohol abuse 516–17
angina pectoris 288
body image alteration 69–70
cervical carcinoma 843, 844–6
chronic illness management in community 88
colorectal cancer 488–9
diabetes mellitus 581–2, 584–5
elderly people 44–5
assessment 52–3
grief process 72–3
hiatus hernia 452
Hodgkin's disease 407–8
hypothyroidism 590–1
leukaemia 416
myocardial infarction 294–6
needle phobia 153
obesity 549–50
pneumonia 343, 344
sickle cell disease 394
suicide 985–6
undernutrition in hospitalized patient 551–2
urinary incontinence 650
urinary retention 652
Catabolism 538, 622, 625
Cataract 771–5
clinical features 771
degenerative 771
developmental (congenital) 771
extraction procedures 771–2
complications 774–5
extracapsular 771–2
intracapsular 772
postoperative care 772–4
intraocular lens implantation 772, 773–4
patient care 772
spectacles/contact lenses 773

Cataract glasses 773, 774
Catecholamines 566
Cauda equina 673
Caudal anaesthesia 174
CD4 142
Ceftriaxone 830
Cell cycle 204
Cell division 195
Cell membranes
drug transport 98–9
receptors 103
Cell-mediated immune response 129
Central hearing loss 751
Central nervous system 665, 669–74
drug access 98, 102
Central obesity 547
Central venous access 413–14, 415
Central venous catheters 205, 413, 414
care plan 415
Central venous ports 208
Central venous pressure (CVP)
measurement 269
renal function impairment 620
Cephalic phase of gastric secretion 439
Cerebellar ataxia 680
Cerebellum 671
Cerebral abscess 742
Cerebral aneurysm 688–9
clinical features 689
investigations 689
management 690
nursing care 690–2
prognosis 689–90
subarachnoid haemorrhage 689–90
Cerebral angiography 685
Cerebral artery bypass 687
Cerebral atherosclerosis 686
Cerebral contusion/laceration 700
Cerebral cortex 670
Cerebral dominance 670
Cerebral function assessment 678
Cerebral perfusion pressure 697
Cerebral thrombosis/embolism 687
Cerebrospinal fluid (CSF) 672–3
circulation 673
specimen collection *see* Lumbar puncture
Cerebrovascular accident *see* Stroke
Cerebrovascular disorders 677, 686–97
Cerebrum 670
Cerumen 748
impacted 753
Cervical carcinoma 840–3
case study 843, 844–6
human papilloma virus 197, 840
precursor stages 840
screening 25–6
staging 840–1
treatment 841–3
Cervical carcinoma in situ 840
Cervical collar 718, 907
Cervical dysplasia 842
human papilloma virus 831
Cervical mucus
ferning 816
menstrual cycle changes 804
ovulation-related changes
infertility investigations 816
rhythm contraception method 815
sperm immunological cross-hostility 817
spinnbarkeit 816
Cervical plexus 675
Cervical polyp 838
Cervical smear 840
grading 841
Cervical spinal injury 720

Cervical suture 823
Cervix 801
congenital anomalies 810
menstrual cycle changes 804
Chain of infection 135–6
Chalazion 770
Chemical burns 934
first aid 940
Chemical carcinogenesis 196
Chemical disinfection 139
Chemical eye injury 777
Chemical sterilization 139
Chemoreceptor trigger zone 442
Chemotaxis 127, 376
Chemotherapy 203–8
adjuvant/neoadjuvant 204
administration 204–5
ambulatory 208, 860–1
devices 205, 208
breast cancer 859–62
administration 860–1
metastatic disease 865
colorectal cancer 488
definitive treatment 203–4
historical aspects 203
Hodgkin's disease 405–7
leukaemia
acute 398–400
chronic lymphocytic 401
chronic myeloid 401
lung cancer 353
multiple myeloma 409
non-Hodgkin's lymphoma 408
palliative 204, 239
preventive rehabilitation 241
salvage treatment 204
second primary malignancy 208, 397
side effects 399
spinal cord compression 234
superior vena cava obstruction 234
treatment regimens 204
tumour lysis syndrome 233
see also Cytotoxic agents
Chest drainage 355–8
closed (water-seal) system 355–7
indications for clamping 358
pneumothorax management 354
removal of drain 358
responsibilities/precautions 357–8
Chest pain
cardiovascular disease 262, 275–7
angina pectoris 285–8
anxiety reduction 277
coronary heart syndrome 285
drug treatment 276–7
early recognition 276
heart failure 311
management goals 275
myocardial infarction 289
oxygen therapy 276
reduction of demand on heart 277
causes 263
non-cardiac 262
Chest radiography 340
cardiovascular disease 266
Chest wall trauma 358
Chewing (mastication) 437, 438
Cheyne–Stokes respiration 336, 693
Children
arterial blood pressure 253
burn injuries 937
capacity to consent 169
immune response 136
pain experience 114
preoperative foods/fluids 170

Chlamydia trachomatis 126, 828, 829, 830
  non-specific urethritis 790
  prostatitis 789
Chlorambucil 401, 406
Chloramphenicol 753
Chloroform 622
Chloroquine 527, 908
Chlorphenamine (chlorpheniramine) 429, 952
Choking 369, 996
Cholangitis 529
Cholecystectomy 528, 529
Cholecystitis 528–9
Cholecystography 512
Cholecystokinin–pancreozymin 440, 509
Cholecystostomy 529
Choledochitis 529
Choledochoduodenostomy 529
Choledochojejunostomy 529
Choledocholithiasis 529
Choledochostomy 529
Cholelithiasis 386, 528
Cholestasis 522
Cholesteatoma 754
Cholesterol 255, 541, 569, 686
Cholinesterase 676, 677
CHOP chemotherapy 408
Chordae tendinae 248
Chorea 677
Choreiform movements 680
Choriocarcinoma 203
Choroid 759
Choroid plexus 669, 673
Christmas disease (haemophilia B; factor IX deficiency) 418
Chromium 199
Chromosomal mutation 196
Chronic illness 6, 82–91
  barriers to change 89–90
  definition 82–3
  living with chronic conditions 83, 87–8
  prevention in older people 54
  primary care management 75, 83–7
    call/recall systems 84
    educational processes 88–9
    evaluation (audit) 85–7
    nurses' role 87–90
    setting up register 83–4
    trajectory model 83, 89
Chylomicrons 255, 538
Chymotrypsin 439
Ciclosporin 402, 640, 909
Ciliary body 759
Ciliary muscles 760
Cimetidine 102, 439, 455
  adverse effects 107
Ciprofloxacin 790, 919
Circle of Willis 672
Circulating nurse (surgical team) 176
Circulation
  burn injuries 938
  cardiopulmonary resuscitation 307–8
  postoperative care 189
    immediate care 181–2
  trauma assessment 872
Circulatory overload, transfusion reactions 430
Circulatory system 247–54
  ageing changes 47, 48
  physical examination 259–63
  physiology 250–4
  pulmonary 248
  structures 247–50
  systemic 248
Circumcision 788, 789

Cirrhosis 521–6
  causes 521–2
  clinical features 522
  complications 523–5
  education for lifestyle modification 526
  liver tissue changes 521
  nursing management 525–7
  portal hypertension 522, 523
  treatment 522–3
    liver transplantation 528
Cisternal puncture 685
Citric acid (Krebs) cycle 538, 539
Clarithromycin 455
Cleaning procedures 139–40
Cleft palate 447
Climacteric 804
Clindamycin 919
Clinical drug trials 108
  cytotoxic agents 204
Clitoris 783, 804
Clodronate 233
Clomethine (mustine) 406
Clomifene 818
Clonidine 863
Clonogenic assay 200
Closed questions 35
Clostridium difficile 467
Clostridium tetani 126, 742
Clostridium welchii 897
Clot formation 377, 378
Clotting factors *see* Coagulation factors
Co-analgesics 231–2, 866
Co-codamol 97
Co-proxamol 404
Coagulation disorders 417–23
  coagulation factor deficiencies 418–22
  liver disease 513
  renal disease 620–1
Coagulation factor concentrates 427
Coagulation factor deficiencies 418–22
Coagulation factors 377
  liver synthesis 508
  vitamin K-dependent 420
Coarctation of aorta 281
Cocaine 968, 969
  crack cocaine 969–70
Cocci 125
Cochlea 748
Code of professional Conduct 5, 8–9, 13, 14, 33
Codeine 97, 119, 468, 481
Coeliac disease *see* Gluten-sensitive enteropathy
Cognitive behavioural therapy
  group programmes 122
  maintenance of gains 122
  pain management 121–2
Cognitive function
  ageing changes 49
  anaemia 392, 393
  endocrine disorders 568
  following intracranial surgery 716
  liver disease 514
  renal function impairment 620, 628, 636
    acute renal failure 624, 625, 626
  stroke (cerebrovascular accident) 693, 694
Cognitive restructuring 121
Cognitive status assessment 679
Coitus interruptus 816
Cold application
  rheumatoid arthritis 907
  skin lesions 952
Cold autoimmune haemolytic anaemia 386
Cold exposure, arterial occlusive disease 326

Cold and flu remedies 97
Coliforms 126
Collagen (connective tissue) disease 916–18
  vascular purpura 420
Collecting tubules 611, 612
Colles' fracture 872, 896
Colon
  ascending 437
  descending 437
  functional aspects 440
  sigmoid 437
  transverse 437
Colonic resection 489
  critical pathway 490–3
  discharge advice 489–90, 493–4
Colonoscopy
  colorectal cancer 487, 488
  inflammatory bowel disease 480
Colorectal cancer 487–94
  case study 488–9
  clinical features 467, 488
  contributing factors 487
  diagnosis 488
  discharge advice 489–90, 493–4
  incidence 487
  metastases 487
  prevention 494
  screening 488, 494
  treatment 488
    colonic resection 489, 490–3
Colostomy 487, 494, 495–6
  colorectal cancer 488
  community support 503
  complications 503
  divided 496
  double-barrelled 496
  drainage appliance selection 498–9
  ileostomy comparison 496
  irrigation 499
  loop 496
  medication use 502–3
  nursing assessment 497
  nutrition alterations 500, 502
  permanent 495
  postoperative assessment 498
  preoperative preparation
    physical 497
    psychological 496
  psychosocial adjustment 500
  self-care
    activities 502
    education 501–2
  sexual function 500–1
  skin care 499–500, 502
  temporary 495
Colour of extremities 323
Colposcopy 842
Coma *see* Consciousness level alteration
Comedo (blackhead) 949
Commensal organisms 126
Commissural tracts 671
Committee on Medical Aspects of Food and Nutrition Policy (COMA) report 543
Common cold 126
Communication 29–39
  ageing changes 47
  assessment frameworks 32–3
  barriers 30–4
  breaking bad news 68, 162
  care of suddenly bereaved 68
  decision to withhold cardiopulmonary resuscitation 309
  environmental factors 31
  ethnic minority groups 23

health education 30–1, 32, 33
hearing impaired people 752–3
importance for patient care 29–30
listening skills 31, 32
multiple sclerosis 734
Parkinson's disease 735
reflecting skills 33
stroke 695
tracheostomy patient 364, 366
unpopular patient 38–9
ventilated/intubated patients 362
visually impaired people 768
Communication skills 34–9
active listening 35–6
asking questions 35
empathy 36–7
handling emotion 37–8
non-verbal aspects 35
silence 36
starting interview 34–5
Community care 6
elderly people 42–3
resources for hearing impaired people
753
see also Primary health care
Community children's nurses 79
Community learning disabilities nurses 79
Community mental health nurses 79
Community nursing
infection prevention 141
specialist nurses 78–80
terminal cancer care 240
Complement system 127, 373
Complementary therapies
cancer 219–20
older people 54
Complete (third degree) heart block 293, 303
Compliance
cardiovascular patients 271
health education 21–2
psychological reactance 90
Computed tomography (CT) 160–1
liver disorders 511
neurological disorders 683
phaeochromocytoma 608
pituitary disorders 600
renal system 617
respiratory disorders 340
stroke (cerebrovascular accident) 693
Computerized information 6
Concussion 699–700
Condom 788, 811–12
Conduction system 249, 251
regulation of activity 252
Conductive hearing loss 750
Condylomata acuminata (genital warts)
790–1, 829, 830, 831
Cone biopsy 841–2
Cones 759
Confidentiality 8
Congenital cardiovascular defects 280–2
circulatory blood flow resistance 281
left-to-right shunts 280–1
management in adulthood 280
right-to-left shunts 281–2
Conjunctiva 759
Conjunctivitis 769
Connecting (internuncial) neurone 666
Connective tissue (collagen) disease 420,
916–18
Connective tissues, drug absorption 98
Consciousness 682
Consciousness level alteration
acute renal failure 624
consent for treatment 169–70

eye care 712
faecal incontinence 713
fluid balance 712
head injury 703, 706
nursing care 711–13
heart failure 311
intracranial pressure elevation 708,
709–10
joint movement 712
metabolic causes 703
mouth care 712
nutrition 712
positioning 712
postoperative ventilation adequacy 181
protection from injury 712
restlessness 709–10
sensory stimulation 713
skin care 713
spinal cord injury 718
stroke (cerebrovascular accident) 692,
693
urinary catheterization 712–13
Consciousness level assessment 682, 703–5
Consensual pupil reaction 763
Consent form 169, 171, 172
Constipation 443, 465, 469–71
Alzheimer's disease 731
assessment 470
bladder surgery postoperative prevention
659
cancer 239, 240
chemotherapy side effects 208
nursing care 225
cardiac patients 273
causes 469–70
colonic 469
colorectal cancer 488
fracture patient in traction 886, 888
immuncompromised patient 412
intestinal obstruction 486
management 470–1
multiple sclerosis 734
opioid side-effects management 232–3,
239
Parkinson's disease 736
rectal (dyschezia) 469
spinal cord injury 722
Consumer expectations 21
Contact dermatitis 953
Contact lenses 766
after cataract extraction 773
Contaminated materials disposal 137
Context of care 1, 7, 8
Continence mechanism, women 835, 838
Continent ileal urinary pouch 656–7
Contingency management, urinary
incontinence 649
Continuity theory 50
Continuous ambulatory peritoneal dialysis
(CAPD) 629–31
complications 630–1
dialysis cycles 630
nursing care 631
peritoneal catheters 630
Continuous hyperfractionated accelerated
radiotherapy (CHART) 209–10
Continuous intracranial pressure
monitoring 682
Contraception 788, 811–16
methods 811–16
nursing responsibilities 811
Contracts for health education 22
Contractures
multiple sclerosis 734
spinal cord injury 723

Contrast media 160, 161
Contrast venography 327
Control of Substances Hazardous to
Health (COSHH) Guidelines (1988)
204
Controlled hyperventilation 701
Convalescence 130
Convergence 761
Cooperation see Compliance
Cooper's ligaments 847
Coordination of care 12
Coordination testing 680
Coping self statement 122
Core gender identity 783
Corn 950
Cornea 759, 760
Corneal transplantation (keratoplasty)
776–7
Coronary artery bypass surgery (CABG)
292, 314–15
complications 315, 317–18
Coronary artery catheterization 267
Coronary artery system 249–50
Coronary atherosclerosis 285
see also Ischaemic heart disease
Coronary care units 291
Coronary heart disease see Ischaemic heart
disease
Coronary heart syndrome 285
Corpus albicans 801
Corpus luteum 800–1
Corrosive oesophageal burns 448
management 449
Corticospinal tract (pyramidal tract) 674,
677
Corticostriatonigral degeneration see
Huntington's disease
Corticotrophin-releasing hormone (CRH)
562, 566
Cortisol 566
Cough 335
cardiogenic pulmonary oedema 262
Counselling 6
family involvement in cancer care 239
pre-investigative tests 162–3
Coup/contrecoup injury 698
[51]Cr-labelled EDTA clearance test 616
Crackles (rales; crepitations) 339
Cranial nerves 674
assessment 678–9
Craniectomy 713
Cranioplasty 713
Craniotomy 713
Creatine phosphokinase
MB isoenzyme 291
myocardial infarction 290–1
Creatinine clearance test 616
Creatinine serum level 616
acute renal failure 621
Credé, manoeuvre 649, 722
Crepitation, fractures 876
Crepitations (crackles; rales) 339
Cricopharyngeal (upper oesophageal)
sphincter 436
Criminal abortion 826
Crisis intervention 63, 64
phases of crisis 65
sudden death see Sudden death
Crista acustica 749
Critical incidents 7
chronic illness management in
community 88
ileostomy 504–5
needlestick injuries 521
non-Hodgkin's lymphoma 431–2

Critical incidents (*contd*)
pressure ulcers 957–8
reflection 1001
traditional diets 557–8
urine specimen collection 163
Critical pathway approach 10, 12
Crohn's disease 385, 478–9
clinical features 479
quality of life impact 481–2
contributing factors 479
diagnostic investigations 480–1
diarrhoea 466, 467, 481, 482, 485
extragastrointestinal manifestations 480
ileostomy 494
incidence 479
ulcerative colitis comparison 479–80
see also Inflammatory bowel disease
Cross-infection control 133–4, 137–40
burns injuries 943–4
community nursing 141
diarrhoea 468–9
disinfection procedures 138, 139
isolation procedures 134
key measures 140
kidney transplant patients 639
levels of decontamination 138
neutropenic patients 398, 412, 413
operating theatre 172
sexually transmitter disease 791, 832
standard precautions 134
sterilization procedures 138, 139
surgery 178–9
transmission-based precautions 134, 135
universal blood/body fluid precautions 140, 141, 518, 520, 791, 832, 951
viral hepatitis 518, 520
Crush injury 622
Crust (scab) 950
Cryoprecipitate 427
Cryptococcosis 729
Cryptorchidism 787, 795
Cultural issues
diet 554–7
eating behaviour 545
health education 22–3
pain experience 114
views of health 15–16
Culture for infectious agents identification 131
Cushing's disease 600
hypertension 320
Cushing's syndrome 568, 604, 607
causes 607
clinical features 607
management 607
Cyanosis
cardiovascular disorders 262
postoperative 181
respiratory disorders 334
Cyclic adenosine monophosphate (cAMP) 561
Cyclical neutropenia 396
Cyclophosphamide 136, 225, 406, 408, 409, 417, 654, 859, 909, 917
Cyclopropane 174
Cystectomy 656, 657
Cystic fibrosis 79
Cystitis 653
radiotherapy side effects 214
Cystocele 833, 835, 837
Cystometrography 647
stress incontinence 837
Cystoscopy 617, 656
Cystostomy 657, 658, 659
patient education 659–60

Cystotomy 657
Cytomegalovirus 639, 729, 730
blood/blood products screening 423, 425
Cytotoxic agents
classification 204
clinical trials 204
handling/disposal 204–5
hypersensitivity reactions 233
mode of action 204
side effects/toxicities 206–7, 208, 225
tumour resistance 204
Cytotoxic (T8) T lymphocytes 129

D-Dimer test 327
Dacarbazine 225, 406
Dalteparin 328
Danazol 821
Dapsone 342
Dark adaptation 761–2
Day surgery 190–1
discharge criteria 191
patient selection 191
Deafness *see* Hearing loss
Deamination 539, 540
Debridement
burns 942
pressure ulcers 932
Decerebrate rigidity 681
Decorticate rigidity 681
Decubitus ulcer *see* Pressure ulcers
Deep tendon reflexes 669
assessment 681
Deep vein thrombosis 327–8
arthroplasty 914
complications 327–8
diagnosis 327
postoperative 189
prophylaxis 328
risk factors 327
treatment 328
Defaecation 437
promotion techniques 471
see also Bowel elimination
Defibrillation 293, 306
advanced cardiac life support 308
ventricular fibrillation 301
ventricular tachycardia 298
Degenerative joint disease 910–16
Degenerative nervous system disorders 678, 728–39
Dehiscence 188
Dehydration
acute renal failure 622
infection 132, 133
intestinal obstruction 486
intracranial pressure reduction 702
nursing of terminally ill 553
preoperative preparation 169
Delerium 314
Delerium tremens 962
Deliberate self-harm 982, 986–7, 988
assessment of repetition risk 987
calcaneal fracture 894
see also Suicide
Dementia 49
Demography 41–2
Dendrites 666
Denham pin 880
Denial
advanced cancer patient 239
body image alteration response 70–1, 236
breast cancer 864
chronic illness 89
communication skills 38

grief response 61, 62, 63, 68, 235
myocardial infarction 290
Dental care 446–7
Dental caries 444, 540
immuncompromised patient 412
radiotherapy side effects 214
Dental health 540
Dental infection/abscess 444
Dentures 712
endotracheal intubation 362
immunocompromised patient 412
preoperative removal 171
Deontological world-view 13
Dependence 962
physical 962
psychological 962
Depo-Provera 814
Depolarization
myocardial cells 251, 264
nerve function 667
Depressant drugs, misuse of 967, 970–2
Depression
cancer patients 238, 240
dying patient 63, 235, 240
elderly people 49
fracture patient in traction 889
grief response 61, 63, 235
learned helplessness 115
pain experience 115
rheumatoid arthritis 905
Dermatitis 952, 953–4
contact 953
exfoliative 953
Dermis 925, 926
Dermoid cyst 839
Desmopressin (DDAVP) 420
Detrusor muscle 614, 615, 835
instability 645, 835
Development, Erikson's theory 49
Developmental crises, grief reaction 63–4
Dexamethasone 232, 417, 709
Dextropropoxyphene 119
Diabetes insipidus 602–3
Diabetes mellitus 6, 82–3, 568–88
blood glucose monitoring 579–80
sampling devices 156
cardiovascular risk 254, 257, 570
stroke 686
case studies 581–2, 584–5
characteristics 568–9
chronic pancreatitis 533
complications 569–70
erectile dysfunction (impotence) 787
foot ulcers 570
macrovascular degenerative changes 570
microvascular degenerative changes 569–70
neuropathy 570
renal function impairment 627
retinopathy 569, 581, 776
epidemiology 568–9
ethnic minority groups 16
glycaemic control 572
assessment 579–80
health education 25
health monitoring 581
hypertension 570
hypoglycaemic episodes 572, 580, 587–8
risk-taking behaviour 90
insulin deficiency 569
management 571–6
diet 571–2, 573, 578
foot care 579
illness episodes 578

insulin therapy 572–5, 578
  oral hypoglycaemic drugs 575, 578
  physical activity 575–6, 579
  skin care 579
  travel arrangements 578–9
metabolic emergencies 580–1, 585–8
  diabetic ketoacidosis 580, 583–4, 585–6
  hyperosmolar non-ketotic coma 580, 586–7
microalbuminuria 569, 570, 579
obesity association 547, 548, 568, 570
patient/family education 576–81
  learning needs assessment 576–7
  teaching plan development 577
  teaching plan implementation 577–81
preoperative preparation 169
prevention
  primary 570
  secondary 570–1
primary care management 83, 84, 85, 88
register of patients 83, 84
secondary 568
support services 581
type I (insulin-dependent) 568, 569, 578
type II (non-insulin-dependent) 568, 569, 578
urine monitoring 579
urine tests 157
Diabetic identification card 581
Diabetic ketoacidosis 580, 583–4, 585–6
  consciousness level alteration 703
Diabetic neuropathy 570
Diabetic retinopathy 569, 581, 776
Diagnostic imaging see Imaging investigations
Dialysate 629, 631
Dialysis 629–34, 917
  acute renal failure 624
  methods 629
Diamorphine (heroin) 119, 276, 968, 970
  withdrawal profile 979
Diaphragm contraception 812
Diaphysis 871
Diarrhoea 443, 465–9
  assessment 467
  cancer patients
    chemotherapy side effects 208, 399, 862
    nursing care 226
    radiotherapy side effects 211, 214
  causes
    extrinsic 467
    intrinsic 466–7
  colorectal cancer 488
  infectious illness 132, 133
  inflammatory bowel disease 466, 467, 481, 482, 485
  management 467–9
    drug treatment 468
  renal function impairment 620
Diastole 251
Diastolic blood pressure 253
  auscultation 260
Diazepam 460, 624, 866, 968
Dichloralphenazone 171
Dietary causative factors
  breast cancer 848–9
  carcinogenesis 196
  constipation 469
  diarrhoea 467
  gastritis 452, 453
Dietary fibre 104, 469, 470, 494, 540
  intake recommendations 543

Dietary modification
  anaemia 392
    iron deficiency 384
  cardiovascular disease 279
  cardiovascular risk modification 255–6
    guidelines 256
  chronic pancreatitis 533
  colorectal cancer prevention 494
  constipation 470–1
  diabetes mellitus management 571–2, 573, 578
  diarrhoea 468
  faecal impaction 472
  hypertension 320–1
  ileostomy/colostomy patient 500
  malabsorption 475
  peptic ulcer 455
  stomach/duodenal disorders 460
    gastric resection patients 464
  weight reduction programme 549
Dietary reference values 542, 543
Diethylstilbestrol 843–5, 846, 847
Digestive enzymes 437, 439
Digestive processes 437–41
Digoxin 83, 273, 279, 297, 301, 302, 303, 310, 312
Dihydrocodeine 119
Dilated cardiomyopathy 282
Diphenoxylate 468
Diplopia 761, 777
Direct observations 11
Disaccharides 540
Discharge criteria following day surgery 191
Discharge preparations 190
  acute renal failure 626–7
  burns injuries 947
  hip replacement surgery 914
  rheumatoid arthritis 910
  skin disorders 953
  stroke (cerebrovascular accident) 696–7
Disease-modifying antirheumatic drugs (DMARDS) 908
Disengagement theory 50
Disinfection procedures 138, 139
Dislocation 873
Disopyramide 297, 299
Dissecting aortic aneurysm 322
Disseminated intravascular coagulation 386, 421–2
  management 422
Distal convoluted tubule 611, 612
District nurses 79
Diuretics
  cardiac disease 273, 314
  cirrhosis 522
  pulmonary oedema 310
  respiratory failure 361
Diverticulitis 466
Divided colostomy 496
DNA replication errors 195
DNA viruses 126
  carcinogenesis 196–7
Do not attempt resuscitation (DNAR) 309
Dobutamine 273, 312
Doderlein's bacillus 800
Dopamine 273, 312
Doppler echocardiography 265
Doppler ultrasound
  arterial occlusive disease 324
  carotid arteries assessment 683
  varicose veins 326
Dorsal column medial lemniscal pathway 112
Dorzolamide 771

Dose–response curve 104
Double-barrelled colostomy 496
Down's syndrome 397
Doxazosin 792
Doxorubicin (adriamycin) 406, 408, 859
Doxycycline 790
Drains
  postoperative care 187
  see also Chest drainage; Gastric drainage
Dreams 682
Dressings
  burns injuries 945
  moist compresses for skin lesions 952
  pressure ulcers 932, 933
Dressler's syndrome 293
Drift testing 680
Drug detoxification 508
Drug overdose 39
  consciousness level alteration 703
Drug–enzyme interactions 102
Drug-induced haemolytic anaemia 386
Drug–receptor interactions 102–4
  qualitative aspects 102–3
  quantitative aspects 103–4
Drugs 95
  absorption 98–9
    blood flow 99
    molecular size 98
    solubility 98–9
  administration 95–7
    buccal/sublingual 101
    intramuscular 101
    intravenous 101
    local 99–100
    oral 100–1
    principles 97–8
    rectal 101
    subcutaneous 102
    transdermal 102
  adverse effects (toxicity) 103, 107–8
  bioavailability 102
    oral 101
  central nervous system access 98, 102
  classification/naming 97
  combinations 97
  discovery/development process 108
  elimination 105
  enzyme induction 107
  enzyme inhibition 107
  first-pass metabolism 101
  functional groups 98, 103, 107
  half-life 107
  influence on clinical investigation results 152
  interactions 107, 108
  metabolism 105–7
    active metabolites 106
    phase 1 reactions 106
    phase 2 reactions 106
  mode of action 102
  nurse education 96, 97
  placebo effects 102, 104–5
  plasma protein binding 102
  preoperative history-taking 168
  preoperative preparation 171
  therapeutic index 103
  therapeutic window 103
  tolerance 103, 119
  see also Pharmacology
Dry mouth, nursing of terminally ill 553, 554
Dual-energy X-ray absorption 919
Duct ectasia 854
Duct papilloma 854
Ductal carcinoma in situ 855

Duffy blood group 425
Dumping syndrome 458
Duodenal disorders 452
  history-taking 458–9
  management 459–62
Duodenal obstruction, acute pancreatitis
  531
Duodenal ulcer 452
  pain 454
  see also Peptic ulcer
Duodenum 436
Duplex ultrasound
  arterial occlusive disease 324
  deep vein thrombosis 327
Dura mater 669
Dwarfism 600
Dying patient 59–73
  cancer terminal care 235, 239–41
    family involvement 239
  dehydration 553
  spiritual issues 240–1
  stages of grief 62, 63, 235
  withholding of nutritional support 552–3
Dying trajectory concept 235
Dyschezia (rectal constipation) 469
Dysfunctional grieving 60
Dysfunctional uterine bleeding 819–20
Dysgeusia 224
Dysmenorrhoea 819
Dyspareunia 808
Dysphagia 447, 448, 449, 450
  causes 447
  gastrointestinal disorders 442
  iron deficiency anaemia 383
  neurological disorders 447
  radiotherapy side effects 214
Dysphasia 678
Dyspnoea see Breathlessness
Dystonic movements 680
Dysuria 644, 645

Ear 748–9
  disorders 749, 753–6
    see also Hearing loss
  physical examination 750
Early postoperative ambulation 187, 188,
  189
Eating behaviour 545
Eating disorders 550, 551
Ecchymosis 876
Echocardiography 265
Echymosis (bruise) 422
Ecstasy
  (3,4-methylenedioxymethamfetamine;
  MDMA) 968
Ectopic beats (premature beats;
  extrasystoles) 298–9
Ectopic pregnancy 826
  acute tubal rupture 826–7
Eczema 100, 953–4
Editronate 233, 920
Effector 668
Efferent (motor) neurone 666
Ejaculation 784
  spinal reflex arc 784
Elastic compression stockings 189
  deep vein thrombosis 328
  varicose veins 326, 327
Elderly people 6, 41–55
  alcohol consumption problems 966–7
  assessment 51–3
  burn injuries 937
  case study 44–5
  demography 41–2
  drug absorption 99

empowerment/re-enablement approach
  43, 52
exercise 554
  cardiovascular patients 275
femur neck fracture 890
  care pathway approach 892
  institutionalization following 891
fractures 873–4
health/social care 42–5
  equity issues 45–7
  health/wellness promotion 53–5
  National Service Framework 43–4
  total population approach 54
immune system changes 136
normal ageing 47–51
nutrition 554
pain experience 114
person-centred assessment 46
professional nursing skills 53
renal function impairment 621
screening health assessment 54
sociological perspectives 50–1
standards of services 43–4
stereotyping 43, 44, 46
  see also Ageing
Elective surgery 165
Electrical burns 934
Electrical devices, urinary incontinence
  management 649–50
Electrocardiography (ECG) 263–5
  ambulatory (Holter technique) 264–5
  bedside monitoring 264
  exercise (stress test) 265
  hyperkalaemia 623
  myocardial infarction 290
  telemetry monitoring 264
Electroencephalography (EEG) 684
  stroke 693
Electrolyte balance
  burn injuries 937
  consciousness level alteration 703
  inflammatory bowel disease 484–5
  intestinal obstruction 486, 487
  postoperative care 184–5
  preoperative preparation 169
  renal function 612, 613–14
    impaired 619–20, 628, 634–5
  respiratory disorders 341
Electromyography (EMG) 684
Electrophysiological studies, cardiac
  arrhythmias 268–9
Electroretinography 763
Elemental feeding 484
Elliptocytosis, hereditary 386–7
Embolism
  acute arterial occlusion 322, 323
  atrial fibrillation 301
  post-myocardial infarction 293
Emergency contraception 815
  sexual assault victim 810
Emergency surgery 165
  preoperative preparation 171
Emergency treatment
  consent 169–70
  fractures 877
  head injury 705
  spinal cord injury 717, 718
  see also First aid
Emetic (vomiting) centre 442
Emetine 527
Emmetropia 760
Emollients 952
Emotional patients, communication skills
  37–8
Empathy 8, 36–7

Employment
  older people 42
  rheumatoid arthritis patients 910
Employment contract, nurse accountability 5
Empowerment 17, 18
  elderly people 43
Empyema 354
Encephalitis 742
Endarterectomy 325, 687
  postoperative care 687
  preoperative preparation 687
Endemic disease 135
Endocardium 248
Endocrine disorders 561–610
  signs/symptoms 567–8
Endocrine glands 561, 562
  ageing changes 48
Endocytosis 98
Endometrial biopsy 816
Endometrial carcinoma 843
Endometrial polyp 838
Endometriosis 820–1
  hysteroscopy 821
  laparoscopy 820
  treatment 821
Endometrium 801
  menstrual cycle changes 801
Endorphins 112, 118
Endoscopic retrograde
  cholangiopancreatography (ERCP)
  511–12, 529
Endoscopy 160
  cancer diagnosis 201
  nursing care 454
  peptic ulcer 454
Endosteum 870
Endotracheal intubation 361–3
  extubation 363
  general anaesthesia 173
  indications 362, 369
  insertion procedure 362–3
Endotracheal tube 362
Enema 471
  cleansing 170, 472
  oil retention 472
Energy metabolism 538
  obesity 548
Energy requirements 543, 544
Energy value of nutrients 540
Enkephalins 112
Entamoeba histolytica 527
Enteral drug administration 100
Enteral (nasogastric tube) feeding
  acute pancreatitis 532
  procedure 460
  unconscious patient 712
Enterohepatic circulation 105, 106
Enterokinase 440
Enucleation of eyeball 778
Environment
  cleaning 139
  external 8
  focus of nursing 7–8
  health promotion 17
  immuncompromised patient 411, 413
  internal 7–8
  pressure ulcers 833
  reservoirs of infection 136
Environmental Protection Act (1990) 137
Enzyme inducing drugs 107
Enzyme inhibitors 103, 107
Enzymes 103
  digestive 437, 439
Eosinophils 375, 376
Epicardium 248

Epidemic disease 135
Epidemiology 135
Epidermis 925, 926
Epididymitis 789
Epidural anaesthesia 174, 175
Epilepsy 677, 690, 739–42
  antiepileptic drugs 741
  automatism 739
  care during seizure 740–1
  causes 739
  classification 739
  incidence 739
  patient education 741
  primary care management 82, 84
  psychosocial support 741–2
  seizure types 739–40
Epiphyseal (growth) plate 871
Epiphysis 871
Epirubicin 859
Epistaxis (nosebleed) 757
Epithelial drug absorption 98
Epsilon-aminocaproic acid 690
Epstein–Barr virus 403, 417
Equipment decontamination 138
Equity of health care 76, 77
Erectile dysfunction (impotence) 786–7
Ergocalciferol 920
Erikson's model of
    developmental/situational crises 63
Erikson's theory of development 49
Erosion (excoriation) 950
Erythema 949, 951
  radiotherapy side effects 211
Erythroblastalis fetalis 379
Erythrocyte apheresis 395, 396
Erythrocyte count, normal values 341
Erythrocyte disorders 380–96
Erythrocyte excess (polycythaemia) 395
Erythrocyte sedimentation rate 131
Erythrocytes (red blood cells) 373
  destruction in liver 508
  haematological values 381
  life cycle 375
  terminology for microscopic examination
      380
Erythrogenin (renal erythropoietic factor)
    614
Erythromycin 324
Erythropoiesis 373–4
  abnormalities 382–5
  nutritional requirements 374–5
Erythropoietin 374, 395, 612, 614
Eschar 945
Escharotomy 941
Escherichia coli 135, 477, 527, 641, 789
Escherichia coli type 0157 136, 466–7
  verocytotoxin 467
Esotropia 777
Essential amino acids 540, 541
Essential fatty acids 541
Estimated average requirements (EAR)
    542, 543
Ethambutol 352
Ethanol 107
  see also Alcohol consumption
Ether 174, 199
Ethical issues 6, 13–14
  advocacy 67
  assisted fertility techniques 818
  health education 25, 26
  organ donation 638
  withholding of cardiopulmonary
      resuscitation 308–9
  withholding of nutritional support
      552, 553

Ethmoid sinuses 757
Ethnic minorities 6
  cardiovascular risk 255
  communication issues 23, 30
  diabetes mellitus 568, 627
  end-stage renal failure 627
  health education 23
  health status 15–16
  pain experience 114
  stereotyping 31
  traditional diets 555–7
    critical incident 557–8
    religious influences 556
Ethylene glycol 622
Ethylene oxide sterilization 139
Etomidate 702
Eupnoea 336
European Code against Cancer 199, 200
Eustacian (auditory) tube 748
Evacuation enema 170
Evaluation of care plan 12
Evening primrose oil 852
Evidence-based practice 9
Evisceration
  eyeball 778
  postoperative wound 188
Ewing's sarcoma 203
Exchange theory 50
Excisional biopsy 202
Excoriation (erosion) 950
Exenteration of eyeball 778
Exercise 90
  acute renal failure 626
  arterial blood pressure 253
  burns injuries 945
  cardiovascular disease 270, 274–5, 286
    rehabilitation 293
  cardiovascular risk modification 254, 257
  COMA report recommendations 544
  consciousness level alteration 712
  constipation 471
  diabetes mellitus 575–6, 579
  elderly people 554
  hypertension 321
  influence on blood test values 157
  limb amputation 901
  osteoarthritis 911
  osteoporosis 920
  peripheral vascular disease 325–6
  postoperative care 186–7
  preoperative preparation 169
  pressure ulcer wound care 833
  respiratory failure 361
  rheumatoid arthritis 907
  visual impairment 768
  weight reduction programme 549
  see also Activity intolerance
Exercise electrocardiography (stress test)
    265
Exfoliative cytology 201
Exfoliative dermatitis 953
Exhalation, drug excretion 105
Exocrine glands 561
Exocytosis 98
Exophthalmic goitre see Hyperthyroidism
Exotropia 777
Expressive (motor; Broca's) aphasia 678
Extended Nurse Prescribers' Formulary
    96
Extension 872
External auditory meatus 748
External chest compression 307–8
External ear 748
External fixation 878
  see also Plaster cast

External skeletal fixation 878
  postoperative care 886
  preoperative preparation 885–6
Extracorporeal shockwave lithotripsy
    (ESWL) 643
Extradural haematoma 700
Extradural space 669
Extrapyramidal system (tracts) 677
Extrasystoles (ectopic beats; premature
    beats) 298–9
Extrinsic ocular muscles 759
  convergence 761
  functional assessment 762
Exudate 354
Eye care 767
  Parkinson's disease 736
  unconscious patient 712
Eye disorders 769–78
  see also Visual impairment
Eye examination 762–4
  electroretinography 763
  extraocular muscle function 762
  eye reflexes 762–3
  fluorescein staining 763
  gonioscopy 764
  intraocular pressure measurement 763
  macroscopic 762
  ophthalmic 763
  routine 765–6
  slit-lamp microscopy 763
  terminology 766
  visual acuity 763
  visual field measurement (perimetry)
      763
Eye injury
  chemical damage 777
  first aid treatment 767
  foreign body 777
  lacerations 777
  prevention 766–7
Eye neoplasms 778
Eye reflexes 760
  assessment 762–3
Eyeball
  anterior/posterior cavities 759
  fluid system 759–60
  structure 759
Eyelids (palpebrae) 758–9
Eyes 758–61
  movement 759

Facial (VII) nerve assessment 679
Factor VIII concentrate 427
Factor VIII deficiency (haemophilia A) 418
Factor VIII replacement therapy 418–19
  complications 419
Factor IX concentrate 427
Factor IX deficiency (haemophilia B;
    Christmas disease) 418
Faecal diversion see Colostomy; Ileostomy
Faecal drug excretion 105
Faecal fat test 511
Faecal impaction 466, 471–2
  management 472
  spinal cord injury 722
  stroke 693
  urinary incontinence 645
Faecal incontinence 443, 466, 472–3
  assessment 472
  management 472–3
  stroke 692, 693
  unconscious patient 713
Faecal occult blood 443
  colorectal cancer screening 488
Faeces 440

Fallopian tubes, menstrual cycle changes 804
Familial cancer patterns 196, 197
Familial cardiovascular risk 255
Familial polyposis coli 495
  colorectal cancer risk 487
Family involvement 8
  cancer care 238–9
    terminal phase 239, 240
  cardiovascular patient care 271, 277–8
  dying patient, presence/absence at time of death 67–8
  head-injured patient rehabilitation 716
  health education 21
  immuncompromised patient care 412–13
  presence during cardiopulmonary resuscitation 309
  spinal cord injury 724–5
  sudden death, support needs 64
  support for elderly people 42
Fanconi anaemia 397, 401
Fasciculations 680
Fat, dietary 541
  intake recommendations 543
  stroke risk 686
Fat digestion 437, 440, 508
Fat embolism 892
Fat metabolism 538–9
  insulin actions 567
  liver 508
Fat storage 539
Fatal Accident Enquiry 61
Fatigue
  cancer patients
    chemotherapy side effects 208
    nursing care 226, 227
    radiotherapy side effects 214
  diabetes mellitus 569
  endocrine disorders 568
  heart failure 311
  myocardial infarction 289
Fatty acids 541
Fears
  arterial blood pressure effect 253
  cancer patients 237–8
  cardiovascular patients 270
  communication skills 38
Female condom (femidom) 812
Female reproductive system disorders 797–867
  assessment 805–6
  congenital anomalies 810–11
  genital organ displacements/relaxations 832–7
  infections 828–36
    sexually transmitted 829–32, 833, 834, 835, 836
  nursing interventions 807
  physical examination 806
  tumours 838–46
Female reproductive tract 797–805
  development 797–8
  external genitalia 797, 799
Femidom (female condom) 812
Femoral cast brace 893
Femoral catheter 632
Femur neck fracture 890–2
  assessment 890–1
  extracapsular 890
  internal fixation 882, 883, 884, 891
  intracapsular 890
  nursing care 891–2
Femur shaft fracture 879, 892–3
Fentanyl 99, 119–20
Ferritin 375, 384

Fertility
  cancer patients 236
    radiotherapy side effects 212
  multiple sclerosis 733
  renal function impairment 628
Fertilization 782, 800, 801
Festination gait 735
Fetal haemoglobin (HbF) 387, 388
Fetor hepaticus 514
Fever 128
  following intracranial surgery 716
  infection 130, 132
  intracranial pressure elevation 708, 710
  management 132–3
  myocardial infarction 289
  renal infections 620
  respiratory disorders 335
  seizures 739
Fibrin 377, 421
Fibrinogen 372, 373, 377
Fibrinogen degradation products (FDPs) 421, 422
Fibrinolysis 378
Fibroids (uterine myomas) 838–9
Fibrous joints 871
Fidelity 13
Fight or flight response 675
Finasteride 792
Fine needle aspiration cytology, breast disorders 852–3
Finger prick blood specimens 156
First aid
  burn injuries 939–40
  eye injuries 767
First degree atrioventricular block 302
First-pass metabolism 101
Fissure 950
Fissures of cerebrum 670
Fixed traction 879
Flaccidity 680
Flail segment 335, 358–9, 360
Flapping tremor 514
Flatulence 443
  postoperative care 184
Flexion 872
Flucloxacillin 101
Fludarabine 401
Fludrocortisone 605, 609
Fluid balance
  acute pancreatitis 532
  adrenal surgery 609
  bladder surgery 659
  burn injuries 937, 941–2
  consciousness level alteration 712
  diabetes insipidus 602
  diarrhoea management 468
  heart failure 311, 313–14
  inflammatory bowel disease 482, 484–5
  intestinal obstruction 486, 487
  intracranial pressure elevation 708, 710
  intracranial surgery 713
  limb amputation 900
  postoperative assessment 180
  postoperative care 184–5
  preoperative preparation 169
  renal function 613
  renal function impairment 619–20, 621
    acute renal failure 624
    chronic renal failure 627–8, 634–5
  syndrome of inappropriate antidiuretic hormone (SIADH) 603
  urinary diversion procedures 661–2
Fluorescein staining 763
Fluoroscopic examination

inflammatory bowel disease 480
respiratory disorders 340
5-Fluorouracil 225, 488, 861
Fluticasone 99
Focal (partial) seizures 739
Folic acid 374, 375, 441, 474
  dietary sources 383
Folic acid deficiency anaemia 385
Follicle-stimulating hormone (FSH) 562
  functions 563
  menopause 804
  menstrual cycle 801
  ovarian proliferative response 800
  spermatogenesis 782
Food groups 544–5
Food poisoning 136
Foot care, diabetes mellitus 579
Foot ulcers, diabetes mellitus 570
Forced vital capacity (FVC) 340
Foreign body
  aspiration 368–9
  eye injury 777
Fovea centralis 759
Fractures 874–96
  assessment 873
  causes 874
  clinical features 875–6
  complications 876–7
  emergency care 877
  healing 876–7
    delayed 876
  local tissue response 874–5
  malunion 876
  multiple myeloma 408, 410
  non-union 876
  osteoporosis-related 920
  rehabilitation 885, 889
  systemic response 875
  treatment 877–82
    external fixation 878
    internal fixation 882
    open (compound) fractures 882
    reduction 877–8
    traction 878–82
  types 874, 875
Frequency 644, 645
Fresh frozen plasma (FFP) 425, 427
Friction burns 934
Frigidity 808
Frontal lobes 671
Frontal sinuses 757
Fructose 572
Frusemide 282, 622
Full-thickness burns 936
  healing 945
Functional residual capacity (FRC) 340
Fundus oculi (optic disc) 759
Fungal infection 410
Fungi 126
Funnel-shaped chest 337

Gag reflex 669, 712
Gait abnormalities 680–1
Galactocele 854
Gallbladder 508–9
Gallbladder disease 507, 528–30
  nursing care 525–30
  terminology 528
Gallstones see Cholelithiasis
Gamete intrafallopian transfer (GIFT) 818
Gamma globulin 373
Gamma hydroxybutyrate (GHB) misuse 970
Gamma-glutamyl transferase 510

Ganglia 675
Gangrene 323
Gas gangrene 897, 898
Gaseous exchanges 333
Gastrectomy
  stomach cancer 458
  subtotal 455–6
Gastric cancer 457–8
Gastric drainage 462–3
  acute pancreatitis 532
  removal of tube 463
Gastric emptying 438
Gastric enzymes 435, 436, 439
Gastric glands 438
Gastric intubation 171
Gastric juice 435, 436, 439
  bactericidal activity 127
  regulation of secretion 439
Gastric lipase 439
Gastric motility 438
Gastric phase of gastric secretion 439
Gastric resection
  plus vagotomy 456
  subtotal gastrectomy 455–6
Gastric surgery 455–6
  dumping syndrome following 458
  information for patient 464
  nutritional deficiency following 464, 473,
    474
  postoperative care 462
    fluid/nutritional intake 463–4
      gastric drainage 462–3
      respiratory function 463
  preoperative care 462
Gastric ulcer 452, 457
  pain 454
  see also Peptic ulcer
Gastric varicosities *see* Oesophagogastric
  varices
Gastrin 439, 534, 567
  peptic ulcer aetiology 453
Gastritis 452–3
  causes 452
  chronic 453, 457
  clinical features 452–3
  peptic ulcer 453
Gastroduodenostomy 456, 458
Gastroenterostomy 456
Gastrointestinal disorders 435–505
  clinical features 441–4
  upper gastrointestinal tract 444–64
Gastrointestinal haemorrhage 422,
  443–4
  peptic ulcer haemorrhage 456–7
Gastrointestinal tract 435–7
  absorption 441
  ageing changes 47, 48
  digestive processes 437–41
  local drug administration 99–100
  motility 437
  radiotherapy side effects 211
Gastrojejunostomy 456, 458
Gastrostomy feeding 461
  complications 461
Gate control theory of pain 112–13, 118,
  120
Gaucher's disease 522
Gaviscon 448
Gel floatation pads 931
Gemprost 825
Gender differences
  cardiovascular risk 255
  pain experience 113–14
Gender dysphoria (transsexuality) 786
Gender identity 783, 786, 807

General anaesthesia 173
Generalized seizures 739
Generic (non-proprietary; approved)
  medicines 97
Genetic assessment 162–3
Genital herpes 832
Genital warts (condylomata acuminata)
  790–1, 829, 830, 831
Genomic mutation 195
Gentamicin 622, 752
Geographical variation, influence on clinical
  investigation results 152
Gerontological nurse specialist 53
Giant breast fibroadenoma 854
Giardiasis 126
Gigantism 568, 600
Gingivitis 444
Glandular fever (infectious mononucleosis)
  403–4
Glasgow Coma Scale 703, 704, 705
Glaucoma 770–1
  acute angle-closure 770–1
  open-angle (chronic) 770
Glibenclamide 575
Gliclazide 575
Glipizide 575
Glitazones (thiazolidinediones) 575
Globulins 372, 373
  liver function assessment 510
Glomerular filtration 105
Glomerular filtration rate (GFR)
  612–13
  measurement 616–17
Glomerulonephritis 136, 622, 627, 641
  causes 641
  clinical features 641
  management 641
Glomerulus 611
  blood supply 612
  filtration processes 612–13
Glossitis
  iron deficiency anaemia 383
  nursing care 393
  vitamin B_{12} deficiency (pernicious
    anaemia) 384
Glossopharyngeal (IX) nerve assessment
  679
Glucagon 439, 509, 567
  functions 567
Glucocorticoids 566
  nutrient metabolism 539, 540
Gluconeogenesis 566
Glucose
  metabolism 538
  renal handling 613
Glucose-6-phosphate dehydrogenase
  (G6PD) deficiency 387
Gluten-sensitive enteropathy (coeliac
  disease) 385, 420
  dietary modification 475
  malabsorption 474
Gluteraldehyde sterilization 139
Glycated haemoglobin (HbA1$_c$) 580
Glycerine suppositories 471, 472
Glyceryl trinitrate 101, 102, 276, 285, 286,
  483
  tolerance 103
Glycogen 508, 538
Glycogenesis 508
Glycolysis 538
Glycosuria 569
Goal setting 11–12
Goitre 447, 588, 590
  toxic/exophthalmic *see* Hyperthyroidism
Gold compounds 908

Gonadotrophin-releasing hormone (GnRH)
  562
  female reproductive function 800
    menstrual cycle 801
  male reproductive function 782
Gonadotrophins, infertility treatment 818
Gonioscopy 764
Gonorrhoea 790, 829, 830
Goserelin 862
Gout 395, 916
Graafian follicle 800
Graft-versus-host disease 217
Gram staining 158–9
Gram-negative bacteria 125, 158
Gram-positive bacteria 125, 158
Granulocyte concentrates 425
Granulocytes 375
Graves' disease *see* Hyperthyroidism
Gray (Gy) 209
Grey matter 670, 673
Grief 59–73
  abortion 823, 824
  anticipatory 60, 63
  cancer patients 235
  case study 72–3
  determinants/predictors 61
    historical antecedents 62
    mode of death 61–3
    personality variables 62
    relationship 62
    social variables 62–3
  dysfunctional 60
  life transitions 59, 63–4
  multiple sclerosis 733
  normal process (uncomplicated) 60–1
  nursing issues 60
  paralysis 724
  stages model 62, 63, 235
  sudden death 61, 64–8
  see also Loss
Groshong type catheter 205
Group cognitive behavioural therapy 122
Group instruction, preoperative preparation
  168
Group protocols 96
Grown Up Congenital Heart (GUCH) teams
  280
Growth disorders 568
Growth (epiphyseal) plate 871
Growth hormone 562, 871
  functions 564
    nutrient metabolism 539, 540
  hypersecretion 600–10
  pulsatile release 152
Growth hormone release-inhibiting
  hormone (GHRIH) *see* Somatostatin
Growth hormone-releasing hormone
  (GHRH) 562
Guedel airway 709
Guided imagery 122
Guillain–Barré, syndrome (acute infective
  polyneuropathy) 360, 744
Guilt
  communication skills 38
  grief reaction 61, 62
Gumma 791, 831
Gynaecomastia 514
Gyri 670

H_2 antagonists 361, 439, 453
  peptic ulcer 455
Habitual abortion 822
Haemarthrosis 423
Haematemesis 422, 443
Haematocrit, normal values 341

Haematological disorders 371–432
Haematoma 423
  postoperative 187–8
Haematopoiesis 373
  radiotherapy side effects 211
Haematopoietic growth factors 374, 376
Haematuria 619
Haemodialysis 629, 631–4
  nursing care 633–4
    postdialysis responsibilities 634
    predialysis responsibilities 633–4
    responsibilities during dialysis 634
  patient education 633–4
  psychosocial aspects 633
  vascular access 631–2
Haemoglobin 336, 373, 374
  adult types 387
  anaemia 380
  fetal (HbF) 387, 388
  normal values 341
  oxygen saturation 336–7
  oxygen transport 373
  release from burn injuries 937
  structural aspects 387
Haemoglobin H disease 387–8
Haemoglobin S (HbS) 388
Haemoglobinopathies 387–91
Haemolytic anaemia 386–91
  acquired 386
  inherited 386–91
Haemolytic disease of newborn 386
Haemolytic jaundice 513
Haemolytic transfusion reactions 428–9
Haemophilia 418–20
  care/healthcare services 419–20
  clinical features 418
  clotting factor administration 418–19
    complications 419
    viral infection transmission 419
  inheritance 418
  management 418–20
  patient education 419
Haemophilia A (factor VIII deficiency) 418
Haemophilia B (factor IX deficiency;
  Christmas disease) 418
Haemophilus influenzae 742
Haemopneumothorax 354, 359
Haemorrhage 422
  acute pancreatitis 531
  acute renal failure 622
  postoperative 181–2
Haemorrhagic disease of newborn 420
Haemorrhagic disorders 417–23
  history-taking 422
  nursing care 423, 424
  physical examination 422–3
  platelet disorders 417
  see also Coagulation disorders
Haemorrhagic telangiectasia, hereditary
  420
Haemorrhoids 326, 514
Haemostasis 377–8
Haemothorax 354
Hair 926
Hair loss (alopecia)
  cancer patient nursing care 226
  chemotherapy side effects 208, 400, 861
  radiotherapy side effects 211, 213
Hair removal, preoperative 170
Half-life 107
Hallucinogens 967, 972
Halo traction 720
Haloperidol 233, 736
Hamilton Russell traction 880, 881, 889,
  891, 893

Handwashing 137, 141
  immuncompromised patient care 412,
    413
Haptens 107
Hashimoto's thyroiditis (autoimmune
  thyroid disease) 588
Hay fever 757
Head injury 697–716
  assessment 700–1
  brainstem lesions 703
  cerebral perfusion pressure 697
  classification 698
  clinical features 706–7
  closed/open 698
  consciousness level alteration 703, 706,
    711–13
    airway management 711–12
    monitoring 711
  consciousness level assessment 703–5,
    706
  coup/contrecoup 698
  emergency care 705
  herniation (coning) 697–8
  imaging investigations 701
  intracranial pressure elevation 697–8,
    700, 701–3, 707–11
  intracranial pressure monitoring 701
  loss of consciousness 700
  mechanisms 700
  post-traumatic amnesia 700
  primary 699–700
  pupillary signs 698
  rehabilitation 716
  secondary events 700–1
  space-occupying lesions 703
  surgery *see* Intracranial surgery
Head lice 955
Headache
  cerebral aneurysm rupture (subarachnoid
    haemorrhage) 689, 691
  head injury 700, 706
  intracranial pressure elevation 707, 708,
    710
  renal function impairment 620, 627
  stroke 692, 693
Heaf test 131, 341
Health Action Zones 54
Health Belief Model 22
Health concept 4, 14–16
  definitions 14, 16
  focus of nursing 7, 8
Health education 16–17, 18, 30–1
  chronic illness 88–9
  communication skills 30–1, 32, 33
  compliance 21–2
  contracting 22
  cultural aspects 22–3
  effectiveness monitoring 21
  ethical issues 25, 26
  expectations on nurses 21
  goals 18–19
  health promotion approaches 18
  patient teaching 18–26, 89
    learning goals establishment 25
    learning needs identification 24–5
    teaching plan 25
  safer sex 19, 20
  stages of change model for changing
    behaviour 23–4
  substance misuse 981–2
  see also Patient education/instruction
Health Improvement Programmes 54
Health promotion 6, 12, 14–17
  behavioural change approach 18
  educational approach 18

  elderly people 53–5
  empowerment approach 18
  medical/preventive approach 17–18
  oral health 446
  osteoporosis prevention 920
  social change approach 18
  substance misuse 981–2
Health and Safety at Work Act (1974) 204
Health visiting 80
Healthcare services
  elderly people 42–3
  primary health care delivery approach 76
Healthcare system 4–7
  changes in delivery 5–7
Hearing 748
  ageing changes 47
  auditory pathway 749
  evaluation 750
  pitch/intensity of sound 749
Hearing aids 752
Hearing loss
  acquired 751
  assessment 750
  causes 750–1
  central 751
  classification 750–1
  clinical aspects 751
  communication skills 752–3
  community resources 753
  conductive 750
  congenital 751
  prevention 751–2
  sensorineural (perceptive deafness) 750–1
Heart 248–9
  chambers 248
  conduction system 249, 251
  contraction cycle (cardiac cycle) 251–2
  coronary artery system 249–50
  electrical activity 251, 263–4
  physiology 250–3
  regulation of activity 252–3
  size assessment 266
  valves 248–9
  walls 248
Heart block 301–3
  atrioventricular
    complete 303
    first degree 302
    second degree 293, 302–3
  sinoatrial 302
Heart failure 271–4, 309–14
  acute renal failure 624
  blood pressure 261, 318
  compensatory mechanisms 309
  decompensated 309
  definition 309
  diagnosis 311
  epidemiology 309
  left-sided 310
  management 271, 311–14
    afterload/preload reduction 311–12
    associated problems 273–4
    cardiac contractility enhancement 312
    drugs 273, 312, 313
    fluid accumulation reduction 312,
      313–14
    myocardial workload reduction 271–3,
      311, 312
  post-myocardial infarction 293
  right-sided 310
  symptoms 310–11
Heart murmur 263
Heart rate 251, 252
  ageing changes 47
  myocardial infarction 289

Heart sounds
abnormalities 262–3
auscultation 261
Heartburn 442, 447
Heat application, rheumatoid arthritis 907
Heat production 508
Heel prick blood specimens 156
Heimlich manoeuvre (abdominal thrusts)
369, 996
Helicobacter pylori
chronic gastritis 453
eradication 455
peptic ulcer 455
stomach cancer 457
Helminths 126
Helper (T4) T lymphocytes 129
HIV infection 142
Hemiplegia 681, 696
Heparin 102, 189, 292, 314, 324, 328, 376,
417, 508, 694, 695, 914
haemorrhagic complications 420–1
Hepatic artery 507
Hepatic coma 514, 523
Hepatic vein 507
Hepatitis
cirrhosis 522
interferon treatment 507
toxic 521
viral 517–21
Hepatitis A 517
contacts 520
diagnostic tests 511
treatment 519
Hepatitis B 517–18
blood/blood products screening 423
contacts 520
diagnostic tests 511
transmission
blood products 419
sexual 791
sharps injury 138
treatment 519
vaccination 138, 520–1
Hepatitis C 518
blood/blood products screening 423
diagnostic tests 511
haemophiliacs 419, 420
transmission
blood products 419
sharps injury 138
treatment 519
Hepatitis D 518
diagnostic tests 511
Hepatitis E 518
diagnostic tests 511
Hepatocellular jaundice 513
Hereditary elliptocytosis 386–7
Hereditary haemorrhagic telangiectasia
420
Hereditary spherocytosis 386–7
Herniation (coning) of brain tissue 697–8
Hernioplasty 788
Heroin *see* Diamorphine
Herpes simplex virus 126, 729, 957
anogenital infection 790, 932
cervical smear abnormalities 841
mouth ulceration in cancer patients
223
vaccine 832
Hesitancy 644, 645
benign prostatic hyperplasia 792
Hiatus hernia 450–2
case study 452
causes 450
classification 451

clinical features 451
diagnosis 451
management 451–2
rolling (paraoesophageal) 451
sliding 451
Hiccup (hiccough; singultus) 443
Hickman catheter 205, 413, 861
High altitude 374
influence on clinical investigation results
152
secondary polycythaemia 395
High-density lipoproteins (HDLs) 255
Hip:waist ratio 547
Hip dislocation 897
Hip fracture 882
Hip prosthesis 914
Hip replacement surgery 912–14
discharge preparations 914
hip prosthesis dislocation prevention
913
infection prevention 913
postoperative care 913–14
preoperative preparation 913
Histamine 112, 376, 439
peptic ulcer aetiology 453
Histological examination, cancer diagnosis
200–1
Histoplasmosis 126
HIV infection/AIDS 6, 126, 136, 141–7, 785,
807, 812, 829
AIDS dementia complex 729
antiviral therapy 147
blood/blood products screening 423
clinical disease 144–5
CDC classification 143
children 145, 147
women 145
degenerative neurological disease 728,
729–30
diagnostic testing 144, 145
haemophiliacs 419, 420
health education 19–20
neoplasms 144, 146
Kaposi's sarcoma 956
non-Hodgkin's lymphoma 405
opportunistic infections 144, 146, 342
nervous system 729
skin 957
pathophysiology 142
pre-test counselling 163
progression 144
rape victims 809, 810
screening in pregnancy 162
seroconversion 144
transmission 142
blood products 419
high-risk behaviours 143
intravenous drug use 147
sharps injury 138
vascular myelopathy 729
Hodgkin's disease 404
case study 407–8
chemotherapy 203, 405–7
clinical features 404
investigations 405
nursing care 408
radiotherapy 405, 407
Rye classification 404
staging 405
Holistic care 7, 30
Holter technique (ambulatory
electrocardiography) 264–5
Homan's sign 189, 328
Homograft (allograft) 637
Hordeolum (stye) 769–70

Hormonal anticancer agents 204
breast cancer 862
menopausal symptoms 863
metastatic disease 865
Hormone replacement therapy (HRT) 805,
848, 920
Hormones 561
liver metabolism 508
mechanism of action 561
regulation of secretion 562
target organs 561
trophic 562
Hospital acquired (nosocomial) infection
136–7
endogenous 137
exogenous 137
pneumonia 342
preventive measures 137–40
Hospital Anxiety and Depression (HAD)
Scale 290
Hot flushes 805
Hot-air ovens 139
24-Hour ambulatory electromyography
(EMG) 684
24-Hour urine collection 158, 616
Human leucocyte antigen (HLA) typing
216
kidney transplantation 637, 638
Human papilloma virus 796
cervical carcinoma 840
carcinogenesis 197
cervical dysplasia 831
cervical smear abnormalities 841
genital warts (condylomata acuminata)
790–1, 830, 831
Human T-lymphocytic virus (HTLV-1) 397
Human tissue disposal 137
Humeral neck fracture 895
Humeral shaft fracture 895–6
Hunger 545
Huntington's disease (corticostriatonigral
degeneration) 736–7
Hyaluronic acid 912
Hydatidiform mole 827
Hydraulic lifts 932
Hydrocele 792
Hydrocephalus 690
Hydrochloric acid secretion 435, 436, 439
peptic ulcer 453
regulation 439
Hydrocortisone 429, 481, 605, 606, 608,
609, 908
Hydronephrosis 643
Hydrophilic molecules 98
Hydrophobic molecules 98
Hydrops fetalis 387
Hydroxychloroquine 908, 917
Hydroxycobalamin 385
Hydroxyurea 395, 401
Hyoscine (scopolamine) 171, 756
Hyperaldosteronism 607–8
Hypercalcaemia
cancer patients 233–4
hyperparathyroidism 598
metastatic disease 866
multiple myeloma 409
nephrolithiasis 643
Hypercapnia 252
Hyperextension of head for surgery 177
Hyperglycaemia 567
diabetes mellitus 569
phaeochromocytoma 608
Hyperkalaemia
acute renal failure 623
ECG changes 623

Hyperlipidaemia, cardiovascular risk 254, 255–6
Hypermetropia (long-sightedness) 760
Hyperosmolar agents, head injury 701
Hyperosmolar non-ketotic coma 580
Hyperparathyroidism 453, 587, 598
Hyperpnoea 336
Hypersensitivity reactions see Allergic reactions
Hypertension 318–21, 568
  alcohol consumption 321
  associated organ damage 318–19
  cardiovascular risk 254, 255, 318
  cerebral aneurysm association 689
  definition 318
  diabetes mellitus 570
  dietary modification 320–1
  drug treatment 321
  exercise 321
  intervention thresholds 319
  management 320–1
  microangiopathic haemolytic anaemia 386
  phaeochromocytoma 608, 609
  primary (essential; idiopathic) 319
  primary health care management 82, 84
    audit 85, 86, 87
  renal function impairment 627
  secondary 320
  smoking cessation 321
  stress reduction techniques 321
  stroke risk 686
  symptoms 320
Hyperthyroidism 588, 591–7
  causes 591
  clinical features 591–2
    eye changes 592
  diarrhoea 467, 468
  drug treatment 592
  nursing care 592–4
  radiation treatment 592
  surgery 592, 594–7
Hypertrophic cardiomyopathy 282–3
Hypertrophic scarring 950
  burns injuries 946
Hyperuricaemia 233
Hyperuricaemic nephropathy 233
Hyperviscosity syndrome 409
Hypocalcaemia
  hypoparathyroidism 597, 598
  seizures 739
Hypogeusia 224
Hypoglossal (XII) nerve assessment 679
Hypoglycaemia 99, 567
  consciousness level alteration 703
  diabetes mellitus 572, 580, 587–8
    Somogyi effect 588
  insulin-secreting islet cell tumour 534
  seizures 739
Hypoparathyroidism 597–8
Hypophysectomy 603–4
Hypophysis see Pituitary gland
Hypostatic pneumonia 342
Hypotension, postoperative 181, 189
Hypothalamus 671
Hypothyroidism 588–91
  case study 590–1
  causes 588–9
  clinical features 589–90
  diabetes mellitus 569
  nursing care 590
  primary 588
  treatment 590
Hypotonia 680

Hypoventilation, postoperative 181, 188
Hypovolaemic shock 991
  burn injuries 937, 938, 941–2, 946
  treatment 994
Hypoxia
  anaemia 382
  brain cell sensitivity 672
  cardiovascular disorders 252, 262
  erythropoiesis regulation 374
  seizures 739
Hysterectomy 821
  cervical carcinoma 842
    nursing care 842–3
Hysterosalpingography 816–17
Hysteroscopy 821
Hysterotomy 825

Ibuprofen 908
Icterus see Jaundice
Identification bracelet 172
Idiopathic thrombocytopenic purpura (ITP) 417
Ileal conduit (ureteroileostomy) 657
Ileal continent urinary pouch 656–7
Ileal pouch (continent ileostomy) 494, 495
Ileoanal reservoir 494, 495, 499
Ileocaecal valve 437, 439
Ileostomy 487, 494–5
  care 499
  colostomy comparison 496
  community support 503
  complications 503
  critical incident 504–5
  drainage appliance selection 498–9
  medication use 502–3
  nursing assessment 497
  nutrition alterations 500, 502
  postoperative assessment 498
  preoperative preparation
    physical 497
    psychological 496
  psychosocial adjustment 500
  self-care
    activities 502
    education 501–2
  sexual function 500–1
  skin care 499–500, 502
Ileum 436
Illicit drugs
  Class A 968
  Class B 968
  Class C 968
  depressants 967, 970–2
  hallucinogens 967, 972
  information sources 972–3
  short/long-term effects 968
  stimulants 967, 968–70
  street names 968
Imagery, pain management 122
Imaging investigations 159–61
  arterial occlusive disease 324
  biliary tract disorders 511–12
  cancer diagnosis 200
  cardiovascular disorders 265–8
  head injury 701
  inflammatory bowel disease 480–1
  intestinal obstruction 487
  liver disorders 511–12
  neurological disorders 683
  pancreatic disorders 511–12
  pituitary gland disorders 600
  respiratory disorders 340
  subarachnoid haemorrhage 689
  urinary system 617–18

Immobility
  muscle wasting, fracture patient in traction 887
  pressure ulcer risk 927
Immune cells 129
Immune neutropenia 396
Immune response 128, 129
  cancer causation 197
  cell-mediated 129
  elderly people 136
  humoral 129
  infants 136
  nutritional status associations 136
  pregnancy 136
  primary/secondary 129
  stress effects 136
Immune thrombocytopenia 417
Immunization 141
Immunocompromised patient
  kidney transplant patients 639
  leucocyte disorders 410
  see also HIV infection/AIDS
Immunoglobulin
  classes 129, 130
  structure 129
Immunoglobulin A (IgA) 129, 130, 438
Immunoglobulin D (IgD) 129, 130
Immunoglobulin E (IgE) 129, 130
Immunoglobulin G (IgG) 129, 130
Immunoglobulin M (IgM) 129, 130
Immunosuppressive drugs 136
Immunosuppressive therapy
  aplastic anaemia 402
  idiopathic thrombocytopenic purpura 417
  inflammatory bowel disease 481
  kidney transplant patients 639, 640
  rheumatoid arthritis 909
Imperforate anus 486
Imperforate hymen 810–11
Implantable cardioverter defibrillator (ICD) 283, 306
Implantation 801
Implanted central venous ports 208
Implementation of care plan 12
Impotence (erectile dysfunction) 786–7
In vitro fertilization (IVF) 818
Incisional biopsy, cancer diagnosis 202
Incompetent cervical os 823
Incubation period 129–30
Incus 748
Indometacin 453, 908
Indwelling urinary catheterization
  bladder surgery postoperative care 658
  catheter management 653
  patient education 659–60
  spinal cord injury 722
Indwelling urinary catheters 655
Inequalities in health 15
  elderly people 45–7
Inevitable abortion 822
  management 823
Infarction 289
Infection 125–48
  acute/chronic 130
  arthroplasty postoperative care 913
  barriers 127
  bone 918–19
  burn injuries 938, 943–4
  chain 135–6
  clinical assessment 132
  clinical features 130
  community prevention measures 141
  course of disease 129–30
  definition 125

dental pulp 444
diagnostic procedures 130–2
 collection of specimens 131–2
diarrhoea 466–7
epidemiology 135
female reproductive tract 828–36
fever 128, 130
hospital acquired (nosocomial) 136–7
host defences 127–9
 non-specific 127–8
 specific immune response 128, 129
leucocyte/lymphatic disorders 410
 early identification 413
 preventive interventions 411–13
local 130
male reproductive tract 788–9
nervous system 742–3
patient management 132–5
 nursing interventions 132–3
portals of entry 136
predisposing host factors 136
preoperative preparation 169
prevention of spread 133–5
 isolation procedures 134–5
primary/secondary 130
systemic 130
traction pin site 887
transfusion reactions 429–30
transmission 136
see also Cross-infection control
Infectious agents 125–6
 host interactions 126–9
 identification 131
 virulence 126
Infectious mononucleosis (glandular fever)
 403–4
Infective endocarditis 284
Infective polyneuropathy, acute
 (Guillain–Barré, syndrome) 360, 744
Infertility 816–18
 causes 816
 diagnostic procedures 816–17
 incidence 816
 treatment 818
Inflammatory bowel disease 136, 478–85
 colorectal cancer risk 487
 diarrhoea 466, 467, 481, 482, 485
 drug treatment 481
 fluid and electrolyte replacement 482,
  484–5
 nursing care 482–5
 nutrition 482, 483
  elemental feeding 484
  parenteral 483–4
 patient education 485
 psychosocial needs 482, 485
 quality of life impact 481–2
 sexual function 485
 surgery 481
 see also Crohn's disease; Ulcerative colitis
Inflammatory heart lesions 283–4
Inflammatory intestinal disorders 476–85
Inflammatory joint disease 901–10
Inflammatory response 127
 burn injuries 937–8
 capillary permeability enhancement 98
 fever 128
 infection 130
Influenza 126, 127
Information management 6
Information for patient see Patient
 education/instruction
Informed consent 26, 162
 blood/blood products transfusion 430
 cardiopulmonary angiography 267

children 169
clinical investigations 153–4
emergency treatment 169–70, 171
endoscopy 454
invasive neurodiagnostic procedures 684
preoperative preparation 315
surgery 169–70, 171
tracheostomy 364
Infratentorial surgery 713
Infusion 101
Inguinal hernia 788
Inhalation anaesthetic agents 174
Inhibin 800
Injections
 intravenous administration route 101
 needle phobia 115
 'pen' devices 573–4
Inner ear (labyrinth) 748–9
Inotropic agents 273, 312
Instruction see Patient education/instruction
Insulin 439, 509, 538, 567
 actions 573
 deficiency
  acute pancreatitis 531
  diabetes mellitus 569
 functions 567
Insulin resistance 568, 569
Insulin therapy 102, 572–5, 578
 administration 573–5
 complications 575
 hypoglycaemia 99
 preparations 572–3
  biphasic 573
  intermediate-acting 573, 574
  long-acting 573, 574
  rapid-acting 573, 574
Insulin-secreting islet cell tumour 534
Intensive care unit 180
Intention tremor 680
Interactionist model of health 14, 15
Intercapillary glomerulosclerosis
 (Kimmelstiel–Wilson syndrome) 569
Interdisciplinary (integrated) primary
 health care team 82
Interferon 127–8
Interferon alpha treatment
 chronic myeloid leukaemia 401
 hepatitis 507, 519
Intermittent catheterization 649, 654, 655
 spinal cord injury 722
Intermittent claudication 323, 324
 exercise 325–6
Internal capsule 671
Internal carotid arteries 672
 endarterectomy 687
Internal fixation 882
 femur neck fracture 891
 intramedullary nailing 892
 postoperative care 890
 preoperative preparation 889–90
International normalized ratio (INR) 324,
 328, 421, 694
Internuncial (connecting) neurone 666
Interstitial cell-stimulating hormone
 (ICSH) 562
Intertrigo 851
Intervention strategies 11–12
Intestinal atresia 485
Intestinal juice (succus entericus) 440
Intestinal obstruction 485–7
 causes 485–6
 clinical features 486–7
 diagnostic investigations 487
 postoperative 184
 treatment 487

Intestinal phase of gastric secretion 439
Intra-aortic balloon pump 288
Intra-arterial cytotoxic drug administration
 205
Intracavitary cytotoxic drug administration
 205
Intracerebral haemorrhage 700
Intracranial haematoma 690
Intracranial haemorrhage 700–1
Intracranial pressure elevation
 assessment 707–8
 bowel elimination 710
 cardiac function abnormalities 708, 710
 consciousness level alteration 708, 709–10
  restlessness 709–10
 controlled hyperventilation 701
 fluid balance 702, 708, 710
 head injury 697–8
 headache 707, 708, 710
 hyperosmolar agents 701
 hyperthermia 708, 710
 intracranial haemorrhage 700
 intracranial neoplasms 727, 728
 intracranial surgery 713, 715
 nursing care 707–11
 nutrition 708, 710
 personal hygiene 708, 711
 respiratory status optimization 708, 709
 sedatives 702
 signs/symptoms 700, 702
 skin integrity maintenance 710
 stroke 693
 surgery 702–3
 urinary catheterization 710, 711
 ventricular drainage 711
Intracranial pressure monitoring 682, 701
Intracranial surgery 713–16
 complications 713
 infection prevention 713, 715–16
 intracranial pressure elevation 713, 715
 postoperative care 713–14
 preoperative preparation 713
 procedures 713
 residual neurological deficit 716
Intramammary lymph nodes 854
Intramedullary nailing 892
Intramuscular administration route 101
Intraocular lens implantation 772
Intraocular pressure 759–60
 measurement 763
Intraocular surgery 772–3
Intraocular tumours 778
Intratentorial cranial compartment 669
Intrathecal cytotoxic drug administration
 205
Intrauterine device (IUD) 813–14
 progestogen-only device 814
Intravenous administration route 101
 cytotoxic agents 205
 drug misuse, HIV infection transmission
  147
Intravenous anaesthetic agents 174
Intravenous infusion
 blood sampling procedure 157
 emergency surgery 171
Intravenous pyelography (IVP) 617
Intravenous urography (IVU) 617
Intrinsic factor 384, 464
Intussusception 485, 486, 487
Inverted nipples 851–2
Investigations (laboratory tests) 151–63
 factors influencing values 152–3
 future development 162–3
 information for patient 153, 154
  giving bad news 162

Investigations (laboratory tests) (contd)
  informed consent 153–4
  nursing knowledge 154–5
  patient anxiety 153, 154
  patient care 153
  pre-procedure preparation 155–6
  preoperative 168
  rationale 152
  reference values 152
  specific procedures 156–61
Involucrum 918
Iodine deficiency 588–9
Iodine-131 therapy 592
Ipratropium bromide 350, 351
Iris 759
  pupillary constriction/dilatation 760–1
Iron 374–5
  dietary sources 383, 393
  gastric resection-related deficiency 464
  liver metabolism 508
Iron deficiency anaemia 383–4, 420
Iron supplements 384
Irritable bowel syndrome 467, 473
Irritant contact dermatitis 953
Irritation, carcinogenic potential 196
Ischaemic heart disease 254
  cardiac surgery 314–15
  diabetes mellitus 570
  epidemiology 254
  exercise 90
  primary health care management 83, 84, 85
  register of patients 83, 84
  risk factors 254–8
Islet cell tumour 534
Islets of Langerhans 509, 566–7
  alpha cells 567
  beta cells 567
  delta cells 567
  F cells 567
Isograft 637
Isolation procedures 134–5, 141
  white cell disorders 411
Isoniazid 352
Isoprenaline 302, 303
Isosorbide dinitrate 276
Isosorbide mononitrate 276

Jacksonian seizure 739
Jarisch–Herxheimer reaction 832
Jaundice 509, 510, 512–13
  acute pancreatitis 531, 532
  haemolytic 513
  hepatocellular 513
  obstructive 513
  pruritus 513
Jaw fracture 445–6
Jaw thrust 718
Jehovah's witnesses 430
Jejunostomy feeding 461
Jejunum 436
Joint capsule 871
Joint disease
  degenerative 910–16
  inflammatory 901–10
  metabolic 916
Joint injuries 896–7
Joint replacement surgery
  hip 912–14
  knee 914
  osteoarthritis 912
Joints 871–2
  classification 871
  movement 872, 873
Judgemental attitudes 9, 33, 39

Jugular venous pressure (JVP) 620
Junctional arrhythmia 296
Justice 13, 25
Juvenile chronic arthritis (Still's disease) 902
Juxtaglomerular cells 612

Kanamycin 622
Kanga pants 649
Kaposi's sarcoma 144, 956
Kegel exercises 648
Kell blood group 425
Keloids 950
Keratin 925
Keratitis 775–6
Keratoconus 776
Keratolytic agents 952
Keratoplasty (corneal transplantation) 776–7
Kernig's sign 689
Ketamine misuse 970
Ketones 152, 539, 569, 585
Ketosis 539
  diabetes mellitus 569
Key clinical principles 93
Kidney
  ageing changes 48, 49
  blood supply 612
  disorders see Renal disorders
  function see Renal function
  structure 611–12
Kidney transplantation 637–41
  complications 640–1
  donor 638
  immunological factors 637–8
  immunosuppression 639
  nursing care 639–40
  patient education 640
  procedure 638–9
  recipient 637
  rejection 640
  tissue typing 638
Kimmelstiel–Wilson syndrome (intercapillary glomerulosclerosis) 569
Kirschner wire 880
Klebsiella 641
Knee joint 872
Knee prosthesis 914
Knee replacement surgery 914
Koch continent ileostomy 494
  care 499
Krebs (citric acid) cycle 538, 539
Kupffer cells 508
Kussmaul's breathing 336, 620
Kyphosis 337

Labia 783
Laboratory tests see Investigations
Labyrinth (inner ear) 748–9
Lacrimal system 759
Lacrimation 759
Lactase deficiency 474
Lactate dehydrogenase
  liver function assessment 510
  myocardial infarction 291
Lactobacillus 126
Lactose 540
  intolerance 474, 475
Lactulose 100
Language problems 23, 30
Lansoprazole 439, 448, 455
Laparoscopy
  endometriosis 820
  infertility investigations 816–17
Large intestinal disorders 465
  inflammatory 476–85

Large intestinal motility 440
Large intestine 437
  digestive processes 440–1
  electrolyte/water absorption 440
  microorganisms 441
Laryngeal mask airway
  general anaesthesia 173
  mouth-to-mouth ventilation 307
Laryngeal oedema 368, 369
Laryngeal spasm 368, 369
Larynx 333
  obstruction 368
Lateral position 177
Latex fixation test 905
Laxatives 99, 412, 469, 470, 471
  bulk-forming 471
  diarrhoea 466
  emollient 472
  intracranial pressure elevation 710
  osmotic 471
  postoperative care 186
Lead 622, 739
  shielding 210
Learned helplessness 115
Learning barriers 89
Learning disability
  community nurse specialists 79
  consent for treatment 170
Learning needs 24–5
  chronic illness management 89
  preoperative preparation 167
Left bundle branch block 302
Left heart catheterization 267
Left ventricular end-diastolic pressure 252
Left-to-right shunts 280–1
Leg exercises, preoperative instruction 166, 167, 168
Legal aspects
  documentation 12
  nurse accountability 5
  organ donation 638
  refusal to give care 9
  therapeutic abortion 824
  withholding of nutritional support 552
Leiomyoma
  oesophagus 449
  uterus 838–9
Lens 759, 760
Leucocyte count
  infection 130
  pancreatitis 511
  respiratory disorders 341
Leucocyte disorders 396–416
  central venous access 413–14, 415
  history-taking 410
  immunosuppression 410
    infection prevention 411–13
  laboratory investigations 411
  nursing management 410–15
  physical assessment 410–11
Leucocytes 373, 375–6
  functions 376
  haematological values 382
Leucocytosis 396
Leucopenia 396
  cancer patients 208, 221
Leucoplakia 444–5, 950, 952
Leucopoiesis 376
Leucorrhoea 829
Leucotriene receptor agonists (LTRAs) 346
Leucovorin 488
Leukaemia 397–401
  acute 398–400
    case study 400
    lymphoblastic 203, 216, 398

management 398–400
  myeloid 398
aetiology 397–8
bone marrow transplantation 216
case study 416
chronic 400–1
  lymphocytic 401
  myeloid 216, 400–1
classification 397
incidence 397
individual response 416
thrombocytopenia 417
viral carcinogenesis 196–7
Levamisole 488
Levator palpebrae 759
Levodopa 102
Levonorgestrel
  emergency contraception 815
  implant system 814
  intrauterine system 814
Lice (pediculosis) 955
Lichenification 950
Lidocaine (lignocaine) 298, 299
Life events 60
Life transitions ("life's milestones") 64
  developmental crises 59, 63–4
Lifestyle factors 8
  health promotion 17
Lifestyle modification
  cardiovascular patients 270–1, 278–9
  chronic renal failure 636–7
  cirrhosis 526
  hypertension 320–1
Light adaptation 761
Limb prosthesis 901
Lindemann's characteristics of bereaved 61
Linear analogue anxiety scale 290
Linen decontamination 138
Lip-reading 753
Lipase 437, 439, 440
  serum level 531
Lipid-lowering drugs 256, 292
Lipogenesis 508
Lipophilic drugs 98, 102
Lipoproteins 255
  liver function assessment 511
Listening skills 31
  active listening 35–6
  calming angry patient 38
Lithalopaxy 657
Lithium 84
Lithotomy position 177
Liver 507
  amino acids metabolism 539, 540
  carbohydrate metabolism 538
  drug metabolism 105–7
    first-pass effect 101
  function 508
Liver abscess 527
Liver biopsy 512
Liver disorders 507–34
  alcohol-related risk 514–17
  biopsy 512
  bleeding tendency 513
  clinical features 512–14
  consciousness level alteration 703
    hepatic coma 514, 523
  history-taking 509–10
  imaging investigations 511–12
  laboratory investigations 510–11
  malabsorption 473
  physical examination 510
  portal hypertension 514
Liver function tests 510–11
  viral hepatitis 518, 519

Liver neoplasms 527
Liver transplantation 519, 527–8
Liver trauma 527
Living conditions 17
Lobectomy 353
Local health groups 78
Local infection 130
Local infiltration anaesthesia 173
Long bones 870, 871
Long-sightedness (hypermetropia) 760
Loop colostomy 496
Loop of Henlé 611, 612
  function 613
Loperamide 468
Loss 59–73
  body image alteration response 69–71
  Bowlby's theory (three phases) 71
  impact 69
  normal (uncomplicated) grief 60–1
  nursing issues 60
  phases of response 61
  types 59
  see also Grief
Low air loss beds 932
Low molecular weight heparin 328
Low-density lipoproteins (LDLs) 255
  diabetes mellitus 569
Lower motor neurones 677
Lower oesophageal (cardiac) sphincter
  436
Lower reference nutrient intake (LRNI)
  542
Lower respiratory tract 333
LSD (lysergic acid diethylamide) 972
Lumbar plexus 675
Lumbar puncture 684–5
  stroke 693
Lumbar spinal injury 720
Lumpectomy (wide local excision) 856–7
Lund and Browder burn chart 935, 938
Lung biopsy 341
Lung cancer 353–4
Lung volumes 339
Lungs 333
Luteinizing hormone (LH) 562
  functions 564
    male 782
  menopause 804, 805
  menstrual cycle 801
  ovarian response 800
Luteinizing hormone-releasing hormone
  (LHRH) agonists 862
Lymph node biopsy 341
Lymph nodes 129, 371
Lymphatic disorders 403–16
  central venous access 413–14, 415
  history-taking 410
  immunosuppression 410
    infection prevention 411–13
  laboratory investigations 411
  nursing management 410–15
  physical assessment 410–11
Lymphatic tissue 129
Lymphatics 129
Lymphoblasts 376
Lymphocytes 375
Lymphoedema 858–9
Lymphomas 404–8
  individual response 416
  staging (Ann Arbor classification) 405,
    406
  viral carcinogenesis 197
Lymphopenia 396
Lysergic acid diethylamide (LSD) 972
Lysozyme 127, 438

McBurney's point 476
McGill Pain Questionnaire 118
McLaughlin nail and plate 882
Macrophages 376
  HIV infection 142
  microbial infection 126
  phagocytosis 127
Macule 949
Magic mushrooms 968, 972
Magnesium hydroxide 455, 471
Magnetic resonance angiography 324
Magnetic resonance imaging (MRI)
  cardiovascular disease 265–6
  neurological disorders 683
  pituitary disorders 600
  renal system 618
  see also Magnetic resonance angiography
Malabsorption 473–6
  assessment 474
  clinical features 473
  digestive disorders 473–4
    diarrhoea 466
  drug-induced 474
  dysfunctional absorbing cells 474
  enzyme deficiencies 474
  folic acid deficiency 385
  following gastric surgery 473
  gluten-sensitive enteropathy 474
  management 474–6
  vitamin B_{12} deficiency 384
Malaria 126, 388, 417
Maldescent of testes 781, 787–8, 795
Male rape 787
Male reproductive system 781, 782
  accessory glands 782
  development 781
  duct system 782
Male reproductive system disorders
  781–96
  assessment 784
  congenital anomalies 787–8
  impact on patient 784–5
  infection 788–9
    sexually transmitted 790–2
  nursing interventions 785
Male sexual dysfunction 786–7
Malignant tumours 197–8
  see also Cancer
Malleolar fracture 893–4
Malleus 748
Malunion 876
Mammography 852
Mannitol 701
Mantoux tuberculin skin test 131, 341
Marfan syndrome 322
Marsupial (Kanga) pants 649
Maslow's classification of needs 11
Massage, cancer patient care 237, 866
Mastalgia (breast discomfort) 852
Mastectomy 855, 856, 865
Mastication (chewing) 437, 438
Mastoid cells 748
Mastoidectomy 755
Mastoiditis 754–5
Maxillary sinuses 757
Measles 126, 751
Mechanical ventilation 367–8
  indications 367
  intracranial pressure elevation 709
  postoperative 181
  spinal cord injury 721
Mediastinal lymph gland enlargement
  447
Medical models for health promotion
  17–18

Medicines
classification/naming 97
see also Drugs
Medroxyprogesterone acetate 814, 843, 862
Medulla oblongata 671
Megakaryocytes 376
Megaloblastic anaemia *see* Vitamin B$_{12}$
deficiency
Meglitinides 575
Meibomian glands 758
Melaena 422, 443
Melanin 925
Melanocyte-stimulating hormone (MSH)
925
Melanocytes 925
Melanoma 948, 956, 957
intraocular 778
tumour vaccines 217
Melphalan 409
Memory B cells 129, 375
Menarche 800
Menière's disease/syndrome 755
Meninges 669
Meningitis 678, 742–3
assessment 742
clinical features 742
nursing care 743
Meningococcal meningitis 742
Meningococcal septicaemia 386
Meniscal injury 897
Menisci 872
Menopause 804–5
breast changes 848
hormone replacement therapy (HRT) 805
osteoporosis 919
Menstrual cycle 801, 802, 803–4
breast changes 847
breast surgery timing 856
disorders 818–21
hormonal feedback 801
length 803–4
luteal phase 800
ovarian changes 800
perimenopausal changes 803–4
proliferative phase 800
uterine changes 801
Menstruation 801
disorders 818–21
Mental illness
community nurse specialists 79
consent for treatment 170
elderly people 49
Mercury bichloride 622
Mesenteric artery thrombosis/occlusion 486
Mesentery 437
Metabolic joint disease 916
Metabolic rate 565
Metabolism 538–40
Metastases 197
bone 923
breast cancer 865–7
colorectal cancer 487
liver 527
spinal cord compression 234
stomach cancer 458
Metered dose inhalers 99
patient teaching 351
Metformin 575
Methadone 968, 971
maintenance programmes 979
withdrawal profile 979
Methicillin 622
Methicillin-resistant *Staphylococcus aureus*
(MRSA) 132, 133, 134
Methotrexate 225, 385, 408, 522, 827

Methylamfetamine 968
3,4-Methylenedioxymethamfetamine
(MDMA; ecstasy) 968
Metoclopramide 184, 460
Metronidazole 324, 455, 831
Miconazole 444
Microalbuminuria 569, 570, 579
Microangiopathic haemolytic anaemia 386
Micrometastases 198
Microscopic infectious agent identification
131
Micturition 615
fracture patient in traction 886, 888
Mid-arm circumference (MAC) 547
Mid-stream urine specimen (MSU) 158,
616
Midbrain 671
Middle ear 748
Mifepristone 825
Migraine 99
Mineral micronutrients 542
Mineralocorticoids 566
Minute ventilation (minute respiratory
volume) 339–40
Misoprostol 455
Missed abortion 822
management 822–3
Mithramycin 233
Mitral regurgitation 293, 315
Mitral stenosis 283
Mitral valve 248
Mittelschmerz 818–19
Mixed lymphocyte culture 216
Mixed nerves 674
Mobitz type I (Wenckebach) second degree
atrioventricular block 293, 302
Mobitz type II second degree
atrioventricular block 293, 302
Moist compresses for skin lesions 952
Moisturizers 948–9
Mondor's disease 854
Moniliasis *see* Candidiasis
Monitoring 12
Monoblasts 376
Monocytes 376
phagocytosis 127
Monoplegia 681
Monosaccharides 540
Monounsaturates 541
Montelukast 346
MOPP chemotherapy 406
Moral conduct principles 13
Morbidity, socio-economic factors 15
Morphine 67, 102, 119, 189, 866
cancer pain management 230
tolerance 119
withdrawal syndrome 119
Mortality, socio-economic factors 15
Motivational interviewing 980
Motor cortex 670, 671, 677
Motor (efferent) neurone 666
Motor end plate 667, 677
Motor (expressive; Broca's) aphasia 678
Motor function assessment 679–81
Motor nerves 673
lower motor neurones 677
upper motor neurones 677
Motor neurone disease (amyotrophic lateral
sclerosis) 728, 737–8
Motor system 677
Mouth 333, 435
changes due to gastrointestinal disorders
443
digestive processes 438
health promotion 446

Mouth cancer 445, 447
Mouth care
acute pancreatitis 532
intubated patient 362, 363
renal function impairment 635
acute renal failure 626
tracheostomy patient 366
unconscious patient 712
variceal bleeding 525
Mouth disorders 444–7
history-taking 446
management 446–7
physical examination 446
Mouth-to-mouth ventilation 307
Movement abnormalities 677, 680
Movement assessment 680
fine abnormalities (fasciculations) 680
gross abnormalities 680
Mucositis
chemotherapy side effect 208, 399, 861
nursing care 221, 223–4
radiotherapy side effect 211, 213
Mucous membrane barriers to infection
127
Mucus 127
gastrointestinal secretion 435, 436, 437,
440
Multidisciplinary primary health care team
81–2
Multiple interrelated problems 4
case study 3–4
Multiple myeloma 408–10
clinical features 408–9
hypercalcaemia 409
hyperviscosity syndrome 409
investigations 409
management 409
nursing care 409–10
pain 408, 409
renal function impairment 409
thrombocytopenia 417
Multiple peripheral neuritis (polyneuritis)
744
Multiple sclerosis 728, 731–4
aetiology 732
assessment 732
clinical features 732
early remissions 733
elimination pattern alterations 734
incidence 732
mobility 734
nursing care 733–4
patient education 733
Mumps 126, 445
orchitis 789
Muscle
action at joints 872
nervous control of contraction 677
strength assessment 680
tone assessment 679–80
Muscle relaxants 175
endotracheal intubation 362
Muscular dysfunction
multiple sclerosis 734
myasthenia gravis 738
Parkinson's disease 735, 736
Musculoskeletal disorders 869–923
trauma assessment 872–4
Mutation, carcinogenesis initiation 195–6
Myasthenia gravis 728, 738–9
Myasthenic crisis 739
Mycobacteria tuberculosis 126
skin tests 131
Mycoplasma pneumoniae 126
Mycoplasmas 126

Mycoses 126
Myelin sheath 667
Myelinated nerves 667, 674
Myeloblasts 376
Myelodysplastic syndromes 385
Myelography 685
Myocardial infarction 254, 288–96
  acute myocardial reperfusion 292
  anterior wall 289
  biochemical markers 290, 291
  cardiac arrhythmias 291
  complications 292–3
    risk stratification 293
  coronary care unit management 291
  determinants of survival 289
  diabetes mellitus 570
  diagnosis 290–1
  electrocardiogram (ECG) changes 290
  inferior wall 289
  lateral wall 289
  myocardial workload reduction 291–2
  nursing management case study 294–6
  posterior wall 289
  rehabilitation 293–4
  right ventricular 289
  serum enzyme markers 290–1
  silent 289
  symptoms 289–90
    control 291–2
Myocardial reperfusion therapy 292
Myocardial rupture 293
Myocardium 248
  blood supply 250
    disorders 285–96
  contractility 252
  contraction 250–1
  electrical activity 251
  electrophysiology 251
  hypertrophic response to hypertension
    318
  radionuclide imaging techniques 266
Myoclonic seizures 739–40
Myoclonus 680
Myoglobin
  myocardial infarction 291
  release from burn injuries 937
Myomectomy 839
Myometrium 801
Myopia (short-sightedness) 760
Myringotomy 754

Naevi (spider angiomas) 514
Naloxone 119
Narcotics Anonymous (NA) 981
Nasal cannulae 312, 350
Nasal cavity 756
Nasal foreign body 368
Nasal passages obstruction 368
Nasal sinuses 757
  disorders 757–8
Nasal surgery 758
Nasogastric tube feeding *see* Enteral feeding
Nasopharyngeal cancer 197
Nateglinide 575
National Institute for Clinical Excellence
  (NICE) 43
National Service Frameworks (NSFs)
  audit criteria/standards 86
  Coronary Heart Disease 247, 254, 256,
    292
  elderly people's services 43–4
  registers of patients 84
Natural killer cells 127
Nausea/vomiting
  acute pancreatitis 530

burn injuries 937
cancer 240
  chemotherapy side effect 208, 861
  nursing care 221, 223, 239
  radiotherapy side effect 211, 214, 399
drug adverse reactions 100–1
drug treatment 460
gastrointestinal disorders 442
head injury 700
infection 130
intestinal obstruction 486, 487
myocardial infarction 289
nursing interventions 459–60
opioid side-effects management 233
peptic ulcer 454
postoperative care 184
renal function impairment 620, 627
stroke 692, 693
Nebulizers 99
Needle biopsy 202
Needle phobia 115
  case study 153
Needlestick injury
  critical incident 521
  viral hepatitis transmission 520
  see also Sharps injury
Neisseria gonorrhoeae 126, 127, 789, 790, 828,
  830
Neisseria meningitidis 126
Neomycin 752, 753
Neostigmine 738
Nephrolithiasis (renal calculi) 568, 643–4
  ileostomy patient 503
Nephron 611–12
Nephrotic syndrome (nephrosis) 627, 642
  treatment 642–3
Nephrotoxic agents 622
Nerve impulse 666–7
Nerve tracts 673–4
Nerves 673–4
Nervous system 665–78
  ageing changes 47, 48
  disorders 665–744
    degenerative 728–39
    infections 742–3
  neoplasms 677, 726–8
  organization 665, 666
  trauma 677
Neufeld nail 882
Neurilemma (sheath of Schwann) 674
Neurogenic bladder 645
Neurogenic intestinal obstruction 486
Neurogenic shock 991
  treatment 993
Neuroglia 669
Neurological disorders 447, 685–6
Neurological function assessment 678–85,
  687, 688
  cerebral function 678
  cognitive status assessment 679
  consciousness 679
  continuous intracranial pressure
    monitoring 682
  cranial nerves 678–9
  diagnostic tests 682–5
    invasive 684–5
    non-invasive 683–4
  motor function 679–81
  reflexes 681–2
  sensory function 681
  sleep 682
Neuromuscular defects, stroke 692, 694,
  695–6
Neuromuscular junction 667, 677
Neuromuscular transmission 677

Neurone 666
Neuropsychological tests 684
Neuroticism, pain experience impact 114
Neurotransmitters 667, 668
  autonomic nervous system 675–6
  pain 112
Neutropenia 396–7
  benign idiopathic 396
  chemotherapy side effect 398, 861
  cyclical 396
  immune 396
  management 397
    infection prevention 411
Neutrophils 375, 376
The New NHS, Modern Dependable 77
New variant Creutzfeldt-Jacob disease
  423
NHS and Community Care Act (1990) 77
NHS Direct 6
NHS National Plan 43, 76, 78
NHS organizational structure 77–8
  Northern Ireland 78
  Scotland 78
  Wales 78
NHS walk-in centres 6
Nicotine 967
Night blindness 761
Nikolsky's sign 954
Nipple 847
Nitrates 83, 310
  chest pain 276
Nitrogen mustard 225
Nociceptors 111
Nocturia 619, 627
  benign prostatic hyperplasia 793
Nodule 949
Non-caloric sweeteners 572
Non-Hodgkin's lymphoma 404–5
  AIDS-related 405
  clinical features 405
  critical incident 431–2
  investigations 405
  nursing care 408
  REAL classification 405
  staging 405
  treatment 408
Non-maleficence 13, 25, 26
Non-myelinated nerves 674
Non-proprietary (generic; approved)
  medicines 97
Non-specific urethritis 790
Non-starch polysaccharides 540
Non-steroidal anti-inflammatory drugs
  (NSAIDs) 101, 460
  back pain 921
  cancer pain 866
  gastritis 452
  osteoarthritis 912
  Paget's disease (osteitis deformans) 921
  pain management 118–19
  peptic ulcer 453, 455
  rheumatoid arthritis 908
  systemic lupus erythematosis 917
Non-sulphonylurea insulin secretagogues
  575
Non-union 876
Non-verbal communication 35
  active listening 35–6
Noradrenaline 566, 675
Normal body flora 125, 126, 127
  large intestine 441
  pathogenic potential 135
Norplant 814
Northern Ireland, NHS organizational
  structure 78

Norton scale 928
Nose 333, 756–7
  disorders 757–8
  physical examination 757
Nosebleed (epistaxis) 757
Nosocomial infection see Hospital acquired
  infection
Numerical rating scales, pain assessment
  118, 229
Nurse practitioner role 9
Nurse Prescribers' Formulary 96
Nurse–patient interaction 7, 8, 9, 13, 22
  alienation 90
  older persons 52
  sexual issues 785–6, 807
Nursing 3–26
  accountability 4, 5, 9
  autonomy 5
  central concepts 7–9
  delivery of care 9–12
  focus on caring 7
  specialization 6, 9
  statutory control 5
Nursing care plan 12
Nursing process 9–10
Nutrients 540–2
  determinants of intake 545
  dietary reference values 542, 543
  energy values 540
  factors influencing intake 545
  food groups 544–5
  healthy eating recommendations 542–5
Nutrition 537–8
  acute leukaemia management 399
  bladder surgery postoperative care 659
  burns injuries 946
  cancer patients 225
  cirrhosis 526
  consciousness level alteration 712
  cultural factors 554–7
  deficiency anaemias prevention 383, 392,
    393–4
  diarrhoea management 468
  elderly people 554
  gastrostomy 461
  history-taking 547
  immunocompromised patient 412
  inflammatory bowel disease 482, 483–4
  intracranial pressure elevation 708, 710
  jejunostomy 461
  limb amputation 900
  multiple sclerosis 734
  nasogastric tube (enteral) feeding 460
  osteoporosis 920
  Parkinson's disease 735, 736
  patient education 545
  postoperative care 184–5, 188
  pressure ulcer healing promotion 931
  renal function impairment 629, 635
    acute renal failure 625–6
    dialysis patients 634
  requirements 540–2
    recommendations 543–4
  rheumatoid arthritis 905, 909
  skin care 948
  skin disorders 953
  spinal cord injury 722–3
  stomach/duodenal disorders 460–1
    gastric surgery postoperative care
      463–4
  thyroid surgery postoperative care 596
  tracheostomy patient 366
  urinary diversion procedures 661–2
  variceal bleeding 525
  visual health 765

see also Dietary causative factors; Dietary
  modification
Nutritional disorders 537–58
  gastric resection patients 464
Nutritional status
  assessment 537, 545–7
    physical examination 546–7
  chronic obstructive airway disease
    348–9, 350–1
  immune system function 136
  infectious illness 132, 133
  influence on clinical investigation results
    152
  preoperative preparation 168–9
Nutritional support, withholding treatment
  552–4
Nystagmus 679, 755
Nystatin 444, 829

Obesity 547–50
  arterial blood pressure 253
  assessment 548
  cardiovascular risk 254, 257
  case study 549–50
  causes 548
  central 547
  definition 547
  diabetes mellitus 547, 548, 568, 570
  endocrine disorders 568
  health risks 547–8
  nursing management 548–9
    weight reduction programme 549
  preoperative weight reduction 169
  prevalence 547
  surgical risk 169
Objective measurements 11
Oblique muscles 759
Obstipation 486
Obstructive jaundice 513
Obstructive pulmonary disease, chronic
  (COPD) 343, 345
  activity intolerance 348, 350
  breathing pattern 347–8, 350
  definition 343
  information needs 349, 351
  management 345, 349–52
    primary care 84
    teaching about drug therapy 351–2
  nutrition 348–9, 350–1
  secondary polycythaemia 395
  smoking cessation 90
Occipital lobe 670
Occlusive incontinence devices 650
Occupational hazards
  bladder cancer 656
  carcinogenic chemicals 196, 199
  eye injury prevention 765, 766
  hearing loss prevention 751, 752
  infection in healthcare workers 137
  leukaemia 397
  radiation 210
  radiography 160
Occupational health nurses 79–80
Ocular hypertensive damage 319
Oculocardiac reflexes 669
Oculomotor (III) nerve assessment 679
Oedema
  burn injuries 937, 938, 945
  cardiovascular disease 260, 262, 272–3,
    310
  liver disease 514
  localized skin swelling 951
  renal function impairment 619, 621, 628
    acute renal failure 624
Oesophageal achalasia 448

Oesophageal atresia 448
Oesophageal carcinoma 449–50
Oesophageal disorders 447–52
  assessment 450
  causes 447
  clinical features 447
  congenital abnormalities 448
  diseases of neighbouring structures 447
Oesophageal echocardiography 265
Oesophageal neoplasms 449–50
  benign 449
Oesophageal stenosis 448
Oesophageal surgery 450
Oesophageal trauma 448–9
Oesophageal ulcer 454
Oesophagitis
  nursing care 223
  radiotherapy side effects 214
Oesophagogastric varices 326, 450, 514
  bleeding 523–5
Oesophagoscopy 450
Oesophagus 436
Oestrogen 798, 800, 801, 871
  adrenal cortex 566
  breast responses 848
  fat metabolism 539
Off-pump cardiac surgery 314
Ofloxacin 790
Olfaction (smell sensation) 756
  disturbances 758
Olfactory (I) nerve 756
  assessment 678
Olfactory region 756
Oliguria 618
  acute renal failure 622
Omeprazole 439, 448, 455
Ommaya reservoir 205
Oncogenes 196
Oncological emergencies 233–4
Oocytes 798, 800
Open questions 35
Open-angle glaucoma 770
Operating theatre 172
  cross-infection control 172
  patient reception 172–3
  patient transfer 172
  postoperative 180
Operative site preparation 170
Ophthalmic examination 763
Opioid receptor subtypes 119
Opioids 101, 119, 393, 468, 481
  cancer pain 230–1, 239, 866
  misuse
    substitute prescribing 979
    withdrawal symptoms 979
  sickle cell crises 389
  side effects
    constipation 225, 239
    management 232–3
  tolerance 103
  withdrawal symptoms 962
Opsonization 127
Optic chiasma 760
Optic disc (fundus oculi) 759
Optic (II) nerve 760
  assessment 678–9
Oral administration route 100–1
  opioids for cancer pain 230
Oral cavity see Mouth
Oral contraceptive 812–13, 848
  drug interactions 107
  prothrombin time influence 152
  side effects 812, 813
    major complications 813
    secondary hypertension 320

Oral hygiene
  immuncompromised patient 411–12
  see also Mouth care
Oral hypoglycaemic drugs 575, 578
Oral mucous membranes, infectious illness
      132, 133
Oral surgery 447
Oral thrush (moniliasis) 444
Orbit 758
Orchidopexy 788
Orchitis 789
Organ of Corti 748
Orgasm 783, 784, 804
Oropharyngeal airway 361–2
Orthopnoea 336
  cardiovascular disease 262, 272
Orthoptics 778
Ossification 871
Osteitis deformans (Paget's disease) 921
Osteitis fibrosa cystica
      (von Recklinghausen's disease) 598
Osteoarthritis 910–15
  assessment 911
  clinical features 911
  epidemiology 910
  exercise 911
  pain relief 911–12
  pathophysiology 910–11
  surgery 912
    joint replacement 912–14
Osteoblasts 870
Osteoclasts 870
Osteocytes 870
Osteomalacia 921
  gastric resection patients 464
Osteomyelitis 897, 918–19
  antibiotic therapy 919
Osteoporosis 919–20
  ageing changes 47
  management 920
  risk factors 919
  spinal cord injury 723
Osteosarcoma 897
Osteotomy 912
Otitis externa 753
Otitis media
  acute 753–4
  chronic 754
Otoliths 748
Otosclerosis 755
Otoscope (auriscope) 750
Ototoxic drugs 751, 752
Our Healthier Nation 16, 537, 542, 543
Ovarian ablation 862
Ovarian agenesis 810
Ovarian carcinoma 839
Ovarian cysts 839
Ovarian follicles 798, 800
Ovarian tumours 839–40
Ovary 798, 800–1
  perimenopausal changes 804
Over the counter (OTC) medicines 97
Ovulation 800, 801, 803
  infertility investigations 816
  timing 815
Ovum 800
Oxygen therapy
  cardiovascular disease 273, 312
  chest pain 276
  chronic obstructive airway disease
        350
  head injury 711
  intracranial pressure elevation 709
  postoperative 181
  pulmonary embolism 189

respiratory failure 361
  severely burned patient 940
Oxygen transport 373
Oxytocin 564

p53 196
P wave 264
P–R interval 264
Pacemaker 251
  regulation of activity 252
Pacing catheters 268
Packed red cells 425
Paget's disease of bone (osteitis deformans)
      921
Paget's disease of breast 855
Pain
  abdominal *see* Abdominal pain
  acute 115
    assessment methods 116–18
  age-related differences 114
  biliary colic 513
  cancer *see* Cancer pain
  chest *see* Chest pain
  chronic 115, 116
    depression/anxiety 115
    psychological approaches 121, 122
  cognitive-evaluative component 112
  ethnic differences 114
  fractures 875
  gastrointestinal disorders 441–2
  gate control theory 112–13, 118, 120
  gender differences 113–14
  liver disease 513
  motivational-affective component 112
  multiple myeloma 408, 409
  neurotransmitters 112
  pathways 111–12
  peptic ulcer 453–4
  pleural disorders 358
  postoperative *see* Postoperative pain
  psychological factors 113, 114–15
  receptors 111
  referred 112–13
  renal function impairment 620
  respiratory disorders 335
  role of meaning in experience 115–16
  sensation 926
  sensory-discriminative component 112
  skin lesions 950
  spinal cord injury 723
  trauma assessment 872
Pain assessment methods 116–18
  questionnaires 118
  unidimensional rating scales 116–18
Pain relief 118–22
  amputation 900
  anaemia 392, 393
  analgesic drugs 118–20
  arthroplasty 914
  bone metastatic disease 923
  burn injuries 938, 942
  femur neck fracture 891
  osteoarthritis 911–12
  pancreatitis
    acute 531
    chronic 533
  patient-controlled analgesia 120, 183–4,
        389, 463, 891, 942
  peptic ulcer 454, 455
  physical approaches 118
  postoperative *see* Postoperative pain
    relief
  psychological approaches 120–2
    cognitive behavioural therapy 121–2
    imagery 122

information provision 121
    relaxation 122
  rheumatoid arthritis 905, 908
  sickle cell crises 389, 393
Palliative cancer surgery 203
Palmar erythema 514
Palpebrae (eyelids) 758–9
Palpitations 262, 273
Pamidronate 233, 409, 598, 866
Pancreas 507, 509
  endocrine *see* Islets of Langerhans
  exocrine functions 509
Pancreatic carcinoma 533–4
Pancreatic disorders 530–4
  alcohol-related risk 514–17
  history-taking 509–10
  imaging investigations 511–12
  laboratory investigations 510–11
  physical examination 510
Pancreatic duct 509
Pancreatic enzymes 509
  serum levels 510
  supplements 474, 533
Pancreatic juice 439–40
Pancreatic polypeptide 567
Pancreatic pseudocyst 531
Pancreatitis 511, 530–3
  acute 530–3
    case study 531
    cause 530
    clinical features 530–1
    complications 531
    management 531–3
  chronic 533
Pancytopenia 396
Pandemic disease 135
Panhypopituitarism (Simmonds' disease)
      600, 601–2
Papaveretum 183
Papovavirus 729
Papule 949
Paracetamol 97, 118, 404, 753, 866, 912
Paradoxical respiration 359
Paralysis 681
  grief reaction 724
  spinal cord injury 717, 718
  stroke 692, 694, 695–6
Paralysis agitans *see* Parkinson's disease
Paralytic ileus 476, 486, 487, 531
  postoperative care 184
  spinal cord injury 717, 722
Paranasal sinuses 757
Paraoesophageal (rolling) hiatus hernia 451
Paraphimosis 789
Paraplegia 681, 717, 721, 723
Paraprotein 408, 409
Parasitic skin infection 955–6
Parasitic worms (helminths) 126
Parasympathetic nervous system 675
Parathyroid glands 565
  disorders 597–8
  function assessment 597
Parathyroid hormone (PTH) 565, 871
Parenteral drug administration 100
Parenteral nutrition
  acute pancreatitis 532
  acute renal failure 626
  inflammatory bowel disease 483–4
  unconscious patient 712
Parietal lobe 670
Parietal peritoneum 437
Parkinsonian crisis 736
Parkinson's disease (paralysis agitans) 677,
      728, 734–6
  nursing care 735–6

Parkinson's gait 680
Parotid glands 435
  inflammation 445
Paroxysmal atrial tachycardia 297
Partial cystectomy 656, 657
Partial (focal) seizures 739
Partial sight 768
  see also Visual impairment
Partial thromboplastin time (PTT) 324, 328
Partial-thickness burns 936
  healing 945
Passive immunity 141
Pasteurization 139
Patch intracutaneous (prick) tests 949
Patches, transdermal drug delivery 102
Patellar reflex 668
Patent ductus arteriosus 281
Pathogens 125
  reservoirs of infection 135
Pathological reflexes 669
Patient
  focus of nursing 7
  goals/objectives of care plan 11
  nurse accountability 5
  participation in health care 6–7, 34
Patient education/instruction 7, 8, 30
  Alzheimer's disease 731
  anaemia 394
  bereavement 67, 68
  bone metastatic disease 923
  breast cancer 864
  burn injuries 939
  cancer 235–6
  cardiac surgery 318
  cardiovascular disorders 278–9
  chronic illness 88–9
    objective disagreement 90
  chronic respiratory disease 349, 351–2
  cirrhosis 526
  clinical investigations 153, 154
  communication skills 34
  cystostomy/indwelling urinary catheter
    management 659–60
  diabetes mellitus 576–81
  epilepsy/anticonvulsant medication 741
  ethical aspects 13–14
  gastric surgery 464
  haemodialysis 633–4
  haemophilia 419
  immunocompromised patient 412–13
  inflammatory bowel disease 485
  internal sources of radiation 215
  intracranial surgery 713
  isolation precautions 135
  kidney transplant patient 640
  limb amputation 901
  malabsorption 475–6
  neurological diagnostic tests 682–3
  nutrition 545
  pain management 121
  postoperative care 190
  preoperative preparation 166, 167–8
  pressure ulcers 934
  renal failure
    acute 626–7
    chronic 636
  rheumatoid arthritis 904, 905
  skin disorders 953
  skin grafts 945
  sudden death 64
  systemic lupus erythematosis 918
  tracheostomy patient 364
  urinary diversion 662
  urinary incontinence 651
  see also Health education

Patient-centred health education 18
Patient-controlled analgesia 120, 183–4, 891
  burns injuries 942
  gastric surgery 463
  sickle cell crises 389
Patient-held records 12
Patronizing attitudes 33
Peak expiratory flow rate (PEFR) 340
  measurement 337
  monitoring for asthma management
    346, 347
Peak flow meters 337
Pearson knee flexion piece 881
  pressure sores 887
Pediculosis (lice) 955
Pelvic floor exercises 648, 837
Pelvic fracture 894–5
Pelvic inflammatory disease 828, 830
Pemphigus 952
Penicillin 132, 284, 832
  resistance 134
Penile cancer 796
Penile clamp 650
Penile erection 784
  during delivery of nursing care 786
  spinal reflex arc 784, 786
Penile prosthesis 787
Penis 783
Pentamidine 342
Pepsin 439, 440
  peptic ulcer 453
Peptic ulcer 453–7
  assessment 454–5
  causes 453
  clinical features 453–4
  diagnosis 454
  endoscopy 454
  haemorrhage 456–7
  management 455–6
  pain 453–4
  perforation 457
  pyloric obstruction 457
Peptidase 437
Perceptive deafness (sensorineural hearing
  loss) 750–1
Percutaneous endoscopic gastrostomy
  (PEG) 461
  complications 461
Percutaneous liver biopsy 512
Percutaneous renal biopsy 618
Percutaneous transluminal coronary
  angioplasty (PTCA) 286–8, 292, 315
Perfusion lung scan 340
Pericardial effusion 866
Pericardial tamponade 284, 317
Pericarditis 284
  post-myocardial infarction 293
Pericardium 248
Perimetry (visual field measurement) 763
Periodontal disease 444
Periosteum 870
Peripheral arterial pulses 260
  arterial occlusive disease 323
Peripheral blood stem cell transplants 217
Peripheral facial paralysis (Bell's palsy) 743
Peripheral nerve block 173
Peripheral nerve disorders 743–4
Peripheral nervous system 665, 674–5
Peripheral vascular disease 87, 323
  limb amputation 897
Peripherally inserted central catheter
  (PICC) 205, 413
Peristalsis 438, 440
  stimulation for regular bowel elimination
    470, 472

Peritoneal catheters 630
  complications 631
Peritoneovenous shunt 523
Peritoneum 437
Peritonitis 477–8
  causes 477
  clinical features 477–8
  complicating continuous ambulatory
    peritoneal dialysis (CAPD) 630–1
  intestinal obstruction 486
  postoperative 184
Perkin's traction 880–1
Pernicious anaemia *see* Vitamin B$_{12}$
  deficiency
Persistent vegetative state 552
Personal dimensions 66
Personal hygiene
  diarrhoea management 468
  faecal incontinence 473
  head injury 713
    intracranial pressure elevation 708,
      711
  immunocompromised patient 411
  multiple sclerosis 734
  preoperative preparation 170–1
  skin care 948
  spinal cord injury 723
  urinary tract infection prevention 654
Personality characteristics, cardiovascular
  risk 254, 257
Petechiae 422
Pethidine 119, 463, 531, 643
Phacoemulsification 771
Phaeochromocytoma 320, 608
Phagocytosis 127, 376
Phantom limb 112, 900, 901
Pharmacodynamics 96
  drug interactions 108
Pharmacokinetics 96
  drug interactions 108
Pharmacology 95–109
  nurse education 96, 97
  terminology 103
  see also Drugs
Pharmacotherapy 95
Pharyngeal suction 181
Pharyngitis 447
Pharynx 333, 436
  obstruction 368
  swallowing (deglutition) 438
Phase 1 clinical trials 108, 204
Phase 1 reactions 106
Phase 2 clinical trials 108, 204
Phase 2 reactions 106
Phase 3 clinical trials 108, 204
Phase 4 clinical trials 108
Phenothiazines 736
Phenoxybenzamine 608
Phentolamine 609
Phenylbutazone 453
Phenytoin 107, 385, 743
Philadelphia chromosome 397, 401
Phimosis 789
Phlebothrombosis 328
Phlebotomy (venesection) 395
Pholcodine 97
Phosphorylation 538
Physical dependence 962
Physical examination 11
Phytomenadione 420
Pia mater 669
Picture scales, pain assessment 118
Pigeon chest 335, 337
Pilocarpine 771
Pilot drug studies ('open' trials) 108

Pinna (auricle) 748
Pinworm 126
Pioglitazone 575
Pituitary gland (hypophysis) 562–4
 anterior lobe (adenohypophysis) 562–4
 hormones 599
 posterior lobe 564
Pituitary gland ablation 603–4
Pituitary gland disorders 598–604
 diagnostic investigations 600
 history-taking 598–9
 physical examination 599–600
 radiological studies 600
Placebo effects 102, 104–5
Plain film tomography, respiratory disorders 340
Plantar reflex 669
Plaque 950
Plasma 372
 fresh frozen preparations (FFP) 425, 427
 oncotic pressure 373
Plasma cells 129, 375
Plasma proteins 372–3
 liver synthesis 508
Plasmapheresis 409
Plaster cast 878
 drying 882
 neurovascular monitoring 884–5
 patient care 882, 883–5
 removal 885
Platelet apheresis 395, 396
Platelet concentrates 425
Platelet disorders 417
Platelet transfusion 399
Platelets (thrombocytes) 373, 376–7
 haematological values 382
Pleural aspiration (thoracocentesis) 354, 355, 358, 359
Pleural biopsy 342
Pleural disorders 354–8
 chest drainage 355–8
 respiratory function assessment 354–5
Pleural effusions 354
 metastatic disease 866
Pleural friction rub 339
Plexuses 675
Plummer–Vinson syndrome 383
Pneumocystis carinii pneumonia 144, 147, 342
Pneumonectomy 353, 354
Pneumonia 342–3
 case study 343, 344
 clinical features 342
 postoperative 181, 188
Pneumothorax 354
 following breast fine needle aspiration 853
Podophyllin 791, 831
Point mutation 195
Polarization, nerve function 667
Poliomyelitis 360, 742
Political economy theory 50–1
Political lobbying 18
Polycystic kidney disease 627, 644, 689
Polycythaemia 395
 high altitude adaptation 152
 primary/secondary 395
Polycythaemia rubra vera 395
Polydipsia 568
 diabetes mellitus 569
Polymorphonuclear leucocytes 127
Polyneuritis (multiple peripheral neuritis) 744
Polyphagia
 diabetes mellitus 569
 endocrine disorders 568

Polysaccharides 540
Polyunsaturates 541
Polyuria 568, 619, 645
 diabetes mellitus 569
Pons varolii 671
Porphyria 157
Portal hypertension 514, 522, 523
Portal vein 507
Positioning
 burns injuries 945
 chronic obstructive airway disease 350
 head injury
  intracranial pressure elevation 709, 710
  unconscious patient 712
 heart failure 271–2, 313
 hip prosthesis dislocation prevention 913
 peripheral vascular disease 325
 post-intracranial surgery 715
 post-thoracic surgery 354
 pressure ulcer wound care 833
 rheumatoid arthritis 906
 surgery 176–7
 tracheostomy patient 365
 variceal bleeding 525
 visual impairment 768
Positive reinforcement 649
Positive-pressure ventilation 367–8
 assisted 367–8
 biphasic intermittent positive airway pressure (BIPAP) 368
 controlled 367
Post-marketing surveillance (phase 4 drug trials) 108
Post-pump psychosis 314
Post-traumatic amnesia 700
Post-traumatic stress disorder 66
Postcoital test 816–17
Posterior pituitary 564
 hormones 564, 599
Postoperative care 179–90
 activity levels 186–7, 189
 adrenal gland surgery 609
 amputation 898–9
 anxiety 184, 190
 bladder surgery 658–60
 breast surgery 858
 cardiac surgery 315, 316–17
 cataract surgery 772–4
 circulation 189
 continuing care 182–90
 discharge preparation 190
 drains 187
 early ambulation 187, 188, 189
 elimination 185–6
 endarterectomy 687
 evaluation criteria 190
 evisceration 188
 external skeletal fixation 886
 flatulence/abdominal distension 184
 fluid/electrolyte balance 184–5
 gallbladder/biliary tract disease 529–30
 gastric surgery 462–4
 hip replacement surgery 913–14
 immediate postoperative period 180–2
  assessment 180, 182
  breathing 181
  circulation 181–2
  evaluation criteria 182
  injury prevention 182
 intensive care unit 180
 internal fixation 890
 intracranial surgery 713–14
 intraocular surgery 772–3
 keratoplasty (cornea transplantation) 777

 nausea/vomiting 184
 nutrition 184–5
 oesophageal surgery 450
 pain control *see* Postoperative pain
 pituitary gland ablation 604
 potential problems 183
 preoperative information for patient 167
 preparations to receive patient 180
 recovery room 179–80
 respiratory complications 188–9
 return of patient to surgical unit 182
 spinal surgery 725–6
 stoma surgery 498
 thoracic surgery 354
 transfer from operating theatre 180
 urinary diversion 661–2
 urinary retention 652
 vascular access for haemodialysis 633
 vascular complications 189
 ventilation 188–9
 vital signs assessment 167
 wound care 187–8
Postoperative pain 183
 assessment 183
 cardiac surgery 318
 preoperative information for patient 167–8
Postoperative pain relief 183–4
 gastric surgery 463
 patient-controlled analgesia 120
 thyroid surgery 595
Postural reflexes 669
Posture abnormalities 681
Povidone-iodine 944
PQRST assessment tool
 cardiovascular symptoms 258
 cough 335
 pain evaluation 116
  cancer pain 228
 skin disorders 948
 visual disorders 762
Practice nurses 79
Practice profile 83
Pravistatin 256
Prednisolone 231, 401, 406, 408, 481, 640, 908
Prednisone 481, 908, 952
Pre-eclampsia 386
Prefrontal areas 671
Pregnancy
 breast changes 847, 848
 HIV screening 162
 immune system changes 136
 radiography hazards 160
 rheumatoid arthritis impact 904
Preload 252
Premature (ectopic) beats (extrasystoles) 298–9
Premature ejaculation 786
Premedication 171, 173
Premenstrual syndrome 819
Premotor cortex 671
Preoperative preparation 165–72
 amputation 898
 anxiety management 165–7
 bladder surgery 657–8
 cardiac surgery 315
 emergency surgery 171
 endarterectomy 687
 evaluation criteria 172
 external skeletal fixation 885–6
 faecal diversion 496, 497
 gallbladder/biliary tract disease 529
 gastric surgery 462
 hip replacement surgery 913

Preoperative preparation (*contd*)
  immediate preoperative period 170–1
    elimination 170
    foods/fluids 170
    local site preparation 170
    medication 171
    patient notes 171
    personal care 170–1
  information for patient 166, 167–8
  informed consent 169–70
  internal fixation 889–90
  intracranial surgery 713
  laboratory investigations 168
  oesophageal surgery 450
  physical 168–9
  pituitary gland ablation 603
  premedication 173
  psychological 165–8
  thoracic surgery 353–4
  thyroid surgery 594
  urinary diversion 660–1
Pre-retirement courses 50
Prescription-only medicines (POMs) 97
Pressure area support devices 931
Pressure sensation 926
Pressure ulcers 136, 926–34
  assessment 930–1
  cardiac patients 273
  causes 926–7
  critical incident 957–8
  debridement 832
  dressings 932, 933
  environmental factors 833
  epidemiology 927
  fracture patient in traction 886, 887–8
  grading system 930, 931
  head injured patient 706, 710, 713
  nursing care 931–3
    mechanical devices 931–2
  nutritional support 931
  patient/family education 934
  prevention 929–30
  risk areas 929
  risk factors 927
    assessment scales 927–9
  spinal cord injury 721
  stroke patients 693
  surgical treatment 833
  wound care 932–3
Pressure ultrasound, deep vein thrombosis 327
Pressure-controlled ventilators 367
Pressure-reducing mattresses 932
Presynaptic terminal 666
Preventive health promotion approach 17–18
Primary aldosteronism 604
Primary biliary cirrhosis 522
Primary care: delivering the future 76
Primary Care Cooperatives (PCCs) 78
Primary Care Groups (PCGs) 76, 77
Primary Care Trusts (PCTs) 76, 77, 78
Primary health care
  activities 76, 78
  chronic illness management 75–91
  definition 75–6
  healthcare delivery approach 76, 78
  level of care 76, 78
  organizational aspects 77–8
  philosophy of care 76, 77, 78
  practice profile 83
  specialist nurses 78–80
Primary health care team 80–2
  full 80, 81
  functional 80, 81
  interdisciplinary/integrated model 82

  intrinsic 80–1
  multidisciplinary model 81–2
Primary intention healing 187
Primary nursing 10
Prinzmetal angina 285
Priority setting 11
  healthcare for elderly people 45
Probenecid 105
Problem identification 11
Procainamide 301
Procarbazine 406
Prochlorperazine 460, 756
Proctoscopy 488
Pro-drugs 106
Progesterone 798, 801
  adrenal cortex 566
  breast responses 848
Progestogen pill (mini-pill) 812
Progestogen-only emergency contraception 815
Progestogen-only intrauterine device 814
Progestogens
  breast cancer 862
  endometriosis 821
  intramuscular slow release preparation 101
Projection tracts 671
Prokaryotes 125
Prolactin 562, 848
  functions 564
Prolactin release-inhibiting hormone (PIH) 562
Promoting Better Health 77
Prompted voiding 649
Prone position 177
Propantheline 531
Propofol 173, 174, 191, 702
Propranolol 102, 301
Proprietary medicines 97
Propylthiouracil 592
Prostaglandin E 112
Prostaglandins 825
Prostate carcinoma 794–5
Prostate gland 782, 783
Prostate-specific antigen (PSA) 794
Prostatectomy 794, 795
Prostatic massage 789
Prostatitis 789
Protamine sulfate 324
Protective incontinence pads 649
Protective reflexes 669
Protein digestion 437, 440
Protein intake 168, 541–2
  recommendations 544
  renal function impairment 629, 635
    dialysed patient 625
Protein metabolism 539–40
  insulin actions 567
  liver 508
Proteinases 439
Proteinuria 619
Proteolytic enzymes 437, 440
Proteus 641, 643
Prothrombin time
  liver function assessment 511
  oral contraceptive use 152
Proto-oncogenes 196
Proton pump inhibitors 439
  peptic ulcer 455
  reflux oesophagitis 448
Protozoa 126
Proximal convoluted tubule 611, 612, 613
Pruritus 950
  haemolytic anaemias 386, 393
  jaundice 513

polycythaemia 395
renal function impairment 620, 628
topical drug preparations 952
Pseudoephedrine 97
Pseudomonas 224, 944
Pseudomucinous cystadenoma 839
Psilocin 972
Psilocybin 972
Psoriasis 100, 952, 954–5
Psychiatric illness/substance misuse dual diagnosis 975
Psychological aspects
  age-related changes 49
  eating behaviour 545
  pain experience 113, 114–15
    management approaches 120–2
  preoperative preparation 165–8
Psychological dependence 962
Psychoneuroendocrine immunology 136, 235
Psychosis, register of patients 84
Psychosocial support
  breast cancer 864
  cardiac rehabilitation 293
  epilepsy 741–2
  fracture patient in traction 889
  haemodialysis 633
  limb amputation 900
  rheumatoid arthritis 909–10
  sexual assault 810
  skin disorders 951
  spinal cord injury 724–5
  visual impairment 767–8
Ptosis 679
Puberty 781, 800
Pubic lice 955
Public health measures 16, 17
  infection prevention 141
Public health nursing 80
Pulmonary angiography 340
Pulmonary artery pressure (wedge pressure) measurement 269
Pulmonary catheterization 267
Pulmonary congestion 262
Pulmonary embolism 323, 327–8
  arthroplasty 914
  post-myocardial infarction 293
  postoperative 189
Pulmonary emphysema 345
Pulmonary function tests 339–40
Pulmonary oedema 262
  burn injuries 937, 941
  left-sided heart failure 310
  oxygen therapy 312
  transfusion-related acute lung injury (TRALI) 430
Pulmonary stenosis 281
Pulmonary valve 249
Pulse 253–4
  arterial occlusive disease 323
  cardiovascular system assessment 260, 261
  renal function impairment 620
Pulse oximetry 336–7
Pulsus alternans 261
Pulsus bigeminus 261
Pulsus paradoxus 261
Punch biopsy of cervix 841
Pupil 759
  constriction/dilatation 760–1
Pupillary reflexes 669, 760
  assessment 762–3
  consensual reaction 763
Purkinje fibres 249, 251
Purpura 422

Pus 127
Pustule 949
Pyelonephritis 622, 627, 641–2
Pyloric obstruction 457
Pyloric sphincter 436
Pyloroplasy with vagotomy 456
Pyramidal tract (corticospinal tract) 674, 677
Pyrazinamide 353
Pyridostigmine 738

Quadrantectomy 856
Quadriplegia (tetraplegia) 681, 717, 721, 723
Quality assurance, health education 21
Questioning skills 35
Questionnaires, pain assessment 118
Quinidine 297, 301
Quinine 417

Rabies 742
Radial nerve palsy 896
Radiant heat burns 934
Radiation
  biological effects 209
  breast cancer risk 848
  carcinogenesis 196, 397, 401
  effects on tissues/organ systems 210–11
  monitoring badges 210
  safety principles 210
  shielding 210
  tissue sensitivity 209
Radioactive iodine treatment 592
Radioactive waste 160
Radiography 159–60
  contrast media 160
  hazards 160
  musculoskeletal trauma assessment 874
Radioisotope treatment see Brachytherapy
Radionuclide (radioisotope) scan 160
  cardiovascular disorders 266
  kidney 617
  liver 512
  perfusion lung scan 340
Radionuclide venography 327
Radiotherapy 208–15
  administration 209–10
  bladder cancer 657
  brachytherapy see Brachytherapy
  breast cancer 863–4
    metastatic disease 865
  cancer control 208
  cervical carcinoma 842
  colorectal cancer 488
  continuous hyperfractionated accelerated radiotherapy (CHART) 209–10
  curative 208
  dose
    fractionation 209
    tissues/organ system effects 210
  gastrointestinal system effects 211, 213–14
  haematopoietic system/bone marrow depression 211, 213
  hair loss 211, 213
  Hodgkin's disease 405, 407
  intracranial neoplasms 728
  lung cancer 353
  mode of action 209
  multiple myeloma 409
  non-Hodgkin's lymphoma 408
  nursing care 212–15
    patients receiving internal radiation 214–15, 216
  palliative 208–9, 239

reproductive system effects 212
respiratory system effects 211–12
side effects 210, 211–12
  acute effects 210
  late effects 210–11, 212
  systemic 212
skin reactions 211, 213
superior vena cava obstruction 234
teletherapy (external beam radiotherapy) 209
treatment planning 209
urinary system effects 214
Rales (crackles; crepitations) 339
Randomized controlled trials (phase 3 drug trials) 108, 204
Ranitidine 102, 361, 439, 455, 474, 723
Rape trauma syndrome 808–9
  male rape 787
  see also Sexual assault
Rating scales, pain assessment 116–18
  cancer pain 229
Rationing, healthcare for elderly people 45
Raynaud's disease 323, 917
Reassurance 33–4
  body image alteration response 71
Receptors 103
  desensitization (downregulation) 103
  drug interactions 102–4
  hormones 561
  nervous system 668
Recommended daily amounts (RDAs) 542
Reconstructive surgery
  breast 857–8
  cancer care 203
Records 12–13
  blood/blood products transfusion 428
  cancer pain management 229
  clinical investigation results 162
  preoperative preparation 171
  skin disorder care strategies 953
  teaching plan 25
Recovery room 179–80
Rectal administration route 101
Recti muscles 759
Rectocele 833, 837
Rectum 437
Reduction of fractures 877–8
Reference nutrient intake (RNI) 542
Reference values 152
Referral 12
Referred pain 112–13
  gastrointestinal disorders 441–2
Reflecting skills 33
Reflection 1001
Reflex arc 668
Reflexes 667–9
  neurological function assessment 681–2
Reflexology 54
Reflux nephropathy 627
Reflux oesophagitis 448
  hiatus hernia 451
Refraction 760, 769
Refractive errors 760, 769
Refusal of blood transfusion 430
Regional anaesthesia 173
  advantages/disadvantages 175
  anaesthetic agents 175
  methods 173–4
  procedure 175–6
Register of chronically ill patients 83–4
Regurgitation 447
  gastrointestinal disorders 442
  reflux oesophagitis 448
Rehabilitation
  burns injuries 946–7

cancer patients 241
elderly people (re-enablement approach) 52
fractures 885, 889
head injury 716
limb amputation 901
myocardial infarction 293–4
spinal cord injury 725
stroke 695–7
visual impairment 768–9
Reiki 54
Reiter's syndrome 790
Rejection 640
Relatives see Family involvement
Relaxation techniques
  hypertension 321
  nausea/vomiting 459
  pain management 122
    cancer pain 866
    chest pain 277
    preoperative instruction 167–8
Religious influences
  rites following abortion 824
  traditional diets 556
Renal artery stenosis 627
Renal biopsy 618
Renal calculi see Nephrolithiasis
Renal colic 568
Renal disorders 611–63
Renal drug clearance 105
Renal erythropoietic factor (REF; erythrogenin) 614
Renal failure, acute 621–7
  acute pancreatitis 531
  burn injuries 937
  causes 622
  clinical features 622–3
    diuretic phase 623
    recovery phase 623
  complications 623–4
  drug responses 625
  intrarenal 622
  management 624
  nursing care 624–7
  patient education for discharge 626–7
  postrenal 622
  prerenal 622
Renal failure, chronic 621, 627–44
  causes 627
  clinical features 618–21, 627–9
  consciousness level alteration 703
  conservative treatment 629
  diabetes mellitus 569–70
  dialysis 629–34
  end-stage 628–9
  hypertension 318–19, 320
  multiple myeloma 409
  nursing care 634–7
  stages 627
  systemic lupus erythematosis 917
Renal function 612–14
  assessment 615–18
    blood tests 616
    renal function tests 616–17
    urine 615–16
  endocrine 612, 614
  filtration 612–13
  tubular reabsorption 105, 613–14
  tubular secretion/excretion 105, 614
Renal function tests 616–17
Renal neoplasms 644
Renal pelvic tumours 644
Renal pelvis 611
Renin 439, 612, 614
Repaglinide 575

Repolarization
myocardial cells 251, 264
nerve function 667
Reproductive system
ageing changes 48, 49
disorders in female 797–867
disorders in male 781–96
radiotherapy side effects 212
Reservoir of infection 135
Residual urine 644, 645, 647
Residual volume (RV) 340
Respiration
accessory muscles 337–8
assessment 335–6
chest excursion on inspiration 338
chest movements 337
Respiratory disorders 333–69
bacteriological studies 341
biopsy 341–2
functional assessment 338
pulmonary function tests 339–40
initial assessment 333–7
respiration 335–6
laboratory investigations 340–1
localized airway obstruction 368–9
lower respiratory tract 342–61
physical examination 337–8
breath sounds 338–9
postoperative complications 188–9
radiology 340
radiotherapy side effects 211–12
spinal cord injury 721
stroke 693
Respiratory failure 360–1, 703
Respiratory infection 132, 133
Respiratory rate 335
Respiratory stimulants 361
Respiratory system 333, 334
ageing changes 47, 48
local drug administration 99–100
Responsibility 5
Rest see Bedrest
Rest pain 323
Resting membrane potential 667
Resting tremor 680
Restricted lung expansion 358–60
Restrictive cardiomyopathy 283
Retching 442
Retention of urine 644, 645
with overflow 645
Reticular activating system 671
Retina 759
assessment 763
Retinal detachment 775
Retinoblastoma 778
Retirement 42, 50
Retrograde pyelography 617
Retroverted/retroflexed uterus 832–3, 836
Reverse Trendelenburg position 177
Rhesus (Rh) blood group 378–9
blood donations typing 425
haemolytic disease of newborn 386
rhesus D factor 378, 379
sensitization prevention 379, 823
Rheumatic fever 283–4
Rheumatic heart disease 283–4
Rheumatoid arthritis 136, 901–10
assessment 903–4
classification 902, 903
clinical features 902, 903
coping responses 903
diagnostic procedures 904–5
discharge preparations 910
drug therapy 908–9
exercise 907

extra-articular features 902
heat and cold application 907
joint assessment 904
joint protection 909
joint splinting 906–7
nursing management 905–10
nutrition 905, 909
pain relief 908
pathophysiology 902
patient education 904, 905
pregnancy impact 904
primary care management 84
psychological well-being 909–10
rest 906
self-care abilities 903, 909
surgical procedures 907
Rheumatoid factors 901, 904
latex fixation test 905
Rheumatoid nodules 902
Rhinitis 757
Rhodopsin (visual purple) 761, 765
Rhonchi (wheezes) 339
Rhythm method 815
Rib fracture 358, 876
Riboflavin 441
Rickettsiae 126
Rifampicin 352
Right bundle branch block 302
Right heart catheterization 205, 267
Right ventricular infarction 289
Right-to-left shunt 281–2, 360
Rigidity 680
Ringworm 126
Rinne test 750
RNA viruses 126
carcinogenesis 196–7
Rods 759, 761
Rofecoxib 908
Role theory 50
Rolling (paraoesophageal) hiatus hernia 451
Rosiglitazone 575
Rotating beds 932
Rotator cuff tear 897
Roundworm 126
Rule of Nines 935–6

Saccula 749
Sacral plexus 675
Safe intake 542
Safer sex 518, 520
guidelines 791–2
health education 19, 20
Safety studies (phase 1 drug trials) 108, 204
Salbutamol 346, 351, 361
Saliva 438
Salivary amylase (alpha-amylase) 438
Salivary gland 435
obstruction 445
tumour 445
Salmetrol 346
Salmonella 136, 466, 467
Salmonella typhimurium, multiresistance 134
Salt intake recommendations 544
Sarcoptes scabiei 955
Satiation 545
Saturated fats 541, 543
Scab (crust) 950
Scabies 955–6
Scalds 934
Scales, skin 950
Scalp, local drug administration 100
Scar 950
hypertrophic 946, 950

Schiller test 841
Schilling test 384
School nurses 79
Sclera 759
Scleroderma 918
Sclerotherapy 326
variceal bleeding 524
Scoliosis 337, 358
Scope of Professional Practice 9
Scotland, NHS organizational structure 78
Screening 160–2
cancer 199–200
breast 852
cervical 25–6
colorectal 488, 494
hearing loss 750
older people 54–5
Scrub practitioner 176
Scurvy see Vitamin C deficiency
Sebaceous glands 925, 926
Seborrhoeic dermatitis 952
Seborrhoeic keratosis 952
Sebum 925
Second degree atrioventricular block 302–3
Mobitz type I (Wenckebach) 302
Mobitz type II 293, 302
Second messengers 561
Secondary sex characteristics 800
Secretin 440
Sedation
opioid side-effects management 233
preoperative preparation 171
Segmental lung resection 353
Seizures
acute renal failure 624
see also Epilepsy
Self-care activities
chronic illness 88–9
health education 19
older people's lifestyles 54
rheumatoid arthritis 905, 909
Self-harm see Deliberate self-harm
Semen 782
Semen analysis 817
Semen penetration assay 817
Semicircular canals 749
Semilunar valves 248–9
Seminal vesicles 782, 783
Sengstaken–Blakemore tube 523, 524
Senile keratosis 952
Senna 100
Sense of control, cancer patients 238
Sense organ disorders 747–78
Sensorineural hearing loss (perceptive deafness) 750–1
Sensory (afferent) neurone 666
Sensory aphasia 678
Sensory cortex 670
Sensory deficits
ageing changes 47, 48
multiple sclerosis 734
stroke patients 696
Sensory function assessment 681
Sensory nerves 673
Sensory pathway 747
Sensory receptors 747
Sensory system 677, 747
Sepsis, leucocyte disorders 410
Septic abortion 826
Septic shock 126, 991
treatment 992
Septicaemia 130
Sequestrum 918
Serotinin 112
Serous cystadenoma 839

Sex determination 781, 797, 799
Sex role imagery 783
Sexual acting out during delivery of nursing
    care 786, 807
Sexual assault 808–9
    acute reaction 809
    assessment procedure 809
    phases of response 809
    pregnancy prevention 810
    psychological support 810
    treatment 810
Sexual behaviour 783
Sexual counselling 808
Sexual function
    cancer patients 236
    chronic renal failure 636–7
    disorders
        female 808
        male 786–7
    endocrine disorders 568
    spinal cord injury 724
    stoma patients 500–1
    urinary diversion surgery 660
    urinary tract infection prevention
        following intercourse 654
Sexual harassment 786
Sexual response 783–4
    associations with nursing care 785–6, 807
    excitement phase 783
    female 804
    male 784
    orgasm 783, 784, 804
    plateau phase 783, 804
    resolution phase 783
Sexuality 782–3
    following breast cancer 864–5
    inner feelings/doubts 786, 807–8
    object choice 786, 807
    sexual aim 786
    variations 786, 807
Sexually transmitted disease 785, 806, 812
    clinical pathway 833
    cross-infection control 791, 832
    drug therapy 835
    female 829–32
    follow-up 836
    history-taking 830
    male 790–2
    nursing management 791, 832
    physical examination 834
    risk factors 830
    safer sex guidelines 791–2
Sharps
    disposal 137, 138
    handling 138
Sharps injury 156–7
    management 138
Shave
    head 713
    preoperative 170
Sheath of Schwann (neurilemma) 674
Shigella 466, 467
Shock 991–4
    acute pancreatitis 530, 532
    acute renal failure 622
    burn injuries 937, 938, 941–2
    femur shaft fracture 892
    intestinal obstruction 486
    postoperative 181
    treatment 992–4
Shock lung *see* Adult respiratory distress
    syndrome (ARDS)
Short bowel syndrome 474
Short-sightedness (myopia) 760
Shoulder dislocation 896–7

Sickle cell disease 388–91
    care interventions 389, 390–1
    case study 394
    clinical features 388–9
    crises 389
    nursing management issues 389, 391
    patient education 394
    social support 391
Sickle cell trait 388
Sideroblastic anaemias 385
Sigmoidoscopy
    colorectal cancer 488
    inflammatory bowel disease 480
Sildenafil 787
Silence 36
Silent myocardial infarction 289
Silent thrombosis 328
Silver sulfadiazine 943, 944
Simmonds' disease (panhypopituitarism)
    600, 601–2
Sims–Huhner postcoital test 816–17
Simvastatin 256
Single-photon emission computed
    tomography (SPECT) 683
Singultus (hiccup; hiccough) 443
Sinoatrial block 302
Sinoatrial node 249, 251
Sinus arrhythmia 296
Sinus bradycardia 298
Sinus tachycardia 293, 296–7
Sinuses *see* Nasal sinuses
Sinusitis 758
Sitting position, cardiovascular disease
    272–3, 313
Situational (accidental) crises 63–4
Skeletal traction 880–2
    balanced 881
    Buck's 880, 881
    Hamilton Russell 880, 881, 889, 891, 893
    Perkin's 880–1
Skin 925–6
    ageing changes 47, 48
    bactericidal secretions 127
    barriers to infection 127
    functions 926
    health promotion 947–8
    local drug administration 100
    normal microbial flora 125, 126
    radiotherapy side effects 211, 213
Skin biopsy 949
Skin cancer 956–7
    sunlight exposure 196, 948, 956
Skin care 925–58
    anaemia 392, 393
    cirrhosis 526
    diabetes mellitus 579
    peripheral vascular disease 325
    peristomal 499–500, 502
    pressure ulcers prevention 929–30
    renal function impairment
        acute renal failure 626
        chronic renal failure 635
    spinal cord injury 721
    unconscious patient 713
Skin disorders 948–58
    clinical manifestations 949–51
    diagnostic tests 949
    discharge preparation 953
    documentation 953
    history-taking 948
    local care 951–2
    nutrition 953
    patient education 953
    physical examination 948–9
        skin survey 948

    physical therapy 952
    psychological support 951
    risk factors 949
    systemic therapy 952–3
    topical drug preparations 952
Skin grafts
    burns injuries 944–5
    donar site care 945
    patient education 945
Skin lesions
    primary 949–50
    secondary 950
Skin patches 102
Skin pigmentation changes 568
Skin tests 131
Skin traction 880
Skin-fold thickness 547
Skull fracture 699
Skull radiography 683
Sleep
    assessment 682
    paradoxical (desynchronized) 682
    preoperative preparation 169
    slow-wave (normal) 682
    spinal cord injury 724
Sliding hiatus hernia 451
Slit-lamp microscopy 763
Slow ventricular tachycardia 297
Small bowel resection 474
Small intestinal cancer 488
Small intestinal disorders 464, 473–6
    inflammatory 476–85
Small intestinal motility 439
Small intestine 436–7
    absorption 441
    digestive processes 439–40
Smell sensation 756
    disturbances 758
Smith–Petersen nail 882, 883
Smith's fracture 896
Smoke inhalation injury 936, 938
Smoking 336, 397, 656, 961, 967
    addiction 967
    carcinogenesis 196
    cardiovascular risk 254, 256
    chronic arterial occlusive disease 323
    impact on health 967
    lung cancer 353
    mouth cancer 445
    peptic ulcer 453
    stroke 686
Smoking cessation 90, 256–7, 967
    arterial occlusive disease 326
    cardiovascular disorders 279
    chronic obstructive airway disease 345
    preoperative/postoperative period 167,
        189
Sneeze reflex 669
Snellen chart 763
Social care for elderly people 42–3
Social change health promotion approach
    18
Social–positivist model of health 14, 15
Sodium
    renal function 613–14
    restriction
        heart failure 314
        hypertension 320–1
    retention 262
    salt intake recommendations 544
Solvents abuse 970–1
Somatostatin 509, 562, 567
    functions 567
Somogyi effect 588
Sorbitol 572

Space-occupying brain lesions 703
Spacer devices 99
    patient teaching 351
Spasticity 680
    multiple sclerosis 734
Specialist nursing practice 6, 9
    community nursing 78–80
    elderly people's services 53
Specimen collection 131–2, 156
    bacterial culture/sensitivity 158
    blood 156
    influence on clinical investigation results
        152–3
    sputum 341
    urine 157, 158, 616
Spectacles 766
    after cataract extraction 773, 774
    strabismus (squint) treatment 778
Speech, ageing changes 47
Speech dysfunction 678
    Parkinson's disease 735, 736
    stroke 692–3
Speech reading 753
Speech training 753
Sperm 782
    banking 398
    motility 782
Sperm count 782
Spermatocele 792
Spermatogenesis 781–2
Spermicidal preparations 812
Sphenoid sinuses 757
Spherocytosis, hereditary 386–7
Sphincter of Oddi 440, 508, 509
Sphygmomanometer 260
Spider angiomas (naevi) 514
Spinal anaesthesia 173–4
Spinal cord 673
Spinal cord compression
    cancer patients 234
    metastatic disease 866–7
    spinal cord injury 717
Spinal cord degeneration 384
Spinal cord injury 717–26
    acute phase care 719–20
    assessment 719
    body temperature regulation 724
    cervical spine 720
    complications 723–4
    compression 717
    effects 717
    emergency care at scene of accident 717,
        718
    long-term care 720–5
        bladder training programme 722
        bowel training programme 722
    lumbar spine 720
    mechanisms of injury 717
    pain 723
    paralysis 717, 718
    psychosocial support 724–5
    recovery of function 717
    rehabilitation 725
    sexual function 724, 784
    sleep disturbance 724
    surgical procedures 719
    thoracic spine 720
    transection 717
    trauma assessment 872
Spinal nerves 673, 674–5
    anterior roots 675
    posterior roots 675
Spinal radiography 683
Spinal shock 717
Spinal surgery 725–6

Spinoreticular tract 111–12
Spinothalamic tract 111, 674
Spiritual issues, cancer patients 240–1
Spirochaete 125
Spirometry 339
Spironolactone 312
Spleen 129
Splenomegaly
    inherited haemolytic anaemias 386
    liver disease 514
Splints
    burns injuries 945
    rheumatoid arthritis 906–7
Spores 125
Sputum 335, 341
Squamous cell carcinoma 956, 957
Squint see Strabismus
ST segment 264
Stages of change model 23–4
    patient teaching process 24–5
    substance misuse interventions 978, 981
Staghorn calculus 643
Standard isolation precautions 134
Stapes 748
Staphylococcus 126, 466, 467, 527, 641
Staphylococcus aureus 126, 828, 829, 918, 944
    enterotoxin C 828
    enterotoxin F 828
    infective endocarditis 284
    methicillin resistance 132, 133, 134
Starches 540
Starflower oil 852
Starling's law of the heart 252
Starvation 539
    preoperative 170
State-Trait Anxiety Inventory (STAI) 290
Statins 256, 292
Status epilepticus 740
Statutory control 5
Steapsin 439, 440
Steatorrhoea 473
    chronic pancreatitis 533
Stein–Leventhal syndrome 839
Steinmann pin 880
Stem cell transplantation 402–3
    allogenic 402–3
    autologous 402
    complications 403
    procedure 403
Stem cells 373
Stents
    angina management 287
    myocardial infarction management 292
Stepping gait 680
Stereotactic fine needle aspiration cytology
    853
Stereotyping 31, 32, 39
    elderly people 43, 44, 46
Sterilization
    female 814–15
    male (vasectomy) 788
Sterilization procedures (cross-infection
    control) 138, 139
Steroid hormone receptors 561
Steroid therapy 98–9
    Addison's disease (adrenocortical
        insufficiency) 605
    cancer pain 866
    chronic lymphocytic leukaemia 401
    co-analgesic actions 231
    immunosuppressive actions 136
    inflammatory bowel disease 481
    inhaled 98, 99, 346, 347, 351
    intracranial neoplasms 728
    peptic ulcer aetiology 453

respiratory failure 361
rheumatoid arthritis 908–9
skin disorders 952
systemic lupus erythematosis 917
topical administration 100
Still's disease (juvenile chronic arthritis)
    902
Stimulant drugs of misuse 967, 968–70
Stoma care 499
    skin integrity maintenance 499–500,
        502
    urinary diversion 661
        body image 662
        patient education 662
Stoma care nurse 496, 498
Stoma formation
    drainage appliance selection 498–9
    nursing assessment 497
    postoperative assessment 498
    preoperative preparation 497
    psychological preparation 496
    siting 497
Stoma obstruction 503
Stoma patients
    community support 503
    self care
        activities 502
        education 501–2
        equipment 502
Stoma prolapse 503
Stoma retraction 503
Stomach 436
    digestive processes 438–9
        cephalic phase 439
        gastric phase 439
        intestinal phase 439
    disorders 452–8
        history-taking 458–9
        management 459–62
Stomach cancer 457–8
Stomatitis 444, 447
    iron deficiency anaemia 383
    see also Mucositis
Stool softening agents 471
Storage diseases 522
Story telling 51
Strabismus (squint) 761, 777–8
    convergent (esotropia) 777
    divergent (exotropia) 777
    paralytic/non-paralytic 777–8
    treatment 778
Strangulated hernia 485, 486, 487
Strangury 645
Streptococcus 527, 641, 918
    rheumatic fever 283, 284
Streptococcus pneumoniae 126, 918
    meningitis 742
    penicillin resistance 134
Streptokinase 292
Streptomycin 353, 751
Stress
    cancer associations 197
    diarrhoea 467
    immune response effects 136
    inflammatory bowel disease 482
    management
        hypertension 321
        stomach/duodenal disorders 461–2
    peptic ulcer 453
Stress incontinence 645
    investigations 835–7
    treatment 837
    women 835–7
Stress test (exercise electrocardiography)
    265

Stress ulcers
  burn injuries 937
  spinal cord injury 722
Stridor 339
  postoperative 181
Stroke (cerebrovascular accident) 6, 686–97
  cerebral artery bypass 687
  cerebral atherosclerosis 686
  cerebral thrombosis/embolism 687
  clinical manifestations 692–3
  complete 686
  diagnostic procedures 693
  discharge planning 696–7
  endarterectomy 687
  in evolution 686
  haemorrhagic 686
  incidence 686
  monitoring 693
  nursing care 694–7
  rehabilitation 46, 695–7
  risk factors 686
Stroke volume 252
Structuralist model of health 14–15
Structured medical history 11
Struvite calculi 643
Stye (hordeolum) 769–70
Subarachnoid haemorrhage 689, 700
  grading 690
  intracranial complications 690, 692
  management 690
  nursing care 690–2
  prognosis 689–90
Subarachnoid space 669
Subclavian catheter 632
Subcutaneous administration route 102
  opioids for cancer pain 230
Subcutaneous tissue 925, 926
Subdural haemorrhage 700
Subdural space 669
Subjective assessment 11
Subjective views of health 15
Sublingual administration route 101
Sublingual glands 435
Submaxillary glands 435
Substance misuse 961–88
  assessment 975–7
    aims 975
    in-depth 976–7
    screening 976
    triage (emergency screening) 975
  biopsychosocial explanation 962–3
  detoxification programmes 979
  health promotion/health education
    981–2
  hepatitis prevention 518
  illicit drugs 967–73
    classification 968
  interventions 977–82
    aims 977–8
    behavioural change model 978, 981
    motivational interviewing 980
    relapse prevention 980–1
    substitute drugs prescribing 978–9
  multidisciplinary team approach 973
  self-help groups 981
  services 973–5
    Accident and Emergency departments
      974–5
    primary care 974
    shared care 973–4
  severe mental illness dual diagnosis 975
  suicide association 982, 983
  terminology 962
  withdrawal symptoms 979
Substance P 112

Succus entericus (intestinal juice) 440
Sucralfate 455
Suction
  intracranial pressure elevation 709
  intubated patient 363
  tracheostomy patient 365
Suction dilatation and curettage 824
Sudden death
  absence of bereaved at time of death
    67–8
  cardiac 254
  external support 64–5
  grief reaction 61
  impact on status of bereaved 66
  information provision 64
  inner coping resources 65
  loss response 70–1
  phases of crisis framework 65
  proactive nursing response 66, 67
  resuscitation attempts, presence of
    relatives 67, 68
  viewing body 66–7
Sugars 540
  intake recommendations 543
Suicide 982–6
  associated substance misuse 982, 983
  attempted see Deliberate self-harm
  case study 985–6
  definitions 982
  duty of care 985
  grief reaction 62, 64–8
  prevention 985
  risk assessment 984, 985
  risk factors 982–3
  risk-mitigating factors 984
Sulci 670
Sulfadiazine 622
Sulfasalazine 468
  inflammatory bowel disease 481
Sulfinpyrazone 324, 325
Sulphonamides 521, 622
Sulphonylureas 575
Sunlight exposure see Ultraviolet radiation
Sunscreens 948, 956
Superficial burns 936
Superficial reflexes 669
  assessment 681–2
Superior colliculus 760
Superior vena cava obstruction 234
Supine position 177, 272
Supportive measures 12
Suppositories 170
Suprapubic catheterization 653
Supratentorial cranial compartment 669
Supratentorial herniation 698
Supratentorial surgery 713
Surgery 165–91
  anaesthesia 173–6
    respiratory function 178, 179
  elective 165
  emergency 165
  infection prevention 178–9
  informed consent 169–70
  operating theatre procedures 172–3
  patient position 176–7
  physical injury risk/risk minimization
    178, 179
  postoperative management see
    Postoperative care
  potential problems 177–8
  preparation see Preoperative preparation
  surgical team personnel 176
Substitute drugs prescribing 978–9
Sustained-release formulations 100, 101
Swallowing (deglutition) 437, 438

Swallowing difficulty see Dysphagia
Swan–Ganz catheter 269
Sweat 926
Syme's amputation 898
Sympathetic nervous system 675
Sympathetic ophthalmia 778
Synapses 667, 668
Synchronous video pressure flow
    cystourethrography 647
Syncope 254
Syndrome of inappropriate antidiuretic
    hormone (SIADH) 603
Syngeneic bone marrow transplantation
    216
Synovial fluid aspiration 904
Synovial joints 871–2
  movement 872
Synovial membrane 872
Syphilis 322, 791, 831–2
  blood/blood products screening 423
  gumma 791, 831
  primary/secondary/tertiary stages 791,
    831
Systemic infection 130
Systemic lupus erythematosis 916–18
  clinical features 917
  nursing management 917–18
Systemic sclerosis 918
Systole 251
Systolic blood pressure 253
  auscultation 260
  cardiovascular disorders 261

T lymphocytes 129, 375, 376
  graft-versus-host disease 217
T wave 264
Tachycardia 296–7
Tachypnoea 335, 336
Tamoxifen 862
Tampon use 829
Tapeworm 126
Tarsal plate 758
Taste sensation 757
  alteration in cancer patients 224–5
Teaching plan 25
Team nursing 10
Teamwork
  benefits 80
  primary health care 80–2
Technetium imaging
  liver 512
  lung 340
  myocardial imaging 266
Telangiectasia 950
Telemetry, ECG monitoring 264
Teleological world-view 13
Teletherapy (external beam radiotherapy)
    209
Temazepam 171, 968
Temperature sensation 926
Temporal lobe 670
Tendon of insertion 872
Tendon of origin 872
Tendon reflexes 669
Tenesmus 214
Tension pneumothorax 354
Tentorial herniation 698
Tentorial notch (tentorial incisura) 669
Tentorium cerebelli 669
Teratoma 839
Testicular cancer 203, 795
Testicular descent 781
Testicular self-examination 795
Testicular torsion 792
Testosterone 540, 781, 782

Tetanus 126, 742
Tetrabenazine 736
Tetracyclines 467, 952
Tetralogy of Fallot 282
Tetraplegia (quadriplegia) 681, 717, 721, 723
Thalami 671
Thalassaemia 387–8
Thallium myocardial imaging 266
Thecal cells 800
Therapeutic abortion 824–6
    early 824–5
    late 825
    legal aspects 824
    nursing care 825–6
Therapeutic index 103, 104
Therapeutic measures 12
Therapeutic window 103
Thiamine 441
Thiazolidinediones (glitazones) 575
Thiopental sodium 173
Third degree (complete) heart block 293, 303
Thomas' splint 879, 881
    pressure sores 887, 888
Thoracic spinal injury 720
Thoracic surgery
    lung cancer 353
    postoperative care 354
    postoperative thoracic expansion restriction 358
    preoperative care 353–4
Thoracocentesis (pleural aspiration) 354, 355, 358, 359
Thoracoplasty 358
Thorax
    inspection 337
    physical examination 337–8
Thought monitoring 121, 122
Threatened abortion 821
    management 822
Thromboangiitis obliterans (Buerger's disease) 323
Thrombocytopenia 417
    cancer patients 208, 221
Thrombolytic therapy 247, 264
    myocardial infarction 273, 292
Thrombophlebitis 328
    postoperative 189
    spinal cord injury 723
Thrombosis
    acute arterial occlusion 322, 323
    arthroplasty 914
    polycythaemia 395
    preventive postoperative lower limb exercises 167
Thrombotic thrombocytopenic purpura 386
Thymectomy 738
Thymus 129
Thyrocalcitonin see Calcitonin
Thyroglobulin 564
Thyroid disorders 588–97
    assessment 588
    clinical features 589
    primary care management 84
Thyroid gland 564–5
Thyroid surgery 592
    complications 596
    follow-up care 596–7
    postoperative care 595–7
    postoperative pain relief 595
    preoperative preparation 594
    recovery room care 594–5
    wound healing 595–6

Thyroid-stimulating hormone (TSH) 562, 565
    functions 564
Thyroid-stimulating immunoglobulins (TSI) 591
Thyrotoxicosis see Hyperthyroidism
Thyrotrophic-releasing hormone (TRH) 562, 565
Thyroxine (T$_4$) 565, 871
    nutrient metabolism 539, 540
    thyroid replacement therapy 590
Tibial plateau fracture 893
Tibial shaft fracture 893
Tic douloureux (trigeminal neuralgia) 743
Tics 680
Tidal volume (V$_t$) 339
Tietze's syndrome 854
Timed forced expiratory volume (FEV$_1$) 340
Timolol 771
Tinnitus 755
Tissue plasminogen activator (tPA) 292
Tissue typing 638
Tissue valve homografts 315
TNM system 201–2
Tobramycin 622
Tolerance, pharmacological 103, 119, 962
Tongs 720
Tongue 435
Tonic seizures 740
Tonsillar herniation 698
Tonsillitis 447
Tonsils enlargement 368
Toothache 444
Toothbrushing 446–7
Tophi 916
Topical anaesthesia 174
Topical drug preparations 952
Touch 36
    cancer patient care 235, 237
    complementary therapies 54
    sensation 926
    sexual issues 785–6
        acting out 786
    sexual response 783
Toxaemia 130
Toxic epidermal necrolysis syndrome 953, 954
Toxic goitre see Hyperthyroidism
Toxic hepatitis 521
Toxic shock syndrome 126, 828–9
Toxins, bacterial 126
Toxoplasmosis 136, 729
Trace elements 542
Trachea 333
    obstruction 368–9
Tracheo-oesophageal fistula 448
Tracheostomy 363–7
    care 364–7
        assessment 365
        fluids/nutrition 366
        humidification of inspired air 366
        position 365
        suction 365
    communication 364, 366
    emergency 369
    extubation 366–7
    home care 367
    indications 363
    mouth care 366
    procedure 363–4
        equipment 364–5
        preparation 364–5
    tube care 365–6
    wound care 365–6

Tracheostomy tubes 363, 364
Traction 878–82
    balanced 879–80, 881
    fixed 879
    nursing care 886–9
    rehabilitation following 880
    skeletal 880–2
    skin 880
Tranexamic acid 690
Transamination 540
Transcutaneous electrical nerve stimulation (TENS) 118, 866
Transdermal administration route 102
Transferrin 375
Transfusion reactions 185, 428–30
    allergic 429
    circulatory overload 430
    febrile non-haemolytic 429
    haemolytic 428–9
        acute reaction management 429
        acute renal failure 622
        delayed 429
    infection 429–30
    lung injury 430
Transfusion-related acute lung injury (TRALI) 430
Transient ischaemic attack 686, 687
Transitions see Life transitions
Transjugular intrahepatic portosystemic shunt (TIPS) 525
Transjugular liver biopsy 512
Transmission-based isolation precautions 134, 135
Transposition of great vessels 282
Transsexuality (gender dysphoria) 786
Transudate 354
Transurethral resection of prostate (TURP) 651, 657, 792–3, 795
    postoperative care 658
Transvestitism 786
Trauma assessment 872–4
    radiography 874
Traumatic amputation 898
Traumatic death, grief reaction 61
Travel arrangements
    chronic renal failure 637
    diabetes mellitus 578–9
Treadmill test 338
Tremors 680
Trendelenburg position 177
Trendelenburg test 326
Treponema pallidum 791
Trichomoniasis 126, 830–1
Tricuspid atresia 282
Tricuspid regurgitation 315
Tricuspid valve 248
Tricyclic antidepressants 233
Trigeminal (V) nerve assessment 679
Trigeminal neuralgia (tic douloureux) 743
Triglyceride 255, 538, 539, 541
Trigone 614
Tri-iodothyronine (T$_3$) 565
    thyroid replacement therapy 590
Trimethoprim–sulfamethoxazole 342
Trochlear (IV) nerve assessment 679
Trophic hormones 562
Trophoblast tumours 827
Tropical sprue 385
Troponins 291
Tru-cut biopsy, breast disorders 853
Trypsin 439, 440
Tubal ligation 814–15
Tuberculin skin test 131, 341, 352
Tuberculosis 14
    diagnosis 352

disease process 352
incidence 352
pulmonary 352–3
renal 642
risk factors 352
skin tests 131, 341, 352
treatment 352–3
Tubotympanic perforation 754
Tumour lysis syndrome 233
Tumour markers 201
Tumour resistance 204
Tumour suppressor gene mutation 196
Tumour vaccines 217
Tumours from main tissue types 201
Tuning fork tests 750
Turner's syndrome (XO) 810
Turning frames 932
Tympanic membrane 748
perforation 754
Type A behavioural pattern 257

Ulcer 950
Ulcerative colitis 479
clinical features 479
quality of life impact 481–2
contributing factors 479
Crohn's disease comparison 479–80
diagnostic investigations 480–1
diarrhoea 466, 467, 481, 482, 485
extracolonic manifestations 480
ileostomy 494
incidence 479
see also Inflammatory bowel disease
Ultrasound 159
biliary tract disorders 511
breast examination
(sonomammography) 852
deep vein thrombosis 327
gynaecological examination 827–8
liver disorders 511
urinary system 617
Ultraviolet radiation 926
skin cancer 196, 948, 956
skin protection 948
therapy 952
Unconscious patient see Consciousness level
alteration
Undernutrition 550–4
causes 550
hospitalized patients 551
case study 551–2
nursing interventions 550–1, 555
withholding of nutritional support
552–4
United Kingdom Central Council for
Nursing, Midwifery and Health Visiting
(UKCC) 5
Code of Professional Conduct 5, 8–9, 13,
14, 33
Scope of Professional Practice 9
Universal blood/body fluid precautions 140,
141, 518, 520, 791, 832, 951
Unpopular patient 38–9
Unstable angina 285
Unwanted drug effects 107–8
Upper gastrointestinal tract disorders
444–64
Upper motor neurones 677
Upper oesophageal (cricopharyngeal)
sphincter 436
Upper respiratory tract 333
obstruction see Airway obstruction
Uraemia 619, 621
chronic renal failure 627
diarrhoea 467, 468

nutrition 625–6
seizures 739
Urea formation 508, 540
Urea nitrogen serum level 616
Ureteric colic 643
Ureteric tumours 644
Ureteroileostomy (ileal conduit) 657
Ureters 614
Urethra 614–15
Urethritis 653
radiotherapy side effect 214
Urethrocele 833
Urethrovesical resuspension 650
Urgency 644, 645
Uric acid serum level 616
Urinalysis 615–16
infertility investigations 816
urinary incontinence 647
Urinary bilirubin levels 511
Urinary casts 619
Urinary catheterization 652–3
burn injuries 941
catheter care 653, 655
emergency surgery 171
fracture patient in traction 888
intracranial pressure elevation 710, 711
postoperative 185
preoperative 170
spinal cord injury 722
unconscious patient 712–13
urinary incontinence management 649
urinary retention 652–3
urinary tract infection 654–5
urine specimen collection 158
see also Indwelling urinary catheterization
Urinary diversion 650, 656–7, 660–2
bladder cancer management 656
body image 662
postoperative care 661–2
preoperative preparation 660–1
Urinary drug excretion 105
Urinary incontinence 645–51
Alzheimer's disease 731
assessment 646–8
behavioural interventions 648–9
causes 645–6
clinical diagnostic measurements 647
drug treatment 648
external urinary drainage devices 649–50
functional status evaluation 647
history-taking 646
information for patient 651
multiple sclerosis 734
nursing intervention 650–1
case study 650
Parkinson's disease 736
pelvic floor exercises 648
physical examination 647
prevalence 645
protective pads 649
spinal cord injury 722
stroke 692, 693
surgery 650
voiding record/diary 648
Urinary meatus 615
Urinary outflow obstruction 645
Urinary output monitoring
burn injuries 937, 941
postoperative 185
Urinary retention 651–3
assessment 652
benign prostatic hyperplasia 792
case study 652
causes 651
fracture patient in traction 886, 888–9

multiple sclerosis 734
spinal cord injury 721–2
urinary tract infection prevention 654
Urinary tract 611–15
disorders 644–62
urine changes 644
voiding symptoms 644–5
Urinary tract infection 126, 136, 645,
653–5
causes 654
clinical features 654
prevention 654
treatment 654
urine tests 157
Urinary urobilinogen 511
Urine 614
bacteriological examination (urine
culture) 616
colour 615, 619
composition 614, 619
urinary tract disorders 644
osmolality 617
output measurement 615
pus 619
regulation of concentration 613
specimen collection 616
critical incident 163
24-hour 158, 616
volume abnormalities 618–19
Urine flow studies 647
Urine tests 157–8
diabetes mellitus 579
specimen collection procedures 158
technique 157
Urobilinogen 511
Urodynamic investigations 647
stress incontinence 835–6
Ursodeoxycholic acid 522
Urticaria 950, 952–3
Uterus 801
congenital anomalies 810
menstrual cycle changes 801
myomas (fibroids) 838–9
prolapse 833–4, 837
retroversion/retroflexion 832–3, 836
Utricle 749
Uveal tract 759
Uveitis 775

Vagina 783
congenital anomalies 810
menstrual cycle changes 804
pubertal changes 800
sexual response 804
Vaginal balloon 650
Vaginal carcinoma 843–4, 846
Vaginal discharge 829
Vaginal douche 815
Vaginal examination 806
Vaginal pessary 832
Vaginismus 808
Vaginitis 829
Vaginosis 829
Vagotomy 456
Vagus (X) nerve assessment 679
Valsalva manoeuvre 722
Valvular atresia 282
Valvular heart disease 283
infective endocarditis 284
rheumatic fever 283–4
surgery 315
Valvular incompetence/regurgitation 283
Valvular stenosis 283
Vancomycin-resistance enterococci 134
Vanillylmandelic acid (VMA) 608

Variceal bleeding 523–5
    balloon tamponade 523–4
    monitoring 525
    sclerotherapy 524
    supportive measures 525
    surgery 524–5
    vasopressin infusion 524
Varicella zoster virus 729, 957
Varicocele 326, 792
Varicose veins 326–7
Vascular access for haemodialysis 631–2
Vascular endothelial drug absorption 98
Vascular myelopathy 729
Vascular purpura 420
Vascular surgery 325
Vascular system 250
    disorders 318–29
        postoperative 189
Vasectomy 788
Vasoconstriction, haemostasis 377
Vasodilators 273, 312
Vasopressin see Antidiuretic hormone
Vegetarian diet 555, 556
Veins 250
    valves 250
Venepuncture technique 156–7
Venesection (phlebotomy) 395
Venous blood pressure 253
    cardiovascular disorders 261
    measurement 269
Venous congestion 310
Venous disorders 326–8
Ventilation 333
    intracranial pressure elevation 708, 709
    postoperative care 188–9
    restricted lung expansion 358–60
    severely burned patient 940–1
Ventilation perfusion mismatching 360
Ventricles 248
Ventricular arrhythmias 296
Ventricular drainage 711
Ventricular ectopic beats 299
Ventricular fibrillation 293, 301, 307
Ventricular septal defect 281
Ventricular tachycardia 297–8, 307
Venturi mask 361
Venules 250
Veracity 13
Verapamil 297, 301, 303
Verbal rating scales, pain assessment 116
Vertebral arteries 672
Vertigo 755
Very low-density lipoproteins (VLDLs) 255
Vesicle 949
Vesicular breath sounds 338
Vestibular dysfunction 755
Vestibule of inner ear 748
Vestibulocochlear (auditory) nerve (VIII) 748, 749
    assessment 679
Vibrio 125
Vibrio cholerae 467
Victim blaming 17
Villi of intestinal mucosa 437
    absorption 441
Vinblastine 225, 406
Vincristine 225, 406, 408, 417
Vinyl chloride 196, 199
Viral hepatitis 517–21
    assessment 519
    clinical features 518–19
    contacts 520
    diagnosis 519
    follow-up 521
    nursing care 519–21

prevention 518, 520–1
    treatment 519
Viral infection 126
    carcinogenesis 196–7
    dormancy 126
    host resistance 127–8
    leucocyte disorders 410
    transmission in blood products 419
Virulence 126
Visceral peritoneum 437
Visceral reflexes 669
Vision 758
    ageing changes 47
    dark adaptation 761–2
    focusing mechanism 760–1
        accommodation 760
        convergence 761
        pupillary modification 760–1
        refraction 760
    impulse pathway 760
    light adaptation 761
Visual acuity assessment 763
Visual analogue scales, pain assessment 116, 117
Visual disorders 762–78
    assessment 762–4
    clinical features 762, 764–5
    eye examination 762–4
    history-taking 762
Visual fields 760
    measurement (perimetry) 763
Visual impairment 764–9
    causes 765
    communication problems 768
    continuous assessment 768
    environmental safety 768
    feeding assistance 768
    glasses/contact lenses 766
    incidence 765
    objective manifestation 764–5
    patient care 767–8
    positioning 768
    preventive approaches 765–6
    psychosocial issues 767–8
    rehabilitation 768–9
    subjective manifestation 764
    sympathetic ophthalmia 778
Visual purple (rhodopsin) 761, 765
Vital capacity (VC) 339
Vital signs 693
    postoperative assessment 180
    renal function impairment 620
        acute renal failure 624
Vitamin A 508, 761, 765
Vitamin B 168, 765
Vitamin B$_{12}$ 374, 375, 508
    deficiency 384–5, 457, 464
    dietary sources 383, 393
    malabsorption 474
Vitamin C 168, 374, 375, 393, 765
    deficiency (scurvy) 385, 420
Vitamin D 508, 926
    deficiency 464
    malabsorption 474
    renal metabolism 612
    supplements 920, 921
Vitamin E 508
Vitamin K 126, 441, 508
    deficiency 420
    phytomenadione therapy 420
Vitamins 542
    intake recommendations 544
    small intestinal absorption 441
Vitrectomy 775, 776
Vitreous haemorrhage 776

Vitreous humour (vitreous body) 759
Volume-controlled ventilators 367
Voluntary movement 677
Volvulus 485, 486, 487
Vomiting see Nausea/vomiting
Vomiting (emetic) centre 442
Von Gierke's disease 522
Von Recklinghausen's disease (osteitis fibrosa cystica) 598
Von Willebrand factor 420
Von Willebrand's disease 420
Vulvar varicosities 326

Wales, NHS organizational structure 78
Walking cast 878
Warfarin 279, 301, 315, 324, 328, 694
    drug interactions 102, 324
    haemorrhagic complications 324, 420–1
    monitoring 421
Warm autoimmune haemolytic anaemia 386
Warts 197, 952
Waste categories 137
Waste disposal 137–8, 141
    blood products 428
    radioactive waste 160
Waterlow scale 928
Weber's test 750
Wedge lung resection 353
Weight loss
    cardiovascular disease 262
    chemotherapy side effect 399, 400
    gastrointestinal disorders 442–3
Weight reduction programmes 314, 549
Wenckebach (Mobitz type I) second degree atrioventricular block 293, 302
Wertheim's hysterectomy 842
Wheal 949
Wheezes (rhonchi) 339
    postoperative 181
Whipple's operation 533
White matter 670, 673
Whole blood 425
Withdrawal symptoms 962, 979
    alcohol 962
    opioids 119, 962
Withholding of cardiopulmonary resuscitation 308–9
Withholding of nutritional support 552–4
    clinical factors 552–3
    ethical issues 552, 553
    legal aspects 552
    provision of nursing care 553–4
Working for patients 77
Wound care 925–58
    burn injuries 942–3
    postoperative 187–8
    pressure ulcers 932–3
Wound dehiscence 188
Wound healing 187
    ageing changes 47, 48
    burns injuries 944–5
    thyroid surgery 595–6
Wound infection 126
    postoperative 187
Wrist fracture 896

Xerosis 620
Xerostomia (dry mouth) 213, 223, 240

Yellow card system 107

Zidovudine 144
Zollinger–Ellison syndrome 453, 534